NEUROSURGERY SELF-ASSESSMENT

NEUROSURGERY SELF-ASSESSMENT

Questions and Answers

Rahul S. Shah, BSc(Hons), MBChB(Hons), MRCS(Eng)
Specialty Registrar in Neurosurgery and
Wellcome Trust Clinical Research Fellow
University of Oxford
Oxford, UK

Thomas A.D. Cadoux-Hudson, DPhil, FRCS, MB BS
Honorary Consultant Neurosurgeon
Department of Neurosurgery
Oxford University Hospitals NHS Trust
Oxford, UK

Jamie J. Van Gompel, MD
Associate Professor of Neurosurgery and Otolaryngology
Mayo Clinic College of Medicine
Rochester, MN, USA

Erlick A.C. Pereira, MA, BM BCh, DM, FRCS(Neuro.Surg), SFHEA
Senior Lecturer in Neurosurgery and Consultant Neurosurgeon
Atkinson Morley Neurosciences Centre, St George's Hospital
St George's, University of London
London, UK

Foreword by

Edward C. Benzel, MD
Chairman, Department of Neurosurgery
Center for Spine Health, Cleveland Clinic
Cleveland, OH, USA

For additional online content visit **ExpertConsult.com**

ELSEVIER
Edinburgh London New York Oxford Philadelphia St Louis Sydney Toronto 2017

ELSEVIER

Notices

Knowledge and best practice in this field are constantly changing. As new research and experience broaden our understanding, changes in research methods, professional practices, or medical treatment may become necessary.

Practitioners and researchers must always rely on their own experience and knowledge in evaluating and using any information, methods, compounds, or experiments described herein. In using such information or methods they should be mindful of their own safety and the safety of others, including parties for whom they have a professional responsibility.

With respect to any drug or pharmaceutical products identified, readers are advised to check the most current information provided (i) on procedures featured or (ii) by the manufacturer of each product to be administered, to verify the recommended dose or formula, the method and duration of administration, and contraindications. It is the responsibility of practitioners, relying on their own experience and knowledge of their patients, to make diagnoses, to determine dosages and the best treatment for each individual patient, and to take all appropriate safety precautions.

To the fullest extent of the law, neither the Publisher nor the authors, contributors, or editors, assume any liability for any injury and/or damage to persons or property as a matter of products liability, negligence or otherwise, or from any use or operation of any methods, products, instructions, or ideas contained in the material herein.

ISBN: 978-0-323-37480-4

Printed in China

Last digit is the print number: 9 8 7 6 5 4 3 2 1

Content Strategist: Lotta Kryhl
Content Development Specialist: Humayra Rahman Khan
Project Manager: Srividhya Vidhyashankar
Design: Miles Hitchen
Illustration Manager: Lesley Frazier
Marketing Manager: Rachael Pignotti

Contents

PART V
FUNCTIONAL NEUROSURGERY

PART VI
PERIPHERAL NERVE SURGERY

PART VII
PEDIATRIC NEUROSURGERY

FOREWORD

Neurosurgery Self-Assessment: Questions and Answers by Shah, Cadoux-Hudson, Van Gompel and Pereira is a true masterpiece. All neurosurgeons need 'refreshers'; some for certification, some for maintenance of certification, and others for the mere need to 'keep up'. With over 1000 questions and 700 images available both in print and interactively online, this volume provides an extensive coverage of neurosurgery from top to bottom, and all points in between. Multiple choice questions are used to test foundation of knowledge and, most importantly, educate.

We, as adults, OR As adults, we learn most efficiently and effectively when our minds are exercised and stressed. When multiple modalities are employed (such as questions, answers and explanations), learning becomes more efficient, with a greater long term retention of the newly acquired information. This becomes particularly relevant to those who are to soon be 'tested' in the form of certification or maintenance of certification examinations. Reading, thinking, answering, and then the contemplation of answers and their rationales makes the multiple choice question strategy employed by the authors particularly relevant to modern day foundational neurosurgery information acquisition and retention.

I commend the authors for their tried and true, but uncommonly used, approach to education. It takes the agony out of reading a chapter. It minimizes the laborious efforts required to gather information via searches and other strategies. It brings the art and craft of neurosurgery to life in an enjoyable and relatively painless format. Finally, it provides a near complete coverage of the field – at least as complete as is humanly possible in the space afforded.

So, whether you have an impending examination, or you simply desire to 'spiff up' on your neurosurgical foundations, this book is for you. Use it as one might use a bedside novel. Use it to prepare. Use it to simply stay at the top of your field. This book can truly fulfill all of these needs – and much, much more.

Ed Benzel

Preface

Neurosurgical training is delivered worldwide with the goal of producing a surgeon who is safe for independent practice. Today, neurosurgical residents and their trainers are trying to achieve this goal in the face of reduced working hours, increasing demand on services, individual surgeon outcome publication, and increasing litigation, to name but a few challenges. In this environment, the value of targeted learning materials and advanced surgical simulation is clear. The content of this question book aims to reflect the evolving expectations placed on residents in an age of evidence-based practice, subspecialization, and multidisciplinary teams: one must also be familiar with allied specialties advancing just as fast as our own.

As a counterpoint to currently available self-assessment books, we have organized questions by the highly specific topic areas outlined in most modern neurosurgical textbooks and training curricula. Furthermore, most questions are accompanied by in-depth answers and, where appropriate, suggestions for further reading. We hope this will enable junior trainees to use it as a learning aid and for focused revision prior to rotating onto particular neurosurgical firms. For senior trainees or those about sit their examinations who require a mix of questions (in terms of both topic and difficulty), this is provided by the interactive question bank accessed via the online Inkling platform and smartphone app. This book consists of single best answer (SBA) and extended matching item (EMI) questions constructed according to the guidelines from the US National Medicine Licensing Board and the UK Joint Committee on Intercollegiate Examinations, to enable the user to become familiar with the respective formats before the exam. While SBA- and EMI-style questions are not yet universal in postgraduate neurosurgical examinations across the world, we hope all trainees find them valuable and cost-effective for self-study.

Finally, I would like to thank Elsevier—their support has ensured that this book could also serve as a comprehensive and representative catalogue of commonly examined clinical images and investigation results in a single resource for neurosurgical residents. I hope you enjoy using it!

Rahul S. Shah
Oxford
July 2016

How to Pass Neurosurgical Examinations

LEARNING BY MULTIPLE CHOICE QUESTIONS

The World Federation of Neurosurgical Societies estimates that there are 30,000 neurosurgeons worldwide. In the United States, there are approximately 3500 board certified neurosurgeons and 800 neurosurgical residents. In the United Kingdom, there are close to 300 consultants and 200 trainees, with a total of approximately 8000 qualified neurosurgeons and trainees in Europe. Due to international collaboration through research and education, neurosurgical training curricula have become increasingly standardized across most countries. Both UK and US-style examinations are well established in other countries (e.g. India and Brazil, respectively), and recently developed training programs in Africa have based their examinations on the UK format. Additionally, the need for already qualified neurosurgeons to demonstrate continuing professional development for revalidation purposes has also increased the demand for courses and objective self-assessment tools in neurosurgery.

Although the duration of postgraduate neurosurgical training varies by country, completion of training usually requires the candidate to pass both written and oral examinations set by the relevant national training board or committee. For the written examinations, questions are generally multiple choice and cover the basic and clinical sciences; short answer and essay questions are used in some regions. Topics include neuroanatomy, neurophysiology, neuropharmacology, critical care, fundamental clinical skills, neuroradiology, neuropathology, neurology, neurosurgery, and other disciplines deemed suitable and important (e.g. statistics, medical law, medical ethics). Questions relating to clinical neurosurgery also cover the main subspecialties, including trauma, neuro-oncology, skull base and pituitary surgery, vascular neurosurgery, spinal surgery, pediatric neurosurgery, peripheral nerve surgery, and functional/epilepsy/pain surgery.

For the vast majority of multiple choice questions (MCQs) in this book, we provide a detailed explanation of the correct answer with references to current evidence-based data where appropriate. Like the real examinations, questions test the reader's knowledge of basic and clinical neurosciences and neurosurgery, and are arranged by topic to be useful to doctors in neurology, neuroradiology, and neuropathology, and medical students. Illustrations include anatomical pictures, graphs, tables, radiology images, and histology slides in questions and answers where required.

We suggest the following approach to using this book and learning by MCQs:

- Firstly, start early! Learning throughout one's training will lead to reinforcement and consolidation of deep knowledge not easily forgotten. Use books like this at the beginning, middle, and end of training, and relate them to your clinical practice.
- Secondly, let this book be a guide to consolidate the information learnt. Annotate material from other resources like comprehensive textbooks. Use the "red," "amber," and "green" gradings to distinguish between lower-yield and more difficult questions and high-yield easy questions. Make connections between different subspecialties and general principles, and focus on material most likely to be tested. Remember that this is neither a comprehensive review book nor a panacea for inadequate preparation in the last few months before the exam.
- Thirdly, prime your memory by returning to challenging and annotated questions in the final days before the exam. This book can serve as a useful way of retaining key associations and refreshing important facts fresh in your memory for the exam. Finally, contribute to the book to enable active learning. Email us if you find errors or see ways in which the book can be updated.

HOW TO TACKLE SINGLE BEST ANSWER (SBA) AND EXTENDED MATCHING ITEM (EMI) QUESTIONS

Test performance is influenced not just by your knowledge but also by your test-taking skills. You can improve your performance by honing your test-taking skills and strategies well in advance of the exam so that you can concentrate on the information and your knowledge during the test itself. The following strategies may be useful.

Try to deal with each question in turn, identifying it as easy, workable or impossible from your own perspective; our green, amber, and red classification provides an approximate examiner's guide to difficulty for someone having completed their neurosurgical training. Aim to answer all the easy questions, resolve the workable ones in reasonable time, and make quick educated guesses at any apparently impossible ones. There are different techniques for question reading that include reading the stem, thinking of the answer, and turning to the choices or skimming the answer choices and the last part of the question before returning to the stem. Try different techniques to see what work best for you and yields the highest marks. Our online testing area should help with that.

Set a good pace for answering the questions. Divide the total time for the exam by the number of questions and be strict with yourself. If you are taking too long then mark the question, pick your best answer, and come back to it later if you have time at the end. Avoid burnout by practicing timed tests to develop endurance. Use extra time to check marked questions. Never give up—take a short one-minute break and come back to the test if too disheartened.

Answer all test questions—even if it means guessing! Whereas in the past many neurosurgical examinations were negatively marked, that process has largely been superseded by only positively marked exams, so there is no harm in an educated or instinctive guess, or even just a blind punt. If you have to guess, go on a hunch and pick an answer you are vaguely familiar with rather than something you have never heard of.

COMPUTER-BASED TESTING

The UK FRCS (Neurological Surgery) examination has been using computer-based testing for several years, the American Board of Neurological Surgery moved to a web-based format for the Primary Examination in 2015, and the EANS Part 1 remains a pencil-and-paper test. The UK exam takes place in dedicated test centers found in most cities in front of desktop computers with headphones, pencil, and paper available, and the software is controlled by a mouse. Residents taking the US examination use certified laptops provided by the residency program. Both have high-quality, distinct images, and sometimes include audio and video material.

Given the artificial environment of computer-based testing, it is important to become familiar with it before the actual exam. Most examination boards offer a downloadable or interactive mock examination with a few sample questions to familiarize yourself with the environment. Skipping the tutorial on the exam day sometimes adds extra time to answer the actual questions in the test itself. Learn how to mark questions, go back to them and if there are any rules preventing going back to previous blocks. Become familiar with how to view images and spot the icons for playing audio and video clips. Be vigilant that some multipart questions prevent changing the answer to the first part of the question once the second part has been revealed.

US, UK, AND EUROPEAN NEUROSURGICAL EXAMINATION STRUCTURE

MCQ tests generally form the first part of most neurosurgical examinations, with the subsequent parts being a combination of oral and clinical examinations. The 2015 ABNS Primary Examination consisted of 350 questions (in 6 h 45 min), while the UK FRCS Written Examination is in two parts, the first consisting of 135 SBA questions (in 2 h) and the second part of 110 EMI questions (in 2.5 h). The European Association of Neurosurgical Societies Part 1 examination consists of approximately 200 MCQs to be answered in 3 h. Questions in all three examinations cover neuroanatomy, neurobiology, neuropathology, neurology, neuroradiology, clinical neurosurgery (including subspecialties), fundamental clinical skills, and other disciplines deemed suitable and important.

The marking of such MCQ examinations is now quite standardized and relies upon principles of statistics and psychology. Many examination boards use the modified Angoff method, whereby experts are briefed then allowed to take part or all of the test with the performance levels in mind. They are then asked to provide estimates for each question of the proportion of minimally acceptable candidates that they would expect to get the question correct. The final determination of the cut score is then made by averaging the estimates. Controversial questions—those that polarized the candidates' answers between two answers or those that candidates scoring highly overall got wrong whereas those scoring poorly overall got right—are scrutinized and potentially removed from the overall scoring at examiners' standard setting meetings. It is good practice for a trainee representative who has sat the examination to participate in the whole process.

Whereas the written examination explores an applicant's knowledge in various relevant disciplines, the oral examination explores knowledge and judgment in clinical neurosurgical practice after an applicant has been an independent practitioner. The oral examination is accomplished in a series of face-to-face examinations. The applicant is presented with a series of clinical vignettes using real patients, clinical descriptions, radiographs, computerized images, anatomical models, and/or diagrams. The examiners grade the applicant on specific tasks including diagnostic skills, surgical decision-making, and management of complications.

STANDARDS FOR INDEPENDENT NEUROSURGICAL PRACTICE

The credibility of professional examinations taken at the end of surgical training rests on their ability to satisfy patients and colleagues that those passing have attained a minimum standard of basic and applied science knowledge and clinical decision-making to practice independently. Oral examinations are crucial in this process as they assess communication skills, clinical skills, and decision-making and professionalism in a high-pressure environment. In contrast, MCQs focus on assessing knowledge and analytical and decision-making skills. More clinically integrative questions test higher orders of Bloom's taxonomy and are more effective than simple factual questions in assessing and developing the clinical problem-solving skills of trainee surgeons.

Patients fundamentally wish for their treating surgeon to be as independent as possible in order to maximize their chances for an excellent outcome. Therefore, when setting minimum standards for independent practice, an expert peer group of examiners is accountable to patients, other neurosurgeons and healthcare professionals, and the general public. Postgraduate medical examinations have therefore generally evolved to become as standardized and fair as possible, while maintaining rigor, expanding, and adapting as trends change in clinical practice.

PART I
BASIC SCIENCE

CHAPTER 1

NEUROANATOMY

SINGLE BEST ANSWER (SBA) QUESTIONS

1. From inferior to superior (i.e. ascending), what is the 4th branch of the external carotid artery in the neck?
   a. Maxillary artery
   b. Occipital artery
   c. Facial artery
   d. Lingual artery
   e. Posterior auricular artery

2. The pathway best describing how sympathetic fibers of the autonomic nervous system exit the spinal cord is:
   a. Via the dorsal roots and white rami communicans
   b. Via the ventral roots and white rami communicans
   c. Via the dorsal roots and gray rami communicans
   d. Via the ventral roots and gray rami communicans
   e. Via the ventral roots and spinal nerves

3. The left vertebral artery usually arises from the:
   a. Arch of the aorta
   b. Brachiocephalic trunk
   c. Left common carotid
   d. Left subclavian artery
   e. Costocervical trunk

4. Hemiballismus results from lesioning which basal ganglia target?
   a. Globus pallidus interna
   b. Subthalamic nucleus
   c. Substantia nigra pars reticularis
   d. Striatum
   e. Pedunculopontine nucleus

5. Lesion of which structure increases extensor tone?
   a. Dentate nucleus
   b. Pedunculopontine nucleus
   c. Red nucleus
   d. Ventral tegmentum
   e. Superior olive

6. Which one of the following drain into the cavernous sinus?
   a. Superior ophthalmic vein
   b. Superior petrosal sinus
   c. Inferior petrosal sinus
   d. Basal vein of Rosenthal
   e. Vein of Labbé

7. Persistent trigeminal artery is commonly:
   a. Found in 3-5% of people
   b. Found to connect to the proximal basilar artery
   c. Found to branch off from the ICA just proximal to the meningohypophyseal trunk
   d. Found to have a vascular abnormality in approximately 50% of cases
   e. Found in conjunction with internal carotid artery aplasia

8. The afferent loop of the Hering-Breuer inflation and deflation reflexes is mediated by:
   a. CN XIII
   b. CN IX
   c. CN X
   d. CN XI
   e. C2

9. Which one of the following nerves is outside the annulus of Zinn?
   a. Abducens
   b. Nasociliary
   c. Trochlear
   d. Oculomotor (superior division)
   e. Oculomotor (inferior division)

10. The C2 vertebra has how many secondary ossification centers?
   a. 2
   b. 3
   c. 4
   d. 5
   e. 6

11. A line drawn between the highest point of the iliac crests across the back usually denotes:
   a. L1/2 interspace
   b. L2/3 interspace
   c. L3/4 interspace
   d. L4/5 interspace
   e. L5/S1 interspace

12. Which one of the following is labeled X in the image below?

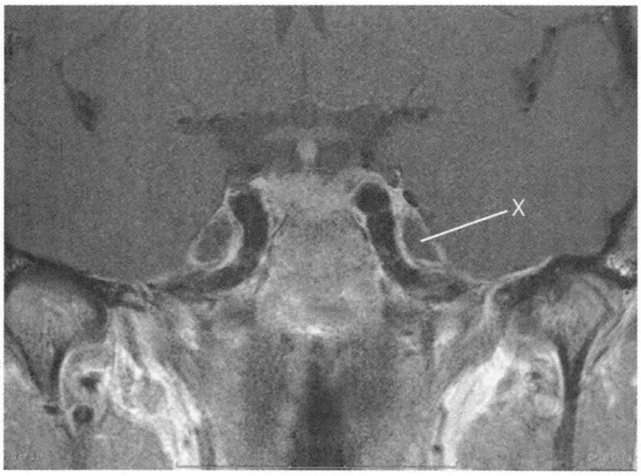

   a. Ophthalmic division of the trigeminal nerve
   b. Meckel's cave
   c. Oculomotor nerve
   d. Maxillary division of trigeminal nerve
   e. Abducens nerve

13. Which one of the following statements about the sympathetic nervous system is FALSE?
   a. Innervation of thoracic viscera arises from T1-T4 spinal segments
   b. Splanchnic nerves are unmyelinated
   c. Preganglionic fibers enter the sympathetic chain via white rami communicans
   d. Sensory afferent fibers are important for visceral pain sensation
   e. Preganglionic fibers synapse in either the sympathetic chain or prevertebral ganglia

14. Nervi erigentes are responsible for:
   a. Inhibition of the external anal sphincter
   b. Inhibition of the internal vesicle sphincter
   c. Inhibition of the internal anal sphincter
   d. Inhibition of the external vesicle sphincter
   e. Inhibition of the rectal muscles

15. Parasympathetic sensory afferents terminate in which one of the following?
   a. Nucleus ambiguus
   b. Solitary nucleus
   c. Edinger-Westphal nucleus
   d. Red nucleus
   e. Superior colliculus

16. Which one of the labels in the diagram below of the internal auditory canal identifies the facial nerve?

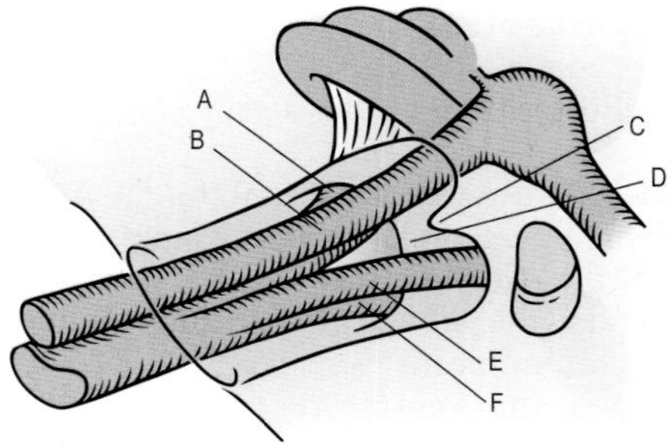

17. Blood supply to the posterior pituitary gland arises from branches of which internal carotid artery segment?

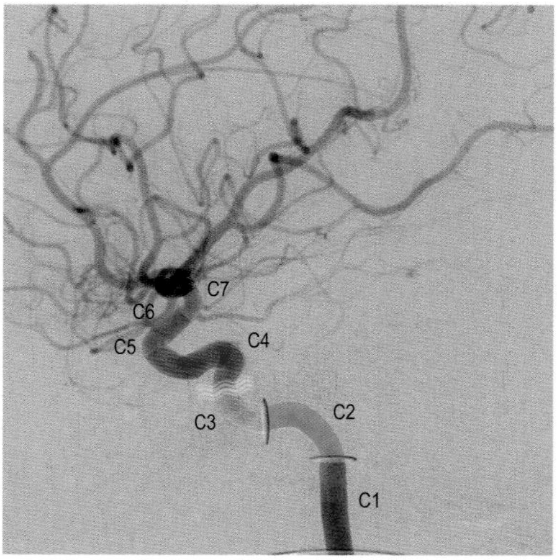

a. C1 (Cervical)
b. C2 (Petrous)
c. C3 (Lacerum)
d. C4 (Cavernous)
e. C5 (Clinoid)
f. C6 (ophthalmic/supraclinoid)
g. C7 (communicating)

QUESTIONS 18–25

Additional questions 18–25 available on ExpertConsult.com

EXTENDED MATCHING ITEM (EMI) QUESTIONS

26. **Cavernous sinus imaging:**

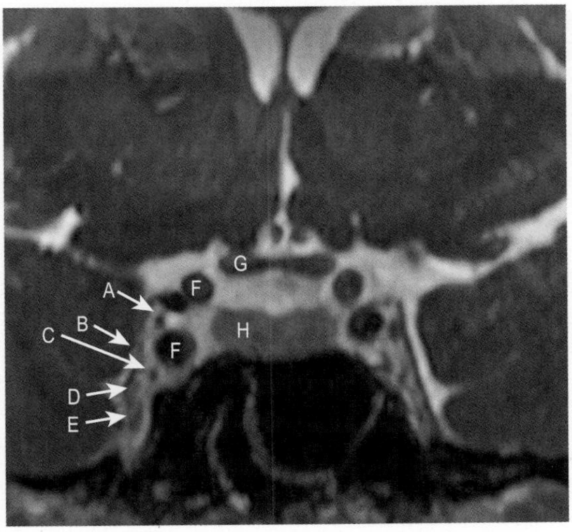

For each of the following descriptions, select the most appropriate answers from the image above. Each answer may be used once, more than once or not at all.

1. Right optic nerve
2. Oculomotor nerve
3. Abducens nerve

27. **Internal auditory canal:**

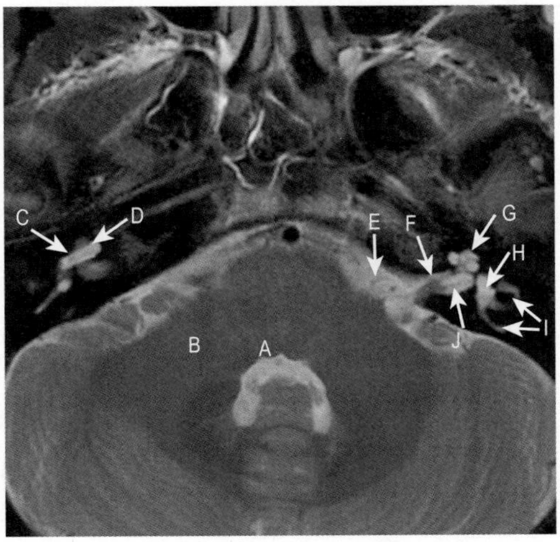

For each of the following descriptions, select the most appropriate answers from the image above. Each answer may be used once, more than once or not at all.

1. AICA
2. Basal turn of cochlea
3. Cochlear nerve

28. **Cavernous sinus anatomy:**

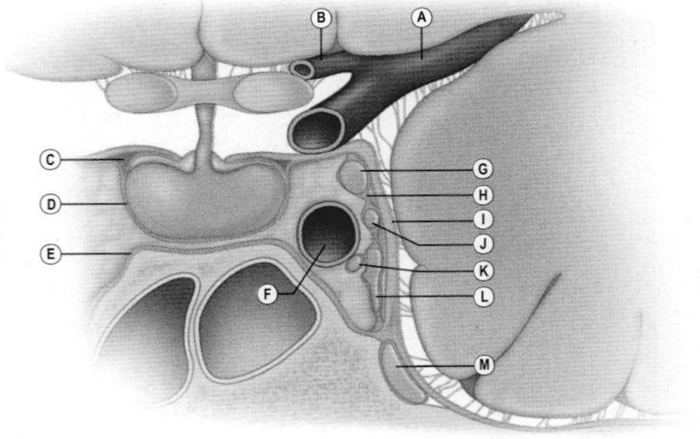

For each of the following descriptions, select the most appropriate answers from the diagram above. Each answer may be used once, more than once or not at all.

1. ACA
2. Maxillary division of CN V (V2)
3. Oculomotor nerve (III)

29. **Internal auditory canal:**

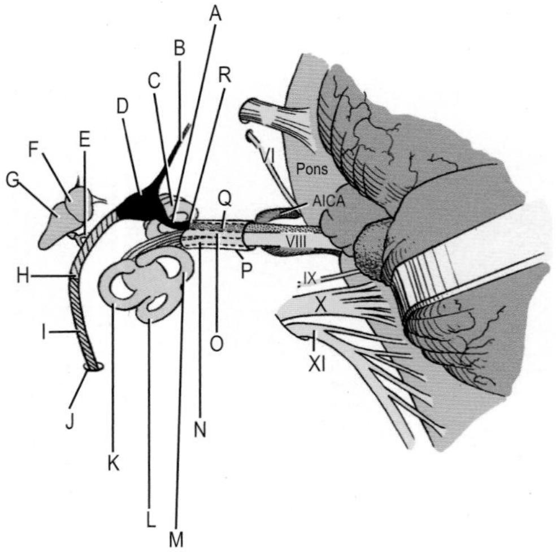

For each of the following descriptions, select the most appropriate answers from the image above. Each answer may be used once, more than once or not at all.

1. Facial nerve
2. Superior vestibular nerve
3. Greater superficial petrosal nerve
4. Posterior semicircular canal

30. **Internal auditory canal:**

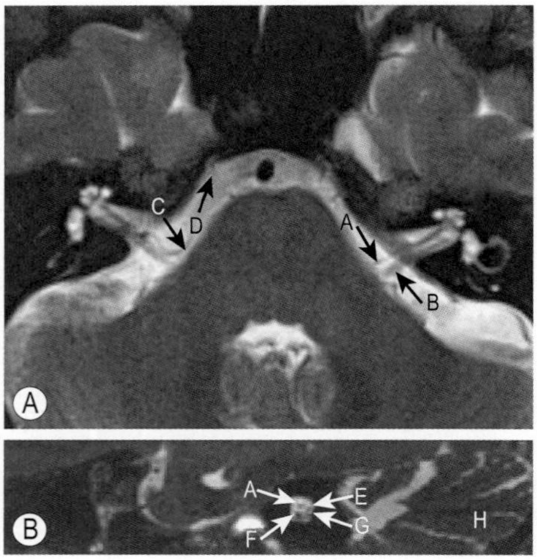

For each of the following descriptions, select the most appropriate answers from the images above. Each answer may be used once, more than once or not at all.

1. Anterior inferior cerebellar artery
2. Vestibulocochlear nerve
3. Facial nerve

31. **Basal Ganglia:**

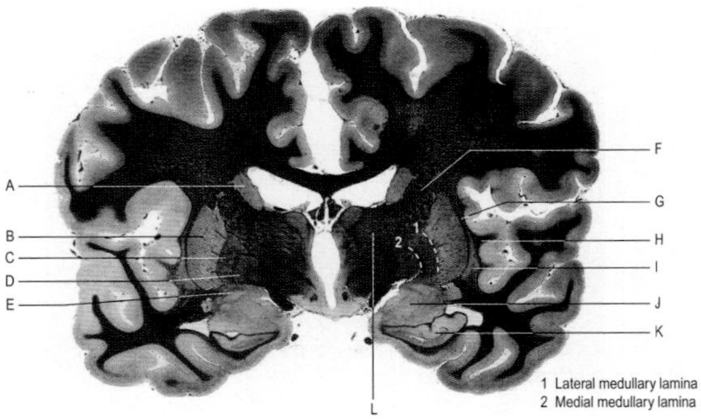

For each of the following descriptions, select the most appropriate answers from the image above. Each answer may be used once, more than once or not at all.

1. Caudate nucleus
2. Claustrum
3. Globus pallidus interna
4. Internal capsule
5. Putamen

32. **Projection and association tracts:**

a. Central tegmental tract
b. Lamina terminalis
c. Median forebrain bundle
d. Stria medullaris
e. Stria terminalis
f. Postcommissural Fornix
g. Nucleus of the diagonal band of Broca (vertical limb)
h. Retinohypothalamic tract
i. Supraopticohypophyseal tract
j. Tuberoinfundibular (tuberohypophyseal) tract
k. Trapezoid body
l. Thalamic fasciculus (Forel's field H1)
m. Nucleus of the Diagonal band of Broca (horizontal limb)
n. Mammillothalamic tract
o. Tapetum

For each of the following descriptions, select the most appropriate tracts from the list above. Each answer may be used once, more than once or not at all.

1. Conducts fibers to the posterior pituitary gland
2. Arcuate nucleus to hypophyseal portal system of infundibulum
3. Septal nuclei to hippocampus
4. Connects sepal area, hypothalamus, basal olfactory areas, hippocampus/subiculum to midbrain, pons and medulla
5. Hippocampus to cingulate gyrus

33. **Vascular territories:**
  a. Middle cerebral artery
  b. Basilar artery
  c. Perforators from internal carotid artery
  d. Ophthalmic artery
  e. P2 portion of posterior cerebral artery
  f. Vertebral artery
  g. Superior cerebellar artery
  h. Posterior inferior cerebellar artery
  i. Anterior inferior cerebellar artery
  j. Posterior communicating artery
  k. A2 portion of anterior cerebral artery
  l. P3 portion of posterior cerebral artery
  m. Recurrent artery of Heubner

For each of the following descriptions, select the most appropriate answers from the list above. Each answer may be used once, more than once or not at all.

1. Posterior limb of the internal capsule
2. Medial and lateral geniculate nuclei
3. Anterior limb of internal capsule and head of caudate
4. Posterior pituitary gland
5. Splenium of corpus callosum

34. **Cerebral veins:**

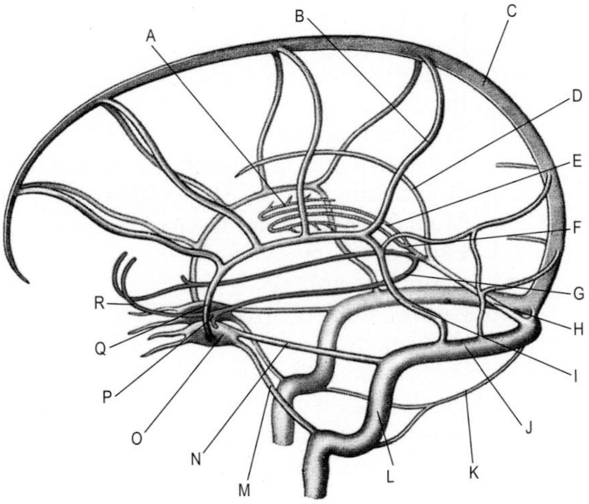

For each of the following descriptions, select the most appropriate answers from the image above. Each answer may be used once, more than once or not at all.

1. Inferior anastamotic vein of Labbé
2. Superficial middle cerebral vein of Silvius
3. Superior anastamotic vein of Trolard
4. Basal vein of Rosenthal
5. Vein of Galen

35. **Offending Artery:**
  a. A1 portion of anterior cerebral artery
  b. Anterior choroid artery
  c. Anterior communicating artery
  d. Anterior inferior cerebellar artery
  e. Basilar arteries
  f. Facial artery
  g. Internal carotid artery
  h. M3 portion of middle cerebral artery
  i. Ophthalmic artery
  j. Posterior cerebral artery
  k. Posterior communicating artery
  l. Posterior inferior cerebellar artery
  m. Superior cerebellar artery
  n. Vertebral artery

For each of the following descriptions, select the most appropriate answers from the list above. Each answer may be used once, more than once or not at all.

1. Glossopharyngeal neuralgia
2. Trigeminal neuralgia
3. Hemifacial spasm
4. Horner's syndrome
5. CN III palsy

36. **Autonomic nervous system:**
  a. Erdinger-Westphal nucleus
  b. Superior salivatory nucleus
  c. Inferior salivatory nucleus
  d. Dorsal nucleus
  e. Ciliary ganglion
  f. Pterygopalatine ganglion
  g. Otic ganglion
  h. Submandibular ganglion
  i. CNII
  j. CNV
  k. Chorda tympani
  l. Vidian nerve
  m. Superior cervical ganglion
  n. Greater petrosal nerve
  o. Lesser superficial petrosal nerve
  p. Auriculotemporal nerve

For each of the following descriptions, select the most appropriate answers from the list above. Each answer may be used once, more than once or not at all.

1. Mediates bronchoconstriction
2. Receives preganglionic parasympathetic fibers via CNIII
3. Postganglionic parasympathetic fibers to parotid gland
4. Preganglionic parasympathetic fibers to the submandibular ganglion
5. Origin of preganglionic parasympathetic fibers transmitted in GSPN IX

37. **Projection and association tracts:**
a. Ansa lenticularis
b. Fasciculus retroflexus
c. Lenticular fasciculus (Forel's field H2)
d. Postcommissural fornix
e. Precommissural fornix
f. Thalamic fasciculus (Forel's field H1)
g. Nucleus of the diagonal band of Broca
h. Mammillothalamic tract
i. Tapetum
j. Uncinate fasciculus
k. Commissure of Probst
l. Central tegmental tract
m. Lamina terminalis
n. Median forebrain bundle
o. Stria medullaris

For each of the following descriptions, select the most appropriate option from the list above. Each answer may be used once, more than once or not at all.

1. Globus pallidus interna to thalamus through internal capsule
2. Globus pallidus interna to thalamus around internal capsule
3. Septal nuclei to amygdala
4. Temporal lobe to occipital lobe
5. Connection between nuclei of lateral lemniscus

38. **Thalamus:**

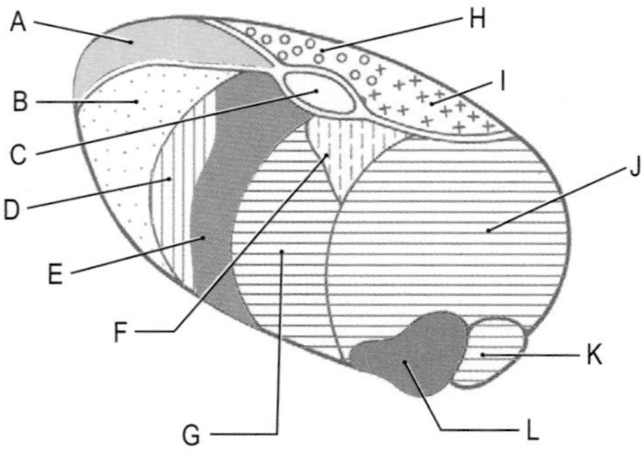

For each of the following descriptions, select the most appropriate part of the thalamus from the image above. Each answer may be used once, more than once or not at all.

1. Pulvinar
2. Ventral anterior nucleus
3. Ventral posterolateral nucleus
4. Lateral geniculate nucleus
5. Medial geniculate nucleus

39. **Thalamus:**

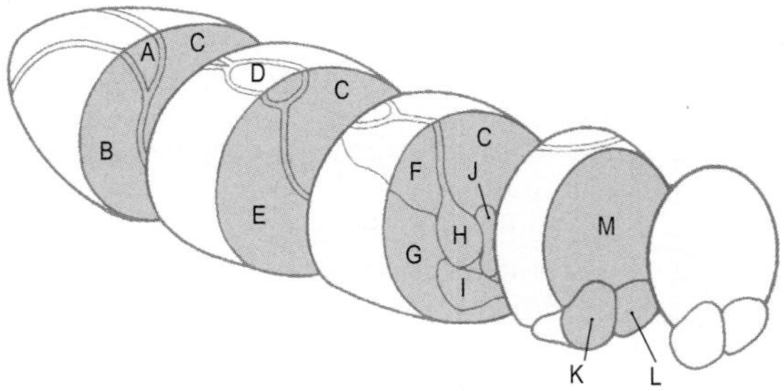

For each of the following descriptions, select the most appropriate part of the thalamus from the image above. Each answer may be used once, more than once or not at all.

1. Receives major input from inferior colliculi
2. Major projection to the primary visual cortex
3. Receives major projections from mammillary body
4. Auditory relay nucleus
5. Contains the area of face representation

40. **Projection and association tracts:**
a. Inferior collicular commissure
b. Cingulate fasciculus
c. Arcuate fasciculus
d. Corpus callosum
e. Posterior commissure
f. Hypothalamospinal tract
g. Brachium conjunctivum
h. Brachium pontis
i. Restiform and juxtarestiform bodies
j. Dorsal longitudinal fasciculus
k. Medial longitudinal fasciculus
l. Uncinate fasciculus
m. Lamina terminalis
n. Commissure of Probst
o. Stria medullaris

For each of the following descriptions, select the most appropriate X from the list above. Each answer may be used once, more than once or not at all.

1. Periventricular hypothalamus and mammillary bodies to midbrain central gray matter
2. Covered with indusium griseum
3. Contains crossing fibers of pretectal nucleus for light reflex
4. Connects Wernicke and Broca's areas
5. Interruption can result in Horner's syndrome

41. For each of the following descriptions, select the most appropriate answers from the image below. Each answer may be used once, more than once or not at all.

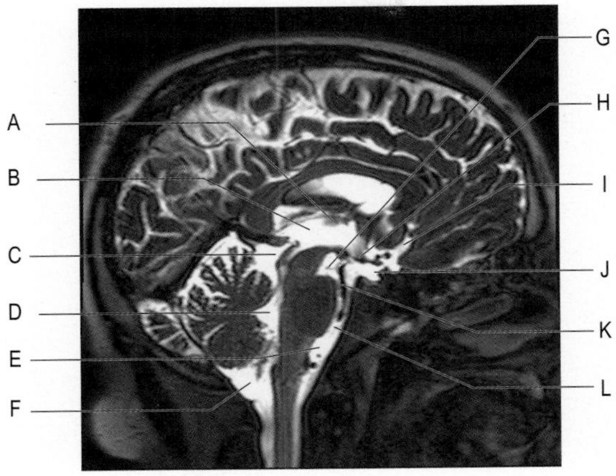

● 1. Cisterna magna
● 2. Interpeduncular cistern
● 3. Chiasmatic cistern

● 42. **Cranial Nerve Nuclei:**

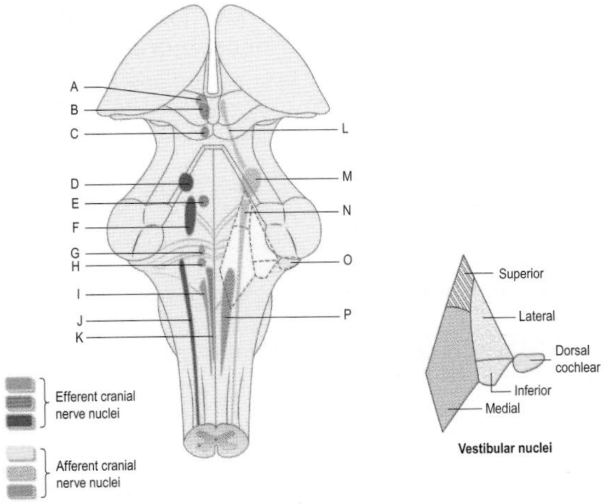

For each of the following descriptions, select the most appropriate answers from the image above. Each answer may be used once, more than once or not at all.
1. Abducens nerve nucleus
2. Principal sensory nucleus of trigeminal nerve
3. Solitary tract nucleus
4. Facial nerve motor nucleus
5. Nucleus ambiguus

● 43. **Sulci and gyri:**

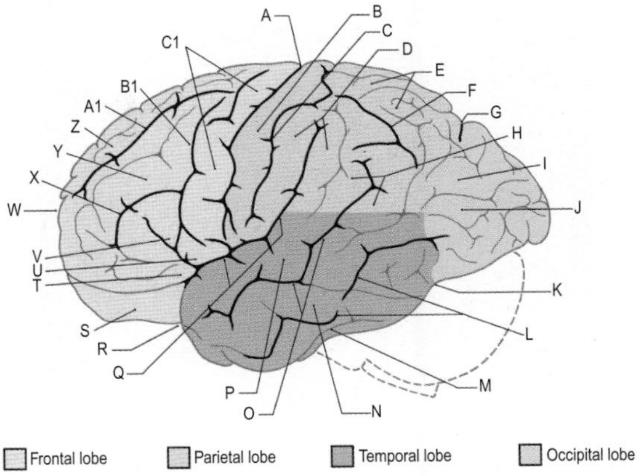

Frontal lobe ☐ Parietal lobe ☐ Temporal lobe ☐ Occipital lobe ☐

For each of the following descriptions, select the most appropriate answers from the image above. Each answer may be used once, more than once or not at all.
1. Angular gyrus
2. Supramarginal gyrus
3. Pars opercularis of inferior frontal grus
4. Middle frontal gyrus
5. Parieto-occipital sulcus

● 44. **Sulci and gyri:**

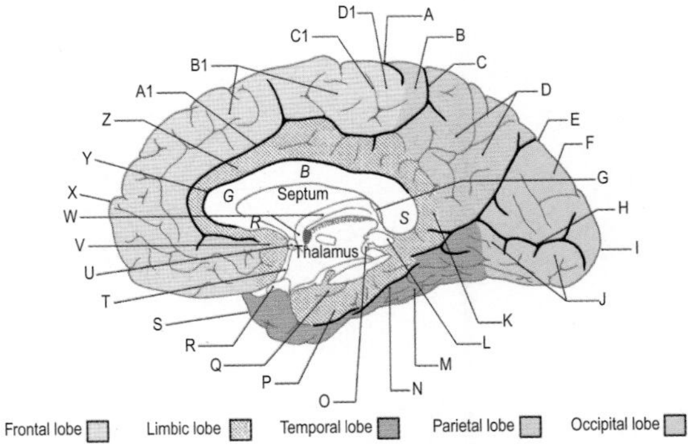

Frontal lobe ☐ Limbic lobe ☐ Temporal lobe ☐ Parietal lobe ☐ Occipital lobe ☐

For each of the following descriptions, select the most appropriate answers from the image above. Each answer may be used once, more than once or not at all.
1. Marginal sulcus
2. Calcarine sulcus
3. Cuneus
4. Collateral sulcus
5. Lamina terminalis

45. **Sulci and gyri:**

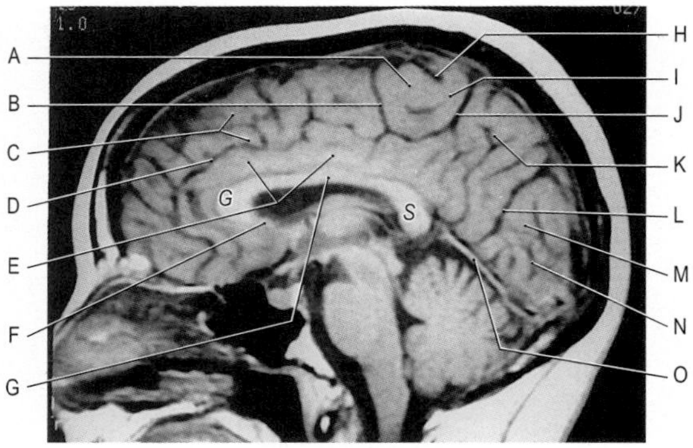

For each of the following descriptions, select the most appropriate answers from the image above. Each answer may be used once, more than once or not at all.

1. Central sulcus
2. Paracentral sulcus
3. Calcarine sulcus
4. Marginal sulcus
5. Precuneus

46. **Fourth ventricular floor:**

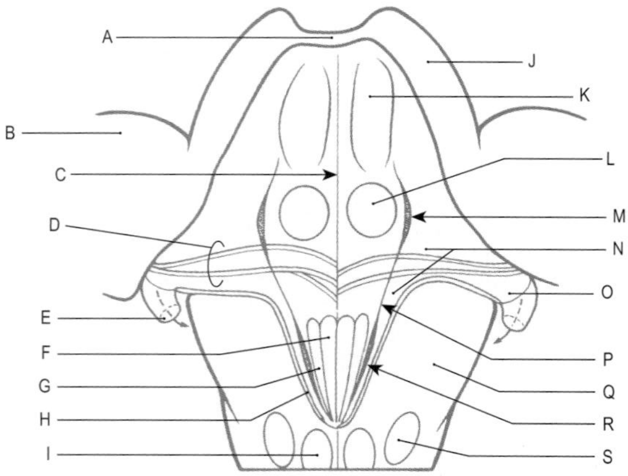

For each of the following descriptions, select the most appropriate answers from the image above. Each answer may be used once, more than once or not at all.

1. Facial colliculus
2. Striae medullaris
3. Sulcus limitans
4. Median sulcus
5. Vagal trigone

47. **Cranial Nerve Nuclei:**

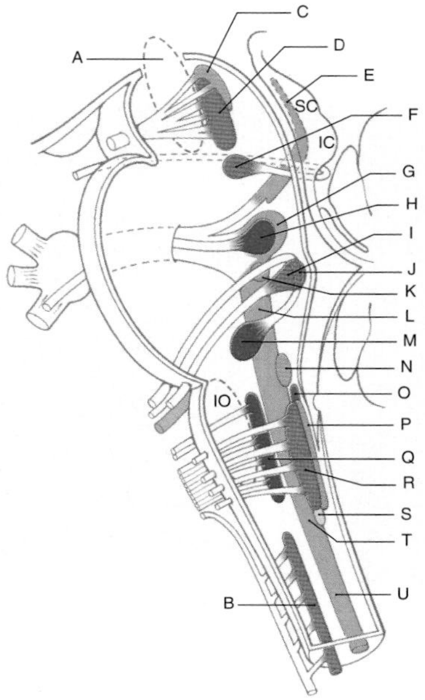

For each of the following descriptions, select the most appropriate answers from the image above. Each answer may be used once, more than once or not at all.

1. Red nucleus
2. Erdinger-Westphal nucleus
3. Oculomotor nucleus
4. Trochlear nucleus
5. Abducens nucleus
6. Facial nucleus
7. Nucleus ambiguus of vagus nerve

48. **Medulla at sensory decussation:**

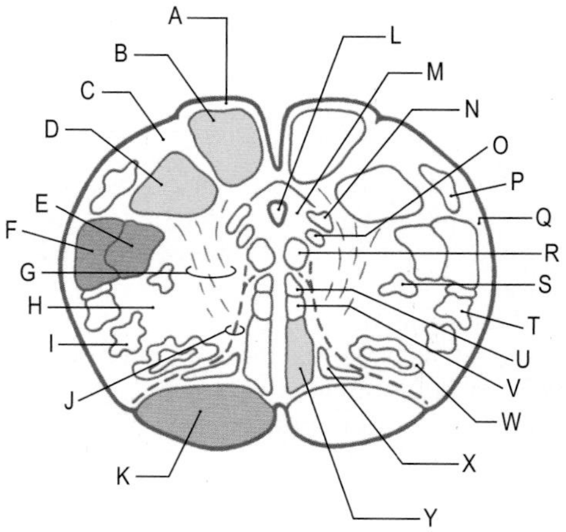

For each of the following descriptions, select the most appropriate answers from the image above. Each answer may be used once, more than once or not at all.

1. Nucleus gracilis
2. Nucleus cuneatus
3. Spinothalamic tract
4. Posterior spinocerebellar fibers

49. **Medulla and vagal nuclei:**

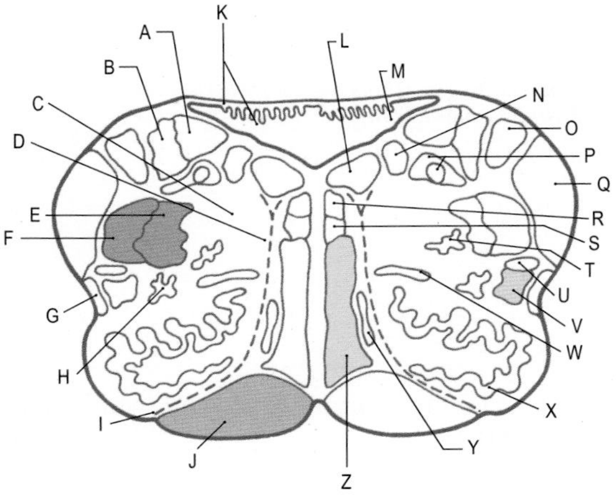

For each of the following descriptions, select the most appropriate answers from the image above. Each answer may be used once, more than once or not at all.

1. Solitary nucleus and tract
2. Dorsal motor vagal nucleus
3. Reticular formation
4. Principal olivary nucleus (inferior olivary nucleus)
5. Medial lemniscus

50. **Rostral medulla:**

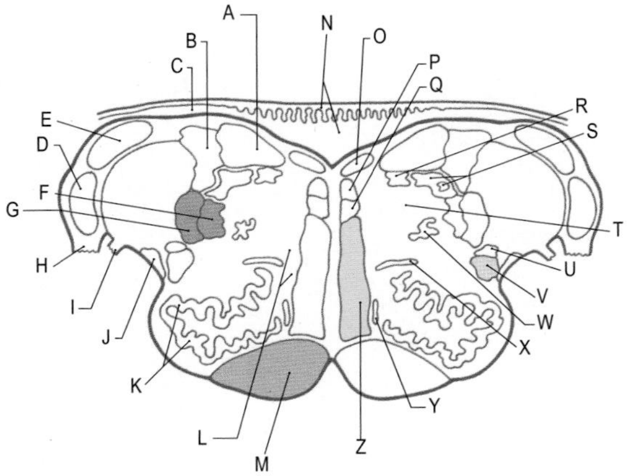

For each of the following descriptions, select the most appropriate answers from the image above. Each answer may be used once, more than once or not at all.

1. Posterior cochlear nucleus
2. Vestibulocochlear nerve
3. Spinal trigeminal nucleus
4. Medial longitudinal fasciculus
5. Nucleus ambiguus

51. **Caudal pons:**

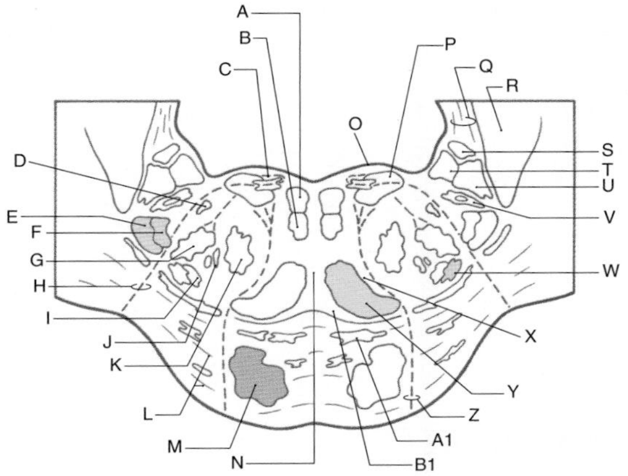

For each of the following descriptions, select the most appropriate answers from the image above. Each answer may be used once, more than once or not at all.

1. Facial nucleus
2. Facial nerve
3. Superior olivary nucleus
4. Abducens nucleus
5. Abducens nerve

52. **Mid-pons:**

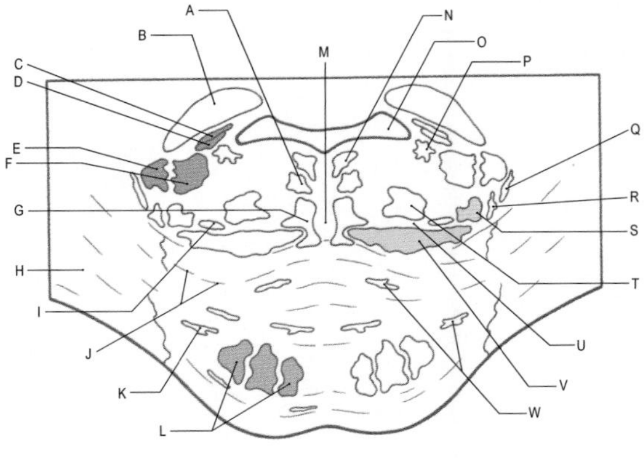

For each of the following descriptions, select the most appropriate answers from the image above. Each answer may be used once, more than once or not at all.

1. Locus ceruleus
2. Corticospinal fibers
3. Principal trigeminal sensory nucleus
4. Fourth ventricle
5. Brachium pontis

53. **Rostral pons:**

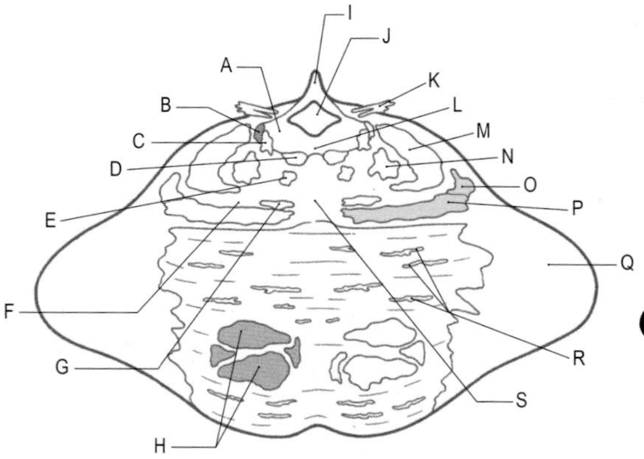

For each of the following descriptions, select the most appropriate answers from the image above. Each answer may be used once, more than once or not at all.

1. Medial lemniscus
2. Medial longitudinal fasciculus
3. Trochlear nerve
4. Central tegmental tract
5. Tectobulbospinal tract

QUESTIONS 54–58

Additional questions 54–58 available on ExpertConsult.com

SBA ANSWERS

1. **c**—Facial artery

The external carotid artery has several branches in the neck (SALFOPSI in ascending order): superior thyroid, ascending pharyngeal, lingual, facial (aka external maxillary), occipital, posterior auricular, superficial temporal, maxillary (aka internal maxillary). It can be distinguished on angiogram (figure) from the ICA, which has no branches in the neck. During EC/IC bypass procedures for Moya Moya disease, anastomosis of the superficial temporal artery to the middle cerebral artery (or less commonly occipital artery to the posterior cerebral artery/posterior inferior cerebellar artery) may be performed.

2. **b**—Via the ventral roots and white rami communicans

3. **d**—Left subclavian artery

Each vertebral artery arises from its ipsilateral subclavian artery. The aortic arch gives off three branches in order: brachiocephalic trunk (or innominate artery), left common carotid and left subclavian arteries (A). The second commonest branching pattern (termed a "bovine arch") is where the left common carotid arises from the brachiocephalic trunk (B).

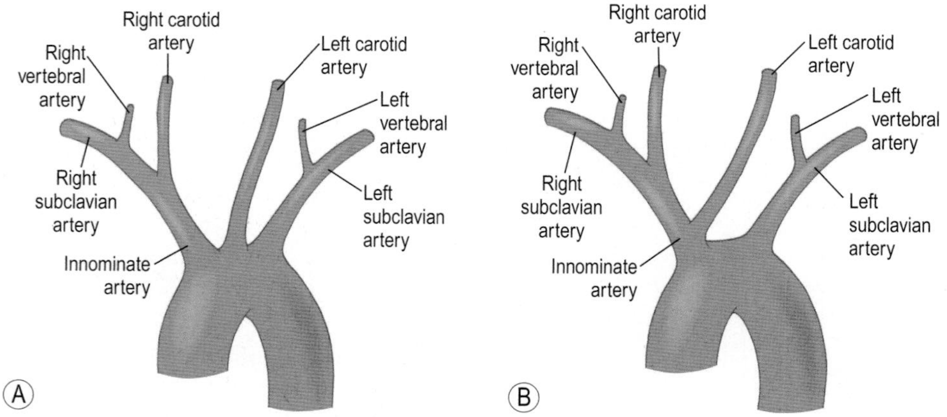

Image redrawn from Layton KF, Kallmes DF, Cloft HJ, Lindell EP, Cox VS. Bovine aortic arch variant in humans: Clarification of a common misnomer. AJNR Am J Neuroradiol 2006;27:1541-1542. In: Low M, Som PM, Naidich TP. Problem solving in neuroradiology. Elsevier.

4. **b**—Subthalamic nucleus

Hemiballismus is a condition characterized by unilateral, involuntary, violent flinging of the limbs. Lesion is based in the contralateral subthalamic nucleus or its connections and due to vascular cause (PCA territory) but can occur in MS. Often settles spontaneously and drug treatment is ineffective.

5. **c**—Red nucleus

Factors normally inhibiting extensor action in the arms and legs are:

(A) Cortical inhibition of lateral vestibular nucleus (vestibulospinal tract) and pontine reticular formation
(B) Red nucleus projections to spinal cord (rubrospinal tract; possibly arms only)
(C) Medullary reticular formation

Disconnection lesion involving red nucleus results in loss of normal inhibition of extension (rubrospinal and medullary reticular formation) and loss of cortical inhibition of extensor action of LVN and pontine RF, producing hyperreflexia and increased extensor tone (decerebrate rigidity). Disconnection lesions above the red nucleus result in extension in legs, but flexion in arms (decorticate rigidity). This is explained as in humans the rubrospinal tract terminates in the cervical spine, meaning intact rubrospinal input could counteract vestibulospinal (extensor) input in the arms but it remains unopposed in the legs.

6. **a**—Superior ophthalmic vein

The cavernous sinus receives the superior and inferior ophthalmic veins, sphenoparietal sinus and the superficial middle cerebral vein (coursing from superiorly to inferiorly in the Sylvian fissure). It drains via superior petrosal sinus (to the junction of the transverse and sigmoid sinuses), inferior petrosal sinus (to the internal jugular vein). Right and left cavernous sinuses are also connected across the midline anterior and posteriorly to the pituitary gland via the anterior and posterior intercavernous sinuses, resulting in the circular sinus. Each cavernous sinus is also connected to the pterygoid venous plexus via small branches in the foramen Vesalii, foramen ovale and foramen lacerum.

7. **c**—Found to branch off from the ICA just proximal to the meningohypophyseal trunk

After the Pcomm, persistent primitive trigeminal artery is the next commonest remnant of the fetal circulation. It is seen in 0.1-0.6% of cerebral angiograms. It connects the cavernous ICA (just proximal to meningohypophyseal trunk) to the basilar artery between superior cerebellar and anterior inferior cerebellar arteries. Its persistence is usually associated with a hypoplastic basilar and vertebral arteries proximal to the anastomosis, as well as a hypoplastic PcommA. Its frequency is explained as the order of regression during embryogenesis is otic/acoustic artery first, then hypoglossal followed by trigeminal. Vascular abnormalities (AVM, aneurysm) is seen in 25%. Characterized by the tau sign (flow void) on sagittal MRI.

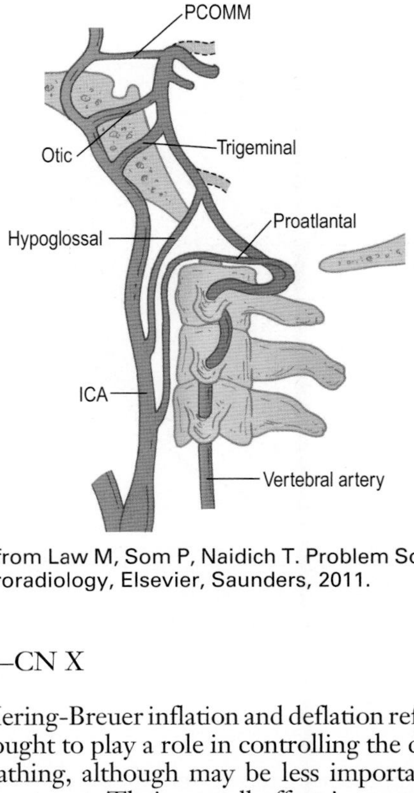

Image from Law M, Som P, Naidich T. Problem Solving in Neuroradiology, Elsevier, Saunders, 2011.

8. **c**—CN X

The Hering-Breuer inflation and deflation reflexes are thought to play a role in controlling the depth of breathing, although may be less important in humans at rest. Their overall effect is to prevent overinflation and extreme deflation of the lungs. The inflation reflex is mediated by pulmonary stretch receptor afferents signaling via CNX during lung inflation to inhibit medullary inspiratory center and the pontine apneustic center, as well as inhibiting cardiac vagal motor neurons resulting in sinus tachycardia. The deflation reflex also acts via CNX and directly activates medullary inspiratory centers, stopping expiration and initiating inspiration.

9. **c**—Trochlear nerve

The Annulus of Zinn (or annular tendon) is a fibrous ring which surrounds the optic nerve, and which is continuous with the dura of the middle cranial fossa. It is divided into upper (superior tendon of Lockwood) and lower (inferior tendon of Zinn) parts which together give rise to the four recti muscles (superior, inferior, medial, lateral) and superior oblique. The remaining two extraocular muscles, inferior oblique and levator palpabrae superioris arise from the maxillary and sphenoid bones respectively. The Annulus of Zinn contains the optic nerve, ophthalmic artery, superior division of CNIII, nasociliary division of CNV1, CNVI, and the inferior division of CNIII.

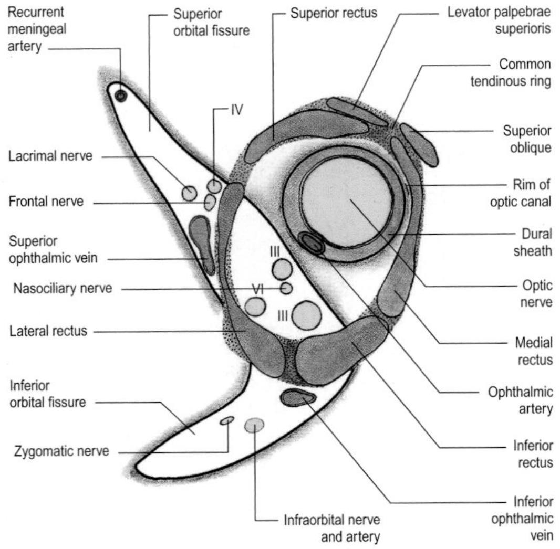

Image from Mancall EL. Gray's Clinical Neuroanatomy: The Anatomic Basis for Clinical Neuroscience, Elsevier, Saunders, 2011.

10. **d**—5

Development of the vertebral column occurs in three stages:

Mesenchymal stage—where somites gives rise to sclerotomes (condensation of mesenchymal cells around notochord and neural tube, divided into a loosely packed upper half and a densely pack lower half) and myotomes. The centrum (primordial vertebral body) forms from the lower half of a cranial sclerotome and the upper half of the immediately caudal sclerotome, such that the intervertebral disc forms at the level opposite the myotome and the vertebral body is at the level between two myotomes.

Cartilaginous stage—chondrification centers appear in the centrum and vertebral arches, causing cartilaginous fusion, and spinous and transverse processes develop from extensions of the chondrification centers in the vertebral arches. Chondrification spreads until a cartilaginous vertebral column is formed.

Bony stage—By the end of the embryonic period each vertebrae usually has three primary ossification centers (centrum and each half vertebral arch), and the cartilaginous connection between the arch and centrum allows growth as the spinal cord enlarges after birth. After puberty, five secondary ossification centers appear—tip of spinous process, tip of both transverse processes and annular epiphyses of the vertebral body.

Vertebra	Primary Ossification Centers	Secondary Ossification Centers
C1 (atlas)	2 × posterior	1 × anterior
C2 (axis)	1 × centrum and 2 × vertebral arch 2 × base of dens (odontoid peg)	1 × tip of dens 1 × ring apophysis 1 × spinous process and 2 × transverse process

11. **d**—L4/5 Interspace

Intercristal line (Tuffier's line)—space between L4 and L5 spinous process, or through L4 spinous process. In infants this is at the L5/S1 level.

12. **b**—Meckel's cave (containing Gasserian ganglion). Axial view in T2 MRI is shown below

Image from Som PM, Curtin HD. Head and Neck Imaging, vol. 2, 5th ed., Elsevier, Mosby, 2011.

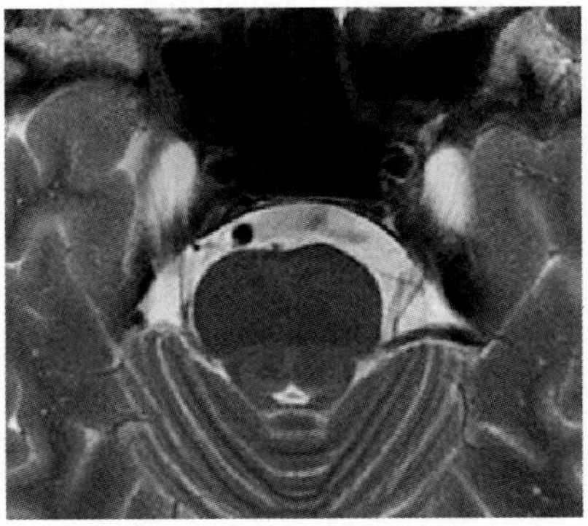

Image from Naidich TP. Imaging of the Brain, Saunders, Elsevier, 2013.

13. **b**—Splanchnic nerves are unmyelinated

Pre-ganglionic sympathetic fibers (myelinated) arise in the lateral horn of gray matter T1-L2 and exit the cord via the anterior (ventral) root then as white rami communicans to reach the sympathetic ganglion. Here they may synapse onto unmyelinated post-ganglionic fibers or pass through unchanged as *splanchnic nerves* (which later synapse in prevertebral ganglia and innervate the viscera). Post-ganglionic fibers exit the sympathetic chain at the same or different level (after ascending or descending), via a gray ramus communicans which relays fibers to an existing spinal nerve. Sympathetic chain runs from the skull base to coccyx on both sides of the vertebral column.

Spinal segments responsible for sympathetic innervation (e.g. vasoconstrictor to skin, pilomotor to hair, sudomotor to sweat glands)

T1-T2: head and neck via ICA/vertebral arteries
T2-T5: upper limb
T1-T4: thoracic viscera via cardiac/pulmonary/esophageal plexus
T4-L2: abdominal viscera via splanchnic nerves to coeliac/hypogastric plexuses (except adrenal medulla which receives a preganglionic fiber which has also traversed the coeliac plexus)
T10-L2: pelvic viscera via splanchnic nerves to pelvic plexus
T11-L2: lower limb

Sympathetic sensory afferents terminate in the intermediate zone of gray matter in the cord and are important in the appreciation of visceral pain.

14. **b**—Inhibition of the internal vesicle sphincter

Sacral parasympathetic outflow:

Anterior (ventral) primary rami of S2, S3 and (occasionally) S4 give off fibers termed pelvic splanchnic nerves or nervi erigentes which join the pelvic sympathetic plexus for distribution to pelvic viscera:

Visceromotor to rectal muscles, inhibitor to internal anal sphincter
Motor to bladder wall, inhibitor to internal vesicle sphincter
Vasodilator fibers to cavernous sinuses of penis/clitoris

15. **b**—Solitary nucleus

Parasympathetic sensory afferents:

Afferent fibers from GI, respiratory, cardiac and mouth/pharynx travelling in CN VII/XI/X terminate in the solitary nucleus of the medulla
Sacral afferents terminate in the S2-S4 gray matter
Important in maintaining visceral reflexes

16. **b**—Facial nerve

The internal auditory canal runs lateral and posteriorly from the porus on the medial surface of the temporal bone to fundus (entry to middle ear). The lateral portion of the internal canal is divided into superior and inferior compartments by the falciform or transverse crest. The superior compartment is further divided into anterior and posterior portions by the vertical crest (Bill's bar). Thus the IAC contains four main neural components in quadrants: the facial nerve (superior and anterior), the superior vestibular nerve (superior and posterior), the cochlear nerve (anterior and inferior), and the inferior vestibular nerve (posterior and inferior). The inferior compartment does not have a bony division for the cochlear and inferior vestibular nerves, but the cochlear nerve leaves the IAC through a multiperforate osseous plate to enter the cochlear modiolus.

Image adapted from Quiñones-Hinojosa A. Schmidek and Sweet's Operative Neurosurgical Techniques, 6th ed., Saunders, Elsevier, 2012.

17. **d**—C4 (cavernous)

Image from Naidich TP. Imaging of the Brain, Saunders, Elsevier, 2013.2. PICA

Bouthillier Classsification of ICA Segments

C1 (Cervical)	Extends from the origin of the internal carotid artery to its entry into the skull base
C2 (Petrous)	Portion of the artery within the carotid canal of the petrous temporal bone. Initially, ascends vertically within the canal (vertical portion) and then turns anteriorly, medially, and superiorly within the canal (genu) and continues horizontally (horizontal portion) toward the petrous apex, where it exits the temporal bone Vidian artery Caroticotympanic artery may (variably)

Continued on following page

Bouthillier Classsification of ICA Segments (Continued)	
C3 (Lacerum)	Begins where the internal carotid artery exits from the carotid canal and extends up to the level of the petroclinoid ligament. Passes over (not through) covered foramen lacerum
C4 (Cavernous)	Begins at the superior aspect of the petroclinoid ligament and includes the portion of the internal carotid artery that courses through the cavernous sinus until the proximal dural ring Meningohypophyseal artery, arises from the posterior genu of C4 and gives rise to three major branches: Inferior hypophyseal artery—posterior pituitary gland Tentorial artery (of Bernasconi and Cassinari) Dorsal clival (meningeal) artery The inferolateral trunk commonly arises from the horizontal portion of C4 and courses laterally to supply CN III, IV, and VI in addition to the trigeminal ganglion and the dura covering the cavernous sinus
C5 (Clinoid)	Short segment between the proximal and distal dural reflections (rings) related to the anterior clinoid process
C6 (ophthalmic/ supraclinoid)	Begins at the distal dural ring/reflection (continuous with the falx) around the anterior clinoid process at which point it is considered to be intradural (in the subarachnoid space) and extends to the origin of the posterior communicating artery Ophthalmic artery typically arises from the medial aspect of the C6 segment and courses with the optic nerve through the optic canal into the orbit. The ophthalmic artery gives rise to multiple ocular, orbital, and extraorbital branches. The ocular branches include the central retinal artery and ciliary arteries Superior hypophyseal artery arises from the medial aspect of C6, anastomoses with its contralateral counterpart, and forms a vascular plexus about the pituitary stalk. This plexus supplies the anterior pituitary gland, tuber cinereum, optic nerve, and optic chiasm
C7 (communicating)	Begins just proximal to the origin of the posterior communicating artery and terminates where the internal carotid artery bifurcates into the anterior and middle cerebral arteries Posterior communicating artery—courses posteriorly through the suprasellar cistern to anastomose with the PCA. Large PCoA size suggests that it directly supplies the PCA territory as a persistent fetal PCA The origin of the PCoA often exhibits a focal enlargement, designated the infundibulum. CN III courses through the suprasellar cistern close to the PCoA, so it is often affected by aneurysms of the PCoA. The anterior thalamoperforating arteries arise from the PCoAs and course superiorly to supply portions of the medial hypothalamus, thalamus, and lateral aspect of the third ventricle Anterior choroid artery arises from the posterior aspect of C7 just above the PCoA. Its long course is divided into three segments. The anterior choroid artery first courses through the suprasellar cistern just medial to the uncus of the temporal lobe (cisternal segment). It then turns laterally and passes through the choroid fissure to enter the temporal horn of the lateral ventricle. Within the ventricle, the anterior choroid artery supplies the choroid plexus and courses posterosuperiorly with the choroid plexus up to and around the pulvinar of the thalamus. In its course, the anterior choroid artery supplies the medial temporal lobe, the optic tract and lateral geniculate body, the dorsal globus pallidus, the inferior half of the posterior limb of the internal capsule, the lateral aspect of the cerebral peduncle, the tail of the caudate nucleus, and the choroid plexus

N.b. Multiple other systems for classifying carotid artery segments exist (e.g. Gibo/Rhoton, Fischer, Ziyal)

ANSWERS 18–25

Additional answers 18–25 available on ExpertConsult.com

EMI ANSWERS

26. 1—g, 2—a, 3—c

Coronal scan through the cavernos sinus. MR contrast-enhanced FIESTA sequence. a, oculomotor nerve; b, trochlear nerve; c, abducens nerve; d, ophthalmic nerve; e, maxillary nerve; f, internal cerebral artery; cavernous segment; g, right optic nerve; h, pituitary gland.

Image from Naidich TP. Imaging of the Brain, Saunders, Elsevier, 2013.

27. 1—e, 2—c, 3—f

Axial T2W MR images at the level of the facial colliculi. a, abducens nucleus; b, superior cerebellar peduncle (brachium conjunctivum); c, basal turn of the cochlea, scala vestibule/scala tympani; d, osseous spiral lamina; e, anterior inferior cerebellar artery (AICA); f, cochlear nerve; g, second turn of cochlea; h, vestibule; i, lateral and posterior semicircular canals; j, inferior vestibular nerve.

Image from Naidich TP. Imaging of the Brain, Saunders, Elsevier, 2013.

28. 1—b, 2—m, 3—g

a, MCA; b, ACA; c, circular sinus; d, Dura propria; e, Periosteal dura; f, ICA; g, Oculomotor nerve (III); h, inner membranous layer; i, Medial temporal lobe dura; j, IV; k, VI; l, V1; m, Maxillary division of CN V (V2).

Image adapted from Yousem DM, Grossman RI. Neuroradiology: The Requisites, 3rd ed., Mosby, Elsevier, 2010.

29. 1—q, 2—o, 3—b, 4—l

a, Labyrinthine segment; b, Greater superficial petrosal nerve; c, Cochlea; d, Geniculate ganglion; e, Stapes; f, Malleus; g, Incus; h, Tympanic segment of facial nerve; i, Vertical (mastoid) segment of facial nerve; j, Stylomastoid foramen; k, Horizontal (lateral) semicircular canal; l, Posterior semicircular canal; m, Superior semicircular canal; n, Inferior vestibular nerve; o, Superior vestibular nerve; p, Internal auditory canal; q, Facial nerve; r, Meatal foramen.

Image adapted from Winn HR. Youman's Neurological Surgery, 4-Volume Set, 6th ed., Elsevier, Saunders, 2011.

30. 1—c, 2—b, 3—a

a, Facial nerve; b, vestibulocochlear nerve; c, anterior inferior cerebellar artery (AICA); d, abducens nerve; e, superior vestibular nerve; f, cochlear nerve; g, inferior vestibular nerve; h, cerebellum.

Image with permission from Naidich TP. Imaging of the Brain, Saunders, Elsevier, 2013.

31. 1—a, 2—i, 3—c, 4—f, 5—b

a, Caudate nucleus; b, Putamen; c, Globus pallidus (External segment); d, Globus pallidus (Internal segment); e, Substantia innominate; f, Internal capsule; g, External capsule; h, Extreme capsule; i, Claustrum; j, Amygdala; k, Hippocampus; l, Thalamus.

Image adapted with permission from Crossman A. Neuroanatomy: An Illustrated Colour Text, 5th ed., Churchill Livingstone, Elsevier, 2015.

32. 1—i, Supraopticohypophyseal tract; 2—j, Tuberoinfundibular (tuberohypophyseal) tract; 3—g, Nucleus of the diagonal band of Broca (vertical limb); 4—c, Median forebrain bundle; 5—f, Postcommissural Fornix

Projection and Association Tracts

A.	Central tegmental tract	Connects rostral solitary nucleus (gustatory) to medial thalamic VPM and red nucleus to inferior olive
B.	Lamina terminalis	Closed rostral end of the neural tube
C.	Median forebrain bundle	Connects septal area, hypothalamus, basal olfactory areas, hippocampus/subiculum to midbrain, pons and medulla
D.	Stria medullaris	Connects the septal area, hypothalamus, olfactory area and anterior thalamus to the habenulum
E.	Stria terminalis	Amygdala to hypothalamus
F.	Postcommissural Fornix	Hippocampus to cingulate gyrus
G.	Nucleus of the diagonal band of Broca (vertical limb)	Septal nuclei to hippocampus
H.	Retinohypothalamic tract	Retinal ganglion cells to suprachiasmatic nuclei and other hypothalamic nuclei (circadian rhythm)
I.	Supraopticohypophyseal tract	Supraoptic/paraventricular nuclei to neurohypophysis (posterior pituitary)
J.	Tuberoinfundibular (tuberohypophyseal) tract	Neuroendocrine neurons from arcuate nucleus to hypophyseal portal system (release dopamine and growth hormone releasing hormone into portal blood which cause anterior pituitary to release prolactin and growth hormone respectively)
K.	Trapezoid body	Ventral cochlear nuclei to contralateral superior olive

Continued on following page

Projection and Association Tracts (Continued)

L.	Thalamic fasciculus (Forel's field H1)	Combination of ansa lenticularis, lenticular fasciculus and cerebellothalamic tract to VA/VL thalamus
M.	Nucleus of the Diagonal band of Broca (horizontal limb)	Connects septal nuclei to amygdala
N.	Mammillothalamic tract	Mammillary body to anterior thalamic nuclei
O.	Tapetum	Corpus callosum fibers connecting temporal to occipital lobes

33. 1—j, 2—e, 3—n, 4—c, 5—m

34. 1—i, 2—q, 3—b, 4—g, 5—f

a, Thalamostriate and choroid veins; b, Superior anastomotic vein; c, Superior sagittal sinus; d, Inferior sagittal sinus; e, Internal cerebral vein; f, Great cerebral vein (Vein of Galen); g, Basal vein; h, Straight sinus; i, Inferior anastomotic vein; j, Transverse vein; k, Occipital sinus; l, Sigmoid sinus; m, Inferior petrosal sinus; n, Superior petrosal sinus; o, Cavernous sinus; p, Deep middle cerebral vein; q, Superficial middle cerebral vein; r, Anterior cerebral vein.

Image adapted with permission from Mancall EL. Gray's Clinical Neuroanatomy: The Anatomic Basis for Clinical Neuroscience, Elsevier, Saunders, 2011.

35. 1—h, Posterior inferior cerebellar artery; 2—g, Superior cerebellar artery; 3—d, Anterior inferior cerebellar artery; 4—g, Internal carotid artery; 5—k, Posterior communicating artery

36. 1—d, 2—e, 3—p, 4—n, 5—d

Parasympathetic motor efferents—This system is divided into cranial and sacral components, and parasympathetic efferents only synapse with postganglionic cells close to or within target viscera (allowing local discrete responses).

Cranial outflow:

- Edinger Westphal nucleus (midbrain)—CN III (preganglionic fibers)—ciliary ganglion—postganglionic fibers to ciliary muscle, sphincter pupillae
- Superior salivatory nucleus (pons)—CN VII branches A) nervus intermedius via greater petrosal nerve to pterygopalatine ganglion and lacrimal gland and B) chorda tympani and lingual nerve to submandibular ganglion for secretomotor to submandibular/sublingual glands
- Inferior salivatory nucleus (medulla)—CN IX via lesser petrosal nerve to otic ganglion then postganglionic in auriculotemporal nerve to parotid gland
- Dorsal nucleus (medulla)—CN X to the plexuses on the walls of respiratory, cardiac and abdominal viscera

37. 1—c, 2—a, 3—g, 4—i, 5—k

Projection and Association Tracts

A.	Ansa lenticularis	Globus pallidus interna around IC to thalamus
B.	Fasciculus retroflexus	Habenulum to midbrain and interpeduncular nuclei
C.	Lenticular fasciculus (Forel's field H2)	Globus pallidus interna through IC to thalamus
D.	Postcommissural Fornix	Hippocampus to cingulate gyrus
E.	Precommissural Fornix	Hippocampus to septal nuclei, hypothalamus, mammillary bodies, anterior thalamus
F.	Thalamic fasciculus (Forel's field H1)	Combination of ansa lenticularis, lenticular fasciculus and cerebellothalamic tract to VA/VL thalamus
G.	Diagonal band of Broca	Connects septal nuclei to amygdala
H.	Mammillothalamic tract	Mammillary body to anterior thalamic nuclei
I.	Tapetum	Corpus callosum fibers connecting temporal to occipital lobes

Continued

J.	Uncinate fasciculus	Anterior temporal lobe to orbitofrontal gyrus
K.	Commissure of Probst	Dorsal nucleus of lateral lemniscus to inferior colliculus
L.	Central tegmental tract	Connects rostral solitary nucleus (gustatory) to medial thalamic VPM and red nucleus to inferior olive
M.	Lamina terminalis	Closed rostral end of the neural tube
N.	Median forebrain bundle	Connects septal area, hypothalamus, basal olfactory areas, hippocampus/subiculum to midbrain, pons and medulla
O.	Stria medullaris	Connects the septal area, hypothalamus, olfactory area and anterior thalamus to the habenulum

38. 1—j, 2—b, 3—g, 4—l, 5—k

a, Anterior nucleus; b, Ventral anterior nucleus; c, Lateral dorsal nucleus; d, Ventral lateral nucleus (oral part); e, Ventral lateral nucleus (caudal part); f, Lateral posterior nucleus; g, Ventral posterolateral and ventral posteromedial nuclei; h, Dorsomedial nucleus (Magnocellular); i, Dorsomedial nucleus (Parvicellular); j, Pulvinar; k, Medial geniculate nucleus; l, Lateral geniculate nucleus.

Image adapted from Haines DE. Fundamental Neuroscience for Basic and Clinical Applications, 4th ed., Saunders, Elsevier, 2013.

39. 1—m, Pulvinar; 2—k, Lateral geniculate; 3—a, Anterior; 4—l, Medial geniculate; 5—i, Ventral posteromedial

a, Anterior (A); b, Ventral anterior (VA); c, Dorsomedial (DM); d, Lateral dorsal (LD); e, Ventral lateral (VL); f, Lateral Posterior (LP); g, Ventral posterolateral (VP); h, Centromedian (CM); i, Ventral posteromedial (VPM); j, Parafascicular (PF); k, Lateral geniculate (LGB); l, Medial geniculate (MGB); m, Pulvinar (P).

Image adapted from Haines DE. Fundamental Neuroscience for Basic and Clinical Applications, 4th ed., Saunders, Elsevier, 2013.

Thalamic Nuclei: Inputs, Outputs and Function

Type	Nucleus	Specific Inputs	Output	Function
Relay	Anterior	Mammillothalamic tract, hippocampus	Cingulate gyrus	Limbic (emotion and memory)
	Lateral dorsal (LD)	Hippocampus (fornix)	Cingulate gyrus	Limbic (memory)
	Ventral anterior, (VA)	Globus pallidus, SN, cerebellum	Premotor (area 6) and PFC	Planning of movement (cortico-subcortico-cortical loop)
	Ventral lateral (VL)	Cerebellum, GP, SN	Primary motor (area 4) and premotor (area 6)	Initiation of movement (cortico-cerebello-cortical loop)
	Ventral intermediate (VIM)	Cerebellum	Primary motor cortex (area 4)	Coordination of movement
	Ventral posterolateral (VPL)	Medial lemniscus (body), spinothalamic tract (body)	Somatosensory cortex (area 1-3)	Somatosensory (body)
	Ventral posteromedial (VPM)	Medial lemniscus (face), spinothalamic tract (face) Central tegmental tract (taste)	Somatosensory cortex (area 1-3) Insula	Somatosensory (head and taste)
	Medial geniculate (MGN)	Brachium of the inferior colliculus	Auditory cortex (area 41,42)	Auditory relay

Continued on following page

Thalamic Nuclei: Inputs, Outputs and Function (Continued)

Type	Nucleus	Specific Inputs	Output	Function
	Lateral geniculate (LGN)	Optic tract	Visual cortex (Area 17)	Visual relay
Association	Dorsomedial (DM)	Prefrontal cortex, olfactory and limbic structures	Prefrontal cortex	Limbic (Emotional response to pain and memory)
	Lateral posterior (LP)	Unknown	Parietal association cortex	Unknown
	Pulvinar	Parietal, occipital, and temporal lobes	Parietal-occipital-temporal association cortex	Visual association
Regulatory	Reticular	Thalamus and cortex	All thalamic nuclei	Attention
	Centromedian (CM)	Brainstem	Putamen and motor cortex	Attention and arousal
	Parafascicular	Brainstem	Caudate nucleus and PFC	Attention and arousal

40. 1—j, 2—d, 3—e, 4—c, 5—f

Projection and Association Tracts

A.	Inferior collicular commissure	Connects the inferior colliculi
B.	Cingulate fasciculus (cingulum bundle)	Cingulate gyrus to entorhinal cortex
C.	Arcuate fasciculus	Wernicke's area to Broca's (temporal, parietal and frontal)
D.	Corpus callosum	Connects both hemispheres. Covered with indusium griseum (supracallosal gyrus) which is a thick layer of unmyelinated fibers arranged as medial and lateral longitudinal striae of Lanscisi
E.	Posterior commissure	Crossing fibers from pretectal nucleus for the consensual light reflex
F.	Hypothalamospinal tract	Hypothalamus to ciliospinal center in intermediolateral column of T1-T2 spinal cord
G.	Brachium conjunctivum	AKA superior cerebellar peduncle
H.	Brachium pontis	AKA middle cerebellar peduncle
I.	Restiform and juxtarestiform bodies	AKA inferior cerebellar peduncle
J.	Dorsal longitudinal fasciculus	Periventricular hypothalamus/mammillary bodies to midbrain central gray matter
K.	Medial longitudinal fasciculus	Optokinetic and vestibularocular reflexes and saccadic eye movements Descending fibers: superomedial vestibular nuclei, tectospinal tract, vestibulospinal tract Ascending fibers: vestibular nucleus to nuclei for III, IV, VI
L.	Uncinate fasciculus	Anterior temporal lobe to orbitofrontal gyrus
M.	Lamina terminalis	Closed rostral end of neural tube
N.	Commissure of Probst	Dorsal nucleus of lateral lemniscus to inferior colliculus
O.	Stria medullaris	Septal area, hypothalamus, olfactory area and anterior thalamus to habenulum

41. 1—f, 2—g, 3—j

a, Massa intermedia; b, Third ventricle; c, Supratectal cistern; d, Fourth ventricle; e, Pontomedullary cistern; f, Cisterna magna; g, Interpeduncular cistern; h, Optic chiasma; i, Cistern of lamina terminalis; j, Chiasmatic cistern; k, Basilar Artery; l, Prepontine cistern.

Image from Standring S (Ed.), Gray's Anatomy, 40th ed., Churchill Livingstone, Elsevier, 2008.

42. 1—e, 2—m, 3—p, 4—f, 5—j

a, Edinger-Westphal nucleus; b, Oculomotor nucleus; c, Trochlear nucleus; d, Trigeminal motor nucleus; e, Abducens nucleus; f, Facial motor nucleus; g, Salivatory nuclei (superior); h, Salivatory nuclei (inferior); i, Dorsal vagal motor nucleus; j, Nucleus ambiguous; k, Hypoglossal nucleus; l, Trigeminal mesencephalic nucleus; m, Trigeminal main sensory nucleus; n, Trigeminal spinal nucleus; o, Dorsal cochlear nucleus; p, Nucleus of tractus solitaries.

Image adapted from Mancall EL. Gray's Clinical Neuroanatomy: The Anatomic Basis for Clinical Neuroscience, Elsevier, Saunders, 2011.

43. 1—h, 2—d, 3—u, 4—y, 5—g

a, Central sulcus; b, Post central gyrus; c, Postcentral sulcus; d, Supramarginal gyrus; e, Superior parietal lobule; f, Intraparietal sulcus; g, Parieto-occipital sulcus; h, Angular gyrus; i, Superior occipital gyrus; j, Inferior occipital gyrus; k, Preoccipital notch; l, Middle temporal sulcus; m, Inferior temporal sulcus; n, Middle temporal gyrus; o, Superior temporal sulcus; p, Superior temporal gyrus; q, Lateral sulcus; r, Temporal pole; s, Orbital surface; t, Inferior frontal gyrus (Pars triangularis); u, Inferior frontal gyrus (Pars opercularis); v, Inferior frontal gyrus (Pars orbitalis); w, Frontal pole; x, Inferior frontal sulcus; y, Middle frontal gyrus; z, Superior frontal gyrus; a1, Superior frontal sulcus; b1, Precentral sulcus; c1, Precentral gyrus.

Image adapted with permission from Haines DE. Fundamental Neuroscience for Basic and Clinical Applications, 4th ed., Saunders, Elsevier, 2013.

44. 1—c, 2—h, 3—f, 4—n, 5—t

a, Central sulcus; b, Posterior paracentral gyrus; c, Marginal sulcus; d, Precuneus; e, Parieto-occipital sulcus; f, Cuneus; g, Hippocampal commissure; h, Calcarine sulcus; i, Occipital pole; j, Lingual gyrus; k, Isthmus of cingulate gyrus; l, Pineal; m, Occipitotemporal gyri; n, Collateral sulcus; o, Posterior commissure; p, Parahippocampal gyrus; q, Uncus; r, Optic chiasm; s, Temporal pole; t, Lamina terminalis; u, Anterior commissure; v, Subcallosal area; w, Fornix; x, Frontal pole; y, Callosal sulcus; z, Cingulate gyrus; a1, Cingulate sulcus; b1, Superior frontal gyrus; c1, Paracentral sulcus; d1, Anterior paracentral gyrus.

Image adapted with permission from Haines DE. Fundamental Neuroscience for Basic and Clinical Applications, 4th ed., Saunders, Elsevier, 2013.

45. 1—h, 2—b, 3—n, 4—j, 5—k

a, Anterior paracentral gyrus; b, Paracentral sulcus; c, Superior frontal gyrus; d, Cingulate sulcus; e, Cingulate gyrus; f, Rostrum of corpus callosum; g, Body of corpus callosum; h, Central sulcus; i, Posterior paracentral gyrus; j, Marginal sulcus; k, Precuneus; l, Parieto-occipital sulcus; m, Cuneus; n, Calcarine sulcus; o, Tentorium cerebelli.

Image adapted with permission from Haines DE. Fundamental Neuroscience for Basic and Clinical Applications, 4th ed., Saunders, Elsevier, 2013.

46. 1—l, 2—d, 3—p, 4—c, 5—g

a, Anterior medullary velum; b, Middle cerebellar peduncle; c, Median sulcus of rhomboid fossa; d, Striae medullares; e, Foramen of Luschka; f, Hypoglossal trigone; g, Vagal trigone; h, Tela choroidea (cut edge); i, Gracile tubercle; j, Superior cerebellar peduncle; k, Medial eminence of fourth ventricle; l, Facial colliculus; m, Superior fovea; n, Vestibular area; o, Lateral recess; p, Sulcus limitans; q, Restiform body; r, Inferior fovea; s, Cuneate tubercle.

Image adapted with permission from Haines DE. Fundamental Neuroscience for Basic and Clinical Applications, 4th ed., Saunders, Elsevier, 2013.

47. 1—a, 2—c, 3—d, 4—f, 5—i

a, Red nucleus; b, Accessory nucleus; c, Edinger-Westphal preganglionic nucleus; d, Oculomotor nucleus; e, Mesencephalic nucleus; f, Trochlear nucleus; g, Principal sensory nucleus; h, Trigeminal motor nucleus; i, Abducens nucleus; j, Internal genu of facial nerve; k, Superior salivatory nucleus; l, Spinal trigeminal nucleus, pars oralis; m, Facial motor nucleus; n, Inferior salivatory nucleus; o, Solitary nucleus (and tract); p, Dorsal motor vagal nucleus; q, Nucleus ambiguous; r, Hypoglossal nucleus; s, Solitary nucleus (and tract); t, Spinal trigeminal nucleus, pars caudalis; u, Substantia gelatinosa (spinal lamina II).

Image adapted with permission from Haines DE. Fundamental Neuroscience for Basic and Clinical Applications, 4th ed., Saunders, Elsevier, 2013.

48. 1—b, 2—q, 3—f, 4—p

a, Gracile fasciculus; b, Gracile nucleus; c, Cuneate fasciculus; d, Cuneate nucleus; e, Spinal trigeminal: Nucleus (pars caudalis); f, Spinothalamic tract; g, Internal arcuate fibers; h, Reticular formation; i, Lateral reticular nucleus; j, Hypoglossal nerve; k, Pyramid (corticospinal fibers); l, Central canal; m, Central gray; n, Solitary nucleus and tract; o, Dorsal motor vagal nucleus; p, Posterior spinocerebellar fibers; q, Accessory cuneate nucleus; r, Hypoglossal nucleus; s, Nucleus ambiguous; t, Anterolateral system; u, Medial longitudinal fasciculus; v, Tectobulbospinal system; w, Principal olivary nucleus; x, Medial accessory olivary nucleus; y, Medial lemniscus.

Image adapted with permission from Haines DE. Fundamental Neuroscience for Basic and Clinical Applications, 4th ed., Saunders, Elsevier, 2013.

49. 1—p, 2—n, 3—c, 4—x, 5—z

a, Medial vestibular nucleus; b, Inferior vestibular nucleus; c, Reticular formation; d, Hypoglossal nerve; e, Spinal trigeminal: Nucleus (pars interpolaris); f, Tract; g, Anterior spinocerebellar tract; h, Lateral reticular nucleus; i, Hypoglossal nerve; j, Pyramid (corticospinal fibers); k, Choroid plexus and fourth ventricle; l, Hypoglossal nucleus; m, Sulcus limitans; n, Dorsal motor vagal nucleus; o, Accessory cuneate nucleus; p, Solitary tract and nucleus; q, Restiform body; r, Medial longitudinal fasciculus; s, Tectobulbospinal system; t, Nucleus ambiguous; u, Rubrospinal tract; v, Anterolateral system; w, Posterior accessory olivary nucleus; x, Principal olivary nucleus; y, Medial accessory olivary nucleus; z, Medial lemniscus.

Image adapted with permission from Haines DE. Fundamental Neuroscience for Basic and Clinical Applications, 4th ed., Saunders, Elsevier, 2013.

50. 1—e, 2—h, 3—f, 4—o, 5—v

a, Medial vestibular nucleus; b, Inferior vestibular nucleus; c, Lateral recess of fourth ventricle; d, Cochlear nuclei: Anterior; e, Cochlear nuclei: Posterior; f, Spinal trigeminal: Nucleus (pars oralis); g, Spinal trigeminal: Tract; h, Vestibulocochlear nerve; i, Glossopharyngeal nerve; j, Anterior spinocerebellar tract; j, Principal olivary nucleus; k, Anterior trigeminothalamic fibers; l, Pyramid (corticospinal fibers); m, Choroid plexus and fourth ventricle; n, Prepositus nucleus; o, Medial longitudinal fasciculus; p, Tectobulbospinal system; q, Inferior salivatory nucleus; r, Solitary tract and nucleus; s, Reticular formation; t, Rubrospinal tract; u, Anterolateral system; v, Nucleus ambiguous; w, Posterior accessory olivary nucleus; x, Medial accessory olivary nucleus; y, Medial lemniscus.

Image adapted with permission from Haines DE. Fundamental Neuroscience for Basic and Clinical Applications, 4th ed., Saunders, Elsevier, 2013.

51. 1—g, 2—h, 3—j, 4—p, 5—z

a, Medial longitudinal fasciculus; b, Tectobulbospinal system; c, Internal genu of facial nerve; d, Superior salivatory nucleus; e, Spinal trigeminal: Tract; f, Spinal trigeminal: Nucleus (pars oralis); g, Facial nucleus; h, Facial nerve; i, Rubrospinal tract; j, Superior olivary nucleus; k, Central tegmental tract; l, Transverse pontine fibers (pontocerebellar); m, Corticospinal fibers; n, Nucleus raphe magnus; o, Facial colliculus; p, Abducens nucleus; q, Inferior cerebellar peduncle: Juxtarestiform body; r, Inferior cerebellar peduncle: Restiform body; s, Vestibular nuclei: Superior; t, Vestibular nuclei: Medial; u, Vestibular nuclei: Lateral; v, Solitary tract and nucleus; w, Anterolateral system; x, Anterior trigeminothalamic tract; y, Medial lemniscus; z, Abducens nerve; a1, Pontine nuclei; b1, Trapezoid body.

Image adapted with permission from Haines DE, Fundamental Neuroscience for Basic and Clinical Applications, 4th ed., Saunders, Elsevier, 2013.

52. 1—p, 2—l, 3—e, 4—o, 5—h

a, Tectobulbospinal system; b, Brachium conjunctivum; c, Mesencephalic tract; d, Mesencephalic nucleus; e, Trigeminal nuclei: Principal sensory; f, Trigeminal nuclei: Motor; g, Reticulotegmental nucleus; h, Brachium pontis; i, Rubrospinal tract; j, Transverse pontine fibers (pontocerebellar); k, Pontine nuclei; l, Corticospinal fibers; m, Nucleus raphe pontis; n, Medial longitudinal fasciculus; o, Fourth ventricle; p, Locus ceruleus; q, Anterior spinocerebellar fibers; r, Lateral lemniscus; s, Anterolateral system; t, Central tegmental tract; u, Anterior trigeminothalamic fibers; v, Medial lemniscus; w, Pontine nuclei.

Image adapted with permission from Haines DE. Fundamental Neuroscience for Basic and Clinical Applications, 4th ed., Saunders, Elsevier, 2013.

53. 1—p, 2—d, 3—k, 4—n, 5—e

a, Periaqueductal gray; b, Mesencephalic tract and nucleus; c, Locus ceruleus; d, Medial longitudinal fasciculus; e, Tectobulbospinal system; f, Anterior trigeminothalamic fibers; g, Rubrospinal tract; h, Corticospinal fibers; i, Frenulum; j, Fourth ventricle-cerebral aqueduct transition; k, Trochlear nerve; l, Posterior raphe nucleus; m, Brachium conjunctivum; n, Central tegmental tract; o, Anterolateral system; p, Medial lemniscus; q, Middle cerebellar peduncle; r, Pontine nuclei; s, Central superior nucleus (of the raphe).

Image adapted with permission from Haines DE. Fundamental Neuroscience for Basic and Clinical Applications, 4th ed., Saunders, Elsevier, 2013.

ANSWERS 54–58

Additional answers 54–58 available on ExpertConsult.com

CHAPTER 2

EMBRYOLOGY

SINGLE BEST ANSWER (SBA) QUESTIONS

1. Which one of the following correctly describes the order of embryological stages of CNS development?
   a. Blastogenesis, gastrulation, dorsal induction, ventral induction, neural proliferation, neuronal migration, and axonal myelination
   b. Dorsal induction, ventral induction, gastrulation, neural proliferation, neuronal migration, and axonal myelination
   c. Gastrulation ventral induction, dorsal induction, neural proliferation, neuronal migration, and axonal myelination
   d. Neural proliferation, gastrulation dorsal induction, ventral induction, neuronal migration, and axonal myelination
   e. Ventral induction, gastrulation, dorsal induction, neural proliferation, axonal myelination, and neuronal migration

2. Which one of the following statements regarding gastrulation is most accurate?
   a. It is the process by which the bilaminar disc is converted into a trilaminar disc
   b. It can result in lipomyelomeningocele if disturbed
   c. It is not dependent on bone morphogenetic protein expression
   d. It starts with closure of the cranial neuropore
   e. It occurs from embryonic days 10-12

3. Which one of the following statements about primary neurulation is most accurate?
   a. Anterior neuropore closure approximately occurs on D19
   b. Disjunction results in formation of the spinal canal below the posterior neuropore
   c. Fusion of the neural folds starts at the anterior neuropore and proceeds caudally in a zip-like fashion until it reaches the posterior neuropore
   d. Notochord induces the overlying ectoderm to differentiate into a flat area of specialized neuroectoderm called the neural plate
   e. SHH/morphogen secretion on D14 causes the neural plate to form median hinge points and start invaginating along its central axis to form a neural groove (with neural folds on either side)

4. Which one of the following statements about secondary neurulation and retrogressive differentiation is most accurate?
   a. Important for the formation of the conus medullaris but not the filum terminale
   b. Involves canalization of a caudal mensenchymal cell mass
   c. Is completed by days 24-26 of embryonic development
   d. Responsible for the formation of thoracic, lumbar, sacral, and coccygeal neural tube
   e. Retrogressive differentiation is a mitotic process

5. Which one of the following statements about ventral induction is most accurate?
   a. It includes development of the primary brain fissure
   b. It includes development of the secondary brain vesicles and brain flexures
   c. It includes formation of the neural plate
   d. It includes formation of the notochord
   e. It includes primary neurulation

6. The disencephalon does not give rise to which one of the following?
   a. 3rd ventricle
   b. Mamillary bodies
   c. Optic vesicle
   d. Posterior pituitary
   e. Superior colliculus

7. Mesencephalon does NOT give rise to which one of the following?
   a. Cerebral aqueduct
   b. Edinger-Westphal nucleus
   c. Pineal body
   d. Red nucleus
   e. Substantia nigra

8. Which one of the following statements about the rhombencephalon is most accurate?
   a. It contains the cerebral aqueduct at its center
   b. It gives rise to diencephalon and myelencephalon secondary brain vesicles
   c. It gives rise to the inferior colliculi and pons
   d. It is separated from the mesencephalon by the isthmus rhombencephalii
   e. Pontine flexure indents the rhombencephalon ventrally

9. Which one of the following statements about cerebellar development is most accurate?
   a. Brainstem input to the cerebellum is via parallel and climbing fibers
   b. Commences at week 15
   c. Golgi cells come to reside in the molecular layer
   d. Granule cells develop axons called Mossy fibers
   e. Granule cells migrate inward past Purkinje cells with the help of Bergmann glia

10. Which one of the following is important in dorsoventral patterning of the neural tube?
    a. BF-1
    b. BMP-4 and BMP-7
    c. EMX1 and EMX2
    d. FGF-8
    e. HOX
    f. SHH

11. Which one of the following best describes cells forming the mantle layer in the developing neural tube?
    a. Ependymal cells
    b. Glioblasts
    c. Neuroblasts
    d. Postmitotic young neurons
    e. Radial cells

12. Which one of the following statements about cerebral cortex formation is most accurate?
    a. Cortical layers are laid down from most superficial to deep
    b. Germinal matrix zone is superficial to the ventricular zone
    c. Intermediate zone contains axons of cortical pyramidal neurons
    d. Migration of cortical pyramidal neurons occurs tangentially
    e. The neocortex usually has four layers in the adult

13. Which one of the following is the first to form in the developing brain?
    a. Anterior commissure
    b. Genu of corpus callosum
    c. Hippocampal commissure
    d. Posterior commissure
    e. Splenium of corpus callosum

14. Which one of the following statements about the developing spinal cord are most accurate?
    a. Alar columns form the intermediolateral horn
    b. Alar columns form the ventral horns
    c. Dorsally the floor plate marks where the paired basal columns meet
    d. Laterally, the alar and basal plates abut at a groove called the sulcus limitans
    e. Ventrally the roof plate marks where the paired alar columns meet

QUESTIONS 15–25

Additional questions 15–25 available on ExpertConsult.com

EXTENDED MATCHING ITEM (EMI) QUESTIONS

26. **Embryological terms:**
    a. Ectoderm
    b. Endoderm
    c. Induction
    d. Mesenchyme
    e. Mesoderm
    f. Neural crest
    g. Notochord
    h. Paraxial mesoderm
    i. Primitive streak
    j. Sclerotome
    k. Somite

For each of the following descriptions, select the most appropriate answers from the list above. Each answer may be used once, more than once or not at all.

1. Population of cells arising from the lateral lips of the neural plate that detach during formation of the neural tube and migrate to form a variety of cell types/structures.
2. The first morphological sign of gastrulation.

3. The process in which one embryonic region interacts with a second embryonic region, thereby influencing the behavior or differentiation of the second region.

27. **Central nervous system formation:**
 a. Diencephalon
 b. Mescencephalon
 c. Metencephalon
 d. Myelencephalon
 e. Prosencephalon
 f. Rhombencephalon
 g. Telencephalon

For each of the following descriptions, select the most appropriate answers from the list above. Each answer may be used once, more than once or not at all.
1. Contains cerebral aqueduct
2. Gives rise to the cerebellar hemispheres

28. **Embryology:**
 a. Days 2-3
 b. Days 4-5
 c. Day 6
 d. Days 8-12
 e. Days 14-17
 f. Day 18
 g. Day 20
 h. Days 24-26
 i. Days 26-28
 j. Day 31
 k. Day 35
 l. Day 42

For each of the following descriptions, select the most appropriate answers from the list above. Each answer may be used once, more than once or not at all.
1. Formation of the neural plate
2. Closure of the posterior neuropore
3. Five secondary brain vesicles

29. **Neurulation:**
 a. Alar plate
 b. Basal plate
 c. Caudal neuropore
 d. Cranial neuropore
 e. Dorsal root ganglion
 f. Neural fold
 g. Neural groove
 h. Notochord
 i. Primary neurulation
 j. Primitive node
 k. Primitive streak
 l. Secondary neurulation

For each of the following descriptions, select the most appropriate answers from the list above. Each answer may be used once, more than once or not at all.
1. Origin of neural crest cells
2. Failure of closure results in spina bifida
3. Structure signaling to midline ectoderm to form neural tube
4. Formed by neural crest cells

30. **Pharyngeal arch derivatives:**
 a. 1st pharyngeal arch
 b. 2nd pharyngeal arch
 c. 3rd pharyngeal arch
 d. 4th pharyngeal arch
 e. 5th pharyngeal arch
 f. 6th pharyngeal arch
 g. Ductus thyroglossus
 h. Foramen caecum
 i. Sinus cervicalis
 j. Tuberculum impar
 k. Tuberculum laterale

For each of the following descriptions, select the most appropriate answers from the list above. Each answer may be used once, more than once or not at all.
1. Common carotid and internal carotid artery and glossopharyngeal nerve
2. Recurrent laryngeal branch of CN X
3. Parts of CN V2 and V3
4. Facial nerve

31. **Disorders of CNS development:**
 a. Adrenoleukodystrophy
 b. Caudal regression syndrome
 c. Dandy-Walker spectrum
 d. Heterotopia
 e. Intradural lipoma
 f. Lipoma of filum terminale
 g. Pelizaeus-Merzbacher disease
 h. Schizencephaly
 i. Segmental spinal dysgenesis
 j. Split cord malformation
 k. Sturge-Weber syndrome
 l. Terminal myelocystocele

For each of the following descriptions, select the most appropriate answers from the list above. Each answer may be used once, more than once or not at all.
1. Disorder of neural proliferation
2. Disorder of notochordal integration during gastrulation
3. Disorder of ventral induction

SBA ANSWERS

1. **a**—Blastogenesis, gastrulation, dorsal induction, ventral induction, neural proliferation, neuronal migration, and axonal myelination.

Below is a simplified timeline of neural development. It is worth noting that different brain regions have a unique course of ontogeny. Late developing structures, including the cortex, hippocampus and the cerebellum set the stage for differential periods of vulnerability to insults in a regionally specific manner. Timings for individual events vary between sources for events beyond ventral induction, but the general sequence is as follows:

Blastogenesis	D1-13	Development from a fertilized embryo into a bilaminar blastocyst implanted in the uterus with amniotic and yolk sacs
Gastrulation	D14-17	It is the process by which the bilaminar disc is converted into a trilaminar disc, including integration of bilateral notochordal anlagen into a single notochordal process and segmental notochordal formation
Dorsal induction	D17-28 (3rd-4th week)	Formation and closure of neural tube (primary neurulation). Development of three primary brain vesicles, and two flexures (D21 mesencephalic and D28 cervical)
Secondary neurulation	D28-D48	Formation of the neural tube caudal to the posterior neuropore (below S2/3) from mesenchyme by cavitation
Ventral induction	5th-10th week	Existing three primary brain vesicles (prosencephalon, mesencephalon, and rhombencephalon) differentiate into five vesicles (telencephalon, diencephalon, mesencephalon, metencephalon, and myelencephalon) and subsequently forebrain, midbrain, and hindbrain structures. Pontine flexure forms on D32
Neural proliferation	6-12 weeks	Neuroblasts (primitive neurons) proliferate in the subependymal zone of the neural tube adjacent to the central canal of the spinal cord or the ventricles of the brain. Glio
Migration (histogenesis)	8 weeks-	Neuroblasts become neurons which then use radial glial cell fibers as scaffolds to reach their eventual destination in cortex or subcortical nuclei. Radial glial cells also have a progenitor function in the late stages of neurogenesis—their asymmetric division produces a new radial glial cell and a postmitotic neuron
Axonal/dendritic outgrowth	16 weeks-	Neuronal arborization and branching in an attempt to establish appropriate connections
Apoptosis	18 weeks-	Approximately 50% of all neurons are eliminated before birth to allow dramatic morphological rearrangements to increase efficiency of synaptic transmission (a second wave of overproduction and elimination occurs later in life during periadolescence)
Synaptogenesis	20 weeks-	Formation of synapses as part of CNS maturation, second wave occurs in periadolescence
Myelination	6 months-adulthood	Axons become insulated with myelin sheaths allowing rapid transmission of action potentials between nodes of Ranvier. Completion of myelination marks maturity of the nervous system
Synaptic elimination/ pruning	12 months postnatally onwards	Competitive elimination of synapses during functional development of each brain region, e.g., 40% reduction in fontal cortex synaptic density between 7 and 15 years of age

2. **a**—It is the process by which the bilaminar disc is converted into a trilaminar disc.

Gastrulation occurs between D14 and D17, and is the process by which the bilaminar disc (consisting of epiblast facing the amniotic cavity and the hypoblast facing the yolk sac) becomes a trilaminar disc with formation of an intervening third layer, the mesoblast (future mesoderm). On day 14 or 15 a strip of thickened epiblast/ectoderm (primitive streak) appears caudally in the midline of the dorsal surface of the embryo to define the craniocaudal axis. The cranial end of the primitive streak forms the primitive (Hendersen's) node, and shows a central depression called the primitive pit. Ectodermal cells start migrating towards the primitive streak, pass inward at the primitive pit to the interface of ectoderm and endoderm, and then migrate laterally to form the mesoderm. The two paired notochordal anlagen (primordia) then fuse in the midline to form a single notochordal process ("notochordal integration"; D16). The primitive node defines the craniocaudal axis, the right and left sides and the dorsal and ventral surfaces of the embryo. Prospective notochordal cells in the wrong craniocaudal position undergo apoptosis maintaining segmental notochordal formation. Multiple signaling molecules, such as bone morphogenetic protein (BMP), fibroblast growth factor (FGF), and Wnt are essential for gastrulation to occur. BMP is very important in establishing the rostrocaudal polarity. In addition, multiple factors and genes are implicated in patterning the primitive body axis (e.g., brachyury, sonic hedgehog (SHH), and HNF-beta genes). Defects in gastrulation (integration or segmental formation) affect development and differentiation of all three primary cell layers and cause abnormalities from the occiput downwards, e.g., split cord malformation (diastematomyelia and diplomyelia), neurenteric, dermoid, and epidermoid cysts, anterior and posterior spina bifida, intestinal malformation, duplication and fistula formation, and anterior meningocele.

3. **d**—Notochord induces the overlying ectoderm to differentiate into a flat area of specialized neuroectoderm called the neural plate

Dorsal induction (3rd-4th weeks; D17-D28) includes primary neurulation, secondary neurulation and formation of the "true" notochord. Primary neurulation involves separation of neuroectoderm in the neural plate from cutaneous ectoderm to form the neural tube (brain and spinal cord) as far caudal as S2/3. The steps are summarized below:

- Neural induction and formation of the neural plate: the notochord induces the overlying ectoderm to differentiate into a flat area of specialized neuroectoderm (neural plate). Relative to Hensen's node, the neural plate expands cranially and narrows/elongates the parts on either side of the primary streak—these areas will form the brain and spinal cord, respectively. This process is regulated by multiple genes, including brachyury and Wnt.
- SHH/morphogen secretion on D18 causes the neural plate to form median hinge points and start invaginating along its central axis to form a neural groove (with neural folds on either side).
- These folds progressively increase in size and flex to approach each other, until they eventually fuse in the midline to form the neural tube (regulated by PAX3 genes). Fusion occurs in a zip-like fashion, probably at multiple sites but first at the level of the 4th somite (future craniocervical junction).
- The cranial end of the neural tube (anterior neuropore) closes first at the site of the lamina terminalis on D24-26, followed by the posterior neuropore on D26-28 to complete primary neurulation. Note that the posterior neural pore is not located at the caudal tip of the neural tube. The caudal part of the spinal cord and the lowest sacrum portion is formed from the solid core of neuroepithelium (tail bud) during secondary neurulation.
- Ectodermal cells progressively disconnecting from the lateral walls of the neural folds during formation of the neural tube differentiate into the neural crest cells (form branchial arch derivatives, dorsal roots/dorsal root ganglia, autonomic ganglia and adrenergic cells).
- Disjunction: Immediately after neural tube closure it becomes separated from the overlying superficial ectoderm (forms the skin) by dorsally migrating mesenchyme (forms meninges, neural arches of the vertebrae and paraspinal muscles).

4. **b**—Involves canalization of a caudal mensenchymal cell mass

The location of the caudal end of the neural plate (posterior neuropore) is approximately at the S3 level. The remaining caudal sacral and coccygeal portions of the neural tube, including the conus medullaris and filum terminale are formed by secondary neurulation and retrogressive differentiation (days 28-48). During secondary neurulation, a secondary neural tube is formed caudad to the posterior neuropore. A caudal cell mass of undifferentiated, totipotential cells initially appears as a result of fusion of neural ectoderm with the lower portion of the notochord. Multiple small vacuoles then appear in the caudal cell mass and progressively coalesce to form a central canal (canalization), which will merge with the canal formed during primary neurulation. Retrogressive differentiation is an apoptotic process in which a combination of regression, degeneration and further differentiation of the caudal cell mass into the tip of the conus medullaris, ventriculus terminalis, and filum terminale.

5. **b**—It includes development of the secondary brain vesicles and brain flexures.

By the end of dorsal induction/primary neurulation the neural tube is closed and three primary brain vesicles (prosencephalon, mesencephalon, and rhombencephalon) are present. During ventral induction (5th-10th weeks of gestation) the primary brain vesicles differentiate into five secondary brain vesicles by day 35 (telencephalon, diencephalon, mesencephalon, metencephalon, and myelencephalon) which then form forebrain, midbrain, and hindbrain structures. Between the 4th and 8th weeks, the brain tube folds sharply at three locations. The first of these folds to develop is the cephalic flexure (between diencephalon and mesencephalon), followed by the cervical flexure between myelencephalon and spinal cord—both flexures are ventral and produce an inverted U shape. The last flexure is dorsally located between metencephalon and myelencephalon (pontine flexure) and changes the shape to an M. By the 8th week, deepening of the pontine flexure has folded the metencephalon (including the developing cerebellum) back onto the myelencephalon. Any insult during this phase affects the development of brain vesicles and the formation of the facial skeleton. Ocular and nasal anomalies are frequently associated with forebrain malformation because the optic placode and forebrain develop at the same time, with subsequent formation of the olfactory vesicle 1 week later. The commonly seen forebrain ventral induction malformations are (1) holoprosencephaly, (2) atelencephaly, (3) olfactory aplasia, (4) agenesis of the corpus callosum, and (5) agenesis of the septum pellucidum (septo-optic dysplasia, cavum vergae and pellucidum). Hindbrain anomalies include vermian dysgenesis (e.g., Dandy-Walker spectrum).

6. **c**—Optic vesicle

The prosencephalon is the most rostral of the three brain vesicles and gives rise to a caudal diencephalon and a rostral telencephalon. A pair of diverticula, known as the telencephalic vesicles, appear dorsally and rostrally, which form the cerebral hemispheres as the central cavities form the lateral ventricles. The posterior part of the prosencephalon becomes the diencephalon, which later develops into the thalami, hypothalamus, epithalamus, optic cups, and neurohypophysis. The central cavity in the region of diencephalon forms the third ventricle. Simultaneously, two lateral outpouchings (optic vesicles) grow from the telencephalon on each side. These optic vesicles form the retina and optic nerve. Cells of the diencephalon and telencephalon originate from the germinal matrix lining of the third and lateral ventricles, respectively. The telencephalon grows rapidly and covers the developing diencephalon, midbrain and hindbrain, because the outer regions grow more rapidly than the floor. This growth of the cerebral hemispheres within the developing cranial cavity gives the characteristic "C" shape to the developing lateral ventricles. The mesenchymal tissue trapped in the midline between the developing hemispheres develops into the cerebral falx.

7. **c**—Pineal body

The mesencephalon undergoes the least amount of change during the expansion from three primary to five secondary brain vesicles, and forms the midbrain. The central cavity decreases in size to form the aqueduct of Sylvius. The neuroblasts from the dorsal alar plates migrate and appear as two swellings that form the superior and inferior colliculi (tectal plate). Some cells of the alar plate also migrate ventrally to form the red nucleus and substantia nigra. The basal plate of the mesencephalon forms the midbrain tegmentum (which include the somatic and general visceral efferent columns, and crus cerebri).

8. **d**—It is separated from the mesencephalon by the isthmus rhombencephalii

With rapid growth of the embryonic brain, the neural tube bends on itself in a zigzag fashion. Two flexures developed initially are the cephalic and the cervical flexures, and these are concave ventrally so the neural tube forms a wide upside-down U-shaped configuration. The mescencephalon and rhombencephalon are separated by a constriction (isthmus rhombencephalii). Around 6 weeks of gestation, the pontine flexure develops dorsally between the two rhombencephalic vesicles—metencephalon (future pons and cerebellum) and myelencephalon (future medulla). This flexure is concave dorsally, thereby converting the shape of the developing neural tube into a broad "M" shape. Hindbrain structures form as follows:

- Pons—develops from a thickening in the floor and lateral walls of the metencephalon.
- Medulla oblongata—develops from the thickened floor and lateral walls of the myelencephalon which is continuous inferiorly with the spinal cord.
- Cerebellum—alar plates of the and rhombic lips of the metencephalon form the cerebellum.

9. **e**—Granule cells migrate inward past Purkinje cells with the help of Bergmann glia

Development of the pontine flexure result in:
- The cranial and the caudal ends of the 4th ventricle approximate together dorsally.
- The rhombencephalic roof plate is folded inward towards the cavity of the 4th ventricle.
- The alar columns are splayed laterally because of the bending of the pons and eventually lie dorsolateral to the basal columns.

Therefore, the roof plate of the developing 4th ventricle remains thin, is wide at its fold/waist and tapers superiorly and inferiorly (diamond shaped). Mesenchyme inserts itself into the roof fold and forms the plica choroidalis (choroid plexus precursor) which divides the roof of the 4th ventricle into a superior anterior membranous area (AMA) and inferior posterior membranous area (PMA). The alar laminae along the lateral margins of the AMA become thickened to form two rhombic lips, which enlarge to approach each other and fuse in the midline dorsally (covering the rostral half of the 4th ventricle and overlapping the pons and the medulla). As the rhombic lips grow to form the cerebellar hemispheres and midline vermis, the AMA regresses by incorporation into the developing choroid plexus. Growth and backward extension of the cerebellum pushes the choroid plexus inferiorly, whereas the PMA greatly diminishes in the relative size compared with the overgrowing cerebellum. Subsequently there is development of a marked caudal protrusion of the 4th ventricle, causing the PMA to expand as the finger of a glove. This Blake's pouch consists of ventricular ependyma surrounded by condensation of the mesenchymal tissues and is initially a closed cavity that does not communicate with the surrounding subarachnoid space of the cisterna magna. The network between the vermis and the Blake's pouch progressively becomes condensed, whereas the other portions about the evagination become rarified resulting in permeabilization of the Blake's pouch to form the foramen of Magendie. The foramina of Luschka also probably appear late into the 4th month of gestation. From superior to inferior, the residual AMA, choroid plexus and residual PMA (i.e., residual rhombencephalic roof plate) form the definitive tela choroidea of the 4th ventricle. Folding, transverse fissure formation and foliation result in anterior lobe (cerebellar vermis and hemisphere above primary fissure), posterior lobe (vermis and hemispheres below primary fissure) and a flocculonodular lobe.

Development of the cerebellar cortex and deep nuclei (dentate, globose, emboliform, and fastigial) occurs as follows:
- Week 8—Metencephalon consists of typical ventricular, mantle and marginal layers and rhombic lips have started to form the cerebellum. The ventricular layer produces four types of neurons forming the mantle layer which will subsequently migrate to the cortex: Purkinje cells, Golgi cells, basket cells, and stellate cells, as well as their associated glia (astrocytes including Bergmann glia, and oligodendrocytes).
- Week 12—Two additional layers form: an external germinal/granular layer derived from the rhombic lips, from which granular cells migrate inwards to form a new internal germinal layer between the ventricular and marginal layers (cells of the mantle layer have now dispersed into the marginal layer where they will form a distinct cortical pattern). External germinal layer also produces primitive nuclear neurons which also migrate inwards to form the deep cerebellar nuclei. Migration of granule cells takes place along Bergman (radial) glia. Purkinje cells migrate toward the cortex, it reels out an axon that maintains synaptic contact with neurons in the developing deep cerebellar nuclei. These axons will constitute the only efferents of the mature cerebellar cortex.
- Week 15—From superficial to deep the cerebellum consists of: external granular layer (persists until approximately 15 months postnatally), Purkinje cell layer, molecular layer (stellate, basket cells), and granular layer (Golgi cells; granule cells and their parallel fibers), white matter (Mossy fibers from brainstem nulcei, climbing fibers from inferior olivary nucleus) and deep cerebellar nuclei.

10. **f**—Sonic hedgehog

Some of the molecular signals patterning brain and spinal cord development include homeobox-containing genes (e.g., HOX, PAX, OTX, EMX). A homeobox is a 180 bp DNA sequence found within genes involved in anatomical development (morphogenesis) and are important in establishing body axes and cellular differentiation:

Homeobox-containing genes coding transcription factors:

- PAX3 and PAX7 are expressed by the entire neural plate.
- Homeotic (HOX) genes control the body plan of an embryo along the craniocaudal axis, e.g., the rhombencephalon is divided into eight segments called rhombomeres, which are regulated by an overlapping HOX gene expression.
- Other homeobox genes are important in establishment of forebrain and midbrain boundaries and are expressed even before the formation of neural fold (e.g., Lim1 and OTX2). Later, once the neural folds and pharyngeal arches appear, additional homeobox genes, including OTX1, EMX1, and EMX2, are expressed in an overlapping pattern to further specify the identity of these brain regions.

Other factors:

- Sonic hedgehog (SHH) is a protein secreted by the notochord and floor plate which downregulates the expression of PAX3 and PAX7 in the midline and ventral half of the neural tube (dorsoventral patterning).
- Wnt signaling pathway is active in the midline and dorsal half of the neural tube (dorsoventral patterning) and axon guidance.
- Bone morphogenetic protein (BMP-4 and BMP-7) are growth factors important in dorsolateral patterning. They are secreted by the adjacent non-neural ectoderm, maintain and upregulate PAX3 and PAX7 expression in the dorsal half of the neural tube which stimulates alar plate formation.
- Fibroblast growth factor-8 is secreted by the anterior neural ridge (an organizing center in the neural plate) which induces expression of the brain factor-1 (BF-1) transcription factor that regulates the development of the telencephalon.

11. **d**—Postmitotic young neurons

Except in the telencephalon, neurogenesis establishes the following architecture of the neural tube (from central to peripheral):

1. Central canal.
2. Ventricular layer—neuroepithelial (radial) cells which give rise to all other layers.
3. Mantle layer—contains cell bodies of postmitotic young neurons which have migrated laterally from the ventricular layer and will form eventual gray matter.
4. Marginal layer—outermost layer contains the axons of neurons in the mantle layer, and will form eventual white matter (folding of the cerebral hemispheres will alter its position to subcortical).

After production of neurons is waning in the ventricular layer, this layer begins to produce a new cell type, the glioblast which differentiate into glia of the CNS—astrocytes and oligodendrocytes. Glia provide metabolic and structural support to the neurons of the central nervous system. The last cells produced by the ventricular layer are the ependymal cells; these line the brain ventricles and the central canal of the spinal cord and produce CSF.

12. **c**—Intermediate zone contains axons of cortical pyramidal neurons

The cerebral cortex is made up of several cell layers (or laminae) that vary in number from three in the phylogenetically oldest parts to six in the dominant neocortex. Compared to the rest of the CNS, cerebral cortex has an "inside-out" arrangement of gray and white matter.

- Proliferating cells of the ventricular layer undergo a series of regulated divisions to produce waves of neurons that migrate peripherally (on radial cell processes spanning the full thickness of the cortex) and establish the neuronal layers of the cortex. The first wave of neurons form a cortical layer is termed the preplate.
- Axons extend from preplate cells back towards the ventricular zone producing an intermediate zone (white matter).
- As neurogenesis proceeds, new neurons are increasingly formed in an accessory germinative zone lying deep to the ventricular zone, called the subventricular (germinal matrix) zone.
- Multiple cortical layers are laid down in a sequence from *deep* to *superficial*, that is, the neurons of each wave migrate through the preceding layers to establish a more superficial layer. This is thought to be mediated by reelin (glycoprotein) secreted by transient Cajal-Retzius cells which migrate to the marginal layer (lamina I) tangentially after being born in a dorsal midline telencephalic structure. As such, after normal cortical histogenesis has been achieved in principle, only lamina II-VI persist in the adult.
- As the production of neurons tapers off, the ventricular layer gives rise to various kinds of glia and then to the ependyma.

More numerous but smaller than the pyramidal neurons are the inhibitory interneurons—the granule cells, which originate in the ganglionic eminences of the ventral telencephalon and migrate dorsally into the cortex via a tangential route.

13. **a**—Anterior commissure

The commissures that connect the right and left cerebral hemispheres form from a thickening at the cranial end of the telencephalon, which represents the zone of final neuropore closure. This area can be divided into a dorsal commissural plate and a ventral lamina terminalis:

- 7th week—anterior commissure forms in the commissural plate and interconnects the olfactory bulbs and olfactory centers of the two hemispheres.
- 9th week—hippocampal (forniceal) commissure forms between the right and left hippocampi.
- 9th week (late)—corpus callosum linking together the right and left neocortices along their entire length. The most anterior part (the genu) of the corpus callosum appears first, and its posterior extension (the splenium) forms later in fetal life.

14. **d**—Laterally, the alar and basal plates abut at a groove called the sulcus limitans.

Cell bodies in subependymal zone: in the spinal cord cells remain near the subependymal zone to form the central gray matter of the spinal cord (mantle layer) and extend axonal processes toward the periphery of the spinal cord.

Axons (white matter) surrounds gray: the surrounding spinal cord white matter is comprised of local and ascending white matter tracts generated in the spinal cord gray matter and descending tracts from supranuclear sources.

Starting at the end of the 4th week, the neurons in the mantle layer of the spinal cord become organized into four plates that run the length of the cord: a pair of dorsal (alar) columns and a pair of ventral (basal) columns. Laterally, the two plates abut at a groove called the sulcus limitans, dorsally the roof plate and ventrally the floor plate (both non-neurogenic). The cells of the ventral columns become the somatic motoneurons of the spinal cord and innervate somatic motor structures such as the voluntary (striated) muscles of the body wall and extremities. The cells of the dorsal columns develop into association neurons receiving synapses from *afferent* (incoming) fibers from the sensory neurons of the dorsal root ganglia, and either synapsing with ipsilateral/contralateral motoneurons to form a reflex arc or it may ascend to the brain. The outgoing (*efferent*) motor neuron fibers exit via the ventral roots. In most regions of the cord—at all 12 thoracic levels, at lumbar levels L1 and L2, and at sacral levels S2-S4—the neurons in more dorsal regions of the ventral columns segregate to form intermediolateral cell columns. The thoracic and lumbar intermediolateral cell columns contain the visceral motoneurons that constitute the central autonomic motoneurons of the sympathetic division, whereas the intermediolateral cell columns in the sacral region contain the visceral motoneurons that constitute the central autonomic motoneurons of the parasympathetic division.

ANSWERS 15–25

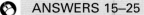

Additional answers 15–25 available on ExpertConsult.com

EMI ANSWERS

26. 1—f, Neural crest; 2—i, Primitive streak; 3—c, Induction (see table of definitions below)

Term	Definition
Ectoderm	Outermost of the three primary germ layers, which forms the neural tube, skin and pigmented cells
Endoderm	Inner most of the three primary germ layers, which forms the respiratory tract, gastrointestinal tract and appendages, urinary tract amongst others
Induction	The process in which one embryonic region interacts with a second embryonic region, thereby influencing the behavior or differentiation of the second region. Most, and perhaps all, tissues require inductive interactions for normal development
Mesenchyme	Loosely associated embryonic cells derived from mesoderm that differentiates into connective or hemopoietic tissue. This is in distinction to epithelial cells, which are tightly connected at specific cell junctions, forming sheets or tubes
Mesoderm	One of the three germ layers, it gives rise to the muscles and skeleton of the body as well as connective tissue, the reproductive and excretory organs and most of the cardiovascular tissue

Continued

Term	Definition
Neural crest cells	Population of cells arising from the lateral lips of the neural plate that detach during formation of the neural tube and migrate to form a variety of cell types/ structures
Notochord	Rod of mesoderm that lies beneath the neural tube along the central midline of the embryo. Derived from the notochordal process. Involved in induction of the neural tube and vertebral bodies, induction of muscle in the somite, and establishment of dorsal-ventral polarity of the neural tube
Paraxial mesoderm	Thick bands of embryonic mesoderm immediately adjacent to the neural tube and notochord. In the trunk, paraxial mesoderm gives rise to somites
Primitive streak	The first morphological sign of gastrulation. Made up of the primitive pit, the primitive node, and the primitive groove
Sclerotome	Portion of the somite that gives rise to the vertebral column and ribs
Somite	Segmented mesodermal structures that first appear at about day 20 by segmentation of the paraxial mesoderm. Gives rise to the axial skeleton of the trunk, all skeletal muscle of the trunk and limbs, and the dermis of the skin of the trunk

Continued

27. 1—b, Mesencephalon; 2—c, Metencephalon

Primary Vesicles (Week 4)	Secondary Vesicles (Week 5)	Adult Derivatives	Ventricles	CN
Prosencephalon	Telencephalon	Cortex—neocortex and hippocampus Striatum (caudate/putamen) Globus pallidus Amygdala Olfactory bulbs	Lateral ventricles	I
	Diencephalon	Alar plate—Thalamus, epithalamus and subthalamic nuclei Basal plate—Midbrain tegmentum, pituitary and hypothalamus Roof plate—pineal body, choroid plexus	3rd ventricle	II
Mesencephalon	Mesencephalon	Roof/alar plate—Midbrain tectum (colliculi) Floor/basal plate—Midbrain tegmentum	Aqueduct	III
Rhombencephalon	Metencephalon	Alar plate—Cerebellum Basal plate—Pons	4th ventricle	IV-VIII
	Myelencephalon	Medulla oblongata	4th ventricle	IX-XII

28. 1—f, Day 18; 2—h, Day 26-28; 3—k, Day 35 Approximate timetable for CNS development is shown below (exact numbers vary depending on source).

Stage	Days	Week
Morula	2-3	1st
Bilaminar disc	4-5	1st
Implantation	6	1st
Amniotic and yolk sacs formed	8-12	2nd
Trilaminar disc with primitive streak	14-17	3rd
Neural plate and groove	18	3rd
Appearance of three primary brain vesicles	20	3rd
Anterior neuropore closure	24-26	4th
Posterior neuropore closure (formation of neural tube)	26-28	4th
Anterior and posterior roots	31	4th-5th
Five cerebral vesicles and developing flexures	35	5th
Primordium of cerebellum	42	6th
Corpus callosum		10th
Cerebellar cortex and Purkinje cells		12th
Dentate nucleus		15th
Primary cerebral fissure		20th

29. 1—f, neural fold; 2—c, caudal neuropore; 3—g, neural groove; 4—e, dorsal root ganglion
30. 1—c, 3rd pharyngeal arch; 2—f, 6th pharyngeal arch; 3—a, 1st pharyngeal arch; 4—b, 2nd pharyngeal arch

Pharyngeal arches consist of a mesenchymal core (mesoderm and neural crest cells) that is covered on the outside with ectoderm and lined on the inside with endoderm. Each arch contains (1) a central cartilaginous skeletal element (derived from neural crest cells); (2) striated muscle rudiments (derived from head mesoderm) innervated by an arch-specific cranial nerve; and (3) an aortic arch artery. Like so many other structures in the body, the pharyngeal arches form in craniocaudal succession: the 1st arch forms on D22; the 2nd and 3rd arches form sequentially on D24; and the 4th and 6th arches form sequentially on D29. The pharyngeal arches of human embryos initially resemble the gill arches of fish, except that they never become perforated to form gill slits.

Arch	Nerve	Artery	Muscle	Bone
1st (Mandibular)	V2 and V3	Maxillary, ECA	Mastication Anterior belly of diagastric Mylohyoid Tensor tympani Tensor veli palatini	Maxilla, mandible, zygoma, temporal bone, incus, malleus, Meckel's cartilage, sphenomandibular ligament
2nd (Hyoid)	VII	Stapedial, hyoid	Muscles of facial expression Buccinator Platysma Stapedius Stylohyoid Posterior belly of diagastric Auricular	Stapes, temporal styloid process, lesser horn and upper body of hyoid, stylohyoid ligament, Reichert's cartilage
3rd	IX	CC/ICA	Stylopharyngeus	Greater horn and lesser body of hyoid, thymus, inferior parathyroids

Continued

Arch	Nerve	Artery	Muscle	Bone
4th	X, superior laryngeal	Right: subclavian Left: aortic arch	Cricothyroid Intrinsic muscle of soft palate (except tensor veli palatine)	Thyroid cartilage, superior parathyroids, epiglottic cartilage
6th	X, recurrent laryngeal	Right: pulmonary Left: pulmonary and ductus arteriosus	Intrinsic muscle of larynx (except cricothyroid)	Cricoid cartilage, arytenoid cartilage, corniculate cartilage, cuneiform cartilage

31. 1—k, Sturge-Weber syndrome; 2—j, Split cord malformation; 3—c, Dandy-Walker spectrum

Gastrulation (notochordal integration)	Gastrulation (segmental notochordal formation)
Dorsal enteric fistula Split cord malformation Neurenteric cyst Dermal sinus*	Segmentation defects Indeterminate/block vertebrae Caudal regression syndrome Segmental spinal dysgenesis
Primary neurulation	**Secondary neurulation**
Myelomeningocele Myelocele Lipomyelomeningocele Lipomyelocele Intradural lipoma Dermal sinus*	Lipoma of filum terminale (fatty filum)/conus Tight filum terminale Persistent terminal ventricle Terminal myelocystocele
Ventral induction	**Neural proliferation**
Holoprosencephaly Septo-optic dysplasia Pituitary anomalies Inferior cerebellar vermis hypoplasia Dandy-Walker spectrum Mega cisterna magna Rhombencephalosynapsis Joubert syndrome	Microencephaly Macroencephaly Neurocutaneous syndromes Aqueduct stenosis
Neuronal migration	**Myelination**
Lissencephaly Heterotopia Pachygyria Schizencephaly Polymicrogyria Agenesis of corpus callosum	Adrenoleukodystrophy Metachromatic leukodystrophy Pelizaeus-Merzbacher disease

*Hemimyelocele and hemimyelomeningocele are considered disorders of both gastrulation and primary neurulation and are extremely rare.

CHAPTER 3

NEUROPHYSIOLOGY

SINGLE BEST ANSWER (SBA) QUESTIONS

1. Which one of the following is NOT a component of the blood-brain barrier?
   a. Capillary endothelial cells
   b. Astrocytic foot processes
   c. Basement membrane
   d. Tight junctions
   e. Microglia

2. Which one of the following regions has an intact blood-brain barrier?
   a. Subforniceal organ
   b. Area postrema
   c. Median eminence
   d. Posterior pituitary
   e. Pineal gland
   f. Subcommissural organ
   g. Organum vasculosum of lamina terminalis

3. Which one of the following statements regarding the area postrema is LEAST accurate?
   a. It is located in the dorsomedial medulla in the caudal part of the fourth ventricle
   b. Its blood supply is mostly from the anterior inferior cerebellar artery
   c. It is a circumventricular organ
   d. It plays a role as a chemoreceptor trigger zone
   e. It expresses 5-HT3 receptors

4. Which one of the following statements regarding the production of CSF by choroid plexus cells is LEAST accurate?
   a. Requires ultrafiltration of plasma to form extracellular fluid at basolateral membrane
   b. Formation is primarily generated by net secretion of Na^+, Cl^-, and HCO_3^- into ventricles
   c. Water is actively pumped into the ventricles via Aquaporin 1 channels in the apical membrane
   d. Active transport of Na^+ into the ventricles via Na^+/K^+ ATPase occurs at the basolateral membrane
   e. Basolateral membrane Na influx via Na^+/H^+ exchange and Na^+/HCO_3^- cotransport channels.

5. Which one of the following statements regarding axonal transport is LEAST accurate?
   a. Large membranous organelles are transported by fast kinesin dependent anterograde transport and dynein dependent retrograde transport
   b. Cytosolic proteins are transported by fast transport
   c. Occurs by retrograde transport
   d. Anterograde transport is dependent upon microtubules and the ATPase kinesin
   e. Rabies virus spreads by retrograde axonal transport

6. Which one of the following statements regarding the concentration of ions in extracellular and intracellular compartments is LEAST accurate?
   a. Extracellular sodium ion concentration is approximately 140 mM (140 mEq/l)
   b. Intracellular potassium ion concentration is approximately 160 mmol/l (160 mEq/L)
   c. Extracellular chloride ion concentration is approximately 110 mM (110 mEq/l)
   d. Intracellular calcium ion concentration is approximately 2 mM (4 mEq/l)
   e. Extracellular bicarbonate ion concentration is approximately 22-26 mmol/l

7. Which one of the following statements concerning the resting membrane potential is most accurate?
   a. Maintenance of the resting membrane potential is an energy dependent process requiring Na/K-ATPase
   b. A membrane is depolarized when there is an increase in separation of the charge across it from baseline
   c. Neurons become depolarized when the charge inside the cell becomes more negative compared to its resting state

d. Hyperpolarization of a cell membrane occurs when the outside of the cell becomes more negatively charged compared to its resting state
e. Resting potential difference across a membrane is not dependent on the separation of charged ions across it

8. Which one of the following statements regarding ion channels is LEAST accurate?
a. Nicotinic AChR is a ligand-gated ion channel
b. NMDA receptor is a ligand-gated cation channel
c. Voltage-gated sodium channels open in response to hyperpolarization of the cell membrane
d. Cyclic AMP is generated by activation of beta-adrenoceptors
e. GABA-B receptor is a ligand-gated ion channel

9. Which one of the following statements regarding the membrane potentials is most accurate?
a. The Nernst equation can be used to calculate the resting membrane potential of a cell
b. The Goldman equation can be used to calculate the intracellular concentration of sodium
c. The equilibrium potential for potassium is approximately +70 mV
d. Equilibrium potential of an ion maintains a unique ion gradient for it exists across a cell membrane
e. At electrochemical equilibrium, the chemical and electrical driving forces acting on an ion are equal and opposite, and no further net diffusion occurs

10. Which one of the following best describes ions responsible for membrane hyperpolarization?
a. Chloride and sodium
b. Chloride and potassium
c. Potassium and sodium
d. Sodium and calcium
e. Sodium only

11. Which one of the following statements regarding the passive membrane properties of neurons is LEAST accurate?
a. The length constant is the distance where the initial voltage response to current flow decays to 1/e (or 37%) of its value
b. Smaller length constant means passive flow of an action potential will stop at a shorter distance along an axon
c. Length constant is greater in unmyelinated and large diameter axons
d. The time constant is a function of the membrane's resistance and capacitance
e. The time constant characterizes how rapidly current flow changes the membrane potential

12. Which one of the following statements regarding the generation of the action potential is LEAST accurate?
a. It is an all-or-nothing, regenerative wave of depolarization
b. It can propagate bidirectionally
c. Repolarization is due to inactivation of sodium channels combined with increased conductance in potassium channels
d. Hyperpolarization occurs due to increases in potassium conductance lasting beyond the point of return to resting membrane potential
e. Repolarization is required for inactivated sodium channels to return to the closed state

13. Which one of the following sites acts as the trigger zone that integrates incoming signals from other cells and initiates the action potential?
a. Soma
b. Dendritic shaft
c. Dendritic spines
d. Axon hillock and initial segment
e. Axon trunk

14. Which one of the following statements regarding phenomena relevant to action potential conduction is LEAST accurate?
a. Accommodation is dependent on postsynaptic receptor phagocytosis
b. Saltatory conduction occurs to high resistance to transmembrane current leak in myelinated segments of nerve
c. Absolute refractory period is due to inactivation of voltage-gated sodium channels
d. Relative refractory period occurs when populations of inactivated voltage-gated sodium channels return to the closed state
e. Unidirectional propagation is function of the refractory periods associated with action potentials

15. Which one of the following synapse types is characterized by gap junctions?
a. Axodendritic synapses
b. Axoaxonic synapses
c. Axosomatic synapses
d. Dendrodendritic synapses
e. Electrical synapses

16. Which one of the following statements regarding neurotransmission at chemical synapses is LEAST accurate?
   a. The action potential stimulates the postsynaptic terminal to release neurotransmitter
   b. Release of the transmitter into the synaptic cleft by exocytosis is triggered by an influx of Ca^{2+} through voltage-gated channels
   c. Postsynaptic current produces an excitatory or inhibitory postsynaptic potential
   d. Neurotransmitters may undergo degradation in the synaptic cleft or be transported back into the presynaptic terminal
   e. Vesicular membrane is retrieved from the plasma membrane after exocytosis

17. Which one of the following statements regarding cholinergic neurotransmission is LEAST likely?
   a. synthesized in nerve terminals from the precursors acetyl coenzyme A
   b. acetylcholinesterase (AChE) hydrolysis Ach into acetate and choline
   c. Nicotinic AChR are a nonselective cation channel complex consisting of five subunits arranged around a central membrane-spanning pore
   d. α-bungarotoxin binds to muscarinic AChRs
   e. mAChRs are metabotropic G-protein coupled receptors

18. Which one of the following statements regarding glutamatergic neurotransmission is LEAST accurate?
   a. At depolarized membrane potentials, an Mg^{2+} blocks the pore of the NMDA receptor
   b. most prevalent precursor for glutamate synthesis is glutamine
   c. glutamine is taken up into presynaptic terminals and metabolized to glutamate by the mitochondrial enzyme glutaminase
   d. Activation of metabotropic GluRs leads to inhibition of postsynaptic Ca^{2+} and Na^{+} channels
   e. AMPA receptors are a type of metabotropic GluR

19. Which one of the following enzymatic conversion pathways is LEAST accurate?
   a. Tyrosine-tyrosine hydroxylase-DOPA (dihydroxyphenylalanine)
   b. DOPA-catechol O-methyltransferase-dopamine
   c. Histidine-histidine decarboxylase-Histamine
   d. Dopamine-Dopamine beta-hydroxylase-Norepinephrine
   e. Tryptophan is converted to serotonin by tryptophan 5-hydroxylase and a decarboxylase

20. Which one of the following statements regarding dopaminergic neurotransmission is LEAST accurate?
   a. Dopamine is loaded into synaptic vesicles via a vesicular monoamine transporter (VMAT)
   b. The neostriatum is the major site of dopaminergic transmission in the brain
   c. Dopamine is derived from norepinephrine
   d. Cocaine inhibits the Na-dependent dopamine transporter
   e. monoamine oxidase (MAO) and catechol O-methyltransferase (COMT)

21. Which one of the following statements regarding GABAergic neurotransmission is LEAST accurate?
   a. Glutamic acid decarboxylase (GAD) conversion of glutamate to GABA
   b. Vitamin B6 is important in the function of glutamic acid decarboxylase
   c. The mechanism of GABA removal from the synaptic cleft is similar to that for glutamate
   d. GABAA and GABAC receptors are ionotropic receptors and are Ca^{2+} conductors
   e. GABAB receptors are metabotropic and increase K conductance

22. Which one of the following areas does the superior temporal gyrus (Heschl's gyrus) primarily receive inputs from?
   a. Centromedian thalamic nucleus
   b. Medial geniculate thalamic nucleus
   c. Dorsomedial thalamic nucleus
   d. Anterior thalamic nucleus
   e. Centromedian-parafascicular nucleus

23. Which one of the following cell types involved in vision is able to generate an action potential?
   a. Ganglion cells
   b. Bipolar cells
   c. Horizontal cells
   d. Rods and cones
   e. Amacrine cells

24. Which one of the following statements regarding cones and rods is LEAST accurate?
   a. In the dark, rods have a high resting membrane potential of about −70 mV

b. In the dark, both rods and cones tonically release glutamate onto synapsing bipolar cells
c. Photon absorption by rhodopsin results in reduced cyclic GMP and hyperpolarization of the rod cell
d. Photon absorption by cone opsin results in reduced cyclic GMP and hyperpolarization of the rod cell
e. Reduced glutamate secretion can cause both hyperpolarization or depolarization in bipolar cells

25. Which one of the following events during visual processing is LEAST accurate?
a. The on-center bipolar depolarizes in response to reduced tonic glutamate release
b. The on-center ganglion cell will produce a burst of action potentials if a spot of light is shone on the receptive field center
c. The ganglion cell that receives its input from an off-center bipolar cell will reduce its firing rate in response a spot of light is shone on the receptive field center
d. The receptive fields of on-center and off-center ganglion cells do not overlap
e. Glutamate released from a cone cell has differential effect in different cells with which it synapses

26. Which one of the following statements about olfaction is LEAST accurate?
a. Bowman glands secrete a fluid that bathes the cilia of the receptors and acts as a solvent for odorant molecules
b. Mucus-coated olfactory epithelium lines the anterodorsal parts of the nasal cavities
c. Binding of odor molecules generates action potentials in a G-protein coupled mechanism
d. Fibers of CN I synapse with the mitral cells of the olfactory bulb
e. Olfactory tract and lateral olfactory stria project to the primary olfactory cortex and amygdala

27. Which one of the following statements regarding taste sensation is LEAST accurate?
a. Receptors for molecules associated with sweet and bitter tastes utilize second messengers
b. Sour and salty-tasting molecules act directly upon the ion channels
c. Taste buds on the anterior two thirds of the tongue send signals through the lingual nerve to the chorda tympani and finally into CN VII (facial)
d. Posterior one-third of the tongue detects bitter and sour tastes and signal through glossopharyngeal and vagus nerves
e. All taste fibers synapse in the nucleus ambiguus

28. Which one of the following statements concerning neurotransmission at the neuromuscular junction is most accurate?
a. It is dependent upon the release of norepinephrine from the nerve ending
b. End plate potential amplitude can be much larger than that of excitatory or inhibitory postsynaptic potentials
c. It is an all-or-none response
d. It is not directly related to the concentration of transmitter released from the presynaptic terminals
e. It is dependent on the opening of ligand-gated calcium channels

29. Which one of the following statements regarding peripheral nerve injury is most accurate?
a. Neuropraxia involves disruption of the myelin sheath only with some evidence of Wallerian degeneration
b. Recovery after neuropraxia is likely to be incomplete
c. Neurotmesis is ideally managed with expectant management
d. Axonotmesis shows Wallerian degeneration distal to injury
e. A dense motor and sensory deficit following a penetrating injury is due to neuropraxia

30. Which one of the following ensures sufficient contraction of the striated portion of intrafusal fibers to enable monitor changes in muscle length?
a. Unmyelinated C fibers
b. 1A fibers
c. Gamma motor neurons
d. Alpha motor neurons
e. General visceral efferent fibers

QUESTIONS 31–45

Additional questions 31–45 available on ExpertConsult.com

EXTENDED MATCHING ITEM (EMI) QUESTIONS

46. **Neurotoxins and other agents:**
   a. 3,4-Methylenedioxy-methamphetamine
   b. Botulinum toxin
   c. Bungarotoxin
   d. Curare
   e. Chlorotoxin
   f. Conotoxin
   g. Ethanol
   h. Phencyclidine (PCP)
   i. Tetraethylammonium (TEA)
   j. Tetrodotoxin (TTX)

For each of the following descriptions, select the most appropriate answers from the list above. Each answer may be used once, more than once or not at all.

1. Uncompetitive NMDA receptor antagonist producing dissociative state
2. Works by presynaptic competitive reuptake inhibition followed by inhibition of VMAT and TAAR1 receptor resulting in synaptic accumulation of monoamines.
3. Neurotoxic peptides isolated from venom of marin cone snail.
4. Blocker of voltage-gated K^+ channels and competitive inhibitor of nicotinic AChRs
5. Blocker of voltage-gated Na^+ channels found in Pufferfish

47. **Neurotransmitters:**
   a. Acetylcholine
   b. Dopamine
   c. Epinephrine
   d. GABA
   e. Glutamate
   f. Glycine
   g. Histamine
   h. L-DOPA
   i. Met-enkephalin
   j. Serotonin
   k. Substance P
   l. Taurine
   m. Tyramine
   n. VIP

For each of the following descriptions, select the most appropriate answers from the list above. Each answer may be used once, more than once or not at all.

1. The immediate precursor of norepinephrine
2. The immediate precursor of dopamine
3. Rate limiting step in the production of this neurotransmitter is tryptophan hydroxylase activity
4. Phenylethanolamine-*N*-methyl transferase is required for production of this transmitter
5. Required in addition to glutamate for co-activation of NMDA receptor, but acts as an inhibitory neurotransmitter via Cl^- channels

48. **Sensory receptors:**
   a. Free nerve endings
   b. Golgi tendon organs
   c. Meissner's corpuscles
   d. Merkel's tactile discs
   e. Nuclear bag fibers
   f. Nuclear chain fibers
   g. Pacinian corpuscles
   h. Pain nociceptors
   i. Peritrichial nerve endings
   j. Ruffini's organs

For each of the following descriptions, select the most appropriate answers from the list above. Each answer may be used once, more than once or not at all.

1. Signal the onset of muscle stretch via A-alpha myelinated fibers
2. Two-point discriminative fine touch
3. Deep pressure and vibration sense

49. **CNS cells:**
   a. Astrocytes
   b. Basket cells
   c. Betz cells
   d. Ependymal cells
   e. Golgi type 2 cells
   f. Granule cells
   g. Martinotti cells
   h. Microglia
   i. Oligodendroglia
   j. Purkinje cells
   k. Schwann cells
   l. Stellate cells

For each of the following descriptions, select the most appropriate answers from the list above. Each answer may be used once, more than once or not at all.

1. These cells are derived from neural crest origin and myelinate neurons of the PNS
2. These cells arise from monocytes (hematopoietic precursor) and thus are the resident macrophages of the CNS. Their function is to protect the CNS. When the brain is damaged or infected, they become activated and multiply quickly to perform functions such as phagocytosis and presenting antigen

3. These cells myelinate neurons within the CNS (one cell myelinates multiple neurons).
4. These are the most abundant and largest of the glial subtypes. Their most notable role is the metabolism and recycling of certain neurotransmitters (glutamate, serotonin, and gamma-aminobutyric acid [GABA]). They also buffer the extracellular potassium concentration, respond to injury (gliosis), and make up the blood-brain barrier
5. These ciliated cells line the cavities of the CNS (ventricular system) in the choroid plexus, where they are involved in the production of cerebrospinal fluid (CSF) and are part of the blood-CSF barrier

50. **Cerebellum:**

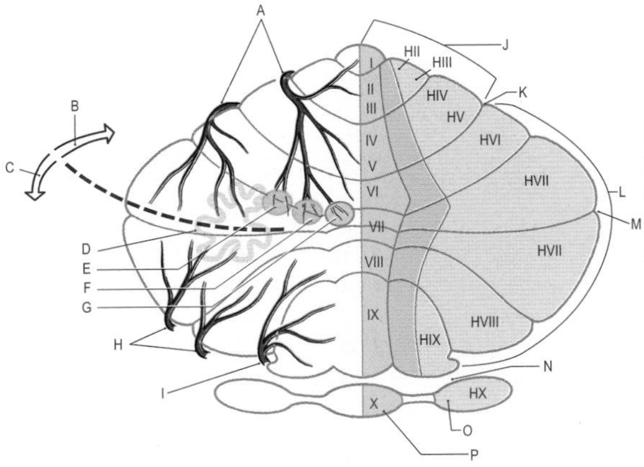

For each of the following descriptions, select the most appropriate answers from the image above. Each answer may be used once, more than once or not at all.

1. Posterior lobe
2. Flocculus
3. Primary fissure
4. Dentate nucleus
5. Anterior inferior cerebellar artery

51. **Cerebellar cortex:**

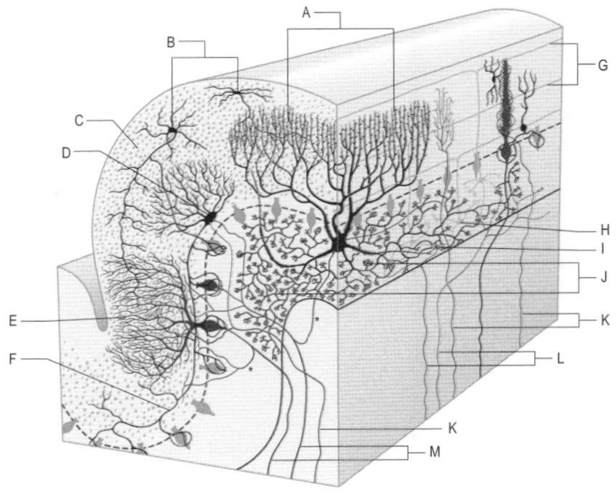

For each of the following descriptions, select the most appropriate answers from the image above. Each answer may be used once, more than once or not at all.

1. Purkinje cell axon
2. Basket cell
3. Climbing fiber
4. Golgi cell
5. Parallel fiber

52. **Hypothalamic-pituitary axis:**

a. ACTH
b. ADH (vasopressin)
c. Cortisol
d. Epinephrine
e. FSH/LH
f. GH
g. TSH
h. Oestradiol
i. Oxytocin
j. Prolactin
k. Testosterone

For each of the following descriptions, select the most appropriate answers from the list above. Each answer may be used once, more than once or not at all.

1. Uterine contractions in labor and milk ejection reflex
2. Renal water conservation
3. Excess may cause galactorrhea

53. **Peripheral nerve:**

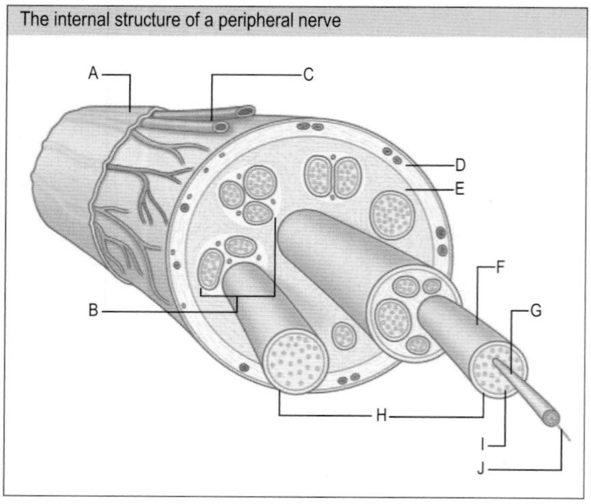

For each of the following descriptions, select the most appropriate answers from the image above. Each answer may be used once, more than once or not at all.

1. Endoneurium
2. Perineurium
3. Mesoneurium
4. External epineurium

SBA ANSWERS

1. **e**—Microglia

2. **f**—Subcommissural organ

The brain regions lacking a blood-brain barrier are the circumventricular organs with neuroendocrine function. They may be sensory organs: subforniceal organ, area postrema, and organum vasculosum of lamina terminalis which can sense levels of various plasma molecules and signal to the autonomic system. Alternatively, they may be secretory organs: median eminence of the hypothalamus, pineal gland, posterior pituitary, and subcommissural organ, which deliver hormones/glycoproteins into the bloodstream in response to neural signals. Overall they form part of feedback loops involved in body water regulation, feeding, thirst, cardiovascular function, immune response and reproductive behavior. The dura and choroid plexus also lack a blood-brain barrier. Generally, lipophilic/hydrophobic substances can cross the BBB (e.g., O_2, CO_2, ethanol, caffeine, nicotine), whereas lipophobic/hydrophilic/large molecules substances cannot.

3. **a**—It is located in the ventral medulla at a position that is caudal to the fourth ventricle

The area postrema is found in the dorsomedial medulla oblongata and can be observed as two convex prominences bulging into the most caudal part of the fourth ventricle. It is a V-shaped structure diverging from an apex at the obex, and receives blood supply from pyramidal branches of the posterior inferior cerebellar arteries which run along its lateral edge. It is thought to be a chemoreceptor trigger zone for vomiting and inhibition of 5-HT_3 receptors here (as well as peripherally on vagal afferents) is effective in reducing the nausea associated with cancer chemotherapy.

4. **c**—Water is actively pumped into the ventricles via Aquaporin 1 channels in the apical membrane

CSF forms in two sequential stages. First, ultrafiltration of plasma occurs across the fenestrated capillary wall into the ECF beneath the basolateral membrane of the choroid epithelial cell. Second, choroid epithelial cells secrete fluid into the ventricle. Fluid secretion into the ventricles is mediated by an array of ion transporters unevenly positioned at the blood-facing (basolateral) or CSF-facing (apical) membranes. Many ionic species are involved in CSF production (e.g., K^+, Mg^{2+}, and Ca^{2+}). However, fluid formation is primarily generated by net secretion of Na^+, Cl^-, and HCO_3^- into ventricles as water molecules follow them passively down a chemical gradient via Aquaporin1 channels in the apical membrane. Na^+ transport into CSF occurs due to active transport via Na^+/K^+ ATPase exchange pump at the apical membrane, and is replaced by basolateral membrane Na influx via Na^+/H^+ exchange and Na^+/HCO_3^- cotransport channels. Transport of Cl^- into CSF occurs via passive diffusion via apical Cl^- selective channels (and possibly $Na^+/K^+/Cl^-$ cotransport), and is replaced at the basolateral membrane in exchange for HCO_3^-. Intracellular HCO_3^- is accumulated by (i) hydration of CO_2 catalyzed by carbonic anhydrase and (ii) influx via basolateral membrane Na/HCO_3^- cotransport, then can enter the CSF at the apical membrane either by anion channel or Na/HCO_3 cotransport. CSF has lower concentrations of K^+ and amino acids than plasma does, and it contains almost no protein.

5. **b**—Cytosolic proteins are transported by fast transport

Nerve cells have an elaborate transport system that moves organelles and macromolecules between the cell body and the axon and its terminals. Axonal transport from the cell body toward the terminals is called anterograde; transport from the terminals toward the cell body is called retrograde. Anterograde axonal transport is classified into fast and slow components. Fast transport, at speeds of up to 400 mm/day, is based on the action of an ATPase protein called kinesin which moves macromolecule-containing vesicles and mitochondria along microtubules. Slow transport carries important structural and metabolic components from the cell body to axon terminals (e.g., cytoskeletal protein components such as actin, myosin, tubulin, and cytosolic enzymes required for neurotransmitter synthesis in the presynaptic terminal) but the mechanism is less clear. Retrograde axonal transport along axonal microtubules is driven by the protein dynein and allows the neuron/cell body to respond to molecules taken up near the axon terminal by either pinocytosis or receptor-mediated endocytosis (e.g., growth factors). In addition, this form of transport functions in the continual recycling of components of the axon terminal (e.g., mitochondria). Retrograde transport of rabies virus allows replication in the cell body and spread to adjacent neurons.

6. **d**—Intracellular calcium ion concentration is approximately 2 mM (4 mEq/l)

	Plasma	Intracellular	Equilibrium Potential
Na^+	140 mM (140 mEq/l)	10 mmol/l (10 mEq/l)	+68 mV
K^+	4.5 mM (4.5 mEq/l)	160 mmol/l (160 mEq/l)	−93 mV
Cl^-	110 mM (110 mEq/l)	9 mmol/l (9 mEq/l)	−86 mV
Ca^{2+}	2 mM (4 mEq/l)	0.0001 mmol/l (mEq)	+129 mV
HCO_3	22-26 mmol/l	10 mmol/l (mEq)	

7. **a**—Maintenance of the resting membrane potential is an energy dependent process requiring Na/K-ATPase

The voltage, or potential difference, across the cell membrane (resting membrane potential) is a result of the separation of positively and negatively charged ions across it, the balance of which is actively maintained by ATP-dependent membrane pumps. At rest, the inside of a cell holds more negative charge than the extracellular fluid outside it. Membrane depolarization is said to occur when the separation of charge across the membrane is reduced from the resting/baseline value (i.e., the inside of cell becomes more positively charged), whereas hyperpolarization is said to occur if the separation of charge is increased (i.e., the inside of the cell becomes more negatively charged than at rest). There is a tendency for ions to passively leak in or out of the cell against their respective electrochemical gradients, hence the requirement for continuously active ATP-dependent membrane pumps to prevent an overall change in the resting membrane potential. The propensity for ion flux across the membrane passively down artificially membrane pump produced and maintained electrochemical gradients is exploited and forms the basis for action potentials during which ion channels open up to allow passive ion flux on a magnitude and time scale at which ATP-dependent membrane pumps cannot prevent, allowing depolarization/hyperpolarization to act as a high fidelity way of information transfer.

8. **e**—GABA-B receptor is a ligand-gated ion channel

Ion channels are transmembrane proteins that permit the selective passage of ions with specific characteristics (size and charge) down their electrochemical gradient by passive diffusion when open. Ion channels are controlled by gates, and, depending on the position of the gates, the channels may be open or closed. The higher the probability that the channel is open, the higher is its conductance or permeability. The gates on ion channels are controlled by three types of sensors:

- Voltage-gated channels have gates that are controlled by changes in membrane potential.
- Second messenger-gated channels have gates that are controlled by changes in levels of intracellular signaling molecules such as cyclic AMP (e.g., beta-adrenoceptors, alpha2-adrenoceptors, M2 muscarinic AChR) or inositol 1,4,5-triphosphate (IP_3; e.g., alpha1-adrenoceptors, M1/M3 muscarinic AChR). In general, G_s/G_i G-protein coupled receptor activation causes adenylyl cyclase to convert ATP to cAMP, which then activates protein kinase A to phosphorylate downstream proteins. In contrast, Gq G-protein coupled receptors cause activation of phospholipase C which hydrolyzes membrane phospholipid (phosphatidylinositol 4,5-bisphosphate; PIP_2) to diacyl glycerol (DAG) and inositol 1,4,5-trisphosphate (IP_3).
- Ligand-gated channels have gates that are controlled by hormones and neurotransmitters. The sensors for these gates are located on the extra-cellular side of the ion channel (e.g., nicotinic AChR allows Na^+ and K^+ passage on binding acetylcholine).

9. **e**—At electrochemical equilibrium, the chemical and electrical driving forces acting on an ion are equal and opposite, and no further net diffusion occurs

The concept of equilibrium potential is simply an extension of the concept of diffusion potential. If there is a concentration difference for an ion across a membrane and the membrane is permeable to that ion, a potential difference (the diffusion potential) is created. Eventually, net diffusion of the ion slows and then stops because of that potential difference. In other words, if a cation diffuses down its concentration gradient, it carries a positive charge across the membrane, which will retard and eventually stop further diffusion of the cation. Equally, if an anion diffuses down its concentration gradient, it carries a negative charge, which will retard and then stop further diffusion of the anion. The equilibrium potential is the diffusion potential that exactly balances or opposes the tendency for diffusion down the concentration difference. At electrochemical equilibrium, the chemical and electrical driving forces acting on an ion are equal and opposite, and no further net diffusion occurs. The Nernst equation is used to calculate the equilibrium potential for an ion at a given concentration difference across a membrane, assuming that the membrane is permeable to that ion. By definition, the equilibrium potential is calculated for one ion at a time. For a given ion X with charge z at 37 °C, the equilibrium potential (Ex) = (−60/z) log10([intracellular concentration of X in mmol/l]/[extracellular concentration of X in mmol/l]). For example, E(Na) = (−60/+1) log10(10/140) = +68.8 mV. Whereas for E(k) = (−60/+1) log10 (140/10) = −87 mV. The Goldmann equation can be used to calculate the exact resting membrane potential based on all the permeable ions across it, but in practice since in neurons 80% of conductance is due to K^+ (residual is 15% due to Na^+ and 5% due to Cl^-), the resting membrane voltage (Vm) of approximately −70 mV is much closer to that of the equilibrium potential for K^+.

10. **b**—Chloride and potassium

Assuming normal intracellular and extracellular concentrations of ions, both potassium and chloride ions have a negative equilibrium potential hence will result in hyperpolarization of the cell if allowed to flow down their electrochemical gradients. Chloride influx into the cell down its electrochemical gradient results in a gain of negative charge, whereas efflux of potassium reflects a loss of positive charge in the intracellular compartment to achieve this. Physiological electrochemical gradients for both sodium and calcium favor influx into the cell, and would cause depolarization due to net gain of positive charge.

11. **c**—Length constant is greater in unmyelinated and large diameter axons

The passive flow of electrical current plays a central role in action potential propagation, synaptic transmission, and all other forms of electrical signaling in nerve cells. For the case of a cylindrical axon, subthreshold current injected into one part of the axon spreads passively along the axon until the current is dissipated (decays) by leakage out across the axon membrane. The decrement in the current flow with distance is described by a simple exponential function: $V_x = V_0 \cdot e^{-x/\lambda}$ where V_x is the voltage response at any distance x along the axon, V_0 is the voltage change at the point where current is injected into the axon, e is the base of natural logarithms (≈2.7), and λ is the length constant of the axon. As evident in this relationship, the length constant is the distance where the initial voltage response (V_0) decays to 1/e (or 37%) of its value. The length constant is thus a way to characterize how far passive current flow spreads before it leaks out of the axon, with leakier axons having shorter length constants. The length constant depends upon the physical properties of the axon, in particular the relative resistances of the plasma membrane (R_m), the intracellular axoplasm (R_i), and the extracellular medium (R_0). The relationship between these parameters is: $\lambda = \sqrt{(R_m/[R_0+R_i])}$. Hence, to improve the passive flow of current along an axon (i.e., slow the rate of decay), the resistance of the plasma membrane should be as high as possible (e.g., myelination) and the resistances of the axoplasm and extracellular medium should be low. Another important consequence of the passive properties of neurons is that currents flowing across a membrane do not immediately change the membrane potential. These delays in changing the membrane potential are due to the fact that the plasma membrane behaves as a capacitor, storing the initial charge that flows at the beginning and end of the current pulse. For the case of a cell whose membrane potential is spatially uniform, the change in the membrane potential at any time, V_t, after beginning the current pulse can also be described by an exponential relationship: $V_t = V_\infty(1 - e^{-t/\tau})$ where V_∞ is the steady-state value of the membrane potential change, t is the time after the current pulse begins, and τ is the membrane time constant. The time constant is thus defined as the time when the voltage response (V_t) rises to $1-(1/e)$ (or 63%) of V_∞. After the current pulse ends, the membrane potential change also declines exponentially according to the relationship $V_t = V_\infty \cdot e^{-t/\tau}$ During this decay, the membrane potential returns to 1/e of V_∞ at a time equal to t. The time constant characterizes how rapidly current flow changes the membrane potential. The membrane time constant also depends on the physical properties of the nerve cell, specifically on the resistance (R_m) and capacitance (C_m) of the plasma membrane such that: $\tau = R_m C_m$. The values of R_m and C_m depend, in part, on the size of the neuron, with larger cells having lower resistances and larger capacitances. In general, small nerve cells tend to have long time constants and large cells brief time constants. Regarding achieving threshold for action potential generation, long time constants favor temporal summation of EPSPs, whereas short time constant allows coincidence detection through spatial summation of EPSPs/IPSPs.

FURTHER READING

Chapter 3 Voltage dependent membrane permeability. In: Purves D, et al. (Eds.), Neuroscience, 3rd ed. MA: Sinauer. p. 60-61.

12. **b**—It can propagate bidirectionally

The action potential, as classically defined, is an all-or-nothing, regenerative, directionally propagated, depolarizing nerve impulse. At rest, the membrane has high K^+ conductance and V_m is near the Nernst equilibrium potential for K^+ (EK). Spread of an action potential from an adjacent area of the membrane brings the membrane potential Em, to a threshold potential (approximately −40 to −55 mV) causing a large increase in Na^+ conductance of the membrane and Na^+ influx such that V_m approaches the Nernst potential for Na^+ (ENa) and the membrane depolarizes. Depolarization causes voltage-gated sodium channels to change from an open to an inactivated state, preventing further rises in membrane potential, and at the same time there is an increase in conductance of delayed-rectifier K channels causing K efflux and movement of V_m towards the equilibrium potential for potassium (repolarization). This increased K^+ conductance usually lasts slightly longer than the time required to bring the membrane potential back to its normal resting level, hence there is an overshoot (hyperpolarization) which subsequently decays. An absolute refractory period for action potential firing is seen when sodium channels are in their inactivated state, but as repolarization progresses more Na channels move from an inactivated to a close state, and thus could be reopened in the presence of a supratheshold stimulus (relative refractory period). The figure below shows the action potential (yellow), and underlying changes in membrane conductance to sodium (purple) and potassium (red) due to opening/inactivation of channels.

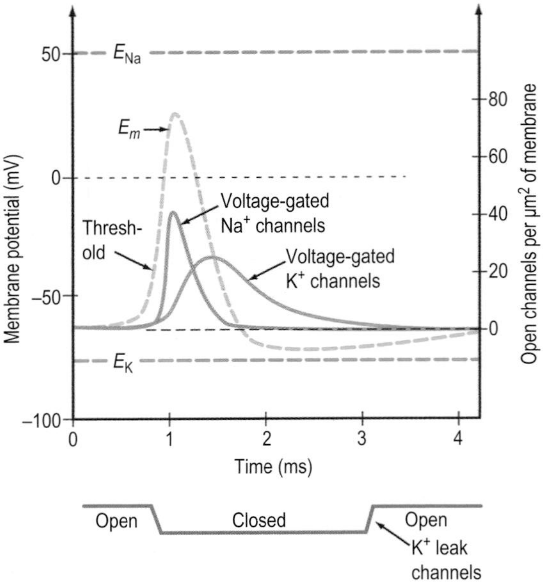

Image with permission from Pollard TD et al. (Eds.), Cell Biology, 2nd ed. Elsevier, 2008.

13. **d**—Axon hillock and initial segment

14. **a**—Accommodation is dependent on post-synaptic receptor phagocytosis

Unidirectional propagation is due to the inactive state of the sodium channel, and this wave of inactivation immediately following the action potential prevents it from reversing direction. Accommodation occurs when subthreshold stimulus will stimulate channels to open, but at a rate that is too slow for there to be a sufficient number of open channels at any one time to fire an AP but sufficient for channel inactivation. Absolute refractory period is the time period immediately after/during the action potential upstroke when most of the neuron's sodium channels are inactivated and cannot be opened to elicit a second action potential. The relative refractory period refers to the period during repolarization when inactivated Na channels return to a closed state and a second action potential can be generated but is more difficult than normal (becomes progressively less difficult to elicit an action potential during the relative refractory period until it returns to normal). Myelination of axons involves wrapping the axon in myelin, which consists of multiple layers of closely opposed glial cell membranes (i.e., oligodendrocytes in CNS, Schwann cells in PNS). Myelination electrically insulates the axonal membrane, reducing the ability of current to leak out of the axon and thus increasing the distance along the axon that a given local current can flow passively such that the time-consuming process of action potential generation occurs only at specific points along the axon, called nodes of Ranvier, where there is a gap in the myelin wrapping (rather than adjacent membrane in a depolarization wave). As it happens, an action potential generated at one node of Ranvier elicits current that flows passively within the axoplasm of the myelinated segment until the next node is reached and another action potential is generated, and the cycle is repeated along the length of the axon. Because current flows across the neuronal membrane only at the nodes, action potentials "leap" from node to node and this is termed salutatory conduction. Myelination greatly speeds up action potential conduction (velocities up to 150 m/s) compared to unmyelinated axons (0.5-10 m/s). (In: Purves D, et al. (Eds.), Neuroscience, 3rd ed. MA: Sinauer.)

15. **e**—Electrical synapses

Electrical synapses only represent a small minority of synapses (**e.g.,** some neuroendocrine cells in hypothalamus) and are characterized by very closely apposed pre and post-synaptic membranes connected by a gap junction. These junctions contain aligned paired channels so that each paired channel forms a pore (larger than those observed in ligand-gated channels) and allows for the bidirectional transmission. Chemical synapse types include:

Axosecretory—axon terminal secretes directly into bloodstream (e.g., hypothalamus)
Axodendritic—axon terminal ends on dendritic spines or shaft (type I excitatory synapse)
Axoaxonic—axon terminal secretes onto another axon
Axoextracellular—axon with no connection secretes into extracellular fluid
Axosomatic—axon terminal ends on cell soma (type II inhibitory synapse, e.g., basket cell onto Purkinje cell)
Axosynaptic—axon terminal ends on presynaptic terminal of another axon

16. **a**—The action potential stimulates the post-synaptic terminal to release neurotransmitter

Neurotransmission at a chemical synapse requires a neurotransmitter to be synthesized and stored in the presynaptic vesicles. The arrival of an action potential at the presynaptic terminal results in depolarization dependent opening of voltage-gated Ca^{2+} channels and calcium influx. Then, there is Ca^{2+} through these channels, causing the vesicles to fuse with the presynaptic membrane in a mechanism mediated by synaptotagmin 1 and SNAP-25 (SNARE) calcium sensitive proteins. The transmitter is then released into the presynaptic cleft (by exocytosis) and binds to receptor molecules in the postsynaptic membrane. This leads to the opening or closing of postsynaptic channels. The resultant current results in an EPSP or IPSP, which causes a change in excitability of the postsynaptic cell. The vesicular membrane is then retrieved from the plasma membrane by endocytosis. If summation of EPSPs or IPSPs exceeds threshold potential at the axon hillock, an axon potential is generated. To prevent repetitive stimulation, neurotransmitters are either degraded in the presynaptic cleft or taken up by endocytosis in presynaptic cell.

17. **d**—α-bungarotoxin binds to muscarinic AChRs

In addition to the action of ACh as the neurotransmitter at skeletal neuromuscular junctions as well as the neuromuscular synapse between the vagus nerve and cardiac muscle fibers, ACh serves as a transmitter at synapses in the ganglia of the visceral motor system, and at a variety of sites within the central nervous system. Acetylcholine is synthesized in nerve terminals from the precursors acetyl coenzyme A (acetyl CoA, which is synthesized from glucose) and choline, in a reaction catalyzed by choline acetyltransferase (CAT). Choline is present in plasma at a high concentration (about 10 mM) and is taken up into cholinergic neurons by a high-affinity Na^+/choline transporter. After synthesis in the cytoplasm of the neuron, a vesicular ACh transporter loads approximately 10,000 molecules of ACh into each cholinergic vesicle. The postsynaptic actions of ACh at many cholinergic synapses terminated by acetylcholinesterase (AChE) hydrolysis Ach into acetate and choline. The choline produced by ACh hydrolysis is transported back into nerve terminals and used to resynthesize ACh. Many of the postsynaptic actions of ACh are mediated by the nicotinic ACh receptor nAChR which is a nonselective cation channels that generate excitatory postsynaptic responses a large protein complex consisting of five subunits arranged around a central membrane-spanning pore. In the case of skeletal muscle AChRs, the receptor pentamer contains two α subunits, each of which binds one molecule of ACh. Because both ACh-binding sites must be occupied for the channel to open, only relatively high concentrations of this neurotransmitter lead to channel activation. These subunits also bind other ligands, such as nicotine and α-bungarotoxin. At the neuromuscular junction, the two α subunits are combined with up to four other types of subunit—β, γ, δ, ε—in the ratio 2α:β:ε:δ. Neuronal nAChRs typically differ from those of muscle in that they lack sensitivity to α-bungarotoxin, and comprise only two receptor subunit types (α and β), which are present in a ratio of 3α:2β. In all cases, however, five individual subunits assemble to form a functional, cation-selective nACh receptor. Each subunit of the nAChR molecule contains four transmembrane domains that make up the ion channel portion of the receptor, and a long extracellular region that makes up the ACh-binding domain. A second type of ACh receptors is activated by muscarine and thus they are referred to as muscarinic ACh receptors (mAChRs). mAChRs are metabotropic and mediate most of the effects of ACh in brain via G-protein signaling. Several subtypes of mAChR are known. Muscarinic ACh receptors are highly expressed in the striatum and various other forebrain regions, where they exert an inhibitory influence on dopamine-mediated motor effects. These receptors are also found in the ganglia of the peripheral nervous system and autonomic effector organs—such as heart, smooth muscle, and exocrine glands—and are responsible for the inhibition of heart rate by the vagus nerve. Nevertheless, mACh blockers that are therapeutically useful include atropine (used to dilate the pupil), scopolamine (effective in preventing motion sickness), and ipratropium (useful in the treatment of asthma). (In: Purves D, et al. (Eds.) Neuroscience 3rd ed. MA: Sinauer.)

18. **e**—AMPA receptors are a type of metabotropic GluR

Nearly all excitatory neurons in the central nervous system are glutamatergic, and it is estimated that over half of all brain synapses release this agent and cause excitotocity in ischemic brain. Glutamate is a nonessential amino acid that does not cross the blood-brain barrier and therefore must be synthesized in neurons from local precursors. The most prevalent precursor for glutamate synthesis is glutamine, which is released by glial cells. Once released, glutamine is taken up into presynaptic terminals and metabolized to glutamate by the mitochondrial enzyme glutaminase. Glutamate can also be synthesized by transamination of 2-oxoglutarate, an intermediate of the tricarboxylic acid cycle. Hence, some of the glucose metabolized by neurons can also be used for glutamate synthesis. The glutamate synthesized in the presynaptic cytoplasm is packaged into synaptic vesicles by transporters, termed VGLUT. Once released, glutamate is removed from the synaptic cleft by the excitatory amino acid transporters (EAATs). Glutamate taken up by glial cells is converted into glutamine by the enzyme glutamine synthetase; glutamine is then transported out of the glial cells and into nerve terminals. In this way, synaptic terminals cooperate with glial cells to maintain an adequate supply of the neurotransmitter. This overall sequence of events is referred to as the glutamate-glutamine cycle. Receptors of these are ionotropic receptors called, respectively, NMDA receptors, AMPA receptors, and kainate receptors. These glutamate receptors are named after the agonists that activate them: NMDA (*N*-methyl-D-aspartate), AMPA (α-amino-3-hydroxyl-5-methyl-4-isoxazole-propionate), and kainic acid. All of the ionotropic glutamate receptors are nonselective cation channels similar to the nAChR, allowing the passage of Na^+ and K^+, and in some cases small amounts of Ca^{2+}. NMDA receptor ion channels allow the entry of Ca^{2+} in addition to monovalent cations such as Na^+ and K^+. As a result, EPSPs produced by NMDA receptors can increase the concentration of Ca^{2+} within the postsynaptic neuron; the Ca^{2+} concentration change can then act as a second messenger to activate intracellular signaling cascades. Another key property is that they bind extracellular Mg^{2+}. At hyperpolarized membrane potentials, this ion blocks the pore of the NMDA receptor channel. Depolarization, however, pushes Mg^{2+} out of the pore, allowing other cations to flow. This property provides the basis for a voltage-dependence to current flow through the receptor and means that NMDA receptors pass cations (most notably Ca^{2+}) only during depolarization of the postsynaptic cell, due to either activation of a large number of excitatory inputs and/or by repetitive firing of action potentials in the presynaptic cell. These properties are widely thought to be the basis for some forms of information storage at synapses, such as memory. Another unusual property of NMRA receptors is that opening the channel of this receptor requires the presence of a coagonist, the amino acid glycine. In addition to these ionotropic glutamate receptors, there are three types of metabotropic glutamate receptor (mGluRs). These receptors, which modulate postsynaptic ion channels indirectly, differ in their coupling to intracellular signal transduction pathways and in their sensitivity to pharmacological agents. Activation of many of these receptors leads to inhibition of postsynaptic Ca^{2+} and Na^+ channels. Unlike the excitatory ionotropic glutamate receptors, mGluRs cause slower postsynaptic responses that can either increase or decrease the excitability of postsynaptic cells. (In: Purves D, et al. (Eds.) Neuroscience 3rd ed. MA: Sinauer.)

19. **b**—DOPA—catechol O—methyltransferase—dopamine

There are five well-established biogenic amine neurotransmitters: the three catecholamines—dopamine, norepinephrine (noradrenaline), and epinephrine (adrenaline)—and histamine and serotonin. Their synthesis is as follows:

- Tyrosine-tyrosine hydroxylase-DOPA (dihydroxyphenylalanine)
- DOPA-DOPA decarboxylase-dopamine
- Dopamine-Dopamine beta-hydroxylase-Norepinephrine
- Norepinephrine-Phenylethanolamine *N*-methyltransferase-Epinephrine
- Histidine-histidine decarboxylase-Histamine
- Tryptophan-tryptophan 5-hydroxylase-5-hydroxytryptophan-Aromatic L-amino acid decarboxylase-Serotonin (5-Hydroxy tryptamine)

20. **c**—Dopamine is derived from norepinephrine

Dopamine is present in several brain regions, although the major dopamine-containing area of the brain is the corpus striatum, which receives major input from the substantia nigra and plays an essential role in the coordination of body movements. Dopamine is also believed to be involved in motivation, reward, and reinforcement, and many drugs of abuse work by affecting dopaminergic synapses in the CNS. In addition to these roles in the CNS, dopamine also plays a poorly understood role in some sympathetic ganglia. Dopamine is produced by the action of DOPA decarboxylase on DOPA. Following its synthesis in the cytoplasm of presynaptic terminals, dopamine is loaded into synaptic vesicles via a vesicular monoamine transporter (VMAT). Dopamine action in the synaptic cleft is terminated by reuptake of dopamine into nerve terminals or surrounding glial cells by a Na^+-dependent dopamine transporter, termed DAT. Cocaine apparently produces its psychotropic effects by binding to and inhibiting DAT, yielding a net increase in dopamine release from specific brain areas. Amphetamine, another addictive drug, also inhibits DAT as well as the transporter for norepinephrine (see below). The two major enzymes involved in the catabolism of dopamine are monoamine oxidase (MAO) and catechol O-methyltransferase (COMT). Both neurons and glia contain mitochondrial MAO and cytoplasmic COMT. Inhibitors of these enzymes, such as phenelzine and tranylcypromine, are used clinically as antidepressants. Once released, dopamine acts exclusively by activating G-protein-coupled receptors. Most dopamine receptor subtypes act by either activating or inhibiting adenylyl cyclase. Activation of these receptors generally contribute to complex behaviors; for example, administration of dopamine receptor agonists elicits hyperactivity and repetitive, stereotyped behavior in laboratory animals. Activation of another type of dopamine receptor in the medulla inhibits vomiting. Thus, antagonists of these receptors are used as emetics to induce vomiting after poisoning or a drug overdose. Dopamine receptor antagonists can also elicit catalepsy, a state in which it is difficult to initiate voluntary motor movement, suggesting a basis for this aspect of some psychoses. (In: Purves D, et al. (Eds.) Neuroscience 3rd ed. MA: Sinauer.)

21. **d**—GABAA and GABAC receptors are ionotropic receptors and are Ca^{2+} conductors

Most inhibitory synapses in the brain and spinal cord use either γ-aminobutyric acid (GABA) or glycine as neurotransmitters. It is now known that as many as a third of the synapses in the brain use GABA as their inhibitory neurotransmitter. GABA is most commonly found in local circuit interneurons, although cerebellar Purkinje cells provide an example of a GABAergic projection neuron. The predominant precursor for GABA synthesis is glucose, which is metabolized to glutamate by the tricarboxylic acid cycle enzymes (pyruvate and glutamine can also act as precursors). The enzyme glutamic acid decarboxylase (GAD), which is found almost exclusively in GABAergic neurons, catalyzes the conversion of glutamate to GABA. GAD requires a cofactor, pyridoxal phosphate, for activity. Because pyridoxal phosphate is derived from vitamin B6, a B6 deficiency can lead to diminished GABA synthesis. Once GABA is synthesized, it is transported into synaptic vesicles via a vesicular inhibitory amino acid transporter (VIATT). The mechanism of GABA removal is similar to that for glutamate: Both neurons and glia contain high-affinity transporters for GABA, termed GATs. Most GABA is eventually converted to succinate, which is metabolized further in the tricarboxylic acid cycle that mediates cellular ATP synthesis. The enzymes required for this degradation, GABA transaminase and succinic semialdehyde dehydrogenase, are mitochondrial enzymes. Inhibitory synapses employing GABA as their transmitter can exhibit three types of postsynaptic receptors, called GABAA, GABAB, and GABAC. GABAA and GABAC receptors are ionotropic receptors, while GABAB receptors are metabotropic. The ionotropic GABA receptors are usually inhibitory because their associated channels are permeable to Cl^-; the flow of the negatively charged chloride ions inhibits postsynaptic cells since the reversal potential for Cl^- is more negative than the threshold for neuronal firing. Like other ionotropic receptors, GABA receptors are pentamers assembled from a combination of five types of subunits (αβγδρ). Benzodiazepines, such as diazepam and chlordiazepoxide, are tranquilizing (anxiety reducing) drugs that enhance GABAergic transmission by binding to the α and δ subunits of GABAA receptors. Metabotropic GABA receptors (GABAB) are also widely distributed in brain. Like the ionotropic GABAA receptors, GABAB receptors are inhibitory. Rather than activating Cl^- selective channels, however, GABAB-mediated inhibition is due to the activation of K^+ channels. A second mechanism for GABAB-mediated inhibition is by blocking Ca^{2+} channels, which tends to hyperpolarize postsynaptic cells. Unlike most metabotropic receptors, GABAB receptors appear to assemble as heterodimers of GABAB R1 and R2 subunits. (In: Purves D, et al. (Eds.) Neuroscience 3rd ed. MA: Sinauer.)

22. **b**—Medial geniculate thalamic nucleus

23. **a**—Ganglion cells

The output of the retina is determined by ganglion cells which can generate action potentials and give rise to optic nerve. The other cell types display graded depolarizing/hyperpolarizing responses and amacrine cells show calcium spikes. In general, 99% of all ganglion cells are concerned with details of image formation and receive input from rods and cones via synaptic relays through the layers of the retina, are involved in circadian rhythms and the pupillary light reflex. The second type, melanopsin-containing ganglion cells, comprise less than 1% of all ganglion cells, are intrinsically sensitive to light and will generate action potentials (even without rods/cones, particularly blue light); are not concerned with image formation, and have connections to the suprachiasmatic and pretectal nuclei maintaining circadian rhythm. This type of ganglion cell explains why those blind due to rod/cone disease (e.g., retinitis pigmentosa) may still have an intact pupillary reflex and maintain circadian rhythm.

24. **a**—In the dark, rods have a high resting membrane potential of about −70 mV

Rod cells are named for the shape of their outer segment, which is a membrane-bound cylinder containing hundreds of tightly stacked membranous discs. In the dark, cGMP levels in the rod outer segment are high facilitating a inward Na and Ca current results in a relatively high resting membrane potential for rod cells, about −40 mV, and at the rod spherule there is tonic release of glutamate. With light, rhodopsin absorbs photons and undergoes a conformational change causing reduced levels of cGMP, causing closure of sodium channels, a wave of hyperpolarization and a transient reduction in this tonic release of glutamate. Cone outer segments also consist of a membranous stack of constantly decreasing diameter (from cilium to tip), giving the cell its characteristic shape. Cone opsin absorbs photons and undergoes a conformational change, resulting in a hyperpolarization of the cell membrane. This hyperpolarization propagates passively to the cone's synaptic ending, the cone pedicle, in the outer plexiform layer. Like rods, cones release the neurotransmitter glutamate tonically in the dark and respond to light with a decrease in glutamate release. There are three types of cones, each tuned to a different light wavelength. L-cones (red cones) are sensitive to long wavelengths, M-cones (green cones) to medium wavelengths, and S-cones (blue cones) to short wavelengths. Because any pure color represents a particular wavelength of light, each color will be represented by a unique combination of responses in the L-, M-, and S-cones. At the posterior pole of the eye is a yellowish spot, the macula lutea, the center of which is a depression called the fovea centralis Cones, which are responsible for color vision, are the only type of photoreceptor present in the fovea. In contrast, rods, which are most sensitive at low levels of illumination, are the predominant photoreceptors in the periphery of the retina. The visual world is a composite formed from a succession of foveal images carrying form and color information supplemented with input from the peripheral retina carrying motion information. Several adaptations of the fovea allow it to mediate the highest visual acuity in the retina. Neurons of the inner layer of retina are actually displaced laterally to the side of the fovea to minimize light scattering on the way to the receptors. In addition, within the fovea, the ratio of photoreceptors to ganglion cells falls dramatically. Most foveal receptors synapse on only one bipolar cell, which synapses on only one ganglion cell. Because each ganglion cell is devoted to a very small portion of the visual field, central vision has high resolution. In other words, the receptive field of a foveal ganglion cell (i.e., the region of stimulus space that can activate it) is small. At the periphery, the ratio of receptors to ganglion cells is high; thus, each ganglion cell has a large receptive field. The large receptive field reduces the spatial resolution of the peripheral portion of the retina but increases its sensitivity because more photoreceptors collect light for a ganglion cell. Lastly, the magnitude of phototransduction amplification varies with the prevailing levels of illumination (light adaptation). At low levels of illumination, photoreceptors are the most sensitive to light. As levels of illumination increase, sensitivity decreases (due to reduction in calcium currents in the rod outer segment), preventing the receptors from saturating and thereby greatly extending the range of light intensities over which they operate.

25. **d**—The receptive fields of on-center and off-center ganglion cells do not overlap

Most of the information in visual scenes consists of spatial variations in light intensity. Each ganglion cell responds to stimulation of a small circular patch of the retina, which defines the cell's receptive field. Turning on a spot of light in the receptive field center of an on-center ganglion cell produces a burst of action potentials. The same stimulus applied to the receptive field center of an off-center ganglion cell reduces the rate of discharge, and when the spot of light is turned off, the cell responds with a burst of action potentials. Complementary patterns of activity are also found for on-center versus off-center cell type when a dark spot is placed in the receptive field center. Thus, on-center cells increase their discharge rate to luminance increments in the receptive field center, whereas off-center cells increase their discharge rate to luminance decrements in the receptive field center. On- and off-center ganglion cells are present in roughly equal numbers. Their receptive fields have overlapping distributions, so that every point on the retinal surface (i.e., every part of visual space) is analyzed by several on-center and several off-center ganglion cells. In practice, silencing on-center ganglion cells in primates caused a deficit in their ability to detect stimuli that were brighter than the background; however, they could still see objects that were darker than the background. These observations imply that information about increases or decreases in luminance is carried separately to the brain by the axons of these two different types of retinal ganglion cells. Having separate luminance "channels" means that changes in light intensity, whether increases or decreases, are always conveyed to the brain by an increased number of action potentials. Because ganglion cells rapidly adapt to changes in luminance, their "resting" discharge rate in constant illumination is relatively low. Although an increase in discharge rate above resting level serves as a reliable signal, a decrease in firing rate from an initially low rate of discharge might not. Thus, having luminance changes signaled by two classes of adaptable cells provides unambiguous information about both luminance increments and decrements. On- and off-center ganglion cells have dendrites that arborize in separate strata of the inner plexiform layer, forming synapses selectively with the terminals of on- and off-center bipolar cells that respond to luminance increases and decreases, respectively. As mentioned previously, the principal difference between ganglion cells and bipolar cells lies in the nature of their electrical response. Like most other cells in the retina, bipolar cells have graded potentials rather than action potentials. Graded depolarization of bipolar cells leads to an increase in transmitter release (glutamate) at their synapses and consequent depolarization of the on-center ganglion cells that they contact via AMPA, kainite, and NMDA receptors. The selective response of on- and off-center bipolar cells to light increments and decrements is explained by the fact that they express different types of glutamate receptors. Off-center bipolar cells have ionotropic receptors (AMPA and kainate) that cause the cells to depolarize in response to glutamate released from photoreceptor terminals. In contrast, on-center bipolar cells express a G-protein-coupled metabotropic glutamate receptor (mGluR6). When bound to glutamate, these receptors activate an intracellular cascade that closes cGMP-gated Na^+ channels, reducing inward current and hyperpolarizing the cell. Decrements in light intensity naturally have the opposite effect on these two classes of bipolar cells, hyperpolarizing on-center cells and depolarizing off-center ones. Retinal ganglion cells are relatively poor at signaling differences in the level of diffuse illumination. Instead, they are sensitive to differences between the level of illumination that falls on the receptive field center and the level of illumination that falls on the surround—that is, to luminance contrast. The center of a ganglion cell receptive field is surrounded by a concentric region (surround) that, when stimulated, antagonizes the response to stimulation of the receptive field center (center antagonism). In practice this means that firing of an on-center ganglion cell is (i) increased above baseline when a spot of light shines on receptive field center, (ii) at baseline when the spot of light is on the center/surround border or outside of the receptive field completely, and (iii) reduced below baseline when shined on the surround alone. Off-center ganglion cells demonstrate surround antagonism. Much of the antagonism is thought to arise via lateral connections established by horizontal cells and photoreceptor terminals (lateral inhibition). Thus, the information supplied by the retina to central visual stations for further processing does not give equal weight to all regions of the visual scene; rather, it emphasizes the regions where there are differences in luminance. In addition to making ganglion cells especially sensitive to light-dark borders in the visual scene, center-surround mechanisms make a significant contribution to the process of light adaptation as background/ambient level of illumination is less important than scaled differences in light intensity. (In Chapter 10 Visual System In: Purves D, et al. (Eds.) Neuroscience 3rd ed. MA: Sinauer.)

26. **b**—Mucus-coated olfactory epithelium lines the anterodorsal parts of the nasal cavities

Smell is detected by olfactory receptor cells, which are situated in mucus-coated olfactory epithelium that lines the posterodorsal parts of the nasal cavities. Olfactory glands (Bowman glands) secrete a fluid that bathes the cilia of the receptors and acts as a solvent for odorant molecules. Olfactory receptor cells (first-order neurons) are stimulated by the binding of odor molecules to their cilia—G protein activation and activation of adenylyl cyclase, a rise in intracellular cAMP with causes opening of a cyclic-nucleotide gated ion channel allowing influx of Na^+ and Ca^{2+} causing neuronal depolarization. The axons of the olfactory receptor cells form CN I (olfactory nerve); these project through the cribriform plate at the base of the cranium to synapse with the mitral cells of the olfactory bulb in olfactory glomeruli. The map of glomerular activation patterns within the olfactory bulb are thought to represent the quality of the odor being detected. The mitral cells of the olfactory bulb are excitatory, second-order neurons. The output axons of the mitral cells form the olfactory tract and lateral olfactory stria, both of which project to the primary olfactory cortex (prefrontal cortex) and the amygdala.

27. **e**—All taste fibers synapse in the nucleus ambiguus

Taste is detected by taste receptor cells, which are located on specialized papillae of the taste buds and are stimulated by taste chemicals. The cellular mechanism for transduction of taste stimuli depends upon the stimulus. Receptors for molecules associated with sweet and bitter tastes utilize second messengers, while those associated with sour and salty-tasting molecules act directly upon the ion channels. Taste buds on the anterior two thirds of the tongue have fungiform papillae and primarily detect sweet and salty tastes. They send signals centrally through the lingual nerve to the chorda tympani and finally into CN VII (facial). Taste buds on the posterior one third of the tongue have circumvallate papillae and foliate papillae, which detect bitter and sour tastes. Most of them send signals centrally through CN IX (glossopharyngeal); however, some located in the back of the throat and epiglottis send signals centrally through CN X (vagus). CN VII, IX, and X synapse with the tractus solitarius (solitary nucleus). Second-order neurons leave the solitary nucleus and project ipsilaterally to the ventral posterior medial nucleus of the thalamus. Neurons from the thalamus project to the taste cortex located in the primary somatosensory cortex. Taste discrimination and perception occur as a result of the comparison of the activation pattern of different groups of taste fibers.

28. **b**—End plate potential amplitude is larger than that of excitatory or inhibitory postsynaptic potentials

An action potential in presynaptic neuron causes calcium influx and release of acetylcholine (ACh) from presynaptic vesicles stored in terminal bouton. Diffusion of ACh occurs across the synaptic cleft and it binds to postsynaptic nicotinic ACh receptors which are ligand-gated ion channels selective for Na^+ and K^+ ions, with subsequent current flow producing membrane depolarization (end-plate potential, EPP). The EPP is a graded potential (rather than an all-or-none response) with an amplitude directly related to the quantity of neurotransmitter (ACh) released from the presynaptic terminals. The amplitude of the EPP can be much greater that of the excitatory and inhibitory postsynaptic potentials in CNS synapses. At the neuromuscular junction, ACh is enzymatically degraded by acetylcholinesterase into acetate and choline. Choline is then taken up by the presynaptic terminal.

29. **d**—Axonotmesis shows Wallerian degeneration distal to injury

At times, it is difficult to tell what form of injury a patient has sustained. Certainly, if a patient has a dense motor and sensory deficit following a penetrating injury, it probably represents a neurotmesis and the patient will benefit from an exploration and nerve repair. On the other hand, if a patient sustained blunt trauma to the upper extremity and now has a partial sensory and motor deficit, it is difficult to know what form of nerve injury they have sustained. Exploration of this wound may not be indicated immediately following the injury and the wait-and-see approach may be more appropriate. Surgical repair may involve end-to-end neurorrhaphy (either epineural repair or fascicular repair with cable nerve grafts), nerve graft reconstruction of peripheral nerve (using donor nerves), neural conduit (e.g., if significant peripheral nerve gap) and less frequently, end-to-side neurorrhaphy.

Classification of Peripheral Nerve Injury

Classification	Grade	Pathology	Return of Function
Neuropraxia	I	Disruption of myelin sheath only. No Wallerian degeneration	Nearly complete in days to weeks
Axonotmesis	II	Disruption of axon only. Wallerian degeneration distal to injury	Nearly complete at a rate of 1 mm/day as endoneurial conduit remain intact (regenerating axons do not need to traverse a coaptation site)

Continued

Classification	Grade	Pathology	Return of Function
	III	Disruption of axon and endoneurial tubes	Variable
	IV	Disruption of axon, endoneurial tubes, and perineurium	Variable
Neurotmesis	V	Disruption of axon, endoneurial tubes, perineurium and epineurium (complete transection)	Incomplete after microsurgical repair due to mismatching of fascicles, scarring at the nerve coaptation site, and loss of axons during regeneration

Adapted from Cederna PS, Chung KC. Nerve Repair and Nerve Grafting, In Guyuron B (Ed.), Plastic Surgery: Indications and Practice, Elsevier, 2009.

30. **c**—Gamma motor neurons

Neuromuscular spindles are stretch receptor organs within skeletal muscles which are responsible for the regulation of muscle tone via the spinal stretch reflex. They lie parallel to the muscle fibers, embedded in endomysium or perimysium. Each spindle contains 2-10 modified skeletal muscle fibers called intrafusal fibers, which are much smaller than skeletal extrafusal fibers. The intrafusal fibers have a central non-striated area in which their nuclei tend to be concentrated. The two types of intrafusal fibers are nuclear bag fiber and nuclear chain fiber. Associated with the intrafusal fibers are branched non-myelinated endings of large myelinated sensory fibers which wrap around the central non-striated area, forming annulospiral endings. Additionally, flower-spray endings of smaller myelinated sensory nerves are located on the striated portions of the intrafusal fibers. These sensory receptors are stimulated by stretching of the intrafusal fibers, which occurs when the (extrafusal) muscle mass is stretched. This stimulus evokes a simple two-neuron spinal cord reflex, causing contraction of the extrafusal muscle mass. This removes the stretch stimulus from the spindle and equilibrium is restored (e.g., knee jerk reflex). The sensitivity of the neuromuscular spindle to stretch is modulated via small gamma motor neurons controlled by the extra-pyramidal motor system. These gamma motor neurons innervate the striated portions of the intrafusal fibers; contraction of the intrafusal fibers increases the stretch on the fibers and thus the sensitivity of the receptors to stretching of the extrafusal muscle mass. During a normal movement, both alpha and gamma motor neurons are co-activated. If only the alpha motor neurons were activated the muscle would contract and the central non-contractile portion of intrafusal muscle fibers would become slack and unable to monitor changes in muscle length. However, where descending inhibition on gamma motor neurons is impaired (e.g., UMN lesion), this can result in exquisitely sensitive stretch receptors and hyperreflexia.

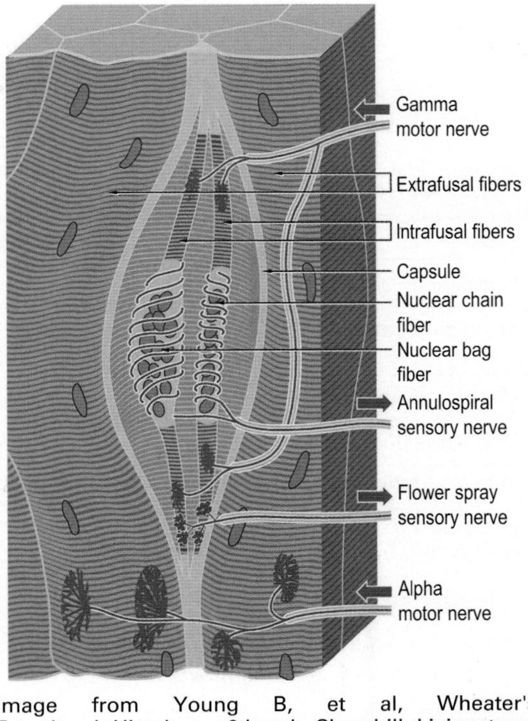

Image from Young B, et al, Wheater's Functional Histology, 6th ed. Churchill Livingstone, Elsevier, 2014.

ANSWERS 31–45

Additional answers 31–45 available on ExpertConsult.com

EMI ANSWERS

46. 1—h, PCP; 2—a, 3,4-methylenedioxy-methamphetamine; 3—f, Conotoxin; 4—i, Tetraethylammonium (TEA); 5—j, Tetrodotoxin (TTX)

Conotoxins include: α-conotoxin inhibits nicotinic acetylcholine receptors at nerves and muscles, δ-conotoxin inhibits the inactivation of voltage-dependent sodium channels, κ-conotoxin inhibits potassium channels, μ-conotoxin inhibits voltage-dependent sodium channels in muscles, ω-conotoxin inhibits N-type voltage-dependent calcium channels. Chlorotoxin is found in the venom of deathstalker scorpion and acts as a Cl^- channel blocker. Botulinum toxin irreversibly blocks release of acetylcholine (ACh) from presynaptic nerve terminal. The α-toxins, including α-bungarotoxin, can produce postsynaptic effects similar to that observed with curare, by binding specifically to the subunits of the nicotinic ACh receptor. Curare competitively antagonises binding of ACh to the postsynaptic nicotinic receptor.

47. 1—b, Dopamine. The conversion of dopamine to norepinephrine comes about by the action of the enzyme dopamine ↓-hydroxylase
 2—h, L-DOPA. The biosynthesis of catecholamines includes the following steps: tyrosine is converted into L-dihydroxyphenylalanine (L-DOPA) by tyrosine hydroxylase. L-DOPA is then decarboxylated by a decarboxylase to form dopamine (and CO_2)
 3—j, Serotonin. Tryptophan is converted to 5-hydroxytryptophan by tryptophan hydroxylase and by 5-hydroxytryptophan decarboxylase into serotonin
 4—c, Epinephrine. Norepinephrine is converted into epinephrine by phenylethanolamine-N-methyl transferase
 5—f, Glycine

48. 1—e, Nuclear bag fibers; 2—c, Meissner's corpuscles; 3—g, Pacinian corpuscles

Types of Sensory Receptors

Type	Modality	Fibers	Tracts
Nociceptors			
Pain/Temperature	Pain (mechanical, thermal, chemical)	A-delta (fast) myelinated C-fiber (slow) unmyelinated	Anterolateral system
Mechanoreceptors			
Free nerve endings	Touch, pressure	A-delta, C-fibers	Anterolateral system
Merkel's tactile discs	Discriminative touch, superficial pressure	A-beta myelinated	Dorsal column-medial lemniscus
Meissner's corpuscles	Two-point discriminative fine touch		
Pacinian corpuscles	Deep pressure and vibration		
Ruffini's corpuscles	Skin pressure/stretch		
Peritrichial nerve endings	Hair movement		
Muscle and tendon mechanoreceptors			
Nuclear bag fibers	Onset of muscle stretch	A-alpha myelinated fibers, muscle spindle afferents, secondary afferents	Dorsal column-medial lemniscus and spinocerebellar
Nuclear chain fibers	Progress of muscle stretch		
Golgi tendon organ	Tendon stretch	A-alpha myelinated fibers	

49. 1—k, Schwann cells; 2—h, Microglia; 3—i, Oligodendrocytes; 4—a, Astrocytes; 5—d, Ependymal cells

Neurons are classified as shown below:

1. Multipolar (several dendrites and one axon) neuron with either a long axon (Golgi type I, e.g., Betz cell, Martinotti cell) or short/no axon (Golgi type II, e.g., interneuron)
2. Bipolar (single dendrite and axon, cell body close to sensory receptor) neuron, e.g., retina, auditory, vestibular, olfactory system
3. Unipolar (single process which is structurally and functionally an axon, cell body far from sensory receptor) neuron, e.g., peripheral sensory afferents

50. 1—l, 2—o, 3—k, 4—d, 5—h

a, Superior cerebellar arteries; b, Superior cerebellar surface; c, Inferior cerebellar surface; d, Dentate nucleus; e, Emboliform nucleus; f, Cerebellar nuclei: Globose; g, Cerebellar nuclei: Fastigial; h, Anterior inferior cerebellar arteries; i, Posterior inferior cerebellar artery; j, Anterior lobe; k, Primary fissure; l, Posterior lobe; m, Horizontal fissure; n, Posterolateral fissure; o, Flocculonodular lobe: Flocculus; p, Flocculonodular lobe: Nodulus.

An unfolded view of the cerebellum showing medial (vermal including nodulus, *gray*), intermediate (paravermal, *green*), and lateral (hemispheric including flocculus, *blue*) zones on the right and their functionally associated deep cerebellar nuclei (fastigial, globose/emboliform, and dentate respectively) on the left in the corresponding color. The general areas of cortex and nuclei served by the cerebellar arteries are also indicated on the left. Roman numerals indicate lobules of the vermis; numerals preceded by H indicate the corresponding lobules of the hemisphere. Note that the IX represents the uvula and HIX the cerebellar tonsil. In general, cerebellar structure is classified by gross anatomical features (anterior, posterior and flocculonodular lobes with primary, horizontal and posterolateral fissures), by organization of cortical projections (vermal, paravermal, hemispheric) and by functional modules (vestibulocerebellum, spinocerebellum, and pontocerebellum).

Image adapted from Haines DE. Fundamental Neuroscience for Basic and Clinical Applications, 4th ed. Saunders, Elsevier, 2013.

51. 1—m, 2—d, 3—k, 4—a, 5—g

A, Dendritic tree of one Golgi cell; b, Stellate cells; c, Molecular layer; d, Basket cell; e, Dendritic tree of one Purkinje cell; f, Axon of basket cell; g, Parallel fibers; h, Granule cell; i, Synaptic glomerulus; j, Ramification of Golgi cell axon in granular layer; k, Climbing fibers; l, Mossy fibers; m, Axons of Purkinje cells.

Afferent projections to the cerebellum arise principally from the spinal cord (spinocerebellar fibers), inferior olivary nucleus (olivocerebellar fibers), vestibular nuclei (vestibulocerebellar fibers) and pons (pontocerebellar fibers). Afferent axons mostly terminate in the cerebellar cortex, where they are excitatory to cortical neurons. Fibers enter the cerebellum through one of the cerebellar peduncles and proceed to the cortex as either *mossy fibers* or *climbing fibers*, depending upon their origin. All afferents originating elsewhere than the inferior olivary nucleus end as mossy fibers. Mossy fibers branch to supply several folia and end in the granular layer, in synaptic contact with granule cells. The axons of granule cells pass towards the surface of the cortex and enter the molecular layer. Here they bifurcate to produce two *parallel fibers* that are oriented along the long axis of the folium. The Purkinje cell layer consists of a unicellular layer of the somata of Purkinje neurons. The profuse dendritic arborizations of these cells extend towards the surface of the cortex, into the molecular layer. The arborizations are flattened and oriented at right angles to the long axis of the folium. They are, therefore, traversed by numerous parallel fibers, from which they receive excitatory synaptic input. Inhibitory modulation of intracortical circuitry is provided by numerous other neurons known as Golgi, basket and stellate cells. The axons of Purkinje cells are the only axons to leave the cerebellar cortex. Most of these fibers do not leave the cerebellum entirely but end in the deep cerebellar nuclei. The other type of afferent fiber entering the cerebellar cortex, the climbing fiber, originates from the inferior olivary nucleus of the medulla. These fibers provide relatively discrete excitatory input to Purkinje cells. At the same time, axon collaterals of climbing fibers excite the neurons of the deep cerebellar nuclei. Purkinje cells utilize GABA as their neurotransmitter, which means that the output of the whole of the cerebellar cortex is mediated through the inhibition of cells in the cerebellar nuclei.

Image adapted from Mancall EL, Gray's Clinical Neuroanatomy: The Anatomic Basis for Clinical Neuroscience, Elsevier, Saunders, 2011

52. 1—i, Oxytocin; 2—b, ADH (Vasopressin); 3—j, Prolactin

Clinical Features of Endocrine Dysfunction

Hormone	Effect	Deficit	Excess
TSH	Production of T3/T4 in thyroid	Hypothyroidism	Hyperthyroidism
ACTH	Adrenal cortex production of cortisol and mineralocorticoids	Secondary adrenal insufficiency	Cushing's disease (most common)
Oxytocin	Uterine contractions in labor, milk ejection reflex		
Prolactin	Lactation	Lactation failure, male reduced fertility, ovarian dysfunction	Galactorrhea, amenorrhea, anovulatory infertility, gynaecomastia, loss of libido, sexual dysfunction
ADH (vasopressin)	Renal water conservation	Diabetes insipidus	SIADH
GH	Stimulate production of insulin-like growth factors	GH deficiency	Acromegaly
FSH	Ovulation in women Sperm production in men	Infertility	
LH	Sex hormone production by gonads	Hypogonadotrophic (secondary) hypogonadism	
Cortisol	Metabolism and stress response	Addison's disease (primary adrenal insufficiency)	Cushings syndrome

53. 1—i, 2—f, 3—a, 4—d

a, Mesoneurium; b, Grouped fascicle; c, Longitudinal vessels on the extrinsic epineurium; d, External epineurium; e, Internal epineurium; f, Perineurium; g, Myelin; h, Fascicle; i, Endoneurium; j, Axon.

Peripheral nerves are composed of connective, vascular, and neural tissue. The connective tissue components include the epineurium, perineurium, and endoneurium. The epineurium consists of loose collagenous connective tissue that either encloses groups of nerve fascicles (external epineurium) or cushions fascicles from external pressure and trauma to prevent injury (internal epineurium). The amount of external and internal epineurium varies greatly among individuals, peripheral nerves, and even within a single nerve. The perineurium surrounds individual nerve fascicles and defines the fascicular pattern of a given nerve: monofascicular, oligofascicular, or polyfascicular. The fascicular pattern of a peripheral nerve has important implications when trying to repair an injured or divided peripheral nerve. The size, quantity, and ultrastructure of nerve fascicles vary greatly along the length of a given nerve. Within the perineurium, individual nerve axons are surrounded by a layer of connective tissue known as the endoneurium. Each nerve has a vascular network along its entire length including arteries, veins, and capillaries. These vascular components of the peripheral nerve are anatomically separated from the neural components of the nerve by a blood-brain barrier. Finally, the peripheral nerve contains myelinated and unmyelinated motor, sensory, and sympathetic nerve fibers. The size and number of axons varies greatly within all nerves. The cell bodies for these nerves fibers are contained within the spinal cord.

Image adapted from Berger RA, Weiss APC. Hand Surgery, Volume 1. Lippincott, Williams and Wilkins, 2003.

CHAPTER 4

NEUROPATHOLOGY I: BASICS

SINGLE BEST ANSWER (SBA) QUESTIONS

1. A 43-year-old South Asian man is brought into the emergency department with generalized seizures and fever >38 (101F). CT head does not show any abnormality. LP is performed with an opening pressure of 22 cm H_2O and CSF analysis shows: WCC 748 (Polymorphs 113, Lymphocytes 635), RBC 28, normal protein and normal glucose. Which one of the following is the most likely cause?
   a. Enterovirus
   b. Listeria monocytogenes
   c. Mycobacterium tuberculosis
   d. Streptococcus pneumoniae
   e. Wegener's granulomatosis

2. A 45-year-old woman presents with sudden onset headache and photophobia. CT head is unremarkable and she undergoes a lumbar puncture. CSF analysis shows WCC 3, RBC 15000 and subarachnoid hemorrhage cannot be excluded due to the presence of oxyhemoglobin. CSF xanthochromia is detected by which one of the following assays?
   a. Fluorescence in situ hybridization
   b. Immunoprecipitation
   c. Light microscopy
   d. Spectroscopy
   e. Western blotting

3. Which one of the following is the most appropriate marker for tumor proliferation?
   a. GFAP
   b. Ki-67
   c. LDH
   d. P53
   e. S100

4. Which one of the following pathologies is most likely to exhibit the finding shown?

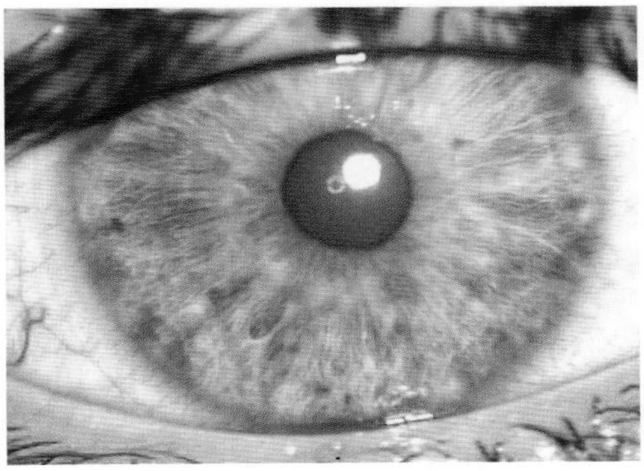

   a. Ataxia telangiectasia
   b. Neurofibromatosis-1
   c. Neurofibromatosis-2
   d. Sturge-Weber syndrome
   e. Tuberous sclerosis

5. Which one of the following is most accurate regarding tumors with 0-6-methylguanine-DNA methyltransferase methylation?
   a. More susceptible to alkylating agents
   b. More susceptible to antimetabolites
   c. More susceptible to antitumor antibiotics
   d. More susceptible to topoisomerase inhibitors
   e. More susceptible to ribunucleotide reductase inhibitors

6. Which one of the following genetic mutations are associated with improved brain tumor prognosis?
   a. Loss of 1p/19q
   b. Loss of 1p/22q
   c. Loss of 1p/10q
   d. Loss of 1p/10q
   e. Loss of 1p/10q

7. Which one of the following types of cerebral edema is seen in malignant hypertension?
   a. Cytotoxic
   b. Hydrostatic
   c. Interstitial
   d. Osmotic
   e. Vasogenic

8. Cerebral ischemia is usually seen when global cerebral blood flow is below:
   a. 60 ml per 100 g tissue per min
   b. 50 ml per 100 g tissue per min
   c. 40 ml per 100 g tissue per min
   d. 30 ml per 100 g tissue per min
   e. 20 ml per 100 g tissue per min

9. Which one of the following descriptions suggest WHO grade II astrocytoma?
   a. Microcystic change
   b. Nuclear atypia and hyperchromasia
   c. >10 mitoses per high power field
   d. Numerous mitoses and anaplasia
   e. Microvascular proliferation or necrosis

10. Which one of the following best describes the finding below?

   a. Ash-leaf (macule)
   b. Café-au-lait spot
   c. Plexiform neurofibroma
   d. Port wine stain
   e. Shagreen patch

11. Which one of the following best describes the finding below?

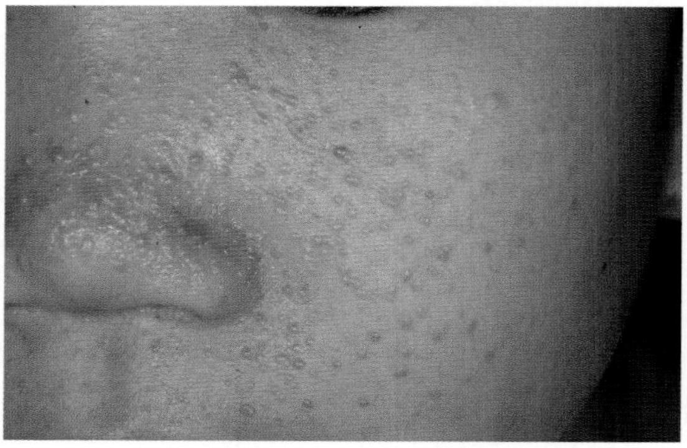

   a. Cowden syndrome
   b. Gorlin syndrome
   c. MEN1
   d. Tuberous sclerosis
   e. Von Hippel Lindau

12. Which one of the following genetic mutations is most likely seen with the finding below?

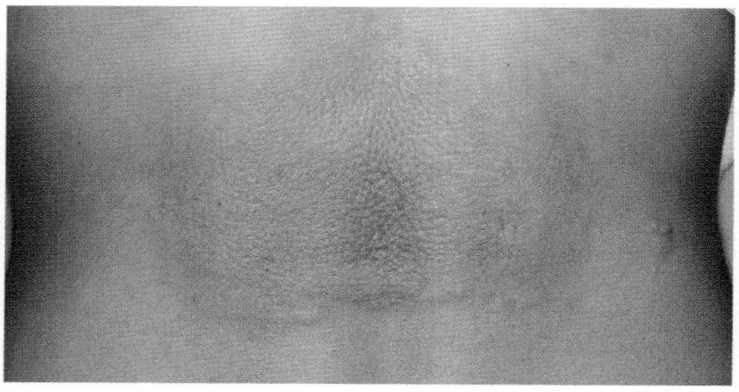

   a. 9q34/16p13
   b. 3p25
   c. 17p13
   d. 9q22
   e. 5q21

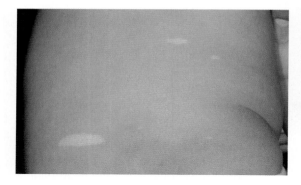

13. Which one of the following best describes the finding shown?

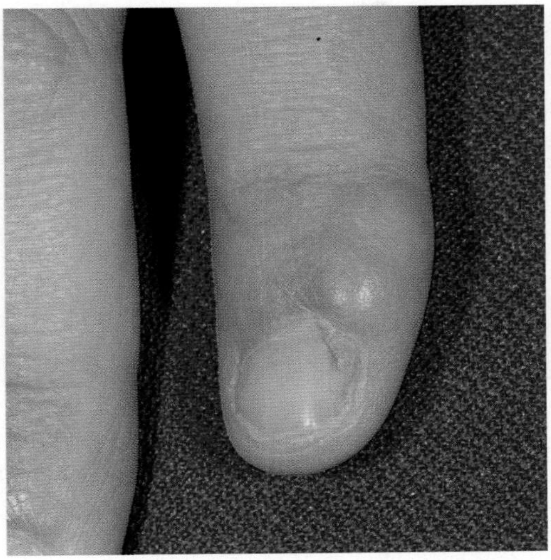

a. Angiofibroma
b. Collagenoma
c. Neurofibroma
d. Neuroma
e. Periungual fibroma

14. Which one of the following findings are most likely associated with the clinical feature below?

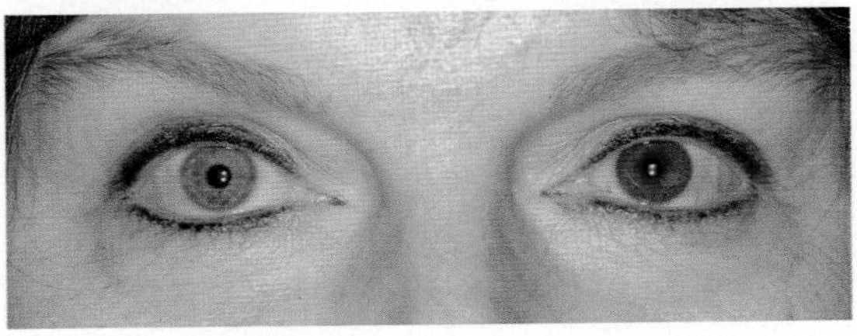

a. Brainstem arteriovenous malformation
b. GI polyps
c. Optic glioma
d. Retinal hamartoma
e. Sensorineural deafness

15. Which one of the following best describes the finding shown?

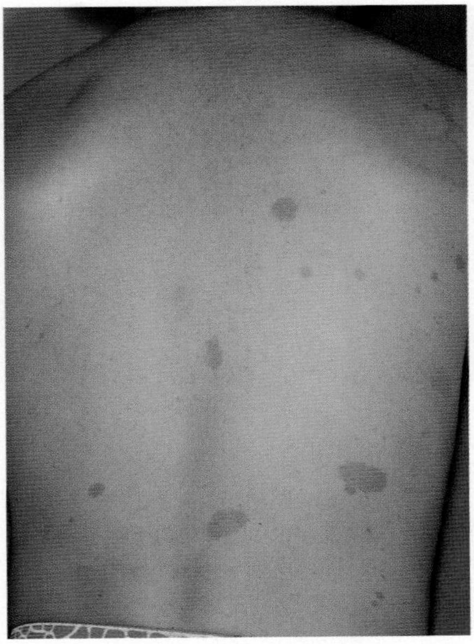

a. Cowden syndrome
b. McCune-Albright syndrome
c. Neurofibromatosis type 1
d. Neurofibromatosis type 2
e. Rhabdoid tumor syndrome

16. Which one of the following best describes the finding shown?

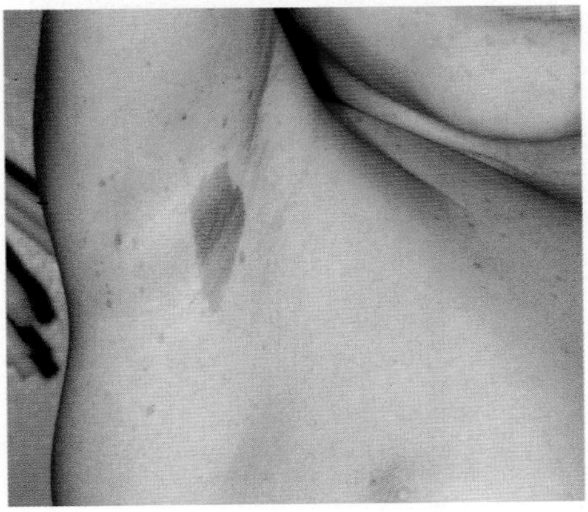

a. Acanthosis nigricans
b. Legius syndrome
c. Muenke syndrome
d. Neurofibromatosis type 2
e. Pfeiffer syndrome

17. Which one of the following best describes the finding shown?

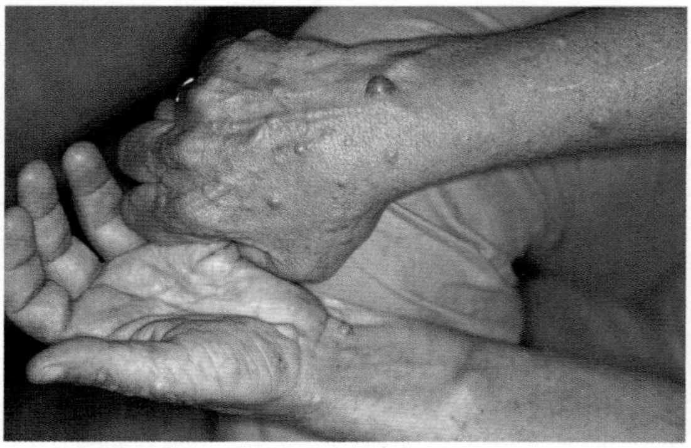

a. Cowden syndrome
b. Legius syndrome
c. Neurofibromatosis type 1
d. Rhabdoid tumor syndrome
e. Tuberous sclerosis complex

18. Which one of the following is most likely in the image shown?

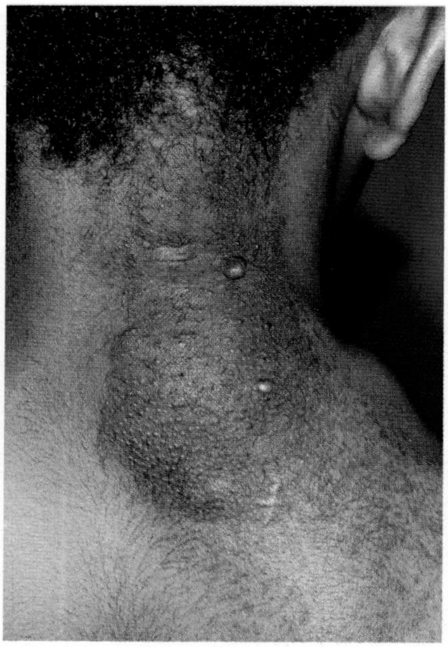

a. Basal cell naevus syndrome (Gorlin)
b. Hereditary Hemorrhagic Telangiectasia
c. Neurofibromatosis type 2
d. Sturge-Weber syndrome
e. Tuberous sclerosis

19. Which one of the following is most likely in the image shown?

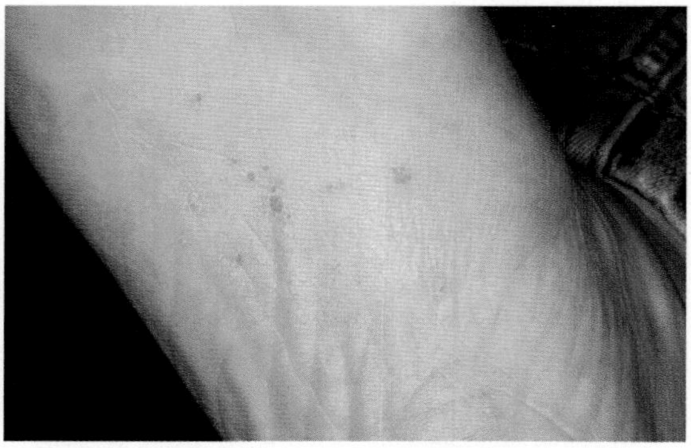

a. Crouzon syndrome
b. Familial adenomatous polyposis syndrome
c. Gardener's syndrome
d. Gorlin syndrome
e. Osler-Weber-Rendu syndrome

20. Which one of the following CNS manifestations are associated with the condition suggested below?

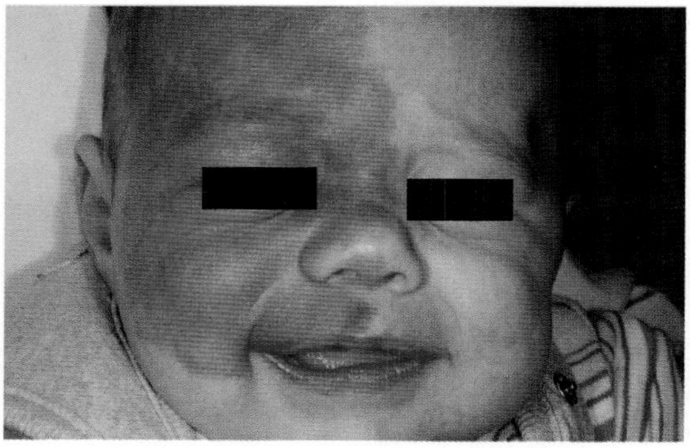

a. Aqueduct stenosis
b. DNET
c. Leptomeningeal angiomatosis
d. Skull base meningioma
e. Sphenoid wing dysplasia

QUESTIONS 21–23

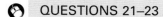

Additional questions 21–23 available on ExpertConsult.com

EXTENDED MATCHING ITEM (EMI) QUESTIONS

24. **Molecular assays of NS tumors:**
    a. B-cell and T-cell receptor gene rearrangement
    b. BRAF-KIAA1549 gene fusion/duplication
    c. Chromosome 1p/19q loss
    d. EGFR gene amplification/10q loss
    e. EWSR1 gene rearrangement
    f. MGMT promotor methylation status
    g. Monosomy chromosome 6
    h. MYC gene amplification
    i. SMARCB1 gene loss/INI1 protein absent
    j. Wnt signaling pathway upregulation

For each of the following descriptions, select the most appropriate answers from the list above. Each answer may be used once, more than once or not at all.

1. Diagnosis of atypical teratoid/rhabdoid tumor
2. Response to alkylating agents in high grade glioma
3. Found in most pilocytic astrocytomas

25. **Tumor syndromes:**
    a. APC
    b. MEN1
    c. NF-1
    d. NF-2
    e. PTCH
    f. PTEN
    g. SMARCB1
    h. TP53
    i. TSC1/TSC2
    j. VHL

For each of the following descriptions, select the most appropriate answers from the list above. Each answer may be used once, more than once or not at all.

1. Gliomas and medulloblastoma
2. AT/RT
3. Hemangioblastoma

26. **Tumor markers:**
    a. Alpha-fetoprotein (AFP)
    b. Beta-2-microglobulin
    c. Beta-human chorionic gonadotropin
    d. CA-125
    e. CA15-3/CA27.29
    f. CA19-9
    g. Calcitonin
    h. CEA
    i. Chromogranin-A
    j. Cytokeratin fragment 21-1
    k. HE-4
    l. LDH
    m. PSA

For each of the following descriptions, select the most appropriate answers from the list above. Each answer may be used once, more than once or not at all.

1. Neuroendocrine tumors
2. Multiple myeloma
3. Liver and germ cell cancers

27. **Cytopathology of neurones and glia:**
    a. Central chromatolysis
    b. Cowdry type A intranuclear inclusions
    c. Flexner Wintersteiner rosette
    d. Hirano Bodies
    e. Homer-Wright rosette
    f. Inclusion bodies
    g. Lewy bodies
    h. Negri bodies
    i. Neurofibrillary tangles
    j. Perivascular pseudorosette
    k. Pick Bodies
    l. Pick Cells
    m. Schiller-Duval bodies
    n. Verocay bodies

For each of the following descriptions, select the most appropriate answers from the list above. Each answer may be used once, more than once or not at all.

1. Schwannoma
2. Ependymoma
3. Retinoblastoma
4. Rabies virus
5. Alzheimer's disease

QUESTIONS 28–29

Additional questions 28–29 available on ExpertConsult.com

SBA ANSWERS

1. **a**—Enterovirus

	Normal CSF	Bacterial meningitis	Viral	Chronic
Pressure	10-20	Normal/increased	Normal/increased	Normal/increased
Appearance WCC (/mm^3)	Clear <5	Turbid/purulent >1000	Clear/cloudy 500-1000	Clear/cloudy <500
Predominant cell type	Lymphocyte	Polymorphonuclear leukocyte	Lymphocytes	Lymphocytes
Protein (mg/dl)	<40	>100-200	Normal or <100	Normal or <100
Glucose	2/3 serum level	Reduced	Normal	Normal or reduced
Lactic acid (mmol/l)	<3.5	>3.5	<3.5	<3.5

2. **d**—Spectroscopy

3. **b**—Ki-67

MIB-1 antibody is directed against the cell cycle-associated antigen Ki-67 expressed in the nucleus of cells that have entered the cell cycle (i.e. exited the G0 (resting) phase). It aids assessment of mitotic figures in order to estimate the proliferative potential and thus aggressiveness of a tumor. Generally grade II gliomas have MIB-1 indices of ~2-5% and glioblastomas of ~>10%. However, tumors with the highest proliferation index are PNETs (~20-60%) and high-grade lymphomas (~40-90%).

4. **b**—Neurofibromatosis-1

Individuals with light irises tend to have orange or brown round Lisch nodules. In an individual with a dark iris, on slit-lamp examination reveals light-colored nodules appear like splattered putty or white paint.

Image with permission from Liu GT, et al. Neuro-Ophthalmology: Diagnosis and Management, 2nd ed., Saunders, Elsevier, 2010.

5. **a**—More susceptible to alkylating agents

Promoter methylation is a mechanism of gene-silencing that occurs spontaneously in many tumor types. MGMT is one of many DNA repair enzymes and in a tumor with MGMT gene silencing by promoter hypermethylation little functional MGMT enzyme is produced. MGMT is particularly effective in repairing DNA damage induced by alkylating chemotherapeutic agents such as temozolomide (TMZ). The less functional MGMT is present in a rapidly proliferating tumor such as GBM, the more effective alkylating agents are likely to be in killing cells off by inducing irreparable cytotoxic DNA damage. Therefore, MGMT methylation status can be used to stratify tumors into likely TMZ-responders and non-responders. It has been shown that GBM patients with a good performance score and MGMT methylation benefit from post-operative combined TMZ and radiotherapy treatment (Further reading *Hegi ME, Diserens AC, Gorlia T. MGMT gene silencing and benefit from temozolomide in glioblastoma, N Engl J Med. 2005 Mar 10;352(10):997-1003*), resulting in a significant survival benefit.

6. **a**—Loss of heterozygosity on Chr 1p and 19q

This is the signature genetic defect in classical oligodendrogliomas (WHO grade II and III). They often occur together and can be the result of a translocation of 1p and 19q [t(1,19)(q10;p10)]. The presence of these mutations typically indicates an improved prognosis particularly for patients with WHO grade III anaplastic oligodendrogliomas (irrespective of treatment). It was also thought that this genetic signature (particularly LOH 1p) was associated with a good response to early PCV chemotherapy resulting in overall improved survival. 1p/19q loss can also occur in mixed oligoastrocytomas. If it is the main genetic abnormality in these tumors, it usually also indicates a somewhat improved prognosis. There are presumed oligodendroglioma tumor-suppressor genes on 1p and 19q, but their specific identity remains unclear.

7. **b**—Hydrostatic

	Cytotoxic	Vasogenic	Hydrostatic	Interstitial	Osmotic
Pathophysiology	Metabolic failure of NaKATPase pump—reversal of osmotic gradient—Net intracellular accumulation of Na and H_2O	Increased vascular permeability	Increased cerebral capillary pressure	Transependymal flow of CSF	Reduced plasma osmolality
Location	ICF	ECF	ECF	ECF	ECF > ICF
Causes	Infarction/ischemia/anoxia, trauma, hypothermia, infection/meningitis	Tumor, abscess, trauma, encephalitis, late infarction	Malignant hypertension,	Hydrocephalus	Dialysis, SIADH, water intoxication
Treatment	Reversal of cause	corticosteroids, reversal of primary insult	Reversal of cause	Treatment of hydrocephalus	Reversal of cause

8. **e**—20 ml per 100 g tissue per min

Normal global cerebral blood flow is 55-60 ml per 100 g of brain tissue per min (i.e. 700 ml/min or 15% of resting cardiac output); more precisely about 70-80 ml per 100 g per min in gray matter and 20-45 ml per 100 g per min in white matter. Physiological and EEG changes associated with different CBF is outlined below:

CBF (ml/100 g/min)	EEG	Physiological
35-70	Normal	Decreased protein synthesis
25-35	Loss of fast beta frequencies	Anaerobic metabolism; neurotransmitter release (glutamate)
18-25	Slowing of background to 5-7 Hz (theta)	Lactic acidosis; declining ATP
12-18	Slowing of background to 1-4 Hz (delta)	Ischemia: Na-K-ATPase pump failure, cytotoxic edema
<10-12	Suppression of all frequencies	Infarction: Calcium accumulation, anoxic depolarization, cell death

9. **b**—Nuclearatypia and hyperchromasia

WHO grade is an independent prognostic factor and currently particularly used in determining need for adjuvant therapies (usually indicated in WHO III/IV lesions). Grade I lesions (pilocytic astrocytomas, meningiomas) are tumors with a low proliferation rate which often can be cured by surgery alone. Grade II lesions are often infiltrative, and in the glioma categories, tend to recur or progress to higher grade lesions (survival generally >5 years). Grade III is generally reserved for tumors with histological anaplasia and brisk mitotic activity; recurrence and progression is the rule (survival 2-3 years). Grade IV lesions are highly aggressive tumors prone to necrosis and relentless progression to within a year if left untreated (note that treatment of some WHO IV lesions such as medulloblastoma and germinoma can be quite successful).

10. **a**—Ash-leaf spot

Tuberous sclerosis. Several lance-ovate (ash-leaf) and thumbprint white macules are noted on this infant's back.

Image with permission from Paller AS, Mancini AJ. Hurwitz Clinical Pediatric Dermatology, 4th ed., Saunders, Elsevier, 2011.

11. **d**—Tuberous sclerosis

Facial angiofibromas ("adenoma sebaceum") are typically 1-4 mm, skin-colored to red, dome-shaped papules with a smooth surface.

Image with permission from Paller AS, Mancini AJ, Hurwitz Clinical Pediatric Dermatology, 4th ed., Saunders, Elsevier, 2011.

12. **a**—9q34 (TSC1)/16p13 (TSC2)

The shagreen patch is characteristically found at the lumbosacral area and has a peau d'orange texture.

Image with permission from Paller AS, Mancini AJ, Hurwitz Clinical Pediatric Dermatology, 4th ed., Saunders, Elsevier, 2011.

13. **e**—Periungual fibroma

Tuberous sclerosis. Periungual and subungual fibromas on the fourth finger of this adolescent boy.

Image with permission from Paller AS, Mancini AJ. Hurwitz Clinical Pediatric Dermatology, 4th ed., Saunders, Elsevier, 2011.

14. **e**—Sensorineural deafness

Waardenburg syndrome is a group of four autosomal dominant disorders characterized by a white forelock (hair depigmentation), heterochromia irides, cutaneous depigmentation and congenital sensorineural deafness. Individuals with the commonest type I have characteristic facial features—broad nasal root, lateral displacement of the medial canthi and lacrimal punctua of the lower lids (dystopia canthorum).

Image with permission from Paller AS, Mancini AJ. Hurwitz Clinical Pediatric Dermatology, 4th ed., Saunders, Elsevier, 2011.

15. **c**—Neurofibromatosis type 1

The presence of six or more café-au-lait spots >0.5 cm in diameter in children and 1.5 cm in adolescents suggests the possibility of NF1, although having café-au-lait spots alone does not allow for definitive diagnosis.

Image with permission from Paller AS, Mancini AJ. Hurwitz Clinical Pediatric Dermatology, 4th ed., Saunders, Elsevier, 2011.

16. **b**—Legius syndrome

Legius syndrome (Neurofibromatosis type 1-like syndrome) is an autosomal dominant RASopathy often mistaken for NF-1. Patients show multiple café-au-lait spots, axillary freckling, lipomas, macrocephaly, learning disabilities among others. It lacks Lisch nodules, bone abnormalities, neurofibromas, optic pathway gliomas and malignant peripheral nerve sheath tumors. Axillary freckling (Crowe's sign) is present in 20-50% of individuals with NF1 and commonly appears between 3 and 5 years of age.

Image with permission from Paller AS, Mancini AJ. Hurwitz Clinical Pediatric Dermatology, 4th ed., Saunders, Elsevier, 2011.

17. **c**—Neurofibromatosis type 1

Neurofibromatosis type 1. Dermal and subcutaneous neurofibromas are rarely found before adolescence. These tumors, which originate from Schwann cells, increase in number progressively thereafter.

Image with permission from Paller AS, Mancini AJ. Hurwitz Clinical Pediatric Dermatology, 4th ed., Saunders, Elsevier, 2011.

18. **c**—Neurofibromatosis type 2

Plexiform neurofibromas are commonly present at birth and can resemble giant café-au-lait spots, although borders are often more irregular. With advancing age, plexiform neurofibromas may enlarge and become more elevated with a firm or "bag of worms" consistency.

Image with permission from Paller AS, Mancini AJ, Hurwitz Clinical Pediatric Dermatology, 4th ed., Saunders, Elsevier, 2011.

19. **d**—Gorlin syndrome

Gorlin (basal cell nevus) syndrome. Shallow erythematous depressions on the plantar surface of an adult female with BCNS (acral pits).

Image with permission from Paller AS, Mancini AJ. Hurwitz Clinical Pediatric Dermatology, 4th ed., Saunders, Elsevier, 2011.

20. **c**—Leptomeningeal angiomatosis

Port-wine stain (PWS) (nevus flammeus). This lesion involves both the V1 and V2 trigeminal dermatomes in this infant with Sturge-Weber syndrome (SWS). Nevus flammeus, or PWS, is a congenital capillary malformation that may occur as an isolated lesion or in association with a variety of syndromes (e.g. SWS, Klippel-Trenauny syndrome, Von Hippel Lindau syndrome, Wyburn-Mason syndrome, amongst others). It is often, but not always, unilateral and the most common site of involvement is the face, although they may occur on any cutaneous surface. SWS (encephalofacial or encephalotrigeminal angiomatosis) is a neuroectodermal syndrome characterized by a PWS in the distribution of the first (ophthalmic) branch of the trigeminal nerve (V1) in association with leptomeningeal angiomatosis (presenting usually with seizures) and glaucoma. Central nervous system disease in SWS: seizures are the most common CNS feature, and often have their onset during the first year of life. The seizures of SWS may be difficult to control, and both early onset and increased seizure intensity are associated with future developmental and cognitive delay. Headaches (including migraines), stroke-like episodes, focal neurologic impairments, cognitive deficits and emotional and behavioral problems, including depression, violent behavior, and self-inflicted injury, are also more common in SWS. Leptomeningeal angiomatosis is a classic component of the syndrome, and lesions are frequently ipsilateral to the cutaneous vascular stain. Cerebral atrophy is a frequent radiologic finding, as is enlargement of the choroid plexus and venous abnormalities. Magnetic resonance imaging is the modality of choice for identifying these changes, although computed tomography scans are better at detecting the classic cortical calcifications, which are also seen. These calcifications follow the convolutions of the cerebral cortex and are characterized by double-contoured parallel streaks of calcification ("tram lines"). Ocular involvement occurs in around 60% of patients with SWS. Glaucoma is the most frequent ocular finding, and it may present at any time between birth and the fourth decade. It may be unilateral or bilateral, with the latter being more common in patients with bilateral facial PWS. Vascular malformations of the eye in patients with SWS may involve the conjunctiva, episclera, choroid, and retina. Other eye findings include nevus of Ota, buphthalmos, and blindness. Dermatologic, neurologic, and ophthalmologic follow-up is indicated and the primary care provider must provide anticipatory guidance and support. Although the primary management for seizures is with pharmacologic agents, surgical therapy may become necessary. Visually guided lobectomy with excision of the angiomatous cortex is considered the primary surgical approach in patient with focal lesions. Hemispherectomy is often advised for patients with intractable seizures and unihemispheric involvement. This radical therapy is often successful, with decreased seizure activity and, in some patients, cognitive and behavioral improvement.

Image with permission from Paller AS, Mancini AJ. Hurwitz Clinical Pediatric Dermatology, 4th ed., Saunders, Elsevier, 2011.

ANSWERS 21–23

Additional answers 21–23 available on ExpertConsult.com

EMI ANSWERS

24. 1—i, 2—f, 3—b

Molecular Target	Principal Assay	Clinicopathological Setting
BRAF-KIAA1549 gene fusion/duplication	PCR/FISH	Found in most pilocytic astrocytomas
Chromosomes 1p/19q—allelic loss	PCR/FISH	Aligns with chemoresponsive/good outcome oligodendrogliomas
EGFR gene—amplification/chromosome 10q—loss	FISH	Found in most small cell astrocytic tumors
MGMT promoter methylation status	PCR	Aligns with response to alkylating agents (e.g. temozolomide) by high-grade gliomas
Wnt signaling pathway—upregulated	IHC for b-catenin	Aligns with low-risk childhood medulloblastoma
Chromosome 6—monosomy	FISH	Aligns with low-risk childhood medulloblastoma
MYC gene—amplification	FISH	Aligns with high-risk childhood medulloblastoma
SMARCB1 gene—loss/INI1 protein—absent *EWSR1* gene—rearrangement	FISH/IHC FISH	Diagnosis of atypical teratoid/rhabdoid tumor Diagnosis of skull/meningeal pPNET/Ewing sarcoma
B cell/T cell receptor genes—rearrangement	PCR	Demonstration of clonal populations of lymphoid cells

25. 1—a: APC (Turcot syndrome), 2—g: SMARCB1 (Rhabdoid tumor predisposition syndrome), 3—j: VHL (Von Hippel Lindau)

Syndrome	Gene Locus	Gene	Type(s) of CNS Neoplasm
Neurofibromatosis type 1	17q11	*NF1*	Neurofibroma, malignant nerve sheath tumor, optic nerve glioma, meningioma
Neurofibromatosis type 2	22q12	*NF2*	Schwannoma, meningioma, ependymoma
Tuberous sclerosis	9q34/16p13	*TSC1/TSC2*	Subependymal giant cell astrocytoma
Von Hippel Lindau	3p25	*VHL*	Hemangioblastoma
Li-Fraumeni syndrome	17p13	*TP53*	Glioma
Gorlin syndrome Turcot syndrome	9q22 5q21	*PTCH* *APC*	Medulloblastoma Astrocytoma, glioblastoma, medulloblastoma
Cowden disease	10q23	*PTEN*	Dysplastic gangliocytoma of cerebellum
Multiple endocrine neoplasia type 1	11q13	*MEN1*	Pituitary adenoma
Rhabdoid tumor predisposition syndrome	22q11	*SMARCB1*	Atypical teratoid/rhabdoid tumor

26. 1—i: Chromogranin A, 2—b: Beta-2-microglobulin, 3—a: Alpha-fetoprotein

Tumor marker	Tumor
Alpha-fetoprotein	Liver, germ cell
Beta-2-microglobulin	Multiple myeloma, CLL, some lymphomas
Beta-human chorionic gonadotropin	Choriocarcinoma, testicular cancer
Cytokeratin fragment 21-1	Lung cancer
CA15-3/CA27.29	Breast cancer
CA19-9	Pancreatic, gallbladder, bile duct, gastric cancer
CA-125	Ovarian cancer
Calcitonin	Medullary thyroid cancer
CEA	Colorectal cancer, breast cancer
PSA	Prostate cancer
HE-4	Ovarian cancer
Chromogranin-A	Neuroendocrine tumors
LDH	Germ cell tumors

27. 1—n: Verocay, 2—j: Pseudorosette, 3—c: Flexner Wintersteiner rosette, 4—h: Negri bodies, 5—i: Neurofibrillary tangles

ANSWERS 28–29

Additional answers 28–29 available on ExpertConsult.com

CHAPTER 5

NEUROPATHOLOGY II: GROSS PATHOLOGY

SINGLE BEST ANSWER (SBA) QUESTIONS

1. Which one of the following is most likely based on the image shown below?

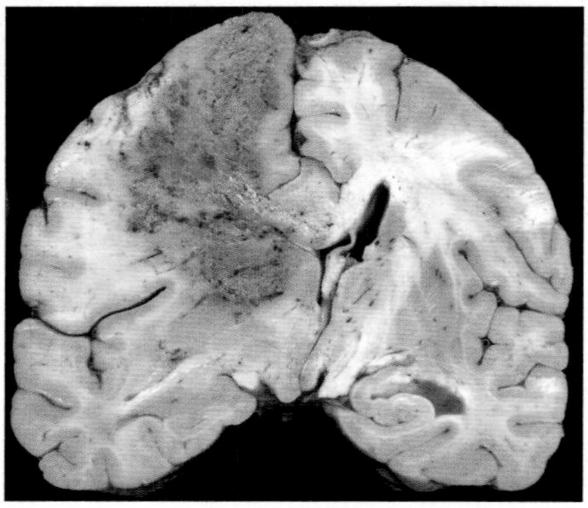

a. Congestive edema
b. Diffuse cytotoxic edema
c. Focal cytotoxic edema
d. Interstitial edema
e. Vasogenic edema

2. Which one of the following is most likely based on the image shown below?

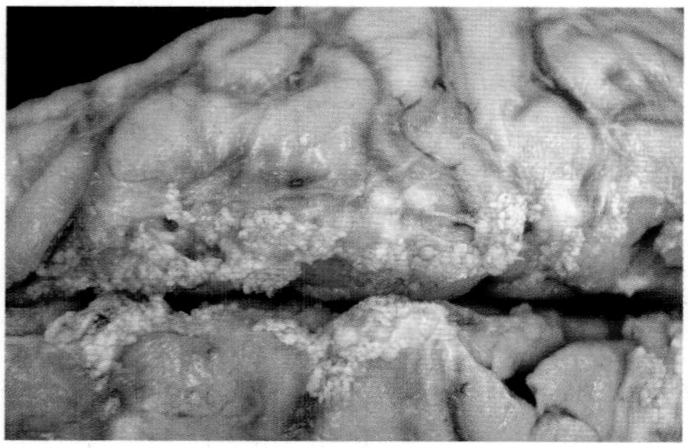

a. Arachnoid granulations
b. Calcification
c. Dural metastasis
d. Meningitis
e. Venous thrombosis

3. Which one of the following is most likely based on the image shown below?

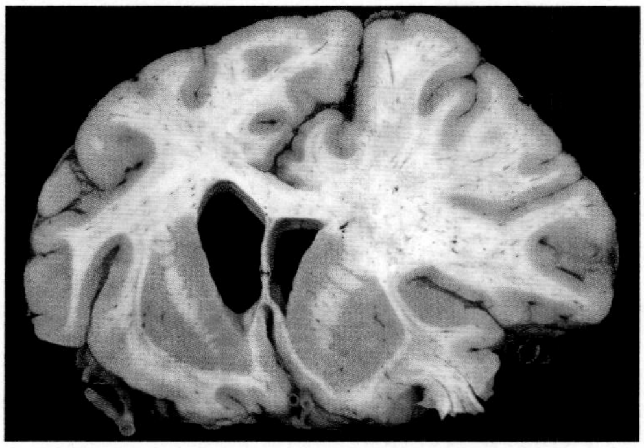

a. Hydrocephalus
b. Subfalcine herniation
c. Tonsillar herniation
d. Transtentorial herniation
e. Upwards herniation

4. Which one of the following is most likely based on the image shown below?

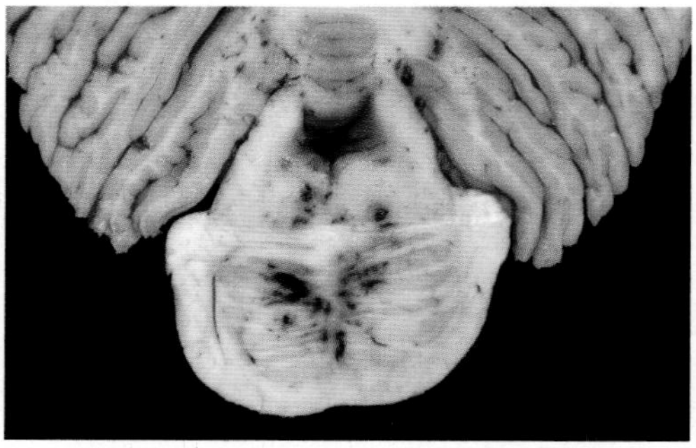

a. Brain stem compression
b. Demyelination
c. Infarction
d. Primary brainstem hemorrhagic stroke
e. Subarachnoid hemorrhage

5. Which one of the following is most likely based on the image shown below?

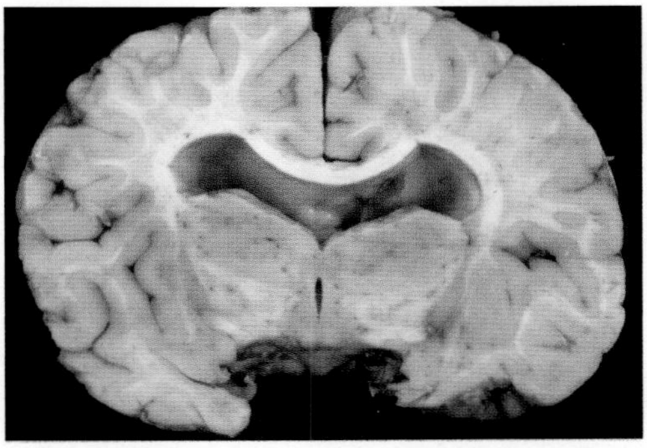

a. Alobar holoprosencephaly
b. Arhinencephaly
c. Lobar holoprosencephaly
d. Semilobar holoprosencephaly
e. Syntelencephaly

6. Which one of the following is most likely based on the image shown below?

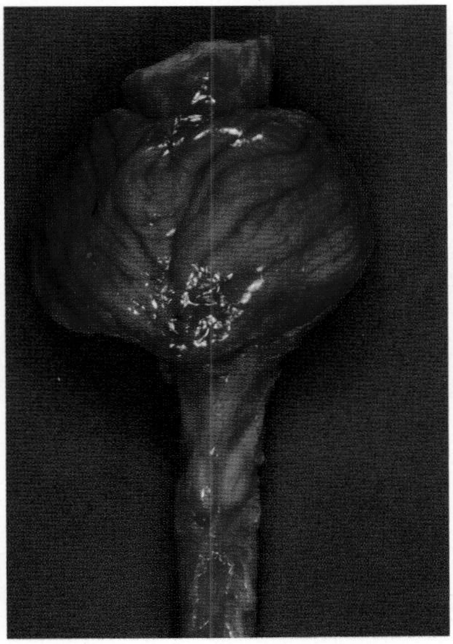

a. Chiari I malformation
b. Chiari II malformation
c. Dandy-Walker Malformation
d. Joubert syndrome
e. Rhombencephalosynapsis

7. Which one of the following is most likely based on the image shown below?

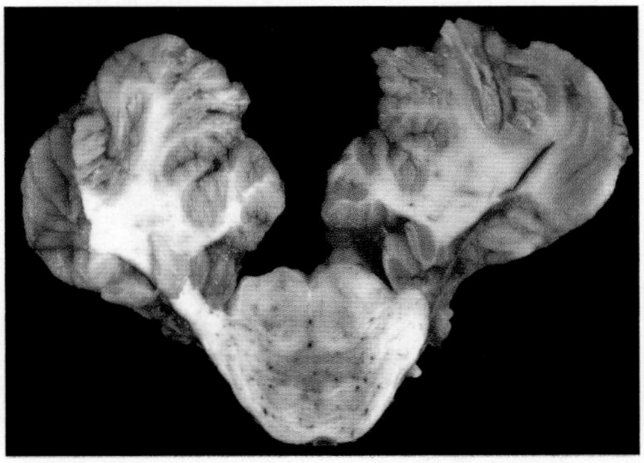

a. Chiari malformation III
b. Craniospinal rachischisis
c. Dandy-Walker malformation
d. Semilobar holoprosencephaly
e. Syntelencephaly

8. Which one of the following is most likely based on the image shown below?

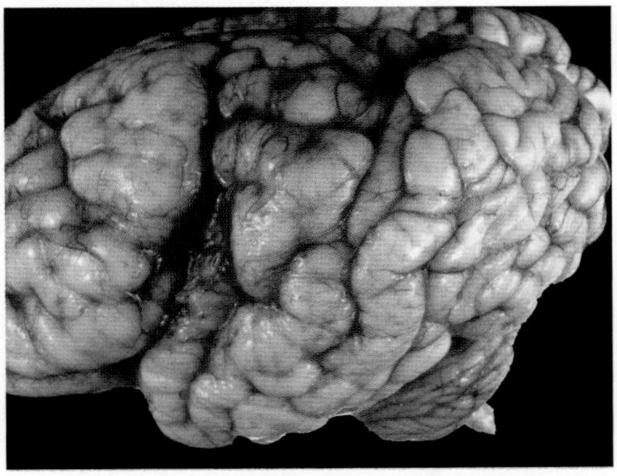

a. Focal cortical dysplasia
b. Lissencephaly type 1
c. Lissencephaly type 2
d. Pachygyria
e. Pick's disease

9. Which one of the following is most likely based on the image shown below?

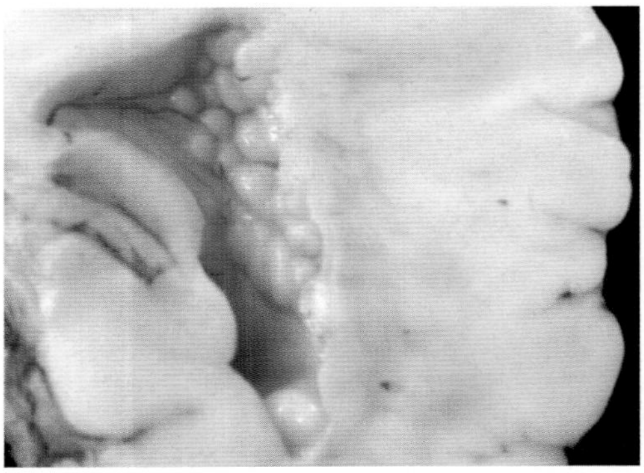

a. Cortical dysplasia
b. Periventricular nodular heterotropias
c. Polymicrogyria
d. Ventriculitis
e. X-linked lissencephaly

10. Which one of the following is most likely based on the image shown below?

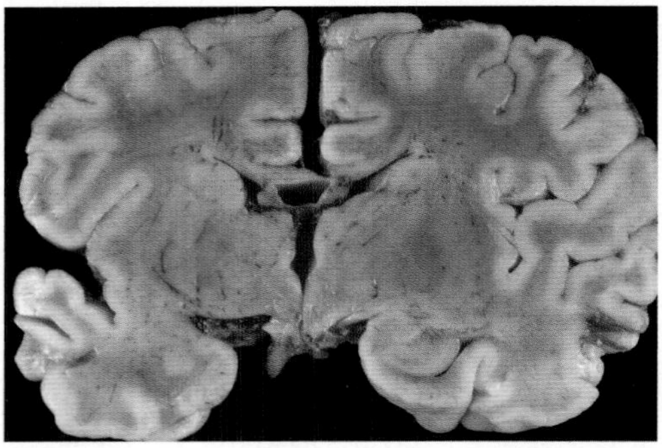

a. Acute diffuse hypoxia
b. Canavan disease
c. Carbon monoxide poisoning
d. Cerebral amyloid angiopathy
e. Pachygyria

11. Which one of the following is most likely based on the image shown below?

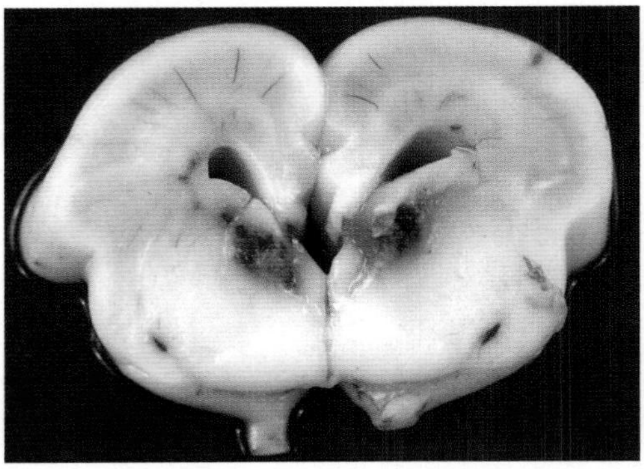

a. Germinal matrix hemorrhage
b. Kernicterus
c. Periventricular leukomalacia
d. Wilson's disease
e. X-linked adrenoleukodystrophy

12. Which one of the following is most likely based on the image shown below?

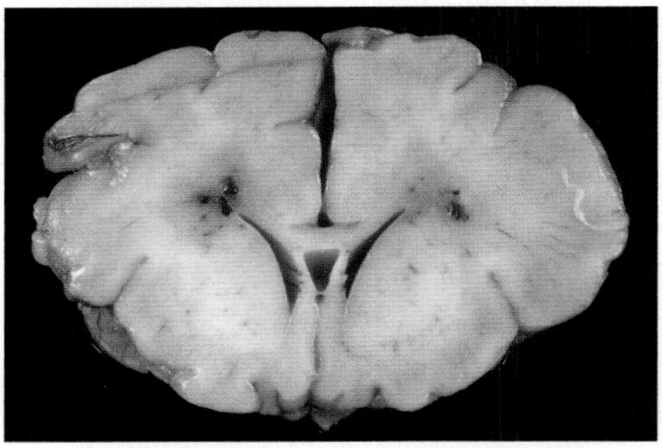

a. Huntington's disease
b. Intraventricular hemorrhage
c. Multiple sclerosis
d. Multiple system atrophy
e. Periventricular leukomalacia

13. Which one of the following is most likely based on the image shown below?

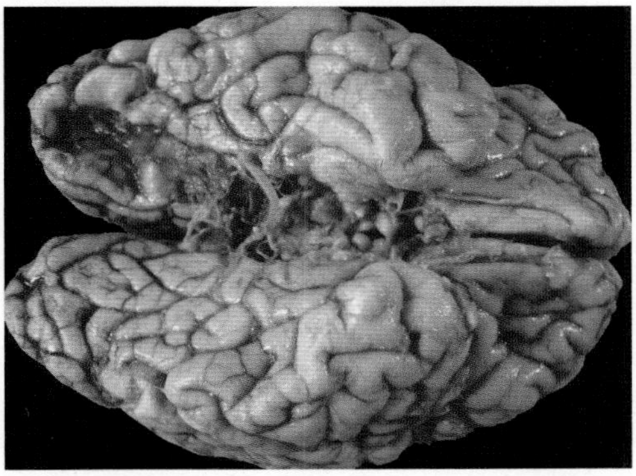

a. Left ACA infarct
b. Left pericallosal infarct
c. Left SCA infarct
d. Right PCA infarct
e. Right pericallosal infarct

14. Which one of the following is most likely based on the image shown below?

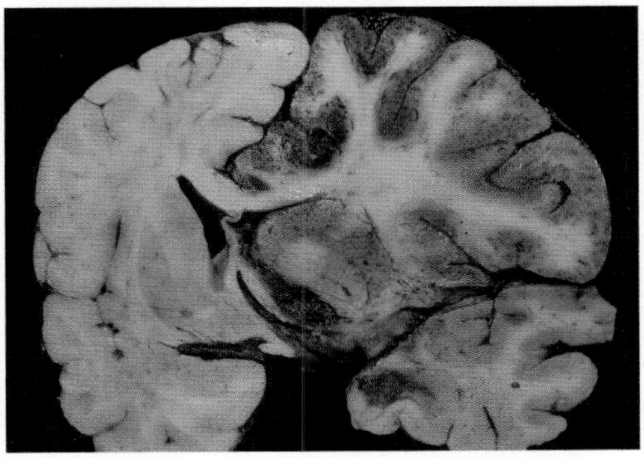

a. Brain contusion
b. CNS lymphoma
c. Malignant infarction
d. Non-accidental injury
e. PRES

15. Which one of the following is most likely based on the image shown below?

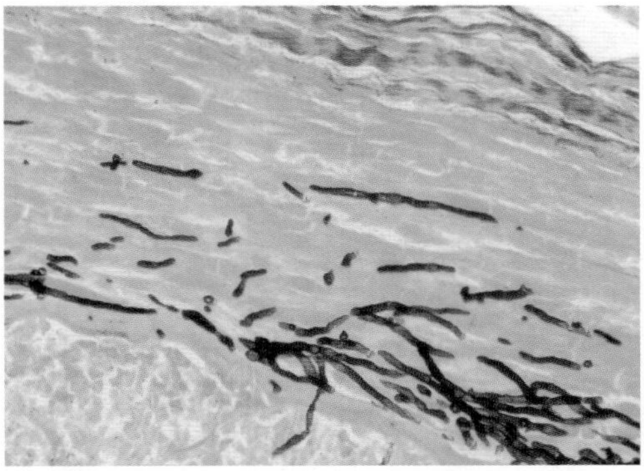

a. Cerebral Toxoplasmosis
b. HSV encephalitis
c. Mycotic aneurysm
d. Rosenthal fibers
e. Tuberculous meningitis

16. Which one of the following is most likely based on the image shown below?

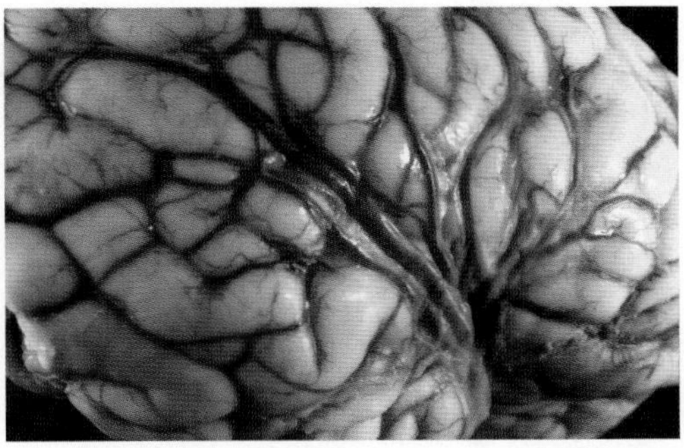

a. Arteriovenous malformation
b. Capillary telangiectasia
c. Caverous hemagioma
d. Developmental venous anomaly
e. Dural arteriovenous fistula

17. Which one of the following is most likely based on the image shown below?

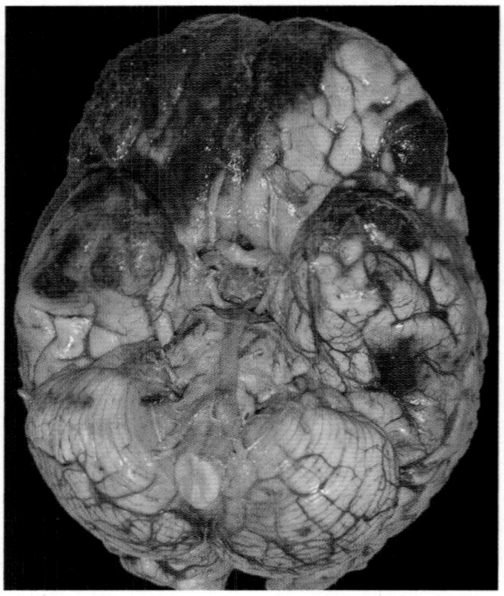

a. Aneurysmal subarachnoid hemorrhage
b. Contrecoup contusion
c. Hemorrhagic stroke
d. Ischemic stroke
e. Vasculitis

18. Which one of the following is most likely based on the image shown below?

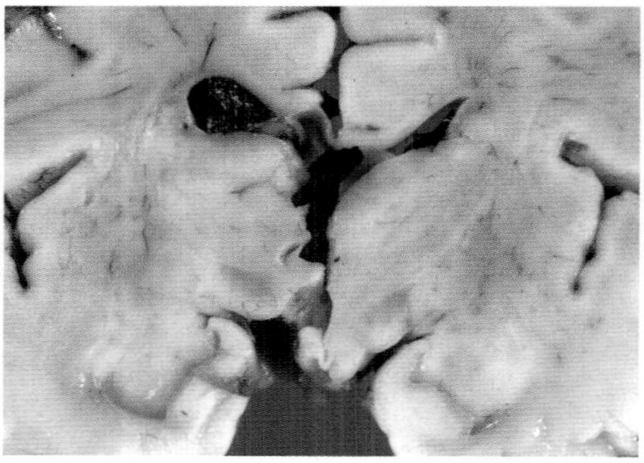

a. Kernicterus
b. Multicystic encephalopathy
c. Pontosubicular necrosis
d. Status marmoratus
e. Ulegyria

19. Which one of the following is most likely based on the image shown below?

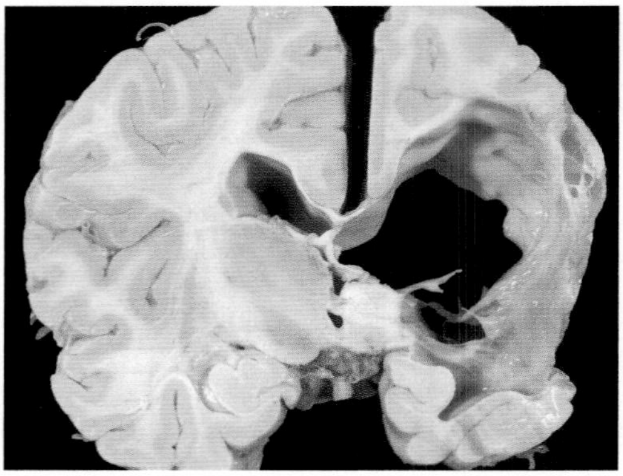

a. Germinal matrix hemorrhage
b. Hydrancephaly
c. Lissencephaly
d. Multicystic encephalopathy
e. Porencephalic cyst

20. Which one of the following is most likely based on the image shown below?

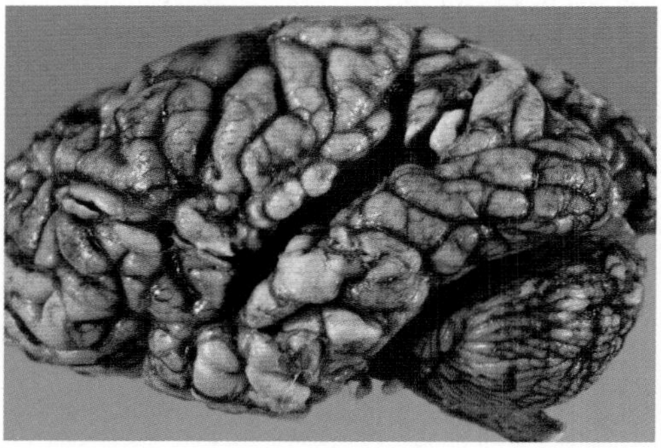

a. Agyria
b. Cobblestone cortex
c. Pachygyria
d. Porencephaly
e. Schizencephaly

21. Which one of the following is most likely based on the image shown below?

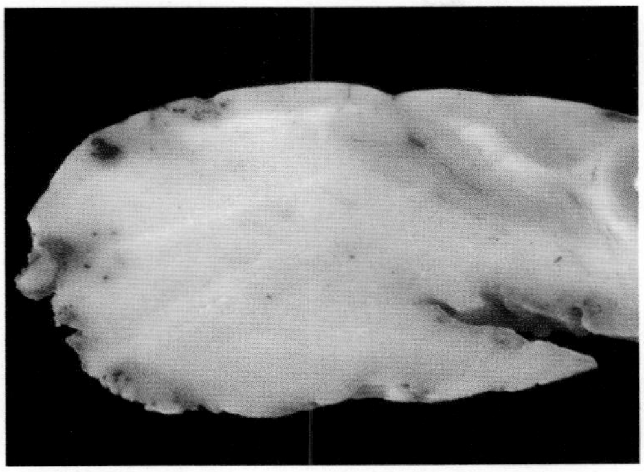

a. Astrocytoma
b. Caseous necrosis
c. Cerebral abscess
d. Cerebral metastasis
e. Tumefactive demyelination

22. Which one of the following is most likely in a patient where the findings shown affect multiple (3 or more) lobes of the brain?

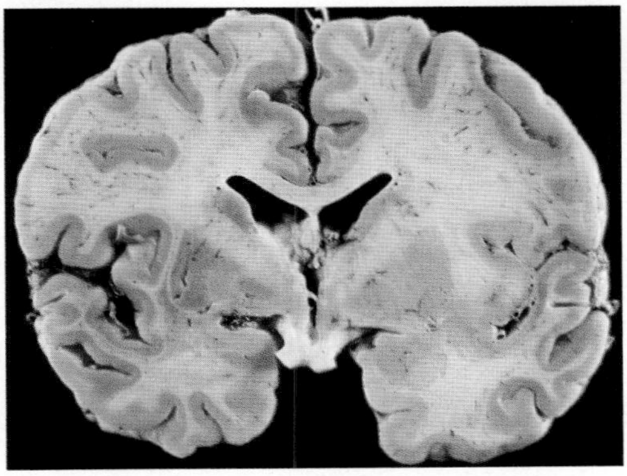

a. Cerebral infarct
b. Gliomatosis cerebri
c. Kernicterus
d. Periventricular leukomalacia
e. Primary CNS lymphoma

23. Which one of the following is most likely based on the image shown below?

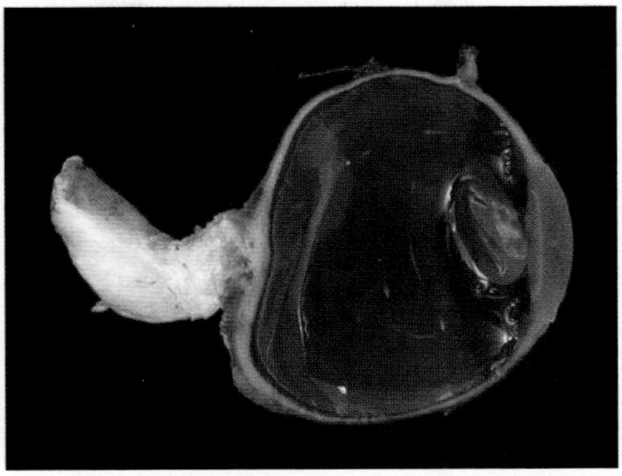

a. Idiopathic intracranial hypertension
b. NF-1
c. Retinal detachment
d. Retinoblastoma
e. Terson's syndrome

24. Which one of the following is most likely based on the image shown below?

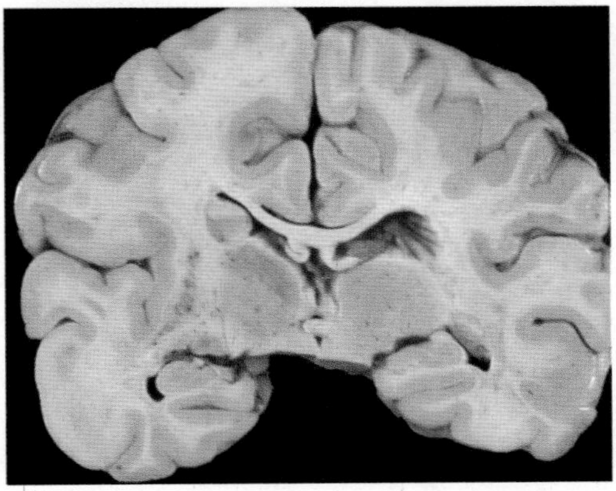

a. Diffuse astrocytoma
b. Germinal matrix hemorrhage
c. Perventricular heterotopia
d. Tuberous sclerosis
e. Von Hippel-Lindau

25. Which one of the following is most likely based on the image shown below?

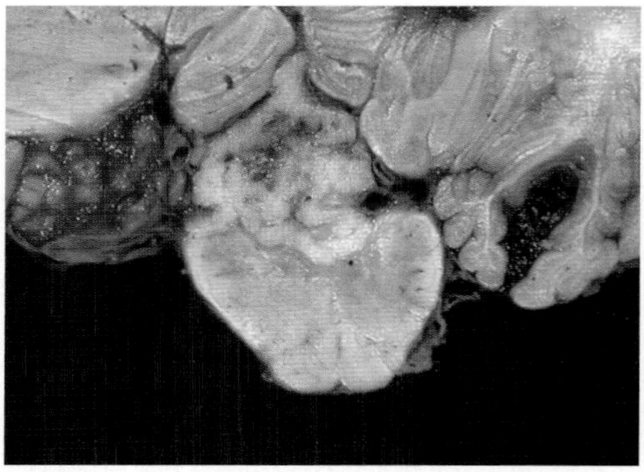

a. Fourth ventricular subependymoma
b. Duret hemorrhage
c. Infarct of cerebellar vermis
d. Myxopapillary ependymoma
e. Tanycytic ependymoma

26. Which one of the following is most likely based on the image shown below?

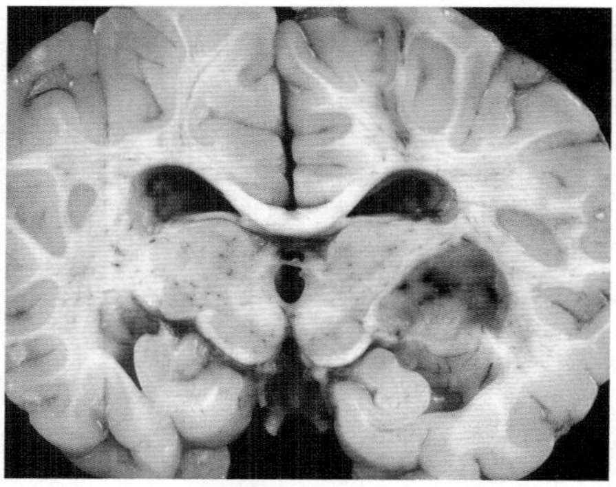

a. Atypical teratoid/rhabdoid tumor
b. Cerebral abscess
c. Choroid plexus papilloma
d. Intraventricular meningioma
e. Mesial temporal sclerosis

27. Which one of the following is most likely based on the image shown below?

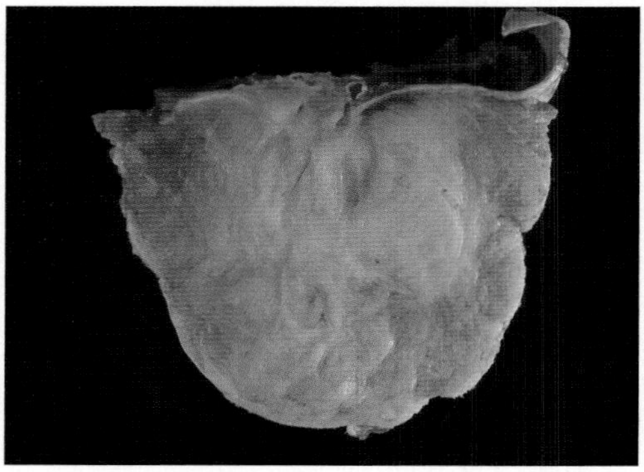

a. Ependymoma
b. Glioblastoma multiforme
c. Meningioma
d. Oligodendroglioma
e. Supratentorial PNET

28. Which one of the following is most likely based on the image shown below?

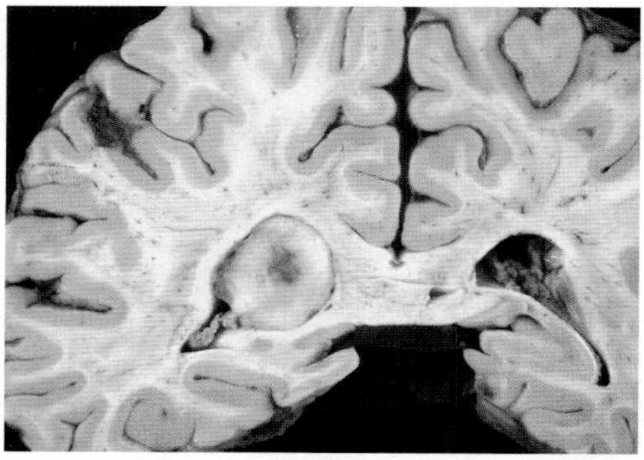

a. Arteriovenous malformation
b. Choroid plexus papilloma
c. Glioma
d. Intracranial aneurysm
e. Meningioma

29. Which one of the following is most likely based on the image shown below?

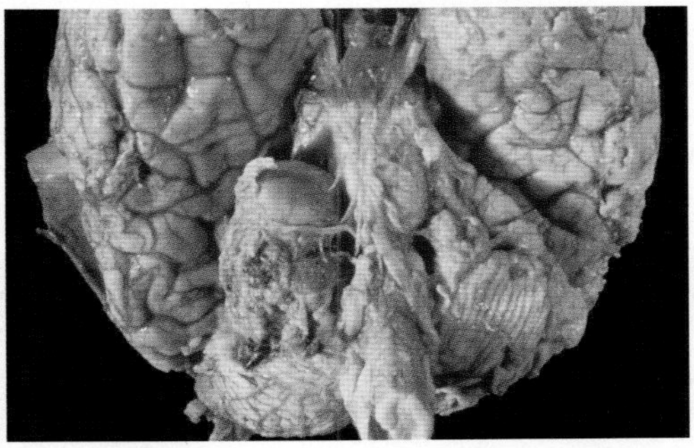

a. Abscess
b. Aneurysm
c. Arachnoid cyst
d. Glioma
e. Schwannoma

30. Which one of the following is most likely based on the image shown below?

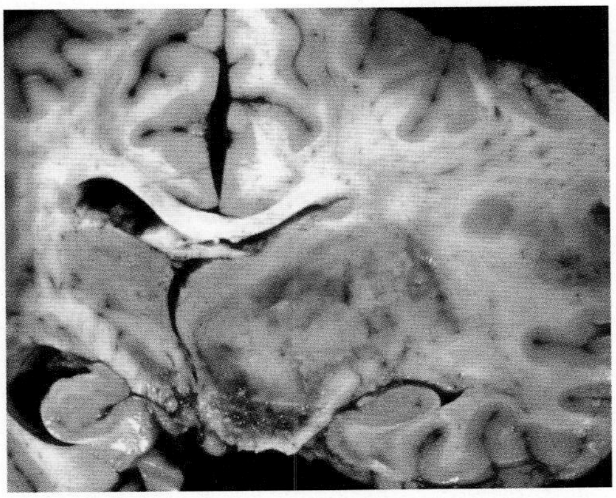

a. Dermoid cyst
b. Diffuse astrocytoma
c. Hemorrhagic stroke
d. Intraventricular meningioma
e. Primary CNS lymphoma

31. Which one of the following is most likely based on the image shown below?

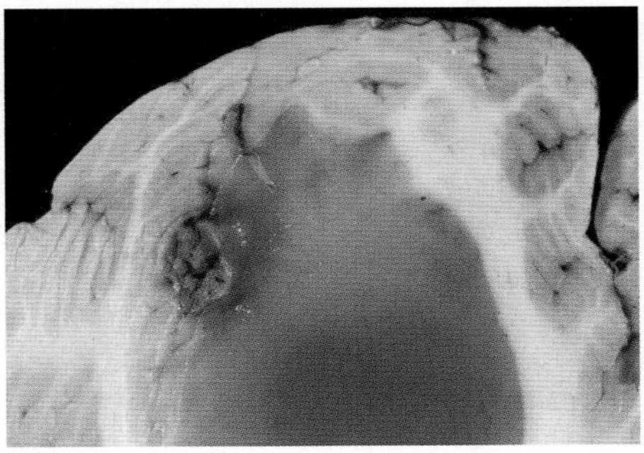

a. Cerebral abscess
b. Cystic Meningioma
c. Ex-vacuo dilatation
d. Germinoma
e. Hemangioblastoma

32. Which one of the following is most likely based on the image shown below?

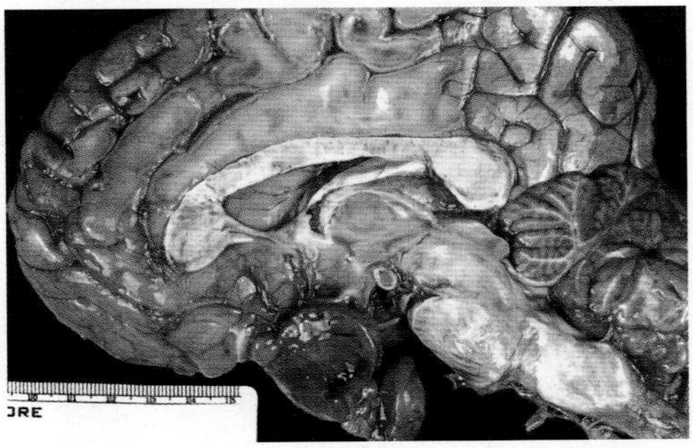

a. Colloid cyst
b. Optic glioma
c. Pineal cyst
d. Pituitary adenoma
e. Sheehan's syndrome

33. Which one of the following is most likely based on the image shown below?

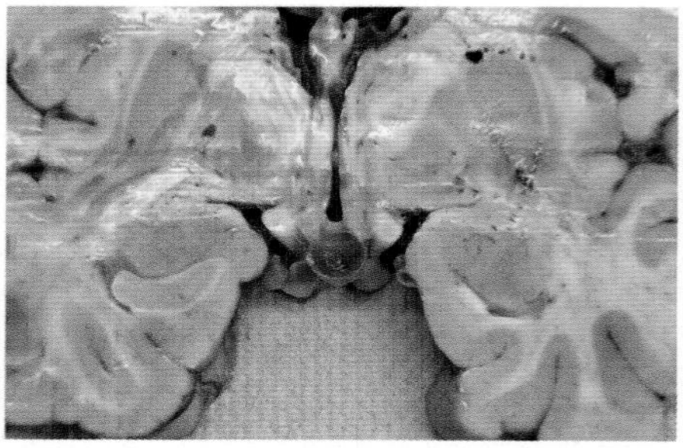

a. Arachnoid cyst
b. Dermoid cyst
c. Epidermoid cyst
d. Pineal cyst
e. Rathke's cleft cyst

34. Which one of the following is most likely based on the image shown below?

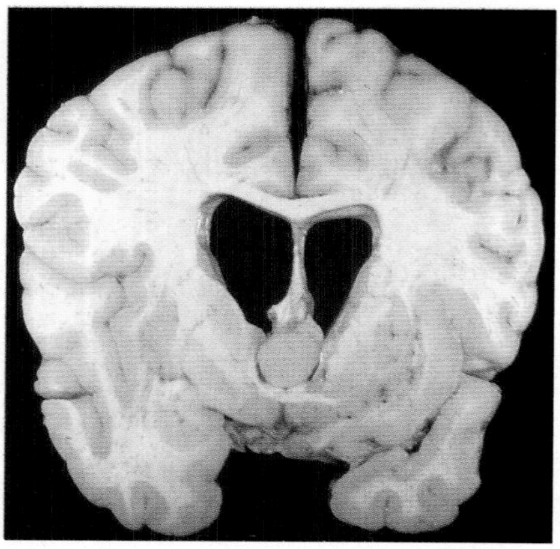

a. Colloid cyst
b. Craniopharyngioma
c. Epidermoid cyst
d. Pituitary adenoma
e. Teratoma

35. Which one of the following is most likely based on the image shown below?

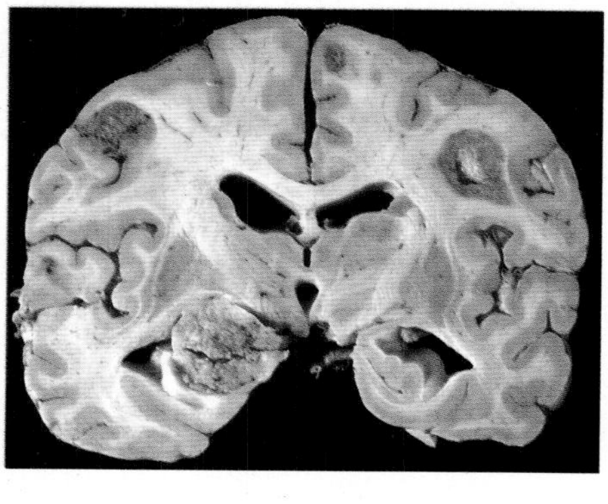

a. Cerebral vasculitis
b. Multifocal glioma
c. Multiple abscesses
d. Multiple metastasis
e. Neurofibromatosis

36. Which one of the following is most likely based on the image shown below?

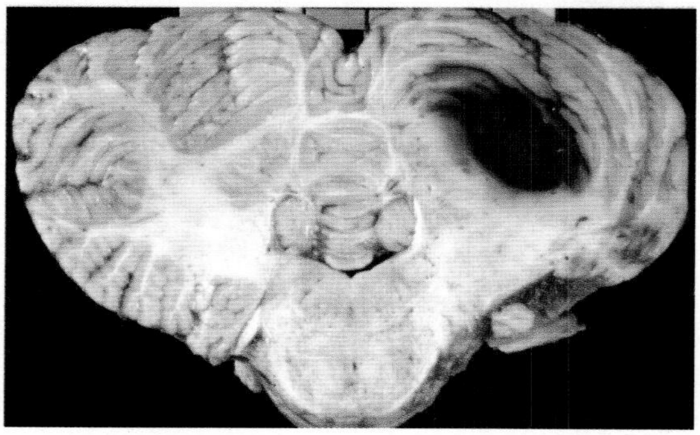

a. Epidermoid
b. Hemangioblastoma
c. Lhermitte-Duclos disease
d. Melanoma
e. Teratoma

37. Which one of the following is most likely based on the image shown below?

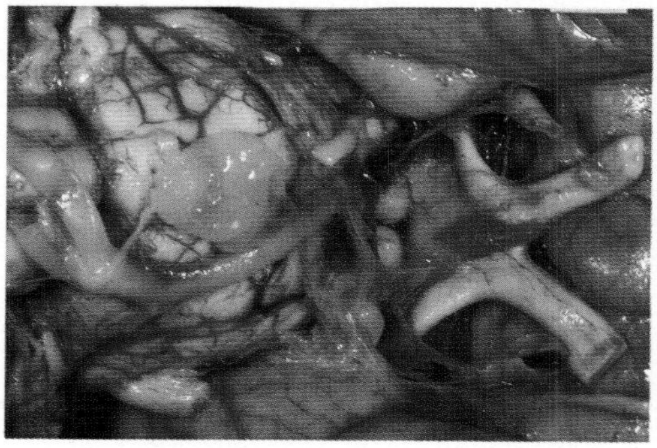

a. Arachnoid villus
b. Choroid plexus
c. Ecchordosis physaliphora
d. PICA aneurysm
e. Schwannoma

38. Which one of the following is most likely based on the image shown below?

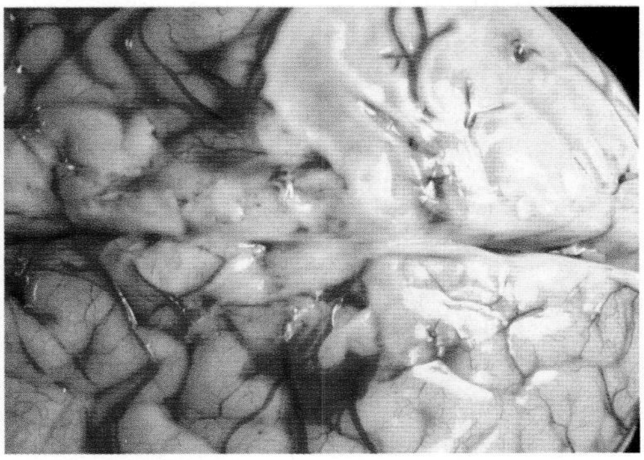

a. Cerebral malaria
b. Cysticercosis
c. Herpes encephalitis
d. Purulent meningitis
e. Subdural empyema

39. Which one of the following is most likely based on the image shown below?

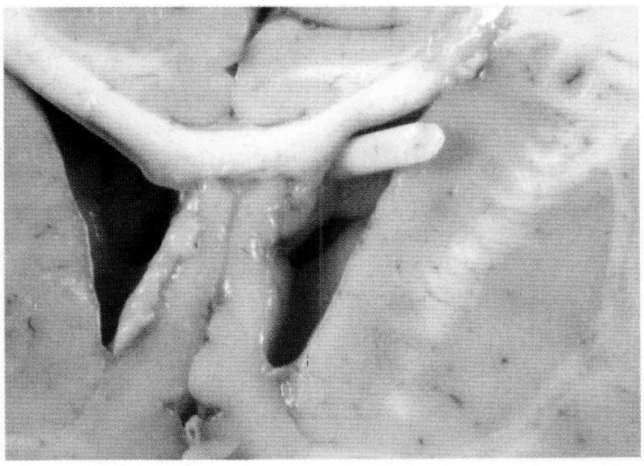

a. Cavum septum pellucidae
b. Periventricular leukomalacia
c. Subependymal giant cell astrocytoma
d. Subependymal heterotopia
e. Ventriculitis

40. Which one of the following is most likely based on the image shown below?

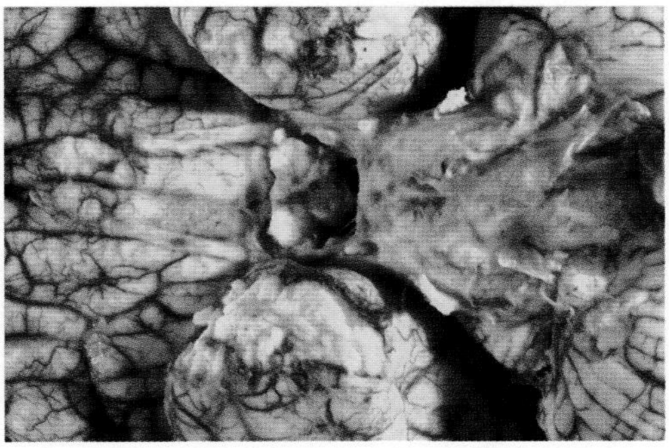

a. Mycobacterium Tuberculosis
b. Pseudomonas
c. Spirochetes (Lyme disease)
d. Staphylococcus aureus
e. Streptococcus pneumoniae

41. Which one of the following is most likely based on the image shown below?

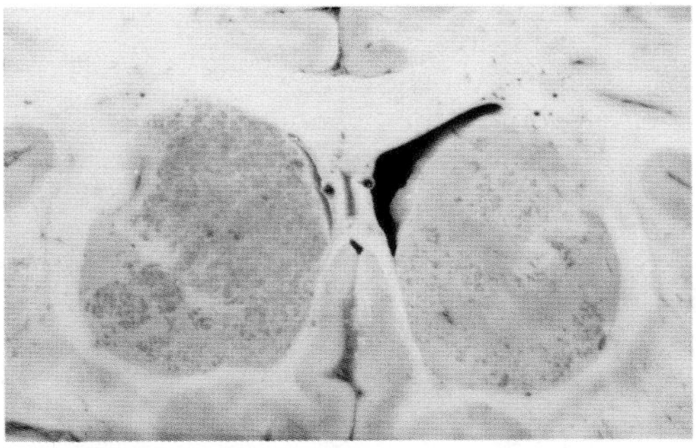

a. Aspergillosis
b. Candidiasis
c. Cryptococcosis
d. Cystercicosis
e. Toxoplasmosis

42. Which one of the following is most likely based on the image shown below?

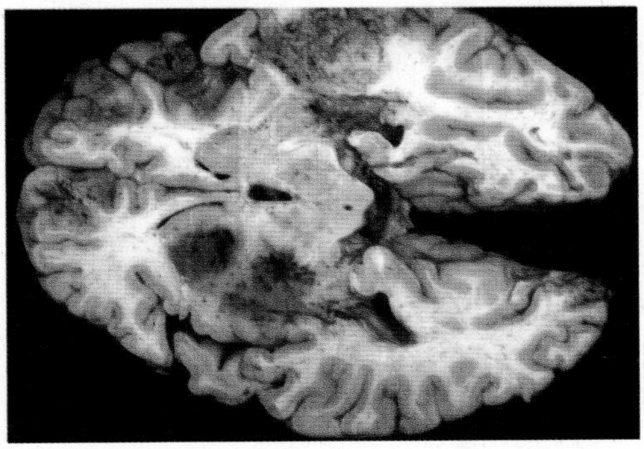

a. Aspergillosis
b. Cerebral abscess
c. Cerebral malaria
d. Hyatid disease
e. Listeria encephalitis

43. Which one of the following is most likely based on the image shown below?

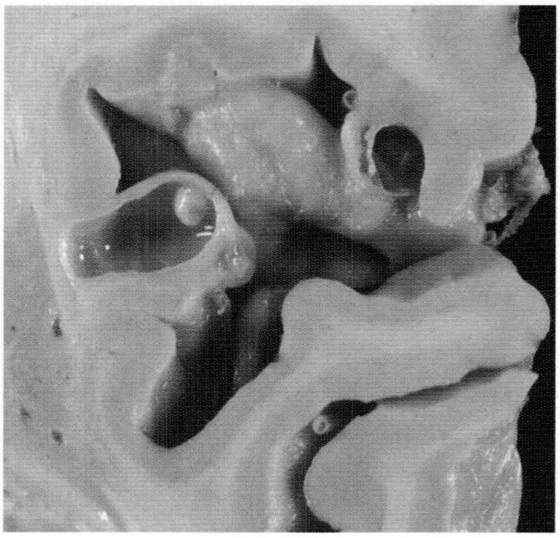

a. Cavernoma
b. Cerebral metastasis
c. Developmental venous anomalies
d. Neurocysticercosis
e. Neuronal migration disorder

44. Which one of the following is most likely based on the image shown below?

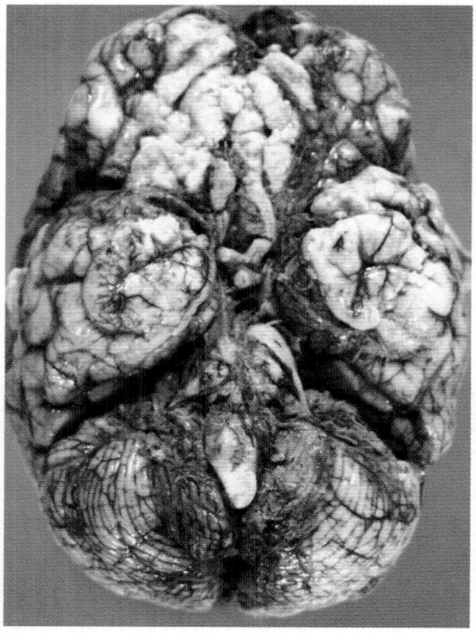

a. Amoebic meningoencephalitis
b. Diffuse subarachnoid hemorrhage
c. Meningeal carcinomatosis
d. Post-radiotherapy change
e. Tuberculous meningitis

45. Which one of the following is most likely based on the image shown below?

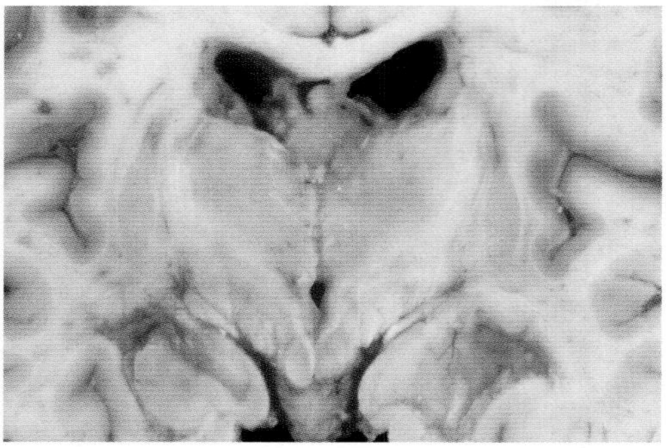

a. CMV ventriculitis
b. HIV encephalitis
c. HSV encephalitis
d. Hypoxic-ischemic encephalopathy
e. TORCH infection

46. Which one of the following is most likely based on the image shown below?

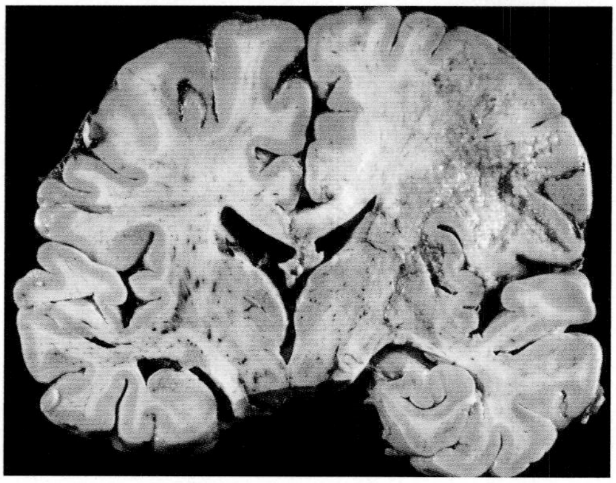

a. Cortical tuber
b. Diffuse astrocytoma
c. Pleomorphic xanthoastrocytoma
d. Progressive multifocal leukoencephalopathy
e. Rabies encephalitis

47. Which one of the following is most likely based on the image shown below?

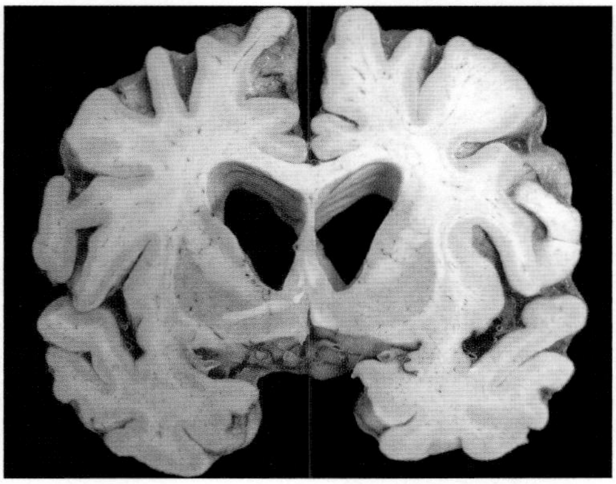

a. Alzheimer's disease
b. Huntington's disease
c. Lhermitte-Duclos disease
d. Parkinson's disease
e. Wilson's disease

48. Which one of the following is most likely based on the image shown below?

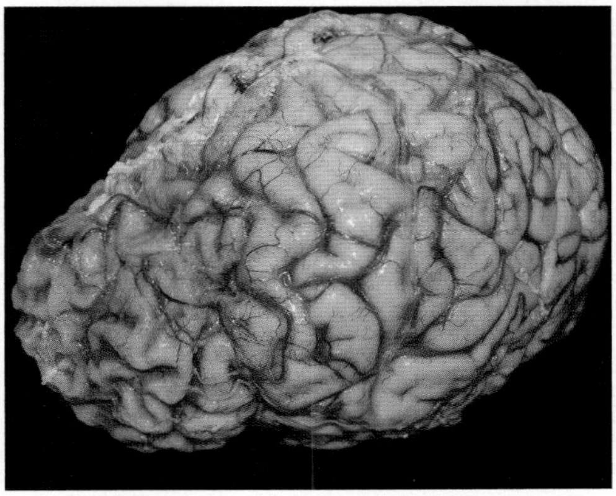

a. Alzheimer's disease
b. Focal cortical dysplasia
c. Lissencephaly type 2
d. Parkinson's disease
e. Pick disease

49. Which one of the following is most likely based on the image shown below?

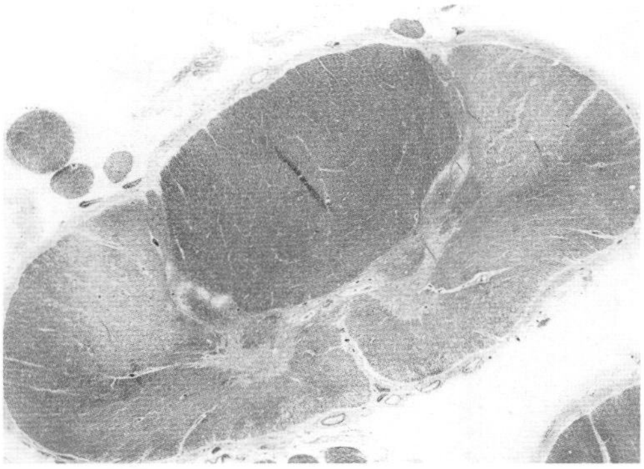

a. Amyotrophic lateral sclerosis
b. Cord infarction
c. Guillain-Barre syndrome
d. Radiation myelopathy
e. Transverse myelitis

50. Which one of the following is most likely based on the image shown below?

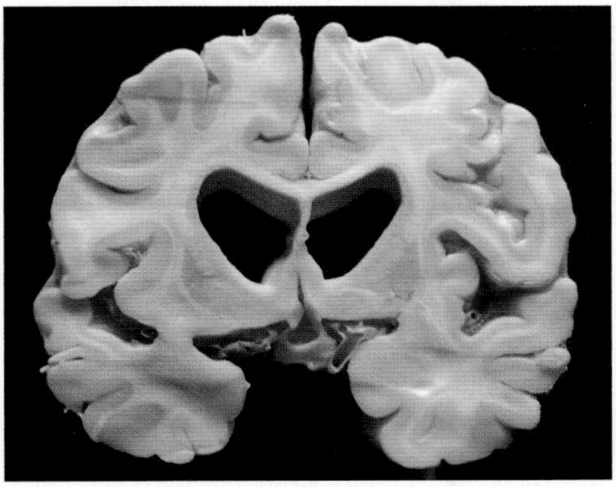

a. Double cortex syndrome
b. Hippocampal atrophy
c. HSV encephalitis
d. Huntington's disease
e. Toxic leukoencephalopathy

51. Which one of the following is most likely based on the image shown below?

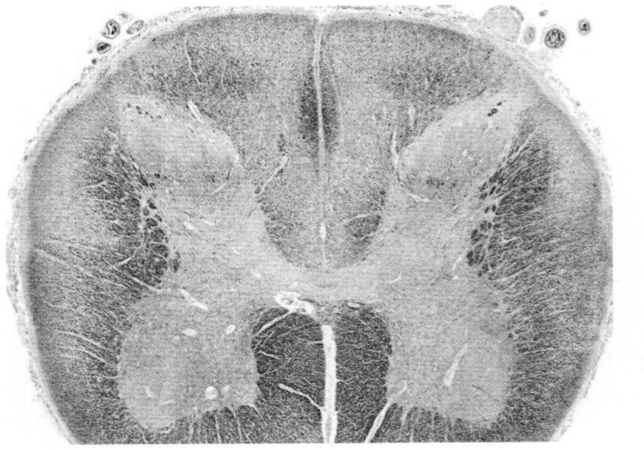

a. Amyotrophic lateral sclerosis
b. Cord infarction
c. Friedreich's ataxia
d. Multiple sclerosis
e. Subacute combined degeneration

52. Which one of the following is most likely based on the image shown below?

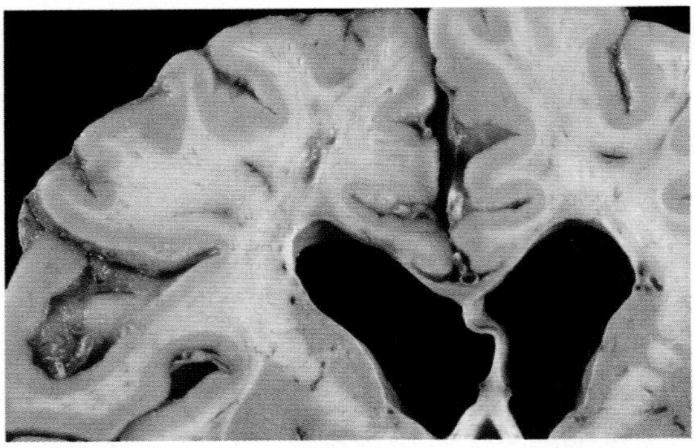

a. Alzheimer's dementia
b. Cortical tubers
c. Periventricular leukomalacia
d. Subependymal heterotopia
e. Vascular dementia

QUESTIONS 53–68

Additional questions 53–68 available on ExpertConsult.com

SBA ANSWERS

1. **e**—Vasogenic edema secondary to GBM. Widened gyri, narrowing of sulci, compression of ventricles may be focal or diffuse. Vasogenic edema often associated with focal lesions, tumors, abscess.

Image with permission from Yachnis AT, Rivera-Zengotita ML. Neuropathology, High-Yield Pathology Series, Saunders, Elsevier, 2014.

2. **a**—Arachnoid granulations. These whitish granular structures are located at the superior medial aspect of the cerebral hemispheres near the sagital sinus. They function in resorption of CS.

Image with permission from Yachnis AT, Rivera-Zengotita ML. Neuropathology, High-Yield Pathology Series, Saunders, Elsevier, 2014.

3. **b**—Subfalcine herniation

In this image, a lesion, not visible in this image (at least the lesion is not), causing significant mass effect in the right frontal lobe has caused right cingulate gyrus herniation under the falx.

Image with permission from Yachnis AT, Rivera-Zengotita ML. Neuropathology, High-Yield Pathology Series, Saunders, Elsevier, 2014.

4. **a**—Brain stem compression.

Duret (secondary) hemorrhage. Hemorrhages of the basis pontis may result from brain stem compression secondary to downward mass effect and herniation from above.

Image with permission from Yachnis AT, Rivera-Zengotita ML. Neuropathology, High-Yield Pathology Series, Saunders, Elsevier, 2014.

5. **c**—Lobar holoprosencephaly.

Two distinct cerebral hemispheres have formed, but there is fusion of inferior-medial structures including the thalamus and mammillary bodies. There is no septum pellucidum.

Holoprosencephaly represents a spectrum of midline patterning defects that involve the forebrain and midline facial structures; brain malformation results from failure of prosencephalon to develop into two telencephalic vesicles. Rare:

1 per 10,000 live births (but 1 in 250 spontaneous abortions); equal gender distribution. Genetic abnormalities (25-50%): trisomy 13 and 18, deletion/duplication 13q, SHH (sonic hedgehog), ZIC2 (zinc finger protein of the cerebellum 2), SIX3, TGIF. Non-genetic: maternal diabetes, retinoic acid, drug/alcohol abuse, hypercholesterolemia. Genetic counseling: risk of recurrence after affected sibling estimated 6%. Presentation variable: arhinencephaly least severe (anosmia, single central incisor), cleft lip/palate, hypotelorism, flat single nostril nose/cebocephaly, microcephaly, hydrocephalus, most severe cyclopsia with proboscis-like structure emanating from forehead. Prognosis depends on type and associated anomalies—high incidence of fetal demise in severe cases, cognitive delay, epilepsy, mental retardation, endocrine abnormalities; less severe cases have normal brain development with mild facial anomalies. Classification:

1. Alobar—complete failure in forebrain separation resulting in single holospheric cerebrum.
2. Semilobar—frontal and parietal lobes appear fused but posterior interhemispheric fissure present.
3. Lobar—only rostral most areas of cerebral hemispheres show fusion.
4. Syntelencephaly (middle hemisphere variant)—hemispheres separated rostrally and caudally except near posterior frontal lobe/parietal lobe.
5. Arrhinencephaly—absent olfactory bulbs, olfactory tracts and gyri recti.

Image with permission from Yachnis AT, Rivera-Zengotita ML. Neuropathology, High-Yield Pathology Series, Saunders, Elsevier, 2014.

6. **b**—Chiari II malformation—small cerebellum with marked tonsillar and vermian herniation.

Chiari malformations are structural defects of the cerebellum and brain stem associated with reduced volume posterior fossa. Incidence 1 per 1000 live births; commoner in females; Chiari type 1 commonest. Presentation: neck pain, balance/incoordination, weakness, numbness, swallowing, hearing, vomiting, insomnia, depression, high pressure headache; asymptomatic (incidental); syringomyelia. Type I is usually asymptomatic—surgery only to reduce symptoms/halt CNS injury, shunting for hydrocephalus in Chiari II. Classification:

1. Type I (commonest): extension of tonsils through FM without brainstem involvement; synringomyelia.
2. Type II ("Arnold-Chiari" malformation): small posterior fossa (low lying torcular herophili; unlike Dandy-Walker) with downward herniation of cerebellar vermis/brainstem into foramen magnum and upward herniation of midbrain (tectal beaking—prominent inferior colliculus) with aqueduct compression causing hydrocephalus (clival hypoplasia). Associated with lumbosacral myelomeningocele.
3. Type III (rare): cerebellar vermis, cerebellar hemisphere and brain stem =/− part of fourth ventricle protrude through foramen magnum; associated with occipital encephalocele.
4. Type IV (rare): cerebellar hypoplasia.

Image with permission from Yachnis AT, Rivera-Zengotita ML. Neuropathology, High-Yield Pathology Series, Saunders, Elsevier, 2014.

7. **c**—Dandy-Walker malformation is characterized by loss of cerebellar vermis with dilatation of fourth ventricle. Incidence 1 in 25,000-30,000. Genetics: possible loci on chromosomes 3 (ZIC1), 6 (ZIC4), 9, partial trisomy 13q, 18, autosomal dominant 2q36; possible association with first trimester infections and warfarin. Presentation: delayed motor development, increasing head circumference, raised ICP, abnormal breathing patterns, associated congenital heart defects, visual problems (nystagmus, cataracts, retinal dysgenesis, coloboma). Prognosis depends on severity of brain and systemic manifestations. Imaging—posterior fossa cyst. Gross pathology: partial or complete absence of cerebellar vermis, posterior fossa cyst continuous with fourth ventricle and congenital hydrocephalus. Other cerebellar vermian malformations include Joubert syndrome (autosomal recessive; vermis agenesis, molar tooth sign as deep interpeduncular fossa with thickened/elongated superior cerebellar peduncles) and rhombencephalosynapsis (fused cerebellar hemispheres, no vermis, associated septo-optic pituitary dysplasia, poly/syndactyly).

Image with permission from Yachnis AT, Rivera-Zengotita ML. Neuropathology, High-Yield Pathology Series, Saunders, Elsevier, 2014.

8. **d**—Pachygyria—enlarged gyri adjacent to sylvian fissure.

Neuronal migration defects result in abnormal cortical development due to abnormal migration of young neurons from periventricular sites of production to the cortex, but also likely to involve dysfunctional stem cell generation, neuronal differentiation, synaptogenesis and functional organization. Rare; neurons and glial cells produced in subventricular zones migrate to cortex in inside out fashion—neurons forming deep cortical layers migrate first then more superficial ones; most migration defects have genetic basis. Presentation: seizures, poor muscle tone/function, developmental delay, mental retardation, failure to grow/thrive, feeding difficulty, microcephaly. Associated dysmorphic facial features or syndactyly depending on cause. Gross classification though can occur in combination:

1. Abnormal proliferation (megancephaly) or apoptosis (microcephaly).
2. Neurons do not migrate away from subventricular zone—subependymal/periventricular heterotopias.
3. Neurons only migrate half way to cortex—subcortical band heterotopias.
4. Neurons reach cortex but abnormal cortical lamination—lissencephaly type 1/pachygyria.
5. Neurons overshoot cortex and end up in subarachnoid space—marginal zone heterotopia (leptomeningeal glioneuronal heterotopia) and lissencephaly type 2 (cobblestone cortex).
6. Late stage migration defects with abnormal cortical organization or neuronal morphology—polymicrogyria and focal cortical dysplasia/microdysgenesis.

Histological classification:

1. Periventricular heterotopia—unorganized nodules of neurons under the ependyma of lateral ventricles; mutation in FNLA gene at Xq28 producing filamin A1 actin binding protein (fatal in males, heterogeneous in females).
2. Lissencephaly type 1 (agyria/pachygyria)—smooth hemispheric surface lacking sulci/gyri and only four cortical layers; mutation in LIS1 gene (17p13), complete loss fatal, partial = seizures + retardation.
3. Lissencephaly type 2 (cobblestone cortex)—neuroglial tissue interrupts pia as it enters subarachnoid space resulting in fine stippling; marked disorganization of neurons, glia and blood vessels.
4. X-linked lissencephaly (double cortex syndrome): subcortical band heterotopia within centrum ovale; mutation of double-cortin gene (DCX; X22.3-q23).
5. Pachygyria—broad gyri and thick cortex with abnormal cryoarchitecture; metabolic CNS disorders.
6. Polymicrogyria—hemispheric surfaces have multiple festoon-like convolutions with four cortical layers only; diffuse or focal, unilateral or bilateral and symmetric or asymmetric; acquired cases CMV infection, hypoxic injury, *in utero* vascular occlusion (in association with schizencephaly); mutation of SRPX2 (bilateral sylvian polymicrogyria), PAX6, TBR2, GPR56.
7. Focal cortical dysplasia-microdysgenesis—focally thickened cortex with disordered cryoarchitecture (large abnormally oriented neurons, hypertrophic astrocytes); for example, cortical tubers (TSC); intractable epilepsy.

Image with permission from Yachnis AT, Rivera-Zengotita ML. Neuropathology, High-Yield Pathology Series, Saunders, Elsevier, 2014.

9. **b**—Periventricular nodular heterotropias.

Image with permission from Yachnis AT, Rivera-Zengotita ML. Neuropathology, High-Yield Pathology Series, Saunders, Elsevier, 2014.

10. **a**—Acute diffuse hypoxia/anoxia. A ribbon effect is produced under conditions of acute hypoxia where the white matter appears diffusely dusky while cortical ribbon appears pale. Periventricular leukomalacia (PVL) encompasses focal necrotic lesions and diffuse white matter gliosis resulting from selective ischemic injury of periventricular white matter during the fetal/perinatal period. Commonest ischemic brain injury in premature infants (4-25%); greatest risk <32/40; hypotension, sepsis, congenital cardiac disease, diaphragmatic hernia, acute chorioamnionitis. Pathophysiology: periventricular white matter is watershed perfusion zone, increased metabolic demand of myelinating white matter, poorly developed autoregulatory mechanisms. Presentation: cerebral palsy (fixed or nonprogressive motor disorder resulting from lesions acquired during fetal/perinatal period; spastic diplegia), quadriplegia in severe PVL, poor suck reflex, developmental delay, coordination problems, vision and hearing impairment. Prognosis depends on severity of brain injury; outcome/cerebral palsy difficult to predict in neonatal period. Emphasis on prevention: good prenatal care, prompt treatment of maternal infection/other conditions. Gross pathology: ribbon effect in acute diffuse hypoxia, cavities in periventricular deep white matter, periventricular lesions may become hemorrhagic.

Image with permission from Yachnis AT, Rivera-Zengotita ML. Neuropathology, High-Yield Pathology Series, Saunders, Elsevier, 2014.

11. **a**—Germinal matrix hemorrhage (16-18 weeks of gestation).

Germinal matrix zone is a fetal periventricular structure that forms between the developing deep cerebral nuclei and ependymal lining; 13-36 weeks gestation; composed of immature neuroepithelial cells and thin walled blood vessels with little supportive stroma. Germinal matrix hemorrhage refers to bleeding into the subependymal germinal matrix zone with or without subsequent intraventricular extension.

Classification:
Grade I—subependymal hemorrhage
Grade II— IVH without HCP
Grade III— IVH with HCP
Grade IV— IPH

FURTHER READING

Papile LA, et al. Incidence and evolution of subependymal and intraventricular hemorrhage: a study of infants with birth weights less than 1500 g. J Pediatr 1978;92(4):529-34.

Risk factors: prematurity (neonates with birth weight 500-750 g at highest risk 45%; affects 20% of neonates weighing <1500 g; rare after 35 weeks; occurs in the first 5 postnatal days: 50% D1, 25% D2, 15% D3, 10% D4 onward), acute chorioamnionitis. Causes: hypertension, venous congestion, hypoxia, traumatic rupture. Presentation: silent/asymptomatic (25-50%), saltatory/gradual (respiratory distress, abnormal eye movements, hypotonia) or catastrophic (acute IVH with bulging fontanelle, split sutures, reduced GCS, focal neurology, hypotension). Sequelae: cerebral palsy, seizures, mental retardation, coma/death, posthemorrhagic hydrocephalus, myelination delay. Mortality: 5% in those with Grade I + II GMH (7% develop hydrocephalus), 20% in Grade III + IV (75% develop hydrocephalus). Management is supportive with intraventricular taps and shunting for those with posthemorrhagic hydrocephalus.

Image with permission from Yachnis AT, Rivera-Zengotita ML. Neuropathology, High-Yield Pathology Series, Saunders, Elsevier, 2014.

12. **e**—Periventricular leukomalacia (hemorrhagic). Areas of periventricular necrosis may undergo extensive hemorrhage.

Image with permission from Yachnis AT, Rivera-Zengotita ML. Neuropathology, High-Yield Pathology Series, Saunders, Elsevier, 2014.

13. **d**—Right PCA infarct. Remote infarct in region of right posterior cerebral artery appears as a depressed, cavitated area.

Image with permission from Yachnis AT, Rivera-Zengotita ML. Neuropathology, High-Yield Pathology Series, Saunders, Elsevier, 2014.

14. 14. **c**—Malignant infarction. A massive right cerebral infarct (recent) resulted in hyperemia, swelling, and right cingulate gyrus herniation.

Image with permission from Yachnis AT, Rivera-Zengotita ML. Neuropathology, High-Yield Pathology Series, Saunders, Elsevier, 2014.

15. **c**—Mycotic aneurysm. Vasoinvasive fungi are revealed by Gomori methenamine silver (GMS) stain.

Image with permission from Yachnis AT, Rivera-Zengotita ML. Neuropathology, High-Yield Pathology Series, Saunders, Elsevier, 2014.

16. **d**—DVA—congenital venous malformation consisting of dilated but fully functional veins of the superficial or subcortical cerebral vasculature. Most common vascular malformation (2% people); accounts for 60% of all CNS vascular malformations; 30% associated with another vascular malformation (typically AVM). Dilated-appearing superficial veins may arise in the region of the Sylvian fissure as shown in the image. Benign lesion not requiring intervention.

Image with permission from Yachnis AT, Rivera-Zengotita ML. Neuropathology, High-Yield Pathology Series, Saunders, Elsevier, 2014.

17. **b**—Contrecoup contusions. The orbital frontal gyri and inferior lateral surfaces of the temporal lobes are typical sites of contrecoup contusional injury.

Image with permission from Yachnis AT, Rivera-Zengotita ML. Neuropathology, High-Yield Pathology Series, Saunders, Elsevier, 2014.

18. **a**—Kernicterus. Yellow discoloration of the subthalamic nuclei with lighter yellow staining of the thalamus and basal ganglia. Neuronal necrosis and yellow staining of deep cerebral and brain stem nuclei associated with infantile hyperbilirubinemia.

Image with permission from Yachnis AT, Rivera-Zengotita ML. Neuropathology, High-Yield Pathology Series, Saunders, Elsevier, 2014.

19. **e**—Porencephaly ("hole in brain"; porencephalic cysts) refers to a spectrum of cystic lesions resulting from loss of neural tissue (encephalomalacia) between the subpial cortical surface and ependymal lining of ventricles. Prevalence <1 per 200,000; thought to result from large vessel occlusion/spasm during gestation (emboli, lupus, maternal cocaine), but familial version due to mutation in COL4A1 gene. Presentation: delayed growth and development, spastic paresis, hypotonia, poor or absent speech, epilepsy, hydrocephalus, mental retardation. Prognosis depends on the size and location of the cyst, and the presence of other abnormalities. Gross pathology: Basket brain—bilateral severe porencephaly with persistence of mesial structures. Porencephalic cysts are lined with white matter, in contrast to schizencephaly, where the cyst is lined with heterotopic gray matter. They are intra-axial, in contrast to arachnoid cysts, which are extra-axial.

Image with permission from Yachnis AT, Rivera-Zengotita ML. Neuropathology, High-Yield Pathology Series, Saunders, Elsevier, 2014.

20. **e**—Schizencephaly is a rare cortical malformation in which gray-matter lined clefts arise near the sylvian fissure, often with adjacent polymicrogyria in the lining dysplastic gray matter. Ependyma and pia mater meet in the cleft at the pial-ependymal seem. Presentation is with seizures, motor and developmental delay. Gross/imaging: may be unilateral or bilateral; open lip/type II (commonest type in bilateral) cleft walls separated and filled with CSF; closed-lip/type I (commonest in unilateral cases) cleft walls are in apposition; frequently associated with septo-optic dysplasia, gray matter heterotopia, absent septum.

Image with permission from Yachnis AT, Rivera-Zengotita ML. Neuropathology, High-Yield Pathology Series, Saunders, Elsevier, 2014.

21. **a**—Astrocytoma. Gross specimen showing an ill-defined lesion with loss of gray-white matter demarcation toward the left of the image.

Image with permission from Yachnis AT, Rivera-Zengotita ML. Neuropathology, High-Yield Pathology Series, Saunders, Elsevier, 2014.

22. **b**—Gliomatosis cerebri. Gross brain section showing subtle effacement of gray and white matter structures. Compare the affected right basal ganglia and surrounding structures with the unaffected left side. Tumor cells were found in contiguous frontal, temporal, and parietal lobes.

Image with permission from Yachnis AT, Rivera-Zengotita ML. Neuropathology, High-Yield Pathology Series, Saunders, Elsevier, 2014.

23. **b**—NF-1 associated optic nerve glioma. Pilocytic astrocytoma causing fusiform enlargement of the optic nerve (left) in a patient with neurofibromatosis type I.

Image with permission from Yachnis AT, Rivera-Zengotita ML. Neuropathology, High-Yield Pathology Series, Saunders, Elsevier, 2014.

24. **d**—Tuberous sclerosis. This gross image is from a patient with tuberous sclerosis that shows a sharply circumscribed subependymal giant cell astrocytoma (SEGA) arising from the lateral wall of the left lateral ventricle. A cortical "tuber" is present in the lower left side of the image.

Image with permission from Yachnis AT, Rivera-Zengotita ML. Neuropathology, High-Yield Pathology Series, Saunders, Elsevier, 2014.

25. **a**—Fourth ventricular subependymoma. Grossly, subependymomas are lobular neoplasms that are well demarcated from adjacent CNS tissue as in this fourth ventricular example situated between cerebellum and medulla. Focal hemorrhage is present.

Image with permission from Yachnis AT, Rivera-Zengotita ML. Neuropathology, High-Yield Pathology Series, Saunders, Elsevier, 2014.

26. **a**—Atypical teratoid/rhabdoid tumor. Grossly, tumors are soft gray, tan, and demarcated from the surrounding brain (right side of image).

Image with permission from Yachnis AT, Rivera-Zengotita ML. Neuropathology, High-Yield Pathology Series, Saunders, Elsevier, 2014.

27. **c**—Meningioma. Meningiomas are typically firm, solid, well-circumscribed neoplasms that are attached to the dura (upper right).

Image with permission from Yachnis AT, Rivera-Zengotita ML. Neuropathology, High-Yield Pathology Series, Saunders, Elsevier, 2014.

28. **e**—This intraventricular meningioma arose from the choroid plexus on the left side. It had histologic features of a fibrous meningioma.

Image with permission from Yachnis AT, Rivera-Zengotita ML. Neuropathology, High-Yield Pathology Series, Saunders, Elsevier, 2014.

29. **e**—Schwannoma. This inferior view of the brain shows a large solid tumor (left) compressing the brain stem at the cerebellopontine angle.

Image with permission from Yachnis AT, Rivera-Zengotita ML. Neuropathology, High-Yield Pathology Series, Saunders, Elsevier, 2014.

30. **e**—Primary CNS lymphoma. Grossly, tumors are located deeply within the cerebral hemispheres in periventricular locations and may contain extensive necrosis.

Image with permission from Yachnis AT, Rivera-Zengotita ML. Neuropathology, High-Yield Pathology Series, Saunders, Elsevier, 2014.

31. **e**—Hemangioblastoma. This image shows a classic gross appearance of a large cerebellar cyst with a hyperemic mural tumor nodule.

Image with permission from Yachnis AT, Rivera-Zengotita ML. Neuropathology, High-Yield Pathology Series, Saunders, Elsevier, 2014.

32. **d**—Large soft tan-brown pituitary adenoma.

Image with permission from Yachnis AT, Rivera-Zengotita ML. Neuropathology, High-Yield Pathology Series, Saunders, Elsevier, 2014.

33. **e**—Rathke's cleft cyst. Grossly, Rathke's cleft cysts have a thin cyst wall and may be adherent to the adjacent infundibular stalk or inferior hypothalamus.

Image with permission from Yachnis AT, Rivera-Zengotita ML. Neuropathology, High-Yield Pathology Series, Saunders, Elsevier, 2014.

34. **a**—Colloid cyst of third ventricle. This colloid cyst fills the third ventricle and obstructs both foramina of Monro causing significant hydrocephalus.

Image with permission from Yachnis AT, Rivera-Zengotita ML. Neuropathology, High-Yield Pathology Series, Saunders, Elsevier, 2014.

35. **d**—Multiple metastasis. Grossly, metastatic tumors are found at the junctions between cortical gray and white matter.

Image with permission from Yachnis AT, Rivera-Zengotita ML. Neuropathology, High-Yield Pathology Series, Saunders, Elsevier, 2014.

36. **d**—Melanoma. Hemorrhagic metastases may be associated with significant mass effect. Metastatic tumors that tend to undergo hemorrhage include renal cell carcinoma, melanoma, and choriocarcinoma.

Image with permission from Yachnis AT, Rivera-Zengotita ML. Neuropathology, High-Yield Pathology Series, Saunders, Elsevier, 2014.

37. **c**—Ecchordosis physaliphora. Gross image of skull base showing the optic chiasm (left center), basilar artery (left), and a focal gelatinous mass adjacent to the basilar artery. Such incidental notochordal rests (remnants) can be seen in 1-2% of autopsies usually located in the retroclival prepontine region, but can be found anywhere from the skull base to the sacrum. Ecchordosis physaliphora arise from remaining notochord cells along the axis of the spine after embryogenesis. Unfortunately, ecchordosis physaliphora and chordoma are histologically indistinguishable, other than by examining the margins, the later demonstrating infiltrative growth.

Image with permission from Yachnis AT, Rivera-Zengotita ML. Neuropathology, High-Yield Pathology Series, Saunders, Elsevier, 2014.

38. **d**—Purulent meningitis. A purulent exudate covers the frontal region of the brain in this superior view. Hyperemia of the superficial blood vessels is also typical.

Image with permission from Yachnis AT, Rivera-Zengotita ML. Neuropathology, High-Yield Pathology Series, Saunders, Elsevier, 2014.

39. **e**—Ventriculitis. The acute purulent leptomeningeal exudate can extend into the ventricular system to cause ependymitis (ventriculitis) that can lead to obstructive hydrocephalus.

Image with permission from Yachnis AT, Rivera-Zengotita ML. Neuropathology, High-Yield Pathology Series, Saunders, Elsevier, 2014.

40. **a**—Mycobacterium Tuberculosis. Thick, grayish exudates are typically located at the base of the brain. Basilar meningitis is commonly TB or cryptococcal, and less commonly syphilis, spirochetes and autoimmune conditions. Risk factors include AIDS and other causes of immunocompromise.

Image with permission from Yachnis AT, Rivera-Zengotita ML. Neuropathology, High-Yield Pathology Series, Saunders, Elsevier, 2014.

41. **c**—Cerebral cryptococcosis. The presence of multifocal gelatinous cysts within the bilateral basal ganglia is a classic pattern of CNS involvement by Cryptococcus in the immunocompromised host.

Image with permission from Yachnis AT, Rivera-Zengotita ML. Neuropathology, High-Yield Pathology Series, Saunders, Elsevier, 2014.

42. **a**—Aspergillosis. Multiple hemorrhagic infarcts resulting from vasoinvasive Aspergillus arose in a child with severe combined immunodeficiency syndrome. Typical lesions are circumscribed, hemorrhagic, and softened.

Image with permission from Yachnis AT, Rivera-Zengotita ML. Neuropathology, High-Yield Pathology Series, Saunders, Elsevier, 2014.

43. **d**—Neurocysticercosis. Grossly two thin-walled cysts (arrows) with scolex present in the larger cyst.

Image with permission from Yachnis AT, Rivera-Zengotita ML.Neuropathology, High-Yield Pathology Series, Saunders, Elsevier, 2014.

44. **a**—Amoebic meningoencephalitis. Gross pathology shows hemorrhagic necrosis of basal frontal lobes, destruction of olfactory bulbs/tracts, cerebral edema, diffuse hemorrhagic meningeal exudate.

Image with permission from Yachnis AT, Rivera-Zengotita ML. Neuropathology, High-Yield Pathology Series, Saunders, Elsevier, 2014.

45. **a**—Cytomegalovirus ventriculitis and encephalitis. Grossly, the ventricular surfaces are discolored and necrotic.

Image with permission from Yachnis AT, Rivera-Zengotita ML. Neuropathology, High-Yield Pathology Series, Saunders, Elsevier, 2014.

46. **d**—Progressive multifocal leukoencephalopathy—CNS demyelinating disease caused by the ubiquitous JC virus (John Cunningham virus; papovavirus/polyomavirus), usually affecting immunocompromised patients (80% HIV; also hematological malignancy, post-transplant, other malignancy). Gross image showing confluence of multiple areas of demyelination to forma unifocal lesion on the right. The adjacent cortical ribbon is spared.

Image with permission from Yachnis AT, Rivera-Zengotita ML. Neuropathology, High-Yield Pathology Series, Saunders, Elsevier, 2014.

47. **a**—Alzheimer's disease. Most cases show diffuse cerebral atrophy with widening of the sulci and narrowing of the gyri. There is also symmetrical ventriculomegaly with blunting of the lateral ventricular angles (ex vacuo hydrocephalus).

Image with permission from Yachnis AT, Rivera-Zengotita ML. Neuropathology, High-Yield Pathology Series, Saunders, Elsevier, 2014.

48. **e**—Pick disease. Characterized by sulcal widening and gyral atrophy in frontal and temporal lobes, but sparing of parietal and occipital lobes.

Image with permission from Yachnis AT, Rivera-Zengotita ML. Neuropathology, High-Yield Pathology Series, Saunders, Elsevier, 2014.

49. **a**—Amyotrophic lateral sclerosis. Lateral corticospinal tract—degeneration manifest by pallor on myelin-stained sections is typical.

Motor neuron disease (or amyotrophic lateral sclerosis) is a progressive neuromuscular disease characterized by degeneration of upper and lower motor neurons resulting in progressive skeletal muscle wasting and weakness leaking to respiratory failure and death. Genetics: most common familial form is AD ALS associated with mutation of copper/zinc superoxide dismutase (SOD1) gene on chromosome 21. Classification: primary lateral sclerosis affects predominantly UMNs, while progressive muscular atrophy affects LMNs. Incidence 2 per 100,000 per year; prevalence 5 per 100,000; mean age of onset for sporadic 60 years; familial cases make up 10%. Presentation: asymmetric extremity weakness, dysphagia and dysarthria; signs of UMN (weakness, hyperreflexia, spasticity) and LMN degeneration (weakness, atrophy, hyporeflexia, fasciculations). Median survival 3-5 years after symptom onset; glutamate inhibitor may slow disease. MRI usually normal but T2 hypointensity of motor cortex. Histology: loss of anterior horn cells, lateral and anterior corticospinal tract degeneration, Bunina bodies, Skein-like inclusion, Lewy-like inclusions, loss of Betz cells in M1/cranial nerve nuclei. Immunohistochemistry: Bunina bodies cystatin-C positive and ubiquitin negative; Differential: spinal muscular atrophy, hereditary spastic paraplegia, myasthenia gravis.

Image with permission from Yachnis AT, Rivera-Zengotita ML. Neuropathology, High-Yield Pathology Series, Saunders, Elsevier, 2014.

50. **d**—Huntington's disease. Huntington's disease is an autosomal dominant neurodegenerative disease characterized by choreiform movements, psychiatric symptoms, dementia and genetic expansion of the trinucleitide (CAG) repeat in the HD gene (chromosome 4p). IAgre range 2-85 (mean 40); incidence 2-4 per 1,000,000 per year, prevalence 5-8 per 100,000; no gender predilection; interaction of mutated Huntington protein with other proteins results in neuronal death. Presentation: insidious onset of chorea, psychiatric symptoms (irritability, depression, anxiety) and cognitive impairment; successive generations have expanded repeats leaded to earlier onset and more severe phenotype (anticipation). Eventually fatal disease. Imaging: striatal and cortical atrophy. Gross appearance: marked atrophy of the caudate nucleus and putamen is associated with enlarged lateral ventricles ("ex vacuo hydrocephalus"). Histology shows striatal atrophy (caudate/putamen) due to degeneration of medium spiny neurons, and reactive gliosis.

Image with permission from Yachnis AT, Rivera-Zengotita ML. Neuropathology, High-Yield Pathology Series, Saunders, Elsevier, 2014.

51. **c**—Friedreich's ataxia. Sections of spinal cord typically show degeneration (pallor) of the posterior columns and lateral corticospinal tracts as shown in this lumbar level. Friedreich's ataxia is an autosomal recessive spinocerebellar degeneration due to mutation of FRDA (frataxin) gene on chromosome 9q—trinucleide repeat (GAA) expansion results in reduced frataxin protein (involved in oxidative phosphorylation and iron homeostasis). Longer repeat size associated with earlier age of onset, increased severity/progression rate and increased neurologic impairment (shows genetic "anticipation"). FA is the commonest hereditary ataxia (50% cases); children and young adults; mean 15 years, 85% before age 20; incidence 2 per 100,000 per year; prevalence 1 in 30,000; rare in Black/Asian populations. Presentation: progressive lower limb and gait ataxia, sensory loss, areflexia, dysarthria; progression of the disease leads to loss of vibration/JPS, areflexia of all extremities, foot deformity, scoliosis, diabetes mellitus, hypertrophic cardiomyopathy/myocardial fibrosis. Prognosis—loss of ambulation within 15 years onset, life expectancy 30-40 years after onset; coenzyme Q and vitamin E may slow disease progression. Gross appearance: brain usually appears normal, but possibly atrophy of cerebellar vermis and dentate nucleus; diffuse atrophy of spinal cord, particularly dorsal and lateral columns. Differential: other hereditary ataxias, hereditary spastic paraplegia, ataxia telangiectasia, acquired ataxias.

Image with permission from Yachnis AT, Rivera-Zengotita ML. Neuropathology, High-Yield Pathology Series, Saunders, Elsevier, 2014.

52. **e**—Vascular dementia. Foci of complete white matter cavitation (upper left) may be evident. There is also marked thinning of the corpus callosum and symmetrical widening of the lateral ventricles because of widespread white matter disease.

Image with permission from Yachnis AT, Rivera-Zengotita ML. Neuropathology, High-Yield Pathology Series, Saunders, Elsevier, 2014.

ANSWERS 53–68

Additional answers 53–68 available on ExpertConsult.com

CHAPTER 6

NEUROPATHOLOGY III: HISTOLOGY

Histological sections shown in this chapter are hematoxylin and eosin stained unless otherwise stated.

SINGLE BEST ANSWER (SBA) QUESTIONS

1. Which one of the following is the main feature demonstrated in this histological section?

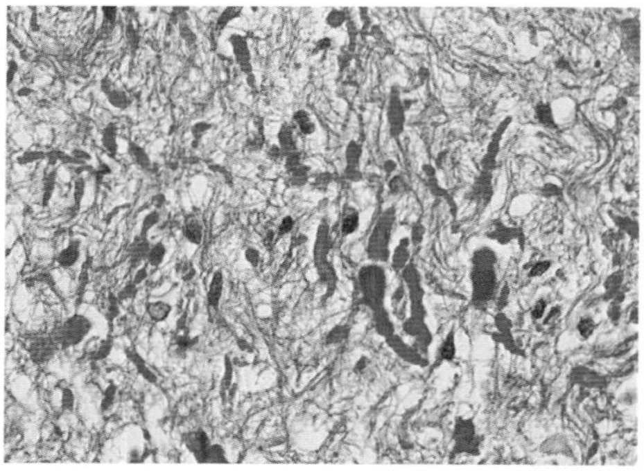

a. Herring bodies
b. Hirano bodies
c. Neuritic plaques
d. Rosenthal fibers
e. Verocay bodies

2. Which one of the following areas in the brain is most likely demonstrated in this histological section?

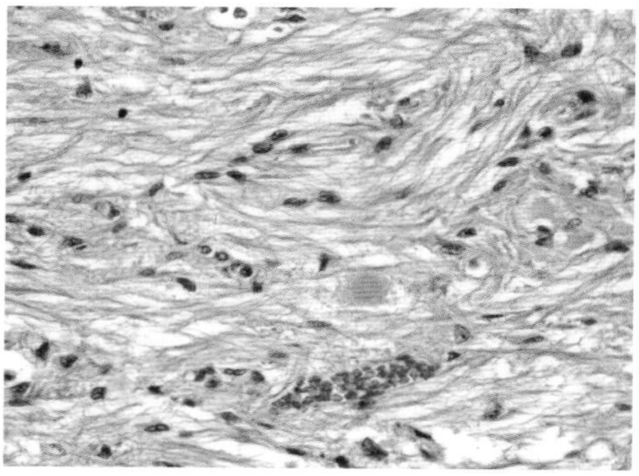

a. Caudate nucleus
b. Cortex
c. Optic nerve
d. Posterior pituitary
e. Thalamus

3. Which one of the following is most likely demonstrated in this histological section?

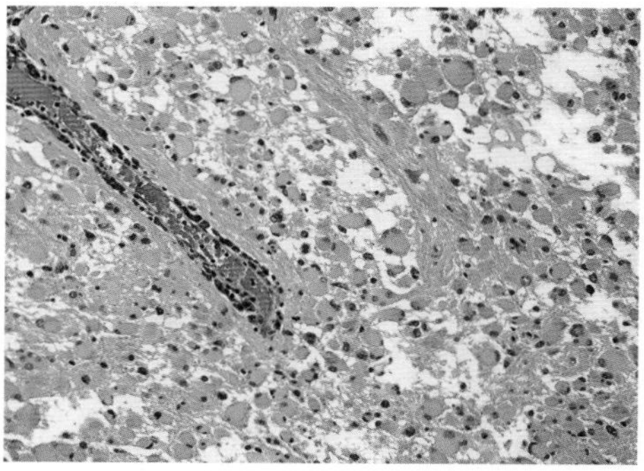

a. Creutzfeldt-Jakob disease
b. Gemistocytic astrocytoma
c. Lymphoma
d. Oligodendroglioma
e. Pineoblastoma

4. Which one of the following is the main feature demonstrated in this histological section?

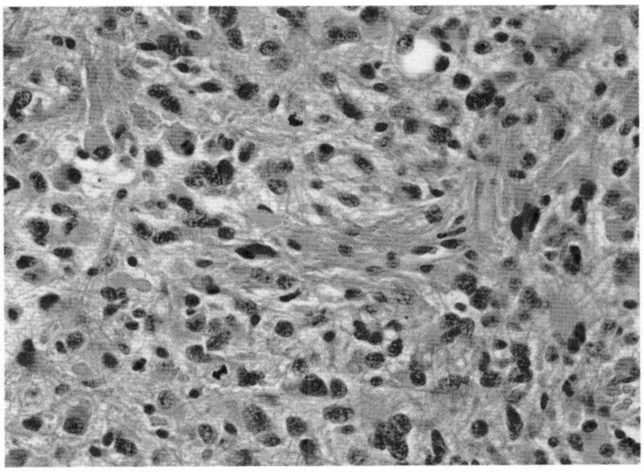

a. Anaplastic astrocytoma
b. Pituitary adenoma
c. Psammomatous meningioma
d. Schwannoma
e. Teratoma

5. Which one of the following is the most likely diagnosis demonstrated in this histological section?

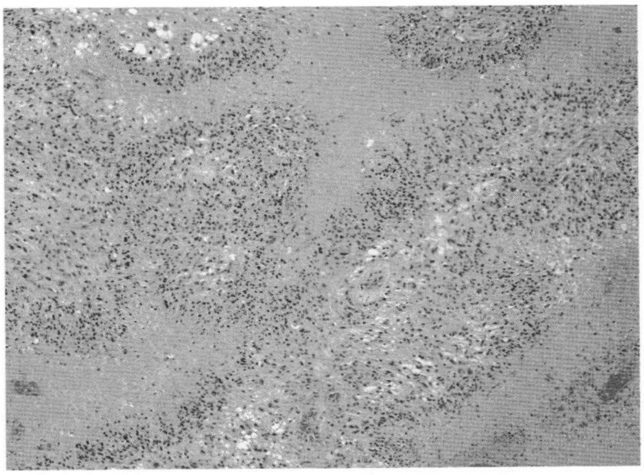

a. Diffuse astrocytoma
b. Germinoma
c. Glioblastoma multiforme
d. Schwannoma
e. Secretory meningioma

6. Which one of the following is the most likely diagnosis demonstrated in this histological section?

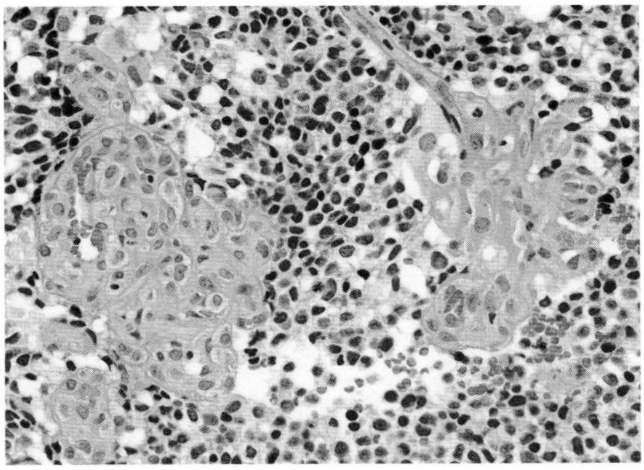

a. Atypical meningioma
b. DNET
c. Glioblastoma multiforme
d. Medulloblastoma
e. Primary CNS lymphoma

7. Which one of the following features is demonstrated in the center of this histological section?

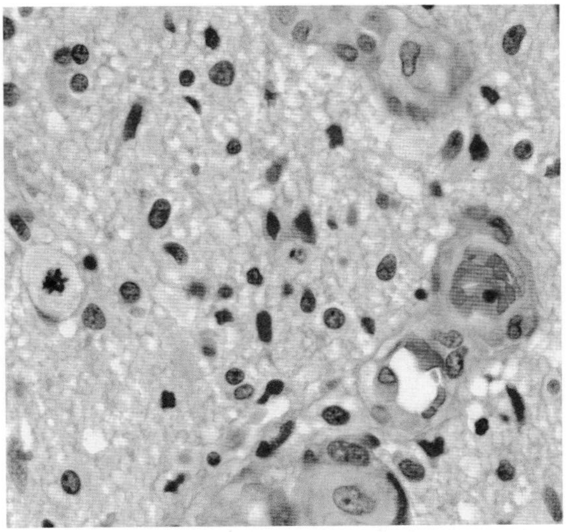

a. Balloon cells
b. Fried egg cells
c. Glomeruloid microvascular proliferation
d. Mitotic figure
e. Pseudopalisading necrosis

8. Which one of the following is the most likely diagnosis demonstrated in this histological section?

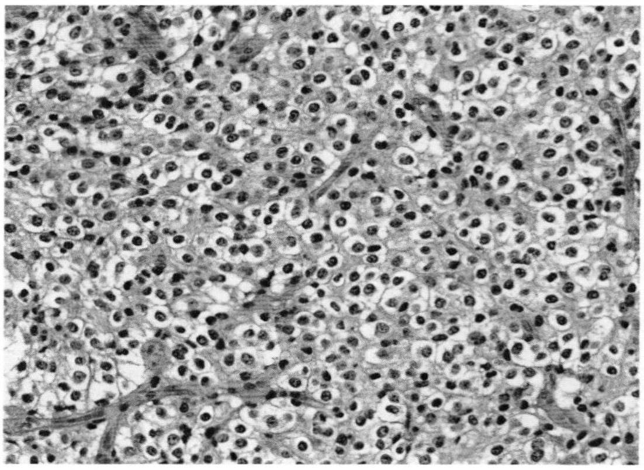

a. DNET
b. Gemistocytic astrocytoma
c. Glioblastoma multiforme
d. Medulloblastoma
e. Oligodendroglioma

9. Which one of the following is the most likely diagnosis demonstrated in this histological section?

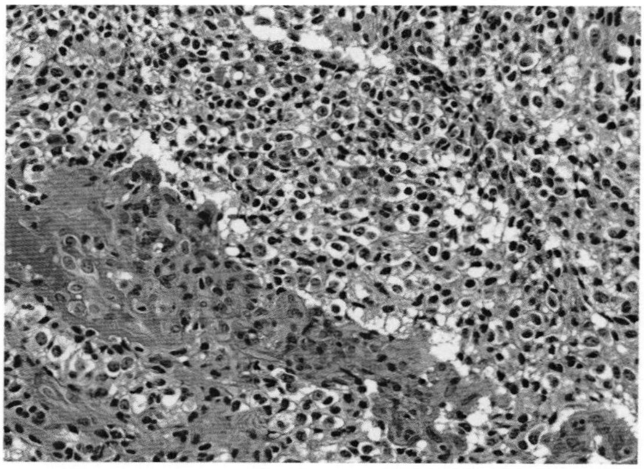

a. Anaplastic astrocytoma
b. Anaplastic oligodendroglioma
c. Glioblastoma multiforme
d. Renal metastasis
e. Secretory meningioma

10. Which one of the following is the most likely diagnosis demonstrated in this histological section?

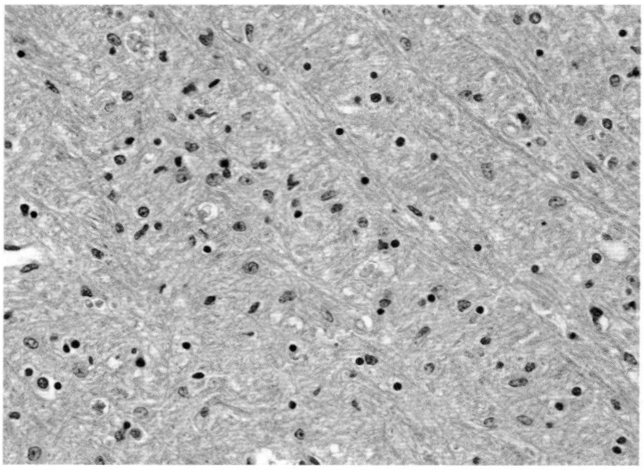

a. Choroid plexus papilloma
b. Gliomatosis cerebri
c. Normal white matter
d. Pineocytoma
e. Teratoma

11. Which one of the following is most likely based on the histology below (low magnification showed microcystic areas)?

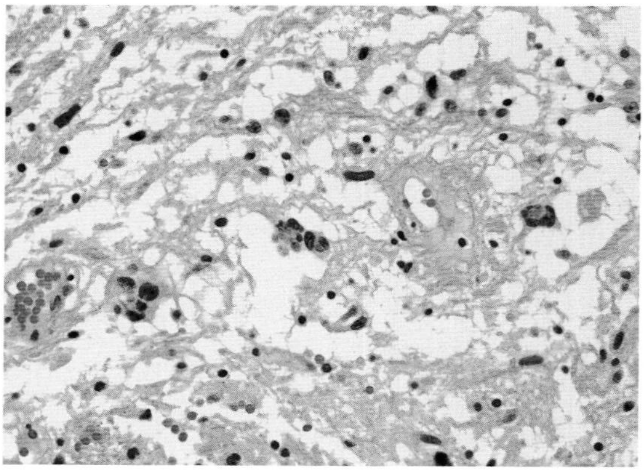

a. Anaplastic oligodendroglioma
b. Ependymoma
c. Fibrous meningioma
d. Medulloblastoma
e. Pilocytic astrocytoma

12. Which one of the following is the most likely diagnosis demonstrated in this histological section?

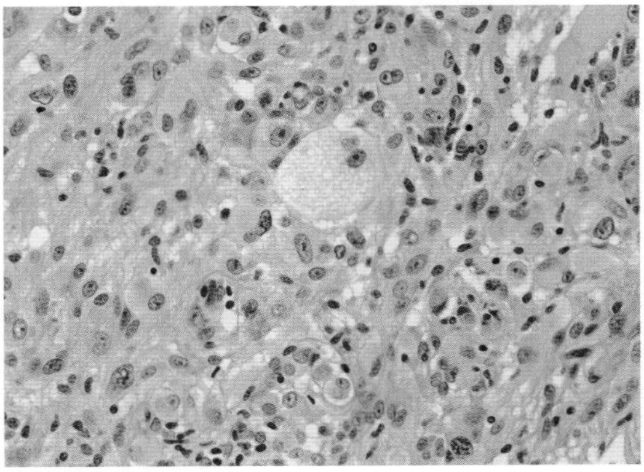

a. Alexander's disease
b. Oligodendroglioma
c. Pleomorphic xanthoastrocytoma
d. Psammomatous meningioma
e. Reactive gliosis

13. This histological section from an intraventricular tumor is most likely to be which one of the following

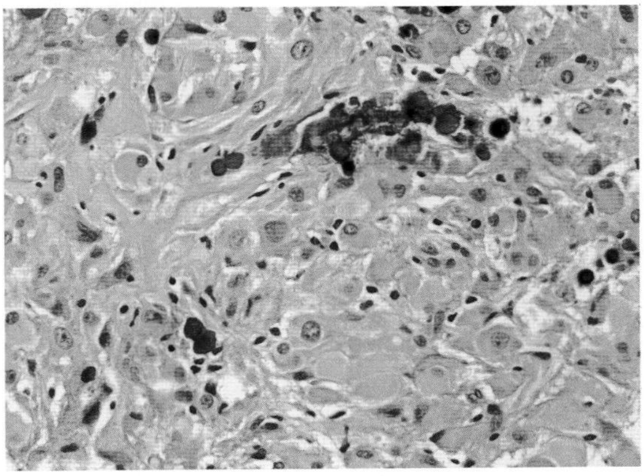

a. Chordoma
b. Choroid plexus papilloma
c. Pineoblastoma
d. Pituitary adenoma
e. Subependymal giant cell astrocytoma

14. This child presented with seizures and a known mutation on chromosome 16p13. A supratentorial lesion was resected with the histological appearance shown below. Which one of the following diagnoses is most likely?

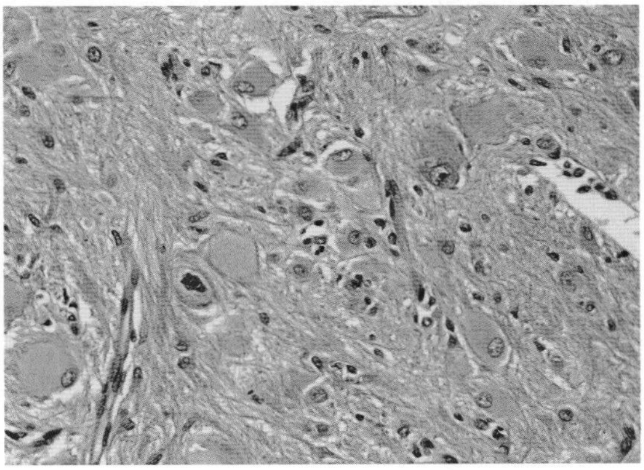

a. Gorlin syndrome
b. NF-2
c. Tuberous sclerosis complex
d. Turcot syndrome
e. Von Hippel-Lindau syndrome

15. Which one of the following is the most likely diagnosis demonstrated in this histological section?

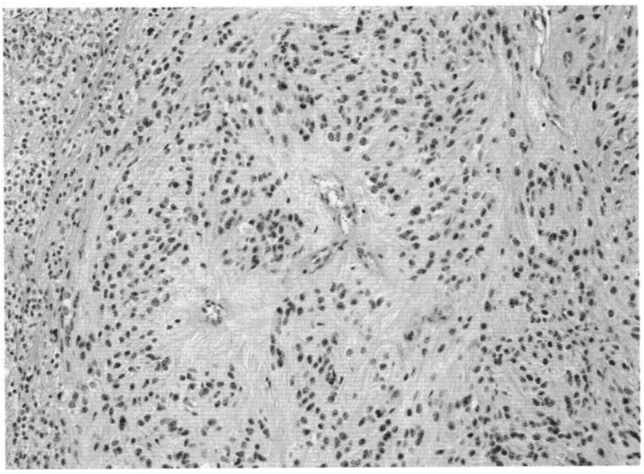

a. Anaplastic oligodendroglioma
b. Ependymoma
c. Glioblastoma multiforme
d. Medulloblastoma
e. Retinoblastoma

16. Which one of the following diagnoses is most likely from this histological section?

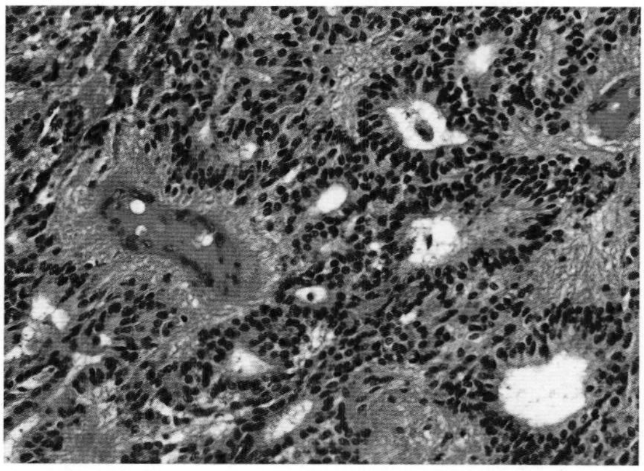

a. Central neurocytoma
b. Chordoid glioma
c. Ependymoma
d. Pleomorphic xanthoastrocytoma
e. Subependymal giant cell astrocytoma

17. Which one of the following is the most likely diagnosis demonstrated in this histological section?

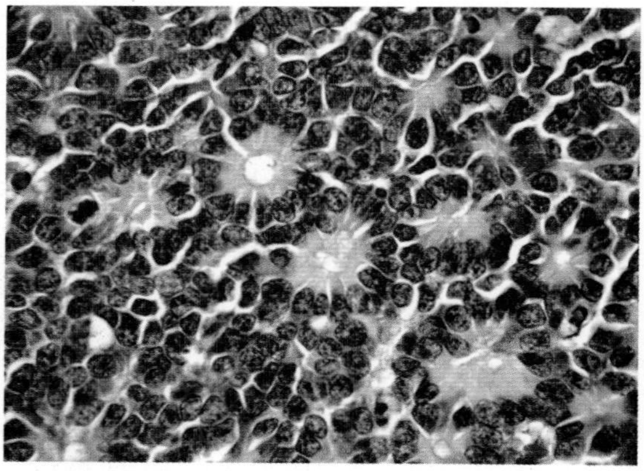

a. Central neurocytoma
b. Ependymoma
c. Pilocytic astrocytoma
d. Pituitary adenoma
e. Retinoblastoma

18. Which one of the following is shown in this histological section?

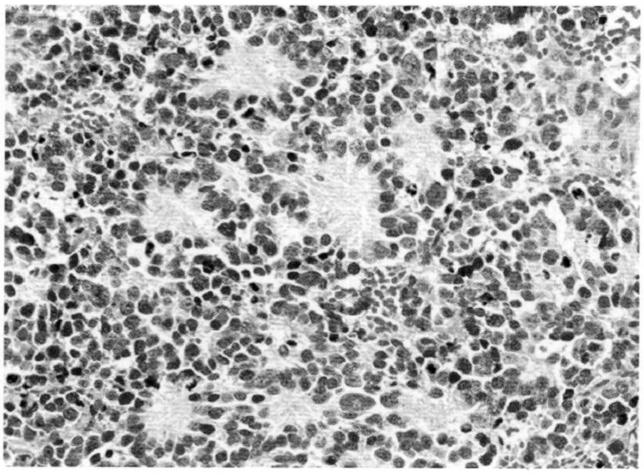

a. Ependymal rosette
b. Flexner-Wintersteiner rosette
c. Homer Wright rosette
d. Neurocytic rosette
e. Perivascular pseudorosette

19. Which one of the following is the most likely diagnosis demonstrated in this histological section?

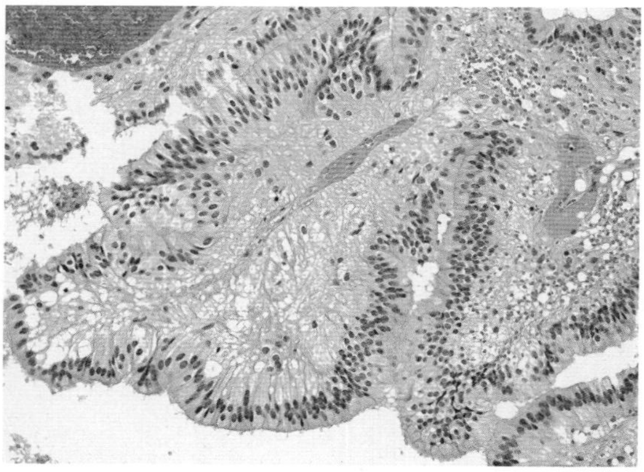

a. Central neurocytoma
b. Craniopharyngioma
c. Germinoma
d. Papillary ependymoma
e. Subependymal giant cell astrocytoma

20. Which one of the following is the most likely diagnosis demonstrated in this histological section?

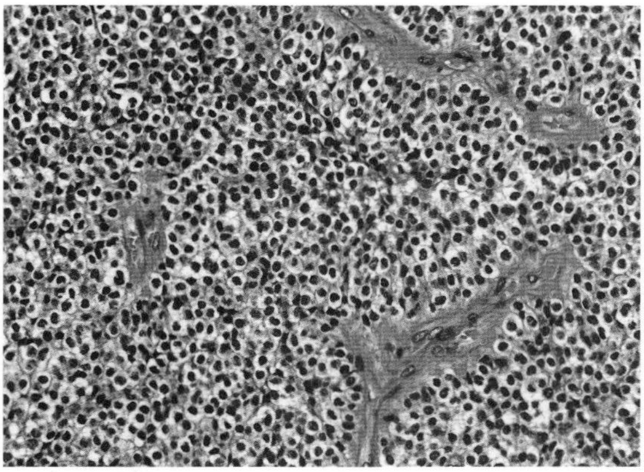

a. Atypical meningioma
b. Choroid plexus papilloma
c. Clear cell ependymoma
d. Glioblastoma multiforme
e. Schwannoma

21. Which one of the following is the most likely diagnosis demonstrated in this histological section from a spinal cord lesion?

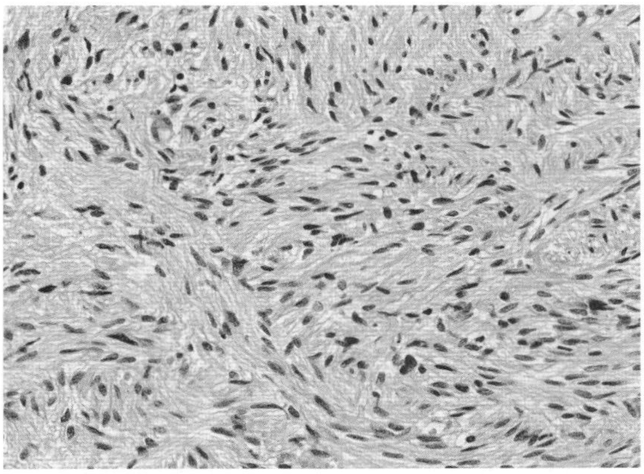

a. Chordoma
b. Oligodendroglioma
c. Pituitary adenoma
d. Retinoblastoma
e. Tanycytic ependymoma

22. Histology of this fourth ventricular tumor extending out of foramen of Luscka laterally is most likely to represent which one of the following?

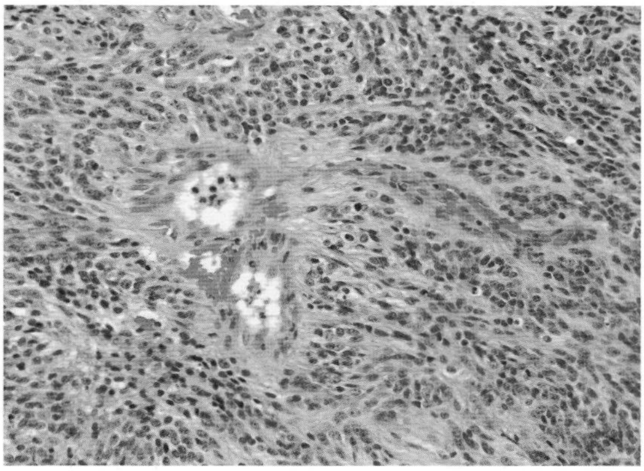

a. Anaplastic ependymoma
b. Atypical teratoid/rhabdoid tumor
c. Pilocytic astrocytoma
d. Pineoblastoma
e. Pontine glioma

23. A 65-year-old male with sciatica undergoes excision of an L3/4 spinal lesion. Which one of the following is most likely based on histological appearances below?

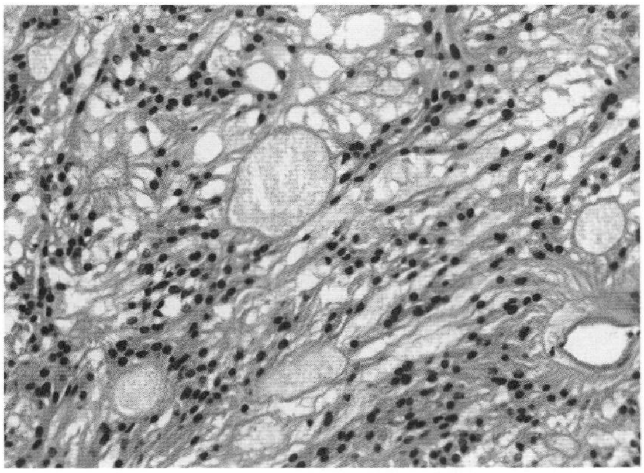

a. Chordoma
b. Gemistocystic astrocytoma
c. Myopapillary ependymoma
d. Pineocytoma
e. Schwannoma

24. Histology of this lateral ventricular tumor in a 65-year-old patient is most likely to represent which one of the following?

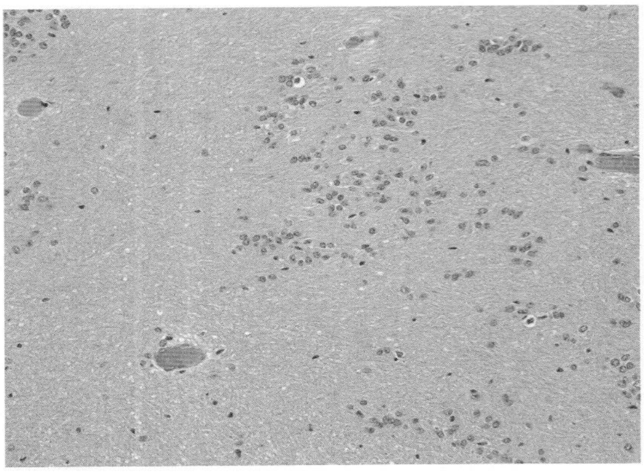

a. Choroid plexus carcinoma
b. Choroid plexus papilloma
c. Ependymoma
d. Meningioma
e. Subependymoma

25. Which one of the following is the most likely diagnosis demonstrated in this histological section from ventricular lesion?

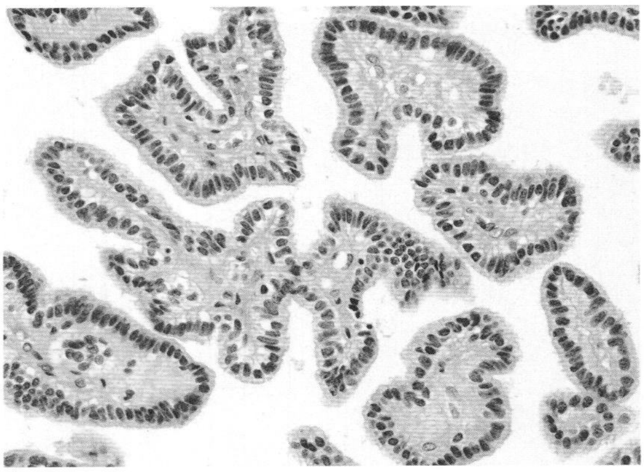

a. Chordoid glioma
b. Chordoma
c. Choroid plexus papilloma
d. Hypothalamic hamartoma
e. Yolk sac tumor

26. Histology of this lateral ventricular tumor in a child with Li-Fraumeni syndrome is most likely to represent which one of the following?

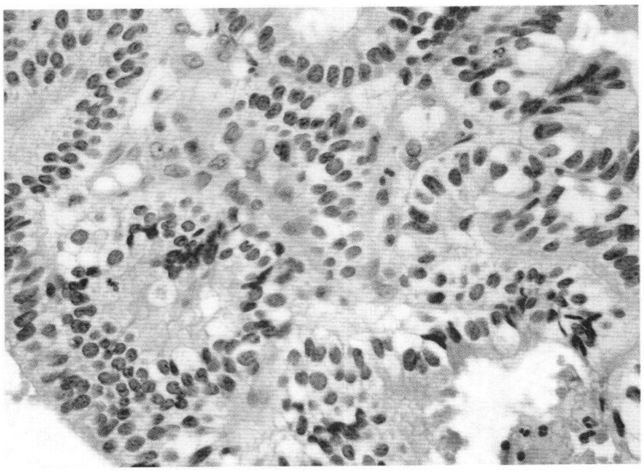

a. Choroid plexus carcinoma
b. Hemangioblastoma
c. Hemangiopericytoma
d. Intraventricular meningioma
e. Subependymal giant cell astrocytoma

27. A 3 year old child with known chromosome 17p loss presents with a posterior fossa tumour with the histological appearance shown. Which one of the following is most likely?

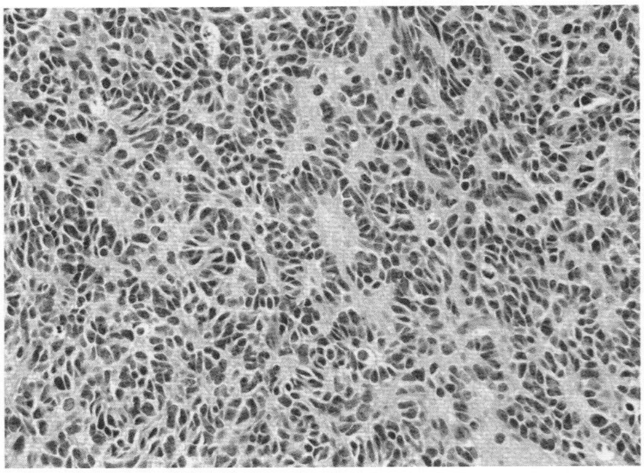

a. Cortical tuber
b. Embryonal carcinoma
c. Gemistocytic astrocytoma
d. Medulloblastoma
e. Meningioma

28. In the context of positive INI-1 staining (not shown), this histological section from a posterior fossa tumor is most likely to represent which one of the following?

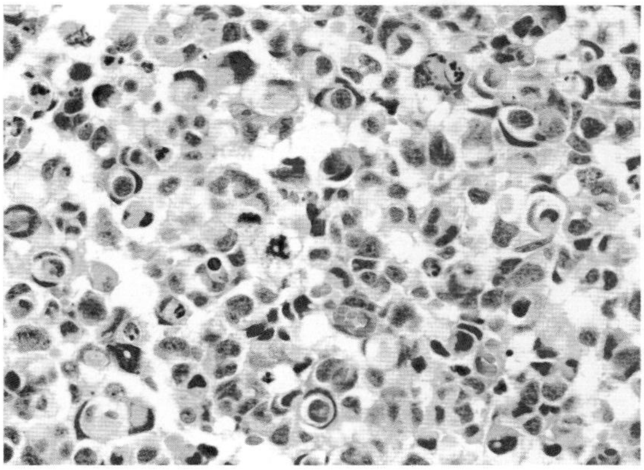

a. Atypical teratoid/rhabdoid tumor
b. Hemangioblastoma
c. Large cell/anaplastic medulloblastoma
d. Nodular/desmoplastic medulloblastoma
e. Pilocytic astrocytoma

29. This INI-1 positive (not shown) tumor arising in the right frontal lobe of a 1 year old is most likely to represent which one of the following?

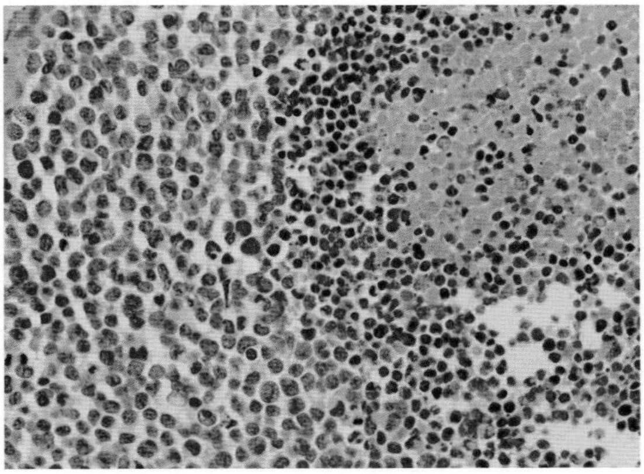

a. Chordoma
b. Germinoma
c. Glioblastoma multiforme
d. Supratentorial primitive neuroepithelial tumor (PNET)
e. Teratoma

30. This histological section from a suprasellar lesion is INI-1 negative but positive for vimentin and epithelial membrane antigen. Which one of the following are most likely:

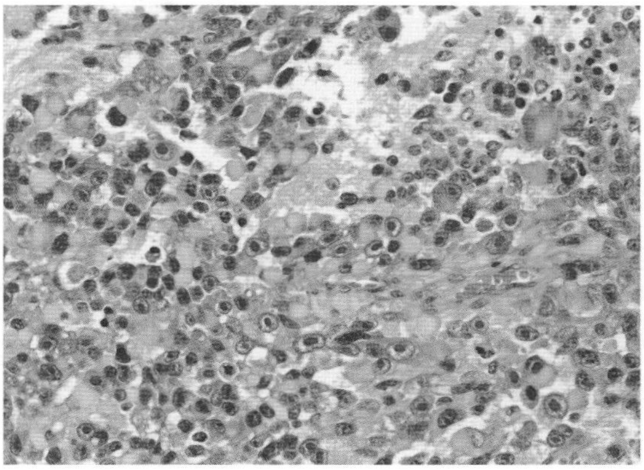

a. Atypical teratoid/rhabdoid tumor
b. Chordoma
c. Craniopharyngioma
d. Pituitary adenoma
e. Pure germinoma

31. Which one of the following is the most likely diagnosis demonstrated in this histological section?

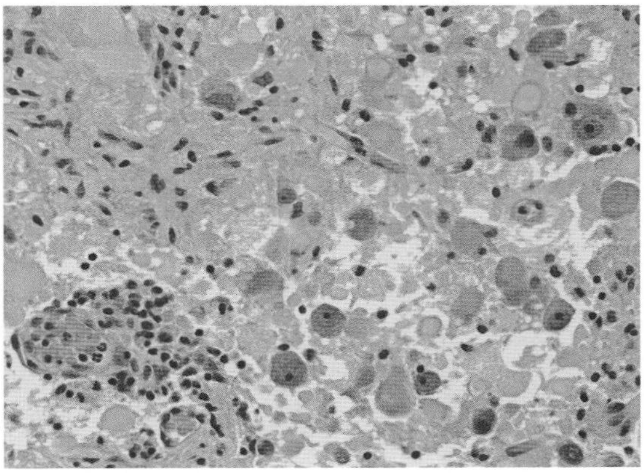

a. Chordoma
b. Ganglioglioma
c. Meningioma
d. Oligodendroglioma
e. Schwannoma

32. Which one of the following is the most likely diagnosis demonstrated in this histological section?

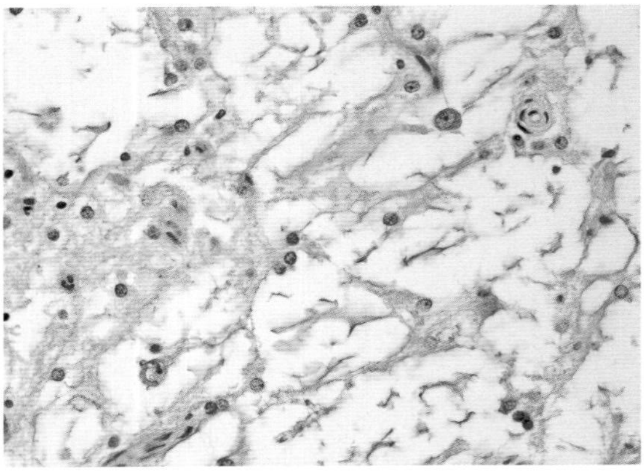

a. Central neurocytoma
b. Dysembryoplastic neuroepithelial tumor
c. Fibrillary astrocytoma
d. Meningothelial meningioma
e. Pineoblastoma

33. Which one of the following is the most likely diagnosis demonstrated in this histological section?

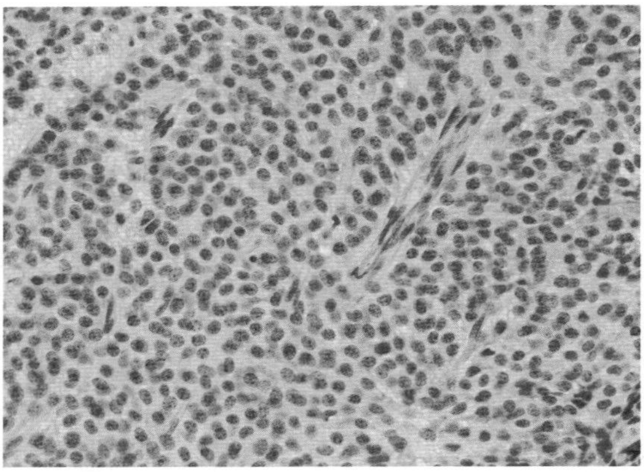

a. Central neurocytoma
b. Chordoma
c. Glioblastoma multiforme
d. Hemangioma
e. Oligodendroglioma

34. Which one of the following is the most likely diagnosis demonstrated in this histological section?

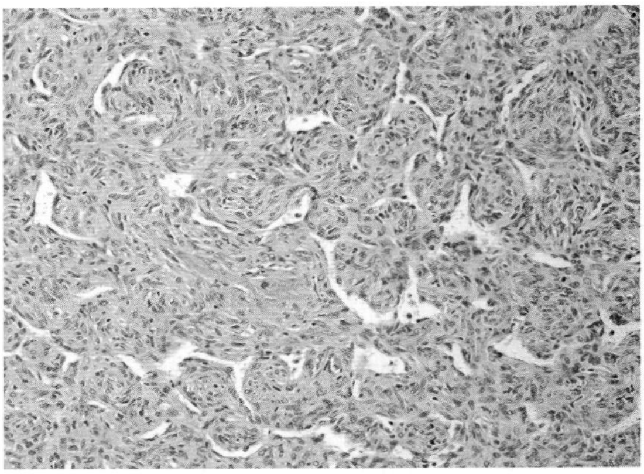

a. Antoni B Schwannoma
b. Hemangioblastoma
c. Hemangiopericytoma
d. Neurofibroma
e. Pilocytic astrocytoma

35. Which one of the following is the most likely diagnosis demonstrated in this histological section?

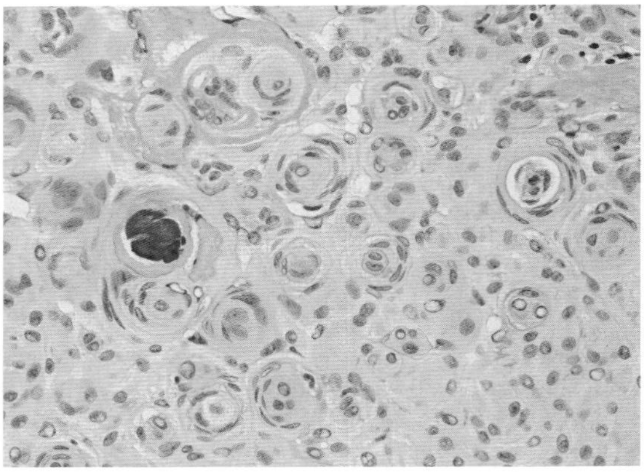

a. Choroid plexus papilloma
b. Glioblastoma multiforme
c. Meningothelial meningioma
d. Pineoblastoma
e. Pituitary adenoma

36. Which one of the following is the most likely diagnosis demonstrated in this histological section?

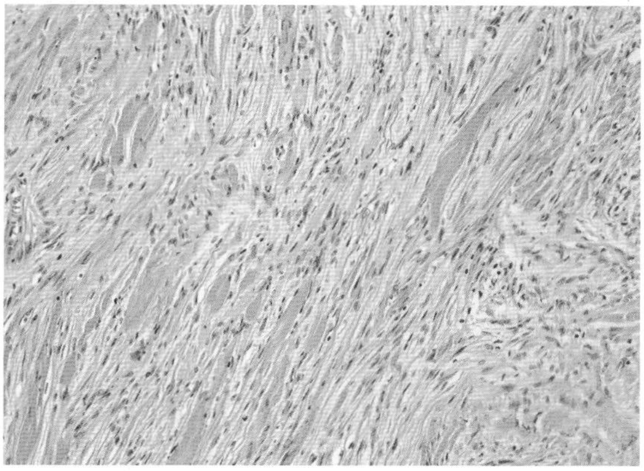

a. Antoni A Schwannoma
b. Fibrillary astrocytoma
c. Fibrous fibroblastic meningioma
d. Malignant peripheral nerve sheath tumor
e. Medulloblastoma

37. Which one of the following is the most likely diagnosis demonstrated in this histological section?

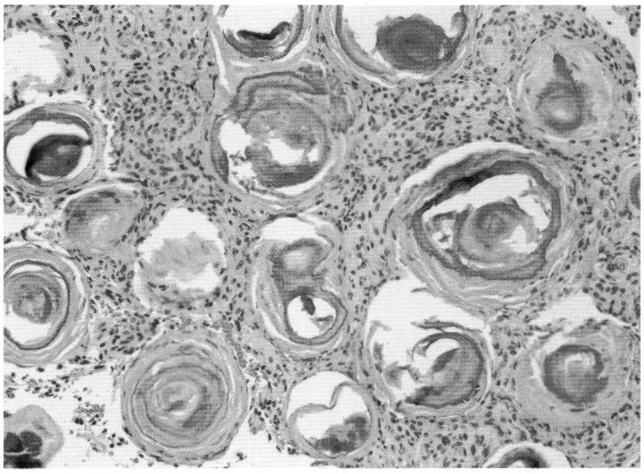

a. Angiocentric glioma
b. Central neurocytoma
c. Chordoma
d. Medulloblastoma
e. Psammomatous meningioma

38. Which one of the following is the most likely diagnosis demonstrated in this histological section?

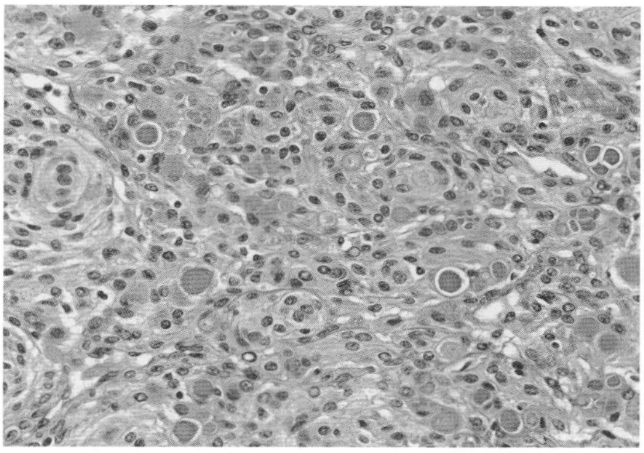

a. Germinoma
b. Glioblastoma multiforme
c. Retinoblastoma
d. Schwannoma
e. Secretory meningioma

39. Which one of the following is the most likely diagnosis demonstrated in this histological section?

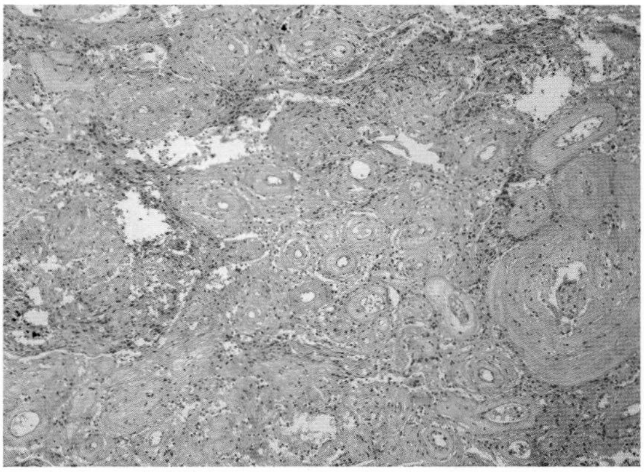

a. Angiomatous meningioma
b. Choroid plexus papilloma
c. Glioblastoma multiforme
d. Hemangiopericytoma
e. Psammomatous meningioma

40. Which one of the following is the most likely diagnosis demonstrated in this histological section?

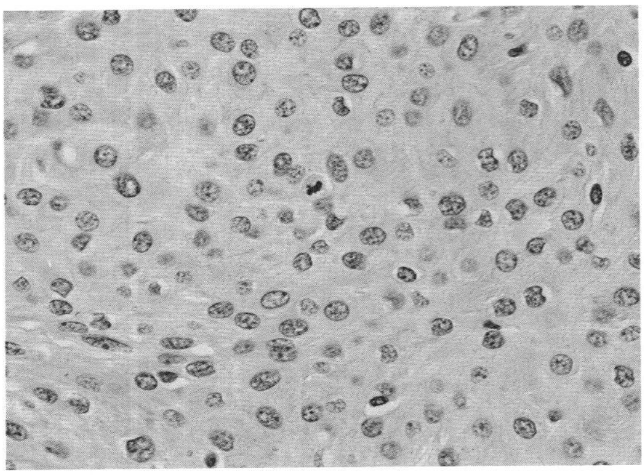

a. Atypical meningioma
b. Atypical teratoid/rhabdoid tumor
c. Diffuse astrocytoma
d. Medulloblastoma
e. Schwannoma

41. Which one of the following is the most likely diagnosis demonstrated in this histological section?

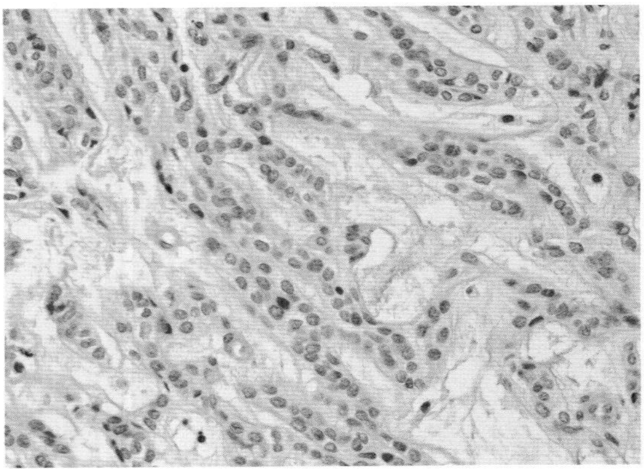

a. Anaplastic astrocytoma
b. Chordoid meningioma
c. Choroid plexus papilloma
d. Oligodendroglioma
e. Pituitary adenoma

42. Which one of the following is the most likely diagnosis demonstrated in this histological section?

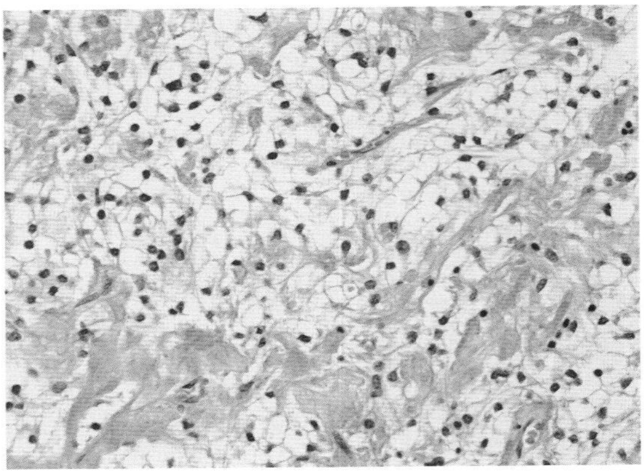

a. Chordoma
b. Clear cell meningioma
c. Gemistocytic astrocytoma
d. Pilocytic astrocytoma
e. Pituitary adenoma

43. Which one of the following is the most likely diagnosis demonstrated in this histological section?

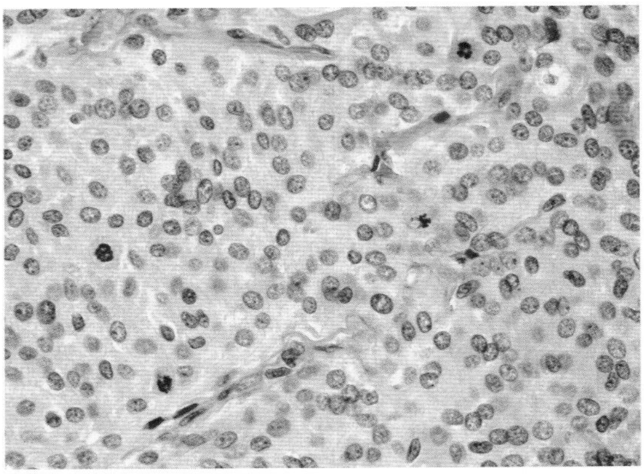

a. Anaplastic meningioma
b. Central neurocytoma
c. Gemistocytic astrocytoma
d. Hemangiopericytoma
e. Medulloblastoma

44. Which one of the following is the most likely diagnosis demonstrated in this histological section?

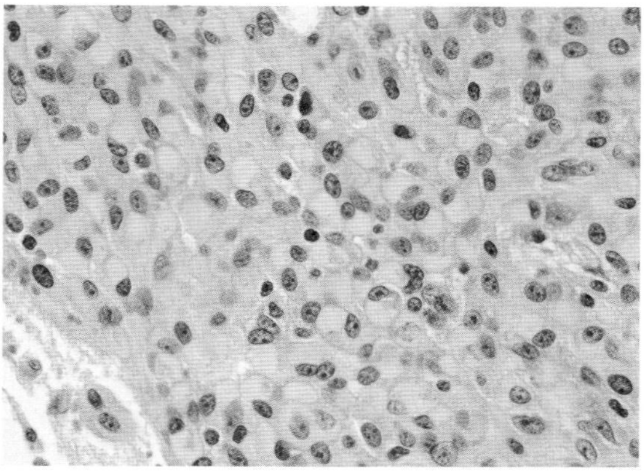

a. Choroid plexus carcinoma
b. Fibrillary astrocytoma
c. Oligodendroglioma
d. Parkinson's disease
e. Rhabdoid meningioma

45. Which one of the following is the most likely diagnosis demonstrated in this histological section?

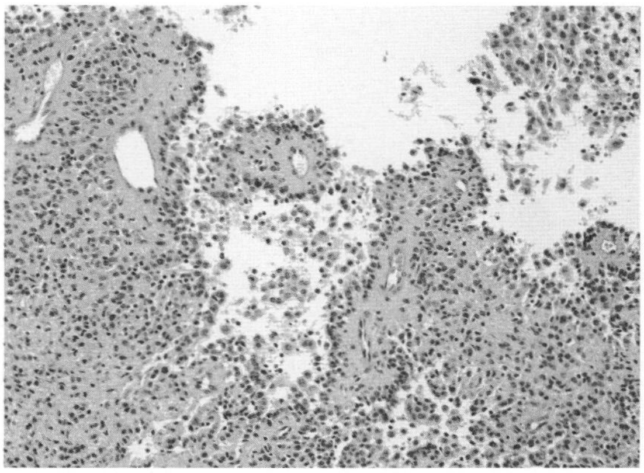

a. Central neurocytoma
b. Choroid plexus papilloma
c. Medulloblastoma
d. Oligodendroglioma
e. Papillary meningioma

46. Which one of the following is the most likely diagnosis demonstrated in this histological section?

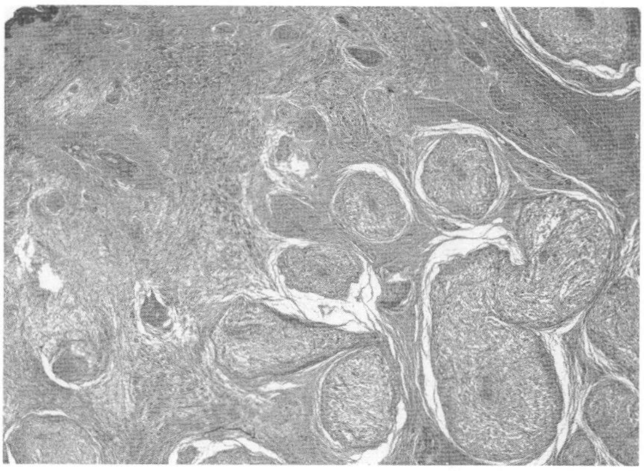

a. Angiocentric glioma
b. Neurofibroma
c. Primary CNS lymphoma
d. Psammomatous meningioma
e. Pseudopsammomatous bodies

47. Which one of the following is the most likely diagnosis demonstrated in this histological section?

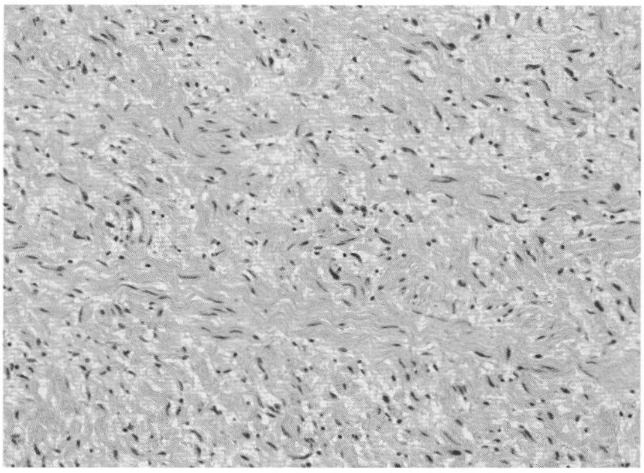

a. Astrocytoma
b. Germinoma
c. Neurofibroma
d. Schwannoma
e. Teratoma

48. Which one of the following is the most likely diagnosis demonstrated in this histological section?

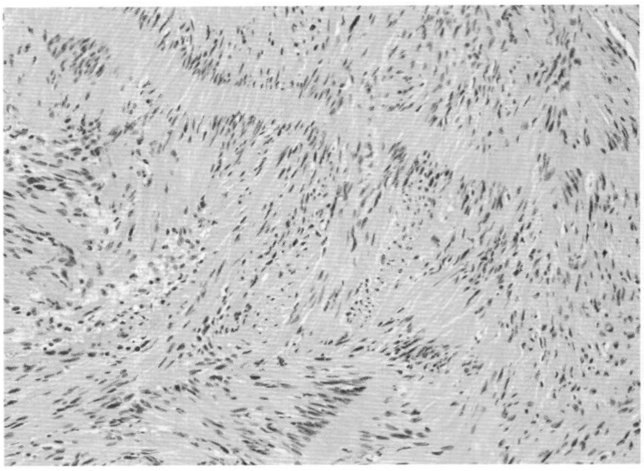

a. Antoni A schwannoma
b. Epidermoid
c. Malignant peripheral nerve sheath tumor
d. Meningioma
e. Neurenteric cyst

49. This dumbbell shaped mass in the spinal cord most likely represents which one of the following?

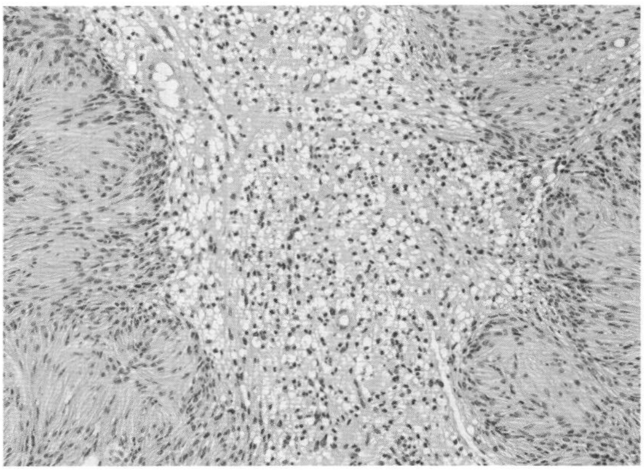

a. Antony B schwannoma
b. Malignant peripheral nerve sheath tumor
c. Myxopapillary ependymoma
d. Neurofibroma
e. Tanycytic ependymoma

50. Which one of the following is the most likely diagnosis demonstrated in this histological section?

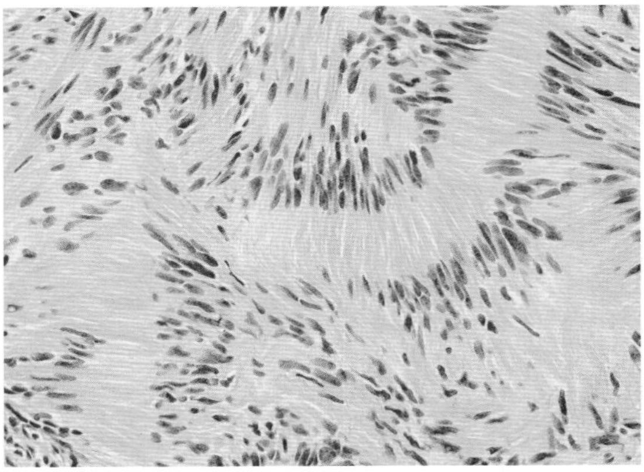

a. Bunina bodies
b. Hirano bodies
c. Lewy bodies
d. Pick bodies
e. Verocay bodies

51. Which one of the following is the most likely diagnosis demonstrated in this histological section?

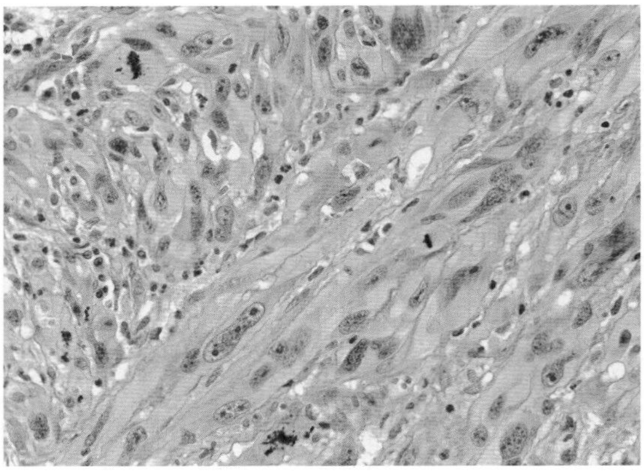

a. Angiocentric glioma
b. Atypical teratoid/rhabdoid tumor
c. Choriocarcinoma
d. Malignant peripheral nerve sheath tumors
e. Secretory meningioma

52. Deep cerebral lesion with the histological appearance shown is most likely to be which one of the following?

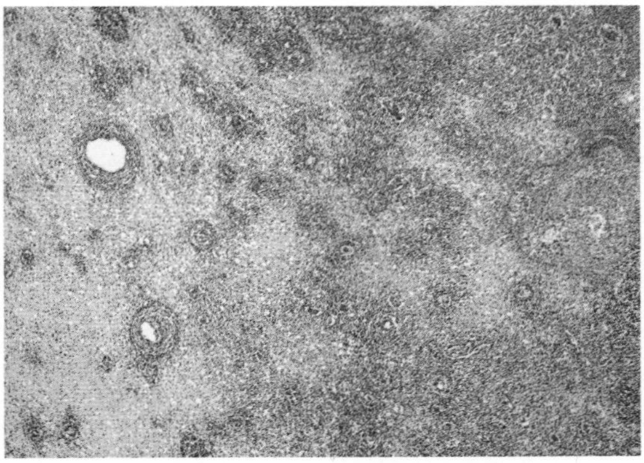

a. Angiofibromatous meningioma
b. Germinoma
c. Hemangiopericytoma
d. Primary CNS lymphoma
e. Toxoplasmosis

53. Which one of the following is the most likely diagnosis demonstrated in this histological section?

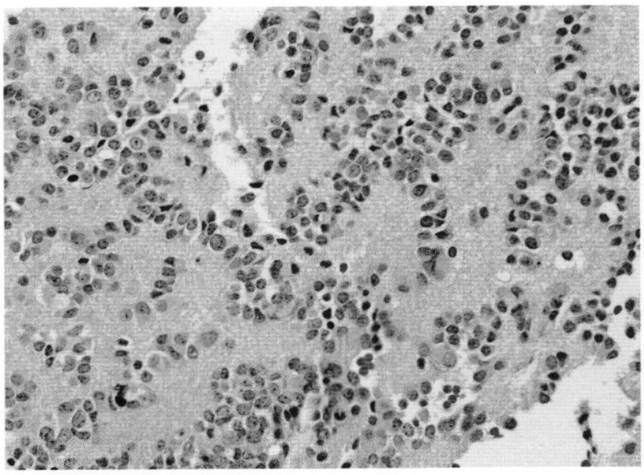

a. Choroid plexus carcinoma
b. DNET
c. Gemistocytic astrocytoma
d. Oligodendroglioma
e. Pineocytoma

54. A pineal region mass with the histological appearance shown is most likely to be which one of the following?

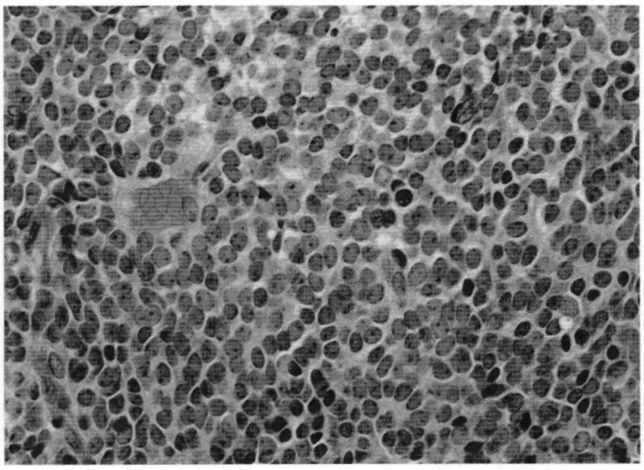

a. Choriocarcinoma
b. Ependymoma
c. Germinoma
d. Pineal parenchymal tumor of intermediate differentiation
e. Teratoma

55. A child with a RB1 mutation develops a supratentorial lesion with the histological appearance shown. Which one of the following is most likely?

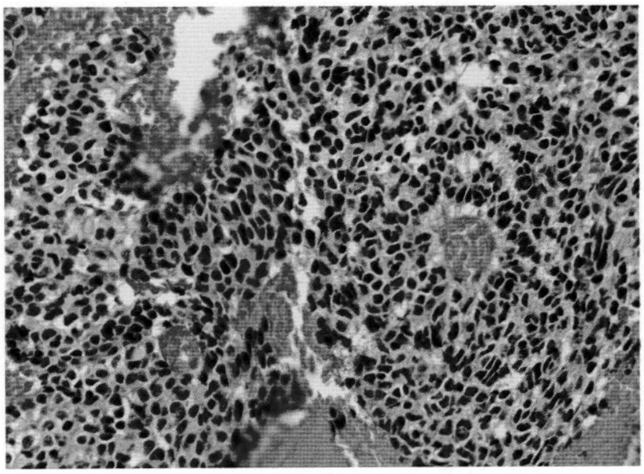

a. Fibrillary astrocytoma
b. Germinoma
c. Pilocytic astrocytoma
d. Pineoblastoma
e. Secretory meningioma

56. Which one of the following is the most likely diagnosis demonstrated in this histological section?

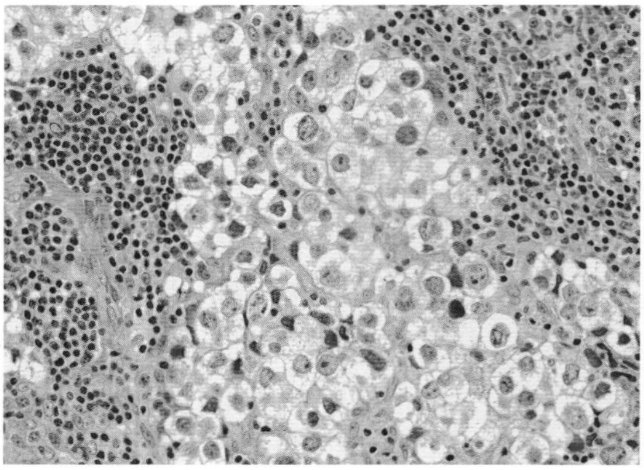

a. Anaplastic astrocytoma
b. Epidermoid
c. Germinoma
d. Hemangioblastoma
e. Oligodendroglioma

57. Which one of the following is the most likely diagnosis demonstrated in this histological section?

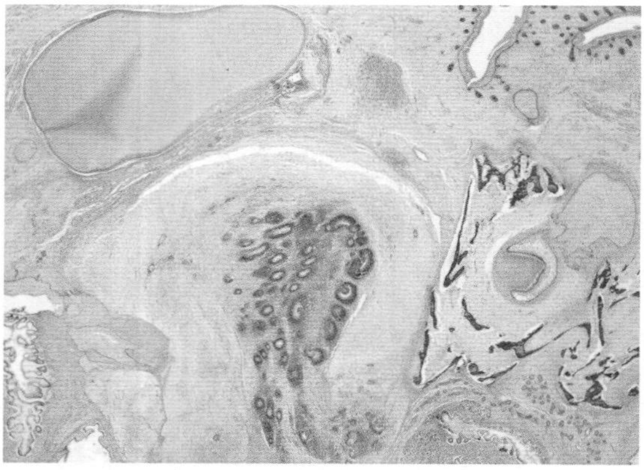

a. AT/RT
b. Chordoma
c. Metastatic melanoma
d. Pituitary adenoma
e. Teratoma

58. Which one of the following is the most likely diagnosis demonstrated in this histological section?

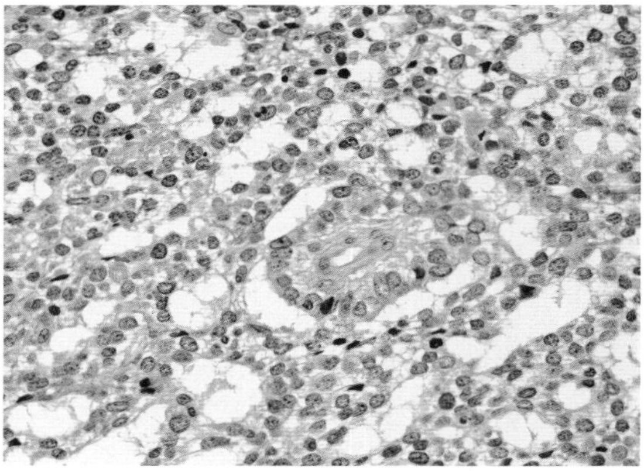

a. Craniopharyngioma
b. Creutzfeldt-Jakob disease
c. Pick's disease
d. Teratoma
e. Yolk sac tumor

59. Which one of the following is the most likely diagnosis demonstrated in this histological section?

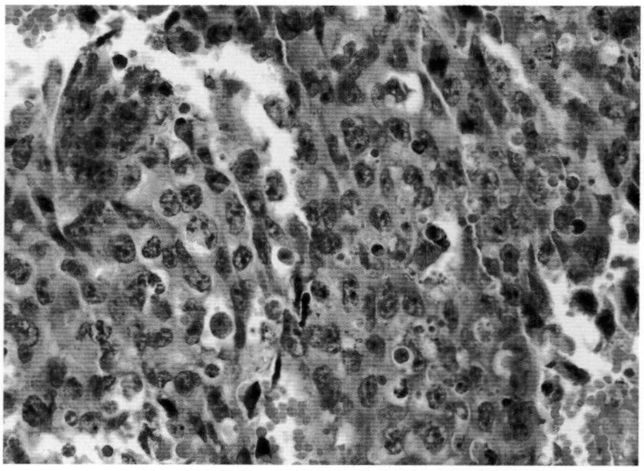

a. DNET
b. Embryonal carcinoma
c. Fibrillary astrocytoma
d. PNET
e. Rhabdoid meningioma

60. Which one of the following is the most likely diagnosis demonstrated in this histological section?

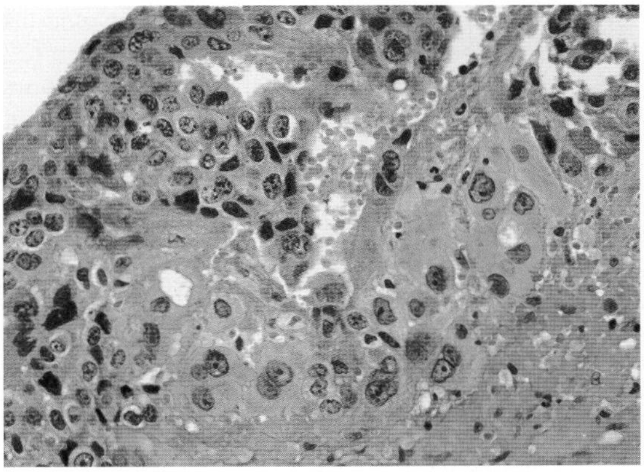

a. Choriocarcinoma
b. Clear cell meningioma
c. Pick bodies
d. Progressive nuclear palsy
e. Renal cell carcinoma metastasis

61. Which one of the following is the most likely diagnosis demonstrated in this histological section?

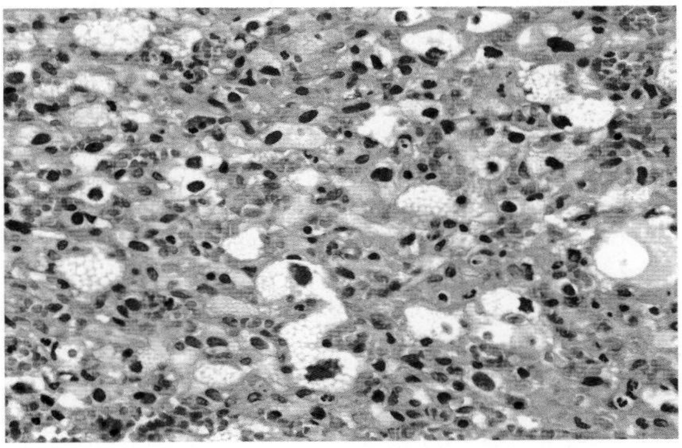

a. Central neurocytoma
b. Hemangioblastoma
c. Neurofibroma
d. Schwannoma
e. Secretory meningioma

62. Which one of the following is the most likely diagnosis demonstrated in this histological section?

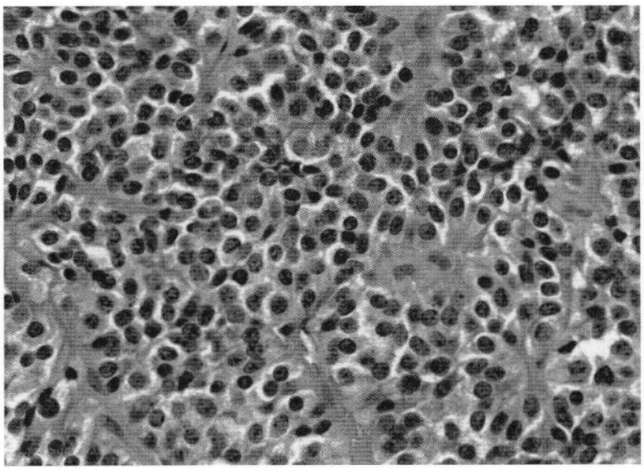

a. Craniopharyngioma
b. Pineocytoma
c. Pituitary adenoma
d. Psammomatous meningioma
e. Teratoma

63. Which one of the following is the most likely diagnosis demonstrated in this histological section?

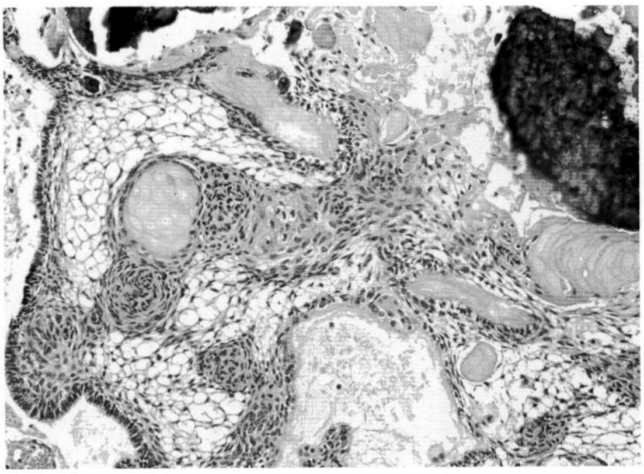

a. Adamantinomatous craniopharyngioma
b. Chordoma
c. Dermoid cyst
d. Pineal parenchymal tumor of intermediate differentiation
e. Rhabdoid meningioma

QUESTIONS 64–81

Additional questions 64–81 available on ExpertConsult.com

SBA ANSWERS

1. **d**—Rosenthal fibers (RFs)

These are intracytoplasmic aggregates of glial fibrillary acidic protein (GFAP) and chaperone proteins. They are bright eosinophilic in H&E-stained sections and cork-screw-like or beaded. Eosinophilic granular bodies are related to Rosenthal fibers and they often occur together. RFs occur most commonly in pilocytic astrocytoma, but may also be seen in Grade I ganglioglioma or Grade II pleomorphic xanthoastrocytoma, and Alexander's disease. They can also be seen in reactive gliosis (piloid gliosis), particularly around chronic lesions in the hypothalamus, spinal cord or cerebellum (e.g., craniopharyngioma, AVM, syrinx, or granulomatous inflammation).

Image with permission from Perry A, Brat DJ. Practical Surgical Neuropathology: A Diagnostic Approach. Churchill Livingstone, Elsevier, 2010.

2. **d**—Posterior pituitary

Posterior pituitary is formed by axonal projections of neurons from the hypothalamus together with primary glial cells and pituicytes, and Herring bodies (eosinophilic axonal dilatations that store neurosecretory peptides) can be seen throughout the posterior gland.

Image with permission from Perry A, Brat DJ. Practical Surgical Neuropathology: A Diagnostic Approach. Churchill Livingstone, Elsevier, 2010.

3. **b**—Gemistocytic astrocytoma

Diffuse astrocytomas are infiltrating glial neoplasm with astrocytic features. WHO grade II. Peak incidence in fourth decade, accounting for 5% of all primary intracranial tumors (10-15% of astrocytic tumors). Genetics: 60% have p53 mutation (90% in gemistocytic) and subset have IDH-1 mutations. Commonly present with seizures and progress to higher grade lesions. Management is surgical resection and radiotherapy. Favorable prognosis with younger age, complete resection, and seizure at presentation. Mean survival 6-8 years. Worse prognosis if older, large size and focal neurological deficit. MRI appearances T1 hypointense, T2/FLAIR hyperintense. Gross appearances of ill-defined lesion with blurring of gray-white matter junction, colored gray/yellow-white without tissue destruction, possibly cystic. Histologically may be fibrillary or gemistocytic. Fibrillary astrocytoma commonest and consists of neoplastic astrocytes in dense fibrillary background, cells often have inconspicuous cytoplasm: "naked" nuclei which can be atypical, with elongation and irregular nuclear contours and often has extensive microcyst formation. Gemistocytic astrocytoma tumor composed of plump, angular cells with eosinophilic, glassy cytoplasm and short, haphazardly arranged processes (gemistocytes; at least 20% are neoplastic) with eccentrically located, round, hyperchromatic nuclei; perivascular lymphocytic infiltrates are common; higher rate of malignant transformation. Immunohistochemistry: GFAP in 100% (not specific), TP53 in >50%, S-100, Ki-67 mitotic index <4%. Histologic differential: reactive gliosis, oligodendroglioma.

Image with permission from Yachnis AT, Rivera-Zengotita ML. Neuropathology, High-Yield Pathology Series, Saunders, Elsevier, 2014.

4. **a**—Anaplastic astrocytoma (WHO III)

Intermediate-grade infiltrating glioma derived from malignant astrocyte-like cells; may arise from lower-grade diffuse astrocytoma, and may progress to glioblastoma. Peak incidence in fifth decade, slight male preponderance; 10% of astrocytic tumors. Genetics: 60% TP53 mutations, 40-60% loss of chromosome 10q, 10-20% PTEN losses, 30-50% p16 losses. Progression from diffuse to anaplastic astrocytoma accompanied by increased seizures and neurologic deficits. Management is biopsy or resection, followed by chemotherapy and radiotherapy. Mean survival 3 years from diagnosis; mean transformation time to GBM is 2 years; better prognosis if young and complete resection; worse prognosis with larger size. MRI: T1 hypointense, T2 hyperintense, but may have foci of gadolinium enhancement. Gross appearances ill-defined without associated tissue destruction. Histology similar to diffuse astrocytoma (fibrillary or gemistocytic) but with increased cellularity and cellular atypia; most important distinguishing feature is presence of mitotic figures. May represent undersampled glioblastoma multiforme in some cases. Staining positive for GFAP, S100, p53 (60%), Increased Ki-67 (MIB1) labeling index 5-10%; mutated IDH-1 in subset of cases. Histologic differential: diffuse astrocytoma, glioblastoma multiforme.

Image with permission from Yachnis AT, Rivera-Zengotita ML. Neuropathology, High-Yield Pathology Series, Saunders, Elsevier, 2014.

5. **c**—Glioblastoma multiforme

This image shows pseudopalisading necrosis. Nuclear palisades may be considered "primary" when they reflect a natural tendency of the nuclei to develop this distinctive pattern of growth or "secondary" when the alignment forms as a response to external influences such as necrosis. The latter have been termed "pseudopalisades": garland-like array of nuclei surrounding a region of necrosis. Palisades are most often seen in (but are not pathognomonic) of schwannomas whereas pseudopalisades are pathognomonic of GBM.

Image with permission from Yachnis AT, Rivera-Zengotita ML. Neuropathology, High-Yield Pathology Series, Saunders, Elsevier, 2014.

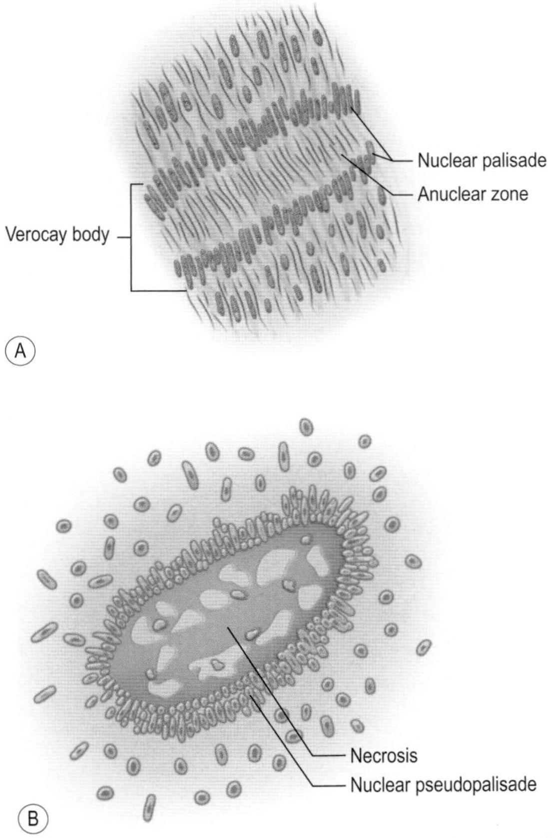

Redrawn with permission from Zülch KJ. Histology of brain tumors. In: Brain Tumors: Their Biology and Pathology. Berlin, Germany: Springer-Verlag, 1986, p. 118-34.

6. **c**—Glioblastoma Multiforme ("glomeruloid tuft" or microvascular proliferation)

This is the most malignant of gliomas, and has astrocytic differentiation; WHO grade IV. Commonest primary brain tumor in adults (15% of all intracranial); accounts for 70% of astrocytic tumors. Mean age at presentation 60 years old, slight male preponderance, rare in children. Most arise rapidly de novo (95%; primary GBM) but some arise from progressive transformation of lower-grade gliomas in younger patients (5%; secondary GBM). Genetics: Primary GBMs show loss of heterozygosity chromosome 10 (70%), epidermal growth factor receptor (EGFR) amplification (40%), p16 deletion (30%), p53 mutation (30%), PTEN mutation (25%), mutated isocitrate dehydrogenase-1 (IDH-1) (<10%); secondary GBMs show mutated isocitrate dehydrogenase-1 (IDH-1) (>80%), loss of heterozygosity chromosome 10 (63%), p53 mutation (60%), EGFR amplification (8%), PTEN mutation (5%). Most occur in subcortical white matter, and may cross corpus callosum into contralateral hemisphere (butterfly glioma). Symptoms present abruptly and progress rapidly, with symptoms of raised ICP, and seizures in 30%. Poor prognosis even with maximal therapy, including surgical resection (complete resection usually impossible given extensive infiltration of tumor) and chemoradiotherapy (Stupp protocol). Prognosis is better in younger patients, those with secondary GBM and tumors with methylated MGMT promotor (respond better to alkylating chemotherapy agents like temozolomide). MRI shows ring/heterogenous enhancement on T1+GAD, central hypointense lesion with zone of surrounding edema on T2. Gross appearance of poorly defined lesion, gray peripherally and yellow/tan necrosis centrally with occasional hemorrhage/cyst. Histology: nuclear atypia, pleomorphism (Figure 1), mitoses, microvascular proliferation (multilayered plump endothelial cells with increased mitotic activity, often forming "glomeruloid tufts"), thrombosis and necrosis (pseudopalisading necrosis is pathognomonic but not always present); "multiforme" indicates, there can be a marked variability between tumors which may be composed of small monotonous cells (small cell glioblastoma), giant cells, gemistocytes, granular cells, and they may rarely have metaplastic epithelial or mesenchymal elements. Immunohistochemistry: GFAP-positive with a high KI-67 (MIB-1) labeling index; p53 immunostaining is positive in tumors with TP53 mutation; mutated isocitrate dehydrogenase-1 (IDH-1)—positive in secondary GBM. Histological differential: anaplastic oligodendroglioma, metastatic carcinoma, lymphoma, radiation necrosis.

Image with permission from Yachnis AT, Rivera-Zengotita ML. Neuropathology, High-Yield Pathology Series, Saunders, Elsevier, 2014.

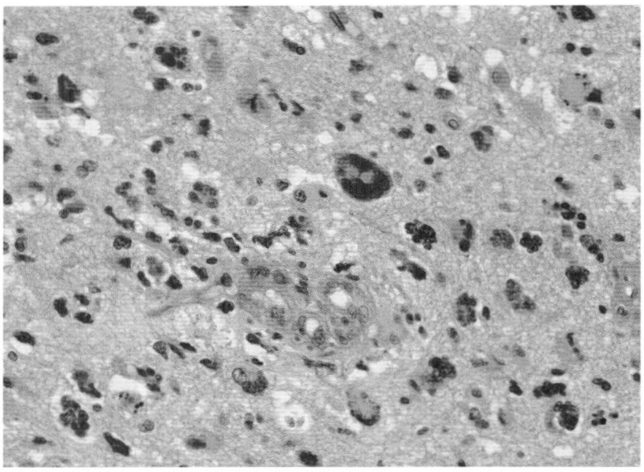

Image with permission from Yachnis AT, Rivera-Zengotita ML. Neuropathology, High-Yield Pathology Series, Saunders, Elsevier, 2014.

7. **d**—Mitotic figure (center—late anaphase)

Mitosis is a continuous process that is traditionally divided into five phases, prophase, prometaphase, metaphase, anaphase and telophase, each stage being readily recognizable with the light microscope (see figure below).

Image with permission from Yachnis AT, Rivera-Zengotita ML. Neuropathology, High-Yield Pathology Series, Saunders, Elsevier, 2014.

8. **e**—Oligodendroglioma

Oligodendrogiomas are diffuse infiltrating gliomas with cells resembling oligodendroglia—WHO grade II. Account for 3% of primary brain tumors and 10% of gliomas; peak in fourth and fifth decades; usually arise in cortex; slight male predominance. Genetics: Isocitrate dehydrogenase-1 (IDH-1) mutations in 75%; 80% have loss of 1p and 19q associated with better prognosis. Presentation: seizures, headache, focal deficit. Imaging: T1 hypointense without contrast enhancement, T2 hyperintense with ill-defined edges; calcification on CT. Gross appearance: soft pink-gray, blurring of gray-white junction; gritty if calcifications. Histology: monomorphic tumor cells with tendency to form small clusters, perinuclear haloes (fried egg appearance) are an artefact of formalin fixation; delicate chicken wire capillary vasculature; perineuronal satellitosis. Immunohistochemistry: GFAP variably reactive, S100 positive, p53 negative, IHD-1 reactive in 75%, Ki67 labeling index variable. Differential: DNET, diffuse astrocytoma, clear cell ependymoma. It should be noted that DNET has cells similar in histology to oligodendroglioma however are arranged in cords and have more superstructure.

Image with permission from Yachnis AT, Rivera-Zengotita ML. Neuropathology, High-Yield Pathology Series, Saunders, Elsevier, 2014.

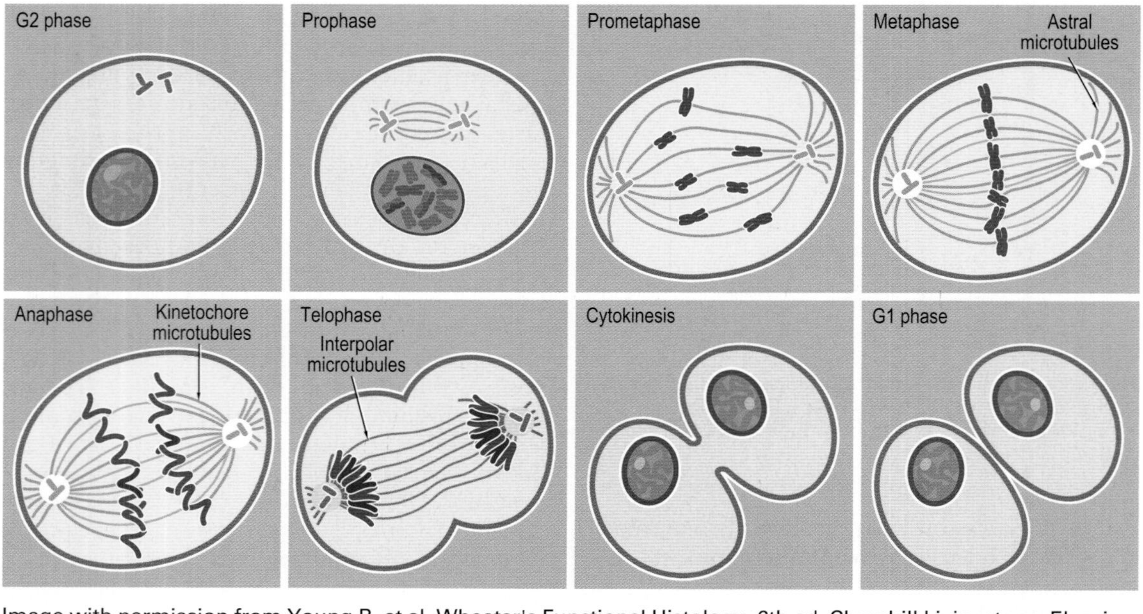

Image with permission from Young B, et al. Wheater's Functional Histology, 6th ed. Churchill Livingstone: Elsevier, 2014.

9. **b**—Anaplastic oligodendroglioma

Anaplastic oligodendroglioma is an oligodendroglial tumor with malignant features—WHO grade III. Accounts for 1% of primary brain tumors and 20-30% of oligodendroglial tumors; peak age 45-50; commonly frontal then temporal cerebrum. Genetics: IDH-1 mutation present in majority; 1p/19q loss in 80% and offers better prognosis. Presentation: seizures; average progression from oligodendroglioma (WHO II) to anaplastic variant is 7 years. Treatment involves surgical resection, radiotherapy and chemotherapy; increased survival in younger patients; median survival 7 years in those with 1p/19q loss, while 3 years in those without. Imaging: as oligodendroglioma but may enhance with contrast. Gross appearance: Well-defined soft pink-gray tumors, may have focal necrosis. Histology: as oligodendroglioma but increased cellularity and pleomorphism, increased mitotic activity, microvascular proliferation, necrosis, gliofibrillary oligodendrocytes and minigemistocytes, focal microcalcifications. Immunohistochemistry: GFAP highly variable, negative p53, mutated IDH-1 positive. Differential: oligodendroglioma (WHO II), anaplastic astrocytoma, small cell glioblastoma.

Image with permission from Yachnis AT, Rivera-Zengotita ML. Neuropathology, High-Yield Pathology Series, Saunders, Elsevier, 2014.

10. **b**—Gliomatosis cerebri

Gliomatosis cerebri is an extensively infiltrating glioma involving at least three lobes of the brain; typically resembles diffuse astrocytoma but occasionally oligodendroglioma—WHO grade III. Peak in fifth decade; bilateral in 75% cases; can arise de novo or secondary to diffuse infiltration by locally infiltrative glioma. Genetics: unclear, some have p53 mutation. Present with seizures, gait disturbance or dementia. Treatment is chemotherapy or whole brain radiotherapy—poor prognosis; favorable factors are young age, good performance status, lower WHO grade and histological subtype. Imaging: diffuse T2 hyperintense lesion, foci of contrast enhancement (multifocal glioma). Gross: blurring/effacement of gray-white junction, gyral widening. Histology: diffusely infiltrating tumor with irregular pleomorphic nuclei consistent with astrocytoma, can have other glial morphologies within same tumor, typically no necrosis/microvascular proliferation. Immunohistochemistry: variable GFAP and S100. Differential: diffuse astrocytoma, anaplastic astrocytoma, oligodendroglioma, progressive multifocal leukoencephalopathy.

Image with permission from Yachnis AT, Rivera-Zengotita ML. Neuropathology, High-Yield Pathology Series, Saunders, Elsevier, 2014.

11. **e**—Pilocytic astrocytoma

Pilocytic astrocytomas are WHO grade I circumscribed, well-differentiated tumors usually presenting as a cystic cerebellar mass but also arise in hypothalamus, optic pathway and brainstem (midbrain tectum or exophytic). Commonest childhood brain tumor; overall accounts for 2% of brain tumors and 6% of gliomas. Average age of diagnosis is 13 years old. Genetics: BRAF gene duplications on chromosome 7q34 lead to KIAA1549:BRAF fusions in 80% of cerebellar, 60% of optic pathway/hypothalamic and 15% of cerebral pilocytic astrocytomas; tumors arising in NF1 have distinct alterations, with loss or mutation in NF1 gene. Presentation can be hydrocephalus (fourth ventricle or aqueduct compression), visual loss (optic pathway) or endocrine dysfunction (hypothalamic). Prognosis is good with approximately 80% survival at 20 years; better prognosis in context of NF1 and worse if supratentorial location. Imaging appearance in cerebellum is a cystic mass with enhancing mural nodule; diffusely enhancing or cystic in hypothalamus; fusiform in optic pathway. Gross appearance is well-demarcated lesion with large cyst and pink-tan, soft mural tumor nodule; may be calcified. Histological appearance is biphasic (dense microfibrillar areas vs loose, microcystic areas), bipolar piloid cells (elongated hair-like cytoplasmic processes), round to oval nuclei, oligodendrogliomatous appearance in some areas, multinucleate cells with clustering of nuclei (pennies on a plate), eosinophilic granular bodies, Rosenthal fibers, microvascular hyperplasia, mitoses are rare. Immunohistochemistry: GFAP positive, S-100 variable, PAS (identifies eosinophilic granular bodies and Rosenthal fibers). Differential: Pilomyxoid variant, diffuse astrocytoma, oligodendroglioma, reactive piloid gliosis (craniopharyngioma, hemangioblastoma, syringomyelia, pineal cysts).

Image with permission from Yachnis AT, Rivera-Zengotita ML. Neuropathology, High-Yield Pathology Series, Saunders, Elsevier, 2014.

12. **c**—Pleomorphic xanthoastrocytoma

Pleomorphic xanthoastrocytoma is a circumscribed astrocytic neoplasm with reticulin deposition and significant pleomorphism (variability of cell/nuclear size, shape and staining) usually found in superficial cortex and involving the meninges. Most are WHO grade II (anaplastic PXA is WHO III). Accounts for <1% all CNS tumors; two thirds occur in those under 18 years. Genetics: BRAF gene (7q34) point mutation (V600E) in two thirds of cases; 50% of lesions will have loss of chromosome 9; multiple other genetic alterations can be found but are not specific. Usually present with prolonged history of seizures. Surgical excision often curative, adjuvant therapy indicated if incomplete resection, recurrent or anaplastic features. Malignant transformation occurs in 15-20%. Favorable prognosis with 80% 5-year and 70% 10-year survival. Imaging appearance is cystic mass with enhancing mural nodule (or solid mass) and meningeal involvement. Gross appearance is firm, well-demarcated solid or cystic mass, often with calcification. Histological appearance: significant cellular and nuclear pleomorphism, spindled cells with astrocytic features, storiform/fascicular growth pattern, multinucleated cells, lipidized tumor cells (in 25%), eosinophilic granular bodies and perivascular lymphocytes; usually very low mitotic rate (no microvascular proliferation or necrosis)—increased mitotic rate (>5 mitoses per high power fields) and necrosis suggestive of anaplastic PXA. Immunohistochemistry: GFAP and S100 positive, neuronal markers (synaptophysin/neurofilament) positive in 25%, Ki67 mitotic index <3%, PAS staining shows eosinophilic granular bodies, reticulin deposition surrounds small groups of tumor cells. Differential: ganglioglioma, glioblastoma variants.

Image with permission from Yachnis AT, Rivera-Zengotita ML. Neuropathology, High-Yield Pathology Series, Saunders, Elsevier, 2014.

13. **e**—Subependymal giant cell astrocytoma

Subependymal giant cell astrocytomas (SEGA) are benign intraventricular neoplasms with astrocytic and neuronal features associated with tuberous sclerosis complex—WHO grade I. Rare (<1% of all brain tumors); seen in 5-15% of TSC patients, usually in first two decades of life. Genetics: TSC is autosomal dominant (but 50% cases arise de novo), 50-90% cases due to TSC2 gene mutation (chromosome 16p13; codes for tuberin) and 10% due to TSC1 mutation (chromosome 9q34; codes for hamartin). Presentation may be due to hydrocephalus as SEGAs arise in lateral ventricle near foramen of Monro (or sometimes third ventricle); seizures are due to cortical hamartomas (tuber) not SEGA; other features of TSC include facial angiofibromas, ungula fibroma, cardiac rhabdomyoma, renal angiolipoma, lymphangiomatosis, retinal hamartomas and hypomelanotic macules. Management is surgical excision (often curative) for primary tumor or recurrence—malignant transformation is rare. Prognosis depends on severity of other TSC manifestations. Imaging appearance is solitary, circumscribed intensely enhancing intraventricular mass. Gross appearance is solid well-circumscribed mass, calcification, spontaneous hemorrhage. Histological appearance: astrocyte-like tumor cells can appear polygonal with glassy eosinophilic cytoplasm, spindled, or epithelioid; cells typically arranged in fascicles or nests separated by fibrillary areas; "ganglioid" cells with neuronal-like features also seen; nuclei with finely granular chromatin and distinct nucleoli; perivascular pseudorosette-like arrangement of tumor cells is frequent; nuclear pleomorphism and multinucleated cells often present; mitotic figures can be present but have no impact on prognosis. Immunohistochemistry: Strong GFAP in subset, S100 reactive, individual cells or processes may be positive for neuronal markers. Differential: central neurocytoma, subependymoma, ependymoma, choroid plexus tumor.

Image with permission from Yachnis AT, Rivera-Zengotita ML. Neuropathology, High-Yield Pathology Series, Saunders, Elsevier, 2014.

14. **C**—Tuberous sclerosis complex

Cerebral cortical hamartomas (tubers): circumscribed areas of disorganized CNS tissue; dystrophic neurons and "balloon cells"; highly associated with seizures. The other CNS lesions seen in TSC are subependymal giant cell astrocytoma (SEGA) and subependymal hamartomatous nodules (candle gutterings).

Image with permission from Yachnis AT, Rivera-Zengotita ML. Neuropathology, High-Yield Pathology Series, Saunders, Elsevier, 2014.

15. **b**—Ependymoma

Ependymomas are a slowly growing tumor arising in the central region of the spinal cord in adults or intraventricular in children—WHO grade II. Represent 5-7% of all CNS tumors. Most common intra-axial spinal cord tumor in adults and third most common posterior fossa tumor in children. Infratentorial ependymomas have bimodal age distribution with first peak in childhood (2-16 years) and second peak at 30-40 years; supratentorial ependymomas have no age predilection. Genetics: 30% incidence of aberration involving chromosome 22, associated with neurofibromatosis type 2 involving tumor suppressor NF2 gene located at 22q12 (distinct from the 22q mutation found in many incidental ependymomas of the spinal cord). Presentation depends on location: infratentorial (hydrocephalus/visual disturbances, ataxia), supratentorial (seizures, focal deficits), spinal cord (motor and sensory deficit). Prognosis is good with overall 60-70% 5-year survival with surgery; best prognosis in adults with spinal cord ependymoma; recurrence is common in children hence goal is gross total resection. Imaging shows well-demarcated masses with variable enhancement on MRI. Gross appearance is soft pink-tan well-circumscribed tumor with occasional hemorrhage/necrosis; fourth ventricular tumors may extend out of foramen of Luscka laterally into subarachnoid space/cistern. Histological appearances: uniform appearance of cells (salt and pepper chromatin), distinctive perivascular pseudorosettes (radially arranged tapering cell processes extending to intratumoral blood vessels) are commoner than true ependymal rosettes (tumor attempting to form little ependymal canal-like channels with central lumen). Variants by location and histology include papillary ependymomas, clear cell ependymomas, tanycytic ependymomas, myxopapillary ependymomas (WHO grade I) and anaplastic ependymomas (WHO grade III). Immunohistochemistry: GFAP-positive perivascular cell processes, dot-like EMA reactivity within inner lining of ependymal rosettes, CD99 (nonspecific), Ki67 mitotic index low <5%. Electron microscopy: luminal cilia and microvilli in ependymal rosettes, zipperlike junctional complexes. Differential diagnosis by location—fourth ventricle tumor in child (medulloblastoma, pilocytic astrocytoma, choroid plexus tumor), adult intra-axial spinal cord tumor (diffuse astrocytoma), supratentorial (central neurocytoma, choroid plexus tumor, astroblastoma).

A fourth type of rosette is the perivascular pseudorosette. In this pattern, a spoke-wheel arrangement of cells with tapered cellular processes radiates around a wall of a centrally placed vessel. Perivascular pseudorosettes are encountered in most ependymomas regardless of grade or variant. As such, they are significantly more sensitive for the diagnosis of ependymomas than true ependymal rosettes. Unfortunately, perivascular pseudorosettes are also less specific in that they are also encountered in medulloblastomas, PNETs, central neurocytomas, and less often in glioblastomas, and a rare pediatric tumor, monomorphous pilomyxoid astrocytomas.

Image with permission from Yachnis AT, Rivera-Zengotita ML. Neuropathology, High-Yield Pathology Series, Saunders, Elsevier, 2014.

16. **c**—Ependymoma—section showing true ependymal rosettes (bottom left) and perivascular pseudorosettes

In contrast to the Homer Wright and the Flexner-Wintersteiner rosettes, the empty-appearing lumen of the true ependymal rosette resembles a tubule lumen and contains no fiber-rich neuropil or central cytoplasmic projections. These tubule-like structures, as well as more elongated versions known as ependymal canals, may represent an attempt by the tumor cells to recapitulate the formation of ventricles with ependymal linings. This rosette provides strong evidence of ependymal differentiation at the light microscopic level. Unfortunately, true ependymal rosettes and canals are found in only a minority of the most well-differentiated ependymomas and most commonly in infratentorial examples.

Image with permission from Yachnis AT, Rivera-Zengotita ML. Neuropathology, High-Yield Pathology Series, Saunders, Elsevier, 2014.

Rosette Type	Associated Tumors
Homer Wright rosette	Neuroblastoma, medulloblastoma, primitive neuroectodermal tumor, pineoblastoma
Flexner-Wintersteiner rosette	Retinoblastoma, pineoblastoma, medulloepithelioma
True ependymal rosette	Ependymoma
Perivascular pseudorosette	Ependymoma, medulloblastoma, primitive neuroectodermal tumor, central neurocytoma, glioblastoma, monomorphous pilomyxoid astrocytomas
Pineocytomatous rosette	Pineocytoma
Neurocytic rosette	Central neurocytoma

Table with permission from Wippold II FJ, Perry A, Neuropathology for the neuroradiologist: rosettes and pseudorosettes. AJNR March 2006;27:488-92.

17. **e**—Retinoblastoma

Flexner-Wintersteiner Rosette—retinoblastoma—tumor cells surrounding central lumen containing cytoplasmic extensions. The tumor cells that form the Flexner-Wintersteiner rosette circumscribe a central lumen that contains small cytoplasmic extensions of the encircling cells; however, unlike the center of the Homer Wright rosette, the central lumen does not contain the fiber-rich neuropil. Like the Homer Wright rosette, the Flexner-Wintersteiner rosette signifies a specific form of tumor differentiation. This contention is supported by electron microscopy where the tumor cells forming the Flexner-Wintersteiner rosette have ultrastructural features of primitive photoreceptor cells. In addition, special staining properties of the rosette lumen resemble those seen in rods and cones. Although this type of rosette is particularly characteristic of retinoblastomas, it may also be seen in pineoblastomas and medulloepitheliomas, where it is similarly thought to represent retinal differentiation.

Image with permission from Gault J, Vander JF, Ophthalmology Secrets in Color, 3rd ed. Mosby, Elsevier, 2007.

FURTHER READING

Wippold II FJ, Perry A, Neuropathology for the neuroradiologist: rosettes and pseudorosettes. AJNR March 2006;27:488-92.

18. **c**—Homer Wright rosette

James Homer Wright (1869-1928), recognized a group of adrenal and sympathetic nervous system tumors, which became known as neuroblastomas. The typical Homer Wright rosette with its central lumen or hub filled with fiber-like processes can also be found in medulloblastomas and histologically similar tumors occurring outside of the cerebellum, designated PNETs. Although the cellular mechanisms responsible for the formation of rosettes within medulloblastomas and the significance of these rosettes are not fully understood, most investigators believe that their presence indicates neuronal differentiation. The delicate fibrillary material found within the central lumen of the Homer Wright rosette is composed of neuropil, which contains primitive neuronal processes or neurites. Although the identification of Homer Wright rosettes in a posterior fossa tumor is nearly pathognomonic of the diagnosis of medulloblastoma, the rosettes are encountered in only a third of these tumors. Moreover, Homer Wright rosettes may be found in other tumors such as supratentorial PNETs and pineoblastomas.

Pineocytomas and central neurocytomas represent well-differentiated neuronal neoplasms with small rounded nuclei, analogous to those normally encountered in the internal granular layer of the cerebellum or the dentate fascia of the hippocampus. Although they likely originate from slightly different precursors, the histologic features of these two tumors are virtually identical, including their tendency to form neuropil-rich rosettes, referred to as pineocytomatous rosettes in pineocytomas and neurocytic rosettes in central neurocytoma. Both are quite similar to the Homer Wright rosette, but they are generally larger and more irregular in contour. As in the other types of rosettes discussed, the presence of pineocytomatous or neurocytic rosettes is generally thought to reflect differentiation of the tumor, in this case neuronal. The cells of the pineocytomatous and neurocytic rosettes are also considered to be much more differentiated than the cells forming Homer Wright rosettes in that the nuclei are slightly larger, more rounded, much less mitotically active, and paler or less hyperchromatic.

Image with permission from Perry A, Brat DJ. Practical Surgical Neuropathology: A Diagnostic Approach, Churchill Livingstone, Elsevier, 2010.

FURTHER READING

Wippold II FJ, Perry A, Neuropathology for the neuroradiologist: rosettes and pseudorosettes. AJNR March 2006;27:488-92.

19. **d**—Papillary ependymoma

Papillary ependymomas is a rare variant with uniform epithelial surfaces along the border with CSF with papillary (nipple-like) or pseudopapillary architecture. Differential: choroid plexus tumor, metastasis.

Image with permission from Yachnis AT, Rivera-Zengotita ML. Neuropathology, High-Yield Pathology Series, Saunders, Elsevier, 2014.

20. **c**—Clear cell ependymomas

This is a mimic of oligodendroglioma but has well-demarcated border with adjacent brain; usually located in cerebral hemisphere of young adults; may behave more aggressively. Electron microscopy shows deep nuclear invaginations in the clear cell variant.

Image with permission from Yachnis AT, Rivera-Zengotita ML. Neuropathology, High-Yield Pathology Series, Saunders, Elsevier, 2014.

21. **e**—Tanycytic ependymomas

These usually arise in the spinal cord as a discrete mass that is well demarcated from the adjacent neural tissue; forms fascicles of highly fibrillated bipolar spindle cells; mimic of diffuse astrocytoma; ependymal rosettes usually absent with only vague pseudorosettes.

Image with permission from Yachnis AT, Rivera-Zengotita ML. Neuropathology, High-Yield Pathology Series, Saunders, Elsevier, 2014.

22. **a**—Anaplastic ependymoma

Anaplastic ependymoma is an malignant ependymal tumor seen most commonly in posterior fossa in children—WHO grade III. Treatment included surgical resection (extent is key predictor of outcome), chemotherapy and radiotherapy. Worse prognosis if <3 years old, incomplete tumor resection and CSF dissemination at presentation. Ependymomatous features (e.g., perivascular pseudorosettes) present, but also malignant features such as increases cellularity, mitoses, microvascular proliferation and pseudopalisading necrosis. Differential: ependymoma, poorly differentiated embryonal tumors, astrocytoma, anaplastic oligodendroglioma.

Image with permission from Yachnis AT, Rivera-Zengotita ML. Neuropathology, High-Yield Pathology Series, Saunders, Elsevier, 2014.

23. **c**—Myxopapillary ependymoma

Myxopapillary ependymoma is a slow growing ependymal tumor commonly arising in the conus medullaris, cauda equina and filum terminale—WHO grade I. Represents 10% of all ependymomas, and 50% of all spinal cord ependymomas; twice as common in men. Presents as chronic back pain, sciatica, sensorimotor deficit and sphincter disturbance. Management is surgical resection (high cure rate), greater than 10-year survival; recurrence may be seen in tumors with nerve root invasion. Imaging shows enhancing, well-demarcated ovoid masses attached to filum terminale. Gross appearance is soft, lobulated, white-tan tumor easily separable from surrounding structures. Histological appearance cuboidal/spindled tumor cells arranged radially around papillary vascular cores, myxoid matrix with microcystic structures. Immunohistochemistry: GFAP positive, S100 and vimentin reactivity, absent cytokeratin activity. Differential: filum terminale region tumors (schwannoma, meningioma, paraganglioma), sacral tumors (chordoma, chondrosarcoma), metastatic adenocarcinoma.

Image with permission from Yachnis AT, Rivera-Zengotita ML. Neuropathology, High-Yield Pathology Series, Saunders, Elsevier, 2014.

24. **e**—Subependymoma

Subependymoma is a benign glial neoplasm usually attached to wall of lateral ventricles near the foramen of Monro or floor of fourth ventricle—WHO grade I. Mean age of presentation approximately 60, mostly incidental on imaging or autopsy, though can present with hydrocephalus. Treatment is total or subtotal resection, with low recurrence. Imaging shows small, nodular, discrete mass (<2 cm), occasional foci of calcification/hemorrhage/cystic change. Grossly distinct from adjacent brain tissue. Histology shows nodular growth pattern, clusters of small bland nuclei within background of eosinophilic fibrillary processes, microcystic change (if in lateral ventricle), vague perivascular pseudorosette-like pattern. Immunohistochemistry shows GFAP-positive cell processes, negative for synaptophysin, low mitotic index. Differential: ependymoma, central neurocytoma, astrocytoma.

Image with permission from Yachnis AT, Rivera-Zengotita ML. Neuropathology, High-Yield Pathology Series, Saunders, Elsevier, 2014.

25. **c**—Choroid plexus papilloma

Choroid plexus papilloma (CPP) is an intraventricular papillary neoplasm—WHO grade I. Represents 0.3-0.6% of brain tumors and 2-4% of pediatric brain tumors (10-20% of brain tumors in <1 year olds). Most common in children <15 years; fourth ventricular CPP shows no age predilection while lateral ventricular CPPs arise in younger patients (<20 years). Location is lateral ventricle (50%) > fourth (40%) > third ventricle (5%). Genetics: Association with SV-40 T antigen; May arise in Aicardi syndrome (sporadic mutation linked to X chromosome; partial or total agenesis of corpus callosum, chorioretinal lacunae, infantile spasms); no mutations in p53 gene unlike choroid plexus carcinoma. Presentation is with increasing head circumference or hydrocephalus. Management is surgical resection and prognosis is good. Imaging appearances of well-circumscribed intraventricular mass, enhancing with gadolinium and T2 hyperintense. Gross appearance of well-defined cauliflower-like mass that may adhere to ventricular wall. Histological appearance: resembles normal choroid plexus but has increased cellularity, nuclear crowding, solid areas and stratification; fibrovascular tissue core surrounded by single layer of columnar-cuboidal epithelium with basally oriented nuclei; atypical CPP (WHO grade II) has increased mitoses, pleomorphism and foci of necrosis. Immunohistochemistry: Immunoreactive to transthyretin, cytokeratins (CK), and synaptophysin; 75% are CK7-positive and CK20-negative; Ki-67 (MIB1) labeling range from 0% to 6%; S-100 staining in 55% to 90% of reported cases; Focal glial fibrillary acidic protein (GFAP) reactivity. Differential: normal/hypertrophy of choroid plexus, choroid plexus carcinoma; ependymoma; metastatic carcinoma.

Image with permission from Yachnis AT, Rivera-Zengotita ML. Neuropathology, High-Yield Pathology Series, Saunders, Elsevier, 2014.

26. **a**—Choroid plexus papilloma

Choroid plexus carcinoma is a malignant choroid plexus neoplasm (WHO grade III; 80%

arise in children). Genetics: Reported association with p53 germline mutation or Li-Fraumeni syndrome; nearly all demonstrate p53 immunoreactivity; no INI-1 mutations despite histologic resemblance to atypical teratoid/rhabdoid tumors. Present with hydrocephalus and focal neurology. Management is surgical resection, chemotherapy and irradiation. Poor prognosis due to CSF dissemination. Imaging: large ventricular poorly defined lesion, edema of adjacent brain. Gross appearance: gray-tan tumor with areas of hemorrhage and necrosis, brain invasion may be evident. Histological criteria (at least four of the following): frequent mitoses (>5 of 10 high power fields), increased cellularity, nuclear pleomorphism, blurring of papillary pattern, necrosis. Immunohistochemistry: Cytokeratin reactivity, less reactive than CPP to S100 and transthyretin, GFAP 20%, EMA negative. Differential: AT/RT, metastatic carcinoma.

Image with permission from Yachnis AT, Rivera-Zengotita ML, Neuropathology, High-Yield Pathology Series, Saunders, Elsevier, 2014.

27. **d—**Medulloblastoma

Medulloblastomas are malignant embryonal tumors (PNET) arising in the posterior fossa of children—WHO grade IV. Commonest PNET—0.5/100,000; peak incidence 5-10 years (adults cluster in 30s); accounts for 20% of brain tumors in children, and is the commonest malignant brain tumor in children. Genetics:

- Classic medulloblastoma: most common genetic alteration: 17p loss with isochromosome 17q formation
- Large cell/anaplastic medulloblastoma associated with C-MYC oncogene amplifications
- Desmoplastic medulloblastoma: PTCH gene mutations (sonic hedgehog pathway)
- Gorlin syndrome (nevoid basal cell carcinoma): autosomal dominant germline mutations of patched gene at 9q22.3 with odontogenic keratocysts, pitting of palms and soles, skeletal anomalies, lamellar calcium deposition in falx cerebri and diaphragma sellae, calcifying ovarian fibromas, and multifocal, early-onset basal cell carcinomas
- Li-Fraumeni syndrome/p53 mutation syndromes
- Turcot syndrome (Type 2): medulloblastoma arises in setting of autosomal dominant adenomatous polyposis of colon resulting from APC mutations on chromosome 5q21 APC
- Rubinstein-Taybi syndrome (with meningiomas and oligodendrogliomas): mutations in CREB-binding protein gene on chromosome 16p13 with cognitive impairment, growth retardation, microcephaly, facies

Presentation is with raised ICP or cerebellar signs—75% arise from vermis and fill the fourth ventricle; 30% show CSF spread with spinal drop metastases at presentation. Management is maximal surgical resection followed by chemotherapy and craniospinal irradiation—overall 5-year survival 65%. Good prognostic factors: 3-22 years old at presentation, gross total excision, no CSF spread, WNT signaling activation (nuclear b-catenin immunoreactivity), TrkC neurotrophin receptor overexpression, balanced 17q, monosomy chromosome 6, nodular/desmoplastic and extensively nodular variants. Poor prognostic factors: <3 years old, subtotal resection, CSF dissemination at presentation, C-MYK/N-MYC amplification, isochromosome 17q (unbalanced), 17p loss, large cell/anaplastic variant (aggressive and extraneural metastasis has been reported). Imaging: solid heterogenous enhancing mass adjacent or extending into fourth ventricle; nodular/desmoplastic variant location in cerebellar hemisphere; extensively nodular variant has enhancing nodules which cluster (look grape-like). Gross appearances: solid masses of friable gray-white tissue involving cerebellar folia and leptomeninges. Histological appearance: small round blue cell tumor composed of sheets of undifferentiated cells with indistinct cytoplasm, hyperchromatic angulated nuclei (molding); frequent mitoses; Homer Wright rosettes in about 40% of cases; apoptosis or necrosis may be present but more prominent in large cell/anaplastic variants; overall architecture may be swirling, fascicular, diffuse; scanty stroma containing small blood vessels (occasional microvascular proliferation). Immunohistochemistry: Most are synaptophysin immunoreactive; nodular foci of neuronal differentiation (synaptophysin, neurofilament); GFAP-positive elements appear to be focally entrapped; positive for INI-1 (hSNF5/SMARCB1) using BAF47 antibody to exclude AT/RT; S-100 may be seen in melanocytic variant; Desmin and myoglobin positivity in myogenic cells; Ki-67 index is variable, but generally >20%. Differential: AT/RT, ependymoma, lymphoma, small cell carcinoma, metastasis, high-grade glioma.

Image with permission from Yachnis AT, Rivera-Zengotita ML. Neuropathology, High-Yield Pathology Series, Saunders, Elsevier, 2014.

28. **c**—Large cell/anaplastic medulloblastoma

Large cell/anaplastic medulloblastomas are typically grouped together and probably represent a spectrum; they share frequent mitoses, apoptotic cells, pleomorphism, cell "wrapping" (seen in section). Large cell medulloblastoma: cells are large with rounded vesicular nuclei, prominent nucleoli, and conspicuous eosinophilic cytoplasm; discohesive with numerous mitotic and apoptotic cells. Anaplastic medulloblastoma: marked variation in nuclear size and shape with some bizarre forms: multinucleated, giant cells, cell wrapping/molding.

Nodular/desmoplastic medulloblastoma: reticulin rich, proliferatively active cellular tumor with nodular reticulin-free "pale islands" Neuronal differentiation in nodules (synaptophysin, neurofilament immunoreactive) Reduced mitotic activity in nodules.

Medulloblastoma with extensive nodularity (previously called "cerebellar neuroblastoma"): more advanced neurocytic maturation with more lobular (nodular), pale areas with neuropil-like stroma.

- Predilection for children <3 years of age with a more favorable prognosis than other subtypes
- Greatly decreased proliferation index, linear pattern of tumor cell nuclei
- Rare maturation to benign ganglioneurocytic or gangliogliomatous elements
- "Neuroblastic" foci: may be found in any given tumor case

Image with permission from Yachnis AT, Rivera-Zengotita ML, Neuropathology, High-Yield Pathology Series, Saunders, Elsevier, 2014.

29. **d**—Supratentorial PNET

Supratentorial/CNS-PNET area heterogenous group of embryonal tumors composed of primitive-appearing neuroepithelial cells expressing neuronal or glial antigens and most commonly arise in cerebral hemispheres. Represent 1-3% of pediatric CNS neuroepithelial tumors; age range 4 weeks to 20 years; in older patients may be mistaken as PNET-like areas within GBM. Present with raised ICP, localizing signs or seizures. Management is chemotherapy (stem cell rescue) and radiotherapy as usually large and non-resectable. Overall 5-year survival 20-30%. Imaging: large enhancing lesions with mass effect, restricted diffusion, calcification. Gross—large soft, tan-gray tumors with areas of necrosis or calcification. Histological appearance: highly cellular with scant cytoplasm, hyperchromatic nuclei with granular chromatin, frequent mitoses, necrosis. Immunohistochemistry: variably positive for neuronal antigens (NF, synaptophysin, NSE, beta-III tubulin), high Ki67 labeling index, positive for INI-1. Differential: AT/RT, germ cell tumors, GBM.

Image with permission from Yachnis AT, Rivera-Zengotita ML. Neuropathology, High-Yield Pathology Series, Saunders, Elsevier, 2014.

30. **a**—Atypical teratoid/rhabdoid tumor

Atypical teratoid/rhabdoid tumors (AT/RT) are high-grade embryonal tumors expressing epithelial, neuronal and mesenchymal lineage antigens—WHO grade IV. Represent 1-2% of all pediatric brain tumors (10% of infant brain tumors); >90% cases in under 5 year olds (mean age 20 months); 1.5-2:1 male preponderance; supratentorial location (cerebrum, suprasellar) slightly more common than infratentorial (cerebellar, CPA with brainstem involvement). Genetics: monosomy/deletions or mutations of INI1 (hSNF5/SMARCB1) gene on chromosome 22q11.2 (INI1 protein functions in chromatin remodeling); rhabdoid predisposition syndrome: germline loss or inactivation of INI1 gene. Presentation usually nonspecific irritable, vomiting, lethargic, headache. Management influenced by CSF dissemination (present in 1/3 at presentation) and age (risks of radiotherapy if <3 years); surgery can confirm diagnosis but is not curative; chemotherapy is mainstay. Poor survival 50% at 6 months; survival >2 years is exceptional. Imaging: T1 hypointense, variable enhancement, diffusion restricting, large, partly cystic/hemorrhagic. Gross: large, soft demarcated mass. Histology: Heterogeneous lesion; rhabdoid cells (large, distinct cell borders with eccentric nuclei, macronucleoli, and prominent pink cytoplasmic inclusions); occasional vacuolization; some areas have overlapping histology with other embryonal tumors (such as medulloblastoma or CNS-PNET); spindled mesenchymal or even myxoid-like components may be prominent; overall architecture can be nested, spindled, sheet-like, or even glandular. Immunohistochemistry: INI1 protein negative (BAF47 antibody), immunoreactive for vimentin and EMA, variably positive for SMA, neurofilament, GFAP, synaptophysin, and cytokeratins (AE1/3; CAM 5.20; Ki-67 [MIB-1] labeling index is typically high [>50%]). Differential: medulloblastoma, supratentorial PNET, choroid plexus tumors, germ cell tumors, high-grade glioma.

Image with permission from Yachnis AT, Rivera-Zengotita ML, Neuropathology, High-Yield Pathology Series, Saunders, Elsevier, 2014.

31. **b**—Ganglioglioma cell tumors

These are well-differentiated CNS tumors with mature neurons (ganglion cells) as a defining feature:

1. Ganglioglioma—ganglion cell tumor with a low grade glial element (WHO grade I)
2. Gangliocytoma—ganglion cell tumor without a glial element (WHO grade I)
3. Anaplastic ganglioglioma—ganglion cells and anaplastic glial elements (WHO grade III)

Represent 4% of primary brain tumors (incidence 0.2/100,000 per year); commoner in children and temporal lobe. Presentation with seizures or location specific symptoms. Management is surgery (>90% 10-year survival), while combination with radiotherapy for inoperable or anaplastic (WHO III) cases. Imaging: variably enhancing solid or cystic tumor, possibly calcified. Gross appearance: demarcated tumor mass with or without cystic change or calcification. Histology: disorganized collection of mature ganglion cells with variable glial background; clusters of mature neurons, with large nuclei, prominent nucleoli in disordered/haphazard arrangements; ganglion cells may exhibit binucleation or have bizarre-appearing nuclei; Rosenthal fibers, eosinophilic granular bodies; perivascular lymphocytes, microcalcifications also can be present; exclude anaplastic features. Immunohistochemistry: synaptophysin, chromogranin, neurofilament reactive neoplastic ganglion cells but NeuN negative; GFAP-positive in astrocytic elements; Ki-67/MIB1 usually low, <2%. Differential: pilocytic astrocytoma, diffuse astrocytoma, DNET, developmental lesion, cortical dysplasia, tuberous sclerosis.

Image with permission from Yachnis AT, Rivera-Zengotita ML. Neuropathology, High-Yield Pathology Series, Saunders, Elsevier, 2014.

32. **b**—Dysembryoplastic neuroepithelial tumor (DNET)

This is a benign neuronal-glial neoplasm arising from gray matter—WHO grade I. Accounts for <1% primary brain tumors; affects children/young adults (mean age 9 years); first seizure usually <20 years of age; supratentorial and cortical origin (temporal > frontal). Present with seizures. Excellent prognosis with surgery—recurrence is rare. Imaging: T1 hypointense, T2 hyperintense non-enhancing lesion located within expanded cortical ribbon. Gross appearance: multinodular or cystic; gelatinous/mucoid mass with discrete margins. Histological: specific glioneuronal element consisting of oligodendrocyte-like cells arranged along bundled axons separated by a myxoid matrix that contains floating neurons; cortical dysplasia may be found adjacent to the neoplasm; eosinophilic granular bodies, bipolar astrocytes; no mitotic figures, necrosis, or endothelial hyperplasia. Immunohistochemistry: floating neurons are positive for synaptophysin/NF/neuron specific enolase; GFAP in astrocytes; S100 in oligodendrocyte-like cells; mucin is Alcian blue positive; Ki67 index <1-2%. Differential: oligodendroglioma, astrocytoma with microcystic change, ganglioglioma/cytoma, papillary glioneuronal tumor, rosette-forming glioneuronal tumor of the fourth ventricle.

Image with permission from Yachnis AT, Rivera-Zengotita ML, Neuropathology, High-Yield Pathology Series, Saunders, Elsevier, 2014.

33. **a**—Central neurocytoma

This is an intraventricular tumor composed of uniform round cells with neuronal differentiation—WHO grade II. Rare 0.25-0.5% of intracranial tumors; peak age 20-40 (rare <10 years or >70 years). Presentation is with raised ICP/hydrocephalus; tumor typically attached to septum pellucidum near foramen of Monro. Good prognosis with complete surgical excision—incomplete excision associated with recurrence/progression; radiotherapy used in some cases. Imaging: enhancing intraventricular mass attached to septum pellucidum (calcified/cystic). Gross appearance: well demarcated, gray friable tumor—calcified/cystic/hemorrhagic. Histology: monomorphic bland appearing cells with oval nuclei and salt and pepper chromatin, background fibrillary neuropil is eosinophilic, mimic of oligodendroglioma, rare Homer Wright rosettes and ganglion cells, perivascular pseudorosettes, perinuclear haloes, rarely anaplastic features. Immunohistochemistry: Synaptophysin/NeuN positive, GFAP for astrocytes, Ki67 low <2%, unlike oligodendrogliomas do not show loss of 1p/19q. Differential: oligodendroglioma, ependymoma, pineocytoma, DNET.

Image with permission from Yachnis AT, Rivera-Zengotita ML. Neuropathology, High-Yield Pathology Series, Saunders, Elsevier, 2014.

34. **c**—Hemangiopericytomas

These are rare dural-based mesenchymal tumors—WHO grade II or III. Account for 0.4% of primary CNS tumors; common between second and sixth decades (mean age 45). Presentation is due to local compression/invasion, commonly headache and seizures or myelopathy (10% arise as spinal lesions). Primary treatment is surgical resection but 90% recurrence rate and metastasis in up to 20%; radiotherapy/radiosurgery in some cases. Imaging: dural-based contrast-enhancing masses. Gross appearance: solid, gray to red/brown tumors with tendency to bleed excessively during surgery. Histological appearance: monomorphous cellular spindle cell tumor with staghorn-like blood vessels, focally storiform architecture, no intranuclear inclusions, no whorls/psammoma bodies, necrosis uncommon; WHO III have >5 mitoses per 10 HPF with moderate to high cellular atypia and cellularity. Immunohistochemistry: tumor cells negative for CD34 but blood vessels positive for CD34, Ki67 index mean 5-10% (up to 40%), reticulin rich, vimentin positive but negative for S100 and EMA. Differential: meningioma, solitary fibrous tumor (positive for CD34, Bcl-2, CD99) meningeal sarcoma, metastasis, meningeal lymphoid tumors.

Image with permission from Yachnis AT, Rivera-Zengotita ML, Neuropathology, High-Yield Pathology Series, Saunders, Elsevier, 2014.

35. **c**—Meningiomas

These are tumors arising from meningothelial (arachnoidal) cells attached to the inner surface of the dura mater—most are WHO grade I. Represent 25-30% of primary intracranial tumors; 1.4% at autopsy; most common in fifth to seventh decades, commoner in females 3:1 (10:1 for spinal meningiomas); multiple in 10%. Genetics: many arise secondary to radiation exposure, deletion of chromosome 22, multiple meningiomas seen in NF2 (22q11-13.1 mutation; Merlin peptide production), DAL-1 loss (18p11.3). Presentation: headache and seizures commonest, but local compression related also. Location: intracranial, intraspinal or orbital; intracranial locations are convexity (half of these parasaggital), olfactory groove, sellar/parasellar (cavernous sinus), petrous ridge, tentorium, posterior fossa; rarely in intraventricular/extradural location. Management is gross total resection; recurrence if not completely excised; radiotherapy/radiosurgery for recurrence or small surgically inaccessible lesions (cavernous sinus). Imaging: circumscribed, isodense/isointense contrast-enhancing lesion with dural tail sign; peritumoral edema due to vascular compromise; calcification or bone formation/hyperostosis on CT. Gross appearance: well-demarcated, firm, rubbery, yellow-tan, round/lobulated mass compressing adjacent brain/spinal cord, invasion of skull/hyperostosis. Histology (commonest meningothelial variant): lobules of uniform cells in a syncytium, whorls and psammoma bodies, bland oval nuclei, fine chromatin with central clearing, nuclear pseudoinclusions. Immunohistochemistry: Positive for vimentin and EMA, S100 variable, 60% progesterone receptor positive (mostly females). Differential: Metastatic carcinoma, schwannoma, solitary fibrous tumor, sarcoma.

Image with permission from Yachnis AT, Rivera-Zengotita ML, Neuropathology, High-Yield Pathology Series, Saunders, Elsevier, 2014.

36. **c**—Fibrous (fibroblastic) meningioma: spindled cells forming interlacing, parallel fascicles with surrounding collagenous stroma; psammoma bodies and whorls uncommon. Differential: Schwannoma (versus fibroblastic meningioma).

Image with permission from Yachnis AT, Rivera-Zengotita ML, Neuropathology, High-Yield Pathology Series, Saunders, Elsevier, 2014.

37. **e**—Psammomatous meningiomas are typically found in thoracic spinal region of middle-aged women. *Psammomatous meningioma*: variant having abundant psammoma bodies; most common in the thoracic spinal cord of middle-aged women. Differential: Reactive process with calcification (psammomatous meningioma).

Image with permission from Yachnis AT, Rivera-Zengotita ML. Neuropathology, High-Yield Pathology Series, Saunders, Elsevier, 2014.

38. **e**—Secretory meningioma: "classic" appearing tumor cells with numerous interspersed intracellular lumina containing eosinophilic secretions (pseudopsammoma bodies); may have abundant mast cells; may have peritumoral edema. Pseudopsammoma bodies of secretory variant are carcinembryonic antigen (CEA) immunoreactive (and periodic acid-Schiff [PAS] positive). Differential: Metastatic adenocarcinoma (versus secretory meningioma).

Image with permission from Yachnis AT, Rivera-Zengotita ML. Neuropathology, High-Yield Pathology Series, Saunders, Elsevier, 2014.

39. **a**—Angiomatous meningioma: predominance of small hyalinized blood vessels; background tumor cells may demonstrate marked degenerative nuclear atypia. Differential: Vascular malformation, hemangioblastoma (versus angiomatous meningioma).

Image with permission from Yachnis AT, Rivera-Zengotita ML. Neuropathology, High-Yield Pathology Series, Saunders, Elsevier, 2014.

40. **a**—Atypical meningiomas

These are those dural-based meningothelial tumors which are WHO grade II (includes atypical, chordoid and clear cell variants). Account for 5-20% of meningiomas; clear cell and chordoid usually affect younger individuals (third decade). Genetics (in addition to classic mutations) losses on 1p, 6q, 10q, 14q, 18q; gains on 1p, 9q, 12q, 15q, 20q. Surgical resection is primary treatment; 30-40% recurrence; radiotherapy/radiosurgery in some cases; 80% 10-year survival; 25% may progress to malignant (anaplastic) meningioma WHO grade III. Gross appearance: larger than benign variants, necrosis and adherence to adjacent brain tissue. Histological appearance: high mitotic index (>4 per 10 HPF) or 3 of hypercellularity/sheet-like growth pattern/small cell formation/macronuclei/necrosis/brain invasion/chordoid features/clear cell features. Immunohistochemistry: Vimentin positive but less consistent EMA. Differential: meningioma (WHO I or III), schwannoma, solitary fibrous tumor, chordoma, metastatic clear cell carcinoma.

Image with permission from Yachnis AT, Rivera-Zengotita ML. Neuropathology, High-Yield Pathology Series, Saunders, Elsevier, 2014.

41. **b**—Chordoid meningioma

This affects younger individuals (mean age 35); slight female predominance; rare association with Castleman disease, iron-refractory anemia, bone marrow plasmacytosis with dysgammaglobulinemia. Chordoid meningioma: usually in supratentorial location; rarely found intraventricular, near the foramen jugulare, and intraorbital; most common presenting symptoms are headache, mental or visual disturbances, and seizures. Chordoid meningioma: chordoma-like tumor with cords, nests, or trabeculae of epithelioid and spindled tumor cells with eosinophilic, often vacuolated cytoplasm; myxoid stroma; foci of typical meningotheliomatous features; foci of chronic inflammation may be prominent. Chordoid meningiomas are typically PAS positive. Differential: Chordoma, other meningioma (versus chordoid meningioma).

Image with permission from Yachnis AT, Rivera-Zengotita ML. Neuropathology, High-Yield Pathology Series, Saunders, Elsevier, 2014.

42. **b**—Clear cell meningioma

Rare variant also affecting children and young adults (mean age 29 years old) although reported at all ages; slight female predominance. Clear cell meningioma: tendency to arise in the cerebellopontine angle or cauda equina; also found along cerebral convexities; may have headache and cranial nerve palsies. Histology: Clear cell meningioma: sheets of polygonal tumor cells with abundant clear cytoplasm, bland round to oval nuclei, separated by bands of collagen and interspersed vessels with perivascular hyalinization; rare mitoses; nuclear pleomorphism and necrosis uncommon. Differential: Metastatic clear cell carcinoma, microcystic meningioma (versus clear cell meningioma).

Image with permission from Yachnis AT, Rivera-Zengotita ML. Neuropathology, High-Yield Pathology Series, Saunders, Elsevier, 2014.

43. **a**—Anaplastic meningiomas

Anaplastic meningiomas (WHO grade III; malignant, papillary or rhabdoid) have markedly increased mitotic activity or frank anaplasia. Account for 1-3% of meningiomas; 50% papillary meningiomas occur in children. Genetics: gains on 17q, losses on 9p (CDKN2A, p14ARF, CDKN2B), losses on 1p, 6q, 14q, 18q. Can occur *de novo*, in tumor recurrence or post-radiation; commonly located at falx or convexity. Treatment is with surgical resection followed by radiotherapy; high recurrence rate (50% in papillary meningioma and 90% in rhabdoid meningioma); extracranial metastasis (20% in papillary meningioma, 10% in rhabdoid). Similar imaging and gross appearance to meningioma, but invasion of adjacent brain/skull and hemorrhage/necrosis. Histopathology: high mitotic rate (>20 per 10 HPF) or frank anaplasia with areas resembling carcinoma/sarcoma/melanoma.

Image with permission from Yachnis AT, Rivera-Zengotita ML. Neuropathology, High-Yield Pathology Series, Saunders, Elsevier, 2014.

44. **e**—Rhabdoid meningioma: >50% of tumor composed of loosely cohesive sheets of large cells with eosinophilic inclusion-like cytoplasm sometimes appearing as globular or whorled filamentous inclusions; vesicular nuclei with prominent nucleoli; other histologic features of malignancy—including increased mitoses, high proliferative indices, and necrosis—should be present; foci of conventional meningioma morphology may be present; concurrent papillary features may be present.

- Focal rhabdoid-like histology in otherwise typical meningioma not sufficient for diagnosis of rhabdoid variant
- Metastatic carcinoma/melanoma, rhabdomyosarcoma, gemistocytic astrocytoma (versus rhabdoid meningioma)

Image with permission from Yachnis AT, Rivera-Zengotita ML, Neuropathology, High-Yield Pathology Series, Saunders, Elsevier, 2014.

45. **e**—Papillary meningioma: discohesive meningothelial tumor cells around fibrovascular papillary or pseudopapillary cores; perivascular pseudorosettes may be apparent; increased mitoses, necrosis, and pleomorphism; brain invasion common. Ependymoma, metastatic carcinoma, astroblastoma, choroid plexus tumor (versus papillary meningioma).

Image with permission from Yachnis AT, Rivera-Zengotita ML. Neuropathology, High-Yield Pathology Series, Saunders, Elsevier, 2014.

46. **b**—Neurofibromas

These are peripheral nerve sheath tumors composed of differentiated Schwann cells, perneurial-like cells (epithelioid myofibroblasts in perineurium), fibroblasts and nerve fibers—WHO grade I. Relatively common sporadic tumor that affects all ages and both genders equally; multiple and plexiform neurofibromas associated with NF1 (mutation on 17q). Presentation: localized painless cutaneous nodule/mass (commonest; sporadic); diffuse cutaneous nodules (extraneural types); plexiform neurofibromas in NF1 (multinodular tangles "bag of worms," enlargement/deformity of plexus or nerve trunk, multiple neurofibromas, >5 café-au-lait spots, axillary/inguinal freckling, optic glioma, Lisch nodules, sphenoid dysplasia). Treatment is surgical resection—sporadic neurofibromas are benign, 3-5% of NF1 plexiform neurofibromas undergo malignant transformation. Gross appearance: firm to soft tan pink with variable myxoid stroma; intraneural tumors are well-circumscribed fusiform shape vs diffusely infiltrating extraneural tumor. Histology: delicate spindle cells in matrix of collagen fibers, mucus, axons; Schwann cells have wavy nuclei; expansion of multiple nerve fascicles in plexiform neurofibroma; vascular unlike schwannomas; nuclear atypia and increased cellularity but mitoses rare; uncommon—pseudo-Meissnerian bodies, melanin pigmentation, dense aggregations of hyperchromatic nuclei. Immunohistochemistry: S100 and vimentin positive, EMA for perineurium, CD34 positive cells (non-Schwann). Differential: malignant peripheral nerve sheath tumor, schwannoma, perineurinoma.

Image with permission from Yachnis AT, Rivera-Zengotita ML. Neuropathology, High-Yield Pathology Series, Saunders, Elsevier, 2014.

47. **c**—Neurofibroma

Image with permission from Yachnis AT, Rivera-Zengotita ML. Neuropathology, High-Yield Pathology Series, Saunders, Elsevier, 2014.

48. **a**—Schwannomas

These are encapsulated nerve sheath tumor composed of differentiated Schwann cells—WHO grade I. Represent 8-10% of intracranial tumors and 30% of spinal tumors; peak incidence in fourth to sixth decade; most are sporadic and solitary; 4% are associated with NF2 or schwannomatosis; no gender predilection. Genetics: bilateral vestibular schwannomas involving CN VIII are pathognomonic for NF2 (22q frameshift mutation of gene coding for tumor suppressor merlin found in 60% of schwannomas); Schwannomatosis syndrome characterized by multiple painful schwannomas in a segmental distribution in absence of other NF2 features; psammomatous/melanotic schwannomas associated with Carney complex (mutation of PRKAR1A gene on chromosome 17q; autosomal dominant disorder characterized by lentiginous facial pigmentation, cardiac myxoma, and endocrine disorders). Presentation: Account for 85% of cerebellopontine angle tumors (most arise from vestibular branch of VIII [acoustic neuroma], occasionally V, VII); intraspinal schwannomas arise from sensory roots. Management is surgical resection for large tumors, radiosurgery possible for small (<2.5 cm); malignant transformation is rare. Imaging: intracranial circumscribed/cystic enhancing mass with extension into the internal auditory canal; spinal schwannomas are generally intradural extramedullary (but occasionally extend into extradural space creating dumbbell shape). Gross appearance: well-circumscribed, occasionally cystic mass, heterogenous cut surface will yellow or hemorrhagic foci. Histology: encapsulated, differentiated Schwann cells form two architectural patterns Antoni A (closely apposed spindled tumor cells with palisading, elongated nuclei; Verocay bodies are alternating parallel rows of nuclear palisades with areas devoid of nuclei occurring within Antoni A) and Antoni B (less cellular areas of loosely arranged tumor cells with indistinct processes and microcystic change); nuclear inclusions, nuclear pleomorphism; hyalinized vessels; larger schwannomas may undergo degenerative change and necrosis. Variants: cellular Schwannoma (hypercellular, Antoni A without Verocay bodies, low mitoses, paravertebral and cranial nerve locations), plexiform Schwanomma (affect skin/subcutaneous tissues of extremities in schwannomatosis) and psammomatous/melanotic schwannoma (50% associated with Carney complex; 10% undergo malignant transformation). Immunohistochemistry: Reactive for S100, Leu-7, calretinin; basement membrane type IV collagen and laminin. Differential by location: CPA—meningioma/epidermoid/ependymoma, spinal—meningioma/myxopapillary ependymoma, skin—neurofibroma, large nerve root—MPNST.

Image with permission from Yachnis AT, Rivera-Zengotita ML. Neuropathology, High-Yield Pathology Series, Saunders, Elsevier, 2014.

49. **a**—Antony B schwannoma

Image with permission from Yachnis AT, Rivera-Zengotita ML, Neuropathology, High-Yield Pathology Series, Saunders, Elsevier, 2014.

50. **e**—Verocay bodies

Image with permission from Yachnis AT, Rivera-Zengotita ML. Neuropathology, High-Yield Pathology Series, Saunders, Elsevier, 2014.

51. **d**—Malignant peripheral nerve sheath tumor (MPNST)

These are high-grade sarcomas arising from peripheral nerve or extraneural soft tissue with nerve sheath differentiation. Represent 5% of malignant soft tissue tumors; over half arise from neurofibromas in NF1 (usually plexiform); sporadic cases peak fifth decade, NF1 associated earlier (second and third decades). Genetics: MPNSTs associated with NF-1 have both NF1 alleles inactivated; alterations in p53, p16, and p27; RB and p53 pathways are altered. Presentation: progressively enlarging painful mass on an extremity; medium to large nerves, sciatic nerve commonest; radicular pain with spinal cord lesions; cranial nerves rare (spontaneously from schwannoma/neurofibroma). Treatment is surgical resection with irradiation, but poor prognosis: 60% mortality (80% for paraspinal lesions), local recurrence 40-65%, metastasis 30-80% (usually lungs), overall 16-39% 5-year survival. Imaging: Inhomogenous contrast enhancement with irregular contours and invasion. Gross appearance: fusiform/globoid, thick pseudocapsule, light tan fleshy tumor with necrosis and hemorrhage. Histology: cellular/hypercellular bipolar spindle cells arranged in herringbone pattern, hyperchromatic nuclei, moderate to marked pleomorphism, mitoses and necrosis. Variants: Epithelioid MPNST, MPNST with mesenchymal differentiation (including Triton tumor), MPNST with glandular differentiation, melanotic MPSNT. Immunohistochemistry: scattered S100 reactivity in 50-70%, p53 reactive, Leu-7 focally positive, Ki67 5-65%. Differential: fibrosarcoma, synovial sarcoma, leiomyosarcoma, melanoma.

Image with permission from Yachnis AT, Rivera-Zengotita ML. Neuropathology, High-Yield Pathology Series, Saunders, Elsevier, 2014.

52. **d**—Primary CNS lymphoma is a malignancy arising independently within the CNS without evidence of systemic lymphoma. Comprise 1-5% of primary brain tumors; peak incidence is in immunocompetent individuals age 55-77 years; increased risk in inherited or acquired immunodeficiency (AIDS, transplant patients, Wiskott-Aldrich syndrome) where it is associated with EBV; HAART therapy has reduced incidence in AIDS patients; 50% of post-transplantation PCNSL occur in first year. Present as focal or multifocal neurologic deficit, neuropsychiatric symptoms, seizures, raised ICP. Survival without therapy is 6 months; treatment is systemic and intrathecal methotrexate chemotherapy with or without whole brain radiotherapy; also rituximab (anti-CD20 monoclonal antibody) and autologous stem cell transplantation. Five-year survival in immunocompetent individuals is 75% (under 60 years) and 20% (over 60)—in general approaches 48 months. HIV-infected patients undergoing HAART and radiation reported median survival 36 months. Imaging: highly variable appearance, usually deep and periventricular location; iso-hyperintense T2, less peritumoral edema than metastasis/abscess, in context of AIDS difficult to distinguish from opportunistic infections, steroids may cause disappearance (glucocorticoids are lymphocytic) but usually returns. Gross appearance: single or multifocal (commoner in immunocompromised) deep lesions, necrosis is present, lymphomatosis cerebri. Histology: 92-98% are aggressive non-Hodgkin B-cell lymphoma (95% are large cell), express pan-B-cell lineage antigens (CD20, CD79a), atypical lymphoid cells, angiocentric growth pattern, mitotic activity, necrosis, background reactive astrocytes; low grade B-cell lymphoma and T cell lymphoma less common. Immunohistochemistry: CD

20, CD79a (CD19 flow cytometry); majority express BCL-6 and BCL-2 (but not indicative of t(14;18) translocation); 90-100% express MUM-1; high Ki 67 index 80%. Differential: glioma, opportunistic infection in immunocompromised individuals, metastasis of systemic lymphoma (meningeal > cerebral).

Image with permission from Yachnis AT, Rivera-Zengotita ML. Neuropathology, High-Yield Pathology Series, Saunders, Elsevier, 2014.

53. **e**—Pineocytoma is a primary pineal parenchymal tumor composed of small, uniform pinealocyte-like cells—WHO grade I. Accounts for 14-60% of pineal parenchymal tumors; mean age 38. Presentation: raised ICP/hydrocephalus from aqueduct compression, Parinaud's syndrome (upgaze palsy, light-near dissociation, convergence/retraction nystagmus, lid retraction/sun setting), brainstem/cerebellar dysfunction, hypothalamic dysfunction. Treatment is surgical resection; 5-year survival 85% (debulking), does not metastasize. Imaging: contrast enhancing, T2 hyperintense. Gross: gray-tan tumor, well demarcated. Histology: pineocytomatous rosettes, sheets of well-differentiated pinealocyte-like cells, low mitotic rate, no necrosis, occasional multinucleate giant cells, ganglion cells. Immunohistochemistry: positive neural markers (synaptophysin, NF, NSE), positive retinal S-antigen and rhodopsin, Ki67 <3%. Differential: normal pineal gland tissue (lobular and contains calcifications), pineal cyst, pineal tumor of intermediate differentiation or pineoblastoma, germ cell tumors, metastasis.

Image with permission from Yachnis AT, Rivera-Zengotita ML. Neuropathology, High-Yield Pathology Series, Saunders, Elsevier, 2014.

54. **d**—Pineal parenchymal tumors of intermediate differentiation define those intermediate-grade malignancies between pineocytoma and pineoblastoma. Account of 20% of pineal parenchymal tumors. Similar presentation and imaging features to pineocytoma. Treatment is resection with 40-75% 5-year survival rate. Gross: solid gray-tan tumor. Histology: diffuse or lobular architecture, moderate/high cellularity, mitotic index <15%, occasional giant cells and Homer Wright rosettes. Immunohistochemistry: positive for neuronal markers, variable for NF, chromogranin, retinal S-antigen and S100. Ki67 index 3-10%. Differential: other pineal parenchymal tumors, germ cell tumors, metastasis, normal pineal gland.

Image with permission from Yachnis AT, Rivera-Zengotita ML. Neuropathology, High-Yield Pathology Series, Saunders, Elsevier, 2014.

55. **d**—Pineoblastoma is an aggressive embryonal tumor of pineal region—WHO grade IV. Accounts for 40% of all pineal parenchymal tumors; present in first two decades of life. Genetics: 3% of patients with bilateral retinoblastoma have pineoblastoma ("trilateral retinoblastoma"; RB1 mutation; pineoblastoma must be concurrent/sequential rather than pineal retinoblastoma metastasis). Treatment is resection and radiotherapy; infiltration into adjacent brain and CSF dissemination is common; median postsurgical survival 24-30 months; prognosis for trilateral retinoblastoma is <1-year survival from diagnosis. Imaging: ill-defined lobular mass >3 cm, heterogenous contrast enhancement. Histology: sheets of densely packed small blue cells, no pineocytomatous rosettes but occasional Homer Wright or Flexner-Wintersteiner rosettes; necrosis/calcification common; high nuclear/cytoplasmic ratio; increased mitotic index. Immunohistochemistry: positive for neuronal markers and retinal-S-antigen. Differential: pineal parenchymal tumors, medulloblastoma metastasis, AT/RT, germ cell tumors, metastasis.

Image with permission from Yachnis AT, Rivera-Zengotita ML. Neuropathology, High-Yield Pathology Series, Saunders, Elsevier, 2014.

56. **c**—Germinoma is a germ cell tumor (resembling testicular seminoma and ovarian dysgerminoma) arising in the pineal or suprasellar region. Account for 3% of pediatric intracranial tumors; 65% of CNS germ cell tumors are germinomatous (i.e., germinomas; lack cellular differentiation), 35% are non-germinomatous (display tissue type differentiation; teratoma, yolk sac, embryonal carcinoma, choriocarcinoma); male predominance; present teens/early 20s. Presentation: 80% are midline pineal (hydrocephalus, Parinaud's) or suprasellar lesions (visual field defect, panhypopituitarism, diabetes insipidus). Given the lack of differentiation in germinomas serum and CSF markers may often be negative. Primary treatment is radiotherapy—10-year survival 85% or more; poorer prognosis with mixed germinoma (germinoma with syncytiotrophoblastic giant cells, mixed germinoma/teratoma). Imaging: hyperdense, enhancing lesions.

Gross: solid, soft tan-white tumor. Histology: biphasic with large neoplastic cells with abundant cytoplasm intermixed with fibrovascular septae harboring lymphocytic infiltrate, occasional granulomas/syncytiotrophoblastic cells/foci of other germ cell tumor. Immunohistochemistry: positive CD117 (c-kit), OCT3/4, SALL4, placental alkaline phosphatase (PLAP); if syncytiotrophoblasts present betaHCG or human placental lactogen may be present. Differential: primary pineal/suprasellar tumor, non-germinomatous germ cell tumors.

Image with permission from Yachnis AT, Rivera-Zengotita ML. Neuropathology, High-Yield Pathology Series, Saunders, Elsevier, 2014.

57. **e**—Teratoma. Numerous germ cell elements are present including cartilage (upper left), squamous epithelium with skin adnexal structures (upper right), bone (lower right), and neuroepithelial elements (center).

Non-germinomatous germ cell tumors (NGGCTs) include teratomas, embryonal carcinomas, yolk sac tumor (endodermal sinus tumor) and choriocarcinomas. Prognosis depends on histological subtype of GTC: good prognosis (pure germinoma, mature teratoma), intermediate prognosis (germinoma with syncytiotrophoblasts, immature teratoma, teratoma with malignant transformation, mixed germinoma/teratoma), and poor prognosis (choriocarcinoma, yolk sac tumor, embryonal carcinoma, mixture of these). Surgical resection of mature teratoma can be curative.

Teratomas are comprised of cells originating from usually all three of endoderm, mesoderm and ectoderm. Intra-axial teratomas are rare but are the commonest cause of fetal brain tumors (25-50%); located in cerebral hemispheres presenting antenatally or in the neonatal period with increased head circumference. Extra-axial (suprasellar or pineal) teratomas are commoner and present in childhood/early adulthood. Mature teratoma contain differentiated skin, brain, cartilage, fat, respiratory/enteric epithelium and may be cystic (n.b. dermoids are ectodermal in origin only hence will not contain fat). Immature teratomas have foci of incompletely differentiated tissue elements including immature neuroepithelium, embryonal mesenchymal tissue, abortive retinal epithelium; malignant transformation of any component can occur. Immunohistochemistry: cytokeratin positive in epithelial elements.

Image with permission from Yachnis AT, Rivera-Zengotita ML. Neuropathology, High-Yield Pathology Series, Saunders, Elsevier, 2014.

58. **e**—Yolk sac (endodermal sinus) tumor.

Yolk sac tumors may have gelatinous appearance Yolk sac (endodermal sinus) tumors: highly variable histology with cuboidal/elongated epithelial cells surrounding fibrovascular cores (Schiller-Duval bodies) or having eosinophilic hyaline globules within cytoplasm. Immunoreactive for AFP, SALL4, glipican-3.

Image with permission from Yachnis AT, Rivera-Zengotita ML. Neuropathology, High-Yield Pathology Series, Saunders, Elsevier, 2014.

59. **b**—Embryonal carcinoma. This highly malignant neoplasm consists of large cells with prominent nucleoli and abundant clear to eosinophilic cytoplasm forming solid sheets, nests, or lining glandlike spaces; frequent mitoses and necrosis. Embryonal carcinoma: positive for cytokeratins, CD30, OCT4, SALL4, PLAP.

Image with permission from Yachnis AT, Rivera-Zengotita ML. Neuropathology, High-Yield Pathology Series, Saunders, Elsevier, 2014.

60. **a**—Choriocarcinoma. These highly hemorrhagic tumors contain neoplastic cytotrophoblastic (left) and syncytiotrophoblastic giant cells (right center). Choriocarcinoma: composed of both neoplastic cytotrophoblastic and syncytiotrophoblastic giant cells with extensive hemorrhagic necrosis. Choriocarcinoma: syncytiotrophoblastic cells positive for β-HCG, HPL, PLAP (variable).

Image with permission from Yachnis AT, Rivera-Zengotita ML. Neuropathology, High-Yield Pathology Series, Saunders, Elsevier, 2014.

61. **b**—Hemangioblastoma is a highly vascularized tumor composed of stromal cells and capillaries. Accounts for 1-2% of intracranial tumors; peaks in third to fifth decade (affects children as part of VHL); mostly sporadic; 25% associated with von Hippel-Lindau disease (autosomal dominant inherited defect in VHL gene on 3p25-p26; multiple hemangioblastomas, renal cell carcinoma, phaeochromocytoma, pancreatic/liver cysts, endolymphatic sac tumor). Presentation: sporadic hemangioblastomas commonest in cerebellum, while those in VHL in cerebellum,

brain stem, spinal cord (associated with syrinx), cerebrum, leptomeninges, retina and peripheral nerves; 10% associated with secondary polycythemia (stromal EPO production). Surgical resection is treatment of choice for these benign lesions; can bleed extensively hence may require preop embolization; multiple lesions and recurrence seen in VHL. Imaging: commonly cystic lesion with contrast-enhancing mural nodule in cerebellum. Gross: circumscribed, non-encapsulated usually cystic with vascularized red mural nodule or yellow from lipid cells. Histology: lipid rich stromal cells with vacuolated cytoplasm ovoid nuclei surrounded by network of capillaries; intratumoral sclerosis/hemorrhage; mitoses/necrosis rare; Rosenthal fibers and reactive gliosis in cyst wall. Immunohistochemistry: Stromal cells positive for NSE, inhibin A, aquaporin 1, S100, CD56, vimentin, GFAP; unlike renal cell carcinoma also negative for CD10, EMA, cytokeratin; capillaries positive for CD31, CD34, and reticulin. Differential: metastatic RCC, pilocytic astrocytoma, endocrine neoplasm.

Image with permission from Yachnis AT, Rivera-Zengotita ML. Neuropathology, High-Yield Pathology Series, Saunders, Elsevier, 2014.

62. **c**—Pituitary adenomas are tumors of the anterior pituitary gland. Represent 10-15% of all intracranial tumors; incidence 0.2-2.8 per 100,000 per year; 20-30% non-functioning, 25% prolactin-secreting, 20% growth hormone, 10% ACTH, 10-15% secrete FSH/LH, 1-3% secrete TSH; occasional bihormonal adenomas, usually prolactin and GH. Genetics: most sporadic; 3% associated with multiple endocrine neoplasia type 1 (11q13 mutation; pituitary, pancreatic and parathyroid tumors). Presentation:
   1. General: headache, facial pain, fatigue, weight loss
   2. Mass effect: bitemporal hemianopia, cranial nerve palsy, stalk effect (prolactin rise without prolactinoma)
   3. Pituitary apoplexy: hemorrhagic necrosis of adenoma—sudden headache, visual loss, Addisonian crisis
   4. Prolactin excess: amenorrhoea, irregular periods, galatorrhoea, infertility in women; hypogonadism, loss of libido, impotence in men
   5. Growth hormone excess: gigantism in children, acromegaly in adults
   6. ACTH excess: Cushing disease
   7. TSH excess: thyrotoxicosis
   8. Gonadotrophins (FSH/LH): amenorrhoea in females, impotence in males

Medical treatment of prolactinomas with dopamine receptor agonist (bromocriptine or cabergoline) and GH-secreting tumors with somatostatin analogs (octreotide). Transphenoidal resection for symptomatic non-functioning lesions or resistant to medical therapy. Radiotherapy for residual tumor, recurrence or invasive. Management of pituitary apoplexy includes glucocorticoids, close monitoring and surgical decompression if vision deteriorating. Imaging: circumscribed, variably enhancing compared to adjacent pituitary, macroadenomas expand the sella. Gross: circumscribed, non-encapsulated tan-brown tumor (microadenoma <10 mm, macroadenoma >10 mm). Histology: loss of normal lobar architecture of anterior pituitary; sheets and cords of monomorphic cells; basophilic granules in ACTH secreting types; eosinophilic cytoplasmic granules (cytokeratins; CAM5.2) in GH-secreting types. Immunohistochemistry: reticulin staining demonstrates loss of architecture; chromogranin, cytokeratin, EMA positive; hormone stains. Differential: pituicytoma, craniopharyngioma, granular cell tumor, sellar meningioma/schwanomma, Rathke cleft cyst, germ cell tumor, metastasis, hypothalamic hamartoma/glioma, carotid cavernous fistula/aneurysm.

Image with permission from Yachnis AT, Rivera-Zengotita ML. Neuropathology, High-Yield Pathology Series, Saunders, Elsevier, 2014.

63. **a**—Adamantinomatous Craniopharyngioma

Craniopharyngiomas are epithelial tumors derived from Rathke's pouch. Accounts for 3% of intracranial tumors; Incidence is 0.5-2.5 per million/year; no gender predilection; adamantinomatous subtype (children; 5-10% of pediatric intracranial tumors) and papillary subtype (exclusively adults). Presents due to local compression in suprasellar region: hypothalamus (endocrine dysregulation/diabetes insipidus), third ventricle (hydrocephalus), optic chiasm (bitemporal hemianopia). General symptoms: cognitive impairment, N&V, somnolence. Management is surgical resection, with $>90\%$ 10-year recurrence free survival depending on extent of resection (limited by adherence to adjacent structures); rare reports of malignant transformation to SCC post-radiotherapy. May need hormone replacement if hypopituitarism. Imaging: suprasellar cystic mass (T1 hyperintense) but occasionally solid enhancing tumor (T1 hypointense). Gross: solid and cystic mass with calcification, motor-oil like material in adamantinomatous type.

Histology:

1. Adamantinomatous: nests and trabeculae of epithelium in lose fibrous stroma, palisading at periphery of tumor, stellate reticulum (loosely arranged epithelium), wet keratin (eosinophilic), cysts, calcification, xanthogranulomatous reaction (cholesterol clefts, foreign body giant cells, inflammation), gliosis/Rosenthal fibers at lesion edges
2. Papillary: circumscribed papillary tumor with fibrovascular cores lined by well-differentiated monotonous squamous epithelium (i.e., no stellate reticulum, wet keratin, calcification, xanthogranulomatous change).

Immunohistochemistry: cytokeratin and focal HCG, CK7, CK20; adamantinomatous subtype associated with beta-catenin mutations resulting in nuclear reactivity. Differential: xanthogranulomatous inflammation, Rathke cleft cyst, epidermoid cyst, metastasis, pilocytic astrocytoma.

Image with permission from Yachnis AT, Rivera-Zengotita ML. Neuropathology, High-Yield Pathology Series, Saunders, Elsevier, 2014.

ANSWERS 64–81

Additional answers 64–81 available on ExpertConsult.com

GLOSSARY

P: chromosome short (petit) arm
Q: chromosome long arm
Myxoid: mucous like
Papillary: with small nipple-like projections
Spindle: cell long and slender
Palisade: row of elongated nuclei parallel to each other
Rosette: ring or garland-like arrangement of nuclei with or without a central channel
Piloid: thin hair-like cells arranged in parallel array
Fibrillary cells: have projecting fibres
Clear cells: have abundant clear cytoplasm
Small cells: primitive-appearing cells with little cytoplasm
Storiform: cartwheel pattern (i.e., radiating out from center)

CHAPTER 7

PHARMACOLOGY

SINGLE BEST ANSWER (SBA) QUESTIONS

1. Which one of the following best describes the main mechanism of propofol sedation?
   a. Cyclo-oxygenase inhibition
   b. Depolarizing neuromuscular blockade
   c. Endocannabinoid activation
   d. Non-depolarizing neuromuscular blockade
   e. Potentiates GABA-A receptor activity

2. Which one of the following combinations of clotting factors are affected by warfarin?
   a. II, IX, X, Protein C
   b. II, VII, IX, X
   c. II, VII, IX, X, Protein C, Protein S
   d. II, VII, X, Protein C
   e. II, VII, X, XII

3. Which one of the following blood tests would you perform to monitor the effect of low molecular weight heparin?
   a. Factor VII
   b. Factor VIII
   c. Factor Xa activity
   d. Prothrombin time
   e. Von Willebran Factor

4. A 75-year-old patient presents with GCS E3V4M5 and due to ICH. INR is 5.0 on warfarin for atrial fibrillation. Assuming you have access to all of the following therapies, which one of the following is the most appropriate next treatment?
   a. Fresh frozen plasma
   b. Protamine
   c. Prothrombin complex concentrate
   d. Recombinant factor VIIa
   e. Vitamin K

5. A patient with a right extradural hematoma fixes and dilates his right pupil on the way to theater. The anesthetist administers 100 ml of 20% mannitol and his pupil normalizes after 2 min. Which one of the following best explains the immediate effect of mannitol?
   a. Autoregulatory vasoconstriction
   b. Diuretic effect
   c. Increased cerebral blood volume
   d. Osmotic effect reducing interstitial brain fluid
   e. Local effect on pupillary constrictors

6. Which one of the following best describes the mechanism of dexamethasone action in reducing cerebral edema?
   a. Reduces cytotoxic edema through nitric oxide inhibition
   b. Reduces cytotoxic edema through VEGF inhibition
   c. Reduces vasogenic edema through VEGF inhibition
   d. Reduces vasogenic edema through upregulation of aquaporins
   e. Reduces vasogenic edema through nitric oxide signaling

7. Propofol-related infusion syndrome is usually characterized by which one of the following?
   a. Acute refractory bradycardia with metabolic alkalosis
   b. Acute refractory bradycardia with metabolic acidosis
   c. Acute refractory bradycardia with respiratory alkalosis
   d. Acute refractory bradycardia with respiratory acidosis
   e. Acute refractory bradycardia with normal acid-base balance

8. Red man syndrome is seen with which one of the following medications?
   a. Levodopa
   b. Procyclidine
   c. Propofol
   d. Rifampicin
   e. Vancomycin

9. Which one of the following is the initial treatment for a dystonic reaction to levodopa?
   a. Adenosine
   b. Bromocriptine
   c. Cyclizine
   d. Procyclidine
   e. Topiramate

10. Which one of the following would you monitor during infusion of an intravenous loading dose of phenytoin?

a. Capillary blood glucose
b. Cardiac monitoring
c. Nystagmus
d. Peak flow rate
e. Urine output

QUESTIONS 11–20

Additional questions 11–20 available on ExpertConsult.com

EXTENDED MATCHING ITEM (EMI) QUESTIONS

21. **Anticonvulsants:**
    a. Acetazolamide
    b. Carbamazepine
    c. Ethosuxamide
    d. Gabapentin
    e. Lacosamide
    f. Lamotrigine
    g. Levetiracetam
    h. Perampanel
    i. Phenytoin
    j. Pregabalin
    k. Sodium Valproate
    l. Topiramate
    m. Vigabatrin
    n. Zonisamide

For each of the following descriptions, select the most appropriate answers from the list above. Each answer may be used once, more than once or not at all.

1. Risk of thrombocytopenia and increased warfarin effect
2. Affect T-type calcium current and used in absence seizures
3. Associated with weight loss

22. **Chemotherapy:**
    a. Bevacizumab
    b. Carmustine (BNCU)
    c. Cisplatin
    d. Erlotinib
    e. Everolimus
    f. Lomustine (CCNI)
    g. Methotrexate
    h. Procarbazine
    i. Tamoxifen
    j. Temozolomide
    k. Vincristine

For each of the following descriptions, select the most appropriate answers from the list above. Each answer may be used once, more than once or not at all.

1. Microtubule inhibitor
2. VEGF inhibitor
3. SEGA treatment
4. Chemotherapy wafer for GBM

23. **Bleeding:**
    a. Abciximab/epitifibatide/tirofiban
    b. Aspirin
    c. Clopidogrel/prasugrel
    d. Dalteparin
    e. Desmopressin
    f. Dipyridamole
    g. Enoxaparin
    h. Fondaparinux
    i. Protamine
    j. Rivaroxiban
    k. Tranexamic acid
    l. Warfarin

For each of the following descriptions, select the most appropriate answers from the list above. Each answer may be used once, more than once or not at all.

1. ADP receptor antagonist
2. Glycoprotein IIa/IIIb antagonist
3. Used preoperatively in factor VIII dysfunction
4. Irreversible cyclo-oxygenase inhibitor
5. Adenosine reuptake inhibitor

24. **Anticoagulants:**
    a. Antithrombin protein
    b. Batroxobin
    c. Citrate
    d. Dabigatran
    e. EDTA
    f. Fondaparinux
    g. Hirudin
    h. Low molecular weight heparin
    i. Rivaroxiban
    j. Unfractionated heparin
    k. Warfarin

For each of the following descriptions, select the most appropriate answers from the list above. Each answer may be used once, more than once or not at all.

1. Synthetic pentasaccharide factor Xa inhibitor
2. Direct inhibitor of factor Xa
3. Direct thrombin inhibitor

25. **Anesthetic drugs:**
    a. Atracurium
    b. Clonidine
    c. Desmopressin
    d. Dobutamine
    e. Fludrocortisone
    f. Glycopyronium
    g. Ketamine
    h. Labetalol
    i. Mannitol
    j. Midazolam
    k. Noradrenaline
    l. Propofol
    m. Remifentanil
    n. Thiopentone
    o. Vasopressin

For each of the following descriptions, select the most appropriate answers from the list above. Each answer may be used once, more than once or not at all.

1. Associated with Ondine's curse
2. Associated with a low serum potassium despite normal total body potassium when chronic infusion used
3. Associated with raised intracranial pressure

26. **Reversal of clotting abnormalities:**
    a. Desmopressin
    b. Factor IX
    c. Factor VIII
    d. Fresh frozen plasma
    e. Platelets
    f. Protamine
    g. Prothrombin complex concentrate
    h. Recombinant factor VIIa
    i. Tranexamic acid
    j. Tranexamic acid
    k. Vitamin K

For each of the following descriptions, select the most appropriate answers from the list above. Each answer may be used once, more than once or not at all.

1. Preoperatively in patients with mild hemophilia A
2. Major hemorrhage in warfarinized patient

SBA ANSWERS

1. **e**—GABA(A) receptor activation. While propofol may have multiple effects, the main mechanism of action is thought to result from activation of GABA(A) receptors, causing increased transmembrane chloride conductance and hyperpolarization of the neuron preventing generation of an action potential.

2. **c**—II, VII, IX, X, Protein C, Protein S. Protein C has a short half-life (8 h) compared with other vitamin K-dependent factors and therefore is rapidly depleted with warfarin initiation, resulting in a transient hypercoagulable state.

3. **c**—Factor Xa activity.

4. **c**—Prothrombin complex concentrate

5. **a**—Autoregulatory vasoconstriction

Mannitol has hemodynamic, osmotic, and diuretic effects. Following a bolus of hyperosmolar mannitol, body water is drawn (including from RBC) in to plasma causing expansion and reduction in blood viscosity (reduction in volume, rigidity, and cohesiveness of RBC). Altered blood rheology reduces cerebral vascular resistance, increases cerebral blood flow and CPP. Autoregulatory vasoconstriction then reduces CBV (to restore normal CPP) and reduces ICP. These immediate rheological effects may also explain why ICP reduction with mannitol occurs in situations where the BBB is not intact. The osmotic effect of mannitol in causing brain shrinkage by drawing water out requires an intact BBB (across which an osmotic gradient can be set up) and can take up to 30 min to develop. Adverse effects of mannitol include hypotension, renal failure (especially if serum osmolality >320) and rebound rise in ICP (penetration of osmotically active solutes into edematous brain reversing osmotic gradient).

6. **c**—Reduces vasogenic edema through VEGF inhibition

Tumor-related disruption in the blood-brain barrier resulting in vasogenic edema is caused by local factors increasing the permeability of vessels (VEGF, glutamate, leukotrienes) and absence of normal tight endothelial junctions in tumor vessels as they grow in response to VEGF and bFGF. In large part, VEGF is responsible for the loss of integrity of the blood-brain barrier in brain tumors. Gliomas, meningiomas, and metastatic tumors all have upregulation of VEGF. VEGF is secreted by tumor cells as well as host stromal cells and binds to its receptors VEGFR1 and VEGFR2, which are located primarily on the surface of endothelial cells. VEGF stimulates the formation of gaps in the endothelium, a process that leads to fluid leakage into the brain parenchyma, thereby resulting in vasogenic edema. Most patients with brain tumors and peritumoral edema can be adequately managed with glucocorticoids. Reduction of intracranial pressure and improvement in neurologic symptoms usually begins within hours. A decrease in capillary permeability (i.e. improvement in blood-brain barrier function) can be identified within 6 h and changes of diffusion-weighted MRI indicating decreased edema are identifiable within 48-72 h. However, adequate reduction in elevated ICP resulting from peritumoral edema may take several days with glucocorticoid therapy alone. Dexamethasone is the standard agent, because its relative lack of mineralocorticoid activity reduces the potential for fluid retention. In addition, dexamethasone may be associated with a lower risk of infection and cognitive impairment compared to other glucocorticoids. The mechanism of action of glucocorticoids for control of vasogenic edema is not fully understood. Dexamethasone has recently been shown to upregulate Ang-1, a strong BBB-stabilizing factor, whereas it downregulates VEGF, a strong permeabilizing factor, in astrocytes and pericytes. Glucocorticoids may also increase the clearance of peritumoral edema by facilitating the transport of fluid into the ventricular system, from which it is cleared by cerebrospinal fluid (CSF) bulk flow.

FURTHER READING

Kim H, Lee JM, Park JS, Jo SA, et al, Dexamethasone coordinately regulates angiopoietin-1 and VEGF: a mechanism of glucocorticoid-induced stabilization of blood-brain barrier Biochemical and Biophysical Research Communications, 2008, 372(1):243-248.

7. **b**—Acute refractory bradycardia with metabolic acidosis

Propofol infusion syndrome (PRIS): acute refractory bradycardia leading to asystole, in the presence of one or more of the following: metabolic acidosis, rhabdomyolysis, hyperlipidemia, and enlarged or fatty liver. There is an association between PRIS and propofol infusions at doses higher than 4 mg/kg/h for greater than 48 h duration. It is proposed that the syndrome may be caused by either a direct mitochondrial respiratory chain inhibition or impaired mitochondrial fatty acid metabolism mediated by propofol. ECG shows new right bundle branch block with convex-curved ("coved type") ST elevation in the right precordial leads (V1 to V3). Risk factors include young age, severe critical illness of central nervous system or respiratory origin, exogenous catecholamine or glucocorticoid administration, inadequate carbohydrate intake and subclinical mitochondrial disease. Hemodialysis or hemoperfusion with cardiorespiratory support has been the most successful treatment.

FURTHER READING

Kam PC1, Cardone D, Propofol infusion syndrome. Anaesthesia 2007 Jul; 62(7):690-701

8. **e**—Vancomycin

Red man syndrome is characterized by a complex of symptoms including: pruritis, urticaria, erythema, angioedema, tachycardia, hypotension, occasional muscle aches, and a maculopapular rash that usually appears on the face, neck, and upper torso. The etiology is thought to be due to a non-immune related release of histamine.

9. **d**—Procyclidine

10. **b**—Cardiac monitoring. During intravenous loading of phenytoin for control of seizures cardiac monitoring is essential due to the risk of bradycardia and heart-block. Elderly patients requiring multiple intravenous doses of phenytoin should also be monitored for purple glove syndrome.

ANSWERS 11–20

Additional answers 11–20 available on ExpertConsult.com

EMI ANSWERS

21. 1—k, Valproate; 2—c, Ethosuxamide; 3—l, Topiramate

Features of Common Antiepileptic Drugs

Drug	Mechanism	Clearance/Half-Life	Side Effects
Carbamazepine	Voltage gated Na channel	Hepatic CYP450 12-17 h	CYP450, hyponatremia, neurotoxicity, leukopenia, aplastic anemia, Stevens Johnson syndrome, hepatitis
Sodium Valproate	Voltage dependent Na channels, increases GABA, T-type Ca current	Hepatic 9-12 h	Weight gain, insulin resistance, thrombocytopenia, hepatotoxicity, teratogenicity, pancreatitis, hyperammonemia
Gabapentin	Voltage dependent Ca channel, GABA(B) reduces glutamate	Renal 4-6 h	Weight gain, sedation
Pregabalin	Voltage gated Ca, glutamate, norepinephrine, substance P	Renal 6 h	Euphoria, myoclonus, weight gain
Lacosamide	Voltage gates Na channels, modulated CRMP-2	13 h	Dizziness, ataxia, blurred vision
Ethosuxamide	T-type Ca current in thalamus	Hepatic 30-60 h	Insomnia, pancytopenia, hyperactivity
Levetiracetam	Binds SV2A and inhibits presynaptic Ca channels	Renal 6-12 h	Aggression, depression
Topiramate	GABA(A) receptors, NMDAR antagonist, weak Ca inhibitor	Renal 20 h	Cognitive impairment, weight loss, mood disturbance, somnolence, metabolic acidosis, renal stones
Phenytoin	Voltage dependent Na channels, synaptic transmission, Ca-calmodulin phosphorylation	Hepatic amine oxidase 7-40 h	Gingival hypertrophy, osteomalacia, teratogenicity, hirsutism, rash/SJS, lymphadenopathy
Phenobarbital	GABA(A) receptor—increase chloride current	Hepatic 24-100 h	Lethargy, cognitive impairment, teratogenic
Perampanel	AMPAR antagonist	Hepatic 100 h	Dizziness, aggression, weight gain
Zonisamide	Voltage dependent Na and T-type Ca channels, CA inhibitor	Hepatic/renal 60 h	Renal stones, anorexia, rash/SJS, agranulocytosis
Lamotrigine	Na channel blocker	Liver glucoronidation, renal excretion, 10-60 h	Rash/SJS, angioedema, multiorgan failure/DIC, somnolence, drug interaction, myoclonus
Vigabatrin	GABA transaminase inhibitor	Renal 6-8 h	Concentric visual field loss, weight gain, depression

22. 1—k, Vincristine; 2—a, Bevacizumab; 3—e, Everolimus; 4—b, Carmustine

Features of Common Antiepileptic Drugs

Chemotherapy Agent	Mechanism	Comments
Bevacizumab (Avastin)	VEGF inhibitor	GBM; hypertension, delayed wound healing, bowel perforation, ICH, thrombosis
Erlotinib	Tyrosine kinase inhibitor (EGFR)	Metastatic non-small cell lung cancer
Carmustine (BNCU)	Alkylating agent	GBM, astrocytoma, medulloblastoma; wafer may cause seizures, cerebral infarction; intravenous may cause N&V, fatigue, respiratory complications/pulmonary fibrosis, bone marrow suppression
Cisplatin	Platinum alkylating agent	Glioma, medulloblastoma, others; minor pancytopenia, ototoxicity, peripheral neuropathy, nephrotoxicity, N+V (carboplatin can cause alopecia)
Everolimus	mTOR inhibitor	GBM, SEGA
Tamoxifen	Estrogen receptor antagonist	Breast cancer
Methotrexate	Dihydrofolate reductase inhibitor	Lymphoma; myelosuppression, mucositis, N+V, nephrotoxic, hepatic fibrosis, pulmonary, neurotoxicity if intrathecal
Lomustine (CCNI)	Alkylating agent	PCV regimen for oligodendroglima/mixed oligoastrocytoma;
Procarbazine	Alkylating agent	PCV regimen for oligodendroglima/mixed oligoastrocytoma; malignant hypertension when taken with tyramine containing food.
Temozolomide	Alkylating agent	GBM; constipation, nausea/vomiting, fatigue, headache
Vincristine	Microtubule inhibitor	PCV regimen for oligodendroglima/mixed oligoastrocytoma; pancytopenia, neuropathy, N+V, mouth ulcers, fatigue

23. 1—c, Clopidogrel; 2—a, Abciximab; 3—e, Desmopressin; 4—b, Aspirin; 5—f, Dipyridamole

24. 1—f, Fondaparinux; 2—i, Rivaroxiban; 3—d, Dabigatran

25. 1—m, Remifentanil; 2—n, Thiopentone; 3—g, Ketamine

26. 1—a, Desmopressin; 2—g, Prothrombin complex concentrate

PART II
CARE OF THE NEUROSURGICAL PATIENT

CHAPTER 8

NEUROLOGY AND STROKE

SINGLE BEST ANSWER (SBA) QUESTIONS

1. An 84-year-old man has been brought into hospital because of self-neglect. He lives alone in a ground floor flat and has daily carer who have found him to be increasingly suspicious, accusing them of stealing and moving his property and becoming physically aggressive. In the past month he had been refusing to let them in. He also seemed to be experiencing auditory hallucinations and had lost weight. Examination was normal except for BMI 19 and MMSE 18/30. Bloods, CXR, urine, cultures normal. CT is shown. Which one of the following is most likely?

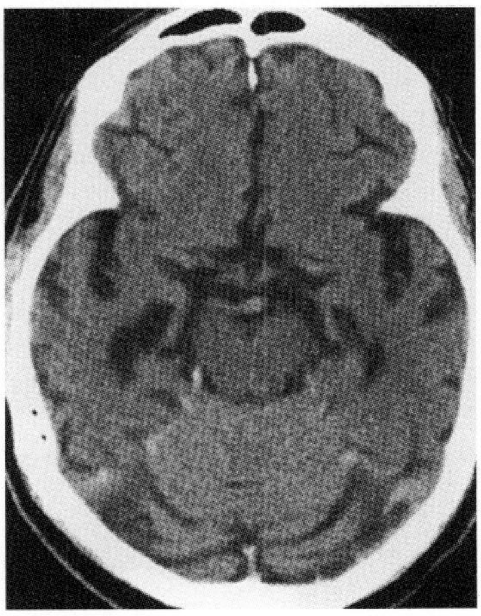

a. Alcoholic hallucinosis
b. Alzheimer's disease
c. Delirium
d. Paranoid schizophrenia
e. Pick's disease

2. A 70-year-old gentleman attends outpatient clinic with his wife. She reports that her husband's behavior has changed and that he has become increasingly forgetful over the past year. He has gained 10 kg of weight over the past 6 months. His wife reports that he has an uncontrollable appetite occasionally eating to the point of vomiting. She also states that he has a lack of interest when the grandchildren visit. Over the last 4 weeks she has noticed that her husband has become more unsteady on his feet having had a number of falls. On examining him in clinic he has impaired word comprehension, reduced safety awareness on mobilizing and a positive palmomental reflex. There is no tremor, rigidity or shuffling gait. MMSE is 22/30. CT head is shown. Which one of the following is most likely?

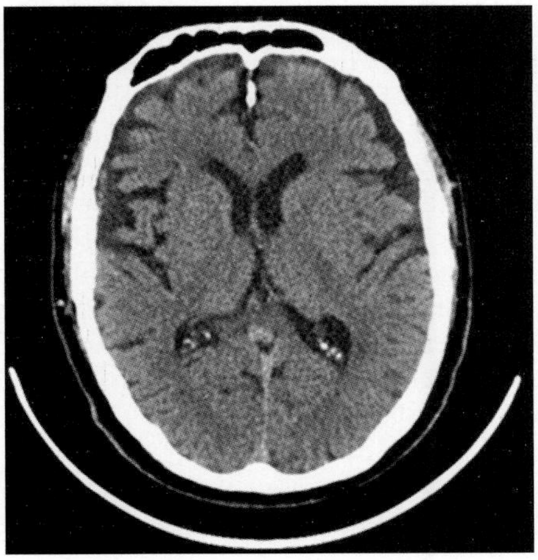

a. Depression
b. Hypomania
c. Pick's disease
d. Lewy body dementia
e. CJD

3. A 64-year-old man presents with a 6 month history of abnormal behaviors which have been noticed by his wife. He has described seeing vivid visual hallucinations of clowns in his living room which sometimes talk to him and appear very real. He believes that he is the head of a circus and is about to go on a world tour although this is not true. At times he is lucid and is fully independent but at other times he is disorientated in time and place and is unable to perform simple tasks such as preparing food and going to the shops. His wife thinks that his mood is also lower since the onset of symptoms. He presented in A+E today because of having a second fall in 2 weeks. There is no history of infective symptoms. He went to see his GP two days ago who thought that he may have a UTI and prescribed trimethoprim. He has a history of stroke 10 years ago and hypertension and takes warfarin, amlodipine, and enalapril. Physical examination is unremarkable except for slightly increased tone on the left side compared to the right. Which one of the following is most likely?
a. Alzheimer's disease
b. Semantic dementia
c. Hypothyroidism
d. Lewy body dementia
e. Schizophrenia

4. A 55-year-old man presents with cognitive decline over a 6-month period. He continues to progress and develops myoclonus and a left hemiparesis. On examination, he is alert and orientated to time and place but appears easily startled every time you start a sentence. There is bilateral finger-nose and heel-shin dysmetria, mild postural tremor and mild speech slurring. Blood tests are normal including thyroid and liver function. Lumbar puncture: WCC < 1, RBC 16, Protein 0.5 g/l, Glucose 3.4 mmol/l, gram stain negative, and no organisms cultured. An EEG demonstrated brief periodic spikes. A MRI head (FLAIR sequence) is shown. Which one of the following is most likely?

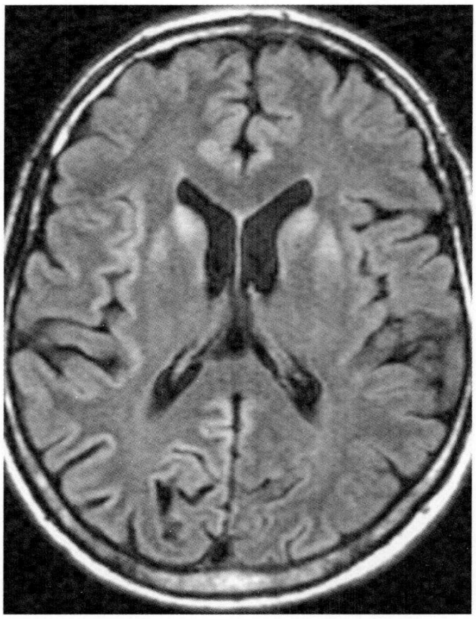

a. Alzheimer's disease
b. Creutzfeldt-Jakob disease
c. Carbon monoxide poisoning
d. Huntington's disease
e. Pick's disease

5. A 81-year-old male experiences progressive cognitive decline over the past 10 years. His wife reports that every 6 months or so she will notice another significant decrease in his functioning. It is now at the point where he is aggressive and has little short-term memory. Past medical history includes hypertension and percutaneous coronary intervention after a myocardial infarction. Examination findings include poor attention and memory, mild left hemiparesis (face, arm, and leg), and brisk reflexes throughout with extensor plantar reflex bilaterally and a shuffling gait. Which one of the following is most appropriate?
a. Referral for subthalamic nucleus deep brain stimulation
b. Treat cardiovascular risk factors
c. Carotid endarterectomy
d. Commence carbidopa/levodopa
e. Commence memantine

6. A 55-year-old man presents with a 2-month history of weakness in his right arm. He has also noticed that his voice has become softer. He is finding it hard to use door handles and open jars. On two occasions his wife has noticed him stumbling whilst walking. On examination he has fasciculations over his right deltoid muscle and wasting of the interossei muscles of the right hand. Power is 4/5 in right shoulder abduction with absent reflexes in the right arm but present elsewhere. Coordination and sensation are normal with a negative Romberg's test. Which one of the following is the most likely diagnosis?
   a. Cervical myelopathy
   b. Diabetic neuropathy
   c. Amyotrophic lateral sclerosis
   d. Multiple sclerosis
   e. Hereditary sensory motor neuropathy

7. An 18-month-old girl presents with leg weakness. Tremors, primarily of the hands, had been noted since 4 months of age. She was crawling by 9 months of age and cruising about the furniture by 12 months. Her language development was normal. Her 4-year-old sister was developing normally. Cranial nerve examination was normal, and specifically, fasciculations of the tongue were not noted. She was able to sit, crawl, and pull to a stand. She could walk holding onto furniture but could not walk independently. Deep tendon reflexes were absent throughout, and there were no Babinski signs. Sensory examination was normal. Which one of the following is the next appropriate test?
   a. Serum ceruloplasmin
   b. Electromyography
   c. Nerve conduction studies
   d. Survival motor neuron gene testing
   e. MRI head

8. A 41-year-old man presents with confusion and headaches for the last few weeks. He was diagnosed with HIV 15 years ago and has been stable on highly active antiretroviral treatment. Other past medical history includes an episode of Pneumocystis jirovecii pneumonia 1 year ago. His latest CD4 count is 29 cells/µl. An MRI (T1 C+) is shown. The enhancing lesions on MRI show increased uptake on Thallium-201 Chloride SPECT scan. Which one of the following is likely to be required?

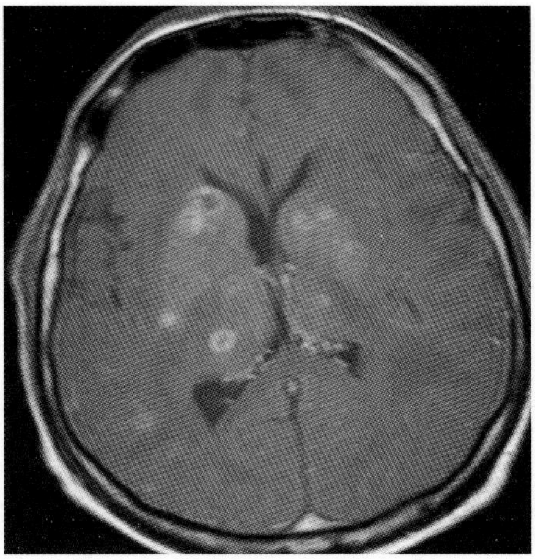

   a. Sulfadiazine + pyrimethamine
   b. Dexamethasone
   c. Methotrexate
   d. Amphotericin B
   e. Image guided aspiration and intravenous antibiotics.

9. A 31-year-old man was diagnosed with HIV 5 years ago and had been taking highly active antiretroviral therapy until 8 months ago when he decided to stop. He had been doing well on highly active antiretroviral therapy, but stopped taking his medications 8 months ago because he thought that he would be better off. Two months ago, he was successfully treated for Pneumocystis carinii pneumonia. He now presents with confusion and speech deficit. His CD4 count is 155/ul. MRI appearances are shown below. CSF PCR is positive for JC virus. Which one of the following is most likely?

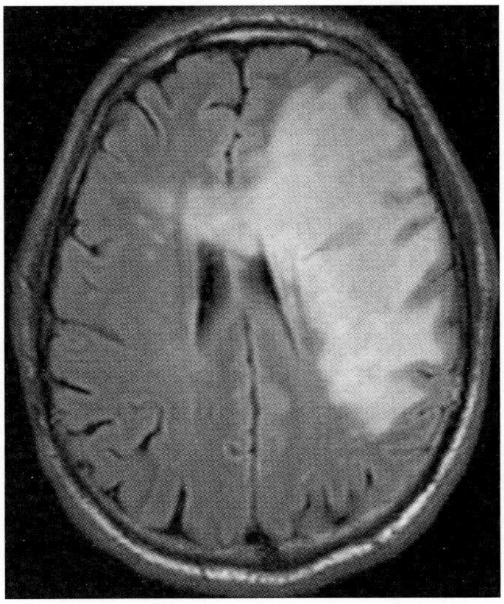

a. Adrenoleukodystrophy
b. Multiple sclerosis
c. Subacute sclerosing panencephalitis
d. Progressive multifocal leukoencephalopathy
e. AIDS dementia complex

10. A 43-year-old man has been having nightly, unilateral, throbbing headaches with the pain focused at the back of his left eye. They have been occurring daily for the past week. The patient recalls having had a similar headache 5 years ago that lasted for several weeks. The patient has noticed that the headache is associated with lacrimation and nasal congestion. Which one of the following would be appropriate next in acute management?
a. Dihydroergotamine
b. Glyceryl trinitrate
c. Indometacin
d. Inhaled 100% oxygen
e. Propanolol

11. A 18-year-old female presents with a severe right-sided throbbing headache associated with nausea, vomiting, and photophobia which failed to respond to ibuprofen. There are no other neurological features in the history. She has been having similar headaches 3-4 times per month for the past year. Her mother had a similar problem. Her examination is normal. Which one of the following would be appropriate next in acute management?
a. Amitriptyline
b. Propanolol
c. Sumatriptan
d. Topiramate
e. Verapamil

12. A 45-year-old man is referred urgently to hospital with a severe headache. The pain had started gradually three days before and was now severe. The patient reported the headache was exacerbated by an upright posture with relief obtained by lying flat. Since the headache started the patient had been unable to stand for more than a few minutes at a time but was reasonably comfortable when lying down. The patient denied any focal neurological symptoms and was constitutionally well. Clinical examination did not demonstrate any focal neurological signs or features of meningism. CT brain: no evidence of intra-axial or extra-axial bleeding; no space occupying lesion; no hydrocephalus. MRI brain with gadolinium: diffuse pachymeningeal enhancement without leptomeningeal enhancement; subtle downward displacement of brain on sagittal views. Which one of the following would be appropriate next in acute management?

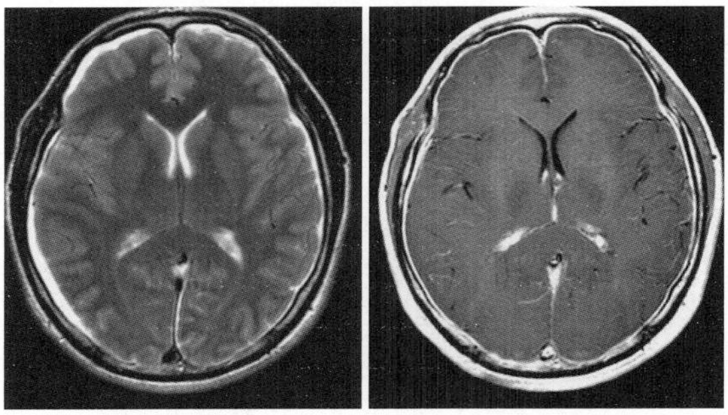

a. Epidural blood patch
b. Flat bed rest
c. Laminectomy dural repair and sealant
d. Lumbar puncture
e. MRI whole spine with STIR

13. A 26-year-old female presents with difficulty walking and complains of problems with her vision in her right eye. She had an episode of diarrhea a week ago, but has no other relevant past medical history apart from problems with her left eye 3 months earlier which had resolved. On examination there is a right relative afferent papillary defect. Visual acuity and color vision are 6/6 (20/20) with 17/17 Ishihara plates on the left, and 6/60 (20/200) with 0/17 Ishihara plates on the right. She reports no diplopia with a full range of eye movements, no facial weakness and normal facial sensation. Fundoscopy was unremarkable. Examination revealed 2/5 power on the left arm and leg in all movements; and 4/5 in all movements in right arm and leg, brisk reflexes bilaterally with extensor plantar responses. There is patchy loss of sensation to cotton wool on right lateral wrist and anterior aspect left lateral shin. Anal tone and saddle sensation are intact. MRI brain is normal and MRI spine (Sagittal T2 +T1 with gad) shown below. CSF shows WCC 12/mm^3, RBC <1/mm^3, Glucose 4.5 mmol/dl, Protein 0.9 g/l, and negative for oligoclonal bands. Which one of the following tests is likely to be positive?

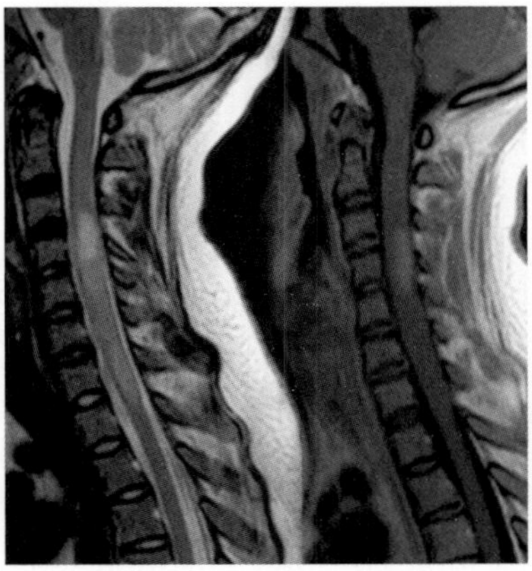

a. Anti-acetylcholine receptor antibody
b. Anti-aquaporin 4 antibody
c. Anti-muscle specific kinase antibody
d. Anti-voltage gated calcium channel antibody
e. Anti-voltage gated potassium channel antibody

14. A 10-year-old girl presents with subacute mental status change and left arm weakness. She had a viral illness 1 week ago. On examination she appears drowsy. She has a left sided hemiparesis with bilateral nystagmus. Fundoscopy reveals papilledema. There are no skin rashes. MRI head FLAIR sequence is shown. MRI spine showed a longitudinally extensive transverse myelitis. Which one of the following is most likely?

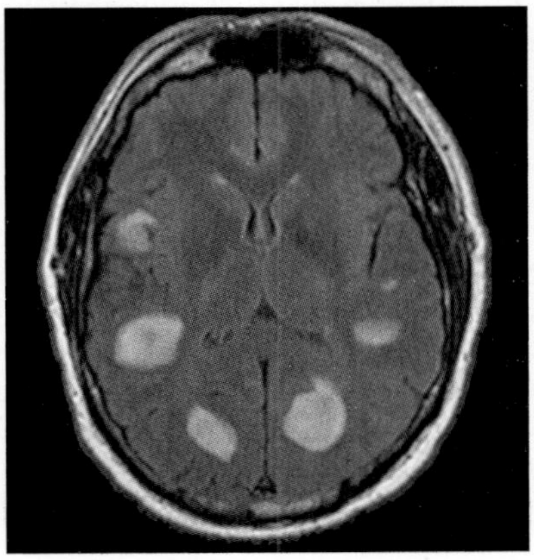

a. Multiple sclerosis
b. Acute disseminating encephalomyelitis
c. Neurosarcoidosis
d. Neuromyelitis optica
e. Systemic lupus erythematosis
f. Lyme disease

15. A 35-year-old female presents with three days of increasing weakness in the right arm and reduced visual acuity in the left eye. She has had a similar episode 2 years ago which she recovered from completely. On examination she has weakness in wrist extension and finger abduction in the left hand and visual acuity in the left eye was measured at 6/24 with an associated reduction in color saturation. Blood tests were unremarkable. Her MRI scan is shown (Axial T1 with contrast and FLAIR). Which one of the following options should be used in acute management?

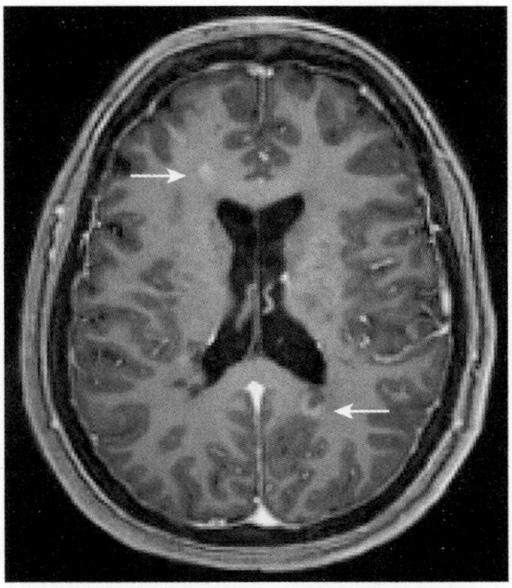

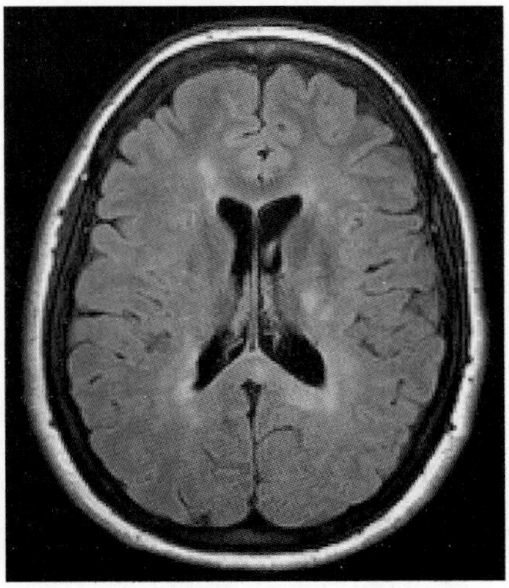

a. Commence high dose oral prednisone and wean over a month
b. IV methylprednisolone
c. Natalizumab infusion
d. Interferon beta
e. Biopsy

16. A 43-year-old female presents with a second episode of loss of sensation in her left anterior thigh and right foot. This is her second episode within the past 4 months. She had recently reported an episode of left anterior shin numbness 1 year ago, when an MRI with gadolinium

demonstrated "spots in her spinal cord" and she was diagnosed with transverse myelitis. Her past medical history also includes ulcerative colitis, diagnosed aged 27 years old and primary sclerosing cholangitis. Routine bloods are normal except for mild derangement of liver function tests. Which one of the following is most appropriate?

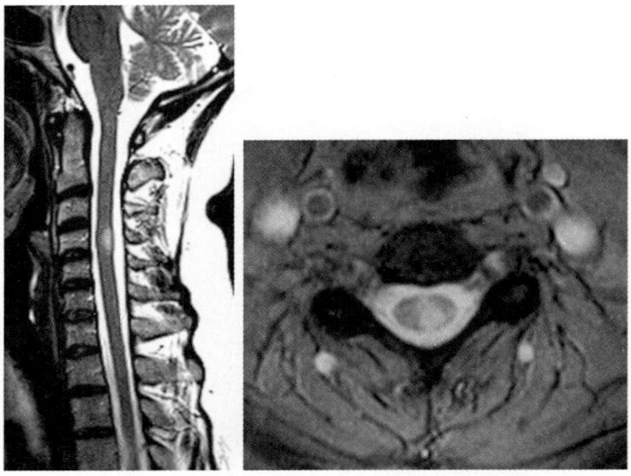

a. Interferon beta
b. Glatiramer acetate
c. Fingolimod
d. Natalizumab
e. Mitoxanthrone

17. A 43-year-old female presents with a 2 week history of mild left arm weakness and headache. MRI was done at presentation (shown). She was discharged on dexamethasone 2 mg twice daily due to her focal neurology with a plan for awake craniotomy and resection. An image guidance scan is repeated one week later but there is no longer any ring-enhancement. Which one of the following is most likely?

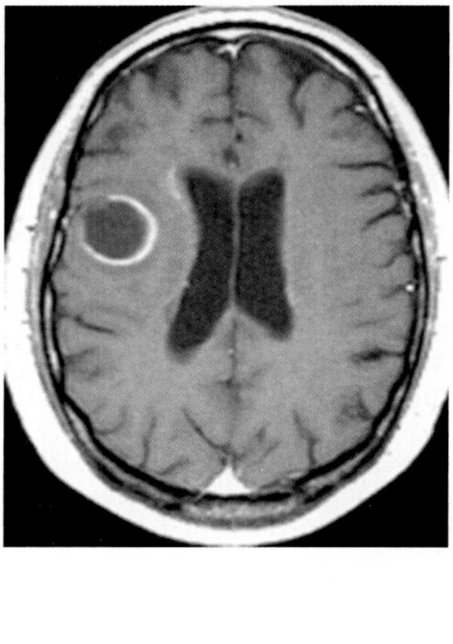

a. Cerebral abscess
b. High grade tumor
c. Metastasis
d. Primary CNS lymphoma
e. Demyelination

18. A 31-year-old female suffered multiple cuts and burns to both arms. On examination there is marked wasting of brachioradialis and the small muscles in both hands, with reduced biceps and brachioradialis reflex. She is weak in both arms, distally more than proximally. Her lower limb and cranial nerve examination is unremarkable. On testing upper limb sensation, vibration and proprioception are intact but there appears to be reduced pain and temperature sensation over the C3/C4/C5 dermatomes. Which one of the following is most likely?
a. Chiari malformation
b. Chronic inflammatory demyelinating polyneuropathy
c. Guillain-Barré syndrome
d. Miller Fisher syndrome
e. Multiple sclerosis

19. A 64-year-old man presents with sudden onset severe headache while watching television, followed by confusion and a tonic-clonic seizure. Past medical history included a 20 pack year smoking history, hypertension, hypercholesterolemia and myocardial infarction two years ago requiring stenting. On examination, GCS M5V4E3 but was protecting his own airway. Pupils were equal and reactive. The patient was spontaneously moving all his limbs and had downgoing plantar reflexes. Cardiovascular, respiratory and abdominal examination was unremarkable. Initial observations were blood pressure 220/115 mmHg, heart rate 89 beat/min, O_2 sats (15 l O_2) 100%, Respiratory rate 19/min, temperature 37.1°C. CT brain is normal and lumbar puncture shows WCC 3/mm^3, RBC 3, protein 0.6 g/l, glucose 5.4 mmol/l, and no xanthochromia. MRI is shown (FLAIR). Which one of the following is most likely?

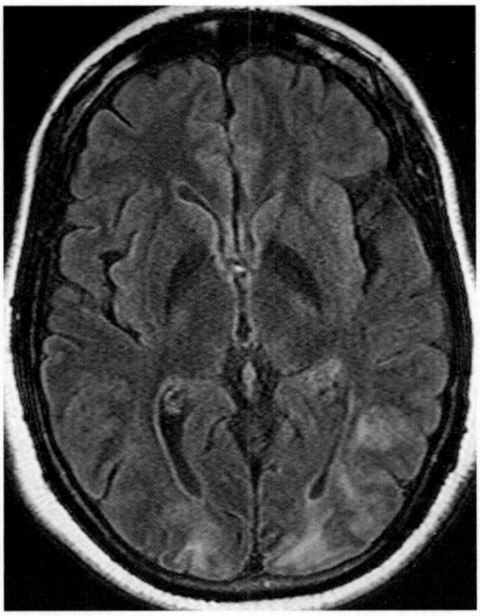

a. Acute disseminated encephalomyelitis
b. Herpes simplex virus encephalitis
c. Multiple sclerosis
d. Posterior circulation stroke
e. Posterior reversible encephalopathy syndrome

20. A 12-year-old boy with Lyme disease and bilateral facial weakness is being treated with a cephalosporin. The child's facial strength improves, but he notices twitching of the left corner of his mouth whenever he blinks his eye. This involuntary movement disorder is probably an indication of which one of the following?
a. Horner's syndrome
b. Marcus Gunn phenomenon
c. Mononeuritis multiplex
d. Parinaud syndrome
e. Recurrent meningitis

21. A 25-year-old woman has progressive gait disorder. The initial physical examination reveals hepatosplenomegaly and left sided ataxia and abnormal finger-nose test. Urinalysis reveals proteinuria and microscopic hematuria. Which one of the following findings is most likely?
a. Neurofibromas
b. Ash leaf spots
c. Retinal telangiectasia
d. Kayser-Fleisher rings
e. Facial angiofibromas

22. A 62-year-old female has discomfort in her limbs and trouble getting off the toilet. She is unable to climb stairs and has noticed a rash on her face. On examination, she is found to have weakness about the hip and shoulder girdle. She has purplish-red discoloration of the skin around her eyes, erythematous discoloration over the finger joints and purplish nodules over the elbows and knees. Which one of the following is the most likely diagnosis?
a. Becker muscular dystrophy
b. Dermatomyositis
c. Inclusion body myositis
d. Myotonic dystrophy
e. Polymyositis

23. A 67-year-old male is investigated for chest pain and painful swallowing progressing over the last few months with no response to proton pump inhibitors. There is no history of weight loss or anorexia or smoking. On examination you note a left-sided partial ptosis, and he reports diplopia on testing extrocular muscle movements. Sustained upward gaze exacerbates his ptosis. There is no limb muscle weakness or sensory disturbance. CXR is shown. Which one of the following tests is likely to be helpful?

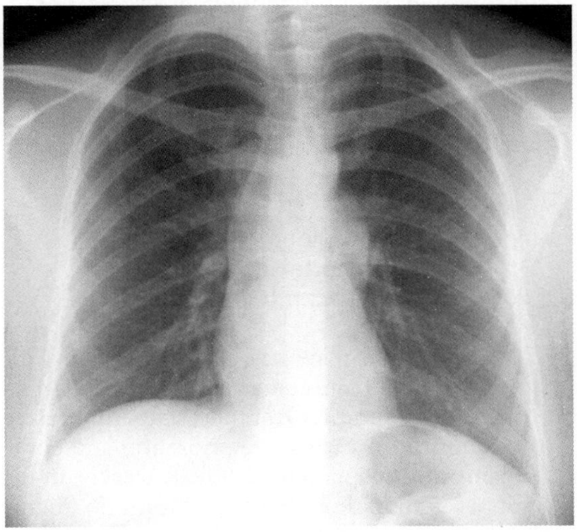

a. Anti-acteylcholine receptor antibodies
b. Anti-GM1 antibody
c. Anti-GQ1b antibody
d. Anti-muscle specific kinase antibody
e. Anti-voltage gated calcium channel antibody

24. A 65-year-old presents with a 3 month history of progressive weakness. She had initially noticed difficulty opening jars, but now also has difficulty walking up stairs. She denied any pain or sensory symptoms. Past medical history included osteoporosis, type 2 diabetes mellitus and hypertension.

On neurological examination there were no fasciculations, tone was normal and sensation was intact. Power was reduced in finger flexion (3/5), wrist flexion (4/5), knee extension (3/5), and hip flexion (4/5) bilaterally. Upper limb reflexes were present but diminished, but the knee jerk was absent and there were flexor plantar responses bilaterally. There was no tenderness over any muscle groups. Cranial nerve examination was unremarkable. Blood results were normal except for CRP 10 mg/l, ESR 41 mm/h, CK 290 u/l. Which one of the following is most likely?
a. Diabetic amyotrophy
b. Inclusion body myositis
c. Polymyalgia rheumatica
d. Polymyositis
e. Chronic inflammatory demyelinating polyneuropathy

25. A 77-year-old male presents with a 2-day history of right temporal throbbing headache. He has had migraines previously but never this severe and usually occipital. There was no other past medical history of note. On examination, his right scalp is tender and a prominent right temporal artery is noted. He is apyrexic with no skin rashes. His blood tests are as follows: Hb 13.1 g/dl, Plt 450 × 10-9/l, WCC 11.5, ESR 85, Na 142, K 4.0., Urea 10, Cr 118 umol/l, CRP 23 mg/l. Which one of the following would you do next?
a. CT angiogram
b. Biopsy
c. Start prednisolone
d. Start azothiaprine
e. Carotid duplex ultrasound

26. A 65-year-old male has been diagnosed with small cell lung cancer and is currently undergoing chemotherapy. Over the last few months he has noticed his vision deteriorating and complains of diplopia. He also feels weaker in his upper limbs although his symptoms do fluctuate. On examination he has mild ptosis of the eyelids bilaterally and a complex ophthalmoparesis affecting both eyes. He also has reduced power proximally in the upper limbs. Which one of the following may be associated with this clinical picture?
a. Anti-Ro antibody
b. Anti-voltage gated potassium channel antibody
c. Anti-voltage gated calcium channel antibody
d. Anti-Hu antibody
e. Anti-GQ1b antibody

27. A 17-year-old girl presents with a second episode on waking earlier in the morning where she could not move at all for 2 h. She reports no loss of consciousness and was aware throughout the episode. There is no other significant past medical history or epilepsy. Routine systemic and neurological examination is normal. A 12 lead ECG demonstrated a jerky baseline with flat T waves. What one of the following is most likely?
a. Andersen-Tawil syndrome
b. Cataplexy
c. Hyperkalemia periodic paralysis
d. Hypokalemic period paralysis
e. Night terror

28. A 10-year-old presents to your neurology clinic reporting 9 months of subtle and gradual onset, progressive lower limb weakness. For the past 18 months, he has noticed a difficulty in keeping up with his peers in PE lessons, which he initially put down to "not being very sporty." However, he feels weak whenever he walks and has particular difficulty getting up from a chair. His appearance is shown below. Formal examination of power is 4/5 bilaterally in shoulder abduction, adduction and normal 5/5 distally. 4/5 is also noted in hip flexion and extension, 4+/5 in knee flexion and extension, 5/5 in ankle plantar and dorsiflexion. The weaknesses demonstrated are not fatiguable and are persistent. Reflexes are present in all areas, plantars are downgoing. He has no other past medical history. What is the likely diagnosis?

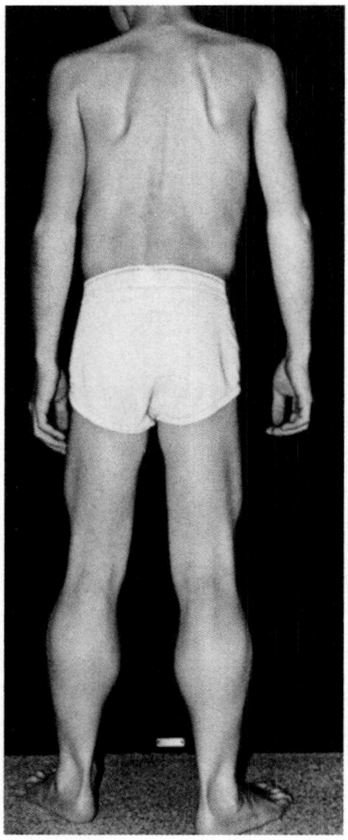

a. Becker muscular dystrophy
b. Duchenne muscular dystrophy
c. Emery-Dreifuss syndrome
d. Facial-scapulo humeral syndrome
e. Limb-girdle dystrophy

QUESTIONS 29–51

Additional questions 29–51 available on ExpertConsult.com

EXTENDED MATCHING ITEM (EMI) QUESTIONS

52. **Alcohol-related neurological disorders:**
a. Alcoholic cerebellar degeneration
b. Alcoholic hallucinosis
c. Alcoholic neuropathy
d. Alcohol withdrawal seizures
e. Beriberi
f. Delerium tremens
g. Marchiafava-Bignami disease
h. Tobacco-alcohol amblyopia
i. Wernicke's encephalopathy
j. Wernicke-Korsakoff syndrome

For each of the following descriptions, select the most appropriate answers from the list above. Each answer may be used once, more than once, or not at all.

1. A 55-year-old male known alcoholic is found confused on a street by a policeman not orientated in time or place. He is able to follow your commands in lifting his upper and lower limbs during his neurological exams. All reflexes were present. He fails to follow your finger with his eyes on cranial nerve examination and you note horizontal nystagmus. His gait is grossly ataxic.
2. A 45-year-old heavy drinker (30 units per day) presents 72 h after his last drink with agitation, and pointing around the room as if having hallucinations. He has a coarse tremor, sinus tachycardia at 120 bpm and sweating.
3. A 60-year-old female is brought in by police as she was wandering and confused. She was disorientated in place and time, did not remember her birthday, was unable to recall three objects after 5 min and identified the hospital cleaner as her father and seemed to recognize people she had never met. On examination pupils were reactive, there was an ophthalmoparesis, nystagmus on attempted horizontal gaze and ataxic gait. Motor and sensory systems were normal.

53. **Poisoning:**
a. Aluminum
b. Arsenic
c. Carbon monoxide
d. Cyanide
e. Ergot
f. Lead
g. Manganese
h. Mercury
i. Organophosphates
j. Thallium

For each of the following descriptions, select the most appropriate answers from the list above. Each answer may be used once, more than once, or not at all.

1. A 34-year-old male working in a felt-processing plant develops tremors, memory disturbances and personality change over the course of months. On examination, he has prominent gait ataxia, limb and facial tremors, and decreased pain and temperature sense in his feet.
2. A 23-year-old volunteers abroad painting houses during a 3-month exchange. Towards the end of the trip he develops weakness in both wrists. On examination, there is bilateral wrist drop without any sensory deficit. An EMG reveals evidence of a peripheral motor neuropathy.
3. A 45-year-old worker in an insecticide factory complains of severe stomach pain. She also has had problems with her memory, excessive drowsiness, and a sensorimotor neuropathy with absent tendon reflexes.
4. A 22-year-old farm worker has seizure. Neurological examination reveals fasciculations and occasional myoclonus. He is ataxic and has absent deep tendon reflexes. A sensory neuropathy is evident in his legs. Ulcers are evident on his fingers and toes. He says his diet was poor and mostly made food from his rye crop.
5. A 38-year-old miner develops a shuffling gait, tremor, and drooling. His speech is difficult to understand and becomes quieter as he talks. On examination, cogwheel rigidity is evident in his arms and legs. His tremor is most evident when his limbs are at rest.

54. **Genetic syndromes with learning disability:**
    a. Angelman's syndrome
    b. Cri du Chat syndrome
    c. Down's syndrome
    d. Fragile X syndrome
    e. Neurofibromatosis
    f. Prader-Willi syndrome
    g. Rett syndrome
    h. Tuberous sclerosis
    i. Velocardiofacial syndrome
    j. Williams syndrome

For each of the following descriptions, select the most appropriate answers from the list above. Each answer may be used once, more than once, or not at all.

1. A 15-year-old boy has moderate mental retardation, attention deficit disorder, a long face, enlarged ears, and macroorchidism. Development has been steady but always at a delayed pace.
2. An 11-year-old girl presents with obesity, excessive and indiscriminate gorging, small hands, feet, hypogonadism and mental retardation.
3. A 7-year-old boy is noted to have characteristic elfin facies, short stature and cardiovascular defects.
4. A 13-year-old boy has a history of thymus abnormalities, ear deformities, cleft palate, cardiac defects and short stature. He has annual blood tests to assess serum calcium.
5. A 5-year-old girl with progressive deterioration in cognitive function and loss of language displays stereotypic hand movements.

55. **Neuropathy:**
    a. Acute intermittent porphyria
    b. Charcot-Marie Tooth
    c. Chronic axonal neuropathy
    d. Chronic inflammatory demyelinating polyneuropathy
    e. Diabetic neuropathy
    f. Hereditary sensory and autonomic neuropathy
    g. HIV neuropathy
    h. Mononeuritis multiplex
    i. Multifocal motor neuropathy with conduction block
    j. Paraneoplastic neuropathy
    k. Paraproteinemic neuropathy
    l. Sarcoidosis
    m. Vasculitis

For each of the following descriptions, select the most appropriate answers from the list above. Each answer may be used once, more than once, or not at all.

1. A 48-year-old male develops weakness of his left wrist extensors and digits over one week, followed by involvement of his right hand and foot over the subsequent 6 weeks. On examination, he has wasting and 2/5 power in the left wrist and digit extensors. There is evidence of clawing of the right ring and little fingers along with wasting of the small muscles of the right hand (except the thenar eminence and the first two lumbricals). He has a right foot drop along with wasting of the anterior tibial and perineal muscles on that side. Fasciculations are seen in all of the areas of weakness. Sensory examination and reflexes are normal, no clonus and a flexor plantar response.
2. A 56-year-old female has a 6 month history of worsening numbness and paresthesias distally in the hands and feet, as well as proximal muscle weakness. Bulbar muscles are normal. An EMG shows multifocal conduction block, slowing of nerve conduction, and minimal loss of amplitude of muscle action potentials. CSF examination shows an elevation in protein, but no increase in the number of cells.
3. A 40-year-old male has a prophylactic dose of phenytoin for 7 days after conservative management of head injury. He presents with confusion, psychosis, abdominal pain, and vomiting. On examination, he is tachycardic, hypertensive, and febrile and appears delirious. His arms are weak and areflexic but sensation is relatively preserved.
4. A 25-year-old woman with a prior history of visual loss in the left eye and a spastic gait develops impaired pain and temperature perception in her feet. She was diagnosed with multiple sclerosis (MS) shortly after her visual loss. Her left fundus reveals optic atrophy, and her facial movements are asymmetric. Chest X-ray reveals large hilar lymph nodes. Mammogram reveals no apparent carcinoma. Serum ACE is positive.
5. A 55-year-old female presents with 3 weeks of bilateral tingling sensation in her medial one and half digits at night. She has noted a clawing of her 4th and 5th digits and she is particularly concerned by the cosmetic elements. She also complains of a left sided foot drop present over the past 8 months. She has also had multiple admissions for surgery to her feet at childhood but she is unaware of further details. On examination, she clinically has a left common peroneal palsy with bilateral thin calves, and loss of sensation in bilateral ulnar nerve territories.

6. A 29-year-old female with Type 1 diabetes mellitus presents with weakness in several muscles in different limbs. The pattern is lower motor neuron and does not fit with any particular peripheral, plexus, or root localization.

56. **Paraneoplastic disorders:**
    a. Dorsal root ganglionopathy
    b. Guillain-Barré syndrome
    c. Hypercalcemia
    d. Lambert-Eaton myasthenic syndrome
    e. Limbic encephalitis
    f. Motor neuron disease
    g. Myasthenia gravis
    h. Opsoclonus-myoclonus
    i. Paraneoplastic cerebellar degeneration
    j. Paraproteinemic neuropathy
    k. Stiff man syndrome

For each of the following descriptions, select the most appropriate answers from the list above. Each answer may be used once, more than once, or not at all.

1. A 67-year-old female has a 2 month history of progressive gait disturbance. On examination, she has dysmetria of the limbs, a wide-based, unsteady gait; and hypermetric saccades. A hard, firm breast lump is discovered.
2. A 70-year-old male with a history of lung cancer develops nausea and vomiting and then becomes lethargic. On examination, he is lethargic but arousable, disoriented, and inattentive. He is weak proximally and has diminished reflexes.
3. A 57-year-old female with a history of smoking has a 3-month history of hip and shoulder weakness. She also complains of xerostomia. There are no sensory symptoms, and she is cognitively intact. On examination, she is orthostatic. There is proximal muscle weakness, but she has increasing muscle strength with repetitive activity of her muscles. Eye movements are normal.
4. A 65-year-old female develops pain and paresthesias in her feet. On examination, she has stocking distribution sensory loss, and mild distal weakness with areflexia. Serum protein electrophoresis reveals a monoclonal gammopathy, and bone marrow biopsy reveals plasma cell dyscrasia.

57. **Hereditary ataxia:**
    a. Abetalipoproteinemia
    b. Ataxia telangiectasia
    c. Ataxia with isolated vitamin E deficiency
    d. Episodic ataxia type 1
    e. Episodic ataxia type 2
    f. Fragile X tremor ataxia syndrome
    g. Friedreich's ataxia
    h. Machado-Joseph disease (SCA3)
    i. Mitochondrial disorders
    j. Spinocerebellar ataxias (SCA1)

For each of the following descriptions, select the most appropriate answers from the list above. Each answer may be used once, more than once, or not at all.

1. A 3-year-old boy presents with gait ataxia, choreoathetoid movements in his right hand and recurrent ear infections or episodes of unexplained fever. On examination he had dilated venules on his ear, mild dysarthria and a wide based ataxic gait. Deep tendon reflexes were absent.
2. A 24-year-old presents with progressive unsteadiness on walking over the past 6 months. Over the past 3 months, he has noticed a lack of articulation with his speech. On examination, his cardiovascular, respiratory and abdominal systems are normal. His finger-nose test is impaired bilaterally and he is unable to tandem walk. He denies any neck stiffness or headache. He has a full range of eye movements. He has absent reflexes in his lower limbs and upgoing plantars bilaterally.
3. A 36-year-old male presents with a 5-year history of increasing, progressive "clumsiness." He cannot write legibly or even hold a key still using either hand to open a door. On examination, his cranial nerves were unremarkable except for mild multidirectional nystagmus at primary gaze. Fundoscopy was normal. Limb examination revealed significant impairment of finger-nose and heel-shin testing. His gait, tone, power, sensation and reflexes were normal with downgoing plantars. A brief mini-mental state examination scored 30/30. Serum ANA was negative.
4. At age 5, a child is noted to have the loss of ankle jerks. At age 10, limb ataxia develops, followed by a peripheral neuropathy. During adolescence, retinitis pigmentosa develops. Peripheral blood smear shows acanthocytosis.

58. **Nutritional deficiency:**
    a. Folate
    b. Niacin
    c. Pyridoxine (vitamin B6) deficiency
    d. Riboflavin
    e. Thiamine (vitamin B1) deficiency
    f. Vitamin A deficiency

g. Vitamin B12 deficiency
h. Vitamin C deficiency
i. Vitamin E deficiency
j. Vitamin D deficiency
k. Vitamin K

For each of the following descriptions, select the most appropriate answers from the list above. Each answer may be used once, more than once, or not at all.

1. A 36-year-old man with tuberculosis is started on therapy with isoniazid, rifampin, and ethambutol. After 2 months his liver enzymes are slightly deranged and he reports pins-and-needles sensations in his feet. Neurological examination reveals preserved power, but hypoactive deep tendon reflexes in the legs and impaired position sense.
2. A 47-year-old known alcoholic female is found wandering and brought to the emergency room. She is disoriented to time, place, and person, but has no external evidence of head trauma. Examination reveals ataxic gait, paresis of conjugate gaze, and horizontal nystagmus. She does not have any ethanol in her bloodstream on testing.
3. A 59-year-old man developed progressive cramping of his legs, gait unsteadiness and paresthesia affecting his hands and feet over 1 year. He has also had some episodes of urinary incontinence. On examination, he has a spastic paraparesis with severe disturbance of position and vibration sense in his legs, absent knee and ankle reflexes. Blood results show a megaloblastic anemia.
4. A 5-year-old boy develops progressive gait ataxia and limb weakness over the course of 3 months. Examination reveals diffusely absent deep tendon reflexes, proximal muscle weakness, ophthalmoparesis, and poor pain perception in the feet. Blood tests reveal elevated creatine kinase levels and evidence of liver disease without features of liver failure.

59. **Leukodystrophies:**
a. Acute disseminated encephalomyelitis
b. Alexander disease
c. CADASIL
d. Canavan disease
e. Cerebrotendinous xanthomatosis
f. Krabbe Disease
g. Metachromatic leukodystrophy
h. Pelizaeus-Merzbacher disease
i. Refsum disease
j. X-linked Adrenoleukodystrophy
k. Zellweger syndrome

For each of the following descriptions, select the most appropriate answers from the list above. Each answer may be used once, more than once, or not at all.

1. Two brothers, 4 and 6 years of age, but not their 9-year-old sister, exhibit limb ataxia, nystagmus, and learning disability, and have abnormally low serum cortisol levels.
2. A 3-month-old boy exhibits nystagmus and limb tremors unassociated with seizures. Over the next few years, he develops optic atrophy, choreoathetotic limb movements, seizures, and gait ataxia. He dies during status epilepticus and at autopsy is found to have widespread myelin breakdown with myelin preservation in islands about the blood vessels. The pathologist diagnoses a sudanophilic leukodystrophy to describe the pattern of staining observed on slides prepared to look for myelin breakdown products.
3. A 17-month-old boy had developed normally until approximately 13 months of age, when he began having progressive gait problems. On examination, the patient is spastic, yet nerve conduction studies (NCS) reveal slowed motor and sensory conduction velocities. Cerebrospinal fluid (CSF) protein is elevated. MRI reveals white matter abnormalities. Leukocyte testing reveals deficient arylsulfatase A activity.
4. A 6-month-old child has a rapid regression of psychomotor function and loss of sight. There is increased urinary excretion of *N*-acetyl-L-aspartic acid.

60. **Sphingolipidosis:**
a. Batten's disease
b. Cerebrotendinous xanthomatosis
c. Fabry disease
d. Gaucher's disease
e. GM1 gangliosidosis
f. Krabbe disease
g. Metachromatic leukodystrophy
h. Neimann-Pick disease
i. Sandhoff's disease
j. Tay-Sachs disease
k. Wolman disease

For each of the following descriptions, select the most appropriate answers from the list above. Each answer may be used once, more than once, or not at all.

1. A 12-month-old develops progressive blindness and delayed cognitive milestones. Fundal examination shows a cherry red spot. There is a deficiency of hexaminosidase A.

2. An 8-month-old boy develops spasticity, head retraction, and difficulty swallowing. There is abnormal accumulation of glucocerebroside and the child will deteriorate and die within 3 years.

61. **Antibodies:**
   a. Anti-muscle specific kinase
   b. Anti-NMDA receptor antibody
   c. Anti-voltage gated calcium channel antibody
   d. Anti-Aquaporin 4 antibody
   e. Anti-Hu (ANNA-1)
   f. Anti-Yo (PCA-1)
   g. Anti-Ri (ANNA-2)
   h. Anti-Tr
   i. Anti-GAD
   j. Anti-voltage gated potassium channel antibody
   k. Anti-TA Ma2
   l. Anti-GQ1b
   m. Anti-myelin associated glycoprotein/sulfated glucoronul paragloboside
   n. Anti-GD1b

For each of the following descriptions, select the most appropriate answers from the list above. Each answer may be used once, more than once, or not at all.

1. Non-paraneoplastic limbic encephalitis
2. Neuromyelitis optica (Devic's disease)
3. Guillain-Barré syndrome
4. Myasthenia gravis
5. Lambert-Eaton myasthenic syndrome

62. **Mucopolysaccharidoses:**
   a. Hunter syndrome
   b. Hurler syndrome
   c. Sanfilippo syndrome A
   d. Sanfilippo syndrome B
   e. Sanfilippo syndrome C
   f. Sanfilippo syndrome D
   g. Maroteaux-Lamy syndrome
   h. Morquio syndrome A
   i. Morquio syndrome B
   j. Natowicz syndrome
   k. Sly syndrome

For each of the following descriptions, select the most appropriate answers from the list above. Each answer may be used once, more than once, or not at all.

1. A 4-year-old is found to have dwarfism, mental retardation, and clouding of his corneas. Tests show an α-L-iduronidase deficiency.
2. A 6-year-old child is diagnosed with X-linked recessive mild learning difficulty due to iduronate sulfatase deficiency.
3. A 7-year-old child presents with severe skeletal dysplasia, short stature. Test shows abnormal accumulation of keratan sulfate secondary to deficiency of galactose-6-sulfate sulfatase.

63. **Mitochondrial disorders:**
   a. Alpers-Huttenlocher syndrome
   b. Ataxia neuropathy syndromes
   c. Chronic progressive external ophthalmoplegia
   d. Kearns-Sayre syndrome
   e. Leber's hereditary optic neuropathy
   f. Leigh syndrome
   g. MELAS
   h. MEMSA
   i. MERRF
   j. NARP

For each of the following descriptions, select the most appropriate answers from the list above. Each answer may be used once, more than once, or not at all.

1. A 19-year-old male presents with diplopia, ataxia, and heart block.
2. A 24-year-old male presents with reduced vision in both eyes over several weeks, and has developed "spasms" of his left hand and complains of palpitations. ECG is suggestive of ventricular pre-excitation.
3. A 34-year-old female with a history of migraines present's with stroke-like episodes affecting her left arm and leg, lactic acidosis, and cognitive impairment.

64. **Dementia:**
   a. Alzheimer's disease
   b. B12 deficiency
   c. Cortical Lewy body disease
   d. Corticobasal degeneration
   e. Creutzfeldt-Jacob disease
   f. Depression
   g. Frontotemporal dementia
   h. HIV dementia complex
   i. Huntington's disease
   j. Hypothyroidism
   k. Neurosyphilis
   l. Normal pressure hydrocephalus
   m. Transient global amnesia
   n. Vascular dementia

For each of the following descriptions, select the most appropriate answers from the list above. Each answer may be used once, more than once, or not at all.

1. A 73-year-old man steps out of the shower on a Saturday evening and is unable to remember that he and his wife have tickets to a play. He asks her repeatedly, "Where are we going"? He appears bewildered, but is alert, knows

his own name, speaks fluently, and has no motor deficits. He has no history of memory disturbance and after 8 h returns to normal.

2. A 50-year-old woman began having double vision and blurry vision 3 months ago and has since had diminishing interaction with her family, a paucity of thought and expression, and unsteadiness of gait. Her whole body appears to jump in the presence of a loud noise. MRI is normal but CSF is positive for 14-3-3 protein.
3. A 17-year-old girl develops mild dementia, tremor, and rigidity. Her father died in his fourth decade of life of a progressive dementing illness associated with jerking (choreiform) limb movements. On exposure to L-dopa, she becomes acutely agitated and has jerking limb movements.
4. A 62-year-old man has had 2 years of progressive memory loss and inappropriate behavior. He has been delusional. More recently, he has developed tremors, myoclonus, dysarthria, and unsteadiness of gait. The CSF shows a lymphocytic pleocytosis, protein of 150, and positive VDRL.
5. A 44-year-old woman presents with inattentiveness, poor concentration, weight gain and lethargy. She has paranoid delusions. There is mild proximal weakness and ataxia. On general examination, she has edema, coarse and pale skin, macroglossia and delayed relaxation of the ankle reflexes.

65. **Syncope:**
   a. Autonomic failure
   b. Cardiac arrhythmia
   c. Carotid sinus syncope
   d. Cerebrovascular steal
   e. Dehydration
   f. Drug-induced orthostatic syncope
   g. Epileptic seizure
   h. Hypoglycemia
   i. Neurally mediated (vasovagal) syncope
   j. Non-epileptic attack disorder
   k. Situational syncope
   l. Structural cardiac disease

For each of the following descriptions, select the most appropriate answers from the list above. Each answer may be used once, more than once, or not at all.

1. A 36-year-old female complianed of a syncopal episode. She described dizziness and fatigue on her way to her bedroom, shortly after she passed out. She regained consciousness after a few minutes, feeling tired and soaked in her sweat. Her PE was normal. Her resting ECG was within normal. Routine laboratory work up was normal. Echocardiography was normal.
2. A 51-year-old female presents to the ER complaining of a sudden syncopal episode while climbing up the stairs. Her PE showed that she is in respiratory distress, BMI of 40, hemodynamically stable, cardiac examination showed normal. Routine laboratory work up was normal. Echocardiography was normal apart from mild MR and mild TR.
3. A 72-year-old with a 10-year history of Parkinson's disease presents with recurrent syncopal episodes on standing up from a sitting position.

66. **Headache:**
   a. Analgesic overuse headache
   b. Atypical facial pain
   c. Cluster headache
   d. Hypnic headache
   e. Migraine with aura
   f. Migraine without aura
   g. Opthalmoplegic migraine
   h. Paroxysmal hemicranias
   i. Postherpetic neuralgia
   j. Retinal migraine
   k. Sinusitis
   l. Short-lasting unilateral neuralgiform headache with conjunctival injection and tearing (SUNCT)
   m. Tension headache
   n. Trigeminal neuralgia
   o. Vertebrobasilar migraine

For each of the following descriptions, select the most appropriate answers from the list above. Each answer may be used once, more than once, or not at all.

1. A 22-year-old complains of regular, right-sided throbbing headaches. Changes in her vision that precede the headache by 20 min include scintillating lights just to the left of her center of vision progressing to a blind spot which then clears before the headache starts. It rarely lasts more than 1 h, but is usually accompanied by nausea and vomiting.
2. A 35-year-old man has severe throbbing pain waking him from sleep at night and persisting into the day. This pain is usually centered about his left eye and appears on a nearly daily basis for several weeks or months each year. He becomes combative and agitated during the onset, but never vomits or develops focal weakness.
3. An 81-year-old man with chronic lymphocytic leukemia develops pain and burning over the right side of his face. Within a few days, a vesiculopapular rash in the

distribution of the first division of the trigeminal nerve appears. The vesicles become encrusted, and the burning associated with the rash abates. Within 1 month the rash has largely resolved, but the man is left with a dull ache over the area of the rash that is periodically punctuated by shooting pains.

67. **Headache:**
   a. Analgesic rebound headache
   b. Aseptic meningitis
   c. Carotid artery dissection
   d. Glioblastoma multiforme
   e. Idiopathic intracranial hypertension
   f. Paroxysmal hemicranias
   g. Post-traumatic headache
   h. Raeder syndrome
   i. Spontaneous intracranial hypotension
   j. Thunderclap headache

For each of the following descriptions, select the most appropriate answers from the list above. Each answer may be used once, more than once, or not at all.

1. An obese 37-year-old woman has had a daily headache, worse in the morning, for 1 year. She has episodes of transient visual obscurations affecting each eye and also hears a pulsatile tinnitus. Examination is notable for bilateral papilledema. MRI is normal.
2. A 42-year-old man presents with a sudden and severe headache associated with nausea during coitus. The headache reaches maximal intensity within 5 s. He has no prior history of headache. Examination is unremarkable. CT head is normal and CSF shows a traumatic tap and cannot exclude subarachnoid hemorrhage. A good quality CT angiogram is negative for aneurysm, dissection or AVM.
3. A 29-year-old man relates that he has had recent headaches only when standing up. The headaches resolve quickly when he lies down and are accompanied by mild nausea. His examination is normal.

68. **Disorders of language:**
   a. Akinetic mutism
   b. Anomic aphasia
   c. Broca's aphasia
   d. Cerebellar mutism
   e. Conduction aphasia
   f. Global aphasia
   g. Mixed transcortical aphasia
   h. Transcortical motor aphasia
   i. Transcortical sensory aphasia (fluent)
   j. Wernicke's aphasia

For each of the following descriptions, select the most appropriate answers from the list above. Each answer may be used once, more than once, or not at all.

1. A 45-year-old woman with chronic atrial fibrillation discontinues warfarin treatment and abruptly develops problems with language comprehension. She is able to produce some intelligible phrases and produces sound quite fluently; however, she is unable to follow simple instructions or to repeat simple phrases. On attempting to write, she becomes very frustrated and agitated. Emergency MRI reveals a lesion of the left temporal lobe that extends into the superior temporal gyrus.
2. A 62-year-old man has had a left hemisphere stroke. He has impaired naming and repetition. His speech is nonfluent. Comprehension is preserved.
3. A 28-year-old woman is hit in the left neck while playing lacrosse. Approximately 2 h later she begins having language difficulties. Her speech is fluent and nonsensical. She cannot understand commands, but repeats well.

SBA ANSWER

1. **b**—Alzheimer's disease

Alzheimer's dementia can present as self-neglect and weight loss, especially when the patient is living alone. Paranoid ideation is also quite common and may be used by the patient as an explanation for symptoms of memory loss (e.g. misplacing items), as is physical aggression whereas auditory and visual hallucinations are less common. Alzheimer's disease is the commonest cause of dementia, and most cases are sporadic; 5% of cases are inherited as an autosomal dominant trait mutations in the amyloid precursor protein (chromosome 21), presenilin 1 (chromosome 14), and presenilin 2 (chromosome 1) genes are thought to cause the inherited form. Risk of Alzheimer's disease is increased in those with the apolipoprotein E allele E4 (present in 20% of population) is 15 times higher than those with two E3 alleles. Mild AD is characterized by minor behavioral changes, loss of memory of recent events (e.g. conversations, events), misplace items, struggle to find the right word in conversation, confused or lose track of day/date, difficulty planning and making decisions, visuospatial impairment, and lose interest in people or activities. Moderate AD will need reminders about self-care, increasingly forgetful, not recognize people, place themselves/others at risk (e.g. miss medication, leave gas stove on), easily upset/angry/aggressive, night-day reversal, agitation, socially inappropriate, delusions/hallucinations. Severe AD is characterized by increasing dependence on others for nursing care, bed/wheelchair bound, weakness, unable to recognize familiar objects/people, incontinence, difficulty eating/swallowing and gradual loss of speech. Death is usually 8-10 years after symptom onset. Pathological changes include widespread cerebral atrophy, particularly involving the cortex and hippocampus. In AD, FDG-PET can show hypometabolism in the temporoparietal regions and/or the posterior cingulum. On microscopy there are cortical plaques due to deposition of type A-Beta-amyloid protein and intraneuronal neurofibrillary tangles caused by abnormal aggregation of the tau protein (excessive phosphorylation). There is also reduced acetylcholine due to damage to ascending forebrain projection, hence acetylcholinesterase inhibitors (donepezil, galantamine, and rivastigmine) as options for managing mild to moderate Alzheimer's disease. Memantine (a NMDA receptor antagonist) is reserved for patients with moderate—severe Alzheimer's disease.

Image with permission from Loevner L. Brain Imaging: Case Review Series, 2nd ed. Mosby: Elsevier, 2009.

2. **c**—Pick's disease

Frontotemporal lobar degeneration (FTLD) is the third most common type of cortical dementia after Alzheimer's and Lewy body dementia. Common features of frontotemporal lobar dementias include: Onset <65 years, insidious onset, relatively preserved memory and visuospatial skills, personality change and social conduct problems. CT shows cortical loss in the frontal and temporal lobes, and FDG-PET/CT shows hypometabolism. There are three recognized types of FTLD:

1. Frontotemporal dementia (Pick's disease). Most common type and is characterized by personality change and impaired social conduct. Other common features include hyperorality, disinhibition, increased appetite, and perseveration behaviors. Focal gyral atrophy ("knife-blade" atrophy) is characteristic of Pick's disease and is localized to frontal and temporal lobes only. Microscopic findings include Pick bodies, gliosis, neurofibrillary tangles, and senile plaques.
2. Progressive non-fluent aphasia (chronic progressive aphasia). Patients have non-fluent speech, they make short utterances that are agrammatic but comprehension is relatively preserved.
3. Semantic dementia: Here the patient has a progressive fluent aphasia but speech lacks content and conveys little meaning. Unlike in Alzheimer's memory is better for recent rather than remote events.

Image with permission from Hinds SR II, Stocker DJ, Bradley YC. Role of positron emission tomography/computed tomography in dementia, Radiol Clin North Am. 2013;51(5):927-34.

3. **d**—Lewy body dementia

Lewy body dementia is an increasingly recognized cause of dementia, accounting for up to 20% of cases. The characteristic pathological feature is alpha-synuclein cytoplasmic inclusions (Lewy bodies) in the substantia nigra, paralimbic, and neocortical areas. The relationship between Parkinson's disease and Lewy body dementia is complicated, particularly as dementia is often seen in Parkinson's disease. Also, up to 40% of patients with Alzheimer's have Lewy bodies. Neuroleptics should be avoided in Lewy body dementia as patients are extremely sensitive and may develop irreversible Parkinsonism. Features include progressive cognitive impairment, Parkinsonism, and visual hallucinations (other features such as delusions and non-visual hallucinations may also be seen). Two out of three are needed for diagnosis. The visual hallucinations are often very vivid. He also has a few supportive features of Lewy body dementia hallucinations in other modalities, delusions, depression and repeated falls. Diagnosis is usually clinical, but SPECT is increasingly used. It is currently commercially known as a DaT scan. Dopaminergic iodine-123-I FP-CIT is used as the radioisotope. The sensitivity of SPECT in diagnosing Lewy body dementia is around 90% with a specificity of 100%. Currently, evidence best supports cholinesterase inhibitors in the treating of Lewy body dementia. It must be remembered that these patients have high sensitivity to neuroleptics so Olanzapine should not be used here.

4. **b**—Creutzfeldt-Jakob disease

Creutzfeldt-Jakob disease is a rapidly progressive spongiform encephalopathy due to accumulation of prion proteins resistant to proteases. Sporadic CJD accounts for 85% of cases whereas 10-15% of cases are familial. The mean age of onset is 65 years, except for new variant CJD which affects younger patients (mean age 25 years). Features include dementia, myoclonic jerks (often stimulus-sensitive), startle response, and less commonly extrapyramidal signs. New variant CJD usually has psychological symptoms such as anxiety, withdrawal and dysphonia. MRI shows high signal on the cortical sulci surfaces (ribboning) and increased signal in putamen and caudate head. EEG shows periodic spikes with sharp waves in sporadic CJD. CSF profile is usually normal but positive for 14-3-3 protein.

Image with permission from Naidich T, Castillo M, Cha S, Smirniotopoulos J. Imaging of the Brain, Saunders: Elsevier, 2013.

5. **b**—Treat cardiovascular risk factors

Vascular dementia is one of the most common causes of dementia after Alzheimer's disease, causing around 15% of cases. The history and findings are most suggestive of a vascular dementia caused by multiple strokes, hence management of stroke risk factors is the primary option as there is no licensed treatment for it. Targeted treatment is made more difficult as there are multiple subtypes of vascular dementia depending on profile of ischemia: multi-infarct (cortical) dementia, small vessel (subcortical white matter) dementia, hypoperfusion dementia (watershed infarcts), hemorrhagic dementia, CADASIL, and mixed vascular-Alzheimer's disease type.

6. **c**—Amyotrophic lateral sclerosis

Motor neuron diseases (MND) result in progressive degeneration of upper motor neurons (Betz cells) and/or lower motor neurons (anterior horn cells). Genetic studies have implicated Cu/Zn superoxide dismutase-1 (*SOD1*) gene in sporadic cases. They rarely presents before 40 years of age. Various patterns/subtypes are recognized including: amyotrophic lateral sclerosis (Lou Gehrig disease), progressive bulbar palsy (bulbar onset ALS), primary lateral sclerosis, spinal muscular atrophy, X-linked spinobulbar muscular atrophy (Kennedy disease) and hereditary spastic paraparesis. ALS is the most common form and may present with limb symptoms (tripping, foot drop, wasting of the small hand muscles, wrist drop) in 75% or bulbar symptoms (slurred speech, hoarseness, decreased volume of speech, aspirating/choking on meals) in 25% of cases. Progression of disease results in muscle atrophy, fasciculations, spasticity, muscle cramps, voice changes, dysphagia, dysarthria, and drooling. Other clues which point towards a diagnosis of motor neuron disease include absence of sensory signs/symptoms, both UMN and LMN symptoms, no cerebellar signs, no ocular signs and abdominal reflexes are usually preserved and sphincter dysfunction is a late feature. MRI is usually performed to exclude the differential diagnosis of cervical cord compression or cranial lesion, and shows T2 hyperintensity (better seen on FLAIR) along the length of the corticospinal tract. The diagnosis of motor neuron disease is clinical, but EMG and nerve conduction studies will show normal sensory conduction with abnormal spontaneous (fasciculation) and evoked muscle potentials. Riluzole is the only drug that has been proven to demonstrate a disease modifying effect in motor neurone disease, increasing survival from diagnosis from 12 to 15 months and should be started; therapies to reduce oxidative stress such as addition of vitamin E and *N*-acetylcysteine (NAC) are not recommended. Non-invasive ventilation is the only other therapy that seems to prolong life expectancy but only if the patient can tolerate greater than 4 h of NIV per day and does not have severe bulbar dysfunction. NIV is recommended when the patient has developed signs of respiratory distress, type 2 respiratory failure, FVC $< 50\%$ or the patient has reported orthopnea/nocturnal hypoventilation. However, patients with severe bulbar palsy or cognitive impairment are excluded. Tracheostomy and long term invasive mechanical ventilation have been used in selected cases with respiratory deterioration despite being largely neurologically intact. Prognosis poor: 50% of patients die within 3 years

7. **d**—Survival motor neuron gene testing

Spinal muscular atrophy is a congenital lower motor neuron disorder manifesting as progressive, symmetric proximal muscular weakness occurring in 1 in 6000 to 1 in 10,000 births (second most common autosomal recessive disease in humans after cystic fibrosis). It is the leading inherited cause of infant death. Spinal muscular atrophy is classified clinically by the age at symptom onset and disease severity into type I (Werdnig-Hoffman disease, acute), type II (intermediate form, usually 7-18 months old and can sit unsupported but can't walk independently), type III (Kugelberg-Welander disease, mildest form, presents >18 months and able to achieve independent walking), and type IV SMA (adult-onset). Spinal muscular atrophy is inherited in autosomal recessive fashion or is sporadic. Mutations or deletions in the telomeric *SMN* (survival of motor neuron) gene occur in most patients. The loss of functional SMN protein results in premature neuronal cell death. The SMN protein has a role in cardiac development. If the history and physical examination suggest spinal muscular atrophy, a positive DNA test for deletion of the survival motor neuron gene eliminates the need for electrophysiological testing and muscle biopsy. However, the *SMN* gene is deleted only in 96% of patients, serum creatine kinase activity may be 1 to 2 times normal. Electromyography reveals large motor units; nerve conduction velocities and sensory conduction times are normal, ruling out motor neuropathies. Muscle biopsy reveals group atrophy of type 1 and type 2 muscle fibers as opposed to the normal checkerboard pattern. In the most severe cases (Type I), children never gain the ability to sit unsupported and severe respiratory problems mean children rarely survive beyond two years of age. Type II SMA may shorten life expectancy, but improvements in care standards mean the majority of people can live long, fulfilling, and productive lives. Survival into adulthood is now expected. Life expectancy is usually unaffected in Types III and IV.

8. **c**—Methotrexate

Common focal cerebral lesions in HIV patients are toxoplasmosis (50%), primary CNS lymphoma (30%), and less commonly cerebral tuberculosis. Typically, PCNSL in immunocompetent individuals (whether HIV positive or not) will appear as a single homogenously enhancing lesion, or spread across the corpus callosum (butterfly pattern) and has a dramatic response to dexamethasone treatment hence is easier to differentiate from infection. In immunocompromised patients, however, imaging appearances of PCNSL are more variable—with smaller lesions and faster growth outstripping blood supply leading to necrosis (ring-enhancing lesions) and making them challenging to differentiate from other ring-enhancing lesions seen in immunocompromised individuals such as toxoplasma (multiple lesions) and tuberculosis (usually only single abscess). Several limitations of diagnostic testing also complicate matters and are worthy of note. Firstly, even when primary CNS lymphoma presents with its classical, homogeneously enhancing imaging appearance a cytological diagnosis is still required before treatment with methotrexate can start. In this scenario, if there is little intracranial mass effect lumbar puncture can be performed and CSF cytology, flow cytometry, PCR for immunoglobin clonal gene rearrangements (to establish monoclonality) and EBV PCR (80% positive in AIDS-related PCNSL). Despite this, CSF is often non-diagnostic and serial samples may be required or alternatively brain biopsy which is the gold standard. Additionally, many patients receive dexamethasone due to raised ICP or focal deficits which (i) further reduces the chance of diagnostic LP and (ii) may cause the lesion to "disappear" and prevent accurate brain biopsy. In those AIDS patients in whom diagnostic uncertainty between cerebral toxoplasma and PCNSL remains after non-diagnostic CSF, brain biopsy should be considered in the context of negative serological screening for toxoplasma and thallium-enhanced SPECT scan results (negative in toxoplasma, positive in PCNSL). Treatment for toxoplasma includes sulfadiazine and pyrimethamine, whereas it is methotrexate chemotherapy for PCNSL (or radiotherapy as second-line therapy).

Image with permission from Tang YZ, Booth TC, Bhogal P, et al. Imaging of primary central nervous system lymphoma, Clin Radiol 2011;66(8):768-77.

9. **d**—Progressive multifocal leukoencephalopathy

Adrenoleukodystrophy, MS, SSPE, are all demyelinating diseases, but PML is the only one linked to JC virus in the context of immunocompromised patients (e.g. AIDS, post-transplantation). Generalized CNS disorders in patients with HIV include viral encephalitis, Cryptococcus meningitis, PML and AIDS dementia complex. Progressive multifocal leukoencephalopathy (PML) results in widespread demyelination due to infection of oligodendrocytes by JC virus (a polyoma DNA virus; papovavirus) resulting in subacute onset of behavioral changes, speech, motor, and visual impairment. On CT this may appear as single or multiple lesions, no mass effect, no enhancement but MRI clearly shows widespread high T2 and FLAIR signal. Encephalitis may be due to CMV or HIV itself rather than HSV. Cryptococcus is the most common fungal infection of CNS and presents with meningism, seizures, and focal neurological deficit with raised CSF pressure on LP and positive India Ink staining. AIDS dementia complex is caused by HIV itself (i.e. HIV encephalopathy/encephalitis) and correlates with high viral loads and the duration of the infection. With the use of HAART, a milder form of cognitive dysfunction, minor cognitive motor disorder (MCMD) has become common. MCMD accounts for approximately 30% of patients with HIV infection, while HIV-associated dementia accounts for less than 10%. Imaging findings include widespread cortical atrophy, ventricular enlargement and white matter damage.

Image with permission from Tan CS, Koralnik IJ. Progressive multifocal leukoencephalopathy and other disorders caused by JC virus: clinical features and pathogenesis. Lancet Neurol 2010;9:430.

10. **d**—Inhaled 100% oxygen

This patient describes features of cluster headache, which is most likely to be terminated with inhalation of pure oxygen within minutes. Cluster headaches usually occur at night when the patient is asleep, and so practical access to the oxygen tank is possible. Propranolol is a β-adrenergic-blocking agent that is useful in the prophylaxis of some vascular headaches, but it is of no value in aborting a cluster headache. Dihydroergotamine suppositories may abort some vascular headaches, but they do not have as obvious an effect in cluster as in classic or common migraine syndromes.

11. **c**—Sumatriptan

This patient has common migraine (migraine without aura). Of the agents listed, only sumatriptan is generally considered of use to abort a headache. The triptans are a group of medications that act as agonists at serotonergic receptors (specifically, the 5HT-1 receptors), and they have been found to be very effective at stopping migraine headaches. Additional agents that might be of benefit in abortive therapy include ibuprofen, aspirin, acetaminophen, isometheptene, or ergotamine. Several medications are effective as prophylactic agents in the treatment of migraine. These include amitriptyline hydrochloride, propranolol, verapamil, and valproate. Verapamil and amitriptyline may be used as prophylactic (preventative) therapy. Most experts recommend initiating prophylactic therapy only when headaches occur at least one to two times per month. Metoclopramide hydrochloride, sumatriptan, and ergotamine tartrate are appropriately used to treat an acute attack of migraine and should not be prescribed on a daily basis. Daily use of these medications can establish a rebound syndrome that results in a chronic daily headache.

12. **a**—Epidural blood patch

The clinical presentation is consistent with spontaneous intracranial hypotension, in particular given the strong relationship of pain to upright posture. The patient has known connective tissue disease and so is at increased risk for this diagnosis. The MRI brain with gadolinium images are characteristic for spontaneous intracranial hypotension and so confirm the diagnosis. Lumbar puncture is often difficult in spontaneous intracerebral hypotension and would not change initial management unless CSF infection needed excluding. Post lumbar puncture headache (PLPH), a common complication of a lumbar puncture (30%) and is thought to be caused by excess leakage of cerebrovascular fluid causing a relatively low intracranial pressure. Risk factors include: factors which may contribute to headache; increased needle size; direction of bevel; not replacing the stylet; increased number of LP attempts; factors that do not contribute to headache; increased volume of CSF removed; bed rest following procedure; increased fluid intake post procedure; opening pressure of CSF; and position of patient. Management is conservative, including administering analgesia and sufficient fluids and caffeine. If this fails to resolve the headache after 72 h an epidural blood patch.

Image with permission from Inamasu J, Nakatsukasa M. Blood patch for spontaneous intracranial hypotension caused by cerebrospinal fluid leak at C1-2, Clin Neurol Neurosurg 2007;109(8):716-19.

13. **b**—Anti-aquaporin 4 antibody

Neuromyelitis optica (NMO; Devic's disease) is monophasic or relapsing-remitting demyelinating CNS disorder Although previously thought to be a variant of multiple sclerosis, it is now recognized to be a distinct disease, particularly prevalent in Asian populations. Features of optic neuritis include unilateral decrease in visual acuity over, poor discrimination of colors, "red desaturation," pain worse on eye movement, relative afferent pupillary defect and a central scotoma. Diagnosis of NMO requires bilateral optic neuritis, transverse myelitis and 2 of the following:

1. Spinal cord lesion involving three or more spinal levels (longitudinally extensive transverse myelitis)
2. Initially normal MRI brain
3. Aquaporin 4 positive serum antibody (positive in 80%)

Adults are especially likely to develop a pattern more typical of relapsing-remitting MS after an initial episode of neuromyelitis optica. Management of acute episodes is with prednisolone or plasma exchange, and recovery from acute optic neuritis usually takes 4-6 weeks. Long term treatment is with immunosuppression (e.g. azothiaprine, rituximab). Disease modifying drugs used in MS are not used in the treatment of NMO.

Image with permission from Sheerin F, Collison K, Quaghebeur G. Magnetic resonance imaging of acute intramedullary myelopathy: radiological differential diagnosis for the on-call radiologist, Clin Radiol 2009;64(1):84-94.

14. **b**—Acute disseminating encephalomyelitis

Acute disseminated encephalomyelitis (ADEM, postinfectious encephalomyelitis) is a demyelinating disease of the brain, brainstem, and spinal cord that is indistinguishable from MS on MRI. It is, however, monophasic, meaning that it occurs acutely on a single occasion and not in a recurrent fashion like MS. It usually develops within days or weeks of a viral illness (e.g. scarlet fever, measles, chickenpox) or immunization. It is characterized by an acute onset of multifocal neurological symptoms with rapid deterioration, which can be fatal if untreated. Non-specific signs such as headache, fever, nausea, and vomiting may also accompany the onset of illness. Motor and sensory deficits are frequent and there may also be brainstem involvement including occulomotor defects. The diagnosis is suggested by the MRI or CT picture of rapidly evolving white matter damage associated with a high ESR and a CSF under increased pressure with elevated red cell and white cell counts and elevated protein content. The CSF glucose content is usually normal. Management involves intravenous glucocorticoids and the consideration of IV immunoglobulins where this fails.

Image with permission from Yachnis AT, Rivera-Zengotita ML. Neuropathology, High-Yield Pathology Series, Saunders, Elsevier, 2014

15. **b**—IV methylprednisolone

Multiple sclerosis is a chronic, predominantly autoimmune demyelinating disease of the central nervous system (CNS) characterized by subacute neurologic deficit (relapses last at least 24 h) correlating with CNS lesions separated in time and space, excluding other possible disease. Peak presentation at 20-40 years. Subtypes include: Relapsing-remitting MS (80%): relapses followed by complete or near-complete recovery, most of which later transition to secondary progressive MS during which there progression of disability with few or no relapses. Primary progressive MS (20%) shows progression of disability from the onset, rarely with relapses. Presentation is with optic neuritis, neurological symptoms related to transverse myelitis (e.g. bladder dysfunction, myelopathy) or intracranial plaques of demyelination. Lhermitte's sign is an electrical sensation radiating down the spine when the neck is passively flexed and is believed to signify spinal cord demyelination. Uhthoff's phenomenon describes the worsening of MS symptoms with higher body temperature (e.g. hot weather, exercise, fever). Eye signs include nystagmus, RAPD (Marcus Gunn pupil), and internuclear opthalmoplegia. Atypical presentations include trigeminal neuralgia, seizures and acute psychiatric disturbance. Diagnosis of MS requires demonstration of lesions disseminated in time and space (McDonald criteria), hence after a single episode it is termed "clinically indeterminate syndrome" (unless there is past medical history and old and newer lesions on MRI). If there are >3 white-matter lesions on MRI the 5-year risk of developing multiple sclerosis is c. 50%. MRI features of demyelinating plaques include T1 hypointense (black holes), T2 and FLAIR hyperintense, and if new/active inflammation they enhance on T1 +GAD sequences. T2/FLAIR imaging may also show linear regions of perivenous demyelination perpendicular to the corpus callosum known as Dawson's fingers. Other investigations include lumbar puncture which may show a raised protein and in 80% positive for oligoclonal bands (in CSF but not in serum) signifying increased intrathecal synthesis of IgG. Visual evoked potentials may be delayed, but well preserved waveform. Treatment in multiple sclerosis is focused at reducing duration of relapses (acute) and reducing the frequency of relapses (disease modifying drugs) as there is no cure. For acute relapses high dose steroids (e.g. oral or IV methylprednisolone) may be given for 3-5 days to shorten the length of an acute relapse, although they do not alter the degree of recovery (i.e. whether a patient returns to baseline function).

Image with permission from Sicotte NL. Magnetic resonance imaging in multiple sclerosis: the role of conventional imaging, Neurol Clin 2011;29(2):343-56.

16. **b**—Glatiramer acetate

Clinical and imaging features (focal lesion that does not exceed two vertebral segments in length and does not affect more than half the cross-sectional area of the cord) suggest relapsing-remitting MS with plaques in the cervical spinal cord. In general, current evidence suggests starting disease-modifying therapy at the point of diagnosis of relapsing-remitting forms of MS since damage continues to occur (based on MRI studies) even between relapses. As such, disease modifying therapy is used in those with "active" relapsing MS defined either as 2 or more relapses in the last 2 years or one recent relapse and/or signs of new lesions on MRI. Interferon beta 1a or 1b can be used in relapsing remitting MS, secondary progressive MS if there are still significant relapses and clinically isolated syndrome, but is contraindicated with deranged liver function. Glatiramer acetate may act as a myelin decoy for the immune system and is not contraindicated in liver dysfunction. Fingolimod is the only oral drug and is a sphingosine 1 phosphate receptor modulator affecting lymphocyte migration that has been proven to reduce number of relapses and slow the rate of number of new MRI lesions. However, it was also associated with increased incidence of varicella zoster, tumor formation, and progressive multifocal leucoencephalopathy (PML) hence reserved for patients who fail 1st line therapies. Similarly, while natalizumab is effective in modifying multiple sclerosis progression, it is also associated with PML and not considered a 1st line treatment. Mitoxanthrone is a chemotherapy agent that inhibits DNA synthesis and repair, associated with significant cardiotoxicity, reserved as last resort. Other problems may also need symptomatic treatment:

- Fatigue—exclude common causes (e.g. anemia, hypothyroid or depression), amantadine, mindfulness training and CBT.
- Spasticity—physiotherapy, baclofen, and gabapentin are first-line. Other options include diazepam, dantrolene, and tizanidine. Botox.
- Bladder dysfunction—ultrasound first to assess bladder emptying. If significant residual volume → intermittent self-catheterization, whereas if no significant residual volume anticholinergics may improve urinary frequency.
- Oscillopsia may respond to gabapentin.

Images with permission from Saraf-Lavi, Efrat, Spine Imaging: Case Review Series, 3rd ed. Saunders, Elsevier, 2014.

17. **e**—Demyelination

Tumefactive demyelination is inflammatory demyelinating disease which presents as a solitary large (>2 cm) focus of demyelination within a cerebral hemisphere with associated edema that may simulate neoplasm or abscess. Presentation is acute (≤3 weeks) with headache, seizures, and focal neurologic deficits. Often it may be a monophasic episode of disease without recurrence, but some may evolve into relapsing-remitting MS. Imaging features in 50% have contrast enhancement in the form of an incomplete ring, without enhancement at junctions with gray matter (or basal ganglia depending on orientation), and there is usually minimal mass effect. Advanced MR imaging techniques may be useful, and the rCBV values are significantly lower than for high-grade glial neoplasms. Management is with high-dose corticosteroid therapy. Radiation or surgical excision of lesions misdiagnosed as tumor will cause additional irreversible neurologic deficits. Equally, ring-enhancing lesions in the setting of MS should not be considered to be TDL—neoplasia and abscess should be excluded first.

Image with permission from Adam A, et al., editors. Grainger & Allison's Diagnostic Radiology, 6th ed. Churchill Livingstone: Elsevier, 2014.

18. **a**—Chiari malformation

The presence of loss of pain and temperature sensation in a "cape-like" distribution is highly suggestive of syringomyelia, which is commonly associated with Chiari I malformation. It may be slowly progressive, cause wasting and weakness of the arms, spinothalamic tract deficit (pain and temperature), loss of reflexes and upgoing plantars, and Horner's syndrome.

19. **e**—Posterior reversible encephalopathy syndrome

Posterior reversible leucoencephalopathy syndrome may present with thunderclap headache, usually followed rapidly by confusion, seizures and visual symptoms. The most common causes of PRES are hypertensive encephalopathy and eclampsia. Hypertension is commonly observed. CT brain and lumbar puncture results are usually normal or near normal. The elevation of CSF protein with hypertensive encephalopathy is variable because intracranial hemorrhage may occur with the hypertensive crisis, but most patients will have moderate increases in CSF protein.

Diagnosis is made by evidence of vasogenic brain edema on MRI brain. PRES is often associated with reversible cerebrovascular vasoconstriction syndrome with vasospasm on cerebral angiography. Management in this case will require blood pressure control in the critical care setting. Other causes of thunderclap headache include aneurysmal subarachnoid hemorrhage, cerebral venous sinus thrombosis, internal carotid artery dissection, pituitary apoplexy reversible cerebral vasoconstriction syndrome, and benign coital headache.

Image with permission from Loevner L. Brain Imaging: Case Review Series, 2nd ed. Mosby: Elsevier, 2009.

20. **b**—Marcus-Gunn phenomenon

Aberrant regeneration of a cranial nerve is not all that uncommon, but it is more often seen after injury to the third nerve than to the seventh. For unknown reasons, the regenerating motor fibers miss their original targets and innervate new destinations. With cranial ALS, facial twitching occurs, but it is not preceded by unilateral weakness, and it is seen as the weakness evolves, not as it remits. Sarcoidosis may produce facial weakness with aberrant regeneration, but this patient's history does not suggest this idiopathic granulomatous disease. There is nothing to suggest that his Lyme disease is recurring, although recurrent meningitis may develop with inadequate treatment.

21. **c**—Retinal Telangiectasias

The association of erythrocytosis with cerebellar signs, microscopic hematuria, and hepatosplenomegaly suggests von Hippel-Lindau syndrome. This hereditary disorder is characterized by polycystic liver disease, polycystic kidney disease, retinal angiomas (telangiectasia), and cerebellar tumors. This is an autosomal dominant inherited disorder with variable penetrance. Men are more commonly affected than women. Although neoplastic cysts may develop in the cerebellum in persons with von Hippel-Lindau syndrome, these usually do not become sufficiently large to cause an obstructive hydrocephalus. Other abnormalities that occur with this syndrome include adenomas in many organs. Hemangiomas may be evident in the bones, adrenals, and ovaries. Hemangioblastomas may develop in the spinal cord or brainstem, as well as in the cerebellum.

22. **b**—Dermatomyositis

Dermatomyositis is an inflammatory disorder causing a symmetrical, proximal muscle weakness and skin lesions. Polymyositis is a variant where skin lesions are not prominent. It may be idiopathic, associated with connective tissue disorders or a paraneoplastic syndrome in about 20% of cases overall. Lung, ovarian, gastrointestinal tract, breasts, and other malignancies can cause it hence a thorough search for a primary is indicated. Skin manifestations include a lilac (heliotrope) rash around the eyes, photosensitive skin, macular rash over back and shoulder, Gottron's papules, nail fold capillary dilatation and flat-topped purplish nodules over the elbows and knees. Other features are proximal muscle weakness with tenderness, Raynaud's syndrome, respiratory muscle weakness, interstitial lung disease and dysphagia/dysphonia.

23. **a**—Anti-acteylcholine receptor antibodies

Myasthenia gravis is an autoimmune damage that occurs at the neuromuscular junction, specifically at postsynaptic membrane acetylcholine receptors. A functional acetylcholine deficiency develops at the synapse because receptors are blocked or inefficient. Myasthenia is more common in women (2:1). Approximately 1/3 of patient have a thymoma (commonest tumor of anterior mediastinum) which can cause death by airway compression or cardiac tamponade. The chest X-ray shows a partially delineated mediastinal mass (anterior mediastinum) with regular borders, bulging the left upper mediastinal contour suggestive of a thymoma. Other associations include thymic hyperplasia and autoimmune disorders (pernicious anemia, autoimmune thyroid disorders, rheumatoid, SLE). Presentation is with ocular weakness (90%) including ptosis, opthalmoparesis generally worse with sustained upward gaze. More severe disease includes limb weakness, difficulty with swallowing, and respiratory difficulties. The key feature is muscle fatigability—muscles become progressively weaker during periods of activity and slowly improve after periods of rest. Patients usually report fatigue that increases as the day progresses. Investigations include single fiber electromyography (high sensitivity 92-100%), CT thorax to exclude thymoma, CK is normal, around 85-90% of patients have antibodies to acetylcholine receptors. In the remaining patients, about 40% are positive for anti-muscle-specific tyrosine kinase antibodies. Tensilon test (intravenous edrophonium) reduces muscle weakness temporarily—not commonly used anymore due to the risk of cardiac arrhythmia. Management includes initiating long-acting anticholinesterases (e.g. pyridostigmine), immunosuppression and thymectomy. Myasthenic crises (severe enough to require intubation) may be triggered by other medications, infection or other physiological stressors and necessitate plasma exchange or intravenous immunoglobulin.

Image with permission from Mattler FA. Essentials of Radiology, 3rd ed. Saunders, Elsevier, 2014.

24. **b**—Inclusion body myositis

Inclusion body myositis is the most common primary myopathy in the elderly manifesting as a slowly progressive weakness, usually affecting finger and wrist flexion initially (but does affect both proximal and distal muscles). Lower limb weakness may also occur with quadriceps. In upper and lower limbs flexors affected more than extensors. Reflexes are usually diminished as in other myopathies. Creatine kinase levels are usually normal or only mildly raised, in contrast to polymyositis (where creatine kinase levels are usually markedly elevated). Associated with cytoplasmic inclusions on muscle biopsy. Muscles are often tender in polymyositis, the distal muscles are usually not affected until the disease is advanced and CK is significantly raised. Diabetic amyotrophy is characterized by painful wasting of the proximal lower limb muscles.

25. **c**—Start prednisolone

Temporal (giant cell) arteritis. is large vessel vasculitis which overlaps with polymyalgia rheumatica (PMR) typically in a patient >60 years old, usually rapid onset with evidence of headache and jaw claudication in many, and visual disturbances secondary to anterior ischemic optic neuropathy in the presence of a tender, palpable superficial temporal artery. In contrast, PMR usually presents with myalgia, morning stiffness in proximal limb muscles (not weakness), lethargy, depression, low-grade fever, anorexia, night sweats with a raised ESR but normal CK. Investigations for temporal arteritis include raised inflammatory markers: ESR >50 mm/hr and CRP may also be elevated, normal CK. Treatment with high dose prednisolone is started on clinical suspicion (due to the risk to vision) while awaiting temporal artery biopsy, and also because histology shows changes which characteristically "skips" certain sections of affected artery whilst damaging others hence a negative temporal artery biopsy does not rule out temporal arteritis. Patients with visual symptoms should be seen the same-day by an ophthalmologist as visual damage is often irreversible. If there is no response to prednisolone the diagnosis should be reconsidered.

26. **c**—Anti-voltage gated calcium channel antibody

Lambert-Eaton myesthenic syndrome (LEMS) is a paraneoplastic myesthenic syndrome associated with small-cell lung cancer where antibodies to voltage-gated calcium channels (VGCCs) have been reported in 75-100%. It presents similarly to myasthenia gravis, with proximal muscle weakness, hyporeflexia and autonomic features but does not show fatiguability of muscle strength—strength actually improves with greater effort.

27. **c**—Hyperkalemia periodic paralysis

Periodic paralysis can be classified into hypokalemic and hyperkalemic periodic paralysis and Andersen-Tawil (long-QT) syndrome, due to mutations in skeletal muscle ion channels. Onset is most commonly in childhood and adolescents, with attacks of paralysis lasting hours and neurological examination is normally unremarkable in between attacks. Diagnosis of hypokalemic periodic paralysis is often made clinically by episodes of paralysis, typically occur at night and may be triggered by carbohydrate meals, in association with low serum potassium but genetic testing can help if known mutations are present. Management is with lifelong potassium supplementation.

28. **b**—Duchenne muscular dystrophy

Duchenne muscular dystrophy (DMD) and Becker muscular dystrophy (BMD) are X-linked recessive disorders caused by mutations in the dystrophin gene on Xp21 (DMD occurs in 1 in 3000-6000 live births; BMD is much less common). Dystrophin is part of a large membrane associated protein in muscle which connects the muscle membrane to actin, part of the muscle cytoskeleton. In DMD there is a frameshift mutation resulting in one or both of the binding sites are lost leading to a severe form while in BMD there is a non-frameshift insertion in the dystrophin gene resulting in both binding sites being preserved leading to a milder form. DMD usually presents with skeletal muscle weakness before the age of 5 years, calf pseudohypertrophy, Gower's sign (child uses arms to stand up from a squatted position) and intellectual impairment (in 30%) which progresses if untreated such that boys become wheelchair-bound by their early teens. Historically, death occurs by age 25 years, primarily from respiratory dysfunction and less often from heart failure. A multidisciplinary treatment approach including steroids, scoliosis surgery, ventilatory support, and cardiac therapy has improved survival. BMD is associated with a more variable presentation of skeletal muscle weakness from the age of 10 onwards and absence of intellectual impairment, and carries a better prognosis, with most patients surviving to the age of 40-50 years. Cardiac involvement is seen in both disorders, and the severity is not correlated with the severity of skeletal muscle involvement. CK is elevated to 5-10 times normal in both. Facioscapulohumeral muscular dystrophy is autosomal dominant and the third most common after the DMD and myotonic dystrophy. Muscle weakness tends to follow a slowly progressive but variable course. The patient initially presents with facial and/or shoulder girdle muscle weakness, which progresses to involve the pelvic musculature. The limb-girdle muscular dystrophies are a group of disorders with a limb-shoulder and pelvic girdle distribution of weakness, but with otherwise heterogeneous inheritance and genetic cause. The onset of muscle weakness is variable but usually occurs before age 30 with complaints of difficulty with walking or running secondary to pelvic girdle involvement. As the disease progresses, involvement of the shoulder muscles and then more distal muscles occurs, with sparing of facial involvement. Emery-Dreifuss muscular dystrophy is a rare X-linked disorder in which skeletal muscle symptoms are often mild but with cardiac involvement that is both common and serious. It is characterized by a triad of early contractures of the elbow, Achilles tendon, and posterior cervical muscles; slowly progressing muscle weakness and atrophy, primarily in humeroperoneal muscles; and cardiac involvement.

Image with permission from Daroff RB, et al., editors. Bradley's Neurology in Clinical Practice, 7th ed. Elsevier, 2016.

ANSWERS 29–51

Additional answers 29–51 available on ExpertConsult.com

EMI ANSWER

52. 1—i, Wernicke encephalopathy. Thiamine deficiency can result in this classic triad of nystagmus, opthalmoplegia and ataxia requiring urgent replacement. 2—f, Delerium tremens. 3—j, Wernicke-Korsakoff syndrome. Represents the addition of anterograde amnesia, retrograde amnesia and confabulation to Wernicke's encephalopathy.

53. 1—h, Mercury; 2—f, Lead; 3—b, Arsenic; 4—e, Ergotism; 5—g, Manganese.

Clinical features of course depend on the precise metal involved but acute poisoning typically include encephalopathy, gastrointestinal upset and myalgia in addition to peripheral neuropathy. Significant sensory neuropathy causing neuropathic pain is commonly prominent.

Environmental Poisoning: Clinical Features

Toxin	Effects	Treatment
Lead	Ataxia and tremor in children exposed to relatively low levels. Chronic exposure routinely impairs psychomotor development and may lead to substantial retardation in very young children. Acute toxicity in children can cause brain edema and may be lethal even with efforts to relieve the intracranial pressure. In adults, it produces a painless bilateral neuropathy often targeting the radial nerve and resulting in a wrist drop abdominal pain, constipation, anemia, basophilic stippling of erythrocyte precursors, and a linear discoloration along the gingival margin (lead lines)	NaEDTA, dimercaprol or *N*-acetyl-penicillamine
Arsenic	Diarrhea, polyneuropathy, gastrointestinal pain, vomiting, shock, coma, renal failure	Dimercaprol Penicillamine
Manganese	Long-term exposure to this metal may produce Parkinsonism but axial rigidity and dystonia may also develop. Chronic poisoning results in polyneuropathy	Levodopa EDTA
Mercury	Depends on route (vapor, ingestion, skin). Vapor toxicity may show fatigue, weakness, abdominal cramp, headache, and fever. Chronic toxicity usually associated with tremors, gingivitis and erethism (behavior change). Other features are peripheral neuropathy, ataxia, visual disturbance	Dimercaprol
Aluminum	Encephalopathy and osteodystrophy in renal dialysis patients	Desferrioxamine
Carbon monoxide	Confusion and headache at carboxyhemoglobin levels of 20% to coma, posturing, and seizures at levels of 50% to 60%. Characteristic of CO poisoning is delayed neurological deterioration occurring 1-3 weeks after the initial event. Typically, this takes the form of an extrapyramidal disorder with Parkinsonian gait and bradykinesia	Pure oxygen, hyperbaric oxygen
Ergot	Ergot is a potent vasoconstricting agent derived from the rye fungus, *Claviceps purpurea*. Ergotism is convulsive (diarrhea, paresthesias, headache) or gangrenous (dry gangrene due to vasoconstriction affecting fingers and toes)	Discontinue ergots, Anti-platelets

Continued

Toxin	Effects	Treatment
Organophosphates	Severe abdominal cramps, blurred vision, twitching, and loss of consciousness bronchospasm and diaphragmatic paralysis	Atropine (muscarinic features) Oximes (nicotinic features) May require intubation and ventilation.
Cyanide	Onset of symptoms is usually rapid and can be within seconds to minutes for inhalation and within an hour for oral exposure. The "classical" presentation is rapid onset of coma, seizures, shock and profound lactic acidosis	Resuscitation and decontamination. Dicobalt edetate, hydroxocobalamin
Thallium	Hair loss, stupor, gastrointestinal distress, seizures, and headaches, as well as a painful, symmetric, primarily sensory neuropathy	Gastrointestinal decontamination Prussian blue or activated charcoal

54. 1—d, Fragile X syndrome; 2—f, Prader-Willi syndrome; 3—j, Williams syndrome; 4—i, Velocardiofacial syndrome; 5—g, Rett syndrome

Genetic Syndromes Associated with Learning Disabilities

Genetic syndrome	Cause	Features
Tuberous sclerosis	Usually sporadic but can be autosomal dominant (Ch 9,11,16)	Skin changes (adenoma sebacium, shagreen patches, ash leaf spots), seizures, cortical tubers, subependymal giant cell astrocytoma, retinal hamartoma, renal angiomyolipoma, cardiac rhabdomyoma
Down's syndrome	Trisomy 21 due to non-dysjunction, translocation, mosaicism	Characteristics include facial appearance, simian crease, clinodactyly, congenital heart defects, GI defects, atlantoaxial instability, dementia, thyroid disorders, diabetes, sleep apnea, hearing loss, and visual problems
Rett syndrome	X-linked defect of methyl CpG-binding protein 2	Most boys die before birth. Girls developmental retardation, mutism, and movement disorder from early childhood, generally during the second year of life. There is loss of previously acquired language skills and effective eye contact, as well as purposeful hand movement. Stereotypic hand movements develop (hand wringing, tapping, patting, and at times hand-mouth movements). Seizures may also occur
Cri du Chat syndrome	Chromosome 5 deletion	High pitched cry, microcephaly, hypotonia, facial features, including widely set eyes (hypertelorism), low-set ears, a small jaw, and a rounded face. Some children with cri-du-chat syndrome are born with a heart defect
Neurofibromatosis	Usually autosomal dominant. May be sporadic (Ch 17+22)	The disorder is characterized by numerous benign Neurofibromas, but also ependymoma, meningioma, schwannoma and childhood chronic myelogenous leukemia
Prader-Willi syndrome Angelman syndrome	70% sporadic (deletion on Ch 15 of paternal origin)	Inheriting the deletion through the mother gives rise to Angelman syndrome, which is characterized by short stature, severe mental retardation, spasticity, seizures, and a characteristic stance. Inheriting the deletion from the father produces the more common Pader-Willi syndrome, which is characterized by obesity, excessive and indiscriminate gorging, small hands, feet, hypogonadism and mental retardation. In rare cases, uniparental disomy involving chromosome 15 produces

Continued on following page

Genetic Syndromes Associated with Learning Disabilities (Continued)

Genetic syndrome	Cause	Features
		PWS when both copies are inherited from the mother and AS when both copies are inherited from the father
Velocardiofacial syndrome (22q11 deletion, DiGeorge syndrome)	Usually sporadic, may be autosomal dominant (microdeletion Ch 22)	Thymus abnormalities, ear deformities, cleft palate, cardiac defects and short stature. Hypocalcemia in adolescence
Fragile X syndrome	X-linked (*FMR-1* gene has expansion of trinucleotide repeats at fragile site on X chromosome). Shows anticipation.	Boys with syndrome have long faces, prominent jaws, large ears, and are likely to be mentally retarded. Affected men have large ears, a high-arched palate, hypotelorism, and large testes. Autism also occurs among affected men
Williams syndrome	Deletion in Chromosome 7	Characteristic elfin facies, short stature, cardiovascular defects, dental problems and GI disorders (among others). Hypercalcemia

55. 1—i, Multifocal motor neuropathy with conduction block (MMNCB). Younger to middle-aged men who develop focal arm weakness in the distribution of a named nerve relatively rapidly (e.g. a week). Over several months additional named motor nerves become involved asymmetrically such that it may resemble MND (MMNCB shows conduction block due to segmental demyelination. MND does not. MMNCB is a demyelinating condition, MND is axonal). Nerve conduction studies help to decide whether a motor neuropathy is axonal or demyelinating. Anti-GM1 antibodies may also be present. MMNCB, Guillain-Barré, and CIDP are all examples of demyelinating neuropathies, all of which therefore respond to intravenous immunoglobulin (IVIG). 2—d, Chronic inflammatory demyelinating polyneuropathy (CIDP). Similar to Guillain-Barré syndrome (acute inflammatory demyelinating polyneuropathy, AIDP), but it takes a slowly progressive or remitting course rather than one of acute onset. It is a poly*radiculo*neuropathy affecting the proximal portions of the nerves where they exit the spinal cord (i.e. nerve root). Because nerve roots are affected, patients experience proximal and distal weakness and sensory loss from the onset. Raised CSF protein may be present due to the inflammatory response affecting nerve roots within the thecal sac. 3—a, Acute intermittent porphyria. A disorder of heme biosynthesis in the liver resulting from increased production and excretion of porphobilinogen and θ-aminolevulinic acid. It is characterized by recurrent attacks of abdominal pain, psychosis, and neuropathy (motor and autonomic). Autonomic neuropathy results in gastroparesis, constipation/pseudoobstruction (hence abdominal pain), and autonomic instability. Attacks may be provoked by drugs, such as barbiturates, anticonvulsants, sulfonamide antibiotics, and estrogens. Treatment is best accomplished with use of intravenous hematin when supportive measures are not adequate or the case is severe. 4—l, Sarcoidosis. Neurosarcoid affects both central and peripheral nervous system, with optic atrophy, facial nerve palsies and peripheral neuropathy. 5—f, Hereditary sensory and motor neuropathy (HSMN, Charcot-Marie tooth disease). HSMN type I autosomal dominant due to defect in *PMP-22* gene (which codes for myelin) resulting in a predominantly demyelinating neuropathy. Features often start at puberty, motor symptoms predominate with distal muscle wasting, pes cavus, clawed toesfoot drop, and leg weakness. HSMN type II is primarily axonal neuropathy. 6—h, Mononeuritis multiplex. In this disorder, individual nerves are transiently disabled over the course of minutes to days, and the recovery of function may require weeks to months. Diabetes is the commonest cause.

56. 1—i, Paraneoplastic cerebellar degeneration. Characterized by subacute, progressive ataxia, dysarthria, and nystagmus. Myoclonus, opsoclonus (irregular jerking of the eyes in all directions), diplopia, vertigo, and

hearing loss may also occur. The most common associated tumor types are small cell carcinoma of the lung, ovarian/breast carcinoma, and lymphoma. Anti-Purkinje cell antibodies (anti-Yo antibodies) may be present in 50%. Paraneoplastic cerebellar degeneration may precede the symptoms of the underlying tumor itself. 2—c, Hypercalcemia. It may be a result of parathyroid-related peptide secreted by the tumor itself (usually lung cancer) or of bone destruction by metastatic disease. The elevated serum calcium decreases membrane excitability, leading to the clinical syndrome of fatigability, lethargy, generalized weakness, and areflexia progressing to coma and even convulsions. Symptoms usually do not occur until levels reach 14 mg/dL (3 mmol/l) or higher. 3—d, Lambert-Eaton myasthenic syndrome (LEMS) shows subacute proximal muscle weakness and spares the bulbar musculature, and is due to presynaptic blockade of voltage gated calcium channels by autoantibodies. A characteristic feature is the increase in strength briefly after repeated muscle activation. Most cases are associated with small cell lung cancer, or in the context of other autoimmune diseases. 4—j, Paraproteinemic neuropathy. Polyneuropathy may occur in up to 15% of patients with multiple myeloma presents as a chronic distal symmetrical sensory or sensorimotor neuropathy. CSF protein may be elevated if there is a chronic inflammatory demyelinating polyneuropathy-like picture. Up to 20% of patients referred for evaluation of polyneuropathy may a *monoclonal gammopathy of undetermined significance*, but a hematologic malignancy may later declare itself.

57. 1—b, Ataxia telangiectasia; 2—g, Friedreich ataxia; 3—j, Spinocerebellar ataxia; 4—a, Abetalipoproteinemia

Hereditary Ataxias: Clinical Features

Hereditary ataxia	Features
Spinocerebellar ataxia (SCA1-SCA10)	Autosomal dominant ataxias many of which are trinucleotide repeat disorders, demonstrate anticipation and tend to present in the third and fourth decades. Frequently associated with pyramidal signs such as hyperreflexia and spasticity. Sensory neuropathy is common, and patients may display dystonia, chorea, or cognitive decline. Machado-Joseph disease (SCA3) is one of the commonest and ataxia, hyperreflexia, nystagmus/ophthalmoplegia, and dysarthria develop early in the disease and may also show a levodopa-responsive rest tremor
Freiderich's ataxia	The most common genetic ataxia (1 in 50,000) and occurs secondary to a GAA repeat located on chromosome 9 (autosomal recessive) but unusually does not demonstrate anticipation. Loss of frataxin affects mitochondrial iron homeostasis, making the cell susceptible to oxidative stress. The typical age of onset is 10-15 years old with gait ataxia and scoliosis followed by progressive loss of neuromuscular function, with the patient wheelchair-bound 10-20 years after symptom onset. Neurological features are absent ankle jerks/extensor plantars, cerebellar ataxia, optic atrophy, spinocerebellar tract degeneration. Other features hypertrophic obstructive cardiomyopathy (90%, most common cause of death) diabetes mellitus (10-20%) and high-arched palate
Ataxia telangiectasia	Ataxia-telangiectasia is the second most common autosomal recessive ataxia, with a frequency of 1 in 100,000 persons. Due to a deficit in the DNA repair pathway, and patients are predisposed to the development of neoplasms. Onset is in early childhood, with postural instability and ataxia first becoming apparent as the child begins to walk. Later, hypotonia, bradykinesia, areflexia, and proprioceptive deficits develop. Chorea may occasionally be seen. The eponymous telangiectasias develop later in childhood. Patients are often wheelchair bound by their second decade, and death usually occurs in the fourth to fifth decade as a result of either pulmonary infection or malignancy. EMG shows a sensory neuropathy and MRI shows cerebellar atrophy
Fragile X-associated tremor ataxia syndrome	Fragile X-associated tremor ataxia syndrome (FXTAS) is characterized by the presence of a permutation for fragile X syndrome (CGG triplet repeat in insufficient number to cause the full fragile X syndrome). It is accompanied by intention tremor, gait ataxia, rigidity, bradykinesia, polyneuropathy, and autonomic manifestations

Continued on following page

Hereditary Ataxias: Clinical Features (Continued)

Hereditary ataxia	Features
Abetalipoproteinamia	Usually becomes symptomatic during early childhood. The peripheral blood smear will exhibit acanthocytes, and the plasma lipid profile will reveal a very low cholesterol and triglyceride content. These are an unusual hematologic findings in patients with ataxia and are often diagnostic. The initial complaints are similar to the spinocerebellar signs of Friedreich disease. Ataxia, areflexia, distal muscle atrophy, intestinal symptoms, loss of vibratory sense; retinitis pigmentosa; steatorrhea (fat malabsorption) resulting in vitamin A, E, K deficiency; acanthocytes on smear. Position sense is lost and extensor plantar responses develop as the disease progresses. Deficits accumulate over the course of years. Vitamin E supplementation may slow the disease's progression
Episodic ataxias	Eight forms of episodic ataxia have been thus far been described (EA1 to EA7 and DYT9), all caused by ion channel mutations. EA1 and EA2 are of particular interest because they arise from defects in the same chromosome (chromosome 19) but have different phenotypes. EA1 is caused by mutations in a potassium channel gene and EA2 by mutations in a voltage-dependent calcium channel. EA1 is characterized by kinesigenic attacks of myokymia and ataxia that last seconds to minutes. EA2 is characterized by non-kinesigenic episodes of ataxia and vertigo that can last days. Although the symptoms of EA1 abate over time, EA2 is a lifetime affliction
Ataxia with isolated vitamin E deficiency	Mimic of Freiderich's ataxia but treatment with vitamin E can slow or reverse the disease

FURTHER READING

Haq IU, Foote, KD, Okun, MS. Clinical overview of movement disorders. In: Winn RH, editor. Youmans Neurological Surgery, 6th ed. Saunders: Elsevier, 2011.

58. 1—c, Pyridoxine deficiency. Patients on antituberculous therapy with isoniazid may develop isolated pyridoxine deficiency and subsequent peripheral neuropathy. 2—e, Thiamine deficiency. Symptoms suggest Wernicke's encephalopathy. 3—g, Vitamin B12 deficiency. Symptoms suggest subacute combined degeneration of the cord. 4—i, Vitamin E deficiency.

Vitamin Deficiency States: Clinical Features

Nutrient	Findings in deficiency	Causes (other than dietary factors)
Thiamine (B1)	Wet beriberi, dry beriberi, Wernicke's encephalopathy, Wernicke-Korsakoff psychosis	Alcoholism, chronic diuretic use, hyperemesis, thiaminases in food
Riboflavin	Magenta tongue, angular stomatitis, seborrhea, chellosis	Alcoholism
Niacin	Pellagra (rare)	Alcoholism, deficiency of Vit B6 or riboflavin or tryptophan
B6 (Pyridoxine)	Seborrhea, glossitis, convulsions, neuropathy, depression, confusion, microcytic anemia	Alcoholism, isoniazid
Folate	Megaloblastic anemia, atrophic glossitis, depression, increased homocysteine	Alcoholism, sulfasalazine, pyrimethamine, triamterene
B12	Megaloblastic anemia, subacute combined degeneration of the spinal cord, increased homocysteine and methylmalonic acid	Pernicious anemia, terminal ileal disease, metformin, acid-reducing drugs
Vitamin A	Xeropthalmia, night blindness, Bitot's spots, follicular hyperkeratosis, immune dysfunction, impaired embryonic development	Fat malabsorption, infection, measles, alcoholism, protein-energy malnutrition (e.g. marasmus, kwashiorkor)

Continued

Nutrient	Findings in deficiency	Causes (other than dietary factors)
Vitamin C	Scurvy (inflamed/bleeding gums, petechiae, ecchymosis, fatigue, joint effusion, poor wound healing)	Smoking, alcoholism
Vitamin D	Rickets	Aging, lack of sunlight, fat malabsorption, deeply pigmented skin
Vitamin E	Peripheral neuropathy, spinocerebellar ataxia, skeletal muscle atrophy, retinopathy	Fat malabsorption, genetic abnormalities of transport
Vitamin K	Coagulopathy (factors I, II, VII, IX)	Fat malabsorption, liver disease, antibiotic use

59. 1—j, X-linked adrenoleukodystrophy. Produces rapidly evolving brain damage in male infants or boys, with survival from onset of symptoms usually limited to 3 years. Long-chain fatty acids accumulate in adrenal cortical and other cells, resulting in adrenal insufficiency and CNS disease. 2—h, Pelizaeus-Merzbacher disease. Leukodystrophy with significant Sudan-staining typically become symptomatic during the first months of life, but survival may extend into the third decade of life. Most affected persons are male. 3—g, Metachromatic leukodystrophy. Sphingolipidosis due to arylsulfatase-A deficiency resulting in accumulation of galactosyl sulfatides. The affected person usually has retardation, ataxia, spasticity, and sensory disturbances usually symptomatic during infancy. 4—d, Canavan disease may produce developmental regression at about 6 months of age, with extensor posturing, rigidity and myoclonic seizures may develop. There is accumulation of *N*-acetylaspartic acid in the blood and urine, but elevated levels in the brain establish the diagnosis.

60. 1—j, Tay-Sachs disease. This is a ganglioside storage disease that occurs more commonly in Ashkenazi Jews than in the general population. The early-onset form will produce macrocephaly and a cherry red spot in the fundus (retinal ganglion cells become distended with glycolipid making retinal pale compared to fovea lacking ganglion cells). Children exhibit mental retardation, seizures, blindness and die prematurely. 2—d, Gaucher disease.

All the sphingolipids are nothing more than lipids that contain a sphingosine moiety. Storage diseases of sphingolipids are mostly autosomal recessive and can lead to CNS degeneration and early death.

Sphingolipidoses: Clinical Features

Sphingolipidosis	Enzyme deficiency	Abnormal accumulation	Features
Niemann-Pick disease	Sphingomyelinase	Sphingomyelin and cholesterol	Autosomal recessive; death by age 3 year
Tay-Sachs disease	Hexaminosidase A	GM_2 ganglioside	Autosomal recessive; death by age 3 year; cherry-red spot on fundus.
Krabbe disease	Galactosylceramide β-Galactosidase	Galactocerebroside	Autosomal recessive; optic atrophy, spasticity, early death
Gaucher disease	β-Glucocerebrosidase	Glucocerebroside accumulation in liver, brain, spleen, and bone marrow	Autosomal recessive; "crinkled paper" appearance of cells, hepatosplenomegaly
Fabry disease	α-Galactosidase A	Ceramide trihexosidase	X-linked recessive
Metachromatic leukodystrophy	Arylsulfatase-A	Galactosyl sulfatide	Autosomal recessive; retardation, ataxia, spasticity, and sensory disturbances; early death

61. 1—j, Anti-voltage gated potassium channel Ab; 2—d, Anti-Aquaporin 4; 3—l, Anti-GQ1b; 4—a, Anti-muscle specific kinase; 5—c, Anti-voltage gated calcium channel Ab

Autoantibody-Associated Neurological Disorders

Antibody	Associated disorders
Anti-acetylcholine receptor antibody (AChR) and anti-muscle specific kinase (MuSK)	Myasthenia gravis
Anti-NMDA receptor antibody	NMDAR-antibody encephalopathy
Anti-voltage gated calcium channel antibody	Lambert Eaton myasthenic syndrome, Paraneoplastic cerebellar degeneration
Anti-Aquaporin 4 antibody	Neuromyelitis optica (Devic's disease)
Anti-Hu (ANNA-1)	Subacute sensory neuropathy, limbic encephalitis, brain stem encephalitis, paraneoplastic encephalomyelitis
Anti-Yo (PCA-1)	Paraneoplastic cerebellar degeneration
Anti-Ri (ANNA-2)	Myoclonus/opsoclonus
Anti-Tr	Paraneoplastic cerebellar degeneration
Anti-GAD	Stiff person syndrome/cerebellar ataxia
Anti-voltage gates potassium channel antibody	Neuromyotonia, limbic encephalitis (non-paraneoplastic)
Anti-Ta/Ma2	Limbic encephalitis (paraneoplastic)
Anti-GQ1b	Guillain-Barré syndrome/Miller-Fisher variant
Anti-myelin associated glycoprotein/sulfated glucoronul paragloboside	IgM Paraproteinemic neuropathy
Anti-GD1b	Paraproteinemic neuropathy, CANOMAD (chronic ataxic neuropathy, ophthalmoplegia, M protein, cold agglutinins, anti-disialosyl antibodies).

62. 1—b, Hurler syndrome; 2—a, Hunter syndrome; 3—h, Morquio syndrome A

Mucopolysaccharidoses are a group of metabolic disorders caused by the absence or malfunctioning of lysosomal enzymes needed to break down glycosaminoglycans forming bone, cartilage, tendons, corneas, skin, and connective tissue. Buildup of glycosaminoglycans collect in the cells, blood and connective tissues cause progressive cellular damage which affects appearance, tissue function and mental development. All are autosomal recessive except for Hunter syndrome. Treatment is with enzyme replacement.

Mucopolysaccharidoses: Clinical Features

MPS	Enzyme deficiency	Accumulated product	Clinical features
Hurler syndrome	α-L-Iduronidase	Heparan sulfate, dermatan sulfate	Dwarfism, facial dysmorphism, Clouding of cornea, mental retardation, hepatosplenomegaly, death by age 10 from respiratory/cardiac complications.

Continued

MPS	Enzyme deficiency	Accumulated product	Clinical features
Hunter syndrome	iduronate sulfatase		Mild form of Hurler syndrome; no corneal clouding, mild mental retardation. X-linked recessive
Sanfilippo syndrome A	Heparan sulfamidase	Heparan sulfate	Initially symptom-free, then progressive intellectual decline/speech delay, hyperactivity and sleep disturbance followed by motor disease. Death in third decade.
Sanfilippo syndrome B	*N*-Acetylglucosaminidase		
Sanfilippo syndrome C	Heparan-α-glucosamidine *N*-acetyltransferase		
Sanfilippo syndrome D	*N*-Acetylglucosamine-6-sulfatase		
Morquio syndrome A	Galactose-6-sulfate sulfatase	Keratan sulfate, chondroitin 6-sulfate	Severe skeletal dysplasia, short stature, cord compression, cardiac abnormalities, corneal clouding, death at an early age.
Morquio syndrome B	β-Galactosidase	Keratan sulfate	
Maroteaux-Lamy syndrome	*N*-Acetylgalactosamine-4-sulfatase	Dermatan sulfate	Normal intellectual development, but shares features of Hurler syndrome.
Sly syndrome	B-glucoronidase	Heparan sulfate, dermatan sulfate, chondroitin 6-sulfate	Hydrops fetalis but those that survive to birth have similar to Hurler syndrome
Natowicz syndrome	Hyaluronidase	Hyaluronic acid	Short stature, periarticular soft tissue masses

63. 1—d, Kearns-Sayre syndrome; 3—e, Leber's hereditary optic neuropathy; 3—g, MELAS

Mitochondrial DNA is inherited maternally, and some of these disorders are thus transmitted from mother to children of both sexes. The mitochondrial disorders, also termed mitochondrial myopathies, encephalomyopathies, or respiratory chain disorders, are a heterogeneous group of diseases resulting from abnormalities in mitochondrial DNA and respiratory chain function, hence manifest in tissue with a high respiratory workload such as brain, retina and skeletal muscle, especially extraocular and cardiac muscle.

Mitochondrial Disorders: Clinical Features

Mitochondrial disorder	Features
Ataxia neuropathy syndromes	Sensory ataxia, neuropathy, dysarthria, ophthalmoplegia (SANDO). May also have epilepsy and myopathy
Chronic progressive external ophthalmoplegia	External ophthalmoplegia, bilateral ptosis. May also show mild proximal myopathy
Kearns-Sayre syndrome	Early onset (<20 years) progressive external ophthalmoplegia, pigmentary retinopathy, and one of: cerebellar ataxia, heart block, CSF protein >1 g/l. Other associations: bilateral deafness, myopathy, dysphagia, diabetes mellitus, hypoparathyroidism, and dementia

Continued on following page

Mitochondrial Disorders: Clinical Features (Continued)

Mitochondrial disorder	Features
Leigh syndrome	Infantile onset of subacute relapsing encephalopathy with cerebellar/brain stem signs. Also associated with basal ganglia lucencies, and maternal history positive
Leber's hereditary optic neuropathy	Subacute bilateral painless visual failure in young men (M:F 4:1, median age 24). Associated with dystonia and cardiac pre-excitation syndromes
MEMSA (myoclonic epilepsy, myopathy, sensory ataxia)	Seizures, cerebellar ataxia, and myopathy. Associated with dementia, peripheral neuropathy and spasticity
NARP (neurogenic weakness with ataxia and retinitis pigmentosa)	Late-childhood or adult onset peripheral neuropathy, ataxia and pigmentary retinopathy. Associated basal ganglia lucencies and sensorimotor neuropathy
MELAS (mitochondrial encephalomyopathy, lactic acidosis, and stroke-like episodes)	Commonest mitochondrial disorder. Presents with stroke-like episodes in those <40 years old, seizures and/or dementia, and lactic acidosis. Associated with diabetes mellitus, cardiomyopathy, bilateral deafness, pigmentary retinopathy and cerebellar ataxia
MERRF (myoclonic epilepsy with ragged-red fibers)	Myoclonus, seizures, cerebellar ataxia and myopathy (ragged-red fibers on biopsy). Associated with dementia, optic atrophy, bilateral deafness, peripheral neuropathy, spasticity and multiple lipomata
Alpers-Huttenlocher syndrome	Hypotonia, seizures, liver failure with/without renal tubulopathy

FURTHER READING

Chinnery PF. Mitochondrial disorders overview. In: Pagon RA, Adam MP, Ardinger HH, et al., editors. GeneReviews Seattle, WA: University of Washington, Seattle; 1993-2015. http://www.ncbi.nlm.nih.gov/books/NBK1224.

64. 1—l, Transient Global Amnesia. Episode of complete and reversible anterograde and retrograde memory loss lasting up to 24 h. Patients have a persistent loss of memory for the duration of the attack, which is characterized by bewilderment and repeating questions, but retained personal identity and ability to perform complex cognitive and motor tasks. TGA usually affects middle-aged or older men and often occurs in the setting of an emotional or other stressor, such as physical or sexual exertion. Although it shares features of transient ischemic attack, it is not associated with an increased risk of stroke. 2—e, Creutzfeldt-Jakob disease. Patients may have ataxia, myoclonus, clumsiness, or dysarthria, as well as diplopia, distorted vision, blurred vision, field defects, changes in color perception, and visual agnosia. Ultimately, cortical blindness may occur. The diagnosis may be supported by the finding of periodic sharp waves at a 1-2 Hz frequency on EEG and the finding of elevated protein 14-3-3 in CSF. 3—i, Huntington's disease. 4—k, Neurosyphilis. General paresis is a chronic, often insidious meningoencephalitis that may be delayed up to 20 years after the original spirochetal infection. Clinically, it manifests as dementia, delusions, dysarthria, tremor, myoclonus, seizures, spasticity, and Argyll Robertson pupils. Other presentations of neurosyphilis include meningitis, meningovascular syphilis causing infarcts, optic atrophy, and tabes dorsalis (characterized by ataxia, urinary incontinence, and lightning pains caused by degeneration of the posterior spinal roots). 5—j, Hypothyroidism in adults may present with headache, dementia, psychosis, and decreased consciousness. Neuromuscular findings are also common, and they include a proximal myopathic weakness and a delay in the relaxation phase of reflexes.

65. 1—i, Neurally mediated (vasovagal) syncope; 2—b, Cardiac arrhythmia; 3—a, Autonomic failure

Classification of Syncope

Classification	Pathophysiology	Discriminating clinical features
Cardiac Syncope		
Arrythmia	Tachyarrhythmia Bradyarrhythmia	Palpitations, HR, ECG, cardiac history, family history, ECHO
Structural cardiac disease	Valve disease Outflow obstruction	Abnormal cardiac exam, ECG, cardiac history, family history, ECHO
Pacemaker malfunction		ECG, pacemaker check
Non-Cardiac Syncope		
Neurocardiogenic Cardioinhibitory Vasodepressor	Exaggerated vagal response to stimulus	Prolonged standing, heat, situational, normal exam, normal ECG, tilt table test
Orthostatic hypotension	Autonomic failure (diabetes, Parkinson's) Drug induced	Change in body position, lying/standing BP, ECG, drop in BP without change in HR. Medication history
Seizure	-	Preceding aura, rhythmic jerking, unresponsive, tongue biting, urinary incontinence, post-ictal period, known epilepsy, Babinski positive, pupillary response
CVA/TIA	Hemorrhage/infarct	Other neurological symptoms, fall due to weakness/ loss of balance rather than syncope
Vertigo	Steal phenomenon BPPV	Room spinning, nystagmus
Others	Hypoglycemia Dehydration	

66. 1—e, Migraine with aura. Classic migraine is usually familial, involves a unilateral, throbbing head pain, and diminishes in frequency with age. The blind spot, or scotoma, that may develop as part of the aura is usually homonymous hemianopia. It typically enlarges and may intrude on the central vision. The margin of the blind spot is often scintillating or dazzling. Homonymous hemianoptic defects of the sort that develop during the aura of a classic migraine indicate an irritative lesion that is affecting one part of the occipital cortex in one hemisphere of the brain. Other focal neurological phenomena may precede classic migraine; the most common are tingling of the face or hand, mild confusion, transient hemiparesis, and ataxia. Fatigue, irritability, and easy distractibility often develop before a migraine. Affected persons usually also have hypersensitivity to light and noise during an attack. 2—c, Cluster headache. *Cluster headache* refers to the tendency of these headaches to cluster in time. They may be distinctly seasonal, but the triggering event is unknown. The pain of cluster headache is usually described as originating in the eye and spreading over the temporal area as the headache evolves. In contrast to migraine, men are more often affected than women, and extreme irritability may accompany the headache. The pain usually abates in less than 1 h. Affected persons routinely have autonomic phenomena associated with the headache that include unilateral nasal congestion, tearing from one eye, conjunctival injection, and pupillary constriction. The autonomic phenomena are on the same side of the face as the pain. 3—i, Postherpetic neuralgia. HZV/VZV may reactivate in immunocompromised patients or the severely ill elderly and result in this neuropathic pain syndrome once the acute infection has settled.

67. 1—e, Idiopathic intracranial hypertension (primary pseudotumor cerebri). Symptoms include headaches, transient visual obscurations, progressive visual loss, pulsatile tinnitus, diplopia, and shoulder and arm pain in obese/overweight females. Papilledema or optic atrophy and occasionally sixth nerve palsies may be present. Diagnoses requires

exclusion of structural (e.g. mass lesion or venous sinus obstruction) or other secondary causes, and opening pressure >25 cm H2O on lumbar puncture. Treatment options include serial lumbar puncture, diuretics, ventriculoperitoneal shunting, and optic nerve sheath fenestration. 2—j, Thunderclap headache. 3—i, Spontaneous intracranial hypotension. Causes of intracranial hypotension include persistent CSF leak after lumbar puncture, head trauma, neurosurgery, or even pneumonectomy (thoracoarachnoid fistula), pituitary tumors, dural tear in the spinal root sleeves, traumatic nerve root avulsion or dehydration.

68. 1—j, Wernicke's aphasia; 2—c, Broca's aphasia, I—Transcortical sensory aphasia

Classification of Aphasias

Fluency	Comprehension	Repetition	Diagnosis	Lesion/Features
Fluent	Good comprehension	Good repetition	Anomic aphasia	Isolated word finding deficit; least localized.
		Poor repetition	Conduction aphasia	Arcuate fasciculus damage.
	Poor comprehension	Good repetition	Transcortical sensory aphasia	White matter underlying Wernicke's area
		Poor repetition	Wernicke's (receptive) aphasia	Posterior lesion. Paraphrasias and neologisms.
Non-fluent	Good comprehension	Good repetition	Transcortical motor aphasia	Frontal white matter lesion.
		Poor repetition	Broca's aphasia	Inferior frontal lobe. Telegraphic speech
	Poor comprehension	Good repetition	Mixed transcortical aphasia	Watershed Infarct affecting speech areas
		Poor repetition	Global aphasia	Large territory infarct.

CHAPTER 9

NEURO-OPHTHALMOLOGY

SINGLE BEST ANSWER (SBA) QUESTIONS

1. The horizontal gaze center is formed by which one of the following:
   a. Pontine paramedian reticular formation
   b. Reticular medial longitudinal fasciculus
   c. Preganglionic Erdinger-Westphal nucleus
   d. Brodman Area 6
   e. Superior colliculus

2. A 25-year-old woman presents with a several week history of diplopia, with an 8 month history of generalized headache which has been particularly bad over the last 2 months. On examination she is obese, has a normal pupillary light reflex and no RAPD. Appearance of fundi are shown. Which one of the following is most likely cause of her complaint?

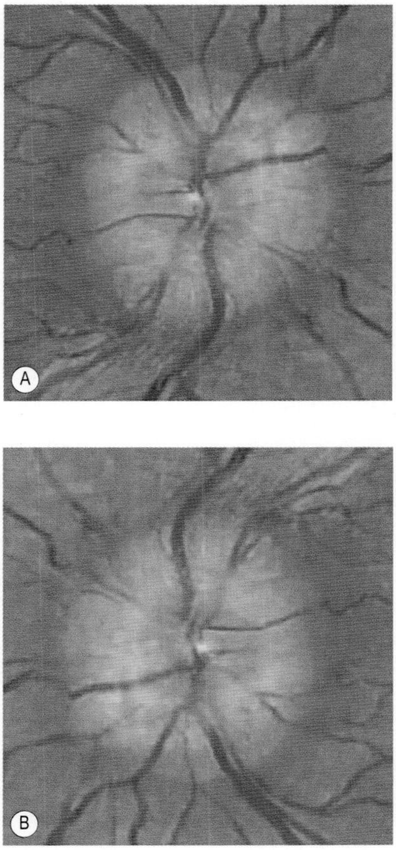

   a. Non-organic disorder
   b. Optic nerve drusen
   c. Optic neuritis
   d. Idiopathic intracranial hypertension
   e. Leber's hereditary optic neuropathy

3. A 50-year-old man complains of 2 days' double vision. Has abducting nystagmus in the right eye and vertical gaze is preserved bilaterally. Which one of the following is most likely?

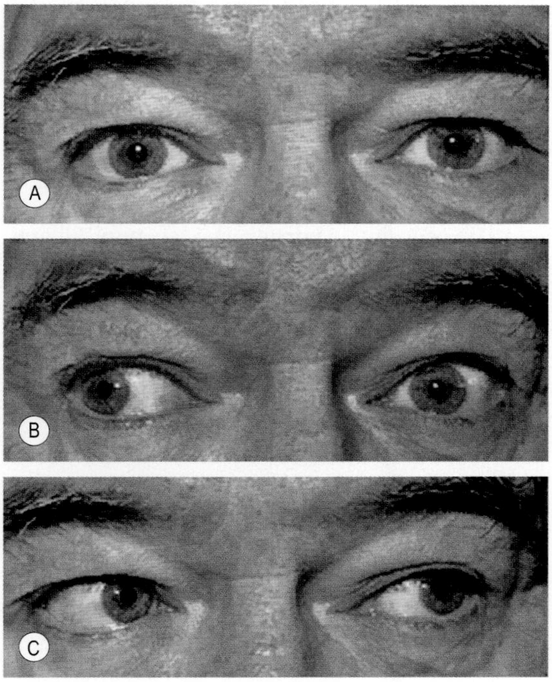

   a. Left internuclear ophthalmoplegia
   b. Orbital apex syndrome
   c. Left incomplete oculomotor palsy
   d. Superior orbital fissure syndrome
   e. Left one-and-a-half syndrome

4. A 53-year-old woman reports drooping of her eyelids for the last 6 months. She experiences diplopia when driving for any extended period of time. Which one of the following is most likely?

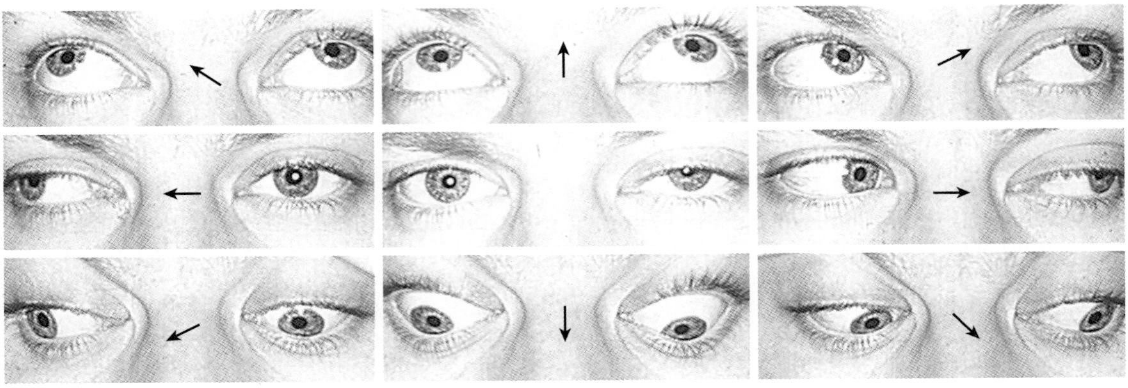

a. Cavernous sinus thrombosis
b. Myasthenia gravis
c. Oculomotor nerve palsy
d. Pituitary apoplexy
e. Thyroid ophthalmopathy

5. Forty minutes after bilateral instillation of 10% cocaine eyedrops, the left pupil dilates, but the right does not.

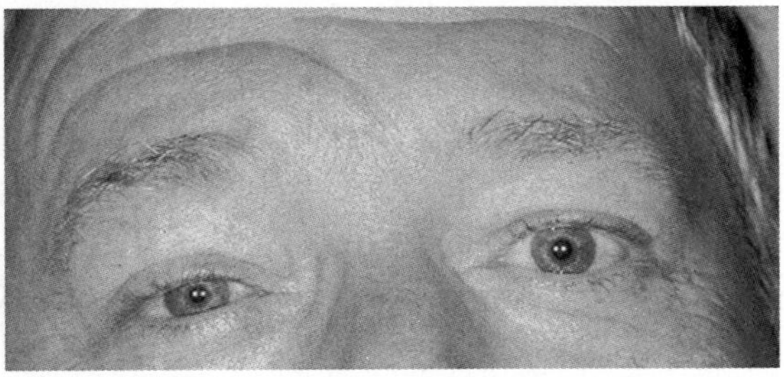

a. Horner's syndrome
b. Myasthenia gravis
c. Oculomotor palsy
d. Trochlear palsy
e. Thyroid ophthalmopathy

6. A 22-year-old female complains of reduced vision and pain in the left eye starting 3 days ago. On examination vision is normal in the right eye but 6/12 (20/40) in the left eye, Left relative afferent pupillary defect, pain when looks to right or left, no redness or photophobia.
a. Arteritic anterior ischemic optic neuropathy
b. Central retinal artery occlusion
c. Iritis
d. Optic neuritis
e. Orbital cellulitis

7. A 34-year-old man present with intermittent diplopia, worse when looking to the left. Examination findings are shown below. Which one of the following is most likely?

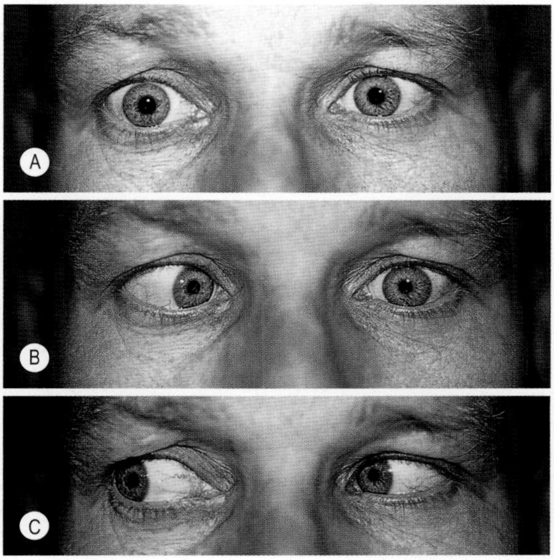

a. Left abducens nerve palsy
b. Left conjugate gaze paresis
c. Left internuclear ophthalmoplegia
d. Left hypotropia
e. Right trochlear palsy

8. On examination, this 15-year-old boy was found to have upgaze paresis, ocular tilt reaction (right superior rectus skew deviation and head tilt), papilledema, and anisocoria. The pupils were moderate in size and poorly reactive to light, but reactive to near stimuli.

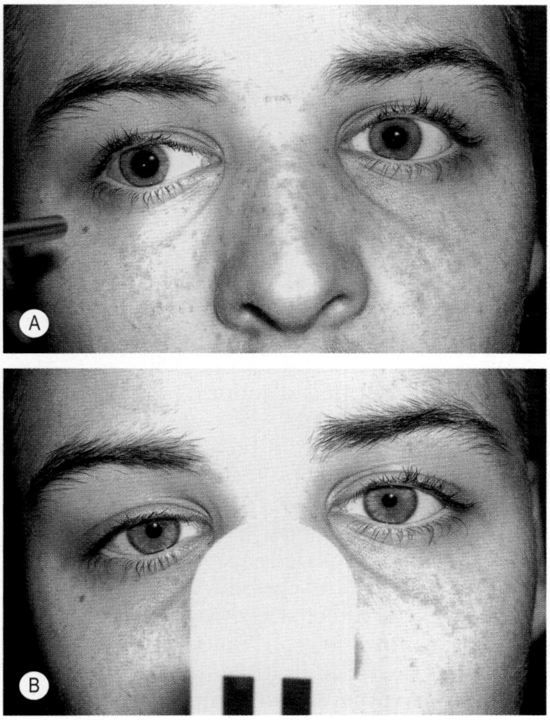

a. Adie's tonic pupil
b. Argyll Robertson pupil
c. Horner syndrome
d. Parinaud syndrome
e. Wallenberg syndrome

9. Which urine test would aid diagnosis in this child?

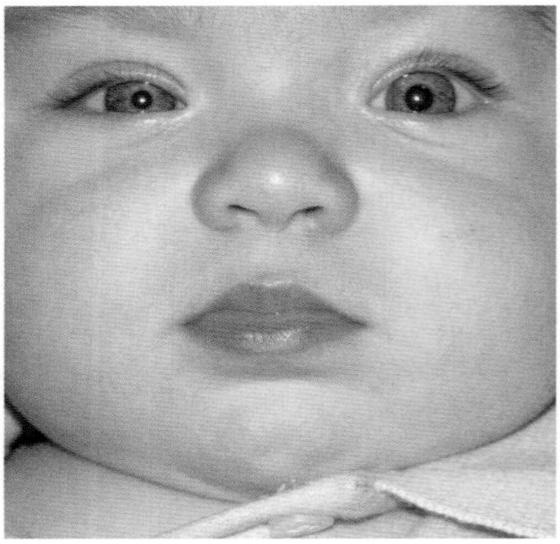

a. Urinary Bence-Jones protein
b. Urinary catecholamines
c. Urinary ketones
d. Urinary casts
e. Urinary protein/creatinine ratio

10. An 82-year-old man had sudden, profound vision loss in his right eye. This was preceded by 2 days of brief episodes of transient vision loss in the affected eye lasting seconds. He also complained of "tender cords" on his scalp, jaw claudication, and weight loss. The erythrocyte sedimentation rate (ESR) was normal and fundoscopy showed a diffusely swollen right optic disc.
a. Anterior ischemic optic neuropathy
b. Iritis
c. Central retinal artery occlusion
d. Central retinal vein occlusion
e. Optic neuritis

11. Which one of the following is the most likely cause of this patient's Horner's syndrome?

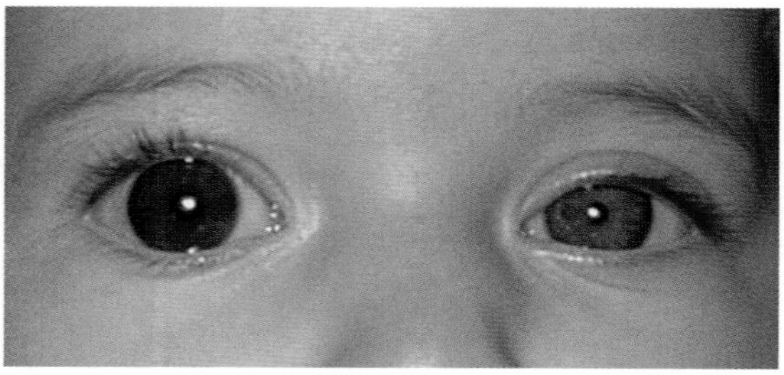

a. Carotid dissection
b. Congenital
c. Neuroblastoma
d. Hypothalamic tumor
e. Cervical cord ependymoma

12. A 54-year-old male presented after being told he had unequal pupils by a colleague. Examination findings are shown to light, accommodation and 30 min after administration of 0.1% pilocarpine to both eyes. Which one of the following is most likely?

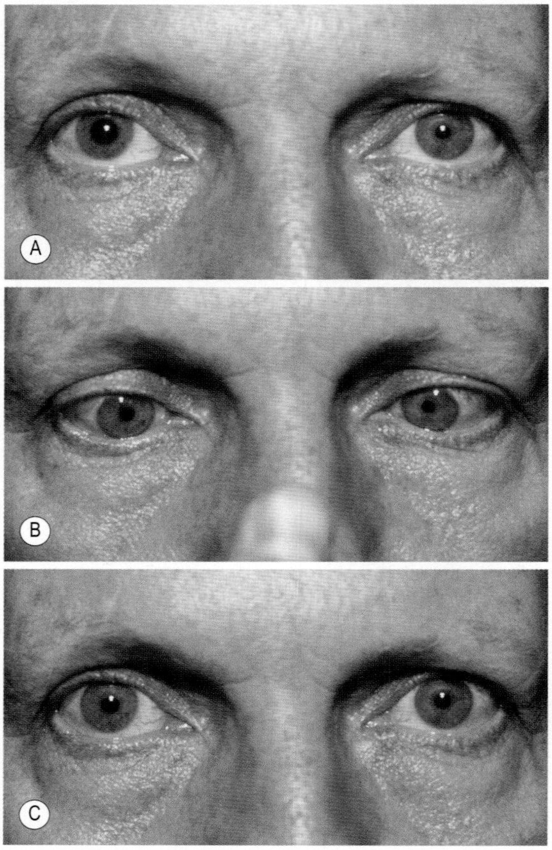

a. Left Argyll Robertson pupil
b. Left Horner's syndrome
c. Right Adie's tonic pupil
d. Right oculomotor palsy
e. Right relative afferent pupillary defect

13. A 69-year-old presented with recurrent falls and unsteadiness. Visual acuity is normal. Examination findings are shown to at rest, to light and to accommodation. Which one of the following is demonstrated?

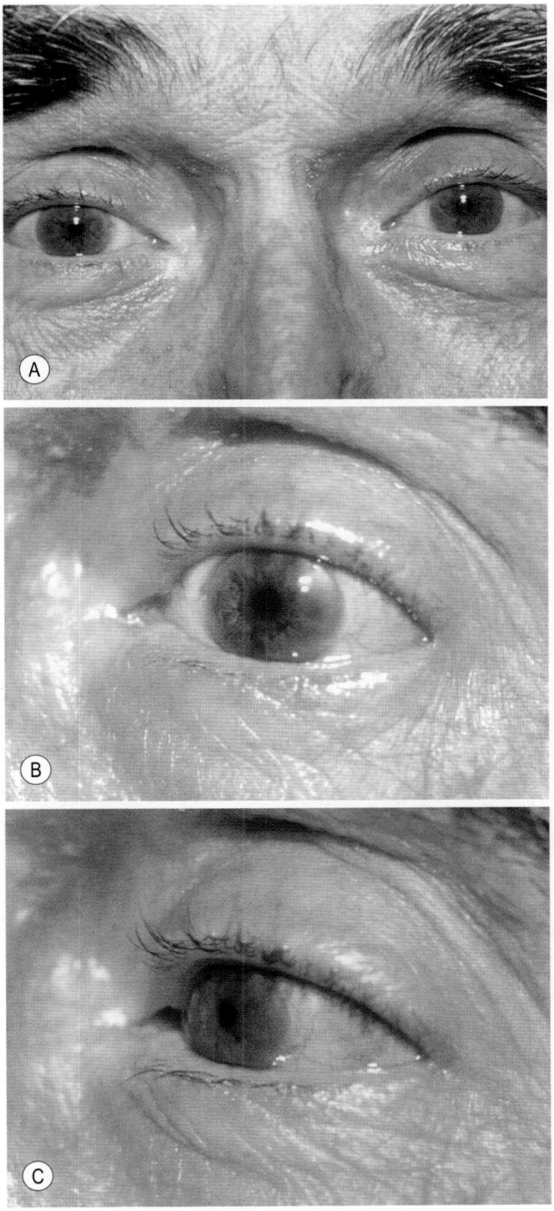

a. Adie's tonic pupil
b. Argyll Robertson pupils
c. Parinaud syndrome
d. Marcus-Gunn pupil
e. Marcus-Gunn phenomenon

14. A 5-year-old child presents with diplopia and numbness over right forehead. Examination findings shown in primary gaze, down gaze, left gaze and right gaze. Which one of the following are most likely?

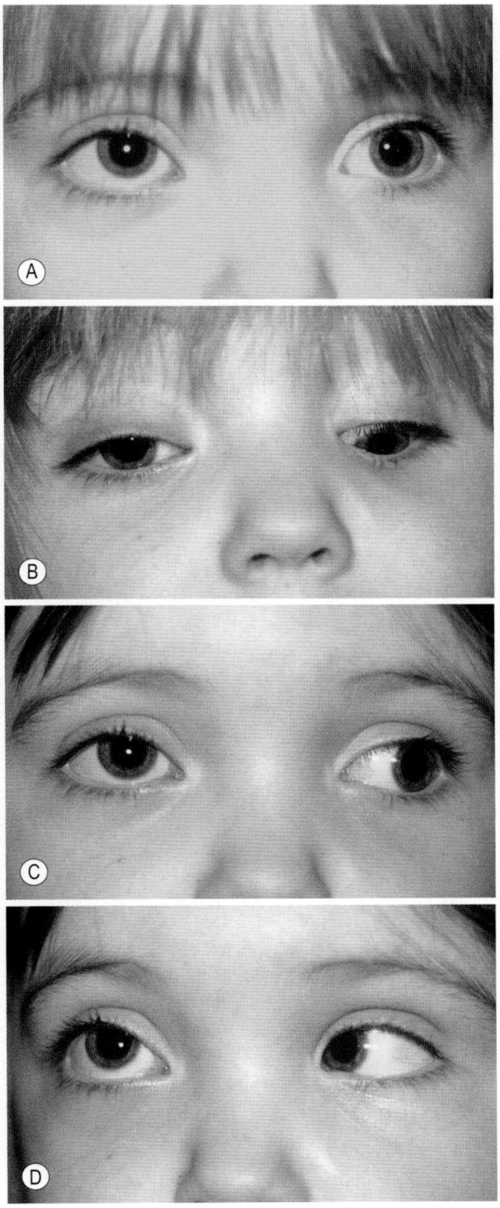

a. Gradenigo's syndrome
b. One-and-a-half syndrome
c. Orbital apex syndrome
d. Parinaud's syndrome
e. Third nerve palsy

15. A 17-year-old presents after a head injury with diplopia, particularly worse when walking down stairs and two images are oblique to each other. Examination findings are shown in right gaze, primary gaze, left gaze, right head tilt, left head tilt and at rest. Which one of the following is most likely?

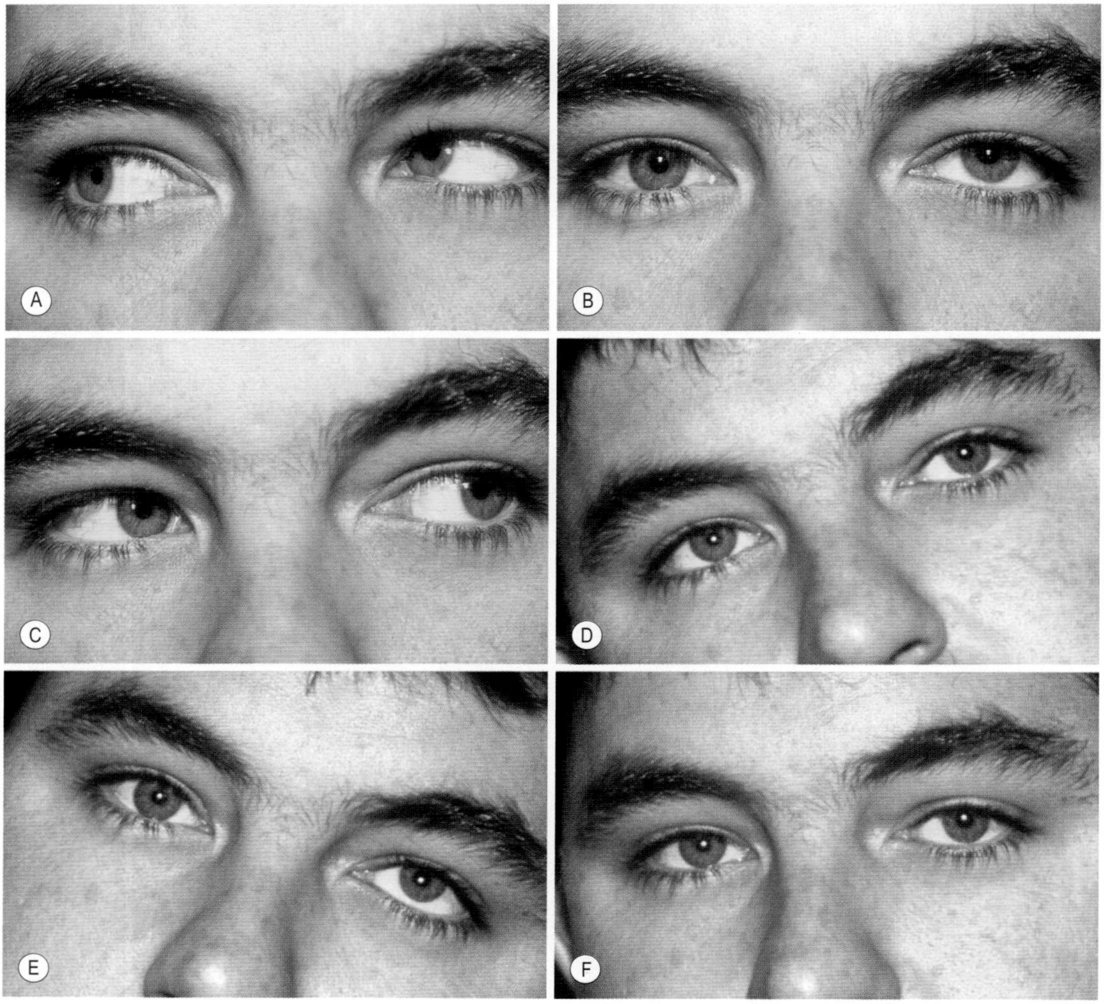

a. Left abducens palsy
b. Left fourth nerve palsy
c. Left hypotropia
d. Right exotropia
e. Right fourth nerve palsy

16. Which one of the following is most likely in the images below?

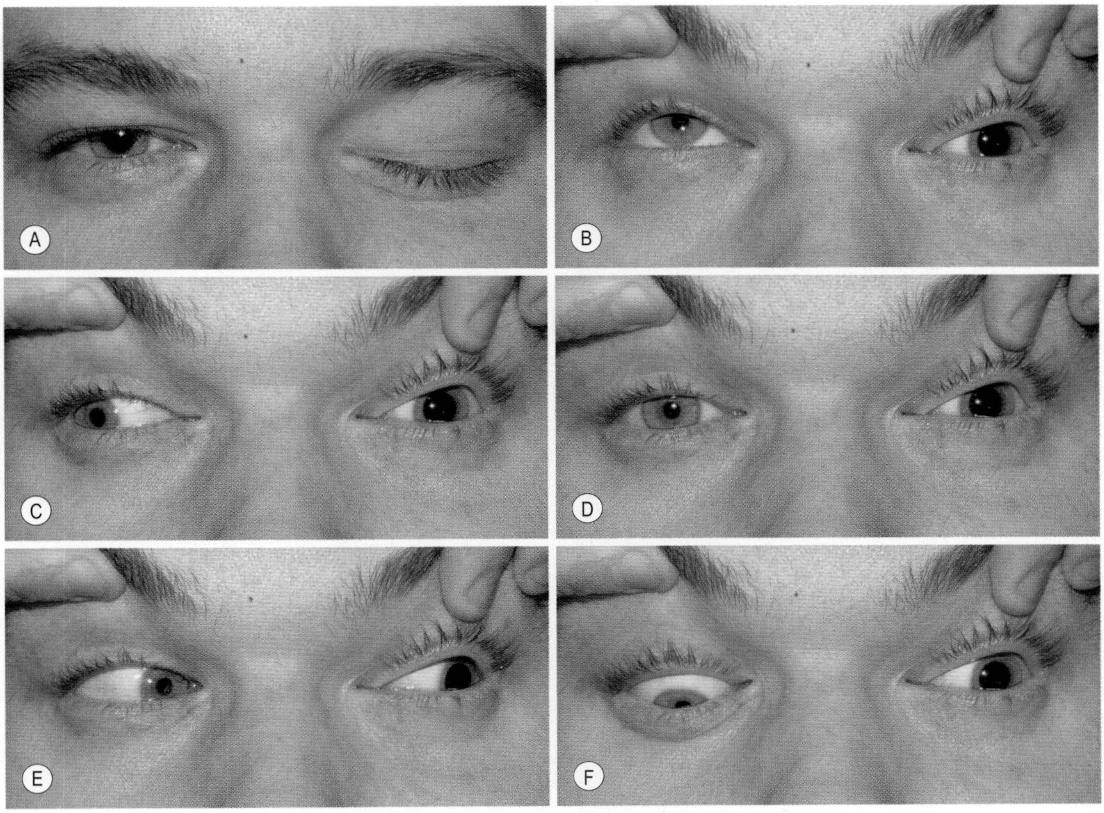

a. Cavernous sinus syndrome
b. Internuclear ophthalmoplegia
c. Left oculomotor nerve palsy
d. Left trochlear nerve palsy
e. Right Horner's syndrome

17. A 45-year-old man presents with bilateral adduction deficit during attempted gaze (with nystagmus of contralateral abducting eye). Adduction is intact during converging (and accommodating) during viewing of a near target. Which one of the following is most likely?

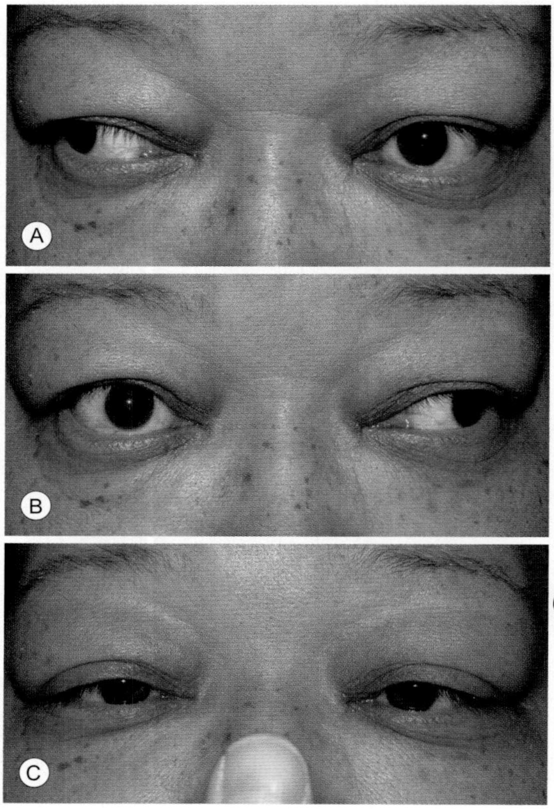

a. Bilateral internuclear ophthalmoplegia
b. Superior orbital fissure syndrome
c. Light-near dissociation
d. Oculomotor neuropathy
e. Myasthenia gravis

18. Which one of the following is the most likely cause?

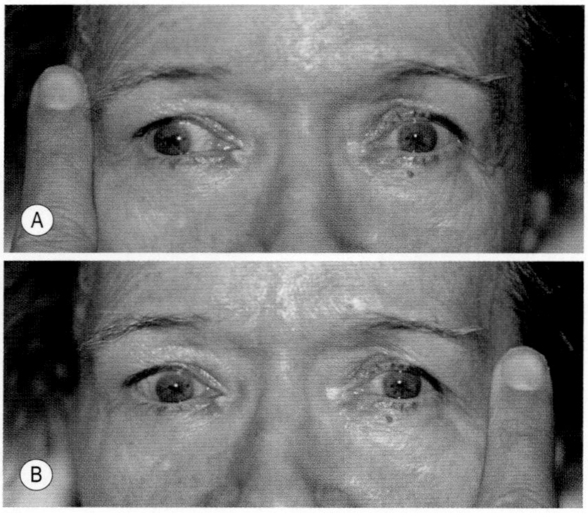

a. Bilateral internuclear ophthalmoplegia
b. Left internuclear ophthalmoplegia
c. Light-near dissociation
d. Left one-and-a-half syndrome
e. Tabes dorsalis

QUESTIONS 19–23

Additional questions 19–23 available on ExpertConsult.com

EXTENDED MATCHING ITEM (EMI) QUESTIONS

24. **Ophthalmoplegia:**
a. Abducens palsy
b. Bilateral internuclear ophthalmoplegia/ WEBINO
c. Cavernous sinus thrombosis
d. Oculomotor palsy
e. Kearns-Sayre syndrome
f. Miller Fisher syndrome
g. Myasthenia gravis
h. One-and-a-half syndrome
i. Orbital apex syndrome
j. Parinaud's syndrome
k. Steele-Richardson-Olszewski syndrome
l. Superior orbital fissure syndrome
m. Thyroid ophthalmopathy
n. Trochlear palsy
o. Unilateral internuclear ophthalmoplegia
p. Wallenberg syndrome

For each of the following descriptions, select the most appropriate answers from the list above. Each answer may be used once, more than once or not at all.

1. An 18-year-old presents with progressive bilateral symmetrical ptosis and ophthalmoplegia, pigmentary retinopathy and cardiac arrhythmia.
2. A 32-year-old presents with ophthalmoplegia, ataxia and areflexia. There is a recent history of diarrheal illness.
3. A 72-year-old admitted with aspiration pneumonia is noted to have impaired downgaze, nuchal rigidity, slurred speech and loss of Bell's phenomenon.

25. **Pupillary abnormalities:**
    a. Aberrant regeneration of oculomotor nerve
    b. Adie's tonic pupil
    c. Argyll Robertson pupil
    d. Holmes-Adie's syndrome
    e. Horner's syndrome
    f. Marcus-Gunn pupil
    g. Pretectal pupil (Parinaud's syndrome)
    h. Physiologic anisocoria
    i. Pupil involving third nerve palsy

For each of the following descriptions, select the most appropriate answers from the list above. Each answer may be used once, more than once or not at all.

1. A 43-year-old presenting with progressive headache and vomiting. Examination reveals light-near dissociation associated with upgaze paresis.
2. A 22-year-old female with right optic neuritis. Swinging flashlight test appears to cause dilatation of the right pupil when light is swung from the left eye to the right eye.

26. **Horner's syndrome:**
    a. Brachial plexus injury
    b. Carotid dissection
    c. Carotid thrombosis
    d. Cavernous sinus lesion
    e. Cluster headache
    f. Head and neck surgery
    g. Hypothalamic injury
    h. Intraoral trauma
    i. Lateral medullary stroke
    j. Midbrain injury
    k. Neuroblastoma
    l. Pancoast tumor
    m. Pontine injury
    n. Small vessel ischemia
    o. Spinal cord lesion

For each of the following descriptions, select the most appropriate answers from the list above. Each answer may be used once, more than once or not at all.

1. A 54-year-old with chronic cough and weight loss presents with a left ptosis and miosis. Hydroxyamphetamine testing dilates the miotic pupil.
2. A 22-year-old with recurrent sinusitis presents with pyrexia, headache and complex bilateral ophthalmoplegia and loss of corneal reflex on the left.
3. A 3-year-old child presents with a right Horner's syndrome. There is no iris heterochromia, no evidence or history of trauma. Urinary catecholamines are increased.

27. **Third nerve palsy:**
    a. Atherosclerosis
    b. Basilar tip aneurysm
    c. Carotid cavernous fistula
    d. Cavernous sinus syndrome
    e. Chordoma
    f. Chronic progressive external ophthalmoplegia
    g. Clival meningioma
    h. Giant cell arteritis
    i. Intraorbital lesion
    j. Peripheral neuropathy
    k. Posterior communicating artery aneurysm
    l. Trauma
    m. Uncal herniation

For each of the following descriptions, select the most appropriate answers from the list above. Each answer may be used once, more than once or not at all.

1. A 21-year-old motorcyclist involved in a road traffic collision where he was thrown 20 ft. He has an obvious right sided scalp laceration and GCS was E2V2M4 at scene. He was intubated and in the ambulance his right pupil dilates to size 6 and is unreactive to light.
2. A 47-year-old type 1 diabetic develops diplopia. On examination he has a left ptosis and weakness of superior rectus. There is no anisocoria or abnormal pupillary reflex.

QUESTIONS 28–30

Additional questions 28–30 available on ExpertConsult.com

SBA ANSWERS

1. **a**—Pontine paramedian reticular formation

Gaze is a complex eye movement that is mainly controlled by the combination of CNs III, IV, and VI. Gaze can be simply classified as lateral, vertical, or conjugate. The frontal eye field (Area 8) and supplementary eye field (Area 6) are regions of the cerebral cortex that control gaze, and they innervate the contralateral paramedian pontine reticular formation (PPRF). Fibers from the PPRF reach the ipsilateral CN VI nucleus and contralateral CN III nucleus through the contralateral MLF to control lateral gaze. Lateral gaze palsies are classified as internuclear ophthalmoplegia (INO), lateral gaze palsy, or one-and-a-half syndrome, and the corresponding lesions are located in the MLF, PPRF, and both MLF and PPRF, respectively. In INO, lesions in the MLF cause ipsilateral eye adduction failure. The contralateral eye can abduct, but with nystagmus. In lateral gaze palsy, lesions in the PPRF cause ipsilateral eye abduction and contralateral eye adduction failure. Lateral gaze to the contralateral side is preserved in these cases. Lesions in both the MLF and the PPRF result in 'one-and-a-half' syndrome with ipsilateral eye abduction and adduction failure and contralateral eye adduction failure. The contralateral eye can abduct, but with nystagmus. The control center for vertical gaze is located at the rostral interstitial nucleus of the MLF, near the CN III nucleus in the midbrain. In addition, it has been suggested that a center for convergence is located near CN III nucleus. A lesion in the midbrain can cause vertical gaze palsy and convergence palsy, and this is known as Parinaud syndrome.

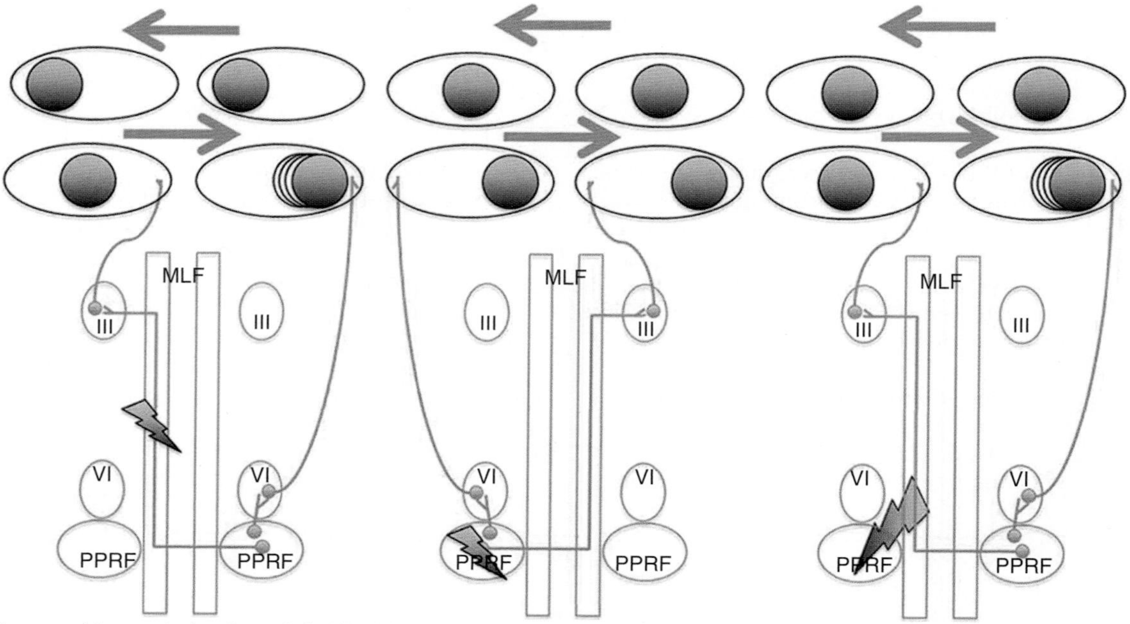

Image with permission from Sakai K, Yokota H, Akazawa K, Yamada K. Brainstem white matter tracts and the control of eye movements, Semin Ultrasound CT MR. Oct;35(5):517-26, 2014.

2. **d**—Idiopathic intracranial hypertension

Elevated intracranial pressure can be transmitted to the optic nerve head and usually results in bilateral optic disc swelling. The optic disc may be markedly elevated, with hemorrhages of the nerve head and surrounding retina. Usually, there is no visual loss acutely, except for enlargement of the physiologic blind spot from elevation and compression of the peripapillary retina. *Chronic papilledema* can cause loss of the peripheral visual field, with central vision affected only very late in its course. IIH typically occurs in obese women between puberty and menopause. Men and non-obese women frequently harbor identifiable causes of elevated intracranial hypertension (e.g. Chiari malformation, occult dural arteriovenous malformation, dural venous sinus occlusion, sleep apnea) and should not be considered to have IIH until an exhaustive clinical investigation confirms that there is no identifiable cause. Fundoscopic features of papilledema are highlighted below.

Papilledema (Common)	Acute	Chronic
Disc elevation	Disc hyperemia	Champagne cork appearance
Venous distension/ tortuosity	Cotton wool spots	Pseudodrusen (gliosis and extruded axoplasm)
Blurred disc margin	Peripapillary hemorrhages	Disc atrophy (pale)
Absent venous pulsations		Venous collaterals Peripapillary subretinal neovascularization

Image with permission from Kaiser PK, Friedman NJ. Case Reviews in Ophthalmology, Elsevier, Saunders, 2012.

3. **a**—Left internuclear ophthalmoplegia

Image with permission from Kaiser PK, Friedman NJ. Case Reviews in Ophthalmology, Elsevier, Saunders, 2012.

4. **b**—Myasthenia gravis

Ocular myasthenia gravis can mimic an isolated or combined neuropathy of CN III (except pupil involvement), IV, or VI, but often presents with diplopia or ptosis that is not easily categorized. Ocular involvement is seen early and may be the only system affected in some patients, with an inability to forcefully close their eyes against resistance. Patients frequently report worsening symptoms as the day progresses and relief after a nap or rest. The diagnosis is sometimes difficult to make because the results of edrophonium chloride (Tensilon) testing, serum acetylcholine receptor antibody assay, repetitive electromyographic nerve stimulation, or trials of pyridostigmine bromide (Mestinon) may be equivocal. The ice test is also a useful screen. Single-fiber electromyography has the greatest sensitivity and specificity but is technically difficult. CT of the thorax is performed to exclude a thymoma.

Image with permission from Kaiser PK, Friedman NJ. Case Reviews in Ophthalmology, Elsevier, Saunders, 2012.

5. **a**—Horner's syndrome

Right Horner's syndrome with right ptosis, miosis and facial anhidrosis due to right lateral medullary infarction. Relative miosis and a slight ptosis (1-2 mm) may result from interruption of the oculosympathetic pathway anywhere along the three-neuron chain: from the hypothalamus to the ciliospinal center of Budge-Waller (C8–T1), across the lung apex to the superior cervical ganglion, or from the superior cervical ganglion by means of the carotid plexus sympathetic nerves to the pupillary dilator. Postganglionic interruption (at or distal to the superior cervical ganglion) is commonly benign or idiopathic, but preganglionic or central oculosympathetic pareses are associated with malignancy in about half the cases.

Pharmacologic evaluation in Horner's syndrome

(1) Apraclonidine 0.5% is a direct alpha receptor agonist. It does not cause pupil dilatation in the presence of an intact sympathetic innervation, but will dilate any pupil with sympathetic denervation. In Horner's it will thus reverse the anisocoria and elevate the ptotic lid.
(2) Cocaine 10% dilates the normal (non-Horner's) pupil by blocking the reuptake of norepinephrine into sympathetic nerve endings producing a prolonged mydriasis over 45 min. Due to the lack of norepinephrine in sympathetic denervated pupil (Horner's) blocking reuptake does not produce a mydriasis. Persistence/worsening of anisocoria establishes the diagnosis.
(3) Hydroxyamphetamine actively releases norepinephrine from adrenergic nerve endings to dilate a normal pupil. In Horner's syndrome due to first- or second-order neuron damage, intact third-order neurons will respond to hydroxyamphetamine as those in a normal pupil and dilate. However, with Horner's due to a third-order (postganglionic) lesion, the damaged nerve endings cannot release norepinephrine and the pupil will not dilate.

Image with permission from Kaiser PK, Friedman NJ. Case Reviews in Ophthalmology, Elsevier, Saunders, 2012.

6. **d**—Optic neuritis

UK (6 m)	6/6	6/9	6/12	6/18	6/24	6/36	6/60
US (20 ft)	20/20	20/30	20/40	20/60	20/80	20/120	20/200

7. **a**—Left abducens nerve palsy

Trauma is a common cause of abducens palsy in all age groups. Acute, painful abducens paresis in a patient 45 years or older who has hypertension or diabetes suggests an ischemic cranial mononeuropathy. Recovery over a period of 2-6 months is the rule. In young patients, abducens palsies may occur as a postviral syndrome, but the clinician must remain alert for the possibility of tumor. Elevation of intracranial pressure can affect the function of one or both VI nerves.

Image with permission from Kaiser PK, Friedman NJ. Case Reviews in Ophthalmology, Elsevier, Saunders, 2012.

8. **d**—Parinaud syndrome

Dorsal midbrain syndrome (*Parinaud's syndrome*) consists of upgaze palsy, convergence spasm or paresis, bilateral mid-dilated pupils with light-near dissociation (poor reaction to light and good reaction to near), and convergence-retraction nystagmus. The nystagmus is unique to this syndrome and consists of rapid convergence with retraction of the globes on attempted upgaze. Common causes include pinealomas, aneurysms of the vein of Galen, and noncommunicating hydrocephalus with distention of the third ventricle and the anterior aqueduct of Sylvius. This syndrome may also occur with stroke as one of the "top of the basilar" syndromes.

Image with permission from Liu GT. Neuro-Ophthalmology: Diagnosis and Management, 2nd ed., Elsevier, Saunders, 2010.

9. **b**—Urinary catecholamines

Horner's syndrome in children may be caused by neuroblastomas, and 50% are adrenal in origin.

Image with permission from Liu GT. Neuro-Ophthalmology: Diagnosis and Management, 2nd ed., Elsevier, Saunders, 2010.

10. **a**—Anterior ischemic optic neuropathy

This is the commonest cause of acute visual loss in older patients, and thought to be due to ischemia in posterior circulation of the gobe—predominantly vessels supplying the optic nerve at its exit from the eye. It is classified as non-arteritic or arteritic, the former being much more common. In all cases of AION, it is vital to determine whether there is any evidence of an arteritic cause (e.g., giant cell arteritis). Untreated giant cell arteritis can cause rapid, sequential, or simultaneous blindness in both eyes. If giant cell arteritis is suspected because of an elevated ESR or CRP, or both, or because of symptoms such as headache, scalp and temple tenderness, myalgias, arthralgias, low-grade fever, anemia, malaise, weight loss, anorexia, or jaw claudication, oral or intravenous steroid treatment should be instituted immediately. In acute cases, the patient may benefit from high-dose intravenous steroids. Biopsy of the temporal artery should follow within days of steroid therapy. In arteritic AION, the visual loss is usually profound, and the optic nerve is often diffusely swollen and pale.

11. **b**—Congenital

Iris heterochromia in idiopathic congenital Horner's syndrome.

Image with permission from Liu GT. Neuro-Ophthalmology: Diagnosis and Management, 2nd ed., Elsevier, Saunders, 2010.

12. **c**—Right Adie's tonic pupil

The right pupil is mid-sized and larger than the left, poorly reactive to light, but reactive to near stimulus (light-near dissociation). It constricted with 0.1% pilocarpine while the left pupil did not indicating denervation hypersensitivity on the right. *Adie's (or Holmes-Adie's) syndrome* which is a symptom complex consisting of tonic pupil(s) and absent deep tendon reflexes and is the commonest cause. Viral or bacterial infection causing inflammation to the ciliary ganglion damages parasympathetic postganglionic input to the eye, and to dorsal root ganglia in the spine. The use of stronger 1% pilocarpine would be effective in constricting normal pupils, as well as third nerve-related mydriasis, tonic pupils, and other pre- and postganglionic parasympathetic disorders because in these cases the receptors at the iris constrictor muscle are either normal or hypersensitive. Pupils dilated with anticholinergic agents such as atropine, tropicamide, or cyclopentolate or sympathomimetic agents such as phenylephrine or neosynephrine, are generally large (> 7-8 mm) and unreactive to light or near stimulation.

Image with permission from Liu GT. Neuro-Ophthalmology: Diagnosis and Management, 2nd ed., Elsevier, Saunders, 2010.

13. **b**—Argyll Robertson pupils

Here the pupils are bilaterally small and show light-near dissociation ("accommodate but do not react"). Apart from pupil size, the other main way of differentiating between Argyll Robertson pupils and Adie's pupil is their speed of constriction to near vision—immediate in the former and slow/prolonged in the latter. In tabes dorsalis (demyelination secondary to syphilis) Argyll Robertson pupils are associated with absent deep tendon reflexes, loss of vibratory sense and proprioception in the lower extremities, and Charcot joints. Lesion locations of the various types of light-near dissociation are outlined below.

Cause of Light-Near Dissociation	Lesion
Adie's tonic pupil	Ciliary ganglion
Optic neuropathy/ Severe retinopathy	Anterior visual pathway
Argyll Robertson pupil	Lesion of midbrain tectum
Parinaud syndrome	Lesion of midbrain tectum
Aberrant regeneration of CNIII	Aberrant innervation of papillary fibers
Peripheral neuropathy	Short posterior ciliary nerves

Image with permission from Liu GT. Neuro-Ophthalmology: Diagnosis and Management, 2nd ed., Elsevier, Saunders, 2010.

14. **c**—Orbital apex syndrome

Cause	Description
Cavernous sinus syndrome	CN III, IV, VI palsy Pain in distribution of V1-2 (and V3 is posterior sinus involved) Horner's syndrome (sympathetic fibers on ICA, VI, V1) Lid malposition (ptosis or lid edema) Mixed CNIII palsy and Horner's gives a small or mid-dilated poorly reactive pupil.
Superior orbital fissure syndrome	As for cavernous sinus syndrome but never has V3 involvement; also no optic nerve involvement
Orbital apex syndrome	Optic nerve (RAPD/visual loss), III, IV, VI, V1 (hypoesthesia in ophthalmic division); proptosis common

Image with permission from Liu GT. Neuro-Ophthalmology: Diagnosis and Management, 2nd ed., Elsevier, Saunders, 2010.

15. **b**—Left fourth nerve palsy

The main causes are head trauma, microvascular infarction, congenital, tumors and demyelination. It is the only cranial nerve which exits the brainstem dorsally (has the longest intracranial course), it decussates to supply the contralateral superior oblique muscle and is enveloped in the anterior medullary velum where it is vulnerable to head trauma. Assessment of a trochlear nerve palsy is challenging, but a three step test is best used:

(1) Which eye is hypertropic in primary gaze?
(2) Is the hypertropia worse in left or right gaze?
(3) Is the hypertropia worse in left or right head tilt?

The *left* hypertropia, which is worse in *right* gaze and *left* head tilt, is consistent with weakness of the left superior oblique muscle. The trochlear nerve innervates the superior oblique muscle and because of its redirection at the trochlea and attachment to the globe it intorts, depresses, and abducts the eye. When the globe is adducted, however, the angle of the muscle's insertion minimizes all actions except pure depression. This fact simplifies clinical evaluation of the superior oblique muscle; the clinician looks at how well the right eye can move down in left gaze and how well the left eye moves down in right gaze. The vital role of the superior oblique muscle in ocular cyclotorsion explains why patients with trochlear palsy often describe diplopia with one image tilted. One can occasionally elicit which fourth nerve is affected by asking the patient to look at a horizontal straight object (e.g. a pen). If the patient sees two images, they can be asked to describe how they intersect. A patient with a unilateral fourth nerve palsy will see a horizontal line and a tilted line below it, intersecting on the side of the abnormal eye (the arrow points to the side of the affected fourth nerve).

Image with permission from Liu GT. Neuro-Ophthalmology: Diagnosis and Management, 2nd ed., Elsevier, Saunders, 2010.

16. **c**—Left oculomotor nerve palsy

The left eye has complete ptosis, defective elevation, absent adduction, a down and out position in primary gaze with a large unreactive pupil, intact abduction, and deficient downgaze. The oculomotor nerve innervates all the extraocular muscles (including the levator palpebrae), except for the lateral rectus (VI) and superior oblique muscles (IV). It also carries parasympathetic efferent fibers to the pupillary sphincter and ciliary muscle through the ciliary ganglion. Complete third cranial nerve palsy produces an eye that is turned down and out (because of remaining function of the superior oblique and lateral rectus muscles) and a dilated pupil with ptosis. Partial or incomplete paresis may present a more confusing picture. The pupillary fibers run superficially in the nerve and are preferentially affected by compression, such as from a posterior communicating artery aneurysm or uncal herniation. Ischemic cranial mononeuropathy of the vasa nervosum of the oculomotor nerve generally shows relative pupillary sparing with the pupil being less affected than motility. Aberrant regeneration after disruption of the axons of the oculomotor nerve may produce clinical signs pupillary constriction or lid elevation with attempted adduction or paradoxical motility. Aberrant regeneration never occurs with an ischemic (diabetic) mononeuropathy and always implies that the nerve has been injured in such a way that the myelin sheath and perineurium have been breached (i.e., aneurysm, tumor, or trauma).

Image with permission from Liu GT. Neuro-Ophthalmology: Diagnosis and Management, 2nd ed., Elsevier, Saunders, 2010.

17. **a**—Bilateral internuclear ophthalmoplegia (INO)

In INO, convergence may or may not be intact. Severe bilateral INOs may also result in a exotropia in primary gaze termed wall-eyed bilateral INO (WEBINO).

Image with permission from Liu GT. Neuro-Ophthalmology: Diagnosis and Management, 2nd ed., Elsevier, Saunders, 2010.

18. **d**—Left one-and-a-half syndrome

On attempted right gaze, the patient has a left internuclear ophthalmoplegia (defective adduction of the left eye and abducting nystagmus of the right eye). On attempted left gaze there is a conjugate gaze paresis so that neither eye can move past midline. This is due to a lesion in the pons affecting the left PPRF and MLF.

Image with permission from Liu GT. Neuro-Ophthalmology: Diagnosis and Management, 2nd ed., Elsevier, Saunders, 2010.

ANSWERS 19–23

Additional answers 19–23 available on ExpertConsult.com

EMI ANSWERS

24. 1—e, Kearns-Sayre syndrome is a form of chronic progressive external ophthalmoplegia (CPEO; mitochondrial myopathies) with onset before the age of 20 years. In addition to ophthalmoplegia, pigmentary retinopathy and complete heart block they may also have cerebellar ataxia, dementia, deafness, short stature and endocrine disturbance.

2—f, Miller Fisher syndrome (variant of Guillain-Barré syndrome),

3—k, Steele-Richardson-Olszewski syndrome (Progressive supranuclear palsy) is an neurodegenerative disorder and included as one of the Parkinson plus syndromes.

25. 1—g, Parinaud syndrome; 2—f, Marcus-Gunn pupil

In the swinging flashlight test, a light is alternately shone into the left and right eyes. Both pupils should constrict equally irrespective of which eye is being illuminated (intact direct and consensual pupillary reflexes). Marcus-Gunn pupil is a relative afferent pupillary defect (RAPD) indicating a decreased pupillary response to light in the affected eye, such that during the test the pupil in the affected eye experiences a relative dilatation during direct illumination.

26. 1—l, Pancoast tumor; 2—d, Cavernous sinus lesion; 3—k, Neuroblastoma

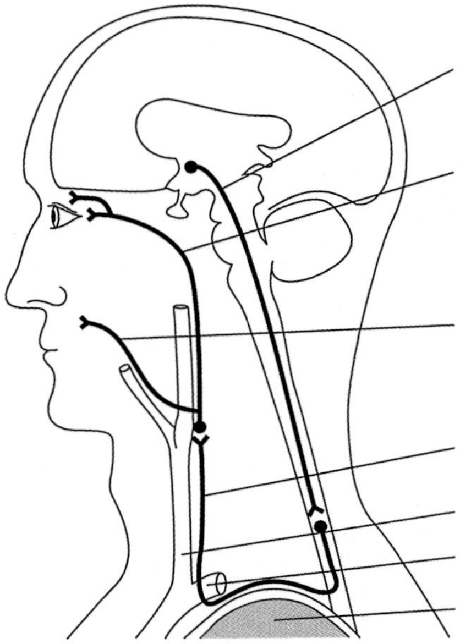

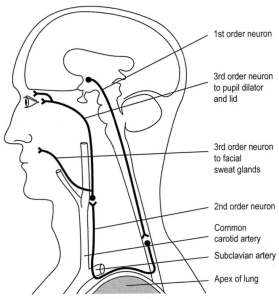

Images with permission from Liu GT. Neuro-Ophthalmology: Diagnosis and Management, 2nd ed., Elsevier, Saunders, 2010.

The sympathetic innervation of the eye consists of three neurons connected in series: first-order neurons, second-order neurons, and third-order neurons. The first-order neurons (central neurons) extend from the posterior hypothalamus to the C8 to T2 level of the spinal cord. The second-order neurons (preganglionic neurons) leave the spinal cord and travel over the lung apex, around the subclavian artery, and along the carotid artery to the superior cervical ganglion. The third-order neurons (postganglionic neurons) diverge and take two paths: Those to the pupil and lid muscles travel along the internal carotid artery through the cavernous sinus to reach the orbit; those to the facial sweat glands travel with the external carotid artery to the face. Lesions in any of these neurons cause Horner syndrome and distinct associated physical signs.

Horner's Syndrome: Clinical Features

Neuron	Cause of Horner's	Associated Symptoms
First-order	CVA MS Vertebral artery dissection	Contralateral hemianesthesia Contralateral hemiparesis VI palsy Wallenberg syndrome
Second-order	Schwannoma Lung/breast tumor Trauma/surgery Epidural anesthetic	Hoarse voice Cough Scapular pain
Third-order	Carotid artery dissection Neck trauma Neck tumors/ inflammation Cluster headache Raeder's paratrigeminal neuralgia Cavernous sinus lesions	Pain Reduced taste Dysphagia Palatal hemianesthesia Headache Involvement of III, IV, V, VI

27. 1—m, Uncal herniation; 2—j, Peripheral neuropathy

Oculomotor (III) Palsy: Causes

Cause	Comments
Infarction	Microvascular infarction usually involves axial portion—pupil spared. Diabetes, hypertension, hyperlipidemia, atherosclerosis.
Nucleus/ fascicular lesion	Weber syndrome Nothnagel syndrome Benedikt syndrome
Subarachnoid space	Posterior communicating artery aneurysm Uncal herniation
Cavernous sinus	Cavernous sinus syndrome involving III, IV, VI, V1 and V2.
Orbit	Superior division—levator palpebrae superioris, superior rectus Inferior division—pupillary constrictor, other recti and inferior oblique

ANSWERS 28–30

Additional answers 28–30 available on ExpertConsult.com

CHAPTER 10

NEURO-OTOLOGY

SINGLE BEST ANSWER (SBA) QUESTIONS

1. Which of the right ear pure tone audiograms shown below most resemble the pattern expected with Meniere's disease?

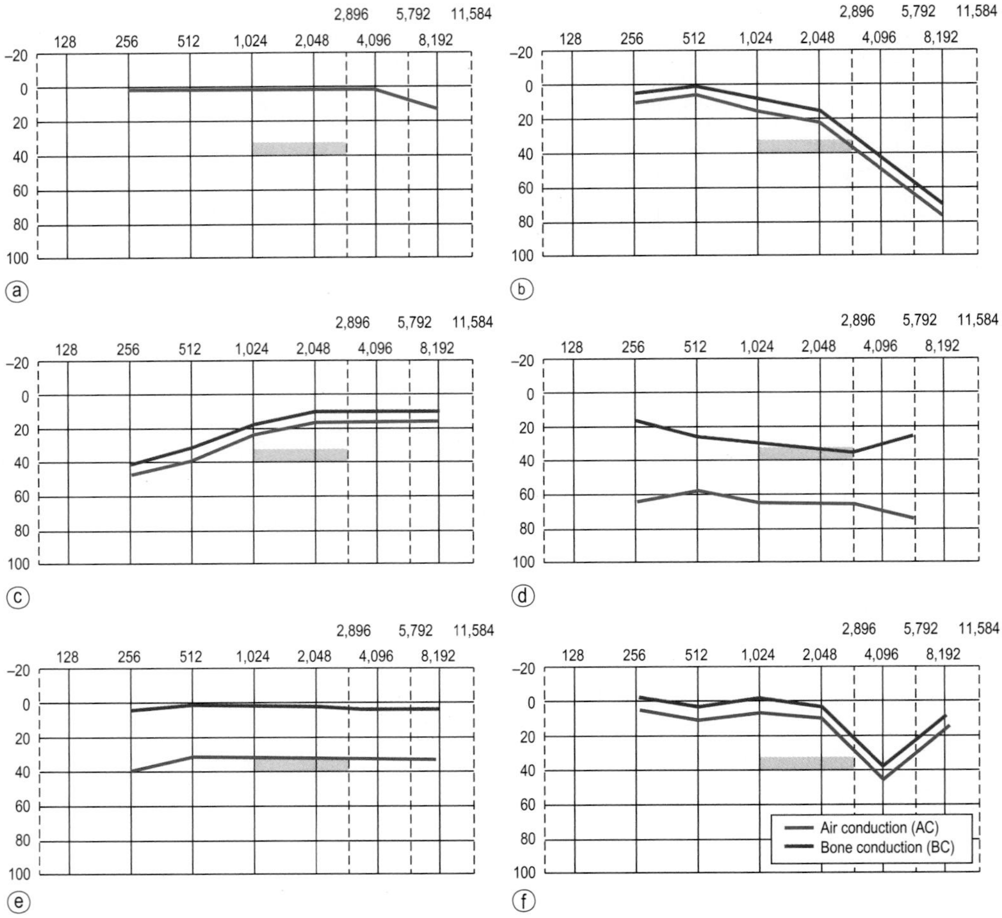

2. Vestibular schwannoma (acoustic neuroma) most commonly affects which one of the following nerves?
   a. Cochlear nerve
   b. Facial nerve
   c. Inferior vestibular nerve
   d. Superior vestibular nerve
   e. Trigeminal nerve

3. Vestibular-ocular reflex elicited during a right head turn is best described by which one of the following?
   a. Relative motion between membranous labyrinth and endolymph causes right horizontal canal cupula to deflect towards the utricle with reflex movement of eyes to left with saccades to right

b. Relative motion between membranous labyrinth and endolymph causes left horizontal canal cupula to deflect towards the utricle with reflex movement of eyes to left with saccades to right
c. Relative motion between membranous labyrinth and endolymph causes right horizontal canal cupula to deflect towards the utricle with reflex movement of eyes to left with saccades to left
d. Relative motion between membranous labyrinth and perilymph causes right horizontal canal cupula to deflect towards the utricle with reflex movement of eyes to left with saccades to right
e. Relative motion between membranous labyrinth and perilymph causes right horizontal canal cupula to deflect away from the utricle with reflex movement of eyes to right with saccades to right

4. In the brainstem auditory evoked response, which one of the following structures gives rise to wave V?
a. Cochlear nerve
b. Inferior colliculus
c. Lateral lemniscus
d. Superior olivary complex
e. Ventral cochlear nucleus

5. A 25-year-old male had occasional difficulty in understanding speech over the telephone with his left ear. Brainstem auditory evoked response is shown for both ears. Which one of the following is most likely?

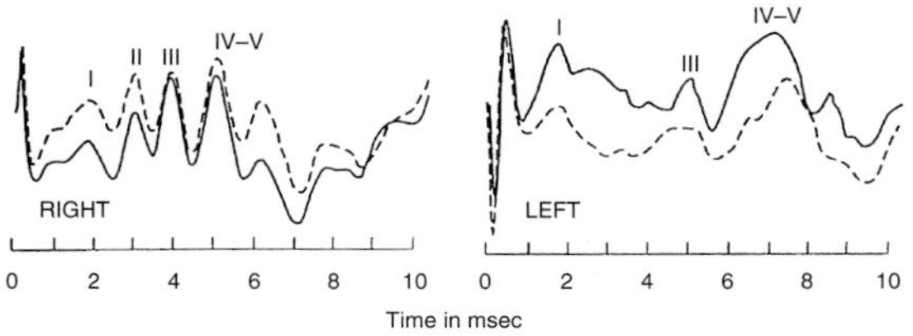

a. Aminoglycoside toxicity
b. Gentamicin ototoxicity
c. Left acoustic neuroma
d. Right cochlear ischemia
e. Right glomus jugulare tumor

6. In which one of the following situations is it NOT appropriate to use intraoperative brainstem auditory evoked response monitoring?
a. Basilar artery aneurysm surgery
b. Microvascular decompression of CN V
c. Posterior fossa surgery
d. Resection of acoustic neuroma in a deaf patient
e. Vestibular neurectomy for intractable tinnitus

7. Damage to hair cells in the basal turn of the cochlea is likely to result in which one of the following?
a. High frequency hearing loss
b. High-intensity hearing loss
c. Low-frequency hearing loss
d. Low-intensity hearing loss
e. Mid-frequency hearing loss

8. Which one of the following sites in the inner ear does gentamicin exert its ototoxic effect?
a. Apical turn of cochlea
b. Cochlear nerve
c. Hair cells
d. Macula densa
e. Striavascularis

9. A 34-year-old female presents with a House-Brackmann grade IV facial palsy. Which one of the following best describes the clinical findings?
a. Complete facial paralysis
b. Obvious asymmetry (not disfiguring); noticeable synkinesis, contracture, or hemifacial spasm; complete eye closure with effort.
c. Obvious weakness or disfiguring asymmetry; normal symmetry and tone at rest; incomplete eye closure.
d. Only barely perceptible motion with asymmetry at rest
e. Slight weakness noticeable on close inspection; slight synkinesis

10. Which one of the following best describes the target region for an auditory brainstem implant?
a. Cochlear nucleus
b. Inferior colliculus
c. Inferior olivary nucleus
d. Superior olivary nucleus
e. Vestibular nucleus

11. A 35-year-old NF-2 patient has sensorineural hearing loss and paresthesia of the posterior aspect of his right ear canal. MRI shows a large cerebellopontine angle tumor. Compression of which one of the following best explains the altered sensation?
a. Facial nerve
b. Glossopharyngeal nerve
c. Inferior vestibular nerve
d. Superior vestibular nerve
e. Vagus nerve

12. Which of the labels below refers to the modiolus?

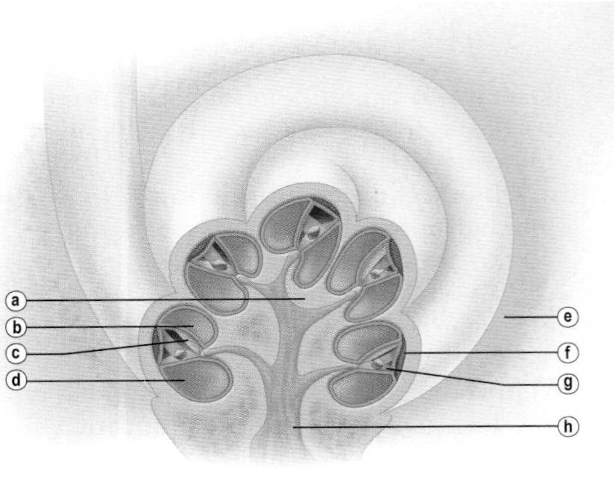

13. Which one of the following is most accurate regarding caloric testing in the right ear?
    a. Cold water irrigation causes endolymph in lateral portion to become dense and fall pulling the right horizontal canal cupula away from the utricle, reducing the firing rate and causes a nystagmus with fast phase to the left.
    b. Cold water irrigation causes endolymph in lateral portion to become dense and fall pulling the right horizontal canal cupula away from the utricle, reducing the firing rate and causes a nystagmus with fast phase to the right.
    c. Cold water irrigation causes perilymph in lateral portion to become dense and fall pushing the right horizontal canal cupula towards the utricle, reducing the firing rate and causes a nystagmus with fast phase away from the stimulus.
    d. Warm water irrigation causes endolymph in lateral portion to become less dense and fall pulling the horizontal canal cupula away from the utricle, reducing the firing rate and causes a nystagmus with fast phase away from the stimulus.
    e. Warm water irrigation causes perilymph in lateral portion to become dense and fall pulling the horizontal canal cupula away from the utricle, reducing the firing rate and causes a nystagmus with fast phase away from the stimulus.

EXTENDED MATCHING ITEM (EMI) QUESTIONS

14. **Audiometry:**
    a. Acoustic reflex
    b. Auditory brainstem evokes response
    c. Electrically evoked auditory potentials
    d. Masking
    e. Otoacoustic emission
    f. Play audiogram
    g. Pure-tone audiometry
    h. Speech recognition threshold
    i. Tympanometry

For each of the following descriptions, select the most appropriate answers from the list above. Each answer may be used once, more than once or not at all.

1. A 9-year-old girl who is struggling to hear in classes at school.
2. A 4-year-old boy whose parents are concerned he can't hear them when not in the same room.
3. A neonate with a family history of sensorineural deafness.
4. A 1-year-old who is being considered for cochlear implantation.

15. **Hearing Loss:**
    a. Acoustic neuroma
    b. Acute otitis media
    c. Genetic
    d. Glue ear (otitis medial with effusion)
    e. Meniere's disease
    f. Meningitis
    g. Noise-induced hearing loss
    h. Ossicular dislocation
    i. Otosclerosis
    j. Ototoxicity
    k. Perilymph fistula
    l. Presbycusis
    m. Tympanosclerosis

For each of the following descriptions, select the most appropriate answers from the list above. Each answer may be used once, more than once or not at all.

1. A 24-year-old man is involved in a road traffic accident and sustains a significant head injury requiring admission to intensive care. After discharge to the ward he reports hearing loss in his left ear. Pure tone audiogram shows a 50 dB conductive hearing loss across all frequencies.
2. A 57-year-old with progressive bilateral hearing loss over several years. Audiogram shows sensorineural hearing loss particularly at the 4 kHz frequency.
3. A 40-year-old woman sustained a head injury following a fall from a pushbike. Since then she has experienced intermittent hyperacusis and fullness in her left ear, with dizziness. These are especially particularly worse after heavy lifting or coughing.

16. **Genetic hearing loss:**
   a. Alport syndrome
   b. Apert syndrome
   c. Crouzon syndrome
   d. Hersh syndrome
   e. Jervell Lange-Nielsen syndrome
   f. Neurofibromatosis type II
   g. Pendred syndrome
   h. Pierre-Robin sequence
   i. Refsum syndrome
   j. Seckel syndrome
   k. Treacher-Collins syndrome
   l. Usher syndrome
   m. Waardenburg syndrome

For each of the following descriptions, select the most appropriate answers from the list above. Each answer may be used once, more than once or not at all.

1. A child with iris heterochromia, hypertelorism and white forelock born with hearing loss.
2. A child with hematuria and high frequency hearing loss
3. A child born with profound deafness and prolonged QT interval.

17. **Dizziness:**
   a. Benign paroxysmal positional vertigo
   b. Central vestibular dysfunction
   c. Head injury
   d. Labyrinthine fistula
   e. Meniere's disease
   f. Migraine
   g. Psychiatric disease
   h. Vertebro-basilar ischemia
   i. Vestibular neuronitis
   j. Vestibular schwannoma

For each of the following descriptions, select the most appropriate answers from the list above. Each answer may be used once, more than once or not at all.

1. A 54-year-old who has had two previous episodes of acute vertigo lasting a few hours only, each preceded by hearing loss, tinnitus and aural fullness in the right ear.
2. A 72-year-old woman who has a 3 month history of vertigo when turning her head in bed, each lasting less than 1 min. Pure tone audiogram shows symmetrical bilateral high frequency hearing loss.
3. A 65-year-old man presenting with progressive unsteadiness, intermittent vertigo and right sided tinnitus. Pure tone audiogram shows asymmetrical right sensorineural hearing loss.

18. **Anatomy:**

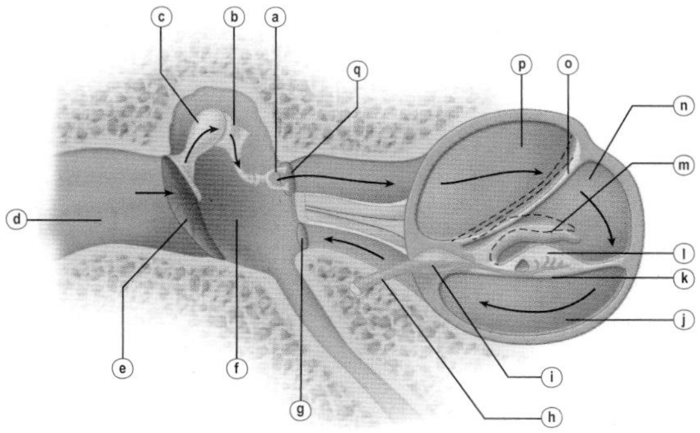

For each of the following descriptions, select the most appropriate answers from the image above. Each answer may be used once, more than once or not at all.

1. Scala vestibuli
2. Scala media
3. Organ of Corti
4. Tectorial membrane
5. Oval window

19. **Cochlear anatomy:**

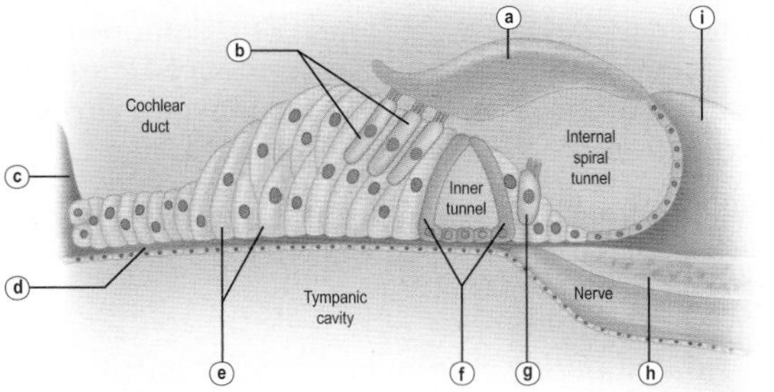

For each of the following descriptions, select the most appropriate answers from the image above. Each answer may be used once, more than once or not at all.

1. Inner hair cell
2. Outer hair cells
3. Tectorial membrane
4. Osseous spiral lamina

20. **Audiogram symbols:**
   a. O
   b. X
   c.]
   d. [
   e. >
   f. <
   g. □
   h. ↘
   i. ↙
   j. Δ

For each of the following descriptions, select the most appropriate answers from the list above. Each answer may be used once, more than once or not at all.

1. Right ear, air conduction, masked
2. Left ear, air conduction, masked
3. Right ear, bone conduction, unmasked

QUESTIONS 21–22

Additional questions 21–22 available on ExpertConsult.com

SBA ANSWERS

1. **c**—Sensorineural hearing loss predominantly of the lower frequencies may be seen in Meniere's disease

a. Normal right audiogram. b. Sensorineural hearing loss: the commonest cause is presbyacusis, with usually high-frequency loss. c. Sensorineural hearing loss predominantly of the lower frequencies may be seen in Meniere's disease. d. Mixed conductive and sensorineural hearing loss: seen in patients with a combination of presbyacusis and middle ear pathology, or in a perilymph fistula. e. Conductive hearing loss: the difference between AC and BC demonstrates the conductive loss. f. Noise-induced hearing loss: commonly affects the frequencies around 4 kHz initially.

Image with permission from Dhillon R, East CA. Ear, Nose and Throat and Head and Neck Surgery, 4th ed. Elsevier, Churchill Livingstone, 2012.

2. **d**—Superior vestibular nerve

Superior vestibular nerve supplies the superior semicircular canal, lateral semicircular canal and the utricle. Inferior vestibular nerve supplies the posterior semicircular canal and saccule

3. **a**—Relative motion between membranous labyrinth and endolymph causes right horizontal canal cupula to deflect towards utricle (and left away) with reflex movement of eyes to left with saccades to right.

4. **b**—Inferior colliculus

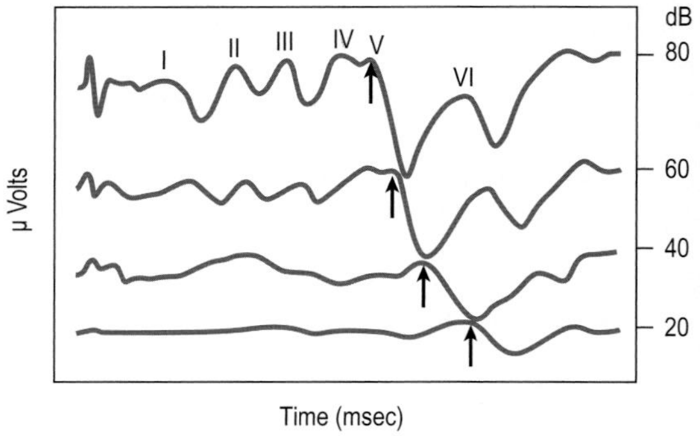

Image with permission from Winn HR. Youman's Neurological Surgery, 4-Volume Set, 6th ed. Elsevier, Saunders, 2011.

The main indication for BAER is when an acoustic neuroma is suspected due to asymmetrical sensorineural hearing loss. BAER testing is more cost effective than MRI, but MRI provides additional information. The most reliable indicator for acoustic neuromas from the BAER is the increased interaural latency in wave V. Sensitivity of BAER for acoustic neuroma is approximately 90%.

Wave	Source
I	Cochlear nerve (first-order neuron)
II	Cochlear nucleus
III	Superior olivary complex (first-order neuron)
IV	Lateral lemniscus
V	Inferior colliculus (first-order neuron)
VI/VII	Not routinely studied—medial geniculate, auditory radiation

5. **c**—Left acoustic neuroma

Preoperative deafness on the operative side eliminates the possibility of recording intraoperative BAEPs. Cases in which BAEPs are commonly monitored include microvascular decompression of cranial nerves (especially V and VII), resection of acoustic neuroma, posterior fossa exploration for vascular or neoplastic lesions, clipping of basilar artery aneurysm, and section of nerve VIII for intractable tinnitus. Changes in BAER can be caused by section/retraction of CNVIII, cerebellum, or brain stem; hypotension and hypocarbia; drilling around the internal auditory canal; irrigation of nerve VIII; severe cerebellar edema; and positioning of the head for retromastoid craniotomy. Patients with transient or persistent increases in latency or decreases in amplitude can be expected to have unchanged or only slight worsening of hearing postoperatively. Patients with complete but reversible loss of BAEP will also have unchanged or mild worsening of hearing postoperatively. Patients with complete irreversible loss of BAEP will most likely have complete or near complete loss of hearing in the ipsilateral ear postoperatively.

Image with permission from Winn HR. Youman's Neurological Surgery, 4-Volume Set, 6th ed. Elsevier, Saunders, 2011.

6. **d**—Resection of acoustic neuroma in a deaf patient

7. **a**—High frequency hearing loss

8. **c**—Hair cells. Gentamicin ototoxicity results in high tone sensorineural deafness through its effects on outer hair cells in basal turn of the cochlea.

House-Brackmann Classification of VII Palsy

Grade	Description
I	Normal facial function
II	Slight weakness noticeable on close inspection; slight synkinesis
III	Obvious asymmetry (not disfiguring); noticeable synkinesis, contracture, or hemifacial spasm; complete eye closure with effort.
IV	Obvious weakness or disfiguring asymmetry; normal symmetry and tone at rest; incomplete eye closure.
V	Only barely perceptible motion with asymmetry at rest
VI	Complete facial paralysis

9. **c**—Obvious weakness or disfiguring asymmetry; normal symmetry and tone at rest; incomplete eye closure.

10. **a**—Cochlear nucleus

11. **a**—Facial nerve

Altered sensation in the posterior aspect of the external auditory canal (Hitzelberger's sign) is secondary to compression of sensory fibers in the nervusintermedius branch of VII.

12. **a**—Modiolus, the conical central axis of the cochlea of the ear.

Image with permission from Lowe JS, Anderson PG. Stevens & Lowe's Human Histology, 4th ed. Elsevier, Mosby, 2015.

13. **a**—Cold water irrigation causes endolymph in lateral portion to become dense and fall pulling the right horizontal canal cupula away from the utricle, reducing the firing rate and causes a nystagmus with fast phase to the left.

EMI ANSWERS

14. 1 = g, Pure-tone audiometry, 2 = f, Play audiometry, 3 = e, Otoacoustic emission testing, 4 = b, Auditory brainstem response

Audiometric Tests

Tympanometry	Relative change in impedance with a change in ear canal air pressure at the plane of the tympanic membrane. The tympanogram provides indirect evidence of the mechanical integrity of middle ear structures
Acoustic reflex	Measurement of the reflex stapedius muscle contraction bilaterally on presentation of an acoustic stimulus. In patients with a retrocochlear site of the lesion (cranial nerve VIII and low brainstem), the acoustic reflex may be elevated or absent
Pure-tone audiometry	For adults and older children (>5 years). Using headphones, each ear is tested individually for air conduction and, if necessary, bone conduction thresholds. The results are usually plotted as a graph. A result of 0 dB (decibels) is the average normal threshold for hearing in young adults
Masking	When a patient has a substantial difference in hearing sensitivity between the two ears, it is necessary to rule out the potential participation of the better hearing ear when testing the poorer hearing ear. Masking is defined as the amount by which the threshold of audibility of a sound is raised by the presence of another (masking) sound
Speech recognition threshold	Measurement of the hearing sensitivity/threshold (in dB) for speech
Speech recognition score	Measurement of the speech recognition (discrimination) ability when presented above the SRT. Those with conductive hearing loss typically score high, whereas those with sensorineural hearing loss show decreased discrimination. When the conductive mechanism is normal but lesions of the auditory system affect the cochlear or retrocochlear structures, the ability to understand the consonant elements of speech is affected. When the cochlear structures are normal but cranial nerve VIII or low-brainstem structures are affected speech recognition can be severely affected. One of the early diagnostic signs of lesions of cranial nerve VIII or the low brainstem is severely reduced speech recognition scores in the presence of mild or moderate pure-tone hearing loss
Brainstem auditory evoked response	Gives objective assessment of hearing thresholds (see earlier discussion)
Otoacoustic emission	Universally used for neonatal screening of hearing. Presentation of an acoustic stimulus to the ear and monitoring of energy in the ear canal allows measurements of emissions from the outer hair cells of the cochlea. In the case of a retrocochlear lesion, when there has been no retrograde degeneration of the outer hair cells, normal OAE can be evoked in the presence of significant sensorineural hearing loss. OAE represents the first available auditory function test with which it may be possible to differentiate neural from cochlear sites of a lesion when the potential exists for each site to be implicated in sensorineural loss. Any middle ear lesion typically precludes measurement of OAE
Electrically evoked auditory potentials	Allow assessment of neural integrity, evaluation of cochlear implant function, and estimation of the psychophysical measures needed to program the cochlear implant speech processor, as well as an indication of performance after cochlear implantation

15. 1 = h, Ossicular dislocation, 2 = g, Noise-induced hearing loss, 3 = k, Perilymph fistula

16. 1 = m, Waardenburg syndrome, 2 = a, Alport syndrome, 3 = e, Jervell Lange-Nielsen syndrome

17. 1 = e, Meniere's disease, 2 = a, BPPV, 3 = j, Vestibular schwannoma

18. 1 = p, 2 = n, 3 = l, 4 = m, 5 = q

Sound waves contact the tympanic membrane, and the acoustic energy is transformed and transmitted to the inner ear through the ossicular chain in the middle ear. Displacement of the oval window by the stapes footplate results in instantaneous transmission of the pressure through perilymph in the scalavestibuli, Reissner's membrane, endolymph, basilar membrane, and perilymph in the scala tympani and in outward displacement of the round window membrane. Hair cell transduction occurs as the basilar membrane containing the organ of Corti moves relative to the tectorial membrane. The plunger-like motion of the stapes in the oval window compresses the perilymph. In the fluid medium of the cochlea, this pressure variation imparts motion to the basilar membrane, causing a wave to travel along it. The basilar membrane is stiffest at its base and becomes progressively more flexible toward its tip. Therefore any given frequency of sound (pure tone) will cause a wave in the basilar membrane that has maximum displacement that is precisely timed and spaced along the membrane. For high tones, this point is close to the base of the cochlea, and for lower frequencies, it is more distal. The response of hair cells to the tone is strongest at the point of greatest displacement. Therefore the position from base to apex along the spiral of the basilar membrane and organ of Corti is directly related to the frequency of the tone that will elicit a response (tonotopy).

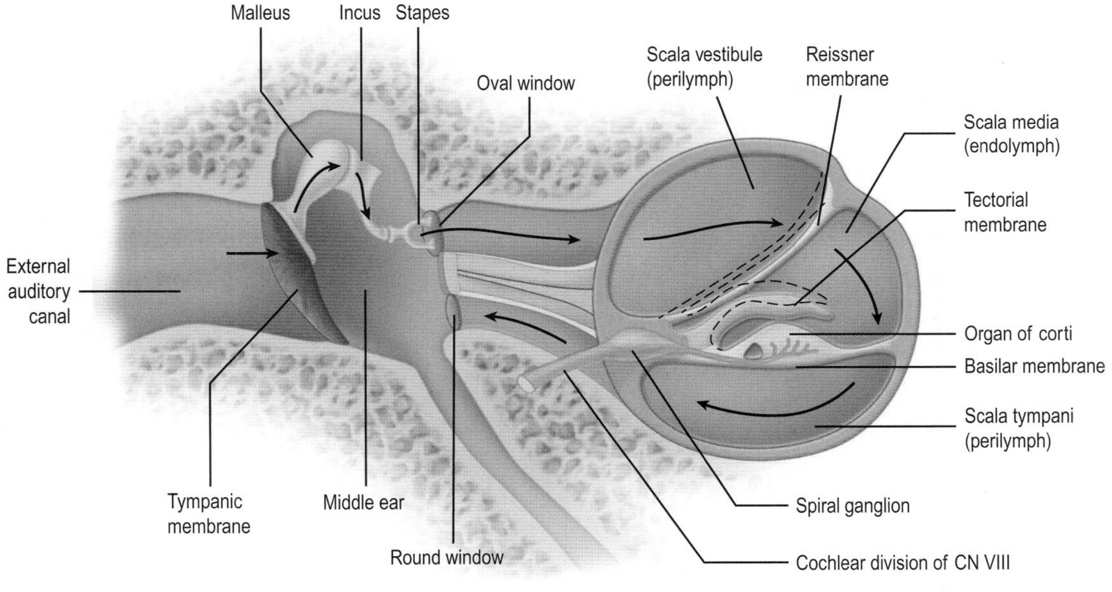

Image with permission from Winn HR. Youman's Neurological Surgery, 4-Volume Set, 6th ed. Elsevier, Saunders, 2011.

19. 1 = g, 2 = b, 3 = a, 4 = h

Inner hair cells are extremely sensitive transducers that convert the mechanical force applied to the hair bundle into an electrical signal. Endolymph, like extracellular fluid, has a high concentration of potassium. In contrast, perilymph, like cerebrospinal fluid, has a high concentration of sodium. The potential difference between the endolymph and the perilymph is maintained by selective secretion and absorption of ions by the striavascularis. As the basilar membrane moves up in response to fluid movement in the scala tympani, the taller stereocilia are displaced against the tectorial membrane. This causes ion channels at the tips of the stereocilia to open, allowing potassium flow down the electrical gradient to depolarize the cell. When a hair cell depolarizes, voltage-gated calcium channels at the base of the cell open, and the resulting influx of calcium causes synaptic vesicles to fuse to the cell membrane and to release a neurotransmitter into the synaptic cleft between the hair cell and the cochlear nerve fibers. The transmitter causes depolarization of the afferent fiber, and an action potential is transmitted along the cochlear nerve fiber.

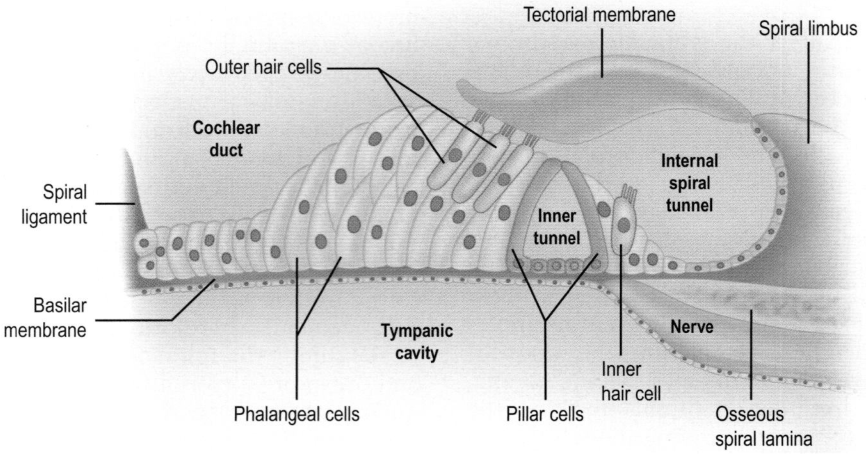

Image with permission from Lowe JS, Anderson PG. Stevens & Lowe's Human Histology, 4th ed. Elsevier, Mosby, 2015.

20. 1 = j, Δ, 2 = g, □, 3 = f, <

	Right ear	Left ear
AC unmasked	O	X
AC masked	Δ	□
BC unmasked	<	>
BC masked	[	]
No response (imposed over other symbol)	↙	↘

ANSWERS 21–22

Additional answers 21–22 available on ExpertConsult.com

CHAPTER 11

NEUROINTENSIVE AND PERIOPERATIVE CARE

SINGLE BEST ANSWER (SBA) QUESTIONS

1. Which one of the following statements regarding cerebral blood flow is LEAST accurate?
   a. Cerebral blood flow to white matter is approximately 25 ml/100 g/min
   b. Total cerebral blood flow is approximately 750 ml/min in adults
   c. Regional cerebral blood flow tends to track cerebral metabolic rate of oxygen consumption rather than cerebral metabolic rate of glucose consumption
   d. Cerebral blood flow to gray matter is approximately 80 ml/100 g/min
   e. Brain tissue accounts for 20% of basal oxygen consumption and 25% of basal glucose consumption

2. Which one of the following statements regarding intracranial compliance is LEAST accurate?
   a. Increase in the volume of one intracranial compartment will lead to a rise in ICP unless it is matched by an equal reduction in the volume of another compartment
   b. Cerebral compliance is equal to intracranial volume displaced divided by the resultant change in intracranial pressure
   c. CSF and CBV compartments normally represent a volume of approximately 1400 ml
   d. Additional intracranial volume is initially accommodated with little or no change in ICP
   e. Once craniospinal buffering capacity is exhausted further small increases in intracranial volume lead to substantial rises in ICP

3. Which one of the following statements regarding the intracranial pressure pulse waveform is most accurate?
   a. Percussion wave, which reflects the ejection of blood from the heart transmitted through the choroid plexus in the ventricles
   b. Third arterial wave is the percussion wave
   c. First wave is the tidal wave which reflects brain compliance
   d. Second wave is the dicrotic wave that reflects aortic valve closure
   e. Intracranial hypertension increase in the peak of the tidal and dicrotic waves

4. Regarding cerebral autoregulation in adults, which one of the following statements is LEAST accurate?
   a. Increasing hypoxia results in increasing cerebral blood flow
   b. Cerebral blood flow is relatively constant over a range of cerebral perfusion pressures from 50 to 150 mmHg
   c. Cerebral blood flow is directly proportional to cerebral perfusion pressure (CPP) when CPP is greater than 150 mmHg or less than 50 mmHg
   d. A pCO_2 of 4.0 kPa (30 mmHg) is associated with an average cerebral blood flow of approximately 50 ml/100 g/min
   e. Cerebral blood flow = cerebral perfusion pressure/cerebral vascular resistance

5. Which one of the following statements regarding control of cerebral vascular tone is LEAST accurate?
   a. CO_2 causes vasoconstriction at low tensions in the blood, and vasodilatation at higher tensions
   b. Alpha2 and beta-1 adrenergic stimulation cause vasodilatation
   c. Prostaglandins PGE2 and PGI2 are vasodilators
   d. Increase in perivascular K+ causes vasodilatation
   e. Thromboxane A2 is a potent vasoconstrictor

6. Maintenance of which one of the following requires the highest proportion of energy expenditure in the brain?
   a. Transmembrane electrical and ionic gradients
   b. Membrane structure and integrity
   c. Synthesis and release of neurotransmitters
   d. Neurogenesis
   e. Axonal transport

7. Immediately below which one of the following regional cerebral blood flow values does the onset of infarction occur if sustained for more than 2-3 h?
   a. Less than 50 ml/100 g/min
   b. Less than 23 ml/100 g/min
   c. Less than 17 ml/100 g/min
   d. Less than 10 ml/100 g/min
   e. Less than 5 ml/100 g/min

8. Which one of the following statements regarding neuroprotection during anesthesia is LEAST accurate?
   a. Burst suppression must be achieved before any neuroprotective effects are seen with barbiturates
   b. Hyperglycemia exacerbates ischemic injury
   c. Mild hypothermia for low-grade aneurysm clipping and for head injury may not be of benefit
   d. Hyperthermia should be treated
   e. Volatile anesthetics reduce the vulnerability of the brain to ischemic injury

9. Which one of the following statements regarding successful strategies for cerebral protection during cerebrovascular surgery is LEAST accurate?
   a. For a given total vessel occlusion time, brief-repetitive occlusions rather than a longer-single occlusion where possible should be the goal
   b. Collateral blood flow can be increased by inducing hypertension (e.g. target MAP 150 mmHg)
   c. Preoperative perfusion imaging to help identify patients who have low cerebrovascular reserve and may be at higher risk for iatrogenic ischemia
   d. Intraoperatively, vessel or graft patency can be confirmed by
   e. IHAST2 trial showed improvement in outcome for clipped ruptured aneurysms (WFNS1 and 2) given mild hypothermia compared to normothermia

10. Which one of the following statements regarding the role of hypothermia in the management of traumatic brain injury is LEAST accurate?
   a. Eurotherm trial showed a significant increase in odds of unfavorable outcome but not death at 6 months in the mild hypothermia group
   b. Two trials of hypothermia therapy in children with TBI have shown no improvement in neurologic or other outcomes one pediatric trial showed a nonsignificant increase in mortality
   c. Eurotherm trial RCT included patients with TBI last 10 days and hypothermia was induced if the ICP climbed above 20 mmHg for 5 min refractory to tier 1 management
   d. Statistically significant increase in the odds of an unfavorable outcome in the group allocated to therapeutic hypothermia
   e. Statistically significant increase in the odds of death at 6 months (HR 1.45 (1.01-2.10)) hence discontinued due to futility

11. A patient in the emergency department has been intubated and ventilated. CT head has shown a right EDH with significant mass effect. His right pupil is larger than the left and the anesthetist is concerned about hemodynamic instability. What ASA grade is this patient?
   a. 1
   b. 2
   c. 3
   d. 4
   e. 5
   f. 6

12. A 27-year-old man undergoes general anesthesia for a hernia repair. As the anesthesia begins, his jaw muscles tense and he becomes generally rigid. He becomes febrile, tachycardic, and tachypneic. Which one of the following treatments is most appropriate?
   a. Atropine
   b. Procyclidine
   c. Succinylcholine
   d. Dantrolene
   e. Thiopental

13. Which one of the following is LEAST likely to be associated with massive blood transfusion?
   a. Iron overload
   b. Hyperkalemia
   c. Hypocalcemia
   d. Hypothermia
   e. Coagulopathy

14. Which one of the following statements regarding intraoperative blood loss management techniques applied in patients refusing blood product transfusion is LEAST accurate?
    a. Meticulous attention to hemostasis and technical blood losses during surgery are not usually important
    b. Phlebotomy should be rationalized
    c. Jehovah's witnesses generally accept prothrombin complex concentrate
    d. Intraoperative cell saver use should be considered if appropriate
    e. DDAVP (vasopressin) can be used as a procoagulant

15. Which one of the following statements regarding the oxygen-dissociation curve is LEAST accurate?
    a. It is sigmoidal due to cooperative binding of oxygen to hemoglobin
    b. The Bohr effect is a shift of the dissociation curve to the left
    c. Reducing pH shifts the oxygen-dissociation curve to the left
    d. The fetal oxygen-dissociation curve is shifted to the left reflecting the increased oxygen affinity of fetal hemoglobin caused by the presence of the gamma subunit of hemoglobin
    e. Increased temperature shifts the oxygen-dissociation curve to the left

16. Which one of the following statements regarding mechanical ventilation is LEAST accurate?
    a. PEEP and CPAP aim to keep alveoli open during inspiration
    b. Delivery of machine breaths may be triggered by time or start of a patients spontaneous breath
    c. SIMV allows patients to breath spontaneously between machine breaths
    d. Patients with sufficient spontaneous respiratory drive can be managed with pressure support ventilation alone
    e. Tidal volume is usually calculated as 6-8 ml/kg of ideal body weight

17. A 70 kg man has lost 1.7 l of blood from a stab wound. Which one of the following is the LEAST likely to be showing?
    a. Respiratory rate 20-30
    b. Narrow pulse pressure
    c. Urine output 5-15 ml/h
    d. Confusion
    e. Pulse rate 120-140 bpm

18. Which one of the following statements regarding shock is LEAST accurate?
    a. Cardiac tamponade is a cause of obstructive shock
    b. Sepsis can cause a distributive shock
    c. Spinal shock can cause bradycardia and hypotension
    d. Hypovolemic shock is managed with restoration of the circulating volume
    e. Neurogenic shock is due to peripheral vasoconstriction

19. Which one of the following is the most appropriate approximate blood volume for a term neonate?
    a. 90-105 ml/kg
    b. 80-90 ml/kg
    c. 70-80 ml/kg
    d. 70 ml/kg
    e. 65 ml/kg

20. A 44-year-old male sustains a major trauma and is found with vomitus in his airway at scene with a GCS on E2V2M4. Primary survey suggests isolated head injury and is admitted to intensive care for medical management of intracranial pressure. ICP is 19 mmHg therefore he is kept sedated and ventilated. On day 2 he starts to desaturate and CXR is performed. PaO_2/FiO_2 ratio is 113 mmHg (15 kPa). TTE is normal and there is no evidence of peripheral edema. Which one of the following is the most likely diagnosis?

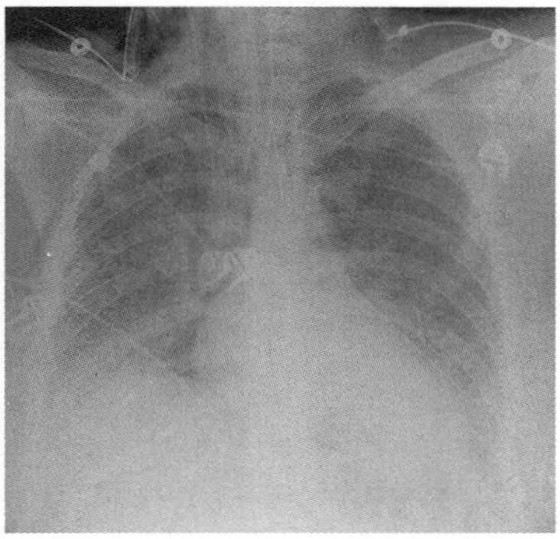

    a. Lower respiratory tract infection
    b. ARDS
    c. ALI
    d. Congestive cardiac failure
    e. Hemopneumothorax

QUESTIONS 21–38

Additional questions 21–38 available on ExpertConsult.com

EXTENDED MATCHING ITEM (EMI) QUESTIONS

39. **Anesthetic agents in NICU:**
    a. Etomidate
    b. Halothane
    c. Isoflurane
    d. Ketamine
    e. Midazolam
    f. Opiates
    g. Propofol
    h. Sevoflurane
    i. Succinylcholine
    j. Vancuronium

For each of the following descriptions, select the most appropriate answers from the list above. Each answer may be used once, more than once, or not at all.

1. Avoided in head injury patients due to rise in $CMRO_2$, CBF and ICP
2. Causes a decrease in $CMRO_2$, CBF and ICP
3. Anticonvulsant effect but no effect on $CMRO_2$, CBF and ICP

40. **Bleeding diatheses:**
    a. Antiplatelets
    b. Disseminated intravascular coagulation
    c. Factor V deficiency
    d. Glanzmann's thrombasthenia
    e. Hemophilia
    f. Liver failure
    g. Thrombocytopenia
    h. Uremia
    i. Von Willebrand's disease
    j. Warfarin or vitamin K deficiency

For each of the following descriptions, select the most appropriate answers from the list above. Each answer may be used once, more than once, or not at all.

1. Normal PT, raised APTT, normal bleeding time, normal platelet count
2. Prolonged PT, prolonged APTT, prolonged bleeding time, reduced platelets
3. Normal PT, Normal APTT, prolonged bleeding time, reduced platelets

41. **Coagulation assays:**
    a. APTT
    b. Bleeding time
    c. Dilute Russell's viper venom time (aRVVT)
    d. Factor V Leiden
    e. Factor VII assay
    f. Factor VIII assay
    g. INR
    h. Mixing (50:50) test
    i. Platelet function assay
    j. Thrombin clotting time

For each of the following descriptions, select the most appropriate answers from the list above. Each answer may be used once, more than once, or not at all.

1. Used to assess fibrinogen deficiency
2. Has largely been replaced by platelet function assays
3. Helpful to determine if prolonged PT or aPTT is due to patient clotting factor deficiency or due to presence of clotting inhibitors
4. Test for lupus anticoagulant

42. **Acid-base balance:**
    a. Acute metabolic acidosis
    b. Acute metabolic alkalosis
    c. Acute respiratory acidosis
    d. Acute respiratory alkalosis
    e. Compensated metabolic acidosis
    f. Compensated respiratory acidosis
    g. Partially compensated metabolic acidosis
    h. Partially compensated metabolic alkalosis
    i. Partially compensated respiratory acidosis
    j. Partially compensated respiratory alkalosis

For each of the following descriptions, select the most appropriate answers from the list above. Each answer may be used once, more than once, or not at all.

1. pH 7.21, pO_2 108 mmHg (14.3 kPa), pCO_2 15 mmHg (1.99 kPa), HCO_3 15 mmol/l, Base Excess −10 mmol/l
2. pH 7.55, pO_2 113 mmHg (15.1 kPa), pCO_2 25 mmHg (3.3 kPa), HCO_3 22 mmol/l, Base Excess +7 mmol/l
3. pH 7.18, pO_2 67 mmHg (8.9 kPa), pCO_2 74 mmHg (9.8 kPa), HCO_3 11 mmol/l, Base Excess −12 mmol/l
4. pH 7.35, pO_2 76 mmHg (10.1 kPa), pCO_2 55 mmHg (7.33 kPa), HCO_3 29 mmol/l, Base Excess −1 mmol/l

43. **Electrolyte disturbance:**
    a. Hypernatremia
    b. Hyponatremia
    c. Hyperkalemia
    d. Hypokalemia
    e. Hypocalcemia
    f. Hypermagnesemia
    g. Hypomagnesemia
    h. Hypophosphatemia
    i. Hyperphosphatemia

For each of the following descriptions, select the most appropriate answers from the list above. Each answer may be used once, more than once, or not at all.

1. Tall T waves progressing to widened QRS complexes
2. U wave
3. Prolonged QT interval

44. **Arrhythmia:**
 a. Amiodarone
 b. Atropine
 c. Bisoprolol
 d. Digoxin
 e. Electrical cardioversion
 f. Flecainide
 g. Furosemide
 h. Lidocaine
 i. Pacemaker
 j. Vagal maneuver plus adenosine
 k. Verapamil

For each of the following descriptions, select the most appropriate answers from the list above. Each answer may be used once, more than once, or not at all.

1. First line for stable ventricular tachycardia
2. First line for narrow complex tachycardia
3. First line for persistent bradyarrhythmia causing symptoms
4. Third degree heart block

SBA ANSWERS

1. **c**—Regional cerebral blood flow tends to track cerebral metabolic rate of oxygen consumption rather than cerebral metabolic rate of glucose consumption

Despite its relatively small size (about 2% of total body mass; adult brain weighs approx 1.4 kg), the high metabolic activity of the brain (20% of basal oxygen consumption and 25% of basal glucose consumption) requires reliable and responsive cerebral blood flow (CBF). The brain receives 15% of cardiac output (750 ml/min in adults) at rest, which equates to an *average* CBF of about 50 ml/100 g/min. Mean CBF values for white and gray matter vary between 20-30 and 75-80 ml/100 g/min, respectively. Regional CBF therefore parallels metabolic activity and varies between 10 and 300 ml/100 g/min. Transmission of electrical impulses by the brain is achieved by energy-dependent neuronal membrane ionic gradients. Increases in local neuronal activity, therefore, are accompanied by increases in the regional cerebral metabolic rate. CBF changes parallel these metabolic changes (i.e. flow-metabolism coupling). However, increases in regional CBF during functional activation tend to track the cerebral metabolic rate of glucose utilization but may be far in excess of that required for the cerebral metabolic rate of oxygen consumption ($CMRO_2$). The regulatory changes involved in flow-metabolism coupling have a short latency (about 1 s) and may be mediated by regional metabolic or neurogenic pathways. In health, flow and metabolism are closely matched, with remarkably little variation in the oxygen extraction fraction (OEF) across the brain despite wide regional variations in CBF and $CMRO_2$.

2. **c**—CSF and CBV compartments normally represent a volume of approximately 1400 ml

The volume of intracranial contents is approximately 1700 ml and can be divided into three physiologic compartments: Brain parenchyma ≈ 1400 ml (80%, of which ≈ 10% is solid material and ≈ 70% is tissue water), Cerebral blood volume (CBV) ≈ 150 ml (10%), CSF ≈ 150 ml (10%). Intracranial pressure (ICP) is the pressure within the intracranial space relative to atmospheric pressure. "Normal" ICP is generally less than 10-15 mmHg and varies with age being lower in infants and children. However, it is rarely constant and is normally subject to substantial individual variations and physiologic fluctuations, for example, with change in position, straining, and coughing. The generalized Monro-Kellie doctrine states that an increase in the volume of one intracranial compartment will lead to a rise in ICP unless it is matched by an equal reduction in the volume of another compartment. Because brain parenchyma is predominantly represented by incompressible fluid, the vascular and CSF compartments play the key role in buffering additional intracranial volume by increasing venous outflow or reducing CBF and by displacing or reducing the amount of intracranial CSF. In infants, an open fontanelle provides an additional mechanism of volume compensation. Because the size of the CBV and CSF compartments is relatively small, many pathologic processes easily lead to increases in ICP by exceeding this compensatory capacity. The dynamic relationship between changes in intracranial volume and pressure can be graphically presented as a "pressure-volume" curve. It is evident from the exponential shape of the curve that additional intracranial volume is initially accommodated with little or no change in ICP (flat part of the curve), but when craniospinal buffering capacity is exhausted (point of decompensation), further small increases in intracranial volume lead to substantial rises in ICP. Intracranial compliance can serve as measure of craniospinal compensatory reserve (position on the pressure-volume curve) and is described by the following equation, in which ΔV is change in volume and ΔP is change in pressure: $C = \Delta V/\Delta P$. Cerebral compliance can be measured directly with invasive devices. A substantial increase in ICP may lead to a reduction in cerebral blood flow (CBF), and this finding triggered interest in estimation of cerebral perfusion pressure (CPP = mean arterial pressure [MAP] – ICP).

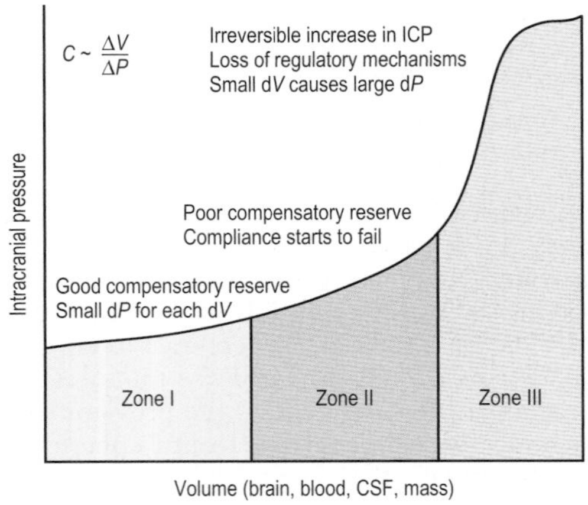

Image with permission from Swaiman K, et al. (Eds.), Swaiman's Pediatric Neurology: Principles and Practice, 5th ed., Elsevier, 2012.

3. **e**—Intracranial hypertension increase in the peak of the tidal and dicrotic waves

Typically, the normal ICP waveform consists of three arterial components superimposed on the respiratory rhythm. The first arterial wave is the percussion wave, which reflects the ejection of blood from the heart transmitted through the choroid plexus in the ventricles. The second wave is the tidal wave, which reflects brain compliance; and finally, the third wave is the dicrotic wave that reflects aortic valve closure. Under physiologic conditions, the percussion wave is the tallest, with the tidal and dicrotic waves having progressively smaller amplitudes. When intracranial hypertension is present, cerebral compliance is diminished. This is reflected by an increase in the peak of the tidal and dicrotic waves exceeding that of the percussion wave

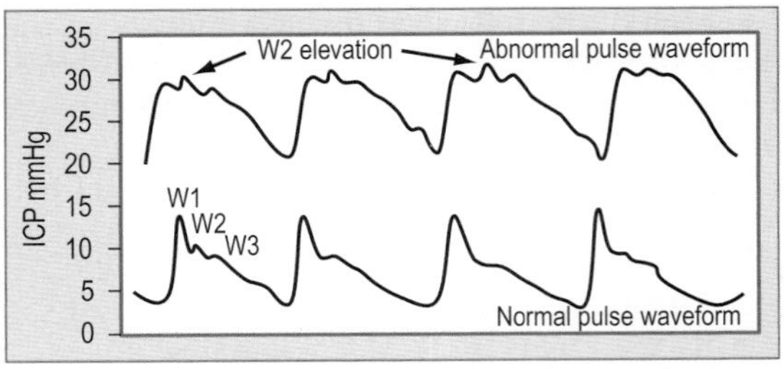

Image with permission from Vincent JL, et al. Textbook of Critical Care, 6th ed., Elsevier, Saunders, 2011.

4. **d**—A pCO_2 of 4.0 kPa (30 mmHg) is associated with an average cerebral blood flow of approximately 50 ml/100 g/min (see graph)

Cerebral blood flow (CBF) is regulated at the level of the cerebral arteriole. It depends on the pressure gradient across the vessel wall (which in turn is the result of CPP) and Pa CO_2 value (which depends on ventilation). Cerebral autoregulation is dominant to ICP homeostasis and keeps CBF constant in the face of changes in CPP or mean arterial pressure (MAP). It does this through alterations in cerebral vasomotor tone (i.e. cerebrovascular resistance [CVR]) such that CBF = CPP/CVR = [MAP – ICP]/CVR. Chronic hypertension or sympathetic activation shifts the autoregulatory curve to the right, whereas sympathetic withdrawal shifts it to the left. Cerebral autoregulation is normally functional for CPP values of 50-150 mmHg and is impaired by intracranial and extracranial (e.g. chronic systemic hypertension) pathologic conditions and anesthetics. Tissue perfusion will decrease proportionally when CPP is below the lower limit of autoregulation (e.g. <50 mmHg if normal autoregulation is intact). Above the upper autoregulation limit, the high CPP causes forced dilation of cerebral arterioles with resultant increases in CBV and ICP, disruption of the blood-brain barrier, reversal of hydrostatic gradients, and cerebral edema or hemorrhage (or both). CBF is proportional to arterial carbon dioxide tension ($PaCO_2$), subject to a lower limit, below which vasoconstriction results in tissue hypoxia and reflex vasodilation, and an upper limit of maximal vasodilation. As such, target pCO_2 in head injury is 4-4.5 kPa (30-35 mmHg), and hyperventilation is avoided as brining CO_2 down further to vasoconstrict can reduce CBV because dangerously low regional CBF and resultant cerebral ischemia can develop. CBF is unchanged until arterial oxygen tension (PaO_2) falls below about 7 kPa (53 mmHg) but rises sharply below that, such that raised ICP may occur in hypoxic individuals. However, the actual threshold may vary based on arterial oxygen content (CaO_2) related primarily to hemoglobin oxygen carriage (and thus oxygen saturation) rather than PaO_2. Because of the shape of the hemoglobin-oxygen dissociation curve, CaO_2 is relatively constant over this range of PaO_2. Below about 7 kPa, CBF exhibits an inverse linear relationship with CaO_2. Hypoxemia-induced vasodilation shows little adaptation with time but may be substantially modulated by $PaCO_2$ levels. Other global factors affecting CBF include hematocrit; sympathetic tone, with β1-adrenergic stimulation causing vasodilation and α2-adrenergic stimulation causing vasoconstriction predominantly in the larger cerebral vessels; and elevated central venous pressure, which may elevate ICP and reduce CPP. Temperature changes CBF by about 5% per 1° C and also decreases both $CMRO_2$ and CBF, whereas autoregulation, flow-metabolism coupling, and carbon dioxide reactivity remain intact. Ischemia results at levels of CBF below 20 ml/100 g/min unless CPP is restored (by increasing MAP or decreasing ICP) or cerebral metabolic demand is reduced (through deepened anesthesia or hypothermia). Increased ICP resulting in reduced CPP is met by cerebral arteriolar relaxation; in parallel, MAP is increased via the systemic autonomic response. As a result, a vicious cycle can be established, particularly in the presence of impaired intracranial homeostasis, as cerebral vessel relaxation increases cerebral blood volume (CBV), thus further raising ICP. In addition, an acute reduction in CPP or MAP tends to acutely increase ICP (the so-called vasodilatory cascade). Reductions in $PaCO_2$ induce vasoconstriction, reducing CBF, CBV, and thus ICP Conversely, hypercapnia increases ICP and should be prevented in the perioperative period. This makes hyperventilation a useful tool for the acute control of intracerebral hyperemia and elevated ICP.

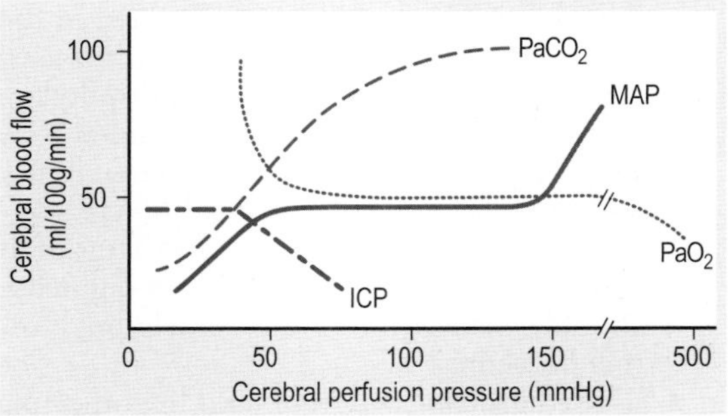

Image with permission from Cottrell JE, Young WL. Cottrell and Young's Neuroanesthesia, 5th ed., Elsevier, Mosby, 2010.

FURTHER READING

Nortje J. Cerebral blood flow and its control. In Gupta K. (Ed.), Essentials of neuroanaesthesia and neurointensive care, Elsevier, Saunders, 2008.

5. **b**—Alpha2 and beta-1 adrenergic stimulation cause vasodilatation

Multiple factors can regulate regional cerebral blood flow. Vasodilatation may be due to beta-1 adrenoceptor stimulation, high pCO_2, nitric oxide, prostaglandins (increase in ECF/CSF during hypotension), perivascular K+ (rises due to hypoxia and seizures), and local adenosine (hypotension and hypoxia). Vasoconstriction may be related to alpha-2 adrenergic stimulation, free calcium ions, thromboxane A2, and endothilin (via action of vascular smooth muscle endothilin A receptors)

6. **a**—Transmembrane electrical and ionic gradients

The human brain accounts for only approximately 2% of total body weight but receives about 15% of resting cardiac output (750 ml/min) and consumes about 20% (150 μmol/100 g/min) of the oxygen and 25% (30 μmol/100 g/min) of the glucose required by the body at rest. This high energy expenditure results mainly from maintenance of transmembrane electrical and ionic gradients (≈60%), but also from maintenance of membrane structure and integrity and the synthesis and release of neurotransmitters (≈40%). Although the energy requirements of the brain are substantial, it has a very small reserve of metabolic substrates. Therefore, normal functioning of the central nervous system is highly dependent on adequate and continuous provision of energy substrates and removal of the waste products of metabolism. Glucose is the brains main substrate for generating ATP, with its oxidation into pyruvate generating 2ATP molecules, but subsequent conversion of pyruvate into acetyl-CoA and oxidation in the citric acid (Krebs) cycle resulting in a net yield of approximately 30 ATP molecules (compared to 2ATP molecules for anaerobic respiration). The brain has a high metabolic requirement for oxygen (40-70 ml O_2/min) that must be met by delivery within blood, which depends on the oxygen content of the blood (typically, 20 ml per 100 ml blood) and blood flow (typically, 50 ml per 100 g brain per minute). Therefore, under normal circumstances, delivery (150 ml/min) is much greater than demand (40-70 ml/min), and around 40% of the oxygen delivered in blood is extracted. This oxygen extraction fraction (OEF) can be increased for short periods when either delivery is reduced or demand is increased. In states of prolonged starvation and in the developing brain, ketone bodies (acetoacetate and β-hydroxybutyrate) can become important metabolic substrates within the brain. In addition, some amino and organic acids can be taken up and metabolized within the brain. Overall, these are minor energy substrates except during periods of metabolic stress, such as during acute hypoglycemia and ischemia. The brain can consume lactate as a substrate, particularly during periods of hypoglycemia or elevated blood lactate.

7. **c**—Less than 17 ml/100 g/min

Cerebral Blood Flow and Ischaemia

CBF	Cell State	Time to Infarction	Consequences
50 (20-80)	Normal	–	Normal
<23	Oligemia	>6 h	EEG slowing
10-17	Penumbra	Several hours	Flatline EEG, absent evoked potentials
<10	Death	Several minutes	Membrane pump failure

Under normal circumstances, CBF is maintained at a relatively constant rate of 50 ml/100 g/min. With a reduction in cerebral perfusion pressure, CBF declines gradually. Physiologic indices of ischemia are not apparent until CBF is reduced to about 20-25 ml/100 g/min; at that time, electroencephalographic (EEG) slowing is apparent. Such slowing indicates that the brain has a substantial blood flow reserve. Below a CBF of 17 ml/100 g/min, the electroencephalogram is suppressed and evoked potentials are absent. It is not until the CBF is less than 10 that ATP energy failure occurs resulting in neuronal depolarization, excitotoxicity, cytotoxic edema and cell death. Within the ischemic territory, the region supplied by end arteries undergoes rapid death and is referred to as the *core*. Surrounding the core is a variable area of the brain called the penumbra. The penumbra is rendered sufficiently ischemic to be electrically silent but has not yet undergone ischemic depolarization. The penumbra is viable for several hours and can be salvaged by restoration of flow. If reperfusion is not established, the penumbra is gradually recruited into the core. Depending on the severity of the injury, blood-brain barrier breakdown occurs about 2-3 days after injury. This permits the entry of plasma proteins into the brain substance, which further increases cerebral edema significantly and is called *vasogenic* edema. The development of post-ischemic edema can be significant enough to result in substantial increases in ICP and neurological deterioration. In the region surrounding the infarction, autoregulation and CO_2 reactivity are re-established in most situations in about 4-6 weeks.

FURTHER READING

Heiss WD, Graf R, The ischemic penumbra, Curr Opin Neurol. 1994;7(1):11-19.

8. **a**—Burst suppression must be achieved before any neuroprotective effects are seen with barbiturates

An anesthetized brain is less vulnerable to ischemic injury. There do not appear to be any differences among anesthetic agents with respect to their neuroprotective efficacy.

- Barbiturates, propofol, and ketamine have been shown to have neuroprotective efficacy. With regard to barbiturates, doses less than those that produce burst suppression of the electroencephalogram achieve the same degree of protection as higher doses do
- Volatile anesthetics reduce the vulnerability of the brain to ischemic injury
- Maintenance of CPP within the normal range for a patient who is at risk for cerebral ischemic injury is essential. Modest increases in blood pressure (5-10%) may be of benefit to those who have suffered from an ischemic insult. Hypotension is deleterious
- Arterial pCO_2 should be maintained in the normal range unless hyperventilation is used for short-term brain relaxation. Prophylactic hyperventilation should be avoided
- Hyperglycemia exacerbates ischemic injury and should be treated with insulin. A reasonable threshold for treatment is 150 mg/dl. If insulin treatment is initiated, blood glucose should be closely monitored and hypoglycemia prevented
- The routine induction of mild hypothermia for low-grade aneurysm clipping and for head injury may not be of benefit. In high-grade SAH patients (WFNS 4-5), the utility of mild hypothermia for purposes of brain protection remains to be defined
- Hyperthermia should be avoided
- Seizures can worsen cerebral injury and should be treated with anticonvulsants

9. **e**—IHAST2 trial showed improvement in outcome for clipped ruptured aneurysms (WFNS1 and 2) given mild hypothermia compared to normothermia

Several strategies may be used in an attempt to provide cytoprotection during cerebrovascular procedures with use of temporary arterial occlusion for dissection of aneurysms and permanent clipping. Limiting the duration of ischemia is probably the most intuitive and direct method of reducing ischemic injury. The duration of focal ischemia that can be tolerated safely without clinically evident sequelae varies between individuals and vascular territories. The current consensus for temporary vessel occlusion is brief repetitive clipping periods, which provides increased safety and less risk for postoperative neurological deficit than a single episode of occlusion does, but variation in other intraoperative parameters means no single occlusion time is accepted as "safe." Collateral blood flow can be increased by inducing hypertension (e.g. target MAP 150 mmHg). Preoperative measurement of flow rates through cerebral vessels can be achieved with perfusion imaging to help the surgeon identify patients who have low cerebrovascular reserve and may be at higher risk for iatrogenic ischemia. Intraoperatively, vessel or graft patency can be confirmed by a number of modalities, including direct microvascular Doppler or transcranial Doppler (TCD) ultrasound, ultrasonic flow probe, intraoperative angiography, EEG, electrocorticography, multimodality evoked potential (MEP) and somatosensory evoked potential (SEP) monitoring, brain tissue oxygenation, and fluorescent angiography (e.g. fluorescein sodium, indocyanine green). Decreasing the metabolic activity of tissue at risk can be achieved by mild hypothermia (33-34.5 °C) and by the use of certain anesthetic agents to induce EEG burst suppression (e.g. pentobarbital, propofol, etomidate). The role of mild hypothermia in neurovascular surgery is less clear after Intraoperative Hypothermia After Aneurysm Surgery Trial (IHAST2), an international double-blind trial in which 1001 WFNS1-3 aneurysmal SAH patients undergoing aneurysm clipping were subjected to mild hypothermia (33 °C at clip placement) versus normothermia (36.5 °C) with no difference in outcome. Hypothermia with circulatory arrest is most often used during aneurysm surgery for giant and complex posterior circulation aneurysms including: those not amenable to endovascular treatment; those with significant intra-aneurysmal thrombus, broad necks, or a projection endangering dissection and preservation of perforators; those adhering to vital structures; and fusiform aneurysms with a distal vessel not suitable for arterial bypass.

10. a—Eurotherm trial showed a significant increase in odds of unfavorable outcome but not death at 6 months in the mild hypothermia group

Induced hypothermia has been a proposed treatment for TBI based upon its potential to reduce ICP as well as to provide neuroprotection and prevent secondary brain injury. Induced hypothermia has been shown to be effective in improving neurologic outcome after ventricular fibrillation cardiac arrest. National Acute Brain Injury Study: Hypothermia II, plus two trials of hypothermia therapy in children with TBI have shown no improvement in neurologic or other outcomes; one pediatric trial showed a nonsignificant increase in mortality. Eurotherm RCT looked at hypothermia in patients with TBI (last 10 days) admitted to a critical care environment with invasive ICP monitoring and an approach to participate was triggered if the ICP climbed above 20 mmHg for 5 min refractory to tier 1 management (usually includes head elevation, encouragement of venous drainage, intubation, sedation and ventilation to appropriate targets). Cooling protocol was a 20-30 ml/kg bolus of cold saline followed by maintenance of hypothermia as they saw fit but directed to a duration of at least 48 h, with additional time as needed to control ICP. Temperature was optional between 32 and 35 °C in the intervention arm, titrated to ICP. All patients were followed up for 6 months and the Extended Glasgow outcome scale (EGOS) was used as the primary outcome measure. From 387 patients, the data committee found a statistically significant increase in the odds of an unfavorable outcome and death at 6 months in the group allocated to therapeutic hypothermia, hence it was discontinued due to futility. Criticisms of this trial include very early use (i.e. tier 2) of hypothermia with high potential variability of subsequent management, inclusion criteria any head injury in previous 10 days, only ICP used as a guide (not CPP).

FURTHER READING

Hypothermia therapy after traumatic brain injury in children. N Engl J Med 2008; 358:2447-2456.

Beca J, et al. Hypothermia for Traumatic Brain Injury in Children-A Phase II Randomized Controlled Trial. Crit Care Med. 2015;43(7):1458-1466.

Clifton GL, et al. Very early hypothermia induction in patients with severe brain injury (the National Acute Brain Injury Study: Hypothermia II): a randomised trial. Lancet Neurol. 2011;10(2):131-139.

Hypothermia for intracranial hypertension after traumatic brain injury. N Engl J Med 2015; 373:2403-2412.

11. **e**—ASA 5

American Society of Anesthesiologists Physical Status classification is as follows: 1—a normal healthy patient (non-smoker, minimal/no alcohol); 2—a patient with mild systemic disease (smoker, pregnancy, obesity); 3—a patient with severe systemic disease (e.g. uncontrolled diabetes/hypertension, alcoholism, dialysis, >3 months since MI/TIA/CVA); 4—a patient with severe systemic disease which is a threat to life (e.g. <3 months since MI/TIA/CVA, ongoing cardiac ischemia, sepsis); 5—moribund patient not expected to survive without the operation (e.g. ruptured AAA, massive trauma, intracranial bleed with mass effect, bowel ischemia with organ failure); 6—declared brain dead patient undergoing organ harvesting.

12. **d**—Dantrolene

Malignant hyperthermia is characterized by acute severe fever, tachypnea, tachycardia, and rigidity, and high mortality rate if left untreated. It is typically precipitated by volatile anesthetics, especially halothane, or muscle relaxants such as succinylcholine. Patients may become severely acidotic and develop rhabdomyolysis. Pathology shows diffuse segmental muscle necrosis. It appears to be a metabolic myopathy in which there is abnormal release of calcium from the sarcoplasmic reticulum and ineffectual uptake afterward. Genetic defects in the ryanodine receptor, involved in calcium flux in the sarcoplasmic reticulum, are responsible for about 10% of cases, although as yet unidentified abnormalities of this or related proteins probably play a role in most cases. It is inherited in an autosomal dominant fashion. Certain other myopathies, including Duchenne muscular dystrophy and central core myopathy, are associated with this condition as well. Treatment consists of discontinuation of anesthesia, administration of dantrolene, which prevents release of calcium from the sarcoplasmic reticulum, and supportive measures.

13. **a**—Iron overload

A massive transfusion is defined as a transfusion equaling the patients' blood volume within 12-24 h. The specific additional problems related to this scenario include:

- Volume overload resulting in non-cardiogenic pulmonary edema
- Thrombocytopenia: following storage there is a reduction of functioning platelets, so that there is a dilutional thrombocytopenia following a large transfusion
- Coagulation factor deficiency (relative)—leading to a coagulopathy if concomitant cryoprecipitate/FFP not also transfused.
- Ineffective tissue oxygenation due to reduced volume of 2,3 bisphosphoglycerate, which does not store well
- Hypothermia unless blood adequately warmed
- Hypocalcemia: Due to chelation by the citrate in the additive solution and may worsen coagulopathy
- Hyperkalemia: Due to progressive potassium leakage from the stored red cells

Types of Transfusion Reaction

Acute (hours)	Delayed (days to weeks)
Acute hemolytic intravascular (ABO)	Delayed hemolytic intravascular
Acute hemolytic extravascular (Rh)	Delayed hemolytic extravascular
Febrile non-hemolytic reaction	Viral infection
Allergy/anaphylaxis	Transfusion graft-versus-host disease
Septic contamination	
Transfusion related acute lung injury	

14. **c**—Jehovah's witnesses generally accept prothrombin complex concentrate

In general, while a hemoglobin (Hgb) between 7 and 8 g/dl appears to have no immediate adverse effect on mortality, there is a clear risk of death in the 30-day postoperative period when hemoglobin fell much below 7 g/dl. Where transfusion is not an option (e.g. Jehovah's witnesses, multiple alloantibodies) the key emphasis is on optimizing hematopoiesis, minimizing bleeding and blood loss (blood conservation), and harnessing and optimizing physiological tolerance of anemia (through application of all available therapeutic resources). Meticulous attention to hemostasis and technical blood losses during surgery (e.g. use of hemostatic surgical devices, fibrin glue and tissue adhesives; controlled hypotension; elevating the surgical field above the rest of the body), minimizing phlebotomy are important. In addition, clarity must be sought (and documented) from the individual about each available blood product and extracorporeal procedure that is acceptable to them in the following groups:

- Allogenic human blood and blood products. Whole blood, RBC, plasma, platelets, white blood cells, blood from specific donors
- Human blood fractions and medications that contain human blood fractions: cryoprecipitate, cryosupernatant, albumin,

plasma protein fraction, human immunoglobulin (e.g. Rh immune globulin, IVIG), plasma derived clotting factor concentrates (e.g. fibrinogen, VIII, IX), tissue adhesive/ fibrin glue
- IV fluids and medications not derived from human blood: hydroxyethyl starch (hetastarch, pentastarch), balanced salt solutions, recombinant clotting factor concentrates (rVIII, rIX, recombinant VIIa), recombinant erythropoietin, antifibrinolytic chemicals (e.g. tranexamic acid, aminocaproic acid), procoagulant chemicals (e.g. DDAVP, vitamin K)
- Extracorporeal techniques for blood conservation or treatment: intraoperative hemodilution, intraoperative blood salvage (cell saver), autologous banked blood (self-donation), cardiopulmonary bypass, chest drainage autotransfusion, plasmapheresis, hemodialysis

15. **b**—The Bohr effect is a shift of the dissociation curve to the left

The sigmoidal shape of the oxygen dissociation curve reflects the progressive nature with which each oxygen molecule binds to hemoglobin such that the binding of one oxygen molecule facilitates the binding of the next. The Bohr effect is a shift of the dissociation curve to the right, signifying a reduction of the oxygen affinity of the hemoglobin molecule and thus a greater tendency to off-load oxygen into the tissues (i.e. in acute or chronically underperfused tissue). This change is caused by increased body temperature, acidosis, chronic hypoxia (increased 2,3-BPG) and hypercapnia. The fetal oxygen-dissociation curve is shifted to the left, reflecting the increased oxygen affinity of fetal hemoglobin compared to maternal hemoglobin molecule and allowing oxygen transfer (gamma subunit instead of the alpha that cannot form covalent bonds with 2,3-BPG).

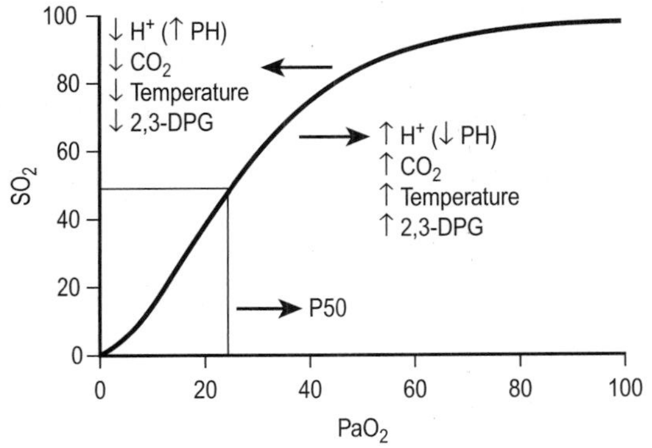

Image with permission from Hayward MP, Medical Secrets, 5th ed., Elsevier, Mosby, 2012.

16. **a**—PEEP and CPAP aim to keep alveoli open during inspiration

Ventilation parameters:
- PEEP (positive end expiratory pressure) or CPAC (continuous positive airway pressure) at the end of expiration to prevent lung atelectasis and improve oxygenation The benefits are redistribution of (1) lung water, (the redistribution of extravascular water leads to improved oxygenation, lung compliance, and ventilation-perfusion matching) (2) increasing FRC (shunting is decreased and thus oxygenation improved) (3) decreasing work of breathing. Patients who benefit are suitable are cardiovascularly stable, do not have raised ICP, and lungs that can be expanded by PEEP, and bilateral lung lesions. PEEP can cause hypotension due to excessive positive pressure. At lower level of PEEP (3-10 cmH_2O) prevents the alveolar collapse, at higher levels reopen or recruit collapsed alveolar unit (alveolar recruitment)
- FiO_2: 1.0% or 100% oxygen during unstable hemodynamic, CPR or initially put on ventilator 0.4-0.5 to prevent hypoxemia (PaO_2 100-50 mmHg) 0.3-0.4 to keep PaO_2 60-80 mmHg or SpO_2 90-92% for patient with high risk for oxygen toxicity e.g. preterm
- Tidal volume: Normally 6-8 cc/kg of ideal body weight e.g. patient who weighs 70 kg, the tidal volume 7 x 70 = 490 cc and look for PIP which is not too high (not more than 50 cmH_2O)
- Inspiratory:Expiratory ratio is 1:2 in normal patients, 1:3 in COPD or asthmatic patient who need longer expired time or reverse I:E ratio for severe ARDS patients
- Respiratory rate 8-25/min to keep normocarbia or permissive hypercarbia. Inspired time 1-2 s depends to respiratory rate. If higher respiratory rate, lower inspired time to keep constant I:E ratio
- Peak flow rate inversely correlate with inspired time and also affects I:E VAC or SIMV, the inspiratory flow rate is usually set at 40-90 l/min

Mechanical Ventilation: Types

	Continuous Mechanical Ventilation (CMV) or "Volume Assist"	Pressure Controlled Ventilation (PCV) or "Pressure Assist"	Pressure Support Ventilation (PSV)	Synchronized Intermittent Mechanical Ventilation (SIMV)
Breath trigger	Time (e.g. 10/min) or patient spontaneous breath sensor (patient draws flow from circuit or creates negative pressure)	Time or patient spontaneous breath	Patient spontaneous breath	Time or patient spontaneous breath
Breath delivery	Fixed flow rate	Fixed pressure	Fixed pressure	Fixed flow rate or pressure
Breath termination (cycling)	Delivered preset Tidal volume	Completed preset inspiratory time	Inspiratory flow decreased to preset percentage of peak flow	Delivered preset tidal volume
Comments	Flow target and frequency that at least equals the preset rate	Pressure target and frequency that at least equals the preset rates	Tidal volume, inspiratory time and frequency are determined by the patient	Patient can breathe spontaneously with or without PSV between machine breaths
Advantages	Not comfortable but delivery of minute ventilation guaranteed	Comfortable, minute ventilation not guaranteed	Comfortable, inadequate minute ventilation if insufficient respiratory drive	Not comfortable but delivery of minute ventilation guaranteed

17. **a**—Respiratory rate 20-30

Classification of Haemorrhagic Shock

	Class I	Class II	Class III	Class IV
Blood loss	<750 ml (<15%)	750-1500 (15-30%)	1500-2000 (30-40%)	>2000 ml (>40%)
Heart rate	<100	100-120	120-140	>140
Blood pressure	Normal	Normal	Reduced	Reduced
Pulse pressure	Normal or widened	Reduced	Reduced	Reduced
RR	14-20	20-30	30-40	>35
Urine output (70 kg male)	Normal (>30 ml/h)	Oliguria (20-30 ml/h)	Oliguria (5-15 ml/h)	Anuria
CNS	Normal	Agitated	Confused	Lethargic

18. **e**—Neurogenic shock is due to peripheral vascoconstriction

Spinal shock refers to complete flaccid paralysis (voluntary and reflex function) below the level of a spinal cord injury, and if between T1-L2 spinal cord segment (i.e. sympathetic outflow) will cause neurogenic shock due to loss of vasomotor tone, and if above T5 may also cause bradycardia.

Features of Different Types of Circulatory Shock

Type of Shock	Mechanism	Causes	Features	Treatment
Hypovolemic	Heart pumping well but not enough circulating volume	Dehydration, hemorrhage, burns	Hypotension, tachycardia, weak thread pulse, cool/pale/moist skin, reduced urine output	Volume replacement
Cardiogenic	Heart failing to pump out blood	Arrhythmia, MI, cardiomyopathy, pericarditis, PE	Hypotension, tachycardia, weak thread pulse, cool/pale/moist skin, reduced urine output, pulmonary edema, tachypnea	Inotropes Pacing PCI
Obstructive	Heart is obstructed from pumping blood	PE, cardiac tamponade, tension pneumothorax	Hypotension, tachycardia, venous congestion	Relieve obstruction
Distributive	Heart pumps well, but there is peripheral vasodilatation	Sepsis, anaphylaxis	Hypotension, tachycardia, tachypnea, flushed skin, fever, reduced urine output	Supportive ABC Antibiotics Epinephrine
		Neurogenic	Bradycardia (if cord injury T5 or above), Hypotension (massive vasodilatation), warm skin below level of injury (loss of vasoconstriction), poikilothermia. Associated spinal shock (loss of voluntary motor and reflex activity below level of injury)	Supportive ABC Atropine for bradycardia Vasopressors for hypotension

19. **b**—80-90 ml/kg

In general, approximate blood volumes are: premature neonate 90-105 ml/kg, term neonate 80-90 ml/kg, child 70-80 ml/kg, male adolescent 70 ml/kg and adolescent female 65 ml/kg.

20. **b**—ARDS

Defined as an acute condition characterized by bilateral pulmonary infiltrates and severe hypoxemia (PaO_2/FiO_2 ratio <200 or 26.6 kPa irrespective of PEEP) in the absence of evidence for cardiogenic pulmonary edema (clinically or pulmonary capillary wedge pressure <18 mmHg). In is subdivided into two stages. Early stages consist of an exudative phase of injury with associated edema. The later stage is one of repair and consists of fibroproliferative changes. Subsequent scarring may result in poor lung function. Causes include infection (>40%), aspiration (30%), trauma (>20%), massive blood transfusion, smoke inhalation, pancreatitis, cardio-pulmonary bypass, burns. Management including treat the underlying cause (e.g. antibiotics if signs of sepsis), aiming for a slightly negative fluid balance, lung/alveolar recruitment maneuvers (e.g. prone ventilation, PEEP), mechanical ventilation strategy using low tidal volumes, as conventional tidal volumes may cause lung injury (only treatment found to improve survival rates).

Image with permission from Khan A, Kantrow S, Taylor DE. Acute Respiratory Distress Syndrome, Hospital Medicine Clinics, 2015, 4(4); 500-512.

ANSWERS 21–38

Additional answers 21–38 available on ExpertConsult.com

EMI ANSWERS

39. 1—d, Ketamine, 2—g, Propofol; 3—e, Midazolam

Physiological Effects of Different Anaesthetic Agents

Drug	$CMRO_2$	CBF	ICP	Anticonvulsant Effect	Comment
Intravenous					
Etomidate	Decrease	No effect	No effect	No	
Propofol	Decrease	Decrease	Decrease	Yes	May reduce CPP
Midazolam	No effect	No effect	No effect	Yes	
Ketamine	Increase	Increase	Increase	No	Neuropsychiatric side effect
Thiopental	Decrease	Decrease	Decrease	Yes	
Inhalational					
Nitrous oxide	Increase	Increase	Increase	No	Muscle rigidity
Desflurane Isoflurane Sevoflurane	Decrease	Increase at MAC 1.0	Increase at MAC 1.0	No	Below MAC 1.0, reduced $CMRO_2$ compensates for vasodilatation
Other					
Succinylcholine	Increase (non-significant)	Increase (non-significant)	Increase	No	Secondary to increased muscle
Vercuronium	No effect	No effect	No Effect	No	
Optiates	Minimal decrease	Minimal decrease	Variable	No	

40. 1—e, Hemophilia, 2—b, Disseminated intravascular coagulation, 3—g, Thrombocytopenia

Effects of Different Bleeding Disorders on Blood Tests

Condition	PT	APTT	Bleeding Time	Platelet Count
Warfarin or Vit K deficiency	Prolonged	Normal or mildly Prolonged	Normal	Normal
DIC	Prolonged	Prolonged	Prolonged	Reduced
Uremia	Normal	Normal	Prolonged	Normal
Aspirin/Clopidogrel	Normal	Normal	Prolonged	Normal
Thrombocytopenia	Normal	Normal	Prolonged	Reduced
Liver failure	Prolonged	Normal or Prolonged	Normal or Prolonged	Normal or Reduced
Von Willebrand's disease	Normal	Normal or Prolonged	Prolonged	Normal
Factor V deficiency	Prolonged	Prolonged	Normal	Normal
Hemophilia	Normal	Prolonged	Normal	Normal
Factor XII deficiency	Normal	Prolonged	Normal	Normal
Glanzmann's thrombasthenia	Normal	Normal	Prolonged	Normal

41. 1—j, Thrombin clotting time, 2—b, Bleeding time, 3—h, 50:50 mixing study, 4—c, Dilute Russell's viper venom time

Common Blood Coagulation Screen Tests

Assay	Description	
Thrombin clotting time (TT)	Thrombin added to anticoagulated (citrate/oxalate tube) blood and time to clot formation measured	Prolonged with heparin, fibrin degradation products and fibrinogen deficiency
Bleeding time	Not a laboratory test—involves making a cut in skin and measuring time for bleeding to stop. Has been replaced by platelet function assays	Prolonged in platelet dysfunction, but also other circumstances where bleeding tendency not reflected in laboratory tests (e.g. uremia)
Platelet function assay	Blood clotting assessed on collagen/epinephrine (Col/Epi) and collagen/ADP membranes. Normal Col/Epi closure time (<180 s) excludes significant platelet function defect. If Col/Epi time prolonged, Col/ADP (Normal <120 s) is automatically performed	Abnormal Col/Epi but normal Col/ADP suggests aspirin induced platelet dysfunction Abnormal Col/Epi and abnormal Col/ADP suggests anemia, thrombocytopenia, von Willebrand disease
INR/PT	Tests extrinsic+common pathway—factors I, II, V, VII and X. Performed by adding tissue factor (III) to anticoagulated sample and measuring time to clot formation. Each batch of tissue factor has differences, hence this is standardized in INR	Prolonged PT due to vitamin K deficiency, warfarin, liver disease or DIC
Activated partial thromboplastin time (aPTT)	Tests intrinsic+common pathway I, II, V, VIII, IX, XI, XII—will be normal despite factor VII or XIII deficiency. Anticoagulated blood (oxalate/citrate sample) mixed with phospholipid, activator and calcium and time to clot formation measured. "Partial" refers to absence of tissue factor (III) from mixture	Prolonged APTT suggests heparin, antiphospholipid antibody, factor deficiency or anti-factor antibodies
Mixing (50:50) study	Plasma of patient with abnormal PT/APTT mixed with normal plasma in 50:50 ratio	Correction of PT/aPTT suggests factor deficiency in patient serum Persistence of abnormal PT/aPTT suggests presence of inhibitor in patient serum (warfarin, heparin, lupus anticoagulant, coagulation factor antibody)
Factor V Leiden	Requires genetic test. Mutated factor V cannot be inactivated by Protein C	
Dilute Russell's viper venom time (aRVVT)	Test for lupus anticoagulant (antiphospholipid antibodies) as venom requires phospholipid for activation	Prolonged aRVVT as antiphospholipid antibodies impair venom activation

42. 1—a, Acute metabolic acidosis, 2—d, Acute respiratory alkalosis, 3—i, Partially compensated respiratory acidosis (Type 2 respiratory failure), 4—f, Compensated respiratory acidosis

Acid-Base Balance

Acid-Base Disturbance	pH	$PaCO_2$	HCO_3	Common Causes
Acute respiratory acidosis	<7.35	High	Normal	Acute Asthma, suffocation
Partly/fully compensated respiratory acidosis	<7.35 or Normal	High	High	COPD, MND
Acute respiratory alkalosis	>7.45	Low	Normal	Pain, type 1 respiratory failure

Continued on following page

Acid-Base Balance (Continued)

Acid-Base Disturbance	pH	$PaCO_2$	HCO_3	Common Causes
Partly/fully compensated respiratory alkalosis	>7.45 or Normal	Low	Low	CNS disturbance, pregnancy
Acute metabolic acidosis	<7.35	Normal	Low	DKA, lactic acidosis; (anion gap present)
Partly/fully compensated metabolic acidosis	<7.35 or Normal	Low	Low	Diarrhea, renal tubular acidosis; (no anion gap)
Acute metabolic alkalosis	>7.45	Normal	High	Vomiting (hypochloremic), primary hyperaldosteronism
Partly/fully compensated metabolic alkalosis	>7.45 or Normal	High	High	Diuresis (hypochloremic), Cushing's syndrome

Mixed or complex acid-base disorders may also occur, and can be diagnosed due to a mismatch in expected compared to actual compensatory changes in ether HCO_3 (in respiratory acidosis or alkalosis) or pCO_2 (in metabolic acidosis or alkalosis).

43. 1—c, Hyperkalemia, 2—d, Hypokalemia, 3—e, Hypocalcemia

Electrolyte Disturbances: Clinical Features

Electrolyte Disturbance	Features	ECG Changes
Hypernatremia	Thirst, restlessness, brisk reflexes, seizures	–
Hyponatremia	Muscle cramp, weakness, raised ICP (confusion, seizures)	Non-ischemic ST elevation
Hyperkalemia	Confusion, hyperreflexia, weakness, paresthesia, ascending flaccid paralysis	Tall T waves progressing to widened QRS complexes
Hypokalemia	Leg cramps, fatigues, weakness, muscle breakdown, paralytic ileus, paralysis, apnea	U wave
Hypercalcemia	Bone pain, flank pain, constipation, hyporeflexic	Shortened QT interval
Hypocalcemia	Paresthesia, tetany, facial nerve twitching (Chvostek's sign), carpopedal spasm (Trousseau's sign), confusion, seizures	Prolonged QT interval
Hypermagnesemia	CNS depression, lethargy, confusion, weakness	Prolonged PR interval, Widened QRS complexes
Hypomagnesemia	Tremor, tetany, myoclonus, seizures	T wave flattening, ST depression, U waves
Hypophosphatemia	Asymptomatic or weakness, bone pain, rhabdomyolysis, altered mental status	–
Hyperphosphatemia	Asymptomatic or signs of hypocalcemia (tetany, Chvostek's)	–

44. 1—a, Amiodarone, 2—j, Vagal maneuver plus adenosine, 3—b, Atropine, 4—i, Pacemaker

FURTHER READING

2015 American Heart Association Guidelines for Cardiopulmonary Resuscitation and Emergency Cardiovascular Care.

CHAPTER 12

INFECTION

Chapter available on ExpertConsult.com

CHAPTER 13

SEIZURES

SINGLE BEST ANSWER (SBA) QUESTIONS

1. Approximately what proportion of patients with epilepsy have medically refractory seizures?
   a. 0-20%
   b. 20-40%
   c. 40-60%
   d. 60-80%
   e. 80-100%

2. Which one of the following is a predictor of spontaneous epilepsy remission?
   a. Abnormalities on neurological examination or developmental delay
   b. Identification of epileptogenic substrate
   c. Inadequate seizure control for greater than 4 years
   d. Persistent epileptiform abnormalities on EEG
   e. Younger age at onset

3. The approximate rate of sudden unexpected death in epilepsy (SUDEP) in patients with medically intractable seizures is which one of the following?
   a. 1 in 200 per year
   b. 1 in 400 per year
   c. 1 in 600 per year
   d. 1 in 800 per year
   e. 1 in 1000 per year

4. A 7-year-old right-handed girl presented with onset of seizures at 3-years old. Typically, her eyes rolled up and she often had either a left or right body twitch. These events lasted 10-12 s and occurred often in activities such as eating or talking. Immediately after these seizures, she spontaneously returned to her baseline. They typically occurred 6-10 times a day. She had been on numerous medications in the past but continues to have frequent breakthrough seizures on a daily basis. EEG shows a 3Hx spike and wave pattern. Which one of the following is most likely?
   a. Breath holding attack
   b. Cardiac syncope
   c. Childhood absence epilepsy
   d. Partial complex seizures
   e. Rolandic epilepsy

5. A 12-year-old boy with diagnoses of attention-deficit disorder and hyperactivity was noted to have "staring episodes" beginning over 1 year before this evaluation. About 6 months earlier, the staring episodes became accompanied by some eye blinking and mouth twitching. He has had one generalized tonic-clonic seizure in the last year. Which one of the following is most likely diagnosis?
   a. Childhood absence epilepsy
   b. Day dreaming
   c. Juvenile absence epilepsy
   d. Neurocardiogenic syncope
   e. Reflex anoxic seizure

6. A 19-year-old man presents with a history of seizures. The first was at age 12 when he got up very early in the morning to play computer games and was found by his mother a few hours later sitting at the computer blinking and unresponsive. Two years later he experiences a generalized tonic-clonic seizure. Currently he has a seizure every 1-3 weeks and can involve a minor jerk of the arms, staring with blinking, or generalized tonic-clonic seizures. He believed that sleep deprivation often precipitated seizures. Which one of the following is most likely diagnosis?
   a. Benign familial convulsions
   b. Benign myoclonic epilepsy in infancy
   c. Epilepsy with myoclonic absences
   d. Juvenile absence epilepsy
   e. Juvenile myoclonic epilepsy

7. Which one of the following abnormalities is demonstrated in the ictal EEG below?

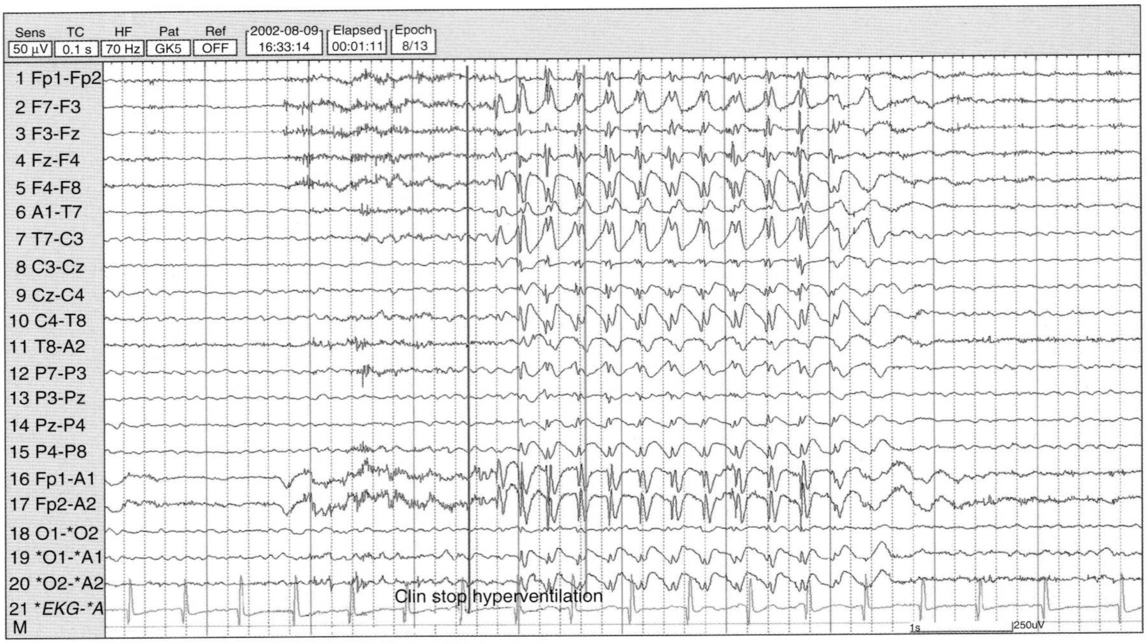

a. 3-Hz spike and wave discharge
b. Hypsarrhythmia
c. Lambda wave
d. Rhythmic temporal theta burst of bdrowsiness
e. Sleep spindles

8. Which one of the following seizure types is classically associated with the pathology shown below?

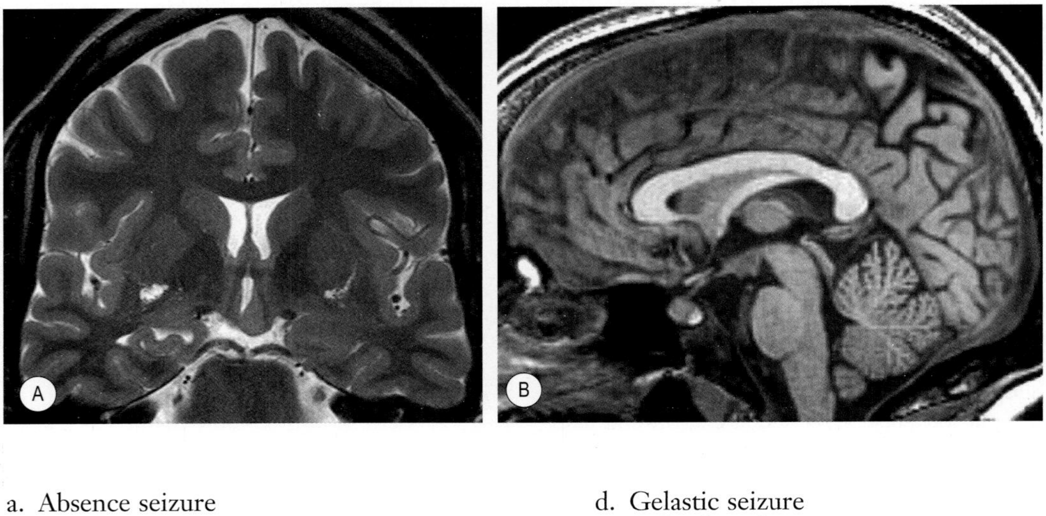

a. Absence seizure
b. Complex partial seizure
c. Focal motor seizure
d. Gelastic seizure
e. Rolandic seizure

9. Background interictal awake EEG in a 10-month-old female infant presenting with clusters of arm abduction and head drop. Which one of the following is most likely?

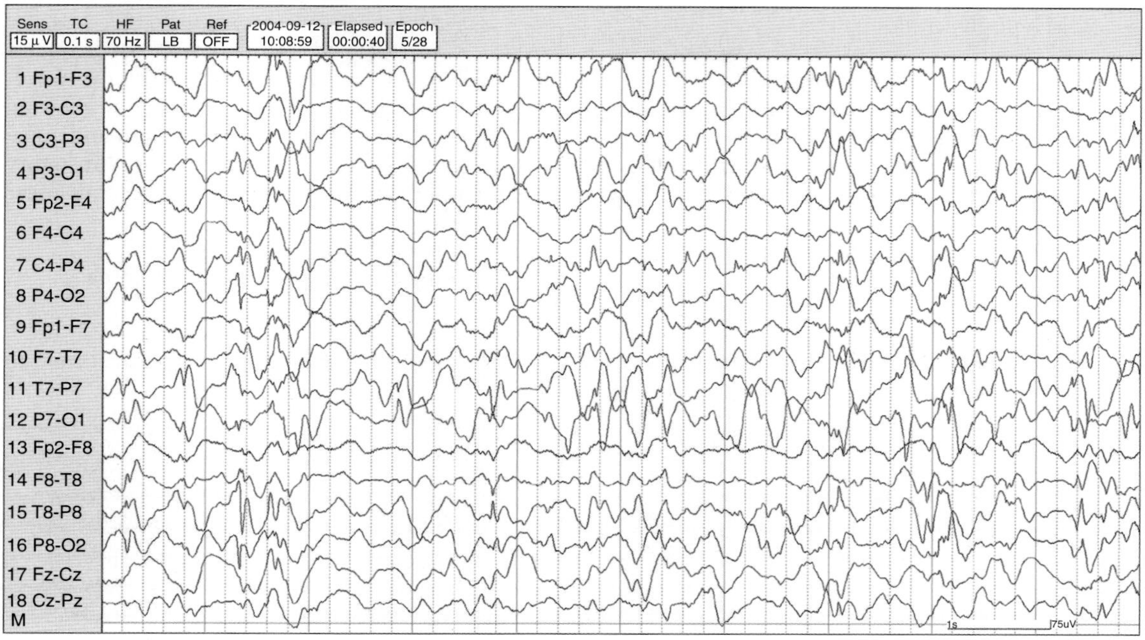

a. Benign Rolandic epilepsy
b. Gelastic epilepsy
c. Landau-Kleffner syndrome
d. Lennox-Gastaut syndrome
e. West syndrome

10. A 12-year-old, right-handed, developmentally delayed boy presented with three seizure types: generalized tonic-clonic, tonic, and atonic. The patient generally had at LEAST three brief seizures (1-10 s) per day of the tonic and atonic types but rarely had generalized seizures. He presented to the emergency department after one generalized tonic-clonic seizure followed by a series of atonic drop attacks concurrent with a streptococcal infection. The patient remained lethargic, and status epilepticus was a concern. Which of the following is the most likely diagnosis?
a. Aicardi syndrome
b. Angelman syndrome
c. Lennox-Gastaut syndrome
d. Otahara syndrome
e. West syndrome

11. When the patient, a young boy, was about age 6½ his mother first noticed an episode in which he failed to respond to her on the telephone. Within 3 months, he had become "deaf" with an auditory aphasia and poor articulation. An EEG during sleep showed continuous epileptiform discharges from the posterior left temporal region. His language markedly improved with valproic acid and prednisone. Which of the following is the most likely diagnosis?
a. Absence seizures
b. Continuous spike and wave during slow-dwave sleep syndrome (CSWS)
c. Landau-Kleffner syndrome
d. Parietal lobe epilepsy
e. Rassmussen's syndrome
f. Temporal lobe epilepsy

12. Which one of the following is the most common cause of neonatal seizures?
    a. Fetal inflammatory response
    b. Hypocalcemia
    c. Hypoglycemia
    d. Hypoxia-ischemia
    e. Pyridoxine-dependent seizures

13. A 24-year-old male presents with episodes characterized by facial (mouth and tongue) clonic movements (which may be unilateral), laryngeal symptoms, articulation difficulty, swallowing or chewing movements and hyper-salivation. Sensory (e.g. epigastric) and experiential (e.g. fear) aura and autonomic (urogenital, gastrointestinal, cardiovascular or respiratory) features are common. Gustatory hallucinations are particularly common. Which one of the following areas may the seizure focus arise?
    a. Cingulate gyrus
    b. Dorsolateral frontal
    c. Fronto-parietal operculum
    d. Frontopolar
    e. Motor cortex
    f. Orbitofrontal
    g. Supplementary sensorimotor area

14. Which one of the following is the likely origin of this secondarily generalized seizure recorded in the EEG below?

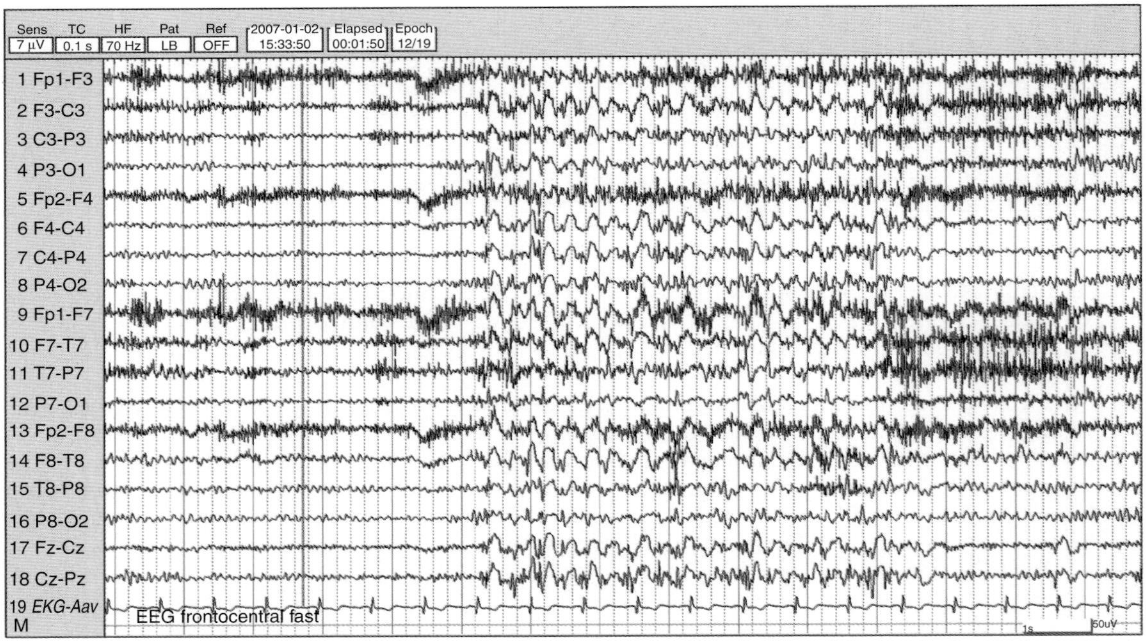

    a. Frontal poles
    b. Mesial temporal lobe
    c. Motor cortex
    d. Occipital
    e. Parietal

15. A 10-year-old right-handed boy presented with episodes of numbness around the mouth, drooling, right-sided facial twitching, and inability to speak on waking up from sleep. There was retained awareness and memory. Episodes were frequently followed by headaches. He experienced several episodes per week lasting up to 1-2 min. Sleep EEG shown below. Which one of the following is most likely?

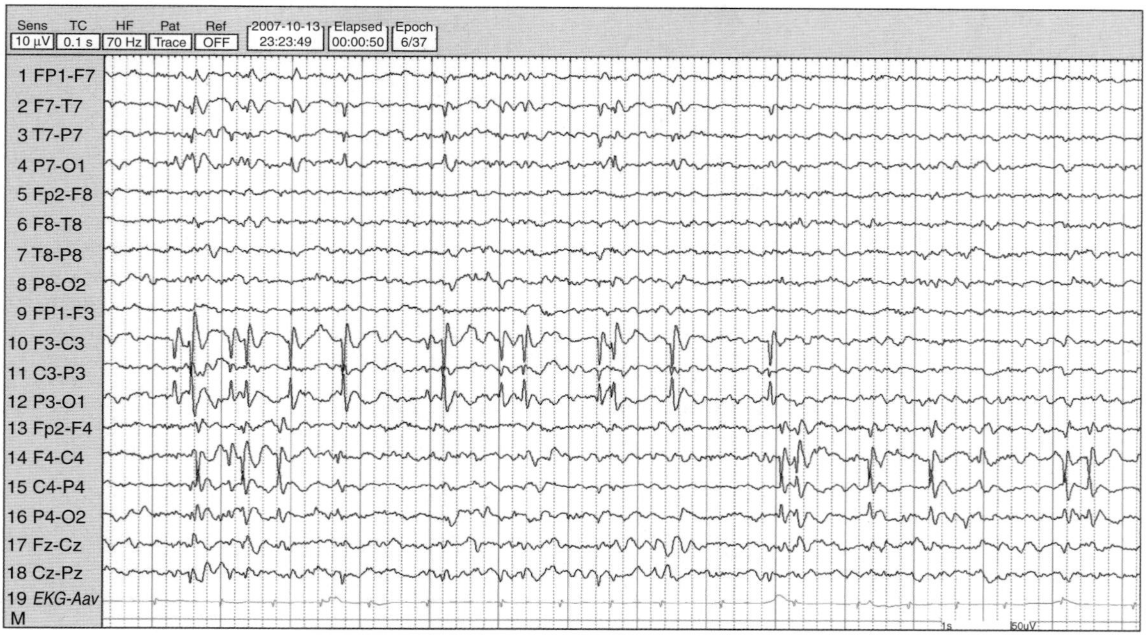

a. Benign Rolandic epilepsy
b. Childhood absence epilepsy
c. Juvenile myoclonic epilepsy
d. Pyridoxine-dependent epilepsy
e. West syndrome

16. A 54-year-old has been experiencing three types of odd episodes for the last few years. The first type involves a wave of non-painful sensation emanating from the left elbow up and down her left arm and then progressing with "electricity" pain marching into her neck and head. This could evolve into a more severe second type of seizure in which the left side became very painful and she felt afraid, had difficulty breathing, and then had clonic activity of the left face and arm with loss of awareness (about 2 per month). The third type was a "hyperawareness" in which she knew something was going to happen and objects looked larger. Which one of the following is most likely?

a. Absence seizures
b. Frontal seizures
c. Mesial temporal lobe seizures
d. Occipital seizures
e. Parietal seizures

17. A 24-year-old female presented with a history of severe migraines as a child associated with nausea and vomiting. She continued to have seizures beginning with flashing lights and colors in the left visual field followed by amaurosis and loss of awareness that might be associated with fumbling automatisms and lip smacking. Which one of the following is most likely?

a. Mesial temporal sclerosis
b. Occipital cortical dysgenesis
c. Parietal meningioma
d. Subependymal giant cell astrocytoma
e. Third ventricular colloid cyst

18. A 37-year-old man was diagnosed at age 25 when he had his first generalized tonic-clonic seizure while bowling. He was then noted to have complex partial seizures during which he would repeatedly respond by saying "what" to all questions, lip smack, and throw up his right arm. He was unaware of any auras and was amnestic for his seizures. Most of his seizures were from sleep with a frequency of about 2 per week. He had been involved in several car accidents secondary to seizures. Which one of the following is most likely?

a. Absence seizure
b. Complex partial seizure
c. Focal motor seizure
d. Generalized tonic-clonic seizure
e. Simple partial seizure

QUESTIONS 19–20

Additional questions 19–20 available on ExpertConsult.com

EXTENDED MATCHING ITEM (EMI) QUESTIONS

21. **EEG terminology:**
    a. Alpha
    b. Beta
    c. Delta
    d. Fast
    e. Gamma
    f. Lambda
    g. Sharp
    h. Slow
    i. Spike
    j. Theta

For each of the following descriptions, select the most appropriate answers from the list above. Each answer may be used once, more than once or not at all.
1. Frequency 8-13 Hz
2. Frequency under 4 Hz
3. Frequency 14-40 Hz

22. **EEG electrode position:**
    a. A1 and A2
    b. C3 and C4
    c. F3 and F4
    d. F7 and F8
    e. Fp1 and Fp2
    f. O1 and O2
    g. P3 and P4
    h. P7 and P8 (or T5 and T6)
    i. Sp1 and Sp2
    j. T7 and T8 (or T3 and T4)

For each of the following descriptions, select the most appropriate answers from the list above. Each answer may be used once, more than once or not at all.
1. Anterior temporal lobe
2. Posterior temporal lobe
3. Superior frontal lobe

23. **Mimics of epilepsy:**
    a. Cardiogenic syncope
    b. Cough syncope
    c. Gastroesophageal reflux
    d. Narcolepsy
    e. Neurally mediated syncope (vasovagal)
    f. Night terrors
    g. Non-epileptiform attack disorder (pseudoseizure)
    h. Paroxysmal dyskinesias
    i. Paroxysmal vertigo
    j. Rages
    k. Reflex anoxic seizure
    l. Shuddering attack
    m. Tic

For each of the following descriptions, select the most appropriate answers from the list above. Each answer may be used once, more than once or not at all.
1. A 2-year-old child accidentally hits his head on the kitchen table when running. He crys, turns pale and collapses to the floor. He starts to respond after 30 s but is groggy.
2. A 6-month-old baby is seen to exhibit paroxysmal dystonic posturing after feeding.
3. A 14-year-old boy starts to feel dizzy then loses consciousness during a car journey on a hot day. He slumps in his seat and his limbs are seen to jerk.

SBA ANSWERS

1. **b**—20-40%

FURTHER READING

Devinsky O. Patients with refractory seizures. N Engl J Med 1999;340(20):1565-70.

2. **e**—Younger age at onset

In general, predictors for low probability of epilepsy remission are (i) symptomatic localized epilepsy secondary to remote CNS injury, (ii) abnormalities on neurological examination or developmental delay, (iii) persistent epileptiform abnormalities on EEG, (iv) older age at onset, (v) inadequate control of seizures for longer than 4 years, (vi) presence of multiple seizure types and frequent generalized tonic-clonic seizures. Seizure duration of over 10 years also decreases likelihood of achieving seizure control in those who undergo epilepsy surgery.

3. **a**—1 in 200 per year

Overall rates of SUDEP in adults is 1 in 1000 and lower in children at 0.2-0.4 in 1000 per year. However, in adults and children with medically intractable epilepsy rates are higher at 1 in 100-200 per year. Cause of death in SUDEP is unclear but thought to be due to seizure related cardiac arrhythmias and/or respiratory compromise. The most reliable risk factor is severity and frequency of seizures (particularly generalized tonic-clonic seizures). Other risk factors include nocturnal seizures, young adult, poor adherence to treatment, earlier age of seizure onset, longer duration of epilepsy, symptomatic epilepsy and male gender.

FURTHER READING

Epilepsy Foundation (www.epilepsy.com/learn/impact/mortality/sudep).

4. **c**—Childhood absence epilepsy

Childhood absence epilepsy is characterized by brief (4-20 s) unresponsive, staring episodes during high-amplitude bisynchronous (generalized) approximately 3-Hz spike and slow wave discharges on ictal EEG (with a normal interictal EEG). Accounts for 8-15% of all childhood epilepsies; onset 4-10 years; history of febrile seizures in up to 30%, family history of epilepsy in 15%; may be induced by hyperventilation. The frequent seizures impair attention and learning and may lead to an inaccurate diagnosis of attention-deficit disorder or daydreaming. The majority have accompanying non-stereotyped motor activity (e.g. blinking, myoclonus of eyelid/mouth, oral automatisms, picking/rubbing movements of hands/feet) and are termed complex absence seizures. Absence seizures usually remit in adolescence, but a significant number of children go on to have generalized tonic-clonic seizures as adults.

5. **c**—Juvenile absence epilepsy

Juvenile absence epilepsy is a type of idiopathic generalized epilepsy. Onset is from age 8 to age 16 years, with a peak occurrence at 10-12 years of age. The frequency of absence seizures in juvenile absence epilepsy is lower than that in childhood absence epilepsy. A higher frequency of generalized tonic-clonic seizures is seen compared with childhood absence epilepsy, and there is an increased probability of epilepsy continuing into the adult years. They also noted that 11% of patients with the disorder report a family history of epilepsy. Absence seizures are predominant. The impairment of consciousness in juvenile absence epilepsy is moderate and not generally as severe as in childhood absence epilepsy. The level of retained consciousness may vary significantly from seizure to seizure in the same patient. Unlike childhood absence epilepsy they may occur once a day or in a cluster in the hour after awakening. The classic clinical feature is "simple absence" with staring and altered alertness (sometimes "complex absence" with blinking or head nodding). Seizures are typically triggered by hyperventilation or sleep deprivation. EEG: Interictal background activity is usual normal, spike and wave slightly faster (3.5-4 Hz).

6. **e**—Juvenile myoclonic epilepsy

Juvenile myoclonic epilepsy comprises 5-10%. It is an idiopathic generalized epilepsy with myoclonic jerks; may also have typical absence seizures, generalized tonic-clonic seizures, or all three seizure types. The majority have myoclonic and generalized tonic-clonic seizures shortly after awakening from sleep. Seizure types have age-specific onset: absence (5-14 years), myoclonic (9-18 years), and generalized tonic-clonic seizures (9-26 years). Sleep deprivation is identified as a precipitating factor in the large majority (>90%) of individuals. The EEG showing paroxysmal spike, polyspike, and wave complexes that may be regular at 3-5 Hz but often are irregular with 2- to 10-Hz components. A photoconvulsive effect on the EEG has been described in at least one third of cases. Hyperventilation less reliably than in childhood absence epilepsy or juvenile absence epilepsy.

7. **a**—3-Hz spike and wave discharges

Image with permission from Werz MA, Pita Garcia IL. Epilepsy Syndromes, Elsevier, Saunders, 2011.

8. **d**—Gelastic seizures

Hypothalamic (or tuber cinereum) hamartomas are associated with gelastic seizures, visual problems, central precocious puberty (increased GnRH) and behavioral change. Gelastic seizures manifest as typically short (<30 s) bursts of uncontrollable laughter with preservation of consciousness.

Image with permission from Loevner L. Brain Imaging: Case Review Series, 2nd ed., Elsevier, Mosby, 2009.

9. **e**—West syndrome

West syndrome is the triad of infantile spasms, hypsarrhythmia on EEG and developmental delay or regression. Onset is typically around 6 months of age (almost all begin within the first year of life); incidence is 1 in 3225 live births. Spasms may involve brief contractions of predominantly flexor or extensor muscle groups ranging from large "jack-knife" type motions to subtle head bobbing. These movements are at times difficult to differentiate from less serious non-epileptic events such as gastroesophageal reflux, colic and benign myoclonus of infancy. Precipitating factors mostly include when falling asleep/waking up, being handled, loud noise, feeding, infection, fever, excitement, hunger and excessive environmental temperatures. Cognitive disorders may include mental retardation, speech delay, autistic features and visuomotor dyspraxia. EEG of hypsarrhythmia consists typically of a diffuse, very high voltage, disorganized, chaotic and asynchronous pattern of multifocal spike and wave discharges. This pattern is seen while the child is both awake and in non-rapid-eye-movement (NREM) sleep. In REM sleep, there is marked reduction or even disappearance of the HA pattern. EEG with simultaneous pyridoxine injection is often performed to rule out pyridoxine-dependent seizures (very rare, <1 in 100,000; treatment is with high doses of vitamin B6). Video-EEG analysis is considered the gold standard to diagnose the spasms, and to assess for focal features of the spasm semiology or EEG tracings. Metabolic screens and LP may help identify cause. MRI should be done to look for surgical lesions. Adrenocorticotropic hormone (ACTH) is effective in the short-term treatment of infantile spasms and in the resolution of HA (takes about 2 weeks with an "all or nothing" response). Vigabatrin indicated for pediatric patients aged from 1 month to 2 years with infantile spasms (but risk of irreversible vision loss; need ophthalmology assessment). If EEG and MRI demonstrate a focal causative lesion surgical resection can be performed, while functional hemispherectomies may be used in more diffuse abnormalities (e.g. Sturge-Weber).

Image with permission from Werz MA, Pita Garcia IL. Epilepsy Syndromes, Elsevier, Saunders, 2011.

10. **c**—Lennox-Gastaut syndrome

Lennox-Gastaut syndrome is characterized by multiple generalized seizure types that are refractory to treatment, cognitive dysfunction, and an interictal slow spike and wave pattern with a slow background on EEG. May be idiopathic or symptomatic (e.g. hypoxic-ischemic, traumatic brain injury). Onset is generally between 2 and 6 years of age. A wide range of behavioral problems will develop in about half of patients. Approximately 25% of patients will have a history of infantile spasms. The most common manifestation is a drop attack. Drop attacks may range from a simple head drop to a fall if proximal legs are involved. Because the drop attack may be due to a tonic, atonic, or myoclonic seizure, video-EEG monitoring may be necessary. Tonic seizures may involve the arms, legs, or whole body. Tonic seizures often occur in sleep. Atonic seizures appear as loss of postural tone of the head or whole body. Clonic (clusters of myoclonus) seizures involving the arms, face, or legs may occur in isolation or in clusters. The EEG shows a bisynchronous spike and wave or polyspikes and wave pattern. Sixty to seventy percent of patients exhibit atypical absence seizures. Hyperventilation does not provoke this seizure type. At least one episode of status epilepticus occurs in more than half of patients over their lifetime. Typical presentations include mental status changes or persistent tonic seizures. Medications are often chosen for the most debilitating seizure type. Broad-spectrum anticonvulsants such as valproic acid have been cited as good choices because of their efficacy in many seizure types. Surgical interventions including vagal nerve stimulator placement and corpus callosotomy have been used in some patients as palliative procedures with varying degrees of success. Lennox-Gestaut is one of the few epilepsies particullarily responsive to deep brain stimulation of the centromedian nucleus (Velasco et al.).

11. **c**—Landau-Kleffner syndrome

Landau-Kleffner syndrome, or acquired epileptic aphasia, is characterized by a progressive verbal agnosia in a child with previous normal language development, paroxysmal EEG abnormalities, and epileptic seizures. Associated symptoms include psychomotor and behavioral disturbances consisting of motor hyperactivity, impulsivity, and aggressive behavior. There is a slight male predominance, and it typically presents at between 3 and 8 years of age. Onset is usually acute and presents initially as difficulty comprehending language, followed by verbal agnosia. Subsequently, expressive language is also affected and may lead to mutism. The EEG background activity during wakefulness is usually normal; severe and variable abnormalities during sleep. Neuroimaging without any structural brain lesion is required for diagnosis. PET scans have demonstrated regions of hypometabolism predominantly in the temporal lobes. Seizures are usually well controlled with traditional antiepileptic drugs but the neuropsychological manifestations have a more variable response. Valproate, clobazam, and ethosuximide, either monotherapy or in polytherapy, are successful in controlling seizures and are occasionally successful in reversing language regression. Carbamazepine, phenobarbital, and phenytoin can lead to worsening of seizures and conversion to electrical status epilepticus during slow sleep because they may increase cortical synchronization. Corticosteroids can provide dramatic improvement in language, cognition, and behavior in some children. In CSWS, seizures are the first symptom in 70-80% of children, followed by neuropsychological regression that may be global or selective regression of cognitive functions, excluding the acquired aphasia characteristic of Landau-Kleffner syndrome.

12. **d**—Hypoxia-ischemia

Hypoxia-ischemia (i.e. asphyxia) is traditionally considered the most common cause associated with neonatal seizures. Intrauterine factors before labor can result in fetal asphyxia without later documentation of acidosis at birth. Both antepartum and intrapartum maternal and placental illnesses associated with thrombophilia, preeclampsia, or specific uteroplacental abnormalities such as abruptio placentae or cord compression may contribute to fetal asphyxial stress leading to metabolic acidosis. Antepartum maternal trauma and chorioamnionitis are additional conditions that also contribute to the intrauterine asphyxia secondary to uteroplacental insufficiency. Intravascular placental thromboses and infarction of the placenta or umbilical cord documented after birth are markers for possible fetal asphyxia. Meconium passage into the amniotic fluid also promotes an inflammatory response within the placental membranes, potentially causing vasoconstriction and resultant asphyxia. Postnatal include persistent pulmonary hypertension of the newborn, cyanotic congenital heart disease, sepsis, meningitis, encephalitis, and primary intracranial hemorrhage are leading diagnoses. Fetal inflammatory response may increase in the risk of unexplained early-onset seizures after intrapartum maternal fever. Other causes include hypoglycemia, hypocalcemia and pyridoxine-dependent epilepsy (rare).

13. **c**—Fronto-parietal operculum

Frontal lobe epilepsy is the second most common localization-related epilepsy, accounting for 20-30% of surgical series. These types of seizures are usually short, occur more frequently during sleep, and tend to cluster. Lateralizing signs include version and unilateral clonic, tonic, or dystonic activity that correlate with contralateral onset. Unless there is secondary generalization, responsiveness persists throughout the seizure. Complex partial seizures of frontal lobe origin are characterized by partial or complete loss of consciousness. Most patients report an initial aura of vague general body sensation or unspecified cephalic aura. The patient initially may develop staring and behavioral arrest. Motor manifestations consist of prominent semi-purposeful automatism. There are frequently bilateral and involve both legs and arms with features of running, pelvic thrusts, and bizarre behavior. Upper extremity automatisms tend to be irregular, involving proximal muscles. Later during the seizures laughing and crying may be observed. Finally, hypermotor activity characterized by complex movements of the proximal segments of limbs and trunks may occur. In contrast, temporal lobe seizures have early and prominent oroalimentary automatism and repetitive upper extremity automatism involving mainly the distal segments. Consciousness is more frequently affected or lost in temporal lobe epilepsy. MRI Abnormalities include encephalomalacia, neoplasm, vascular malformations, cortical dysplasias, and migrational disorders.

Focus	Typical Description
Supplementary sensorimotor area	Bilateral tonic or dystonic postures that are usually asymmetric. Despite vocalization or speech arrest, consciousness is preserved. The typically described fencing posture is rarely seen
Orbitofrontal	Staring, alteration of consciousness, olfactory hallucinations and oral and upper extremity automatisms and autonomic signs. Difficult to distinguish from TLE
Frontopolar seizures	Near-onset head version with associated loss of consciousness
Dorsolateral frontal	Can start with an unspecific aura of cephalic sensation or fear. This is followed by head and eye version and contralateral tonic and clonic activity. If Broca's area is involved, speech arrest or postictal aphasia may be observed
Fronto-parietal operculum	Rolandic seizures are characterized by facial (mouth and tongue) clonic movements (which may be unilateral), laryngeal symptoms, articulation difficulty, swallowing or chewing movements and hyper-salivation. Sensory (e.g. epigastric) and experiential (e.g. fear) aura and autonomic (urogenital, gastrointestinal, cardiovascular or respiratory) features are common. Gustatory hallucinations are particularly common

Continued on following page

Focus	Typical Description
Cingulate gyrus	Usually involve loss of awareness, oral and upper extremity automatism, behavioral alterations, and autonomic manifestations that include tachycardia and tachypnea. In addition, absence-like events are observed with mesial structure foci
Motor cortex seizures	Produce tonic or clonic activity of the contralateral face, arm, or leg depending on the area of origin. Jacksonian march (distal limb to ipsilateral face) is not uncommon especially with involvement of the motor extremity. A postictal Todd's paralysis is occasionally seen

14. **a**—Frontal pole

This ictal EEG begins with attenuation and then low-amplitude fast frequencies frontocentrally (Fp1-F3, Fp1-F7 and Fp2-F4, Fp2-F8) before evolving into more generalized irregular polyspike and wave.

Image with permission from Werz MA, Pita Garcia IL. Epilepsy Syndromes, Elsevier, Saunders, 2011.

15. **a**—Benign Rolandic epilepsy

Benign focal epilepsy with centrotemporal spikes (BECTS; Benign Rolandic epilepsy) is the most frequent focal epilepsy syndrome in childhood. Age at onset ranges from 3 to 13 years of age, and peak incidence is usually around age 8 years. Seizures present usually at night, often shortly after falling asleep or before waking up. The present as somatosensory aura with perioral paresthesias, a sensation of choking, and jaw or tongue stiffness. Hemifacial or hemibody motor seizures, frequently with unilateral clonic, but also tonic or tonic-clonic, activity are seen in up to 34% of patients. Motor features involve the face, lips, tongue, pharynx, and larynx, and this may be associated with speech arrest. Generalized tonic-clonic seizures without focal onset have been described in 54%. The characteristic interictal EEG finding is a distinct high-amplitude, diphasic spike with prominent aftergoing slow wave typically in C3/C4 or T3/T4 electrodes. Spikes are more frequently observed during sleep, and sleep activation of spikes is a salient feature of BECTS. The condition remits spontaneously in almost all patients around the age of 16 years hence indications for treatment include seizures during daytime, repeated generalized tonic-clonic seizures, prolonged seizures, and status epilepticus as well as seizure onset before the age of 4 years. Carbamazepine may control seizures in up to 65% of patients.

Image with permission from Werz MA, Pita Garcia IL. Epilepsy Syndromes, Elsevier, Saunders, 2011.

16. **e**—Parietal seizures

Parietal lobe seizures are infrequent in both medical and surgical cases, representing from 4.4% to 6% of all epilepsies. The etiology of parietal lobe seizures has a strong association with space-occupying lesions, which may include tumors, congenital anomalies, postinflammatory brain scarring, and vascular lesions. As a group, parietal lobe seizures are usually suspected by somatosensory symptomatology at onset. All sensory modalities may be experienced, and often more than one type is perceived in each seizure. The two most common manifestations include paresthetic seizures and painful seizures. Elementary paresthesia is the most common somatosensory perception in seizures. These most commonly are reported as tingling and/or numbness. Other descriptions may be pins and needles, prickling, or a crawling under the skin. Sensation usually starts in a segment of the limb, usually distal, and then spreads to involve the whole extremity in a march-like fashion. Painful seizures are usually experienced in conjunction with other sensory perceptions. They are described as severe, stabbing, throbbing, or cramp-like. The hands are most commonly involved, especially distal, followed by the head, face, and legs.

Less frequent somatosensory seizures of parietal lobe origin include thermal perception, sexual seizures, ideomotor apraxia, and disturbances of body image. Tonic posturing, clonic activity, contralateral version, and hypermotor activity may characterize subsequent spread of the ictal focus to the frontal lobe. If the focus spreads to the temporal lobes it produces automatism and alteration of consciousness. Posterior seizure spread results in visual auras.

17. **b**—Occipital cortical dysgenesis

Occipital lobe epilepsies are uncommon (5%) and identified by the presence of visual phenomena in the early seizure symptoms. In patients with seizures arising from the medial occipital lobe, visual field deficit can be found in 20-40%. The vision loss often is unnoticed by the patient, may be subtle enough to be missed on confrontational testing as part of the neurologic examination, and may require formal visual field testing to be appreciated. The most common auras are simple visual hallucinations (white or colored lights that can be constant, flashing, stationary or moving). Ictal blurring or amaurosis (blindness) is reported in 25-40% of case series and can be described as either a whiteout or blackout. When propagation is infrasylvian and lateral to the temporoparietal visual association areas, complex visual hallucinations and illusions (achromatopsia, micro/macropsia, metamorphopsia, micro/macroproxiopia, or palinopsia) may occur. In contrast, propagation to the mesial temporal lobe may result in reports of rising epigastric sensation, smells, and nausea and complex partial seizures. Suprasylvian parietal spread may lead to reports of somatosensory phenomena such as paresthesias and vertigo. Spread from the occipital lobes may evolve to complex partial seizures typical of temporal origin with prominent oral and gestural automatisms, to lateral frontal lobe with clonic motor activity, or to mesial frontal lobe with tonic seizure manifestations typical of supplementary motor seizures. Apart from focal lesions occipital seizures also occur as part of neurodegenerative disorders such as the progressive myoclonic epilepsies (LaFora body disease, ceroid lipofuscinosis), mitochondrial disorders (MERRF and MELAS) and posterior reversible leukoencephalopathy syndrome.

18. **b**—Complex partial seizures

Most adult focal epilepsies arise from the temporal lobes (60%). Auras (simple partial seizures) and complex partial seizures are the hallmarks of temporal lobe seizures. Unfortunately, patients evolving to complex partial seizures may become amnestic for the aura. Auras of right temporal origin are more commonly remembered than those from the left. Most seizures originate from the mesial temporal structures, including the amygdala and hippocampal formation. The amygdala has associations with emotion and autonomic and olfactory systems. The hippocampus has roles in memory and experiential phenomena. Common auras are described below:

1. The most common aura is a rising epigastric sensation.
2. Fear is common as well and must be distinguished from panic attacks.
3. Experiential auras may include dreamy states, déjà vu, and jamais vu.
4. Sensory auras include smells, which have reliable localization but are actually quite rare. Other sensory manifestations that are not localizing include cephalic sensation, numbness, tingling, and hearing music or phrases. Spread of the seizures to the secondary sensory area that sits in the posterior operculum may produce unusual distributions of sensory symptoms that may be ipsilateral or bilateral.
5. Auras may manifest with autonomic symptoms such as changes in heart rate, piloerection, and urinary urgency.
6. Simple auditory auras such as buzzing, roaring, and muffling usually arise from the temporal neocortex on the superior temporal gyrus near Heschl's gyrus.
7. Complex visual phenomena usually occur from the posterior temporal lobe near the occipital lobe.

Auras often gradually evolve to complex partial seizures. These seizures can be extremely bland with a simple stare and behavioral arrest or can classically have oroalimentary automatisms such as lip smacking, chewing, or swallowing along with gestural automatisms such as picking or fumbling movements. Seizure spread to the frontal lobes may produce proximal automatisms such as bicycling or thrashing. Secondarily, generalized tonic-clonic seizures may also occur, although typically infrequently.

ANSWERS 19–20

Additional answers 19–20 available on ExpertConsult.com

EMI ANSWERS

21. 1—a, Alpha, 2—c, Delta, 3—b, Beta

Alpha	Frequency 8-13 Hz
Delta	Frequency <4 Hz
Beta	Frequency 14-40 Hz
Theta	Frequency 4-8 Hz
Gamma	Frequencies >40 Hz

Continued on following page

Lambda	Diphasic sharp transient occurring over the occipital regions of the head of waking subjects during visual exploration. The main component is positive relative to other areas. Time-locked to saccadic eye movement. Amplitude varies but is generally below 50 mV
Fast	Activity of frequency faster than alpha (i.e. beta and gamma activity)
Slow	Activity of frequency slower than alpha (i.e. theta and delta activity)
Sharp	A transient, clearly distinguished from background activity, with pointed peak at a conventional paper speed or time scale and duration of 70-200 ms
Spike	A transient, clearly distinguished from background activity, with pointed peak at a conventional paper speed or time scale and a duration from 20 to 70 ms

22. 1—d, F7 and F8, 2—j, T7 and T8 (or T3 and T4), 3—c, F3 and F4

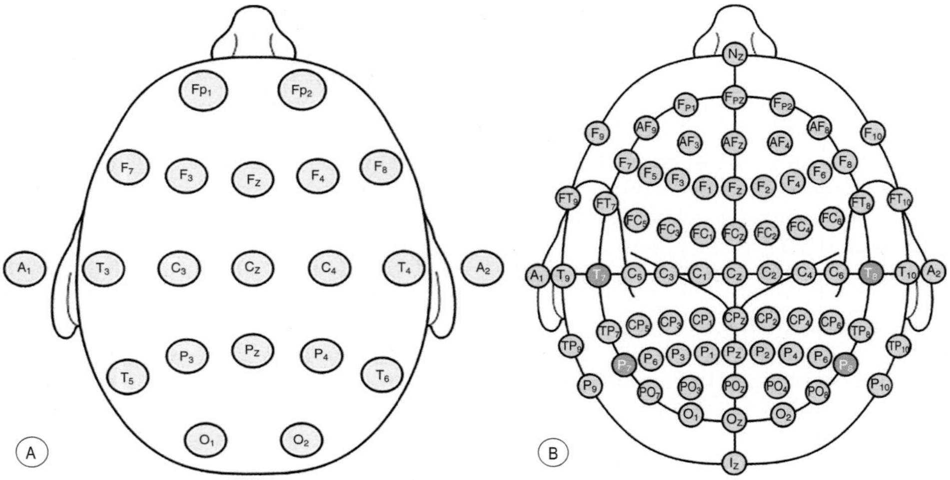

Images with permission from **a**, Libenson MH. Practical Approach to Electroencephalography, Elsevier, Saunders, 2010 and **b**, American Clinical Neurophysiology Society Guideline 5: guidelines for standard electrode position nomenclature. J Clin Neurophysiol 2006;2:107-110.

The electrode nomenclature for the original 10-20 electrode system is shown. This original naming system is still in use in many EEG laboratories. Newer modified version of 10-20 replaces T3 and T4 with T7 and T8, to fit with the 10-10 system (right).

Electrode	Common Name
Fp1 and Fp2	Frontopolar or frontal polar
F7 and F8	Anterior temporal
F3 and F4	Superior frontal
Fz	Frontal midline
T7 an T8 (T3 and T4)	Midtemporal
C3 and C4	Central
Cz	Vertex or central midline

Continued

Electrode	Common Name
P7 and P8 (T5 and T6)	Posterior temporal
P3 and P4	Parietal
Pz	Parietal midline
O1 and O2	Occipital
Sp1 and Sp2	Sphenoidal
A1 and A2	Auricular

Table modified from Libenson MH, Practical Approach to Electroencephalography, Elsevier, Saunders, 2010.

23. 1—k, Reflex anoxic seizure, 2—c, Gastroesophageal reflux, 3—e, Neurally mediated syncope

Reflex anoxic seizure (pallid Breath holding spell)	Common in young children, especially under 2 years. Unexpected stimulus (pain, shock, fright) causes excessive vagal activity—heart and respiration stops transiently and child becomes pale
Cyanotic breath holding spell	Reflex expiration in response to anger/frustration causes child to become cyanotic
Cardiogenic syncope	Syncope resulting from structural or functional cardiac abnormality—no convulsive movements associated
Cough syncope	Prolonged cough spasms (e.g. asthmatic, infection) can reduce venous return and lead to syncope with incontinence
Gastroesophageal reflux	Can lead to paroxysmal dystonic posturing associated with meals due to discomfort
Narcolepsy	Sudden loss of muscular tone secondary to catapexy, usually an emotional trigger, no postictal state or loss of consciousness, EEG shows recurrent attacks of REM sleep
Night terrors	Brief nocturnal episodes of terror without typical convulsive movements, common in ages 4-6
Paroxysmal dyskinesias	Precipitated by sudden movement or startle, no associated change in consciousness
Paroxysmal vertigo	Common in toddlers, triggered by fright/crying—seen to stagger, fall and possibly vomit
Non-epileptiform attack disorder (pseudoseizure)	No EEG changes except movement artefact during episode
Rage attacks/Tantrum	Common in children aged 6-12 years, outburst is explosive and out of proportion to trigger (tantrums are goal directed)
Shuddering attack	Shiver-like movement of the trunk with associated stiffening, neck flexion and arm adduction, each episode lasts seconds and there is no change in consciousness
Vasovagal syncope	Loss of consciousness triggered by postural change, heat or emotion; there is presyncopal dizziness, clouded/tunnel vision before a slow collapse
Tic	Involuntary, non-rhythmic, repetitive movements not associated with impaired consciousness

CHAPTER 14

NEUROradiology

SINGLE BEST ANSWER (SBA) QUESTIONS

1. A patient with severe renal failure but not on dialysis required CT angiogram. In addition to keeping the patient well hydrated, what may be given to the patient to minimize contrast nephropathy?
   a. Hydrocortisone
   b. Magnesium sulfate
   c. N-Acetylcysteine
   d. Ramipril
   e. Sodium bicarbonate

2. Early subacute subdural hematoma (4-7 days old) is most likely to display which one of the following characteristics on MRI?
   a. T1 hypointense, T2 hypointense
   b. T1 hypointense, T2 isointense
   c. T1 hypointense, T2 hyperintense
   d. T1 isointense, T2 hypointense
   e. T1 isointense, T2 hyperintense
   f. T1 hyperintense, T2 hypointense
   g. T1 hyperintense, T2 isointense
   h. T1 hyperintense, T2 hyperintense

3. True diffusion restriction is best assessed by looking at which one of the following MR sequences?
   a. Diffusion tensor imaging
   b. Diffusion weighted image and apparent diffusion coefficient map
   c. Fractional anisotropy map
   d. T2 gradient echo
   e. T1 with gadolinium

4. A ring-enhancing lesion on contrast CT has the below appearance on DWI (C- DWI, D- ADC map) sequence. Which one of the following is of most concern?

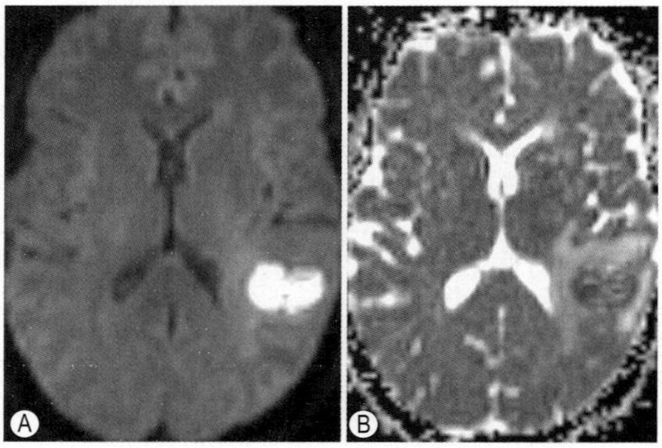

   a. Cerebral abscess
   b. Encephalitis
   c. Glioblastoma multiforme
   d. Metastasis
   e. Radiation necrosis

5. Which one of the following combinations of findings on perfusion weighted MR suggests early infarction
   a. Bright on DWI, low rCBF, long rMTT, low CBV
   b. Bright on DWI, high rCBF, long rMTT, low CBV
   c. Bright on DWI, low rCBF, short rMTT, low CBV
   d. Bright on DWI, low rCBF, long rMTT, high CBV
   e. Dark on DWI, low rCBF, long rMTT, low CBV

6. Which one of the following tracts is most likely depicted in the figure below?

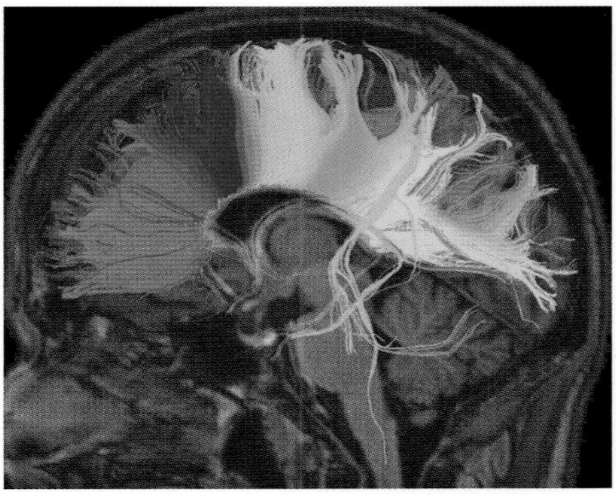

a. Cingulum
b. Corona radiata
c. Corpus callosum
d. U fibers
e. Vertical occipital fasciculus

7. Which one of the following tracts is most likely depicted in the figures below?

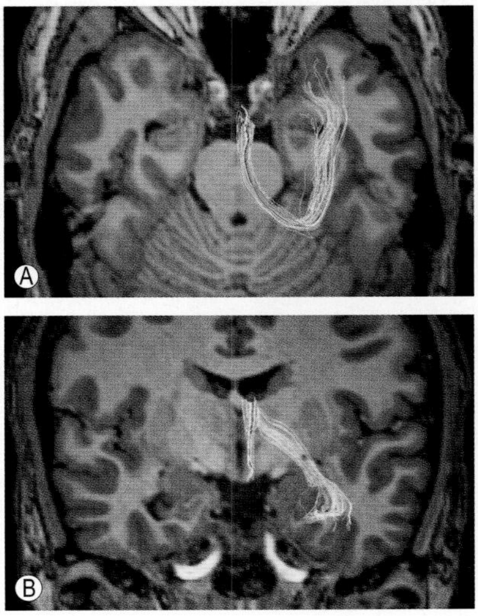

a. Anterior commissure
b. Extreme capsule
c. Fornix
d. Posterior commissure
e. Posterior limb of internal capsule

8. Which one of the following tracts is most likely depicted in the figure below?

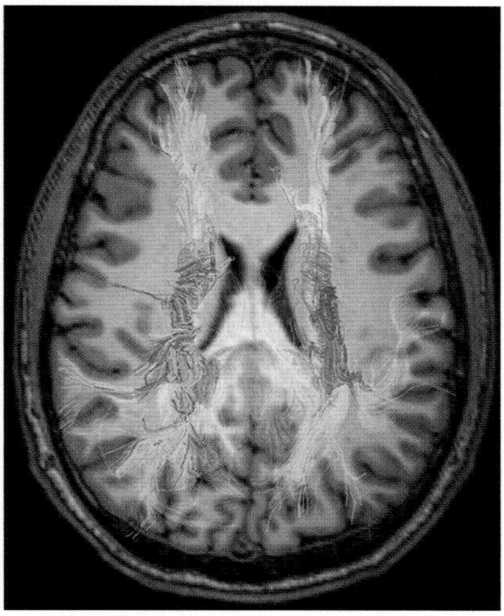

a. Corpus callosum
b. Corona radiata
c. Corticospinal tract
d. Inferior frontooccipital fasciculus
e. Superior frontooccipital fasciculus

9. Which one of the following tracts is most likely depicted in the figure below?

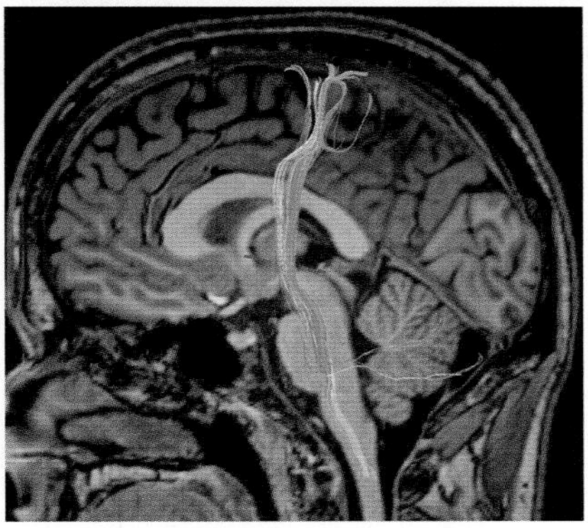

a. Corona radiata
b. Corticospinal tract
c. Medial longitudinal fasciculus
d. Reticulospinal tract
e. Spinothalamic tract

10. Which one of the following tracts is most likely depicted in the figure below?

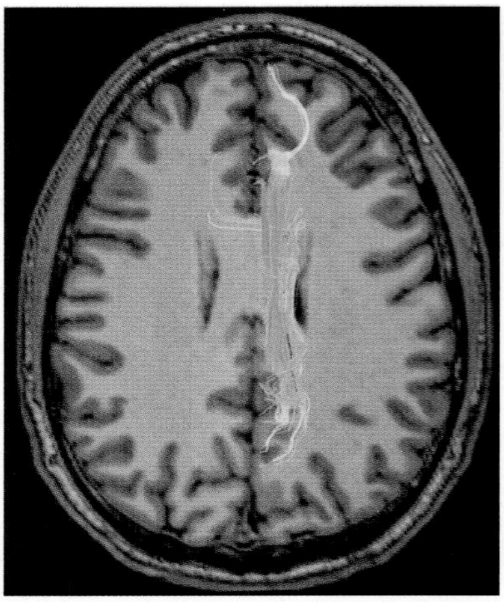

a. Arcuate fasciculus
b. Cingulum bundle
c. Corona radiata
d. Corticospinal tract
e. SFOF

11. Which one of the following tracts is most likely depicted in the figure below?

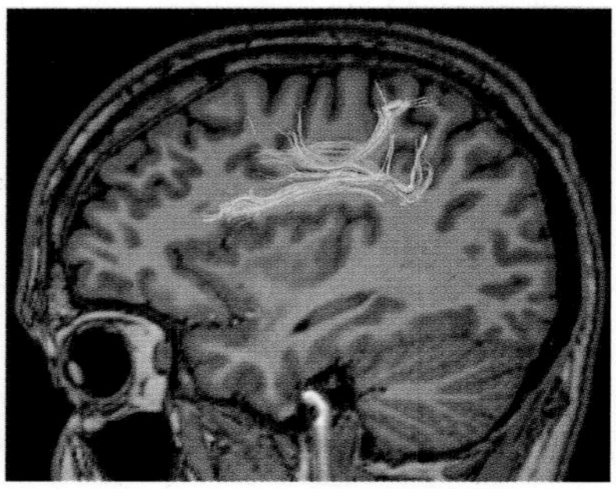

a. Inferior fronto-occipital fasciculus
b. Inferior longitudinal fasciculus
c. Fornix
d. Superior longitudinal fasciculus (II and III)
e. U-fibers

12. Which one of the following tracts is most likely depicted in the figure below?

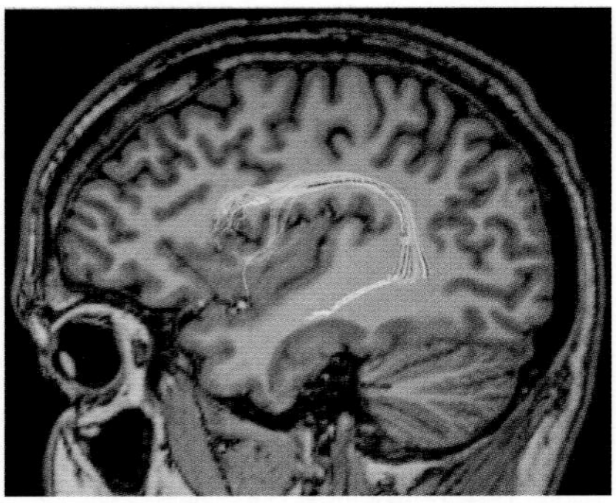

a. Arcuate fasciculus
b. Cingulum bundle
c. Fornix
d. Inferior longitudinal fasciculus
e. Superior longitudinal fasciculus

13. Which one of the following tracts is most likely depicted in the figure below?

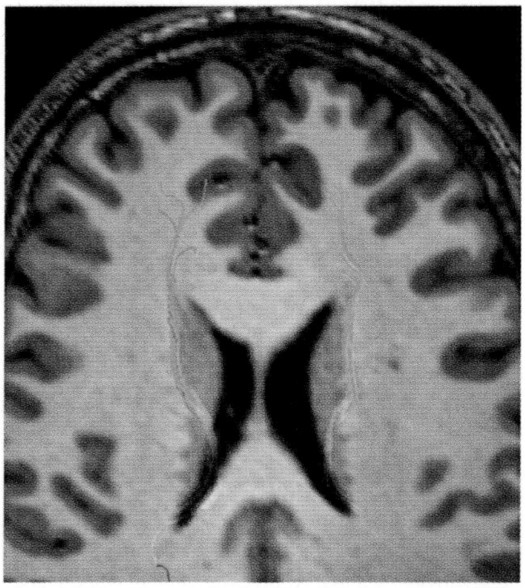

a. Cingulum
b. Posterior commissure
c. Superior fronto-orbital fasciculus
d. Superior longitudinal fasciculus
e. U association fiber

14. Which one of the following tracts is most likely depicted in the figure below?

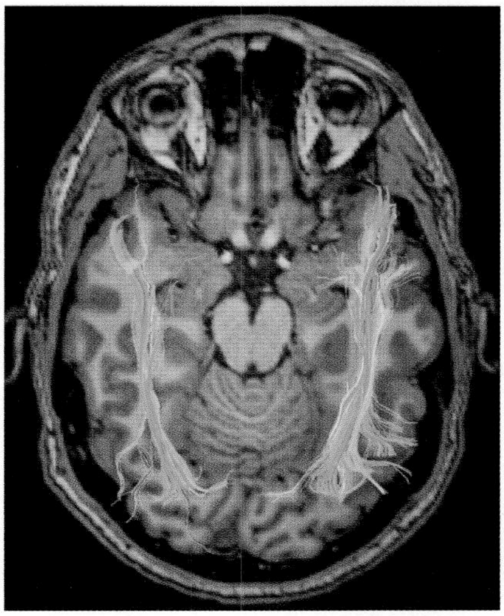

a. Arcuate fasciculus
b. External capsule
c. Fornix
d. Inferior fronto orbital fasciculus
e. Inferior longitudinal fasciculus

15. Which one of the following tracts is most likely depicted in the figure below?

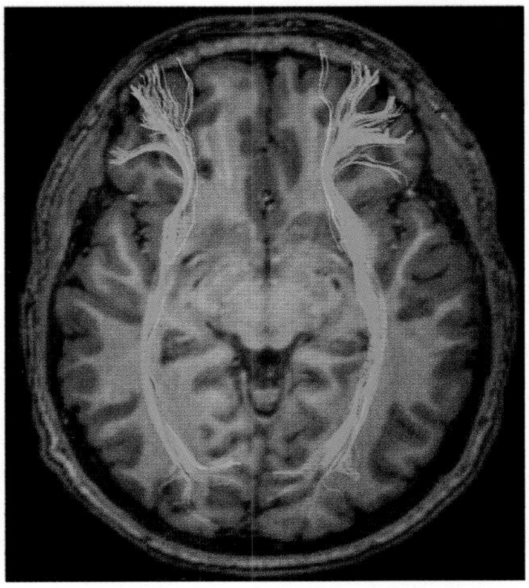

a. Commissure of Probst
b. Corona radiata
c. Inferior fronto orbital fasciculus
d. Inferior longitudinal fasciculs
e. Internal capsule

16. Which one of the following tracts is most likely depicted in the figure below?

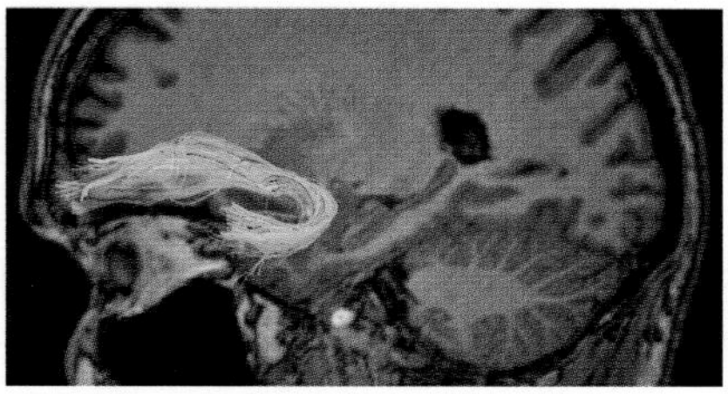

a. Anterior commissure
b. Anterior region of the corona radiata
c. Fornix
d. Optic tract
e. Uncinate fasciculus

17. In MR Spectroscopy, Hunter's angle is best described as which one of the following?

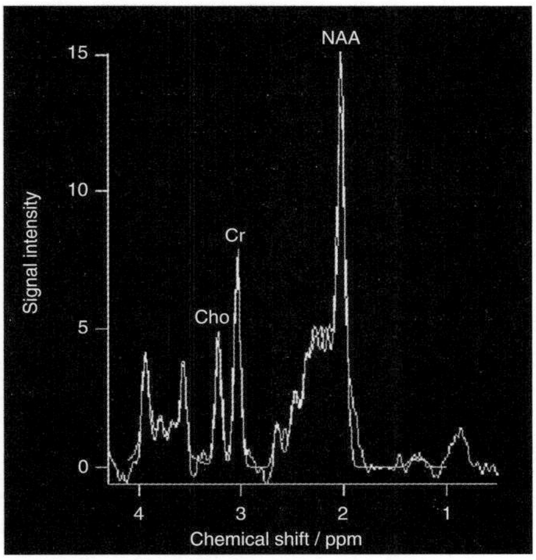

a. The rough angle formed with the x axis when a line is drawn between choline and creatine peaks
b. The rough angle formed with the x axis when a line is drawn between NAA and creatine peaks
c. The rough angle formed with the x axis when a line is drawn between choline, creatine and NAA peaks
d. The rough angle formed with the x axis when a line is drawn between lactate and lipid peaks
e. The rough angle formed with the x axis when a line is drawn between choline and lactate peaks

QUESTIONS 18–26

Additional questions 18–26 available on ExpertConsult.com

EXTENDED MATCHING ITEM (EMI) QUESTIONS

27. **Tractography:**
    a. Anterior commissure
    b. Anterior region of the corona radiata
    c. Arcuate fasciculus
    d. Corticobulbar tract
    e. Corticospinal tract
    f. Cingulum
    g. Cerebral peduncle
    h. Fornix
    i. Inferior fronto-occipital fasciculus
    j. Inferior longitudinal fasciculus
    k. Optic tract
    l. Superior fronto-occipital fasciculus
    m. Superior longitudinal fasciculus
    n. Uncinate fasciculus
    o. Vertical occipital fasciculus

For each of the following descriptions, select the most appropriate answers from the list above. Each answer may be used once, more than once or not at all.
1. Pathway important for recognition of language and appropriate response.
2. Pathway important for object recognition and discrimination, semantic processing and visuospatial processing.
3. Pathway with role in linking object representations to their lexical labels and face recognition.
4. Pathway with role in peripheral vision, visual perception of motion, and visual spatial processing.
5. Pathway with role in initiation of motor activity and higher-order control of body-centered action, spatial attention and gestural components of language and orofacial working memory.

28. **MRI Sequences:**
    a. BOLD Functional MRI
    b. Diffusion tensor imaging
    c. Diffusion weighted imaging (Echo planar)
    d. Fast spin echo
    e. FIESTA
    f. FLAIR CSF suppression
    g. Gradient echo
    h. MR Spectroscopy
    i. Phase-contrast
    j. STIR fat suppression
    k. Susceptibility weighted imaging
    l. T1
    m. T1 with gadolinium
    n. T2
    o. Time of flight

For each of the following descriptions, select the most appropriate answers from the list above. Each answer may be used once, more than once or not at all.
1. CSF flow studies
2. Cavernous malformations
3. Resection of an eloquent temporal glioma in an intact patient presenting with headache
4. Consideration of microvascular decompression for trigeminal neuralgia

29. **Imaging Modalities:**
    a. B-mode Ultrasound
    b. CT intracranial angiogram
    c. CT myelogram
    d. CT venogram cerebral
    e. DAT scan
    f. Doppler ultrasound
    g. FDG-PET CT
    h. Indium-11 Diethylenepentaacetic acid study
    i. MIBG scan
    j. MR perfusion
    k. Somatostatin-PET CT
    l. SPECT
    m. Xenon-133 CT

For each of the following descriptions, select the most appropriate answers from the list above. Each answer may be used once, more than once or not at all.
1. Postoperatively to distinguish between tumor recurrence and radiation necrosis
2. Cisternography
3. Intraoperative localization of spinal cord tumor

30. **MR Spectroscopy:**
    a. Alanine
    b. Choline
    c. Citrate peak
    d. Creatine/phosphocreatine
    e. Gamma-aminobutyric acid
    f. Glucose
    g. Glutamate (Glu)/Glutamine peak

h. Lactate
i. Myo-inositol (ml)
j. N-acetyl aspartate

For each of the following descriptions, select the most appropriate answers from the list above. Each answer may be used once, more than once or not at all.

1. Reference metabolite in MR spectroscopy
2. Marker for cellular turnover
3. Marker for ischaemia and necrosis

31. **Diffusion weighted imaging:**
a. T2 low signal, DWI low signal, ADC low signal
b. T2 low signal, DWI isointense or low signal, ADC low signal
c. T2 low signal, DWI isointense or high signal, ADC low signal
d. T2 low signal, DWI high signal in border and low within lesion, ADC low signal
e. T2 low signal, DWI high signal, ADC high signal
f. T2 isointense signal, DWI low signal, ADC low signal
g. T2 isointense signal, DWI isointense or low signal, ADC low signal
h. T2 isointense signal, DWI isointense or high signal, ADC low signal
i. T2 isointense signal, DWI high, ADC low signal
j. T2 isointense signal, DWI high signal in border and low within lesion, ADC high signal
k. T2 high signal, DWI low signal, ADC high signal
l. T2 high signal, DWI isointense or low signal, ADC low signal
m. T2 high signal, DWI high signal in border and low within lesion, ADC low signal
n. T2 high signal, DWI high, ADC isointense signal
o. T2 high signal, DWI high signal, ADC low signal

For each of the following descriptions, select the most appropriate answers from the list above. Each answer may be used once, more than once or not at all.

1. Epidermoid
2. Arachnoid cyst
3. Ring-enhancing cerebral abscess
4. Ring-enhancing glioblastoma multiforme

SBA ANSWERS

1. **c**—N-acetylcysteine

2. **f**—T1 hyperintense, T2 hypointense

The table below describes the appearance of subdural blood clots on MRI as they age:

Clot Age	T1WI	T2WI	Explanation	Mnemonic*
Hyperacute (4-6 h)	Isointense	Hyperintense	Large amount of diamagnetic oxyhemoglobin which does not affect T1/T2. Appearance due to high water content.	**IB**BY
Acute (7-72 h)	Isointense	Hypointense	Deoxyhemoglobin is paramagnetic and causes T2 effect but not T1	**ID**DY
Early Subacute (4-7d)	Hyperintense	Hypointense	Intracellular methemoglobin is paramagnetic	**BID**DY
Late subacute (1-4w)	Hyperintense	Hyperintense	Hemolysis results in extracellular methemoglobin increasing T2 hyperintensity	**BA**BY
Early chronic (weeks to months)	Hyperintense	Hyperintense	Pool of dilute free methemoglobin surrounded by thin rimmed T2 hypointense wall of ferritin and hemosiderin deposits	
Late chronic (months to years)	Hypointense	Hypointense	Ferritin and hemosiderin diffuse throughout clot	**DU**DU

*I = isointense, B = Bright (hyperintense), D = Dark (hypointense).

3. **b**—A Diffusion weighted image and apparent diffusion coefficient maps

Diffusion restriction is assessed with a diffusion weighted imaging protocol which includes a T2 weighted sequence (low b = 0), diffusion weighted sequence (high b = 1000) and apparent diffusion coefficient map. The b-value parameter identifies the measurement's sensitivity to diffusion and determines the strength and duration of the diffusion gradients. A b value of 0 produces a T2 weighted image for anatomical reference. In the range of clinically relevant b values (i.e. up to 1000) the greater the b value the stronger the diffusion weighting and the higher the contrast in pathogenic regions. A minimum of two b-values must be acquired for an apparent diffusion coefficient map, which is a measure of the strength of diffusion in tissue after eliminating any overlying T2 shine through/contrast effects. T2 shine-through refers to high signal on DWI images that is not due to restricted diffusion, but rather to high T2 signal which "shines through" to the DWI image. T2 shine through occurs because of long T2 decay time in some normal tissue. This is most often seen with subacute infarctions due to vasogenic edema but can be seen in other pathologic abnormalities e.g. epidermoid cyst. To confirm true restricted diffusion one should always compare the DWI image to the ADC. In cases of true restricted diffusion, the region of increased DWI signal will demonstrate low signal on ADC. ADC is a value that measures the effect of diffusion independent of the influence of T2 shine-through. ADC maps thus portray restricted diffusion, such as in ischemic injury, as hypointense lesions relative to normal brain. In contrast, in cases of T2 shine-through, the ADC will be normal or high signal.

4. **a**—Cerebral abscess

Images with permission from Adam A, et al. (Eds.). Grainger & Allison's Diagnostic Radiology, 6 th ed., Elsevier, Churchill Livingstone, 2014.

5. **a**—Bright on DWI, low rCBF, long rMTT, low CBV

6. **c**. The corpus callosum facilitates interhemispheric interactions for communicating and integrating perceptual, cognitive, learned, and volitional information. It is important for the performance of visual and tactile tasks that require transfer of sensory information between the cerebral hemispheres. Commissural fibers crossing through the anterior portion and body of the corpus callosum are essential to perform temporally independent bimanual finger movements. Commissural fibers passing through the posterior corpus callosum play an important role in visual and visuospatial integration. Callosal fibers are also important for higher-order cognition, including normal social, attentional, and emotional function.

Image with permission from Naidich T, Castillo M, Cha S, Smirniotopoulos J. Imaging of the Brain, Elsevier, Saunders, 2013.

7. **c**—Fornix

The fornix is part of the dorsal limbic system and the Papez circuit. It participates in high-level mental processes relevant to episodic memory and emotion. It also provides the main cholinergic input to the hippocampus.

Image with permission from Naidich T, Castillo M, Cha S, Smirniotopoulos J. Imaging of the Brain, Elsevier, Saunders, 2013.

8. **b**—Corona Radiata

The fibers of the corona radiata interconnect the cerebral cortex with the thalamus and brainstem in both directions. From anterior to posterior, they include (1) the thalamic connections to the frontal lobes and the frontopontine motor fibers that pass through the anterior limb of the internal capsule; (2) the thalamic connections to the anterior parietal lobe and the corticonuclear motor projections that pass through the genu; and (3) the thalamic connections to the central parietal and occipitotemporal lobes and corticospinal, corticopontine, and corticotegmental motor fibers that pass through the posterior limb of the internal capsule. The thalamic radiations to and from the cortex are grouped into four thalamic peduncles.

Image with permission from Naidich T, Castillo M, Cha S, Smirniotopoulos J. Imaging of the Brain, Elsevier, Saunders, 2013.

9. **b**—Corticospinal tract

The corticospinal tract is the predominant pathway for the relay of impulses for voluntary skilled movements of the upper extremities, trunk, and lower extremities. It connects pyramidal Giant cells of Betz in layer V of primary motor cortex to alpha motor neurons, decussating in the medulla.

Image with permission from Naidich T, Castillo M, Cha S, Smirniotopoulos J. Imaging of the Brain, Elsevier, Saunders, 2013.

10. **b**—Cingulum

The cingulum bundle is the major component of the dorsal limbic pathway. It is involved in a wide range of motivational and emotional aspects of behavior and participates in spatial working memory. It interconnects the hippocampus and parahippocampal gyrus (critical for memory) with the (1) prefrontal areas (important for manipulating information, monitoring behavior and working memory) and (2) rostral cingulate gyrus (involved in motivation and drive). It can be lesioned or stimulated to treat pain, obsessive compulsive disorder or depression. The limbic system is also important for high-level mental processes relevant to memory and emotion. It is part of the Papez circuit that links the hippocampus, parahippocampal gyrus, mammillary bodies, thalamus, and cingulate gyrus. Other structures subsequently integrated into the limbic system include the amygdala, septal region, and olfactory bulb. These structures have been implicated in dementia, epilepsy, and schizophrenia.

Image with permission from Naidich T, Castillo M, Cha S, Smirniotopoulos J. Imaging of the Brain, Elsevier, Saunders, 2013.

11. **d**—Superior longitudinal fasciculus (II and III)

The SLF is significant for initiation of motor activity and higher-order control of body-centered action. It connects the superior parietal lobule (important for limb and trunk location in body-centered space) with premotor areas (engaged in higher aspects of motor behavior). The SLF is also significant for spatial attention, because it connects the inferior parietal lobule (concerned with visual spatial information) with the posterior prefrontal cortex (important for perception and awareness). Furthermore, the SLF is relevant to gestural components of language and orofacial working memory, because it connects the supramarginal gyrus (concerned with higher order somatosensory information) with the ventral premotor area (containing mirror neurons for action imitation).

Image with permission from Naidich T, Castillo M, Cha S, Smirniotopoulos J. Imaging of the Brain, Elsevier, Saunders, 2013.

12. **a**—Arcuate fasciculus

The classical (direct) arcuate fasciculus interconnects Wernicke's receptive, auditory word processing area in the superior temporal lobe with Broca's speech production area in the inferior frontal lobe. This connection provides for the ability to recognize language and respond to it appropriately. Individuals with more symmetric patterns of connection perform better overall on word tasks of semantic association. It has been considered by some to be the fourth portion of SLF.

Image with permission from Naidich T, Castillo M, Cha S, Smirniotopoulos J. Imaging of the Brain, Elsevier, Saunders, 2013.

13. **c**—Superior fronto-orbital fasciculus

The SFOF is significant for peripheral vision, visual perception of motion, and visual spatial processing. The SFOF connects the superior parietal gyrus (parastriate areas important for peripheral vision and visual appreciation of motion) with the dorsolateral prefrontal cortex of the middle and inferior frontal gyri (necessary for attention)

Image with permission from Naidich T, Castillo M, Cha S, Smirniotopoulos J. Imaging of the Brain, Elsevier, Saunders, 2013.

14. **e**—Inferior longitudinal fasciculus

The inferior longitudinal fasciculus has a role in the ventral visual stream for object recognition, discrimination, and memory. It appears to mediate the fast transfer of visual signals to anterior temporal regions and neuromodulatory back-projections from the amygdala to early visual areas. It likely plays a role in linking object representations to their lexical labels. Face recognition probably depends on the ILF, because disruption of the tract has been implicated in associative visual agnosia, prosopagnosia, visual amnesia, and visual hypoemotionality.

Image with permission from Naidich T, Castillo M, Cha S, Smirniotopoulos J. Imaging of the Brain, Elsevier, Saunders, 2013.

15. **c**—Inferior fronto orbital fasciculus

This fascicle may be a major component of the ventral subcortical "what" pathway important for object recognition and discrimination. The IFOF most likely also has a significant role in semantic processing, because it interconnects the occipital associative extrastriate cortex with the temporobasal region, two areas important to semantic processing. The IFOF also functions in visuospatial processing and enables the interaction between emotion and cognition.

Image with permission from Naidich T, Castillo M, Cha S, Smirniotopoulos J. Imaging of the Brain, Elsevier, Saunders, 2013.

16. **e**—The uncinate fasciculus is a ventral limbic pathway that is critical for processing novel information, for positive/negative valuations of the emotional aspects of data, and for self-regulation. The fibers of the uncinate fasciculus link the rostral superior temporal gyrus (important for sound recognition), the rostral inferior temporal gyrus (important for object recognition), and the medial temporal area (important for recognition memory) with the orbital, medial, and prefrontal cortices (involved in emotion, inhibition, and self-regulation). The uncinate fasciculus may also be critical in visual learning.

Image with permission from Naidich T, Castillo M, Cha S, Smirniotopoulos J. Imaging of the Brain, Elsevier, Saunders, 2013.

17. **c**—The rough angle formed with the *x* axis when a line is drawn between choline, creatine and NAA peaks. Hunter's angle is the formed by a line approximately joining the ascending peaks of the metabolites in MR spectroscopy and is roughly 45°. Myoinositol, Choline, Creatine and N-Acetyl aspartate peaks are ascending in normal spectrum, any alteration in the ascending nature of the peaks means spectrum is abnormal.

Image with permission from Mangrum WI. Duke Review of MRI Principles: Case Review Series, Elsevier, Mosby, 2012.

ANSWERS 18–26

Additional answers 18–26 available on ExpertConsult.com

EMI ANSWERS

27. 1—c, 2—i, 3—j, 4—l, 5—m

28. 1—i, Phase-contrast, 2—k, Susceptibility weighted imaging, 3—a, BOLD Functional MRI, 3—e, FIESTA.

29. 1—g, FDG-PET CT, 2—h, Indium-11 Diethylenepentaacetic acid study, 3—a, B-mode ultrasound

30. 1—d, Creatine, 2—b, Choline, 3—h, Lactate

In order to interpret MRS, one needs to understand the function of the different molecules being measured. **NAA** is synthesized in the mitochondria of neurons, and its function is unknown. Clinically, NAA serves as a marker for the presence of neurons, including neuronal axons in white matter. **Creatine** (Cr) is used clinically as a marker for energy metabolism. Low levels of creatine suggest that the area of interest is highly metabolically active. Creatine is also often assumed to be stable and is used for calculating metabolite ratios (e.g., Cho:Cr and NAA:Cr). **Choline** (Cho) is found in the cell membrane. It serves as a marker for the cellular turnover of a lesion. Choline is elevated both in the setting of increased cellular production, such as in a tumor, and in the setting of cellular breakdown, such as in leukodystrophy and multiple sclerosis. **Lactate** is a marker for anaerobic metabolism. Normally, lactate levels in the brain are so low that they cannot be measured by spectroscopy. Increased anaerobic metabolism, such as with ischemia or tumor necrosis, results in lactate peaks. **Myoinositol** is a sugar. It is absent from neurons but present

Molecule	Chemical Shift	Function	Classic Association (↑ Increased; ↓ Decreased)
Lipids	0.8-1.5 ppm	Fat	↑: Diploic space and subcutaneous fat
Lactate	1.33 ppm	Anaerobic activity	↑: Ischemia, infarction, seizures, metabolic disorders, necrotic tumors
NAA	2.02 ppm	Neuronal/axonal marker	↓ Leukodystrophy, malignant neoplasm, multiple sclerosis, infarction ↑ Elevated in Canavan disease
Creatine	3.02 ppm	Marker of metabolic activity	Assumed to be unchanged and used to calculate ratios (Cho:Cr and NAA:Cr) ↓ Tumors.
Choline	3.22 ppm	Cellular turnover	↑ Increased in tumors, inflammation, infection, multiple sclerosis ...
Myoinositol	3.56 ppm	Glial marker	↑ Gliosis, astrocytosis, Alzheimer's disease

Table with permission from Mangrum WI. Duke Review of MRI Principles: Case Review Series, 2012, Elsevier, Mosby.

in glial cells. It is used as a marker for glial proliferation or an increase in glial size. **Lipids** are markers for fat, as is seen in the subcutaneous tissues or in the diploic space of the calvarium.

Description of Common Spectroscopy Molecules: Their Chemical Shifts, Main Functions, and Classic Associations

31. 1—n, 2—k, 3—o, 4—j

Epidermoids are usually an expansive lesion in the left aspect of the posterior fossa, and despite being solid they demonstrate similar signal intensity to CSF on T2WI, but demonstrate diffusion restriction on diffusion-weighted imaging (high signal DWI, isointense ADC). In contrast, arachnoid cysts may also be seen as a lesion in the posterior fossa demonstrating similar signal intensity to CSF but do not show restricted diffusion (low DWI, high ADC). Cerebral abscess must be considered when a ring enhancing necrotic lesion (usually surrounded by vasogenic edema) demonstrates restricted diffusion (bright DWI, dark ADC). An expansive ring enhancing cystic/necrotic lesion, surrounded by vasogenic edema/infiltrative lesion, demonstrating restricted diffusion and high perfusion in its borders but unrestricted diffusion within the lesion is more consistent with glioblastoma or metastasis. Other highly cellular brain tumors demonstrating restricted diffusion on DWI include lymphoma, medulloblastoma and anaplastic astrocytoma.

CHAPTER 15

Radiotherapy and Stereotactic Radiosurgery

SINGLE BEST ANSWER (SBA) QUESTIONS

1. Which one of the following statements about stereotactic radiosurgery is most accurate?
   a. A high dose of radiation is delivered in a single sitting often to a volume limited target, typically one lesion is treated however more than one can be
   b. It is used to deliver prophylactic craniospinal irradiation
   c. Radiation is delivered in multiple sessions to a single target
   d. Requires a cobalt source for generating ionizing radiation
   e. Requires a copper source for generating non-ionizing radiation

2. Which one of the following utilizes a cobalt-60 source for photon production?
   a. 3D conformal radiotherapy
   b. Carbon-ion therapy
   c. Gamma Knife surgery
   d. Linac-based radiosurgery
   e. Proton beam therapy

3. In radiotherapy planning, which one of the following terms best describes the volume that should be treated to account for the tumor, microscopic spread, and setup errors (systematic and random)?
   a. Clinical target volume
   b. Gross tumor volume
   c. Planning organ at risk volume
   d. Planning target volume
   e. Systematic target volume

4. Which one of the following descriptions does not describe the radiobiological response of common intracranial targets for radiosurgery?
   a. Target volume contains no abnormal tissue and normal tissue shows early radiobiologic effect
   b. Target volume contains no normal tissue and abnormal tissue shows early radiobiologic effect
   c. Target volume is late responding as contains normal and abnormal tissue
   d. Target volume is late responding but only in abnormal tissue and with marked radiobiologic effect
   e. Target volume shows small, early effect on abnormal tissue but bigger, late effect on normal tissue

5. In which one of the following forms of radiation therapy is the Bragg peak utilised to focus treatment and minimise collateral damage to non-targeted structures?
   a. Brachytherapy
   b. CyberKnife radiosurgery
   c. Gamma Knife surgery
   d. Linac-based radiosurgery
   e. Proton beam therapy

6. Which one of the following is not an important biological factor explaining the efficacy of fractionation?
   a. Radiosensitivity
   b. Reassortment (redistribution)
   c. Reduction
   d. Reoxygenation
   e. Repair
   f. Repopulation

7. Stereotactic radiotherapy for brain metastasis is LEAST likely to be appropriate in which one of the following situations?
   a. CNS and systemic progression of disease, with few systemic treatment options and poor performance status
   b. Local relapse after surgical resection of a single brain metastasis
   c. Oligometastases (1-3) metastases especially if primary tumor is known to be radiotherapy resistant
   d. Postsurgical resection of a single BM, especially if 3 cm or smaller and in the posterior fossa
   e. Salvage therapy for recurrent oligometastases (1-3) after WBRT

8. Which one of the following statements regarding radiotherapy for low-grade glioma is most accurate?
   a. Early postoperative radiotherapy increases survival
   b. Early postoperative radiotherapy is associated with better seizure control
   c. Early postoperative radiotherapy is associated with reduced side-effects
   d. Early postoperative radiotherapy results in increased malignant transformation of residual tumor
   e. Early postoperative radiotherapy shows no advantage in time to tumor progression

9. What is the target for stereotactic radiosurgery treatment for trigeminal neuralgia?
   a. Cisternal portion of the trigeminal nerve adjacent to the brainstem
   b. Sensory trigeminal nucleus in pons
   c. Superficial cerebellar artery
   d. Trigeminal ganglion in Meckel's cave
   e. Trigeminal nerve in foramen ovale

10. Which one of the following scenarios describes the most appropriate action taken?
    a. 1 cm Spetzler-Martin grade 3 AVM in the left thalamus treated with embolization followed by stereotactic radiosurgery
    b. 1.5 cm Spetzler-Martin grade 2 AVM in left parietal cortex treated with embolization
    c. 1.5 cm Spetzler-Martin grade 3 AVM in right thalamus treated with stereotactic radiosurgery
    d. 4 cm Spetzler-Martin grade 3 AVM in right frontal lobe treated with stereotactic radiosurgery
    e. 5 cm Spetzler-Martin grade 3 AVM in left temporal lobe treated with surgical excision

11. Which one of the following has not been shown to increase the risk of developing edema after stereotactic radiosurgery for the treatment of meningiomas is most accurate?
    a. Brain-tumor interface $>1\ cm^2$
    b. Clinical treatment volume of $>5\ cm^3$
    c. Location in cavernous sinus
    d. Presence of edema on pretreatment scan
    e. Radiation dose greater than 16 Gy

12. Which one of the following is true of SRS for acoustic neuroma?
    a. Microsurgery is associated with better preservation of serviceable hearing than radiotherapy.
    b. Microsurgery is preferred for lesions smaller than 3 cm.
    c. Radiotherapy is associated with reduced facial nerve and trigeminal nerve toxicity compared to microsurgery.
    d. Stereotactic radiosurgery is more effective than fractionated stereotactic radiotherapy.
    e. Stereotactic radiosurgery is preferred for lesions bigger than 3 cm.

13. What is the risk of secondary neoplasm after SRS at 15 years?
    a. 0.004%
    b. 0.04%
    c. 0.4%
    d. 4.0%
    e. 4.4%
    f. 44%

14. Which one of the following is most accurate about stereotactic radiosurgery for pituitary adenomas?
    a. At doses above 5 Gy, the rate of impaired thyrotropic function at 5 years was 50%.
    b. Contraindicated for tumors within 5 mm of the optic chiasm.
    c. For secretory tumors there is no significant difference in response by tumor subtype.
    d. Improved rates of tumor control are seen when radiation therapy is combined with dopamine agonists.
    e. Radiation-induced hypopituitarism occurs in 10% of patients undergoing SRS.

15. Which one of the following is most accurate about radiation treatment for craniopharyngiomas?
    a. Bleomycin can be used for intracystic irradiation.
    b. Intracystic interferon alpha is utilized to sensitize the cystic component to SRS.
    c. Fractionated conformal radiotherapy is commonly used to treat residual tumour.
    d. SRS with intracystic irradiation is effective for mixed-type tumors.
    e. There is no significant role for radiotherapy in management.

QUESTIONS 16–17

Additional questions 16–17 available on ExpertConsult.com

EXTENDED MATCHING ITEM (EMI) QUESTIONS

18. **Tissue tolerance to radiosurgery:**
    a. Brain lesion 0-2 cm
    b. Brain lesion 2-3 cm
    c. Brain lesion 3-4 cm
    d. Brainstem
    e. Cochlea
    f. Cranial nerves III, IV, VI
    g. Facial nerve
    h. Optic chiasm/nerve
    i. Pituitary
    j. Trigeminal nerve

For each of the following descriptions, select the most appropriate answers from the list above. Each answer may be used once, more than once or not at all.

1. Has a single fraction maximal tolerated dose of 3.7 Gy
2. Has a single fraction maximal tolerated dose of 8 Gy

19. **Indications in stereotactic radiosurgery:**
    a. Arteriovenous malformation
    b. Brain metastasis
    c. Chordoma
    d. Cluster headache
    e. Epilepsy
    f. Glioblastoma multiforme
    g. Glomus jugulare tumors
    h. Low-grade glioma
    i. Meningioma
    j. Obsessive compulsive disorder
    k. Pituitary adenoma
    l. Vestibular schwannoma

For each of the following descriptions, select the most appropriate answers from the list above. Each answer may be used once, more than once or not at all.

1. Treatment targeted at anterior internal capsule bilaterally
2. Latency period of 1-3 years before maximal treatment effect seen
3. Target is cisternal segment of the trigeminal nerve

20. **Radiotherapy and radiosurgery:**
    a. Carbon-ion therapy
    b. Conformal radiotherapy
    c. Fast-neutron therapy
    d. Gamma Knife surgery
    e. Fractionated stereotactic radiotherapy
    f. Intensity-modulated radiotherapy (IMRT)
    g. Linac radiosurgery
    h. Proton beam therapy
    i. TomoTherapy
    j. Volumetric modulated arc radiotherapy
    k. Whole brain radiotherapy (WBRT)

For each of the following descriptions, select the most appropriate answers from the list above. Each answer may be used once, more than once or not at all.

1. Non-conformal photon based therapy with opposed lateral fixed beams
2. Shapes the radiotherapy beams to allow different doses of radiotherapy to be given to different parts of the treatment area and more effectively spare organs at risk
3. Use multileaf collimator in a helmet attached to a stereotactic head frame allowing multiple small beams to deliver high dose to small target small deep lesions

SBA ANSWERS

1. **a**—A high dose of radiation is delivered in a single sitting only to a single target

Radiosurgery usually implies a single outpatient treatment with high dose delivered to a small target, with multiple beams creating a high dose gradient. As no single beam contributes significantly to the cumulative dose the amount of radiation delivered to normal tissues in the beams' paths is minimized while targets less than 4 cm large receive a high dose. Effective radiosurgical treatment of targets larger than 4 cm with would require an unacceptable increase in dose to adjacent normal brain tissue. It can be performed using various devices including linear accelerators, Gamma Knife (GK), and particle beam devices.

2. **c**—Gamma Knife surgery

	LINAC (e.g., CyberKnife)	Gamma Knife	Proton Beam Therapy
Source	Linear accelerator shoots electrons at tungsten target	Cobalt-60 decay	Cyclotron
Rays	X-rays	Gamma rays	Proton
Head immobilization	Stereotactic frame or frameless (fiducials)	Stereotactic frame	Immobilization
	Machine moves around patient during treatment	Equipment stationary	Equipment stationary
Multileaf collimator	In machine	In patient helmet	
Use	Whole body	Intracranial only	Whole body

3. **d**—Planning target volume (PTV)

Gross tumor volume (GTV)	Volume of macroscopic tumor that is visualized on imaging studies
Clinical target volume (CTV)	Volume that should be treated to a high dose, typically incorporating both the GTV and volumes that are assumed to be at risk due to microscopic spread of the disease
Planning target volume (PTV)	Volume that should be treated in order to ensure that the CTV is always treated, including considerations of systematic and random daily setup errors and intertreatment and intratreatment motion
Organ at risk (OR)	Organ whose damage is especially dangerous and where small amount of radiation damage would produce a severe clinical manifestation, e.g., spinal cord. Their radiation sensitivity influences treatment planning or prescribed radiation dose
Planning organ at risk volume (PRV)	Margin added around the OR to account for uncertainties in planning and delivery
Systematic target volume (STV)	Margin added to the CTV to account for systematic errors arising from treatment planning

4. **a**—Target volume contains no abnormal tissue and normal tissue shows early radiobiologic effect

Target volume late responding as contains normal and abnormal tissue	AVM
Target volume late responding but only in abnormal tissue and with marked radiobiologic effect	Benign tumor, e.g., meningioma, pituitary adenoma, vestibular schwannoma
Target volume shows small, early effect on abnormal tissue but bigger, late effect on normal tissue (radiosurgery only indicated in some cases)	Low-grade glioma
Target volume contains no normal tissue and abnormal tissue shows early radiobiologic effect	Metastasis

FURTHER READING

Shrieve DC, et al. Radiosurgery. In: Leibel & Philips Textbook of Radiation Oncology, 3rd ed.

5. **e**—Proton beam therapy

As a photon beam passes through material and is absorbed, the overall intensity of the beam is reduced. In contrast, particles such as protons and ions travel a finite distance, which is termed the range. They deposit a disproportionate amount of energy in the last few millimeters of their path. This large transfer of energy is known as the Bragg peak. The physical depth penetrated by the particles depends on tissue density and the beam's energy.

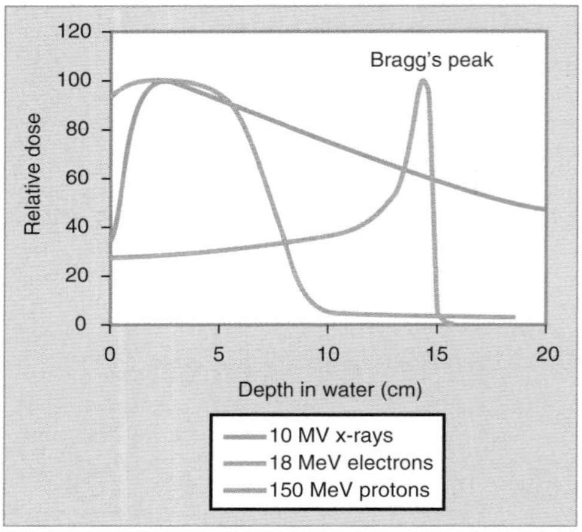

Image with permission from Winn HR. Youman's Neurological Surgery, 4-Volume Set, 6th ed. Elsevier, Saunders, 2011.

6. **c**—Reduction

The five Rs of radiobiology are:

Term	Relevance to Fractionation Efficacy
Repair	Ionizing radiation can cause lethal, sublethal and potentially lethal damage to cells. If radiotherapy is fractionated, sublethal damage can be repaired before the next dose—and this repair occurs more effectively in normal tissue compared to malignant cells (e.g., TP53 mutation). If multiple fractions are to be given on the same day, the repair half-life of the normal tissue must be considered, e.g., 4 h repair half-life in spinal cord therefore separate fractions by 8 h
Repopulation	The increase in cell division that is seen in surviving normal and malignant tissue post-radiotherapy—determines length and timing of course

Continued

Term	Relevance to Fractionation Efficacy
	Normal tissue: at 4 weeks post-radiotherapy in early responding tissue
	Malignant tissue: come tumors show accelerated repopulation at 4-5 weeks—dangerous phenomenon where tumor shows marked increase in growth fraction and doubling time
	Increasing the length of the course to over 4 weeks will thus reduce normal tissue reactions, but increase the risk of accelerated repopulation in the tumor requiring additional fractions
Reassortment/ redistribution	When radiotherapy is given to a population of cells, they may be in different parts of the cell cycle. Cells in S-phase are typically radioresistant, whereas those in late G_2 and M phase are relatively radiosensitive. A small dose of radiation delivered over a short time period will kill a lot of the sensitive cells and less of the resistant cells. Over time, the surviving cells will redistribute the proportion in each cell cycle phase. Surviving cells that now moved into a more radiosensitive phase can now be killed with a second fraction of radiotherapy
Reoxygenation	Radiotherapy works through the production of free radicals (by interaction of photons with water or oxygen) which cause DNA-damage to normal and tumor cells. Normal cells are better able to repair this damage, hence survive better than tumor cells. Tumors can become acutely or chronically hypoxic due to changes in blood supply—reducing the number of free radicals produced during a fraction of radiotherapy and increasing their radioresistance/ reducing radiosensitivity. Fractionating radiotherapy reduces the chances that the cell will be acutely hypoxic during treatments, and gives multiple opportunities for normoxic tumor cells near capillaries to be killed
Radiosensitivity	Refers to the intrinsic radiosensitivity/radioresistance of certain normal and tumor cell types:

Continued

Term	Relevance to Fractionation Efficacy
	Radiosensitive: hematological cells, epithelial stem cells, gametes; hematological and germ cell malignancy
	Radioresistant: myocytes, neurons; melanoma, sarcoma

7. **a**—CNS and systemic progression of disease, with few systemic treatment options and poor performance status

Both surgery and SRS have a proven survival benefit in the management of a single brain metastasis. Typically, surgery is preferred in patients with good performance status, large lesions (>3 cm), or symptomatic tumors with substantial vasogenic edema. In patients who are good candidates for either surgery or SRS, there are no randomized data currently available to indicate which is the preferred treatment modality. In general, the current debate regarding patients with multiple metastases surrounds whether to use WBRT, SRS, or both. Survival, recurrence, focal neurological deficit and neurocognitive outcome are key considerations. Proponents of SRS suggest that highly targeted therapy spares normal brain tissue and preserves neurocognitive function, while WBRT supporters argue that SRS will not treat the invisible micrometastatic foci which will grow to cause neurological deterioration later on. Current practices may be summarized as:

Consider SRS when:

- Oligometastases (1-3) or multiple (4-10) metastases especially if primary tumor is known to be radiotherapy resistant
- Postsurgical resection of a single BM, especially if 3 cm or bigger and in the posterior fossa
- Local relapse after surgical resection of a single brain metastasis
- Salvage therapy for recurrent oligometastases (1-3) after WBRT

Consider WBRT in brain metastasis when:

- CNS and systemic progression of disease, with few systemic treatment options and poor performance status
- Multiple (4-10) brain metastasis especially if primary tumor known to be radiotherapy sensitive (NB current data support SRS use in up to 3 metastasis but there is a growing trend to use it in up to 10)
- Large (>4 cm) brain metastasis not amenable to SRS
- Postsurgical resection of a dominant hemisphere brain metastasis with multiple (4-10) remaining BMs
- Salvage therapy for recurrent BM after SRS or WBRT failure

FURTHER READING

Lin X, DeAngelis LM. Treatment of brain metastases. J Clin Oncol 2015. pii:JCO.2015.60.9503.

Linskey ME, Andrews DW, Asher AL, et al. The role of stereotactic radiosurgery in the management of patients with newly diagnosed brain metastases: a systematic review and evidence-based clinical practice guideline. J Neurooncol 2010;96(1):45-68.

8. **b**—Early postoperative radiotherapy is associated with better seizure control

In a single prospective RCT ($n = 311$) People with LGG who undergo early postoperative radiotherapy showed an increase in time to progression compared with people who were observed and had radiotherapy at the time of progression (mean 5.3 vs. 3.4 years). There was no significant difference in overall survival between people who had early versus delayed radiotherapy; however, this finding may be due to the effectiveness of rescue radiotherapy in the delayed arm (required in 65% of this group). People who underwent early radiation had better seizure control at 1 year than people who underwent delayed radiation. Early radiation therapy was associated with skin reactions, otitis media, mild headache, nausea, and vomiting. There were no cases of radiation-induced malignant transformation of LGG. However, it remains unclear whether there are differences in memory, executive function, cognitive function, or quality of life between the two groups since these measures were not evaluated.

FURTHER READING

Sarmiento JM, Venteicher AS, Patil CG. Early versus delayed postoperative radiotherapy for treatment of low-grade gliomas. Cochrane Database Syst Rev 2015;(6). Art. No.: CD009229.

9. **a**—Cisternal segment of trigeminal nerve

For patients refractory to medications SRS is the least invasive procedure, though microvascular decompression remains superior in candidates fit for surgery. Typical doses are 70-90 Gy in a single fraction directed at the dorsal root entry zone of cranial nerve V near the pons. Initial SRS directed at the gasserian ganglion produced inferior results. Pain relief is experienced with a latency of approximately 1 month. Paresthesia is the most common side effect. Some pain relief (partial or complete) is seen in 60-70% of patients treated.

FURTHER READING

McHaffie DR, et al. Stereotactic irradiation. In: Gunderson Clinical Radiation Oncology, 3rd ed.

10. **c**—1.5 cm Spetzler-Martin grade 3 AVM in right thalamus treated with stereotactic radiosurgery

Arteriovenous malformations (AVMs) harbor a risk of hemorrhage of about 2-4% per year, mortality of 10-15% and morbidity of 50% and given the cumulative lifetime risk treatment is often considered in an asymptomatic patient. Treatment options include observation, embolization, surgery, or stereotactic radiosurgery. Surgery is the treatment of choice, when feasible, as it immediately removes the risk of hemorrhage (compared to the persisting risk of hemorrhage during the latency period between SRS and eventual AVM obliteration). As such, SRS is an approved treatment option for intracranial AVMs that are not treatable via microsurgery. For low-grade deep AVMs smaller than 3 cm, SRS alone can be performed when microsurgery is not possible. Smaller AVMs allow large doses of radiation to be applied safely and thus have a higher obliteration rate. The high dose of radiation presumably unleashes a cytokine cascade that induces fibrointimal reaction, thrombosis, and eventual obliteration of the AVM nidus over 1-3 years (latency period). Given the concomitant increased risks of adverse radiation effects, high doses of radiation cannot be safely used in large AVMs, thereby resulting in a worse obliteration rate. Thus, a multimodal approach consisting of a combination of embolization and SRS has been widely used. Embolization may reduce the size of larger AVMs, making them more amenable to radiosurgery. In addition, intranidal aneurysms and arteriovenous fistulas associated with AVMs not only have a high risk of hemorrhage but are also less sensitive to radiosurgery and can be treated using embolization followed by radiosurgery.

FURTHER READING

Xu F, Zhong J, Ray A, Manjila S, Bambakidis NC. Stereotactic radiosurgery with and without embolization for intracranial arteriovenous malformations: a systematic review and meta-analysis. Neurosurg Focus 2014;37(3):E16.

11. **c**—Location in cavernous sinus

Radiosurgery plays an important role in the treatment of small lesions (<3 to 4 cm) that are surgically inaccessible, such as those in cavernous sinus or posterior parasagittal locations, or those that have been subtotally resected but consistently have been shown to result in high recurrence rates. Two of the largest series that have examined results of SRS are from the Mayo Clinic and the University of Pittsburgh, both of which have shown local control in more than 90% for benign meningiomas at 5 years; doses 12-16 Gy, due to increased risk of edema above this dose.

The most common toxicities include cranial nerve deficits for basal tumors and peritumoral edema for non-basal tumors. The risk of optic neuropathy is very low, with maximum dose constraints to the optic nerves and chiasm of between 8 and 10 Gy. Risk of peritumoral edema is increased by: high dose, a treatment volume of more than 5 cm^3, a brain-tumor interface of >1 cm, the presence of pretreatment edema, and parasagittal location. These factors should be considered when deciding whether or not to include none of the dural tail or only a portion of it within the clinical target volume. Small meningiomas can be controlled with radiosurgery in the majority of patients, with initial results comparable to those of complete resection.

FURTHER READING

McHaffie DR, et al. Stereotactic irradiation. In: Gunderson Clinical Radiation Oncology, 3rd ed.

12. **c**—Radiotherapy is associated with reduced facial nerve and trigeminal nerve toxicity compared to microsurgery

Vestibular schwannomas represent 6-8% of primary intracranial tumors, arising at the point where nerve sheaths are replaced by fibroblasts (Obersteiner-Redlich zone; usually in IAC). Though benign, the lesions can cause severe local symptoms. Typical growth rates are less than 2 mm per year. Common symptoms include unilateral sensorineural hearing loss (>90%), tinnitus, unsteady gait, facial numbness or weakness, mastoid pain, and headaches. Late presentations can include brain stem compression. The typical appearance on T1-weighted MRI with contrast shows a homogenously enhancing mass within the cerebellopontine angle with widening of the internal auditory canal. Treatment options include observation, microsurgical resection, SRS, or fractionated radiotherapy; recommendations are influenced by age, comorbidities, tumor size, presenting symptoms, hearing loss/presence of serviceable hearing, proximity to the brainstem or cochlea, and patient preference. The goals of treatment include maximizing tumor control while preserving hearing and facial nerve and trigeminal nerve function. All interventions (surgery, SRS, FSRT) appear to result in a tumor control probability of more than 90%, and utility is summarized below:

- Microsurgery is preferred for lesions larger than 2.5 cm. The risk of cranial nerve injury with microsurgical resection is highly dependent on tumor size, operative approach (retrosigmoid, middle cranial fossa, or translabyrinthine), and the surgeon's skill and experience.
- SRS is an option for lesions smaller than 2.5 cm. The risk of sensorineural hearing loss is related to the dose of radiation delivered to cranial nerve VIII, the cochlea, and the ventral cochlear nucleus. Compared to microsurgery for similar tumors, SRS shows better serviceable hearing preservation (50-89%) and reduced facial nerve and trigeminal nerve toxicity (<5%).
- Fractionated stereotactic radiotherapy (FSRT) has comparable efficacy with SRS; some series have reported poorer hearing preservation and increased trigeminal nerve injury with SRS.

FURTHER READING

McHaffie DR, et al. Stereotactic irradiation. In: Gunderson. Clinical Radiation Oncology, 3rd ed.

13. **b**—0.04%

FURTHER READING

Patel TR, Chiang VL. Secondary neoplasms after stereotactic radiosurgery. World Neurosurg 2014;81(3-4):594-9.

14. **b**—Contraindicated for tumors within 5 mm of the optic chiasm

Pituitary adenomas represent 10-15% of intracranial neoplasms. Irradiation is generally reserved for patients who have incompletely resected tumors or recurrent disease. Based on the size and location, either SRS or conformal EBRT may be considered. SRS is typically contraindicated for tumors within 3-5 mm of the optic chiasm, respecting a maximum dose constant of 10 Gy or less to the optic nerves and chiasm. Fractionated radiotherapy, used successfully for more than 50 years to treat pituitary adenomas, should be recommended for tumors abutting optic nerve or chiasm and for diffuse or large tumors. Local control using SRS is generally in excess of 90% for non-secretory tumors. Radiation-induced hypopituitarism occurs in more than 50% of patients and is the most common late toxicity. A mean pituitary dose of 15 Gy was found to pose little risk of subsequent thyrotropic, gonadotropic, or adrenocorticotropic function; but at 5 years half of patients had low gonadotropic and thyrotropic function at doses above 17 Gy and low adrenocorticotrophic function at doses above 20 Gy. Dose to the pituitary stalk and hypothalamus may also contribute to hypopituitarism following SRS. For secretory tumors, SRS appears to result in a shorter time to hormone normalization than fractionated radiotherapy. Though tumor control remains high, hormonal remission is seen in 25-75% of patients and depends on the tumor subtype (i.e., prolactinoma, Cushing's disease, Nelson's syndrome, or acromegaly). Cytostatic medical management of secreting pituitary adenomas is often employed, but should be discontinued pre-radiotherapy if symptoms allow because patients receiving octreotide or dopamine agonists show markedly inferior control rates in several series.

FURTHER READING

McHaffie DR, et al. Stereotactic irradiation. In: Gunderson. Clinical Radiation Oncology, 3rd ed.

15. **d**—SRS with intracystic irradiation is effective for mixed-type tumors.

Maximal safe resection is the mainstay of treatment for craniopharyngiomas and leaving residual tumour is often necessary to preserve vision or hypothalamic function. Radiotherapy (RT) has emerged as a valuable adjuvant treatment modality for recurrent or residual craniopharyngiomas. Several radiotherapeutic modalities, including conformal radiotherapy, single-fraction stereotactic radiosurgery, fractionated stereotactic radiotherapy, and proton beam therapy offer reasonable rates of tumor control. With advances in neuroimaging and RT modalities, dose delivery is more accurate and focused, resulting in decreased long-term complication rates over time (hypopituitarism, visual deterioration, cranial nerve deficit, radiation effects). The cystic component of a craniopharyngioma commonly presents a problem for radiation therapy and radiosurgery. Tumor growth and cyst enlargement can be independent: the solid component of the tumor can usually be controlled by radiation while the cystic component may require treatment with one of the following options:

- Stereotactic aspiration (e.g., acute presentation or poor surgical candidate)

- Placement of an Ommaya reservoir allowing intermittent aspiration of a cyst that cannot be completely resected
- Sclerosis of the cyst wall by chemotherapeutic drugs for treatment-resistant cysts (e.g., bleomycin, interferon alpha)
- Internal irradiation (i.e., brachytherapy) with implanted radioisotopes for treatment-resistant cysts (Phosphorus-32)

Although the beneficial effect of radiation in the treatment of craniopharyngiomas has been well recognized, several issues remain sources of significant controversy:

1. On the basis of the complications associated with aggressive resection and the proven efficacy of radiation for craniopharyngiomas, several authors have recommended subtotal resection and RT as an acceptable alternative to gross-total resection. Further support for this approach comes with increasing recognition that while neurological deficits and endocrine dysfunction due to radical resection can be managed, the associated psychosocial consequences for pediatric patients growing into adults significantly affect quality of life.
2. The role of RT immediately after resection without first monitoring for tumor progression (up-front vs. salvage treatment) is debated with early radiotherapy showing some evidence of lower rates of morbidity and improved tumor control in children but not adults.
3. SRS as a primary treatment has shown higher tumor control rates in single-type tumors (solid or cystic) compared to mixed solid-cystic tumors. Solid-type tumors and the solid portions of mixed tumors may be less responsive to brachytherapy than cystic tumors, hence a combination of radioisotope instillation and SRS has been suggested as primary treatment for mixed solid-cystic tumors.

FURTHER READING

Lee CC, Yang HC, Chen CJ, Hung YC, et al. Gamma Knife surgery for craniopharyngioma: report on a 20-year experience. J Neurosurg 2014;121(Suppl.):167-78.

ANSWERS 16–17

Additional answers 16–17 available on ExpertConsult.com

EMI ANSWERS

18. 1—e, Cochlea; 2—h, Optic chiasm and nerves

With increasing international experience with SRS, guidelines for reducing the risk of normal-tissue toxicity have emerged. In general, normal tissues at risk depend on the location of the target volume. These include the brain parenchyma (edema, necrosis), brainstem (edema, necrosis, neuropathy), cranial nerves (neuropathy), and hypothalamic-pituitary axis (hypopituitarism). The interaction of dose and volume irradiated has not been clearly defined for most structures at risk.

Structure	Single-Fraction Dose Constraint
Brain lesion <2 cm	24 Gy (less than 20% risk of serious complication)
Brain lesion 2-3 cm	18 Gy (less than 20% risk of serious complication)
Brain lesion 3-4 cm	15 Gy (less than 20% risk of serious complication)
Brainstem	16 Gy—less than 5% cranial nerve deficit if less than 1/3 brainstem gets 16 Gy
Pituitary	15 Gy—no risk of hypopituitarism below this level
Optic chiasm/nerve	8 Gy—no risk of visual loss below this level
Cranial nerves III, IV, VI	30 Gy
Trigeminal nerve	<12.5-13 Gy
Facial nerve	<12.5-15 Gy
Cochlea	<3.7 Gy
Spinal cord	50 Gy

19. 1—j, Obsessive compulsive disorder; 2—a, AVM; 3—d, Cluster headache (as well as trigeminal neuralgia)

20. 1—k, Whole brain radiotherapy; 2—f, Intensity-modulated radiotherapy; 3—d, Gamma Knife surgery

Radiotherapy can be given externally (external beam radiotherapy) or internally (brachytherapy and radionuclide therapy). External beam radiotherapy can be further divided into photon based (i.e., X-ray) and particle based therapies. The table below describes some terms that usually describe subtle differences in planning or delivery of radiotherapy.

Type	Notes
Radiotherapy	
Conformal radiotherapy (3DCRT)	This uses a device inside the radiotherapy machine to shape the radiotherapy beams to the target in three dimensions (height, width, and depth). The desired cross sectional shape of the beam can be formed using blocks or a multileaf collimator. Beams can be fixed or intensity-modulated
Whole brain radiotherapy (WBRT)	Non-conformal, two dimensional radiotherapy (opposed lateral fixed beams)
Intensity-modulated radiotherapy (IMRT)	Shapes the radiotherapy beams to allow different doses of radiotherapy to be given to different parts of the treatment area. This means lower doses of radiotherapy can be given to normal tissue, hence often used close to organs at risk
TomoTherapy®	Hybrid between CT scanner and IMRT—the radiation source for both radiotherapy and CT imaging can move completely around the patient in a helical arc. CT scans performed immediately before treatment. Highly conformal and precise, conformal avoidance of normal tissue but slower than VMAT. No comparison studies available currently
Volumetric modulated arc radiotherapy (VMAT, e.g., RapidArc®)	Type of IMRT using rotational (arc) delivery. The angle of the beam, the dose rate and the leaf speed are all independently controlled, making this a very accurate form of treatment. Arc therapy treatments also take much less time to deliver than other radiotherapy techniques
Image guided radiotherapy (IGRT)	Refers to any mode of radiotherapy where imaging of the tumor is performed during treatment to ensure treatment precision. Could be between several fractions, immediately prior to each dose (e.g., tomotherapy), or in real-time (e.g., CyberKnife radiosurgery)
Photon (X-ray) radiosurgery	
Gamma Knife®	Use multileaf collimator in a helmet attached to a stereotactic head frame allowing multiple small beams to deliver high dose to small target small deep lesions
Frame-based Linac	Uses stereotactic head frame to and multileaf collimator in the linac radiosurgery machine (with a moving arm)
Frameless Linac (CyberKnife® Robotic Radiosurgery)	Uses a moving couch and a small linear accelerator on a robotic arm to deliver multiple beams of radiation from different angles. It works best on small tumors with well-defined edges. Due to real-time image-guidance it can also adjust the delivery, for example to match the patient's breathing motion
Fractionated stereotactic radiotherapy	Combines the similar dose conformality, precise dose delivery, and steep dose falloff outside the target volume of stereotactic radiosurgery with the radiobiologic advantages of dose fractionation. Fractionation safely treats larger tumor volumes intimate to critical structures such as the optic apparatus
Particle (Hadron) radiosurgery	
Proton beam therapy	Protons deliver a dose of radiation in a much more confined way to the tumor tissue than photons (X-rays, gamma rays). After they enter the body, protons release most of their energy within the tumor region and, unlike photons, deliver only a minimal dose beyond the tumor boundaries. Therefore, especially for smaller tumor sizes, the dose of radiation may conform much tighter to the tumor and there may be less damage to healthy tissue. In particular its use in young children has been increasing, especially where conventional radiotherapy may be contraindicated due to its effects on CNS development
Fast-neutron therapy	Theoretical advantage over photons in low-oxygen (hypoxic) conditions, but interest in the use of neutron therapy has waned because it has shown no advantages in terms of outcome over irradiation with other types of particles
Carbon-ion therapy	Combines the dose-distribution advantages of protons with an increase in biologic effectiveness toward the end of the particle range
Boron-neutron capture therapy	Clinical studies undergoing in recurrent malignant gliomas

CHAPTER 16

NEUROPSYCHOLOGY AND NEUROLOGICAL REHABILITATION

SINGLE BEST ANSWER (SBA) QUESTIONS

1. A 63-year-old male presents as a World Federation of Neurosurgical Societies (WFNS) grade III subarachnoid hemorrhage and undergoes coiling of a basilar tip aneurysm. After a prolonged Intensive Care Unit (ICU) stay, he is ready to be discharged from the ward. He is able to walk with assistance and needs help with toileting and showering. What are his modified Rankin and Glasgow Outcome Scale scores respectively?
   a. mRS 2 and GOS 2
   b. mRS 2 and GOS 3
   c. mRS 3 and GOS 2
   d. mRS 3 and GOS 3
   e. mRS 4 and GOS 3
   f. mRS 4 and GOS 4

2. Which one of the following Karnofsky performance scores is commonly used as a cutoff for functional independence in neuro-oncology?
   a. 40
   b. 50
   c. 60
   d. 70
   e. 80

3. Cerebellar mutism occurs most commonly after resection of which one of the following posterior fossa tumors in children?
   a. Ependymoma
   b. Hemangioblastoma
   c. Medulloblastoma
   d. Meningioma
   e. Pilocytic astrocytoma

4. Cerebellar cognitive affective syndrome does not generally involve which one of the following?
   a. Dysprosodia
   b. Impaired executive function
   c. Mutism
   d. Personality change
   e. Visuospatial impairment

5. Which one of the following domains of cognitive impairment in normal pressure hydrocephalus is LEAST likely to improve with shunt insertion?
   a. Delayed verbal recall
   b. Frontal lobe executive function
   c. Psychomotor speed
   d. Visual memory
   e. Visuoconstructional abilities

6. Which one of the following statements regarding cognitive decline following cranial irradiation for brain metastasis is most accurate?
   a. There is no difference in cognitive decline at 12 months post Whole Brain Radiotherapy (WBRT) compared to controls
   b. There is a greater cognitive decline at 12 months in patients with Stereotactic Radiosurgery (SRS) + WBRT compared to SRS alone
   c. There is a greater cognitive decline at 12 months in SRS alone compared to WBRT alone
   d. There is no difference in cognitive decline at 12 months in patients with SRS + WBRT compared to SRS alone
   e. There is no increase in cognitive decline at 12 months in those receiving 36 Gy of irradiation compared to 25 Gy

7. Which one of the following statements regarding cognitive outcome in aneurysmal subarachnoid hemorrhage in those patients treated with clipping versus those treated with coiling is most accurate?
   a. Cognitive outcomes are poorer in the coiling group overall
   b. Cognitive outcomes are poorer in the clipping group overall
   c. Coiling may offer a superior cognitive outcome in the short term and clipping the superior cognitive outcome in the long term
   d. Cognitive outcomes are poorer in the clipping group for anterior circulation aneurysms

e. Coiling may offer an inferior cognitive outcome in the short term and clipping the inferior cognitive outcome in the long term

8. Which one of the following statements regarding return to work in aneurysmal subarachnoid hemorrhage is most accurate?
   a. Return to previous occupation is approximately 30% in aneurysmal subarachnoid hemorrhage
   b. Return to previous occupation is approximately 40% in aneurysmal subarachnoid hemorrhage
   c. Return to previous occupation is approximately 50% in aneurysmal subarachnoid hemorrhage
   d. Return to previous occupation is approximately 60% in aneurysmal subarachnoid hemorrhage
   e. Return to previous occupation is approximately 70% in aneurysmal subarachnoid hemorrhage

9. Which one of the following is currently seen as the best marker of severity of traumatic brain injury in survivors?
   a. Glasgow coma score
   b. Length of coma
   c. Mechanism of injury
   d. Initial CT scan
   e. Post-traumatic amnesia

10. Neurorehabiliation in the context of stroke is characterized by which one of the following?
   a. Baclofen for dyskinesias resulting from basal ganglia strokes
   b. Botulinum toxin injections to facilitate physiotherapy to the paretic limb (s)
   c. Management in local hospitals by general medical teams to maximize family support in the acute stage
   d. Outpatient management
   e. Task-oriented therapy

11. Neurorehabiliation in the context of spinal cord injury has all of the following goals EXCEPT:
   a. Ensure that required adaptations and equipment are identified and provided
   b. Management of excretion from bowels and bladder
   c. Minimize the risk of preventable complications (e.g. pressure sores)
   d. Recognition and management of autonomic dysreflexia
   e. Routine recruitment into neural stem cell transplantation trials for spinal cord injury

EXTENDED MATCHING ITEM (EMI) QUESTIONS

12. **Neuropsychological tests:**
   a. Affect and personality
   b. Attention
   c. Effort (embedded and free-standing)
   d. Executive functions
   e. Language
   f. Memory
   g. Motor processing
   h. Visuospatial and visuomotor processing

For each of the following descriptions, select the most appropriate answers from the list above. Each answer may be used once, more than once or not at all.
   1. Wisconsin card sorting test
   2. Beck depression inventory
   3. Finger oscillation test

SBA ANSWERS

1. **e**—mRS 4 and GOS 3

mRS	Description
0	No symptoms at all
1	No significant disability despite symptoms; able to carry out all usual duties and activities
2	Slight disability; unable to carry out all previous activities, but able to look after own affairs without consequence
3	Moderate disability; requiring some help but able to walk without assistance
4	Moderately severe disability; unable to walk without assistance and unable to attend to own bodily needs without assistance
5	Severe disability; bedridden, incontinent, and requiring constant nursing care and attention
6	Death

GOS	Term	Definition
1	Dead	No life
2	Vegetative state	Unaware of self and environment
3	Severe disability	Unable to live independently
4	Moderate disability	Able to live independently
5	Mild disability	Able to return to work/ school

2. **d**—70

KPS	Description
100	Normal
90	Capable of normal activity, few symptoms
80	Normal activity with some difficulty, some symptoms
70	Cares for self, cannot work, no normal activity
60	Requires some help, can do most of personal care
50	Requires help often and frequent medical support
40	Disabled, requires special care and help
30	Severely disabled, may need hospital but no risk of death
20	Very ill, requires urgent treatment
10	Moribund, rapidly fatal disease process
0	Dead

3. **c**—Medulloblastoma

Cerebellar mutism is a distinct clinical syndrome described following surgery for posterior fossa tumors both in adults and children but most commonly in children. Its incidence varies from 2% to 40% in different series, particularly with vermian location of the lesion—hence its occurrence particularly after medulloblastoma resection. It consists of diminished speech output, hypotonia, ataxia, and emotional lability. Typically a patient who is initially fine in the first few days postoperatively develops mutism without any corresponding focal neurological signs. The deficit usually recovers with time over a period of a few weeks to 6 months with an immediate return of full words and sentences. Resolution of the muteness is often followed by a period of dysarthria, and more recent studies have demonstrated that persistent impairment of motor speech is common and complete recovery of speech and language is infrequent. The underlying neuroanatomical locus may be the dentatothalamocortical outflow tracts from the cerebellar nuclei through the brainstem.

FURTHER READING

Charalambides C, Dinopoulos A, Sgouros S. Neuropsychological sequelae and quality of life following treatment of posterior fossa ependymomas in children. Childs Nerv Syst 2009;25(10):1313-20.

4. **c**–Mutism

The cerebellum is divided into three parts, based on the arrangement of the afferent fiber projection: the vestibulocerebellum (equilibrium and eye movements), the spinocerebellum (posture, muscle tone, and execution of limb movements), and the pontocerebellum (coordination of skilled movements initiated at a cerebral cortical level). More recently there has been growing appreciation that cerebellar damage can produce cognitive deficits. In patients with right cerebellar injury linguistic processing was impaired, while left cerebellar injury produced visual-spatial defects were noted. Neurpsychological studies have identified a cerebellar cognitive affective syndrome, predominantly in adults:

- Impairments of executive function
- Visual-spatial disorganization and impaired visual- spatial memory
- Personality change with blunting of affect or disinhibited and inappropriate behavior
- Difficulties with language production including dysprosodia, agrammatism, and mild anomia

Mutism is considered to be part of the initial presentation of many children with cerebellar cognitive affective syndrome, but is less common in adults. The major distinction between the two is the chronicity of the symptoms with cerebellar mutism being more transient.

FURTHER READING

Steinlin M, Imfeld S, Zulauf P, Boltshauser E, Lövblad KO, Ridolfi Lüthy A, Perrig W, Kaufmann F. Neuropsychological long-term sequelae after posterior fossa tumour resection during childhood. Brain 2003;126(Pt 9):1998-2008.

5. **b**—Frontal lobe executive function

FURTHER READING

Devito EE, Pickard JD, Salmond CH, Iddon JL, Loveday C, Sahakian BJ. The neuropsychology of normal pressure hydrocephalus (NPH). Br J Neurosurg 2005;19(3):217-24.

6. **b**—There is a greater cognitive decline at 12 months in patients with SRS+WBRT compared to SRS alone

The efficacy of WBRT for treatment of cerebral metastasis is well documented but the establishment of SRS for high precision delivery of radiation has questioned its necessity. Given that survival is comparable between the two modalities, the controversy centers on cognitive and neurological preservation. Supporters of SRS point to evidence suggesting that focal radiation is highly effective in preventing tumor progression in the irradiated volume and that irradiation of normal or near-normal brain tissue increases the risk of cognitive decline in a brain that is already burdened with disease. Equally, proponents of WBRT argue that focal radiation does not address potential micrometastatic foci that are invisible to conventional imaging which, in the absence of radiation treatment, can develop into larger lesions that compromises the patient's neurological and cognitive function. Ultimately, the debate revolves around the trade-off between preserving the function of cerebrum that is not grossly infiltrated with tumor and the harmful effect of tumor growth from micrometastatic foci. In summary:

- Cognitive impairment at 12 months is 12% in control and 41% in prophylactic cranial irradiation (30 Gy)
- Cognitive impairment at 12 months is 62% for 25 Gy and 85% for 36 Gy prophylactic irradiation
- Cognitive impairment at 4 months is 24% in SRS alone vs 52% in SRS+WBRT

FURTHER READING

McDuff SG, Taich ZJ, Lawson JD, et al. Neurocognitive assessment following whole brain radiation therapy and radiosurgery for patients with cerebral metastases. J Neurol Neurosurg Psychiatry 2013;84(12):1384-91.

7. **e**–Coiling may offer an inferior cognitive outcome in the short term and clipping the inferior cognitive outcome in the long term

The majority of studies suggest that clipped versus coiled patients do not differ in the main domains of cognitive and functional outcome. Some (non-randomized) studies suggest a poorer outcome with clipping at 1 year, with greater imaging evidence of focal encephalomalacia and infarction compared to coiled patients. Equally, some studies have shown poorer cognitive function in coiled patients compared to clipped patients at 4-6 months. Further studies/longer term follow up is needed, but each may have different effects on cognitive outcome at different time points since treatment.

FURTHER READING

Al-Khindi T, Macdonald RL, Schweizer TA. Cognitive and functional outcome after aneurysmal subarachnoid hemorrhage. Stroke 2010;41(8):e519-36.

8. **d**–Return to previous occupation is approximately 60% in aneurysmal subarachnoid hemorrhage

FURTHER READING

Al-Khindi T, Macdonald RL, Schweizer TA. Cognitive and functional outcome after aneurysmal subarachnoid hemorrhage. Stroke 2010;41(8):e519-36.

9. **e**—Post-traumatic amnesia

Post traumatic amnesia represents the length of time from injury until return of orientation and continuous memory for events. Its duration has been associated with presence or extent of skull fracture, intracranial hemorrhage, raised intracranial pressure, residual neurological deficits, extent of neuropathology, as well as with longer-term functional outcomes and return to employment. Recent studies investigating individuals surviving to discharge from hospital provide support for post traumatic amnesia as a stronger predictor of longer-term functional outcome, return to employment, and cognitive impairment than Glasgow Coma Score (GCS) or length of coma. It also accounts for more variance in outcome than socio-demographic factors.

FURTHER READING

Ponsford J, Spitz G, McKenzie D. Using post-traumatic amnesia to predict outcome following traumatic brain injury. J Neurotrauma 2015.

10. **e**—Task oriented therapy

The main principles underlying stroke rehabilitation are as follows:

- The patient should be under the care of a specialist stroke rehabilitation unit whilst in hospital, and a specialist stroke rehabilitation service when back in the community.
- Therapy should be task oriented (i.e. practicing an activity is the best way to improve at that activity).
- The patient should be set both short- and long-term goals, and those goals should be relatively challenging and set at the level of activities or social participation.

11. **e**—Routine recruitment into neural stem cell transplantation trials for SCI

Rehabilitation has several general goals in SCI:
- It should aim to minimize the risk of all preventable complications, including through patient education.
- Teach the patient how to manage their impairments and it needs to ensure that all required adaptations and equipment are identified and provided.
- It may need to teach others how to provide additional support to the patient if necessary. In general patients with lesions below the cervical level of the spinal cord can live fully independently, whereas patients with cervical spinal-cord lesions will need assistance to a greater or lesser extent.
- In patients with spinal cord injury particular attention needs to be paid to the management of excretion from bowels and bladder, sexual function, and skin care.
- Medical recognition and management of autonomic dysreflexia (e.g. treat urinary retention, blood pressure control with immediate nifedipine).

EMI ANSWERS

12. 1—d: Executive function, 2—a: Affect and personality, 3—g: Motor processing

A single neuropsychological test may assess multiple domains of neuropsychological performance, hence they may be performed as part of a fixed (e.g. Halstead-Reitan) or flexible battery. Advantages of the fixed battery approach to neuropsychological assessment include: (1) it provides a comprehensive assessment of multiple cognitive domains; and (2) it uses a standardized format that allows the test data to be incorporated into databases for clinical and scientific analysis. Disadvantages of the fixed battery approach include (1) time and labor intensiveness; and (2) a lack of flexibility in different clinical situations; specifically, multiple, nonequivalent data sets exist and specific normative data with TBI patients should be used with caution. Primary advantages of the flexible approach to neuropsychological evaluation include: (1) a potentially shorter administration time; (2) economical favorability; and (3) adaptability to differing patient situations and needs. Disadvantages of the flexible approach include: (1) the need for greater clinical experience; (2) a lack of standardized administration rules for some tests; (3) a potential lack of comprehensiveness; and (4) limitations in establishing systematic databases. A non-exhaustive list of commonly used tests is shown below:

Attention	Trail Making Test, Stroop Test, Digit span (Wechsler Adult Intelligence Scale III and Wechsler Memory Scale III)
Memory	Wechsler Memory Scale III, Rey-Osterrieth Complex Figure Test, California Verbal Learning Test-II, Rey Auditory-Verbal Learning Test
Executive functions	Wisconsin Card Sorting Test, Trail Making Test, Stroop Test, Category Test
Language	Boston Diagnostic Aphasia Examination, Reiten-Indiana Aphasia Screening Test, Word fluency
Visuospatial and visuomotor processing	Facial Recognition Test, Rey-Osterrieth Complex Figure Test
Motor processing	Finger oscillation test, Grooved Pegboard test
Affect and personality	Beck Depression and Anxiety Inventories
Effort (imbedded and free-standing)	Word memory test, tests of memory malingering, dot counting test

FURTHER READING

Podell K, Gifford K, Bougakov D, Goldberg E. Neuropsychological assessment in traumatic brain injury. Psychiatr Clin North Am 2010;33(4):855-76.

CHAPTER 17

Statistics

Chapter available on ExpertConsult.com

CHAPTER 18

PROFESSIONALISM AND MEDICAL ETHICS

SINGLE BEST ANSWER (SBA) QUESTIONS

1. Which one of the following is NOT a required component for assessing an individual's capacity to make a specific treatment decision?
   a. Understand the information
   b. Retain the information for long enough to be able to make the decision
   c. Use or weigh up the information to make the decision
   d. Communicate their decision
   e. Make a rational decision

2. An 8-year-old boy requires a posterior fossa craniotomy for a space occupying lesion. His parents consent to the treatment plan. Which one of the following would you try to establish with respect to the child himself?
   a. Informed consent
   b. Informed assent
   c. Parens patriae
   d. Gillick competence
   e. Coercion

3. A 61-year-old male is admitted with a right frontal space occupying lesion, consistent with a glioblastoma multiforme. His imaging shows a significant amount of edema and midline shift and he is started on high-dose dexamethasone. He is confused with a mild left hemiparesis. His family arrive a few hours later, and you explain that he will need an operation and that the mass is probably cancerous. As you take them back to his bedside, they ask you not to tell their father about the likely diagnosis. Which one of the following principles would be most compromised by operating on him at this point in time?
   a. Autonomy
   b. Non-maleficence
   c. Justice
   d. Beneficence
   e. Futility

4. A 31-year-old female who has been treated for recurrent cerebral metastases from breast cancer presents with multiple new cerebral lesions, including several radiation necrosis lesions from previous radiosurgery. She is mildly drowsy but understands her situation and is competent to make decisions regarding her care. During the consultation palliative care is discussed, but her husband demands that she be treated with any available life prolonging treatment. She says she doesn't want to go through it any more, to which he responds by threatening to leave her if she is just going to give up. Which one of the following principles is potentially at risk in this situation?
   a. Capacity
   b. Voluntariness
   c. Disclosure of relevant information
   d. Authorization
   e. Justice

5. Which one of the following is/are NOT part of the four principles of biomedical ethics?
   a. Autonomy
   b. Utilitarianism
   c. Beneficence
   d. Non-maleficence
   e. Justice

6. A mother does not want her son, a 12-year-old bright, good athlete without neurological deficits, to know that his cerebellar astrocytoma has only been partially removed. She thinks that knowing this fact would place her son in emotional jeopardy, because a second procedure could diminish his sporting abilities. Over time, the follow-up MRI showed a slow but clear progress of the tumor requiring further surgery. Which one of the following ethical principles are most relevant?
   a. Autonomy and beneficence
   b. Beneficence and justice
   c. Autonomy and justice
   d. Justice and non-maleficence
   e. Autonomy and non-maleficence

7. A 45-year-old female presents with WFNS grade I subarachnoid hemorrhage on evening. Vascular imaging reveals a 1.2 cm left supraclinoid internal carotid artery aneurysm. The operating neurosurgeon specializes in functional neurosurgery and elects to perform a clipping the following morning as there is no aneurysm surgeon available for a further 36 h. During the dissection around the aneurysm, an intraoperative rupture occurs and the surgeon struggles to obtain proximal control leading to intraoperative hypotension from blood loss and prolonged cerebral ischemia from temporary clipping. Postoperatively the patient wakes up on the neurointensive care unit with complete hemiplegia and global aphasia. Which one of the following factors is LEAST relevant to this surgical complication?
   a. Task factors
   b. Individual factors
   c. Team factors
   d. Patient factors
   e. Organizational factors
   f. Situational factors

8. A 34-year-old woman has a long history of epilepsy since the age of 24. She only has seizures when she sleeps, and her last seizure was 3 weeks ago. She is known to be compliant with every medication she's been given. She retains the driving license which she applied for last year. Which one of the following is most accurate?
   a. She must stop driving because her seizures are not well controlled
   b. She may be able to continue driving as her seizures only occur during sleep
   c. She must stop driving immediately as she has not been seizure free for 1 year
   d. The doctor must inform the DVLA and stop her driving
   e. She must give up driving indefinitely

9. A 7-year-old boy presents with a reduced GCS and CT head scan shows significant intraventricular hemorrhage and hydrocephalus. You discuss the imaging and the plan for an emergency external ventricular drain with the father but he is not willing to proceed if there is any chance his son will be left a "vegetable." What is the next step in management?
   a. Call social services
   b. Obtain a court order to proceed with surgery
   c. Do not perform surgery as lacking parental consent
   d. Proceed to surgery in the best interests of the child
   e. Keep the child sedated and ventilated on NICU until consent is gained

UK-SPECIFIC QUESTIONS

10. Which one of the following is NOT required for a valid advanced decision?
   a. Mental capacity present when made
   b. It applies to the situation where it is being considered
   c. You must be aged 25 or over
   d. Must be signed by you and a witness if you wish to refuse life-sustaining treatments
   e. Must have been made without harassment by anyone else

11. Frasier guidelines are best described as clarifying circumstances surrounding which one of the following?
   a. Competence of a child to consent to medical treatment without parental involvement
   b. Competence of a child to consent to mental health disorder treatment without parental involvement
   c. Competence of a child to consent to contraceptive advice and treatment without parental involvement
   d. Competence of a child to withhold consent to medical treatment without parental involvement
   e. Competence of a child to withhold consent to mental health disorder treatment without parental involvement

12. You are a junior doctor in the Emergency Department (ED). A 5-year-old boy who has been in ED four times previously this year with several episodes of trauma that did not seem related. Today, the child is brought with a complaint of "slipping into a hot bathtub" with a small burn wound on his lower leg. Which one of the following would you do next?
   a. Admit the child to remove him from possibly dangerous environment
   b. Phone the patient's family doctor
   c. Report your concerns to the local social services
   d. Accept the parent's explanation
   e. Ask the parent whether there has been any abuse

13. A 14-year-old boy presents with precocious puberty and headaches. Cranial imaging reveals a pineal region mass with hydrocephalus. An endoscopic third ventriculostomy is planned and discussed with the family, but the boy refuses to have the operation. He is aware that without surgery, death is likely.

What is the next appropriate step in management?
a. Gain parental consent and proceed to surgery
b. Apply to High Court for wardship
c. Respect the boy's decision and do not operate
d. Proceed to treat in best interests under Mental Capacity Act 2005
e. Call child protection services

14. A 7-year-old boy is a Jehovah's Witness and was involved in a RTA (road traffic accident). He is in hemorrhagic shock and requires emergency blood transfusion but his mother refuses to give parental consent. Which one of the following is the most appropriate next step?
a. Call child protection services
b. Give blood anyway as this is an emergency situation
c. Do not give blood transfusion due to lack of parental consent
d. Contact the courts by telephone
e. Get advice from the Hospital Liaison Committee for Jehovah's Witnesses

15. A 16-year-old girl is a Jehovah's Witness. She refuses a lifesaving blood transfusion. She is aware of and understands the consequences. What is the next step in management?
a. Gain parental consent to give blood
b. Give blood anyway as it is an emergency situation
c. Give blood anyway as she is not competent
d. Do not give blood transfusion but involve courts
e. Call child protection

16. Hilary is a 30-year-old schizophrenic patient. She has an abscess in her chest. But she is refusing treatment for it. She is also refusing to take her medication for schizophrenia for the last 2 weeks. She is thought to have full capacity, and understands the effects and consequences of not being treated for her chest abscess or taking any antipsychotic medication. Which one of the following is true?
a. She can be detained for treatment of both her abscess and her schizophrenia
b. She can be detained for treatment of her abscess only
c. She can be detained for treatment of her mental health disorder only
d. She cannot be detained as she is competent
e. She cannot have capacity as she has a mental health disorder

17. A 44-year-old victim of a car accident with a severe closed head injury was admitted to the ICU. The patient rapidly deteriorated and was declared brain dead within 24 h. He is not on the organ donor register. Which one of the following statements is most accurate?
a. It is not possible for others to consent on behalf of a deceased patient
b. Organ donation is not valid if the potential donor is not on the register
c. It is not possible for children to consent to organ donation even if they are Gillick competent
d. Organ donation is not an option in this situation
e. Family members cannot legally veto organ donation if the patient is on the organ donor register

18. Disclosure of confidential information without patient consent may occur under certain circumstances. Which one of the following is unlikely to meet the criteria for such disclosure?
a. Discussion with a competent patient's family member
b. Terrorist act
c. Notifiable infectious disease
d. Criminal act
e. Significant risk of harm to others

US-SPECIFIC QUESTIONS

19. Which one of the following remains valid when the principal dies?
a. Durable power of attorney
b. Ordinary power of attorney
c. Specific powers of attorney
d. General powers of attorney
e. Last will and testament

20. A patient under your care recently diagnosed with glioblastoma multiforme and undergone gross total resection has threatened to seriously harm their partner, who he believes is having an affair. He is being discharged today, but as you leave the room to seek advice from another colleague regarding his comments you turn to see him place a large serrated kitchen knife into his bag. Which one of the following may become relevant?
a. Tarasoff decision
b. Doctrine of double effect
c. Waiver
d. Virtuism
e. Categorical imperative

21. In the USA, the Emergency Medical Treatment and Active Labor Act makes all of the provisions except for which one of the following?
   a. Transfer of a stable patient for non-emergency care
   b. Right to request a medical screening examination to exclude an emergency medical condition
   c. Transfer of an unstable patient when the treating physician feels the benefits outweigh the risks
   d. Treatment of an emergency medical condition until it is resolved or stabilized
   e. Duty to report inappropriate transfers

22. In those aged under 18 years, which one of the following circumstances would parental consent for treatment still usually be required?
   a. Emancipated minor
   b. Decision regarding birth control
   c. Decision regarding substance abuse treatment
   d. Decision regarding a life or limb-threatening conditions
   e. Decision regarding tethered cord release

EXTENDED MATCHING ITEM (EMI) QUESTIONS

23. **Ethical concepts:**
   a. Autonomy
   b. A positive right
   c. A negative right
   d. Beneficence
   e. A categorical imperative
   f. Justice
   g. Non-maleficence
   h. Virtue ethics
   i. Futility
   j. Utilitarianism

For each of the following descriptions, select the most appropriate answers from the list above. Each answer may be used once, more than once or not at all.

1. The principle of doing good or improving the welfare of patients.
2. The idea that we should create laws that maximize benefit.
3. Respecting decisions made by those capable of making decisions.

24. **Consent:**
   a. Written consent
   b. Valid consent
   c. Invalid consent
   d. Implied consent
   e. Valid advance directive
   f. Invalid advance directive
   g. Gillick competence
   h. Assent
   i. Dissent
   j. Competence
   k. Capacity

For each of the following descriptions, select the most appropriate answers from the list above. Each answer may be used once, more than once or not at all.

1. Doctor tells patient they need a blood test and patient holds out arm and rolls up sleeve.
2. On the insistence of a close relative, an 80-year-old man with advanced dementia signs a form stating he does not want medical treatment if he becomes unwell.
3. A patient with learning difficulties who is unable to read or write has the nature and purpose of a lumbar puncture explained to him in terms which he can understand and agrees to be treated.

25. **Medically assisted dying:**
   a. Suicide
   b. Physician-assisted suicide
   c. Murder
   d. Attempted murder
   e. Voluntary euthanasia
   f. Non-voluntary euthanasia
   g. Involuntary euthanasia
   h. Doctrine of double effect

For each of the following descriptions, select the most appropriate answers from the list above. Each answer may be used once, more than once or not at all.

1. Deliberately ending the life of a person who is incapable of expressing any wishes about whether they want to live or die, motivated by a consideration of that person's best interests.
2. Deliberately ending the life of an elderly person who is gravely ill to make the hospital bed available who can get more use of it.
3. A competent, able bodied person has a progressive illness which will render her incapable at a later stage. She seeks medical assistance for medication with which she may end her own life.
4. A competent patient who is in pain and distress but unable to take his own life asks his doctor to administer a lethal injection.
5. A doctor increases the dosage of painkillers/sedation, at appropriate levels to control symptoms in the knowledge that this may

have a life shortening side effect. The doctor is adamant that she only intends the pain-killing effect of the medication and not side effect.

26. **Ethical theory:**
    a. Altruism
    b. Aristotelian justice
    c. Communitarianism
    d. Consequentialism
    e. Deontology
    f. Hippocratic oath
    g. Libertarianism
    h. Principalism
    i. Utilitarianism
    j. Virtuism

For each of the following descriptions, select the most appropriate answers from the list above. Each answer may be used once, more than once or not at all.

1. To treat equals equally and unequals unequally according to morally relevant inequality.
2. The right not to be killed and to possess property.
3. Take from each according to ability and give to each according to need.
4. A rational person who makes a decision behind a veil of ignorance will look after the least well off.
5. Act to maximize welfare for the greatest number at the least cost.

SBA ANSWERS

1. **e**—Make a rational decision

A lack of capacity can be permanent or temporary and should be assessed in relation to a specific decision to be made. A person with the capacity to consent to therapy should be able to understand the relevant information (treatments purpose, nature, likely effects and risks, chances of success and alternatives to the proposed treatment), retain the information, weigh up the information to make a decision and be able to communicate it in some way. In the UK, the Mental Capacity Act 2005 a might be used to give treatment for physical health problems to someone aged over 16 years who lacks capacity in their best interests (e.g., because of a mental illness, dementia, learning difficulties, unwell).

2. **b**—Informed assent

Historically, children have been thought to lack capacity and are hence unable to provide consent on their own. Typically, decisions were made by their surrogate, usually a parent or guardian, and often without the input of the child. More recently, developmentally capable minors can be allowed to consent on their own, and those without the developmental capacity still participate in the process of decision-making through assent. The American Academy of Pediatrics issued a policy statement in 1995 on assent that should be followed where possible. The process of assent involves (1) helping the child achieve a developmentally appropriate awareness of the nature of his/her condition, (2) telling the child what they can expect from tests and treatments, (3) assessing the child's understanding of the situation and the factors influencing how they are responding, and (4) soliciting an expression of the child's willingness to accept the proposed care. In other jurisdictions (e.g., England, Australia, Canada), this presumption may be rebutted through proof that the minor is "mature" (e.g., "Gillick competent" in the UK) although it is still good practice to also seek parental consent/agreement. Although there is no lower age limit defined for which a child can be deemed Gillick competent, it is unlikely to apply for children under 13 years old. In cases of incompetent minors, informed consent is usually required from a person with parental responsibility. If the person with parental responsibility refuses to consent for a specific treatment and is deemed negligent, medical treatments can be given in the best interests of the child in emergencies or the treating team can make an application to the High Court which can exercise its power as *parens patriae* (legal protector of citizens unable to protect themselves) by making the child a ward of the Court, such that it takes on the responsibility for consenting for the child.

FURTHER READING

American Academy of Pediatrics, Committee on Bioethics. Informed consent, parental permission, and assent in pediatric practice. J Pediatr 1995;102:169–76.

Gillick v. West Norfolk and Wisbech Area Health Authority [1986] AC 112.

3. **a**—Autonomy

This case highlights challenges to the consent process often seen in neurosurgical patients. Firstly, his capacity to make autonomous decisions is compromised because of the effects of his tumor. Therefore, the immediacy of the clinical situation will dictate whether we can afford to wait and see if he regains capacity after a period of dexamethasone treatment or if a surrogate decision maker (e.g., partner, family member) is consulted about what they think the patient would request to have done if they had the capacity. Second, the family has asked that information be withheld from the patient. In a patient with competence or capacity, the withholding of information does not allow the patient to make an informed decision hence any subsequent consent cannot be valid. For patients, full disclosure of relevant information (including risks and benefits) is a right but not a duty—they may not wish to have this information disclosed to them. In this situation they are effectively waiving their right to consent (as valid consent must be informed)—hence it must be well documented and reasons explored. In the case above, while it may be reasonable to withhold certain information while he remains confused, if he regains capacity before any planned operation then an attempt to get informed consent must be made.

FURTHER READING

McDonald P. Informed consent (chapter). In: Ammar A, Bernstein M (Eds.), Neurosurgical Ethics in Practice: Value-Based Medicine. Springer, 2014, p. 54.

4. **b**—Voluntariness

An action such as consenting to a treatment is considered voluntary if it is undertaken freely, without undue influence or coercion from others. However, medical decisions are almost always influenced by the opinion of doctors, family, friends, and past experience or knowledge. Identifying the difference between persuasion which is allowable and under certain circumstance perhaps even obligatory (e.g., if a particular option is clearly in the best interests of a particular patient), and the coercion demonstrated in the husband's threat to leave her if she doesn't want to keep going is key to maximizing patient autonomy.

FURTHER READING

McDonald P. Informed consent. In: Ammar A, Bernstein M (Eds.), Neurosurgical Ethics in Practice: Value-Based Medicine. Springer, 2014, p. 57.

5. **b**—Utilitarianism

There are four principles widely used as a framework for analyzing ethical problems. The four principles must be applied in the appropriate context and should have equal importance (allowing conflicts to arise). They are:

- Autonomy—freedom of the patient to choose and be an advocate for their own health.
- Beneficence—what is considered to be of the patient's best interest.
- Non-maleficence—the harm that may come to a patient because of a specific decision/treatment ("first do no harm").
- Justice—the legal aspects that impact upon the ethical scenarios.

6. **a**—Autonomy and beneficence

When parents request information to be kept from their children, it may be legally permissible, but at the same time compromises the right of the child to autonomy. Therefore, a careful assessment of the following aspects is obligatory:

(1) The ability of the minor to fully understand the situation and to anticipate and evaluate future consequences.
(2) Whether the parental surrogate decision-making is in the best interests of the child or is it obstructing beneficence.

After assessment of these aspects, it is the duty of the physician to form a personal opinion (with help from ombudsmen or other authoritative persons or bodies, as needed), based on the concept of beneficence, and to try to act accordingly to work with the parents to take the right approach.

FURTHER READING

Tan TC, Ammar A. Privacy and confidentiality. In: Ammar A, Bernstein M (Eds.), Neurosurgical Ethics in Practice: Value-Based Medicine. Springer, 2014, p. 63.

Task factors	Clear protocol, information, omission of necessary steps
Individual factors	Mental readiness, technical performance, fatigue
Team factors	Effective communication, leadership, confidence, ability to manage unexpected events
Patient factors	Obesity, anatomical variations, severity of disease, comorbidities
Organizational factors	Appropriate staff, equipment, scheduling/timing of procedure, substitution of team members
Situational factors	Distractions, interruptions, poor equipment design

See Ammar A, Bernstein M. Neurosurgical Ethics in Practice: Value-Based Medicine. Springer.

7. **f**—Situational factors
8. **b**—She may be able to continue driving because she only has sleep seizures

When patients have their first seizure, they should inform the licensing agency and must stop driving. In this case, patient has been diagnosed with epilepsy for at least 10 years and during that time she is only known to have seizures during her sleep. She is also very compliant with her doctor's treatments. Given she has reapplied for the license recently, the licensing agency may be satisfied she does not pose any danger to the public.

UK REGULATIONS KEY POINTS (WWW.EPILEPSY.ORG.UK)

Group 1 Licence (Cars)

- Awake seizures affecting consciousness: allowed when 12 months seizure free after most recent seizure
- Awake seizures not impairing consciousness: allowed if in the last 12 months you have only had seizures which do not affect your consciousness OR if you have only ever had seizures not affecting your consciousness
- Sleep seizure(s): allowed if seizure free or only having sleep seizures for 12 months (and never had seizures while awake) OR awake seizures in the past but only sleep seizures for last 3 years
- Isolated seizure (after being seizure free for 5 years): allowed after 6 months seizure freedom if neurologist thinks another seizure is unlikely and deemed not a risk to the public
- Provoked seizure (e.g., eclamptic, neurosurgery, TIA/stroke): assessed on individual basis

Group 2 Licence (HGV, Minibus, etc.)

- If you have had two or more seizures to regain group 2 entitlements you need to have regained your group 1 licence AND been seizure free for 10 years AND not taken epilepsy medication in the last 10 years
- If you have had 1 isolated seizure the same rules usually apply, but you may be able to regain it if you have been seizure free for 5 years AND off epilepsy medication for 5 years AND assessed as fit to drive by a neurologist
- If you have had a provoked seizure you will be assessed individually

Driving During Antiepileptic Withdrawal/Change

- Change: advised by doctor if need to stop driving and for how long, no need to inform DVLA or return license
- Withdrawal: stop driving during period of withdrawal and for 6 months after

US REGULATIONS (VARIABLE DEPENDING ON STATE; ADAPTED FROM WWW.EPILEPSY.COM)

Ordinary Driver's Licence

Allowed if free of seizures that affect consciousness for a certain period of time, often at least 1 year. Recently, shorter intervals of seizure freedom are being required, for example 3-6 months

Physician usually fills out a form with the date of last seizure, seizure type, and other relevant information. Some states ask for the doctor's recommendation about the person's ability to drive while others leave this to the Department of Motor Vehicles (DVM)

Review and Decision Process

In most states, the medical information and license application is reviewed by the state's DMV. In complex cases, or when the decision is not clear, information is forwarded to a consulting doctor or the state's medical advisory board

Commercial Driver's Licenses

Allowed in people with a history of epilepsy/seizures who have been seizure-free off medication for 10 years

Personal Liability

A person with epilepsy may be civilly or criminally liable for a motor vehicle accident caused by seizures. Liability may occur when a person drives against medical advice, without a valid license, without notifying the state department of motor vehicles of the medical condition, or with the knowledge that he or she is prohibited from driving

See Nashef L, Capovilla G, Camfield C, Camfield P, Nabbout R. Transition: driving and exercise. Epilepsia 2014;55 (Suppl. 3):41–5.

9. **d**—Proceed to surgery as in best interests of the child

In an emergency where you consider that it is the child's best interests to proceed, you may treat the child, provided it is limited to that treatment which is reasonably required in that emergency. Therefore, in this case, the surgery should be performed. In the UK this is governed by the Family Reform Act 1969.

10. **c**—You must be 25 or over to make an advanced decision

An advance decision to refuse treatment (Living Will; advance directive) is legally binding as long as it complies with the Mental Capacity Act 2005, applies to the situation and is valid; it aims to take the place of best interest decisions made for you by other people. Advance decisions are valid if:

- you are aged 18 or over and had the capacity to make, understand and communicate your decision when you made it
- you specify clearly which treatments you wish to refuse
- you explain the circumstances in which you wish to refuse them
- it is signed by you and by a witness if you want to refuse life-sustaining treatment
- you have made the advance decision of your own accord, without any harassment by anyone else
- you haven't said or done anything that would contradict the advance decision since you made it (for example, saying that you have changed your mind)

11. **c**—Competence of a child to consent to contraceptive treatment without parental involvement

The House of Lords case Gillick versus West Norfolk and Wisbech Area Health Authority [1985], was presided over by Lord Scarman and Lord Frasier and regarded legal action taken against the advice given to doctors in a health circular that they could prescribe contraception to minors at their discretion. Victoria Gillick felt prescribing contraception in under 16s was illegal because the doctor would commit an offence of encouraging sex with a minor, and that it would be treatment without parental consent. The case had two main outcomes relevant to health professionals:

1. The concept of "Gillick competence": which declared the parental right to determine whether or not their minor child below the age of 16 will have medical treatment terminates if and when the child achieves sufficient understanding and intelligence to understand fully what is proposed (Lord Scarman).
2. Frasier Guidelines which outline the criteria which must be met for doctors to lawfully provide contraceptive advice and treatment to under 16s without parental consent.

12. **c**—Report your concerns to the local authority social services

The British Medical Association guidance for doctors who have concerns about a child state "where a doctor has a reasonable belief that a child is at serious risk of immediate harm, he or she should act immediately to protect the interests of the child, and this will involve contacting one of the three statutory bodies with responsibilities in this area: the police, the local authority social services or the NSPCC, and making a full report of their concerns."

13. **a**—Gain parental consent and proceed to surgery

UK Regulations Regarding Consent for Treatment

Capacity	Able to Consent to Treatment?	Able to Refuse Treatment?	Can be Treated in Best Interests?	Others Able to Consent for Them?
Adult				
Competent	Yes	Yes (can be rational, irrational or groundless)	No	No
Incompetent	No	No	Yes—Mental Capacity Act 2005	Yes—Court
16- and 17-year-olds				
Competent	Yes—Capacity assumed under Family Law Reform Act 1969	No—decision to withhold consent can be overturned by person with parental responsibility or court	Yes—but need court's authority	Yes—persons with parental responsibility, High Court, specific issues order
Incompetent	No	No	Yes—but may need court's authority if disagreement about MCA 2005	Yes—persons with parental responsibility, High Court, specific issues order
Under 16-year-olds				
Competent	Yes—only if deemed Gillick competent, but if possible also with consent of person with parental responsibility	No—decision to withhold consent can be overturned by person with parental responsibility or court	Yes—but need court's authority	Yes—persons with parental responsibility, High Court, specific issues order
Incompetent	No	No	Yes—but need court's authority	Yes—persons with parental responsibility, High Court, specific issues order

See Shaw M. Competence and consent to treatment in children and adolescents. Adv Psychiatr Treat 2001;7:150–9.

14. **b**—Give blood anyway because this is an emergency situation

Section 8 of the Family Reform Act 1969 states that in an emergency where you consider that it is in the child's best interests to proceed, you may treat the child, provided it is limited to that treatment which is reasonably required in that emergency. Therefore, the child should be given the transfusion. Traditionally, where young children are concerned, the power to give or withhold consent to medical treatment on their behalf lies with those with parental responsibility. Legally, except in an emergency, parental consent is necessary to perform any medical procedure on a child. Two commonly used arguments when parents refuse treatment are parental rights to raise children as they see fit and religious freedom. Courts throughout the Western world recognize parental rights, but these rights are not absolute. Parental rights to raise children are qualified by a duty to ensure their health, safety, and wellbeing. Parents cannot make decisions that may permanently harm or otherwise impair their healthy development. If treatment refusal results in a child suffering, parents may be criminally liable. However, before any harm comes to the child the courts are usually asked to exercise their power under the doctrine of *parens patriae* which allows state interference to protect a child's welfare. This principle applies whether or not the child is in imminent danger, as parents are always required to make decisions in the child's best interests.

FURTHER READING

Wolley S. Children of Jehovah's Witnesses and adolescent Jehovah's Witnesses: what are their rights? Arch Dis Child 2005;90:715–19.

	Child Consent to Transfusion?	Parental Consent to Transfusion?	Plan
Competent (16- or 17-year-old) or Gillick competent (Under 16)	Yes	No	Transfuse
	No	No	In emergency in England/Wales, aim to telephone the court for declaration that treatment is lawful if time permits. The young person must not be allowed to die for want of blood In less urgent cases, aim to persuade child/family, involve Hospital Liaison Committee of the Jehovah's Witnesses
	No	Yes	Transfuse with parental right to consent
Incompetent	N/A	No	Transfuse if in best interest
	N/A	Yes	Transfuse with parental right to consent

See Wolley S. Children of Jehovah's Witnesses and adolescent Jehovah's Witnesses: what are their rights? Arch Dis Child 2005;90:715–19.

15. **d**—Do not give blood transfusion but involve courts

The rights of adolescents to refuse medical treatment vary throughout the world and this judicial inconsistency creates confusion among health-care workers. In England and Wales, mature minors (Gillick competent or over 16) may consent to, but not refuse, treatment, with the courts using the "best interests" test to override the opinions of adolescents. In 1969, the Family Law Reform Act set the age of *consent for* medical treatment at 16 but did not specifically deal with parental-child conflict. The implication, however, is that a child's consent to a procedure overrides parental opinion. The logical inference from *Gillick* is that competent children are competent to both accept and refuse treatment; yet subsequent decisions suggest that a child's refusal may be overridden by a proxy's consent to that treatment and that the child's refusal, while important, may not be conclusive. Where treatment refusal was religion based, there was concern about the child's freedom of choice in the context of a religious upbringing in addition to concerns about whether the child fully grasped the implications of treatment refusal. Thus, while a child's refusal should be considered, it is likely that the court will override the refusal in the child's best interests. In Scotland, although the Age of Legal Capacity (Scotland) Act does not specifically refer to treatment refusal, the inference is that a child deemed competent could refuse, as well as consent to, treatment. In North America, the situation for mature minors is state/province dependent.

16. **c**—She can be detained for treatment of her mental health disorder only

The Mental Capacity Act 2005 can only be used to give treatment to somebody aged over 16 without their consent if that person is assessed as lacking capacity to make a specific decision at that particular time, and if treatment would be in their "best interests." Mostly, the doctor who will be responsible for giving the medical treatment will be responsible for making the "best interests" decision and in order to reach this decision, he or she must work through a process and statutory checklist which is contained in the Mental Capacity Act 2005. If hospital staff want to detain someone for treatment under the Mental Capacity Act, they need to use the "Deprivation of liberty safeguards" procedure. This should not be used to detain someone for treatment for a mental health problem—this is the role of the Mental Health Act 1983 (2007). This law allows people living in England and Wales who have a "mental disorder" to be admitted, detained and treated for their mental disorder in hospital without their consent (even if they have capacity/are competent)—either for their own health or safety, or for the protection of other people. This can be done under various sections of the Mental Health Act 1983 (2007):

MHA Section	Use
Section 2	Admission for assessment and initiation of treatment (up to 28 days)
Section 3	Admission for treatment (up to 6 months)
Section 4	Allows emergency admission when not enough time to organize S2/S3 (up to 72 h)
Section 5(2)	Allows a doctor to stop a voluntary inpatient from leaving hospital (for 72 h)
Section 5(4)	Allows a nurse to stop a voluntary inpatient from leaving hospital (for 6 h)
Section 135	Allows police to gain entry into someone's premises to allow an assessment under the MHA, or to return someone who is absent without leave from hospital
Section 136	Allows police to take someone with a mental disorder from a public place to a place of safety if they think he/she needs immediate care or control

17. **e**—Family members cannot legally veto organ donation if the patient is on the organ donor register

Organ donation is possible posthumously when no prior consent has been given, if a person in a "qualifying relationship" (ranked by the Human Tissue Act 2004) consents to it. It is possible to carry an organ donor card, which will make it much easier to confirm consent to organ donation if it is found on the person, but it is not necessary. According to the Human Tissue Act 2004, it is legal to preserve bodies after death, e.g., by ventilating the patient, to continue perfusion to the organs until consent for donation is established. Competent minors can also consent to posthumous organ donation, and those with parental responsibility should be informed of such a decision by the child. Although relatives can no longer legally veto consent to organ donation, in reality, hospitals will respect the wishes of relatives and organ donation is unlikely to proceed if there is disagreement.

18. **a**—Discussion with a competent patient's family member

The patient needs to give permission for their information to be disclosed to their family, although in some cultures this may not be the norm. All of the other options may require a doctor to disclose information depending on the situation.

19. **e**—Last will and testament

A power of attorney is a document in which one competent person (the principal) appoints another person (the attorney-in-fact) to act for him or her. It becomes invalid when the principal dies and cannot be used to bequeath property upon the death of the principal (this is the function of the last will and testament).

Durable power of attorney	Remains valid even if the principal later becomes mentally incompetent
Ordinary power of attorney	Only valid as long as the principal is capable of acting for themselves and is not valid if they become incompetent
Specific powers of attorney	Gives the attorney-in-fact authority to act for a particular purpose (e.g., to buy or sell a particular piece of property)
General powers of attorney	Gives the attorney-in-fact the authority to do anything the principal could do him or herself
Last will and testament	When a person dies, the executor appointed in the person's last will and testament takes control of the deceased person's property and distributes it according to the instructions in the will. If there is no will (or if the will is invalid), each jurisdiction has intestacy legislation that distributes the deceased person's property to his or her relatives according to a set of rules

20. **a**—Tarasoff decision

Physicians cannot disseminate confidential information about their patient without consent. This principle applies to speaking with families, friends, the court, or other doctors (only communication for the purpose of patient care is acceptable). Exceptions to confidentiality are generally focused on preventing harm and include the following:

1. Tarasoff decision: physician–patient confidentiality must legally be breeched if the patient has threatened to harm another person. The healthcare provider should try to detain the patient, contact the police, and warn the potential victim.

2. Child abuse/elder abuse.
3. Dangerous driving: patients must be reported to the Department of Motor Vehicles if they experience a seizure or otherwise present a danger (e.g., visual loss).
4. Reportable diseases: many diseases must be reported to local authorities (and to the patient's partner in the case of STDs).
5. Waiver: the patient may waive confidentiality so discussions can be held with family members or disclosures made to the insurance company.

21. **a**—Transfer of a stable patient for non-emergency care

Hospitals have three main obligations under EMTALA:

- Any individual who comes and requests must receive a medical screening examination to determine whether an emergency medical condition exists. Examination and treatment cannot be delayed to inquire about methods of payment or insurance coverage.
- If an emergency medical condition exists, treatment must be provided until the emergency medical condition is resolved or stabilized. If the hospital does not have the capability to treat the emergency medical condition, an "appropriate" transfer of the patient to another hospital must be done in accordance with the EMTALA provisions.
- Hospitals with specialized capabilities are obligated to accept transfers from hospitals who lack the capability to treat unstable emergency medical conditions.
- A hospital must report instances when it may have inappropriately received an individual who has been transferred in an unstable emergency medical condition from another hospital.

EMTALA governs how patients are transferred from one hospital to another. Under the law, a patient is considered stable for transfer if the treating physician determines that no material deterioration will occur during the transfer between facilities. EMTALA does not apply to the transfer of stable patients; however, if the patient is unstable, then the hospital may not transfer the patient unless:

- A physician certifies the medical benefits expected from the transfer outweigh the risks OR.
- A patient makes a transfer request in writing after being informed of the hospital's obligations under EMTALA and the risks of transfer.

In addition, the transfer of unstable patients must be "appropriate" under the law, such that (1) the transferring hospital must provide ongoing care within its capability until transfer to minimize transfer risks, (2) provide copies of medical records, (3) must confirm that the receiving facility has space and qualified personnel to treat the condition and has agreed to accept the transfer, and (4) the transfer must be made with qualified personnel and appropriate medical equipment.

22. **e**—Decision regarding tethered cord release

Traditionally, US minors (under 18) have no legal rights and remain under parental jurisdiction until they reach the age of majority. Over the past century, however, legislation has altered this, allowing minors to obtain treatment for specific conditions without parental consent and, in some states, make medical treatment decisions. In general, the need for parental consent should nearly always be respected but in life- or limb-threatening emergencies, treatment should not be delayed despite parental objection. In urgent situations, legal options can be pursued to make the child a ward of the court (e.g., parents cannot refuse life-saving therapy for a minor with cancer). Established exceptions to the need for parental consent in minors are:

1. Emancipated minors: married, serving in the military, self-supporting, or parents to children.
2. Reproductive health: sexually transmitted diseases (STDs), birth control, prenatal care.
3. Substance abuse treatment.

EMI ANSWERS

23. 1—d, Beneficence; 2—j, Utilitarianism; 3—a, Autonomy

Autonomy	Principle that all patients have the right to make their own informed medical decisions for their own reasons. Competent patients have a nearly limitless ability to exercise autonomy even if it means their own death or if it conflicts with their physician's personal ethical principles
A positive right	A right *to be* subjected to an action of another person or group (i.e., oblige action)
A negative right	A right *not to be* subjected to an action of another person or group (i.e., oblige inaction)
Beneficence	Physicians have a duty to do what is best for their patients
Categorical imperative	A rule that is true in all circumstances, which Kant phrased in two ways: 1. Always act in such a way that you would be willing for it to become general law for everyone else to do the same as you in the same situation 2. People should always be treated as valuable in themselves, and not just be used in order to achieve something else
Justice	All people should be treated similarly regardless of age, race, or ability to pay. Medical resources should be allocated fairly
Non-maleficence	Physicians should weigh the relative risks and benefits of an intervention, acknowledging that most treatments have inherent risk and that it may be better to do nothing at all
Virtue ethics	Suggests that the right act is the action a virtuous person would do in the same circumstances. The problem with this is that virtues may vary by culture and historical context
Futility	Futile care can be defined as the initiation or prolongation of "ineffective, pointless, or hopeless" treatments

24. 1—d, Implied consent; 2—f, Invalid advance directive—AD must be made by a person with capacity, be specific and not as a result of coercion; 3—b, Valid consent

25. 1—f, Non-voluntary euthanasia; 2—c, Murder; 3—b, Physician-assisted suicide; 4—e, Voluntary euthanasia; 5—h, Doctrine of double effect

Suicide	The act of trying to intentionally end one's own life
Physician-assisted suicide	Physician provides an individual with the information, guidance, and means to take his or her own life with the intention that they will be used for this purpose
Murder	Where a person of sound mind unlawfully kills another human being, with the intent to kill or cause grievous bodily harm
Attempted murder	In contrast to the offence of murder, attempted murder requires the existence of an intention to kill, not merely to cause grievous bodily harm
Voluntary euthanasia	The intentional killing by act or omission of a dependent human being for his or her alleged benefit at their request (usually to relieve pain or suffering)
Non-voluntary euthanasia	The intentional killing by act or omission of a dependent human being for his or her alleged benefit without them requesting or consenting to it
Involuntary euthanasia	The intentional killing by act or omission of a dependent human being for his or her alleged benefit but against their wishes
Doctrine of double effect	View that it is permissible to cause a harm as a side effect (or "double effect") of bringing about a good result even though it would not be permissible to cause such a harm as a direct means to bringing about the same good end

26. 1—b, Aristotelian justice; 2—g, Libertarianism; 3—c, Communitarianism; 4—e, Deontology; 5—i, Utilitarianism

Aristotelian justice	When individuals receive benefits according to their merits, or virtue: those most virtuous should receive more of whatever goods society is in a position to distribute
Hippocratic oath	Articulates a commitment by the physician to do their best for the patient, cause no harm, and not cause injustice to the patient
Utilitarianism	Says that the best action is that which produces the greatest amount of happiness for the individual, community, or entities concerned, or the best outcome for the largest number of people. Utilitarians are concerned not about intentions or means, but the consequences of adopting the choice
Libertarianism	The rights of individuals to liberty, to acquire, keep, and exchange their holdings, and considers the protection of individual rights the primary role for the state; moral view that agents initially fully own themselves and have certain moral powers to acquire property rights in external things
Communitarianism	This is community-based moral theory in which values are determined by the community and what is best for the community trumps what is best for an individual
Deontology	Duty-based ethics which focus on the intrinsic rightness or wrongness of actions themselves rather than their consequences. In this way, one should do the right thing even if it produces more harm (or less good) than doing the wrong thing
Consequentialism	Action-based ethics which say that at any point in time, the morally right action to take is the one that will produce the best overall consequences. Different theories suggest what good thing should be maximized: utilitarianism (human welfare) and hedonism (human pleasure)
Principalism	System of ethical analysis derived from four principles of common morality: autonomy (free will or agency), beneficence (to do good), non-maleficence (not to harm), and justice (fair distribution of benefits and burdens). Each is a prima facie principle, is equal to all the others, and may override others in different situations, but all remain important in considering execution of decision
Altruism	States that one should choose the action that benefits other's well-being apart from oneself
Virtuism	States that the right action is that which would be done by a virtuous person, i.e., the moral character of the person performing the action is the most important thing in deciding if an action is right

CHAPTER 19

Surgical Technology and Practice

Chapter available on ExpertConsult.com

PART III
CRANIAL NEUROSURGERY

CHAPTER 20

General Neurosurgery and CSF Disorders

SINGLE BEST ANSWER (SBA) QUESTIONS

1. Which one of the following statements regarding intracerebral hemorrhage is LEAST accurate?
   a. Rate of spontaneous intracerebral hemorrhage in a 70-year-old is approximately 0.15% per year
   b. Rate of intratumoral hemorrhage in glioma is 2-4%
   c. Enoxaparin increases the risk of hemorrhage in melanoma and renal cell carcinoma brain metastasis
   d. Risk of recurrent intracerebral hemorrhage after an initial bleed is 3-5% per year
   e. Long-term aspirin therapy reduced the risk of ICH in patients with unruptured intracranial aneurysms

2. Which one of the following statements regarding balancing the risk of thromboembolism with risk of intracranial bleeding is most accurate?
   a. In patient with metallic mitral valve replacement risk of thrombosis off anticoagulation is 8% per year
   b. In a patient with brain metastasis from nonsmall cell lung cancer risk of ICH on LMWH is 35%
   c. In a patient with glioma risk of ICH on warfarin is threefold higher
   d. In a patient with acute ICH and a proximal DVT, the risk of fatal PE off anticoagulation is lower than the risk of recurrent ICH on anticoagulation
   e. In a patient with atrial fibrillation risk of ICH on warfarin is calculated using HASBLED score

3. Which one of the following statements regarding hydrocephalus is most accurate?
   a. Communicating hydrocephalus is usually caused by the presence of intracranial mass lesions
   b. Noncommunicating hydrocephalus is usually treated with spinal CSF diversion
   c. Excess CSF production is likely to produce a communicating, nonobstructive hydrocephalus
   d. Endoscopic third ventriculostomy is appropriate in cases of foramen of Monro obstruction
   e. Ventriculoperitoneal shunts are contraindicated where there is obstruction of CSF entering the cortical subarachnoid space

4. A 75-year-old male having problems with his gait urinary incontinence for the past 6 months, and recently, his short-term memory. When he started to walk he had a “magnetic” gait but normal armswing. Mini-mental state examination was 27/30. His CT head is shown below. Which one of the following is the next appropriate step in management?

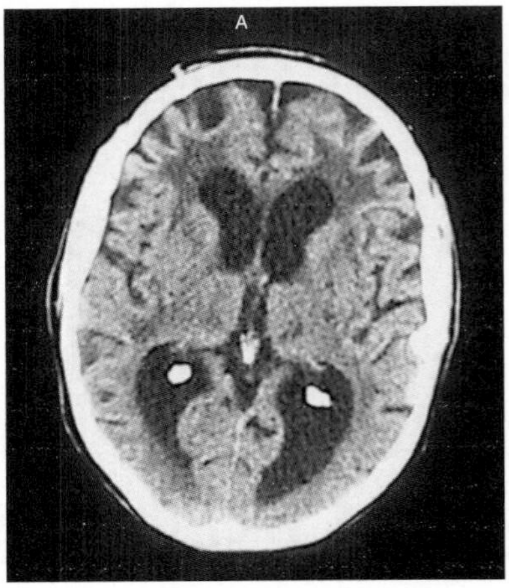

a. Reassure that this is part of normal aging and discharge
b. Amantadine trial
c. ICP monitoring
d. Lumbar puncture tap test
e. Ventriculoperitoneal shunt

5. Which one of the following statements regarding management of idiopathic normal pressure hydrocephalus is most accurate?
a. CSF outflow resistance is normally higher than 13 mmHg/mL/min
b. CSF outflow resistance greater than 18 mmHg/mL/min correlated with shunt responsiveness in NPH
c. Lundberg A waves usually visible during sleep in NPH patients
d. Presence of Lundberg B waves for greater than 80% of ICP monitoring suggests poor outcome with VP shunt
e. External lumbar drainage of CSF carries a lower risk of meningitis compared to lumbar infusion study

6. A 75-year-old man diagnosed with normal pressure hydrocephalus underwent VP shunt insertion 3 months ago. A Codman Hakim Progammable valve was set to 160 mmHg on discharge. CT head today shows no significant change in ventricular size (persistent ventriculomegaly). He reports no significant improvement in his symptoms. You undertake a shunt reservoir tap which records a pressure of 5 cm H_2O in the supine and −10 cm H_2O in the sitting position. Which one of the following statements is the most accurate conclusion?
a. There is evidence of shunt obstruction
b. There is evidence of shunt overdrainage
c. He is likely a shunt nonresponsive NPH patient
d. ICP monitoring as an inpatient is appropriate
e. Adjusting the shunt setting down further should be tried

7. Which one of the following approaches is LEAST likely to be appropriate for management of entrapped 4th ventricle?
a. 4th ventricular-peritoneal shunt
b. Endoscopic Aqueductal stent and lateral ventriculoperitoneal shunt
c. Endoscopic third ventriculostomy and aqueductoplasty
d. Foramen magnum decompression with expansion duraplasty
e. 4th ventricular-cisternal shunt

8. A 3-year-old female presents with headache and transient obscurations of her vision. Which one of the following would you start her on?

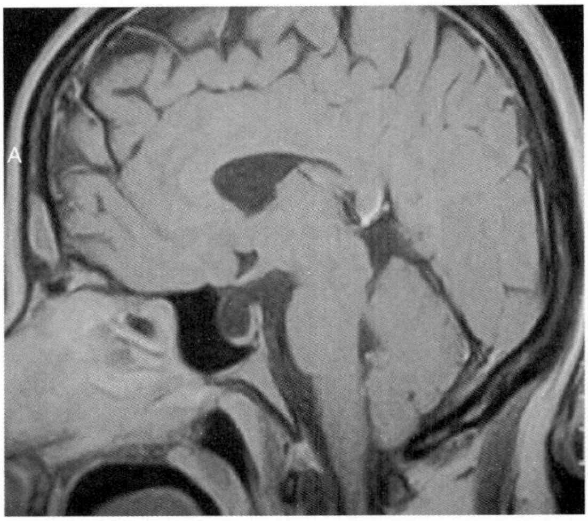

a. Acetazolamide
b. Bromocriptine
c. Corticosteroids
d. Furosemide
e. Topiramate

9. Which one of the following statements regarding surgical management of pseudotumor cerebri is most accurate?
a. Optic nerve sheath fenestration provides better visual outcomes than VP shunt in IIH
b. Choroid plexotomy is routinely used in IIH in patients with recurrent shunt blockage

c. Venous sinus stenting is first line treatment in IIH patients with MRI proven venous sinus stenosis
d. Endoscopic third ventriculostomy is appropriate substitute when optic nerve sheath fenestration is not possible
e. Lumboperitoneal shunt rate failure in IIH is 10%

10. Which one of the following statements regarding hydrocephalus is LEAST accurate?
a. Negative pressure hydrocephalus may be associated with a CSF leak
b. Low pressure hydrocephalus may be due to alteration in transmantle pressure
c. Benign external hydrocephalus usually resolves by 2-years of age
d. Subdural hygromas are difficult to distinguish from chronic subdural hematomas radiologically
e. Normal pressure hydrocephalus is diagnosed using ICP monitoring

QUESTIONS 11–20

Additional questions 11–20 available on ExpertConsult.com

EXTENDED MATCHING ITEM (EMI) QUESTIONS

21. In the endoscopic view during third ventriculostomy shown below (top of picture is anterior, bottom is posterior) which one of the following is the ideal point of fenestration?

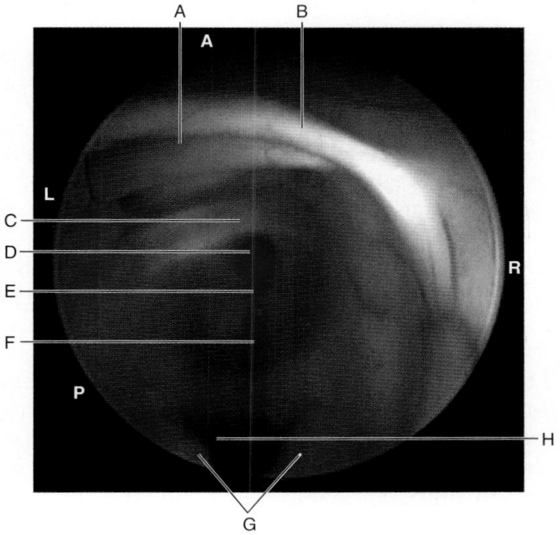

a. Anterior commissure
b. Fornix
c. Chiasm
d. Infundibulum
e. Tuber cinereum
f. Fenestration point for ETV
g. Mammillary bodies
h. Intermammillary space

22. **Operative approaches:**
a. Bifrontal
b. Extended middle fossa
c. Far lateral
d. Interhemispheric
e. Midline suboccipital
f. Orbito-zygomatic
g. Petrosal (retrolabryrinthine)
h. Pterional
i. Retrosigmoid
j. Subfrontal
k. Transphenoidal

For each of the following descriptions, select the most appropriate answers from the list above. Each answer may be used once, more than once or not at all.
1. Approach commonly used for a foramen magnum meningioma
2. Approach commonly used for a large olfactory groove meningioma
3. Approach commonly used for clipping of a pericallosal artery aneurysm
4. Approach commonly used for clipping a AICA aneurysm
5. Approach commonly used for clipping a PICA aneurysm

23. **CSF diversion complications:**
a. CSF pseudocyst
b. Distal catheter migration
c. Infection
d. Intraparenchymal hemorrhage
e. Mechanical obstruction
f. Overdrainage
g. Pseudomeningocele
h. Shunt allergy
i. Shunt disconnection
j. Slit ventricle syndrome
k. Subdural hematoma

For each of the following descriptions, select the most appropriate answers from the list above. Each answer may be used once, more than once or not at all.

1. A 44-year-old female presents after recent shunt insertion with shunt failure and CSF with persistent eosinophilia despite negative cultures

2. A 57-year-old man presents with symptoms of shunt obstruction and nonspecific abdominal pain. His wounds are clean and dry. XR shunt series appears normal

SBA ANSWERS

1. **c**—Enoxaparin increases the risk of hemorrhage in melanoma and renal cell carcinoma brain metastasis

Risk of ICH with and without Antithrombotic Drugs

	Risk of ICH	Risk of ICH with Anticoagulation	Risk of ICH Antiplatelet
General population	0.016-0.033 per year (0.15% per year in 70-year-olds)	0.3-1% per year (INR 2-3)	Excess risk of 0.2-1.2 per 1000-patient-years with aspirin
Unruptured intracranial aneurysm	<7 mm anterior circulation: 0.1% per year 7-12 mm anterior circn: 2.5% per year >13 mm or posterior circulation: 3-20% per year	Paucity of data. Worse outcome of aneurysmal SAH if on warfarin. IV thrombolysis appears safe in acute stroke patients with unruptured intracranial aneurysm	Lower risk of aneurysm rupture in cohort of ISUIA on aspirin
Glioma	2-4%	2-4% (INR well controlled)	
Brain metastasis	15% (NSCLC) to 35% (melanoma/RCC)	No change from baseline (enoxaparin or well controlled warfarin)	
Acute ICH	ICH expansion in first 24 h: 15-38% of patients ICH expansion 24 h-2 weeks: 1-2%	3-5% After 24 h	Unclear
Prior ICH	2-3% per year	3-5% per year	Possibly with lobar ICH
Acute infarction	Unclear	0.9% (warfarin)	0.2% (aspirin) 1% (clopidogrel or dual)

FURTHER READING

Rordorf G, et al. Spontaneous intracerebral hemorrhage: pathogenesis, clinical features, and diagnosis. Uptodate Topic 1133 Version 12.0.

Freeman DW, et al. Risk of intracerebral bleeding in patients treated with anticoagulants. Uptodate Topic 1328 Version 16.0.

Gaasch WH, et al. Complications of prosthetic heart valves. Uptodate Topic 8121 Version 12.0.

Cucchiara BL, et al. Antiplatelet therapy for secondary prevention of stroke. Uptodate Topic 1086 Version 35.0.

Wen PY. Anticoagulant and antiplatelet therapy in patients with brain tumors. Uptodate Topic 5201 Version 17.0.

Alejandro A. Anticoagulant and antiplatelet therapy in patients with an unruptured intracranial aneurysm. Uptodate Topic 1320 Version 8.0.

Wijdicks EFM, et al. The use of antithrombotic therapy in patients with an acute or prior intracerebral haemorrhage. Uptodate Topic 1323 Version 19.0.

Donato J, et al. Intracranial haemorrhage in patients with brain metastases treated with therapeutic enoxaparin: a matched cohort study. Blood 2015; 126(4).

2. **a**—In patient with metallic mitral valve replacement risk of thrombosis off anticoagulation is 8% per year

The use of IVC filters in patients with brain tumors has been associated with substantial complication rates (over 50% experience recurrent VTE, IVC or filter thrombosis, or post-thrombotic syndrome), and the risk of hemorrhage secondary to anticoagulation is not as high as originally feared. The relatively low incidence of intratumoral hemorrhage is a particularly important issue for patients who need anticoagulation for reasons other than VTE (e.g. atrial fibrillation) in whom IVC filter is not appropriate. Although randomized comparisons are not available in brain tumor patients, indirect comparisons from case series suggest that carefully controlled oral anticoagulation with warfarin is reasonably safe and associated with fewer serious complications than routine use of IVC filters.

Balancing the Risk of Venous Thromboembolism with the Risk of ICH

Diagnosis	Risk of Thromboembolic Event off Anticoagulation	Thromboembolism Risk on Antithrombotic	Risk of ICH on Antithrombotic
Glioma	20% risk VTE	Recurrent VTE in all cancer patients at 6 months: Warfarin 17% LMWH 9%	2%—If INR well controlled, not different from glioma patients not on anticoagulation (2-4%)
Brain metastasis	20% risk VTE	Recurrent VTE in all cancer patients at 6 months: Warfarin 17% LMWH 9%	20% significant bleed rate at 1 year—no difference between those treated with enoxaparin and controls, but difference between nonsmall cell lung cancer (15-19%) and renal cell/melanoma (35%)
Mechanical MVR	8% per year	4% per year after 1 month (INR 2.5-3.5)	0.3-1% per year
Bioprosthetic MVR		2.4% per year after 3 months	0.3-1% per year
Prosthetic AVR	1.9% per year after 3 months	N/A	0.3-1% per year
Proximal DVT or nonfatal PE in patient with acute ICH	Risk of fatal PE 25%		Beyond 24 h: 3-5% risk of ICH recurrence
Atrial fibrillation	Calculate using CHAD2vasc score	1-2% per year	0.3-1% per year Calculate all cause risk of major hemorrhage using HASBLED score

FURTHER READING

McKenzie DB, et al. management of patients with mechanical valves and intracerebral haemorrhage. Br J Cardiol 2008;15:145-8.

Donato J, et al. Intracranial haemorrhage in patients with brain metastases treated with therapeutic enoxaparin: a matched cohort study. Blood 2015;126(4).

Rordorf G, et al. Spontaneous intracerebral hemorrhage: pathogenesis, clinical features, and diagnosis. Uptodate Topic 1133 Version 12.0.

Freeman DW, et al. Risk of intracerebral bleeding in patients treated with anticoagulants. Uptodate Topic 1328 Version 16.0.

Gaasch WH, et al. Complications of prosthetic heart valves. Uptodate Topic 8121 Version 12.0.

Cucchiara BL, et al. Antiplatelet therapy for secondary prevention of stroke. Uptodate Topic 1086 Version 35.0.

Wen PY. Anticoagulant and antiplatelet therapy in patients with brain tumors. Uptodate Topic 5201 Version 17.0.

Alejandro A. Anticoagulant and antiplatelet therapy in patients with an unruptured intracranial aneurysm. Uptodate Topic 1320 Version 8.0.

Wijdicks EFM, et al. The use of antithrombotic therapy in patients with an acute or prior intracerebral haemorrhage. Uptodate Topic 1323 Version 19.0.

3. **c**—Excess CSF production is likely to produce a communicating, nonobstructive hydrocephalus

Walter Dandy's classification of hydrocephalus is still commonly used and makes the distinction between communicating (no obstruction in CSF pathway from ventricles to subarachnoid space)

and obstructive (CSF cannot flow from ventricular system to subarachnoid space; "noncommunicating") hydrocephalus as these are the clinically most common and also reflect differing management options. However, almost all hydrocephalus involves an obstruction to CSF flow and it is just the point of obstruction which varies (e.g. within ventricles, arachnoid villi, venous sinus outflow), and true "communicating hydrocephalus" without a point of obstruction would only be produced by overproduction of CSF (e.g. choroid plexus papilloma). A more nuanced system that takes advantage of tremendous advances in imaging is now possible (although developmental forms of hydrocephalus often have multiple points of obstruction):

Hydrocephalus Classification Study Group: Point of Obstruction Model

Point of Obstruction	Differential	Treatments
Foramen of Monro	Tumor, congenital absence, ventriculitis, functional	Shunt (unilateral or bilateral) Endoscopic septostomy
Aqueduct of Sylvius	Tumor, congenital stenosis, secondary	Shunt Endoscopic third ventriculostomy
4th ventricle foramina	Infection, tumor, severe Chiari	Shunt Endoscopic third ventriculostomy Surgical opening
Between spinal and cortical subarachnoid space	Subarachnoid hemorrhage Infection	Shunt Endoscopic third ventriculostomy LP shunt
Arachnoid villi	Subarachnoid hemorrhage Infection	VP or LP shunt
Venous hypertension	Pseudotumor cerebri (PTC) Congenital hydrocephalus Sinus thrombosis	Bariatric surgery for obesity-related PTC VP or LP shunt Anticoagulation Venous sinus stent (debated)

FURTHER READING

Rekate HL. A consensus on the classification of hydrocephalus: its utility in the assessment of abnormalities of cerebrospinal fluid dynamics. Childs Nerv Syst. 2011;27(10):1535-41.

4. **d**—Lumbar puncture tap test

Normal pressure hydrocephalus is a clinical syndrome characterized by gait apraxia (90% of patients), dementia, and incontinence with ventriculomegaly and normal CSF pressure on lumbar puncture. If the gait improves after a single large-volume lumbar puncture (30-50 mL), serial large-volume lumbar punctures can be performed daily for 3 days the diagnosis is probable, and, more importantly, the patient will likely respond to treatment by shunting. In those where lumbar puncture fails or is contraindicated, a ventricular reservoir can be inserted and testing undertaken a few months later. Gait in patients with NPH is described as being "magnetic" in nature, characterized by a broad base and slow, small steps with reduced height clearance as though the feet are "stuck to the floor" but also include unsteadiness, recurrent falls, shuffling, and reduced walking speed (confused with parkinsonism). Urinary incontinence maybe neurological or a consequence of gait disturbance or the cognitive impairment. NPH is estimated to account for less than 5% of all cases of dementia hence commoner causes such as Alzheimer's must be excluded, as well as mimics such as Binswanger's disease (also produces a frontal dysexecutive syndrome). Imaging should show ventricular enlargement not entirely attributable to cerebral atrophy or congenital enlargement (Evans' index >0.3 or comparable measure), bicaudate ratio >0.25, and another supportive feature: enlargement of the temporal horns of the lateral ventricles not entirely attributable to hippocampal atrophy; callosal angle of 40 degrees or greater; evidence of altered brain water content, including periventricular signal changes not attributable to microvascular ischemic changes or demyelination; presence of aqueductal or fourth ventricular flow void on MRI. Current guidelines deal primarily with idiopathic as opposed to secondary NPH, which can occur years after trauma, subarachnoid hemorrhage, intracranial surgery, or meningitis. Continuous ICP monitoring has demonstrated the presence of waves of increased ICP, particularly during rapid eye movement (REM) sleep. It has been suggested that these abnormal CSF pressure spikes, called *B waves*, slowly increase ventricular size by exerting intermittent high pressure on the brain parenchyma that results in ischemic damage. Abnormalities of the aging brain parenchyma may make it more susceptible to these forces. Despite the uncertainty regarding its evolution, NPH is a syndrome that is treatable by CSF diversion (i.e. shunt insertion).

Image with permission from Budson AE. Memory Loss, Alzheimer's Disease, and Dementia, 2nd ed., Elsevier, 2016.

FURTHER READING

Relkin N, Marmarou A, Klinge P, et al. Diagnosing idiopathic normal pressure hydrocephalus. Neurosurgery 2005;57(3 Suppl.):S4-S16, discussion ii-v.

5. **b**—CSF outflow resistance greater than 18 mmHg/mL/min correlated with shunt responsiveness in NPH

There is no single test for idiopathic NPH, but supplementary tests can increase the prognostic accuracy to greater than 90%. A lumbar puncture "tap test" has been shown to produce a specificity of 100% with a sensitivity of 26%, provided that it is performed at a high volume (i.e. withdrawal of 40-50 mL of CSF). Symptomatic improvement after removal of CSF has a high positive predictive value (73-100%) of a probably favorable outcome with shunt placement. It has to be remembered that improvement after a shunt is often delayed in many patients, so a simple tap test would not be expected to reveal all patients who might benefit from a shunt. However, the low sensitivity of the "tap test" precludes using this method as a diagnostic tool for exclusion. Prolonged external lumbar drainage in excess of 300 mL is associated with high sensitivity (50-80%), specificity (80%), and positive predictive value (80-100%), but requires inpatient stay and carries a risk for the complications of nerve root irritation, hemorrhage, and CSF infection. Measurement of CSF outflow resistance (reflecting the capacity of CSF absorption pathways) via a daycase lumbar infusion or ventricular reservoir infusion test with a pressure-volume study is also established. In the Dutch NPH study, outflow resistance greater than 18 mmHg/mL/min had a specificity of 87% and a sensitivity of 46%. Although isolated measurements of CSF pressure in patients with communicating hydrocephalus and NPH may be in the normal range, overnight ICP monitoring may reveal dynamic phenomena such as increased Lundberg "B waves." B waves are slow waves of ICP lasting 20 s to 2 min. The presence of B waves for more than 80% of the period of ICP monitoring is thought to indicate that it is much more likely than not that shunting would be helpful.

FURTHER READING

Marmarou A, et al. The value of supplemental prognostic tests for the preoperative assessment of idiopathic normal-pressure hydrocephalus. Neurosurgery 2005;57(3 Suppl. S2):17-284.

6. **e**—Adjusting the shunt setting down further should be tried

It is the patient in whom the association between clinical findings and ventriculomegaly is uncertain (e.g. NPH) and fails to improve after shunt surgery (or only minimally improves) who represents a clinical challenge. As a result, the failure to improve might be attributed to an incorrect diagnosis, or a shunt nonresponder (e.g. if valve at lowest setting and shunt patency confirmed). If imaging reveals a reduction in ventricular size, a patient should be considered a nonresponder if no clinical improvement occurred. For patients in this scenario who remain with significant ventriculomegaly, strategies for improving drainage should be considered (e.g. removal of antisiphon device, or a programmable valve with a lower pressure limit) as they may have a low-pressure hydrocephalus state. Downward adjustments in valve opening pressure are unlikely to benefit the patient and instead increase the risk of subdural hematoma. Even if shunt flow is documented, one should pursue other interventions as one cannot exclude functional underdrainage. For example, if there is an ASD, remove it. If the patient has a fixed-pressure valve or a flow-restricting valve, change it to an adjustable differential pressure valve (no ASD). It is our observation that ventriculoatrial shunts provide more drainage than ventriculoperitoneal shunts do, and therefore we offer a shunt revision to a ventriculoatrial shunt as well. It is only the case in which the patient has a ventriculoatrial shunt with a differential pressure valve set to 30 mm H_2O or less that an operative intervention is not recommended.

7. **d**—Foramen magnum decompression with expansion duraplasty

Entrapped fourth ventricle has been used to describe the situation in which the fourth ventricle no longer communicates with either the third ventricle and/or the basal cisterns. It is thought that secondary aqueduct stenosis from adhesions, obstruction of the foramina of Luschka or Magendie, or infective debris pooling in the basal cisterns may be responsible for this condition. Patients may have the typical symptoms and signs of hydrocephalus or more atypical symptoms such as lower cranial nerve dysfunction. Patients with prolonged infection or multiple shunt operations are particularly at risk for this syndrome. In cases of hydrocephalus caused by membranous occlusion or short segment stenosis of the aqueduct of Sylvius, endoscopic aqueductoplasty (EA) with and without stenting has been reported. The burr hole for EA is placed more anteriorly than the one for standard ETV. Stenting of the aqueduct may be performed for patients at high risk for aqueductal restenosis or patients with a trapped fourth ventricle. The stent is usually a ventricular catheter with additional holes. Shunted patients with a trapped fourth ventricle often have slit-like lateral ventricles, making them poor candidates for the standard EA so a suboccipital approach for retrograde aqueductoplasty and stenting can be performed. EA restores the physiologic CSF pathways and eliminates the risk for basilar artery injury. There are no arachnoidal adhesions around the aqueduct to interfere with CSF flow. The risk for injuring the hypothalamus is avoided, especially during cases when the floor of the third ventricle is thickened and a considerable amount of force is required to perforate the floor. Strictures at the aqueduct are usually not as tough to penetrate; thus, less force is required for fenestration. A major risk of EA is injuring the periaqueductal gray matter and the floor of the fourth ventricle. Other complications reported, especially in long stenoses, include midbrain injury causing transient or permanent dysconjugate eye movements, Parinaud-syndrome, and cranial nerve palsies. In cases with long stenoses, ETV may be a more appropriate procedure.

8. **a**—Acetazolamide

The pseudotumor cerebri syndrome (PTCS) is a perplexing syndrome of increased intracranial pressure without a space-occupying lesion. annual incidence of pseudotumor cerebri syndrome (PTCS) as 0.9/100,000 in the general population, rising to 3.5/100,000 in women aged 15-44 years and 19.3/100,000 in women aged 20-44 years who weigh 20% or more than their ideal body weight. When no secondary cause is identified (e.g. venous obstruction, endocrine disorders, medications), the syndrome is primary and termed Idiopathic Intracranial Hypertension (IIH). Symptoms include headache, transient visual obscurations, pulsatile tinnitus, visual loss, diplopia. Signs include 6th nerve palsy and papilledema. In addition, for the diagnosis to be made brain imaging must show no structural causes of raised ICP, and lumbar puncture CSF opening pressure >25 cm H_2O in relaxed adults and >28 cm H_2O in a (sedated) child with normal CSF analysis. In the absence of papilledema or 6th nerve palsy, possible diagnosis of PTCS is suggested by MRI showing at least three of: empty sella, flattening of the posterior aspect of the globe, distension of perioptic subarachnoid space (=/- tortuous optic nerve), transverse venous sinus stenosis. The main goal of treatment is preservation of vision. As such, patients presenting with deteriorating vision require more aggressive initial management. General management strategied include weight loss (including bariatric surgery in some cases), salt restriction, acetazolamide, topiramate (headache and causes weight loss), ventriculoperitoneal or lumboperitoneal CSF shunting, optic nerve sheath fenestration and in some cases venous sinus stenting.

Image with permission from Scholes MA. ENT Secrets, 4th ed., Elsevier, 2016.

FURTHER READING

Friedman DI. The pseudotumor cerebri syndrome. Neurol Clin 2014;32:363-96.

9. **a**—Optic nerve sheath fenestration provides better visual outcomes than VP shunt in IIH

Surgery is usually indicated for visual loss or worsening of vision that is attributable to papilledema, rather than chronic headache. The two surgical treatments are optic nerve sheath fenestration (ONSF) and shunting. There have been no prospective, randomized trials of surgical treatments. ONSF as the preferred treatment of visual loss from IIH, perhaps because visual outcomes were better documented with this procedure. ONSF tends to be more effective in acute papilledema than chronic papilledema and is not indicated once the papilledema has resolved. Studies show that bilateral improvement in vision often occurs after a unilateral procedure. The complications of ONSF include failure, ischemic optic neuropathy, transient diplopia, and transient blindness. Because the ventricles are not enlarged in PTCS, lumboperitoneal shunting was previously preferred over ventriculoperitoneal (VP) shunting but usually require multiple revision and failure rate is approximately 50% in PTCS. The most common reasons for revision are shunt obstruction, intracranial hypotension/subdurals, and lumbar radiculopathy. Visual deterioration may be the only sign of shunt failure and may occur even if the shunt is functioning. Other complications include infection, abdominal pain, CSF leak, hindbrain herniation, and migration of the peritoneal catheter. Cisterna magna shunting has been described, but image-guided placement of VP shunts is now favored. Bariatric surgery may be an option for the long-term management of IIH in morbidly obese patients but is not helpful for acute management. Transverse sinus stenosis in association with IIH prompted endovascular stenting as a treatment for the disorder, though there is debate as to whether it is cause or a sign of raised ICP. Despite some positive results, the need for long term anticoagulation has resulted in subdural/epidural hematoma (and also complicates other surgical interventions which may need performing), anaphylaxis, and hearing loss.

FURTHER READING

Friedman DI. The pseudotumor cerebri syndrome. Neurol Clin 2014;32:363-96.

10. **e**—Normal pressure hydrocephalus is diagnosed using ICP monitoring

Other CSF Disorders	
Negative or low pressure hydrocephalus	Rare conditions where patient exhibit features of raised ICP and show ventriculomegaly on imaging despite very low or negative ICP. Clinical suspicion for low- or negative-pressure hydrocephalus should be high when patients with enlarged ventricles have repeated "shunt failures" that do not improve with shunt revisions. Presence of a CSF leak from the cortical subarachnoid space and/or loss of patency between the ventricles and the cortical subarachnoid space (e.g. arachnoiditis, mechanical) may affect transmantle pressure (ventricular pressure—cortical subarachnoid space pressure) and brain turgor, leading to ventriculomegaly and neurological signs
Benign enlargement of subarachnoid space	The course is self-limited, manifesting in the first 6 months of life and resolving spontaneously by 2 years of age and thought to be due to transient mismatch in maturation/ability of arachnoid villi to absorb increasing volumes of CSF being produced
Subdural hygroma	Subdural fluid collection resembling CSF, on similar spectrum as subdural effusion and chronic subdural hematoma
Normal pressure hydrocephalus	Constellation of dementia, incontinence, and gait apraxia with evidence of ventriculomegaly on imaging (without underlying mass lesion) with normal CSF pressure on lumbar puncture

FURTHER READING

Filippidis AS, et al. Negative-pressure and low-pressure hydrocephalus: the role of cerebrospinal fluid leaks resulting from surgical approaches to the cranial base Report of 3 cases. JNS 2012;116(5):1031-7.
Cardoso ER. External hydrocephalus in adults. Report of three cases. JNS 1996;85:1143-7.

ANSWERS 11–20

Additional answers 11–20 available on ExpertConsult.com

EMI ANSWERS

21. f—6. 1—Anterior commissure; 2—Fornix; 3—Chiasm; 4—Infundibulum; 5—Tuber cinereum; 6—Fenestration point for ETV; 7—Mammillary bodies; 8—Intermammillary space

Image with permission from Jandial, R, McCormick PC, Black PM. Core Techniques in Operative Neurosurgery, Elsevier, Saunders, 2011.

22. 1—c, Far lateral; 2—a, Bifrontal; 3—d, Inter-hemispheric, 3—i, Retrosigmoid; 4—c, Far lateral

General Approaches in Neurosurgery

Approach	Positioning	Notes	Indications
Medial subfrontal	Supine, neck flexed, head extended	Frontal bone flap extends to midline. Can also take orbital rim (cranio-orbital approach)	Unilateral tumor or vascular lesion in anterior cranial fossa
Pterional (lateral frontotemporal)	Supine, ipsilateral shoulder elevated 30°, head rotated 30°	extends anteriorly in a curvilinear manner toward the supraorbital rim just above the superior temporal line (key hole), then inferiorly parallel to the supraorbital rim to the frontozygomatic process, then below this and posteriorly (crossing the sphenoid wing) to the squamous portion of the sphenoid bone, and then back up toward the superior temporal line posteriorly	Anterior and middle cranial fossa lesions
Orbito-zygomatic	Supine, ipsilateral shoulder elevated 30°, head rotated 30°	As pterional approach followed by en bloc removal of supraorbital rim, frontozygomatic process posterior half of the body of the zygoma, and the arch of the zygoma in a second osteotomy	Anterior and middle cranial fossa lesions
Extended middle fossa (Anterior petrosectomy)	Supine with head turned contralateral to lesion side	Removal of the petrous apex between the foramen ovale anteriorly, the arcuate eminence of the cochlea posteriorly, and the greater superficial petrosal nerve laterally	Middle/posterior cranial fossa: Petrous apex, superior clival, anterior CPA lesions, posterior cavernous sinus, basilar artery and anterior brain stem
Bifrontal	Supine, neck flexed, head extended	Zygomatic arch to zygomatic arch incision. Extended bifrontal approach involves removal of orbital bar (may cause trigeminocardiac reflex)	Bilateral anterior cranial fossa: Midline tumors Large olfactory groove/ planum sphenoidale/ tuberculum sella meningiomas, large craniopharyngiomas
Interhemispheric	Supine, head slightly flexed or semilateral, head turned 90 deg. to table with 45 deg. upward tilt of vertex	Bipartite box flap crossing midline (ipsilateral half is completely lateral to SSS)	Midline lesions, e.g. distal ACA aneurysm, falcine meningioma, corpus callosum lesion, lateral and third ventricle lesions
Transnasal Transphenoidal	Supine, body flexed, nose in sniffing position	Anterior wall of sphenoid sinus removed followed by sellar floor, can be advanced to include tuberculum sellae and planum sphenoidale	Sellar lesions with or without suprasellar extension or for clival lesions

Continued

Approach	Positioning	Notes	Indications
Petrosal (retrolabryrinthine-middle fossa)	Supine, bolster under ipsilateral shoulder, and 60° head turn contralaterally	C-shaped temporal-occipital craniotomy followed by mastoidectomy. Gives a combined supra and infratentorial exposure. Tentorium and superior petrosal sinus sectioned. In certain cases sigmoid sinus may be divided	Upper 2/3 clivus and anterior brain stem/basilar artery
Midline suboccipital	Prone with head flexed, chin tuck or sitting position (obese, large breasted)	Craniotomy below transverse sinus to lip of foramen magnum. C1 laminectomy may be required for 4th ventricular lesions	Cerebellar hemispheres, midline dorsal medulla/ pons, pineal region
Retrosigmoid suboccipital	Supine, bolster under ipsilateral shoulder, and 90° head turn to floor, vertex tilt as required	Suboccipital craniotomy which also exposes junction of transverse and sigmoid sinus. Bone over sigmoid sinus can be drilled off using diamond burr. neurovascular structures of the temporal bone are avoided at the expense of cerebellar retraction	CPA tumors, cranial nerves V-XI, anterolateral pons, AICA aneurysm, middle 1/3 clivus
Far lateral suboccipital	¾ prone, park bench (lateral decubitus) position, head tucked forward and rotated 120° from vertical and vertex tilted	A suboccipital craniotomy is performed from midline to the sigmoid sinus laterally. The occipital condyle can be drilled down to the hypoglossal canal. A C1 cervical laminectomy is also performed	Lateral and anterolateral foramen magnum, lower 1/3 clivus, PICA aneurysm

23. 1—h, Shunt allergy; 2—a, CSF peudocyst

True shunt allergies are rare. CSF often demonstrates persistent eosinophilia (3-36%), with negative cultures. Recurrent shunt failure is a common presentation. Pathologic examination of the ventricular catheter often demonstrates mechanical obstruction by inflammatory debris consisting of eosinophils and multinucleated giant cells. There are documented cases of immune responses to unpolymerized silicone in the literature. There are several management strategies. One is to consider an endoscopic third ventriculostomy and to remove the offending shunt. A second is to use a shunt system devoid of silicone, such as a polyurethane shunt system or hyperextruded silicone components.

CHAPTER 21

CRANIAL TRAUMA

SINGLE BEST ANSWER (SBA) QUESTIONS

1. Which one of the following approximate ratios for the proportion of traumatic brain injuries that are mild, moderate or severe is most accurate?
   a. 22 : 1.5 : 1
   b. 20 : 3.5 : 1
   c. 20 : 2.5 : 2
   d. 18 : 3.5 : 3
   e. 18 : 4.5 : 2

2. Which one of the following statements regarding the pathophysiology of traumatic brain injury is LEAST accurate?
   a. An acute extradural hematoma is a type of primary brain injury
   b. Diffuse axonal injury is a type of secondary brain injury
   c. Cerebral contusions are a type of primary brain injury
   d. Glutamate excitotoxicity is a type of secondary brain injury
   e. Hypoxia is a cause of secondary brain injury

3. Which one of the following statements regarding prognosis in TBI is LEAST accurate?
   a. Mortality rate in severe TBI (GCS 3-8) is approximately 40%
   b. Hypoxia and hypoglycemia are the extracranial insults which most strongly affect prognosis after TBI
   c. Prognostication based on CT head appearance may be done using Marshall or Rotterdam classifications
   d. Mortality rate in those with mild TBI (GCS 13-15) is <1% overall
   e. Mortality rate at 14 days in those with GCS 13 and bilaterally reactive pupils after a significant, isolated head injury may be up to 30%

4. Which one of the following statements regarding mild traumatic brain injury (GCS 13-15) patients presenting to emergency departments are LEAST accurate?
   a. Loss of consciousness is not a requirement for diagnosis
   b. It is associated with increased glutamate release, and a hyperglycotic and hypermetabolic state in brain tissue
   c. Clinically significant brain injury is present in 10-15% of cases
   d. The majority of patients are symptom free by 7-10 days post-concussion
   e. Approximately 0.5-1% result in death or require neurosurgical intervention due to underlying significant brain injury

5. A football player sustains a head injury during a game. On examination he is GCS 15/15. Which one of the following statements about complications following concussion is most accurate?
   a. Second impact syndrome is a common cause of rapid fatal brain swelling after concussion
   b. The commonest symptoms of post-concussion syndrome are ongoing cognitive impairment
   c. Chronic traumatic encephalopathy is characterized clinically by neurodegeneration
   d. The risk of late seizures (post-traumatic epilepsy) in those with mild traumatic brain injury is thought to be threefold higher in the next 5 years.
   e. Dysfunction of cerebral autoregulation after an initial concussion is thought to underlie the risk for second impact syndrome

6. Which one of the following statements regarding return to play of an athlete who has sustained a concussion is LEAST accurate?
   a. An athlete cannot return to play that day even once concussion symptoms have cleared
   b. Risk of a second concussion is particularly increased in the 10 days following the first concussion
   c. Return to play guidelines are based on risk of second impact syndrome
   d. Have full resolution of their symptoms (off medication) and approval by an LHCP to return to play
   e. Neuroimaging should be obtained based on the presence of risk factors for clinically significant brain injuries

7. In the UK, which one of the following head injury scenarios necessitates a CT scan within 1 h of being identified (NICE head injury guideline CG176)?
   a. More than 30 min of retrograde amnesia of events immediately before the head injury
   b. Loss of consciousness and dangerous mechanism of head injury
   c. Isolated post-traumatic seizure
   d. Amnesia since the injury and history of easily bruising (currently on aspirin)
   e. Loss of consciousness since the head injury and age >65 years

8. Which one of the following statements regarding CT head scanning in those with mild head injury is most accurate?
   a. New Orleans criteria apply to head injured patients with GCS 13-15 and loss of consciousness with no focal deficit on neurological examination
   b. Canadian CT head rule high risk group includes those with GCS 13-15 and are aged 70 or older
   c. Canadian CT head rule medium risk criteria include dangerous mechanism of head injury
   d. Canadian CT head rule medium risk criteria include two or more episodes of vomiting
   e. New Orleans criteria apply to GCS 15 head injured patients without loss of consciousness and with a normal examination

9. Which one of the following statements regarding moderate traumatic brain injury is LEAST accurate?
   a. Include head injuries with GCS 9-13
   b. 30% chance of having a brain lesion (intra- or extra-axial)
   c. Mortality is around 30%
   d. Account for 5-7% of head injury attendances in the emergency department
   e. Includes patients who "talk and die"

10. Which one of the following is a biomarker for traumatic brain injury?
   a. GFAP
   b. TP53
   c. ATRX
   d. VEGF
   e. IDH-1

11. Which one of the following is the LEAST appropriate indication for placement of ICP monitor in TBI?
   a. GCS 3-8 with abnormal CT scan
   b. GCS 3-8 with normal CT scan age >40 years and SBP <90 mmHg
   c. Postoperative period after removal of acute subdural hematoma
   d. GCS of 3-8 and diffuse injury type III (Marshall CT classification)
   e. Diffuse injury type II (Marshall CT classification)

12. A 17-year-old boy is struck on the right side of the head during a sports match. He is dazed initially and is taken off the field despite saying he feels fine. He becomes more sleepy over the subsequent 15 min and an ambulance is called. In the emergency department his GCS is E2V3M5 with a sluggish right pupil and weakness on the left side of his body. CT head is shown. Which one of the following is LEAST likely to be an indication for surgery in this type of pathology?

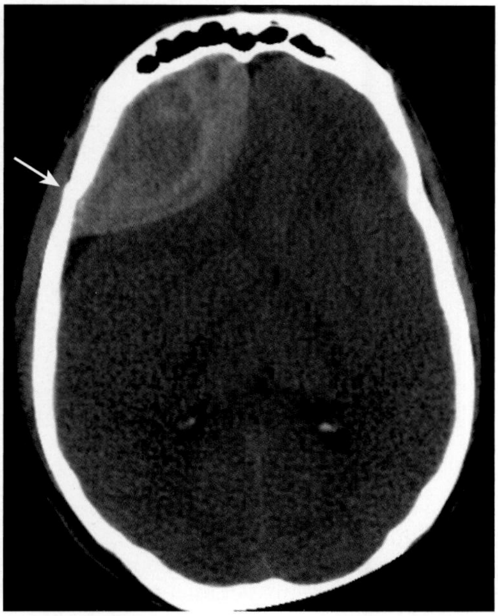

   a. Lesion volume greater than 30 cm^3 with anisocoria and 20 mm maximal thickness
   b. Lesion volume greater than 30 cm^3
   c. GCS 8 or less with evidence of anisocoria
   d. Lesion volume 15 cm^3 with anisocoria but no midline shift
   e. Lesion volume 35 cm^3 with atrophic brain without midline shift

13. A 27-year-old presents to ED after an assault. His GCS is 15/15 but he has evidence of facial fractures involving the frontal sinus and evidence of some CSF rhinorrhea. He is admitted for observation and initial conservative management of CSF leak. On D3 post injury, he developed three episodes of vomiting and became drowsy. On examination he was obtunded and lethargic, but arousable. His BP was 140/90 mmHg, heart rate 59/min, and respiratory rate 20/min and maintained a saturation of 92% on room air. Examination revealed a dilated right pupil whereas the rest of neurological and systemic examination was normal. CT head was repeated (shown). Which one of the following is most appropriate acute management?

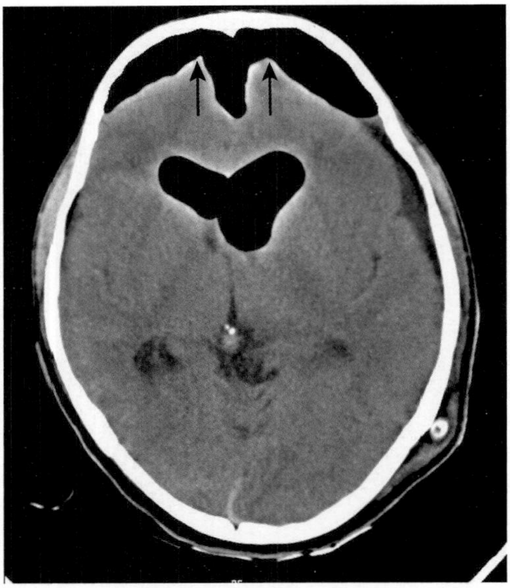

a. High flow oxygen
b. Burr hole decompression
c. Cranialization of the frontal sinus
d. Decompressive craniectomy
e. Minicraniotomy

14. A 57-year-old patient presents with head injury after falling backwards and sudden onset of agitation. Two hours later her blood pressure is 220/110 mmHg, her heart rate is 39 beats per minute, and her consciousness is fluctuating. She is intubated and ventilated. CT is shown. Regarding this type of lesion and its location, which one of the following is LEAST likely to be an indication for surgical evacuation?

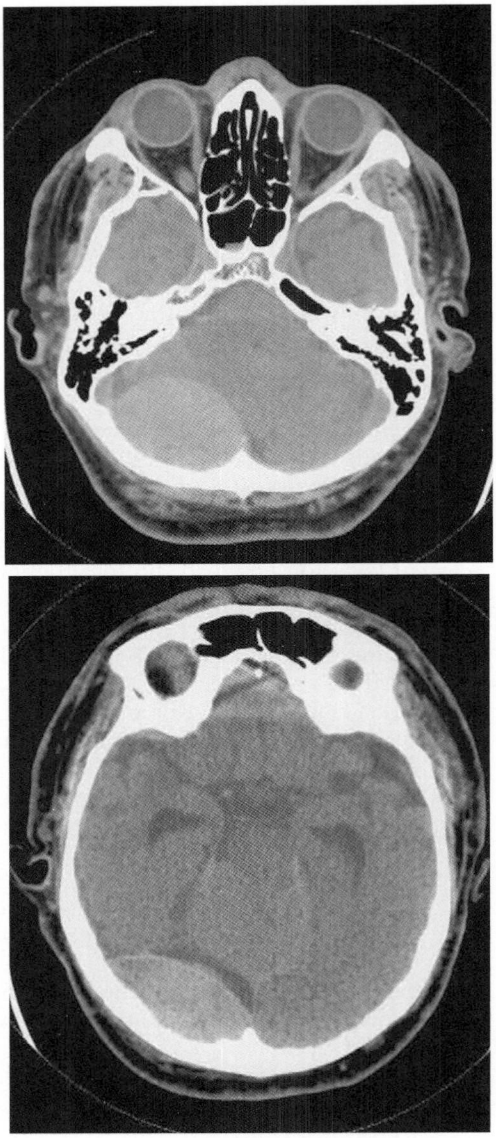

a. Neurological dysfunction or deterioration referable to the lesion
b. Distortion, dislocation, or obliteration of the fourth ventricle
c. Compression or loss of visualization of the temporal horns
d. Presence of obstructive hydrocephalus.
e. Underlying depressed skull fracture

15. A 19-year-old female is involved in a high speed motor vehicle accident and sustained facial injuries from hitting the dashboard. She was GCS 4/15 at the scene and was intubated for transfer. Her pupils are reactive to light. CT head was performed as part of the trauma protocol but did not show any mass lesions or fractures. As this was an isolated head injury a decision was made to wean sedation and assess neurology, but she remained unresponsive. CT is shown below. These are most likely indicative of which one of the following?

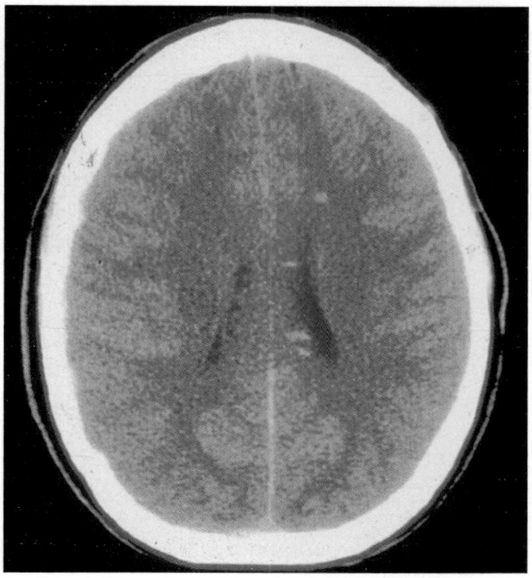

a. Subarachnoid hemorrhage
b. Diffuse axonal injury
c. Cortical contusion
d. Global hypoxic brain damage
e. Cerebral venous sinus thrombosis

16. Which one of the following statements regarding chronic subdural hematomas is LEAST accurate?
a. They form due to separation of the dural border cell layer
b. They may arise secondary to acute subdural hematoma with fails to be resorbed
c. They may arise secondary to repeated hemorrhage into a subdural hygroma
d. They are prone to forming membranes with a tendency to bleed
e. They are more common in females than males at all ages

17. A 72-year-old male develops a worsening headache over the course of 3 weeks. There is no relevant past medical history, except for a minor head injury 6 weeks ago. On examination there is no focal deficit. CT head is shown. In the UK, which one of the following is appropriate next management?

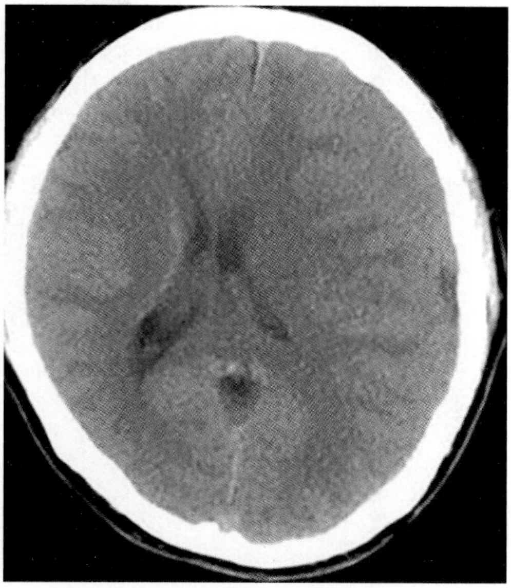

a. Twist drill craniotomy
b. Single burr hole with or without subdural drain
c. Human prothrombin complex concentrate
d. Dexamethasone 2 mg twice daily
e. Minicraniotomy and excision of membranes

18. A 29-year-old is assaulted and is GCS E3V4M5 at the scene. On examination there is significant bruising to the right side of his head with a 5-cm laceration and does not appear to have any focal neurological deficit. He is awaiting a CT scan when you are told he is less responsive. On examination, he is GCS E2V3M4, his right pupil is dilated and on application of painful stimulus appears to only to be moving his left side. Which one of the following is most likely to be responsible for these findings?
a. Transalar (transsphenoidal) herniation
b. Unilateral uncal herniation
c. Ascending transtentorial herniation
d. Tonsillar herniation through the foramen magnum
e. Subfalcine herniation

19. A 45-year-old is involved in a high speed road traffic accident and was GCS E2V3M4 at the scene. He was intubated and ventilated and transferred to a trauma center. En route, his left pupil became sluggish and mannitol was administered. CT head scan is shown. Given the scenario and type of injury shown, which one of the following is the LEAST appropriate indication for surgery according to current guidelines?

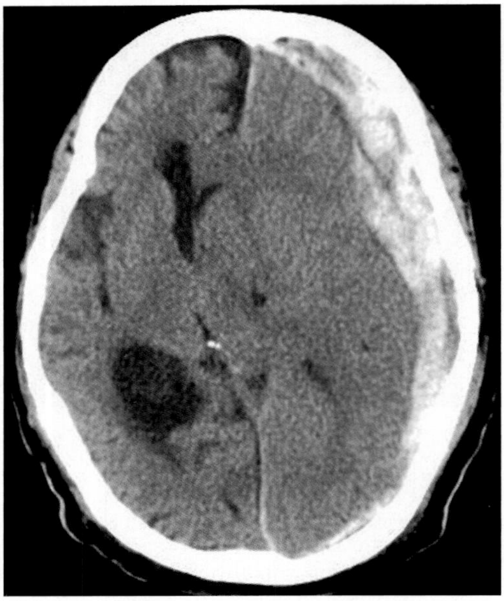

a. Thickness greater than 10 mm
b. Midline shift greater than 5 mm
c. GCS score less than 9, with or without ICP >20 mmHg
d. Documented drop in GCS by 2 or more points since injury
e. Asymmetric or fixed and dilated pupils

20. A 23-year-old female sustains a head injury after accidentally falling from a motorcycle at low speed. She is drowsy at scene and saying inappropriate words, but obeys commands and remained in this state for several hours in the emergency department. CT head showed a small amount of convexity traumatic subarachnoid blood. Which one of the following best reflects her risk of developing post-traumatic epilepsy?
a. <1%
b. 5%
c. 10%
d. 15%
e. 20%

21. Which one of the following statements regarding the lesion shown is LEAST accurate?

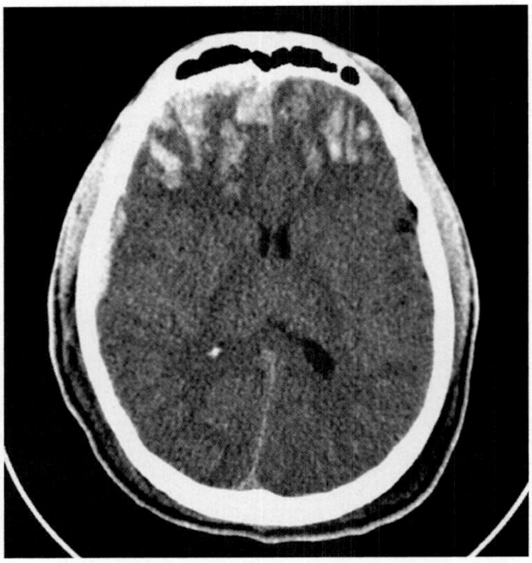

a. Pattern represents about 20% of cases of moderate TBI cerebral contusions
b. Due to acceleration/deceleration injury
c. Associated with ascending transalar herniation
d. Decompressive craniectomy would require cutting the anterior falx
e. Cerebral edema usually peaks between day 5 and 10

22. Which one of the following AP diameters of a decompressive hemicraniectomy flap is the minimum size thought to prevent local complications relating to brain herniation?
a. 10 cm
b. 12 cm
c. 14 cm
d. 16 cm
e. 18 cm

23. Which one of the following statements regarding decompressive craniectomies is LEAST accurate?
a. DECRA trial has shown the utility of early decompressive craniectomy in neuroprotection
b. DECRA trial utilized decompressive craniectomy at tier 2 management of ICP
c. Primary decompressive craniectomy is usually performed during evacuation of an acute subdural hematoma due to concerns regarding brain swelling

d. Secondary decompressive craniectomy is usually undertaken as a last-tier therapy when a patient has intractable intracranial hypertension
e. Level I evidence of the effectiveness of decompressive craniectomy for refractory intracranial hypertension is still lacking

QUESTIONS 24–33

Additional questions 24–33 available on ExpertConsult.com

EXTENDED MATCHING ITEM (EMI) QUESTIONS

34. **Management of ICP:**
    a. Anticonvulsant
    b. Decompressive craniectomy
    c. External ventricular drain and/or hematoma evacuation
    d. ICP monitor
    e. Head up 15°
    f. Hyperosmolar therapy
    g. Midazolam
    h. Normocapnia
    i. Normothermia
    j. Propofol
    k. Thiopentone

For each of the following descriptions, select the most appropriate answers from the list above. Each answer may be used once, more than once, or not at all.

1. Medical therapy only used in highest tier of ICP management
2. Second tier management of raised ICP
3. Surgical procedure considered above tier 3 of ICP management

35. **Continuous Neuromonitoring:**
    a. Brain tissue oxygen tension (PbO_2)
    b. Cerebral perfusion pressure (CPP)
    c. External ventricular drain ICP
    d. Glucose
    e. Glutamate
    f. Glycerol
    g. Invasive microtransducer ICP
    h. Jugular bulb venous oximetry (Svj O_2)
    i. Lactate/pyruvate ratio
    j. Near infra-red spectroscopy
    k. Non-invasive ICP
    l. Pressure reactivity index (PRx)

For each of the following descriptions, select the most appropriate answers from the list above. Each answer may be used once, more than once, or not at all.

1. Assesses changes in the chromophores oxyhemoglobin (HbO_2), deoxyhemoglobin (Hb), and cytochrome oxidase
2. Released from phospholipids
3. Independent marker of increased anaerobic respiration
4. Gold standard for ICP measurement
5. Intact cerebral autoregulation results in a negative value

36. **Complications of decompressive craniectomy and cranioplasty:**
    a. Aseptic bone flap reabsorption
    b. Bone flap depression/cosmetic defect
    c. Bone flap/prosthesis infection
    d. Cerebral abscess
    e. CSF leak
    f. Extradural/subdural empyema
    g. Fall on unprotected cranium
    h. Hemorrhagic progression of contusion
    i. Hydrocephalus
    j. Meningitis/ventriculitis
    k. New contralateral/remote hematoma
    l. New ipsilateral hematoma
    m. Paradoxical herniation
    n. Subdural hygroma
    o. Superficial complications
    p. Syndrome of the trephined

For each of the following descriptions, select the most appropriate answers from the list above. Each answer may be used once, more than once, or not at all.

1. Commonest hemorrhagic complication after decompressive craniectomy
2. Commonest overall reported complication after decompressive craniectomy
3. Commonest complication seen in adult and pediatric autologous cranioplasty

37. **Complications after head injury:**
    a. Carotid-cavernous fistula
    b. Chronic subdural hematoma
    c. Cranial nerve palsy
    d. CSF leak due to skull base fracture
    e. Hydrocephalus
    f. Internal carotid artery dissection
    g. Mucocele
    h. Ossicular disruption
    i. Pituitary dysfunction
    j. Pneumocephalus
    k. Seizures
    l. Subdural hygroma
    m. Traumatic aneurysm
    n. Vasospasm

For each of the following descriptions, select the most appropriate answers from the list above. Each answer may be used once, more than once, or not at all.

1. A 79-year-old presents with a 2-week history of difficulty walking and headache. His wife reports that he seems more confused over the last 2 days. He has a past medical history of hypertension, and takes aspirin and amlodipine. He sustained a fall in the garden 8 weeks ago and hit his head, but did not lose consciousness and not attend the emergency department
2. A 31-year-old presents 2 weeks after sustaining facial trauma after a motorcycle incident which was managed without surgery. Over the last 5 days, she has noticed visual disturbance including double vision, redness of the right sclerae. On examination there is right eye conjunctival injection with corkscrew scleral vessels and proptosis

SBA ANSWERS

1. **a**—22 mild TBI: 1.5 moderate TBI: 1 severe TBI

A World Health Organization (WHO) systematic review of the mTBI literature found that 70-90% of TBI was mild in nature and that hospital-treated mild TBI was approximately 100-300 per 100,000 in the studies it reviewed. However, given the undertreatment and reporting of mild TBI, the WHO estimated that the true yearly incidence was likely 600 per 100,000. Average estimated incidence of TBI in the United States 577 per 100,000, of which 465 per 100,000 were treated in the emergency department and released, 94 per 100,000 were hospitalized and discharged alive, and 18 per 100,000 died. In the UK, every year 1500 per 100,000 of the population attend emergency departments with a head injury, 225-300 per 100,000 are admitted to hospital, 10-15 per 100,000 are admitted to neurosurgical units and 6-10 per 100,000 die from TBI. The aforementioned studies constitute some of the best epidemiological data on incidence of TBI, but the data likely grossly underestimates the incidence of mTBI. European epidemiological studies that calculated a TBI severity ratio of 22 mild TBI: 1.5 moderate TBI: 1 severe TBI (i.e. 90% of TBI is mild). In general, TBI is much more frequent in males than females (1.4:1), highest among young children aged 0-4 (1337 per 100,000) and older adolescence aged 15-19 (896 per 100,000). Older adults aged 75 and above also have a high rate of TBI (932 per 100,000) and they account for the highest rate of TBI-associated hospitalizations (339 per 100,000) and death (57 per 100,000). This pattern of high rates of TBI in early childhood, late adolescence, and in the elderly has been shown in many population-based studies. The relative risk of a second TBI among those with an earlier TBI was 2.8-3 times greater than the non-injured sample. Additionally, in those that sustained a second head injury the risk of sustaining a third head injury was 7.8-9.3 times that of an initial head injury in the population. Alcohol is involved in one third to two thirds of cases, and 20% of those with TBI following motor vehicle collisions.

FURTHER READING

Leo P, McCrea M. Epidemiology. In: Laskowitz D, Grant G, editors. Translational Research in Traumatic Brain Injury. Boca Raton (FL): CRC Press/Taylor and Francis Group, 2016.

Hutchinson PJ, Kirkpatrick PJ. Acute head injury for the neurologist. J Neurol Neurosurg Psychiatry 2002;73(Suppl 1):i3-i7.

2. **b**—Diffuse axonal injury is a type of secondary brain injury

TBI is commonly subdivided into primary and secondary injury. Primary injury results from the mechanical forces on the brain from a combination of direct impact, penetrating injuries and shock waves, and acceleration/deceleration phenomena. Examples of primary injury are diffuse axonal injury, cerebral contusions/hemorrhage, and extra-axial hemorrhage (EDH, SDH, SAH). Secondary brain injury is non-mechanical in nature and due to local (e.g. cerebral edema, regional loss of cerebral autoregulation, anaerobic glycolysis/lactic acidosis, glutamate excitotoxicity) and systemic (e.g. hypoxia, hypotension, hypoglycemia) consequences of the primary injury which aggravate it further. An intermediate set of processes, such as apoptosis and axonal retraction, occur in a delayed fashion (overlapping with time course of secondary injury) but arise from the primary injury. In general, primary brain injury is not treatable (except for hematoma evacuation) and its magnitude is a limiting factor distinguishing survivable from non-survivable brain injury. The major focus of TBI management is thus on limiting/preventing secondary brain injury as much as possible to reduce unfavorable outcomes; this is achieved by ensuring adequate oxygenation/gas transfer, organ perfusion and control of ICP. More recently, tertiary injuries (iatrogenic) have been recognized to contribute to outcome just as strongly as primary or secondary injury. Examples of tertiary injury include complications from a prolonged intensive care unit (ICU) stay (e.g. ventilator-associated pneumonia, line sepsis, decubitus ulcers, or medication administration errors), as well as complications of brain treatment per se, such as transfusion-related acute lung injury, post-operative neurosurgical infections, vasopressor-related ischemia, or hyperosmolar renal failure.

3. **b**—Hypoxia and hypoglycemia are the extracranial insults which most strongly affect prognosis after TBI

Functional recovery from TBI is classified on the Glasgow Outcome Scale and is commonly dichotomized into favorable outcome (5 = good recovery; 4 = moderate disability/independent) versus unfavorable outcome (3 = severe disability/dependent; 4 = vegetative state; 1 = death). The overwhelming majority of patients with mild TBI (GCS 13-15) make a good recovery even though cognitive deficits and symptoms are common in the acute stage, and overall mortality is <1% (reflects the fact that the vast majority of mild TBIs are GCS 15; mortality rate may be up to 30% in those with GCS 13 and reactive pupils but significant brain injury/hematoma on CT head). Mortality rate in moderate TBI is approximately 15% overall. Patients presenting in coma with severe TBI have a 40% mortality rate and a further 20% survive with major disability. Predicting outcome for an individual patient is, however, notoriously difficult and a clear prognosis often emerges only over the days and weeks following injury. MRI of the brain may assist with prognostication of outcome. However, early prognostication and utility in deciding aggressiveness of treatment is plagued by several factors: Inaccurate GCS recording, alcohol/drug intoxication, sedative drugs, intubation (no verbal GCS score), associated trauma preventing assessment of GCS (e.g. maxillo-facial injury), and uncorrected systemic insults (hypotension, hypoxia, hypothermia) which affect consciousness. The IMPACT meta-analysis reviewed reversible insults present on admission and their potential to influence outcome by exacerbating secondary injury. Hypoxia, hypotension (SBP <90 mmHg) and hypothermia (<35 °C) were strongly associated with poor outcomes, with hypoxia and hypotension having synergistic effects. Prognostic models (e.g. IMPACT or CRASH) derived from large prospective datasets have shown that age, severity of primary injury (measured by GCS, pupillary reaction, and CT scan appearances such as traumatic SAH/IVH, cistern effacement, epidural masses, midline shift) and major secondary insults including hypotension, hypoxia and hypothermia are the principal risk factors for death and long-term neurological morbidity. CT appearances alone can also be used for prognostication via Marshall or Rotterdam CT criteria. For illustrative purposes only, CRASH prognostic calculators is shown for isolated head injury (bilateral reactive pupils, CT evidence of petechial hemorrhage, SAH, cistern effacement and MLS without hematoma) scenarios below as ranges of outcome for mild (GCS 13-14), moderate (9-12) and severe (3-8) TBI groups. The CRASH score also incorporates adjustment according to high income (shown) versus low-middle income countries, and GCS 14 or less. IMPACT only considered moderate and severe head injuries (but only motor score is put in) and can be used with or without CT (Marshall) criteria.

	MRC CRASH trial prognosis for a patient with isolated head injury, bilateral reactive pupils, CT evidence of petechial hemorrhage, SAH, cistern effacement/obliteration of third ventricle and midlineshift (but without non-evacuated hematoma) in a high income country		
GCS	Age	Risk of 14-day mortality	Risk of unfavorable outcome at 6 months
Mild (13-14)	≤40 years	14.3-16.4%	38-41.9%
	75-year-old	66.2-69.8%	87.7-89.4%
Moderate (9-12)	≤40 years	18.7-27.2%	45.9-58.1%
	75-year-old	73.1-81.5%	90.8-94.2%
Severe (3-8)	≤40 years	30.5-49.7%	62-78.8%
	75-year-old	83.8-92.1%	95-97.7%

FURTHER READING

The MRC CRASH Trial Collaborators. Predicting outcome after traumatic brain injury: practical prognostic models based on large cohort of international patients. BMJ 2008;336:425.

Predicting outcome after traumatic brain injury: Development and international validation of prognostic scores based on admission characteristics. PLoS Med. 2008;5(8):e165. Website: www.tbi-impact.org.

Kolias AG, Guilfoyle MR, Helmy A. Traumatic brain injury in adults, Pract Neurol. 2013;13(4):228-235.

4. **c**—Clinically significant brain injury is present in 10-15% of cases

Concussion (mild TBI) is a traumatically induced alteration in consciousness (confusion, amnesia with or without an associated loss of consciousness) due to a non-penetrating injury. It usually occurs immediately following the blow or within minutes of it. The majority do not have loss of consciousness hence fail to be recognized. Levels of glutamate rise after concussion and the brain enters a hyperglycotic and hypermetabolic state which may persist for 7-10 days after injury (i.e. the period after which the vast majority of patients are symptom free again), and may make the brain more susceptible to a second impact as altered cerebral autoregulation may produce much more severe sequelae (malignant cerebral edema resistant to treatment and almost certainly fatal). Mild TBI has been classified as GCS of 13-15 (or more recently 14-15 depending on series) but the vast majority are initially GCS 15/15 hence other features must be used to assess risk of further deterioration due to underlying significant brain injury requiring treatment or observation (i.e. a proportion may actually be occult moderate/potentially severe TBI: "talk and die patients" with a lucid interval before deterioration). Clinical grading systems for concussion based on duration/presence of confusion, post-traumatic amnesia and LOC have been used, but key concerns generally focus on the need for and timing of neuroimaging for which more useful rules incorporating these features exist (e.g. Canadian CT head rules, New Orleans Criteria). In a recent systematic review of 23,079 adults presenting with minor head trauma (GCS 13-15 who appear well on examination). The prevalence of severe intracranial injury (subdural, epidural, ventricular or parenchymal hematoma, subarachnoid hemorrhage, herniation, or depressed skull fracture, small intracranial hemorrhages requiring observation in the hospital, neurosurgical evaluation, or operative intervention) was 7.1% (95% CI, 6.8-7.4%) and the prevalence of injuries leading to death or requiring neurosurgical intervention was 0.9% (95% CI, 0.78-1.0%). In those with abnormal CT head not requiring surgery or those with normal CT head but if GCS <15, seizures or coagulopathy inpatient observation for 24 h is recommended due to risk of developing intracranial complications (e.g. cerebral swelling, delayed hematoma) and need for repeat CT head before discharge. In those with normal CT head and normal GCS with none or mild symptoms may be able to be observed at home by a responsible adult aware of signs requiring immediate medical assessment. Further management on discharge relates to post-concussion syndrome, risk of second impact syndrome (particularly return to play guidelines in athletes and contraindications to returning to contact sport), risk of post-traumatic epilepsy and, in those with multiple concussions, risk of chronic traumatic encephalopathy.

FURTHER READING

Easter JS, et al. Will Neuroimaging Reveal a Severe Intracranial Injury in This Adult With Minor Head Trauma?: The Rational Clinical Examination Systematic Review. JAMA. 2015;314(24):2672-2681.

5. **e**—Dysfunction of cerebral autoregulation after an initial concussion is thought to underlie the risk for second impact syndrome

Complications of Concussion (Mild TBI)

Complication	Description
Post-concussion syndrome	Post-concussion symptoms may result from brain injury or from trauma involving head and neck structures. These include headache (commonest), dizziness (including vertigo and nonspecific dizziness), neuropsychiatric symptoms, and cognitive impairment. These typically develop in the first days after mild traumatic brain injury (TBI) and generally resolve within a few weeks to a few months. Post-traumatic vertigo may be due to direct injury to cochlear/vestibular structures, labyrinthine concussion, BPPV, perilymphatic fistulae, vertebral artery dissection amongst others

Continued

Complication	Description
Second impact syndrome	Diffuse cerebral swelling occurs after a second concussion, while an athlete is still symptomatic from an earlier concussion. Some have suggested a similarity with this phenomenon and the shaken baby syndrome. The cause is hypothesized to be disordered cerebral autoregulation causing cerebrovascular congestion and malignant cerebral edema with increased intracranial pressure. The second impact syndrome is a rare and somewhat controversial complication. It is unclear why this is not a more frequently reported occurrence in boxers who seem at very high risk for repeated concussions within a short time span
Chronic traumatic encephalopathy	Defined as a slowly progressive disease (tauopathy) that takes years to decades to develop, often providing a significant latent period between when the neurotrauma occurs and when symptoms develop. It was first described in Boxers, and is thought to be due to repetitive head injury. Clinical features include behavioral disturbances such as impulsivity, depression, and lack of oversight, followed later by cognitive impairment. Pathological criteria include neurofibrillary tangles (NFTs) in a perivascular distribution and within superficial cortical areas with occasional amyloid and TDP-43 protein aggregations. neurotrauma may have many lasting deleterious consequences, including the potential for increased risk and accelerated development of Alzheimer's disease and motor neuron disease
Seizures	Mild TBI is associated with a twofold increase in the risk of epilepsy for the first 5 years after injury. Seizures occurring within the first week of injury are acute symptomatic events and are not considered epilepsy. Half of the seizures consistent with post-traumatic epilepsy will occur in the first year; 80% will occur within 2 years. Prophylactic treatment with anticonvulsants does not prevent post-traumatic epilepsy and is not recommended

6. **c**—Return to play guidelines are based on risk of second impact syndrome

AAN sports concussion guidelines 2013 advised that any athlete suspected of having sustained a concussion should be immediately removed from play to minimize the risk for further injury. The risk of further injury refers to the evidence that a single concussion predisposes to a second one, and this risk of a second concussion is particularly increased in the 10 days following the first concussion. The reason for this increased risk for a second injury is unknown, but given that it mirrors the time taken for >90% of those with concussion to become symptom-free again (i.e. 7-10 days) the most likely hypothesis is that impaired cognition or physical reflexes due to the first concussion increase the player's susceptibility to injury. Due to a lack of robust evidence regarding their respective mechanisms concerns regarding the risks of repetitive head injury (second impact syndrome or chronic traumatic encephalopathy) are not the basis for current recommendations, although the general principle of avoiding a second impact while still symptomatic from the first may be necessary but not sufficient to avoid second impact syndrome based on current concepts regarding its pathophysiology. More specific guidance is outlined below:

- Players who experience symptoms suggestive of concussion, such as blurry or double vision, confusion, dizziness, headache, nausea, memory loss, or other cognitive or behavioral problems, must have full resolution of their symptoms (off medication) and approval by an LHCP to return to play. Supplemental neurocognitive testing, including comparisons with age-matched normal profiles or a patient's baseline profile can be used to aid decision making
- An athlete cannot return to play *that day* if a concussion had been diagnosed, even if symptoms had cleared. This may be inadvertently circumvented if the athlete hides their symptoms and has a normal examination, or player with a witnessed head injury whose concussive symptoms don't appear until after the game (who would have already been exposed to the risk of a second impact)
- Concussion is a clinical diagnosis. In a proportion of those with concussion, a CT head should be obtained based on the presence of risk factors (e.g. Canadian CT head rules, New Orleans criteria) to rule out clinically

important brain injury requiring admission to hospital for observation or neurosurgery

- Athletes with multiple concussions and continued impairment, should undergo formal neurologic and cognitive assessment and be counseled on the risk for developing chronic neurobehavioral or cognitive impairment and retirement recommended (lower threshold for professional vs. amateur athletes)

FURTHER READING

Giza CC, Kutcher JS, Ashwal S. Summary of evidence-based guideline update: evaluation and management of concussion in sports: report of the Guideline Development Subcommittee of the American Academy of Neurology, Neurology. 2013;80 (24):2250-2257.

7. **c**—Isolated post-traumatic seizure

UK NICE Guidelines for CT Head Scan in Patients Presenting with TBI

Risk Factors for Clinically Significant Brain Injury in Those With Head Injury	Actions Required
GCS less than 13 on initial assessment in the emergency department GCS less than 15 at 2 h after the injury on assessment in the emergency department Suspected open or depressed skull fracture Any sign of basal skull fracture (hemotympanum, "panda" eyes, cerebrospinal fluid leakage from the ear or nose, Battle's sign) Post-traumatic seizure Focal neurological deficit More than 1 episode of vomiting	CT head scan within 1 h of any one risk factor being identified
If some loss of consciousness or amnesia since the injury and at least one of the following risk factors: Age 65 years or older Any history of bleeding or clotting disorders Dangerous mechanism of injury (a pedestrian or cyclist struck by a motor vehicle, an occupant ejected from a motor vehicle or fall from a height >1 m or 5 stairs) More than 30 min of retrograde amnesia of events immediately before the head injury	CT head scan within 8 h of head injury
Head injury on warfarin (even without other risk factors)	CT head scan within 1 h

FURTHER READING

National Institute for Health and Clinical Excellence. Head injury (2014) NICE guideline CG176.

8. **c**—Canadian CT head rule medium risk criteria include dangerous mechanism of head injury

Many physicians follow a set of criteria for selecting which patients should receive a head CT following mild TBI (concussion). The Canadian CT Head Rule (CCR) was derived from a study of 3121 patients presenting to 10 Canadian hospitals with a GCS score of 13-15/15 after head injury (excluding those <16 years, bleeding disorders or warfarin, obvious open skull fracture). CT head is mandatory if one or more of the following high-risk criteria for neurosurgical intervention are present: (1) GCS score less than 15 at 2 h after head injury; (2) suspected open or depressed skull fracture; (3) any sign of basal skull fracture (e.g. hemotympanum, "raccoon" eyes, CSF otorrhea/rhinorrhea, Battle's sign); (4) two or more episodes of vomiting; and (5) patient is 65 years of age or older. CT head is also recommended in patients in the medium-risk category who may have clinically important brain injuries that may require admission: (1) greater than 30 min of retrograde amnesia or (2) injury via a "dangerous mechanism" (e.g. motor vehicle accident versus pedestrian, ejection from motor vehicle, fall from greater than 3 feet or down five or more stairs). The New Orleans criteria for CT head in mild TBI applies to emergency department patients with a GCS 15/15 only with LOC and a normal neurological examination. In this situation, CT head should be performed if any one of the following risk factors present: age >60 years, headache, vomiting, drug/alcohol intoxication, persistent anterograde amnesia, post-traumatic seizure, and evidence of trauma above the clavicles. In a recent systematic review of 23,079 adults presenting with minor head trauma (GCS 13-15 who appear well on examination). The prevalence of severe intracranial injury (requiring prompt intervention) was 7.1% (95% CI, 6.8-7.4%) and the prevalence of injuries leading to death or requiring neurosurgical intervention was 0.9% (95% CI, 0.78-1.0%). Features most predictive of severe intracranial injury on CT were examination findings suggestive of skull fracture, GCS score 13/15, 2 or more vomiting episodes, any decline in GCS and pedestrians struck by motor vehicles. Absence of any of the features of the Canadian CT Head Rule (high and medium risk) lowered the probability of severe injury to 0.31% (95% CI, 0-4.7%). The absence of any New Orleans Criteria findings lowered the probability of severe intracranial injury to 0.61% (95% CI, 0.08-6.0%).

FURTHER READING

Pardini J, Bailes JE, Maroon JC. Mild Traumatic Brain Injury in Adults and Concussion in Sports. In Winn HR (ed), Youmans Neurological Surgery, 6th ed., Elsevier, Saunders, 2011.

9. **c**—Mortality is around 30%

TBI with GCS scores of 9-12 is considered moderate, though some now consider those with a GCS of 13 within this category too given that a third have abnormal CT head findings. They account for 5-7% of head injury attendances in the emergency department (22 mild: 1.5 moderate: 1 severe) and affects the young adult population involved in traffic accidents, is associated with alcohol or illicit drugs, and with extracranial injuries. Individuals with moderate TBI have approximately a 30% chance of having a brain lesion (intra- or extra-axial), a 30% chance that such injuries progress in their volume or mass effect (new bleeding, rebleeding, edema) and a 30% chance that these individuals suffer deterioration or worsening in their neurological status. Mortality in moderate TBI is around 15%, >50% have cognitive sequelae and only 20% recover without significant disability. Most "talk and die" patients (i.e. lucid interval; patients presenting with a verbal GCS score ≥3 who were thought to have sustained a survivable head injury who later deteriorate and die to due potentially treatable head injury) should also be in the moderate TBI category. The authors concluded that morbidity and mortality in these patients might be reduced by early diagnosis and more aggressive treatment of raised ICP. More recent studies have shown that patients who "talk and die" are most frequently adult men and the most common mechanisms of trauma are falls, motor vehicle accidents and violence. In these studies, the average GCS at admission to emergency department was 14 and the most frequent intracranial injuries were acute subdural hematoma, diffuse cerebral edema and cerebral contusion. In about 14% of these patients with GCS 13 at admission, initial CT was normal but became abnormal during hospitalization, especially because of development of diffuse cerebral edema. Among the most important factors relating to death are: delays in diagnosis of lesion through CT scan (as initially appear well), delays in the transfer to a specialized center, failure to identify risk factors for deterioration, inadequate prevention of secondary injury, inappropriate correction of underlying coagulopathy and loss of the opportunity for definitive neurosurgical treatment.

10. **a**—GFAP

In future, early biomarkers may facilitate decisions to perform CT head in mild TBI (e.g. improving early identification of patients likely to "talk and die") and later biomarkers to predict prolonged complications or to monitor TBI recovery.

Numerous candidate biomarkers have proven prognostic value with TBI outcome, such as: glial fibrillary acidic protein (GFPA; glial cell injury), unbiquitin C-terminal hydrolase-L1 (UCH-L1; neuronal cell body injury), SBDP150/SBDP145 (spectrin breakdown products; axon and presynaptic terminal necrosis), S100B (Calcium-Binding Protein B; elevated blood and urine levels in glial injury), and NSE (neuron-specific enolase; neuronal injury). However, they generally show low specificity or sensitivity when used individually hence combining biomarkers into a screening panel may provide more information than individual biomarkers (e.g. GFAP/UCH-L1, NSE/S100B).

FURTHER READING

Acute biomarkers of traumatic brain injury: relationship between plasma levels of ubiquitin C-terminal hydrolase-L1 and glial fibrillary acidic protein. J Neurotrauma. 2014;31(1):19-25.

Brain injury biomarkers may improve the predictive power of the IMPACT outcome calculator. J Neurotrauma. 2012;29(9):1770-1778.

Neuron-specific enolase and S100BB as outcome predictors in severe diffuse axonal injury. J Trauma Acute Care Surg. 2012;72(6):1654-1657.

11. **e**—Diffuse injury type II (i.e. cisterns present with midline shift <5 mm and/or lesion densities present, no high or mixed density lesion >25 ml)

The principle of ICP monitoring is to maintain adequate cerebral perfusion and oxygenation to meet metabolic demands. Raised ICP reduces CPP and CBF, which exacerbates secondary injury. Several studies have shown that patients with an ICP <20 mmHg have a reduced risk of neurological deterioration, compared with higher ICPs (ICP ≥25 mmHg). Mortality also increases dramatically from 17% to 47% when an average ICP >20 mmHg. However, Level I and level II evidence suggesting ICP monitoring improves outcome in TBI is lacking. In one randomized trial of ICP versus clinical examination plus imaging, there was no significant improvement in survival between the study groups. Similar findings have been confirmed by other studies that have concluded that ICP-targeted/CPP-targeted intensive care tends to prolong mechanical ventilation and increases therapy intensity without evidence of improved outcome. Nonetheless, ICP monitoring is recommended for the management of severe TBI (GCS 3-8) with abnormal CT scan, and in patients with normal CT scan but >2 of age >40 years, SBP <90 mmHg, decorticate posturing, decerebrate posturing. Indications in those with moderate TBI are less clear, but include: (a) Postoperative period after removal of acute subdural hematoma or multiple cerebral contusion. In these cases, sudden changes in ICP could signal hemorrhages due to decompression or reperfusion, new extra-axial collections or worsening brain swelling. (b) GCS of 9-11 and cerebral contusion (temporal or bifrontal) without surgical intervention. In these instances, ICP monitoring can help recognize progression of the contusions. (c) Diffuse injury type III (Marshall CT classification: cisterns compressed or absent with MLS <5 mm, no high or mixed density lesion >25 ml). Due to the high probability of intracranial hypertension and poor outcome, ICP monitoring in these cases is indispensable. (d) General anesthesia for emergency non-cranial surgery (especially in the presence of conservatively treated intracranial lesions) due to loss of clinical evaluation and potential effects of anesthetics on cerebrovascular autoregulation. (e) Concomitant severe chest trauma requiring deep sedation, high PEEP levels, recruitment maneuvers or prone ventilation which may cause hypercapnia or impair cerebral venous return, causing cerebral vasodilation and increased ICP. (f) Concomitant intra-abdominal compartment syndrome (associated with intracranial hypertension). (g) Prolonged traumatic shock (risk of cerebral edema).

FURTHER READING

Godoy DA, Rubiano A, Rabinstein AA, et al. Moderate Traumatic Brain Injury: The Grey Zone of Neurotrauma, Neurocrit Care. 2016 Feb 29.

12. **e**—Lesion volume 35 cm^3 with atrophic brain without midline shift

The clinical scenario is of a right frontotemporal EDH with a swirling appearance on imaging due to leakage of serum from clot or active bleeding. EDH is seen in 2.7-4% of traumatic brain injury, and 9% of severe TBI. Mortality approximates 10%. Peak incidence of EDH is in the second decade, and the mean age of patients with EDH is between 20 and 30 years of age. EDH can result from injury to the middle meningeal artery (90%), the middle meningeal vein, the diploic veins, or the venous sinuses. Venous epidural less common—usually post fossa, usually pediatric, can extend across tentorium to be both supra and infratentorial (transverse/sigmoid sinus), paramedian/vertex (superior sagittal), middle cranial fossa floor (sphenoparietal sinus). Injury can result in pseudoaneurysm of meningeal artery or a dural AV fistula if both artery and vein lacerated. Presentation is with coma (one third to a half), lucid interval (less than a half) and the remainder remain conscious. Pupillary abnormalities are present in approximately 20-40%. The hematoma volume can be estimated quickly from the head CT scan by using the formula $A \times B \times C/2$, which approximates the volume of an ellipsoid. On the CT slice with the largest area of hemorrhage, A is the greatest hemorrhage diameter and B is the largest diameter perpendicular to A. Giving each slice a value of 1 or 0.5 if the area is >75% or 25-75% of the index slice used to measure A and B, their sum is multiplied by slice thickness in cm to give C. An epidural hematoma (EDH) greater than 30 cm^3 should be surgically evacuated regardless of the patient's Glasgow Coma Scale (GCS) score. An EDH less than 30 cm^3 and with less than a 15-mm thickness and with less than a 5-mm midline shift (MLS) in patients with a GCS score greater than 8 without focal deficit can be managed non-operatively with serial computed tomographic (CT) scanning and close neurological observation in a neurosurgical center, but enlargement occurs in 20% of cases. It is strongly recommended that patients with an acute EDH in coma (GCS score <9) with anisocoria undergo surgical evacuation as soon as possible (i.e. within 1 h). Bilateral EDH is comparatively uncommon entity, accounting for approximately 2-5% of adults with extradural hematoma. Kett-White and Martin classified such cases into two distinct groups: patients with bilateral but separate extradural hematoma located in the convexities, resulting from dura being stripped from the skull independently on both sides, either simultaneously or sequentially; and, more rarely, patients with bilateral extradural hematoma straddling the midline, resulting from injury to the sagittal sinus. Although all identified cases with bilateral extradural hematoma resulting from sagittal sinus injury underwent urgent surgical evacuation, the operative technique varied regarding preserve the midline skull vault and use dural tenting sutures, or—in selected cases—expose the sagittal sinus and attempt primary repair.

Image with permission from Kirmi O, Sheerin F, Patel N, Imaging of the meninges and the extra-axial spaces, Semin Ultrasound CT MR. 2009;30 (6):565–593.

FURTHER READING

Bullock MR, Chesnut R, Ghajar J, et al. Surgical management of acute epidural hematomas. Neurosurgery. 2006;58(3 Suppl):S7-S15; discussion Si-Sv. Review.

Bimpis A, Marcus HJ, Wilson MH. Traumatic bifrontal extradural haematoma resulting from superior sagittal sinus injury: case report. J R Soc Open 2015;6.

13. **b**—Burr hole decompression

Pneumocephalus is the presence of intracranial air, which invariably resolves spontaneously or with conservative treatment. However, clinical deterioration can occur in tension pneumocephalus where a progressive accumulation of intracranial air which cannot escape (ball valve mechanism) exerts mass effect on the brain and can lead to coma, herniation and death. Tension PC is commonly caused by intra or extra-cranial surgeries like drainage of chronic subdural hematoma, craniofacial surgery, otorhinolaryngological procedures, shunt operations/CSF drainage, trauma (fractures through skull base involving air sinuses), meningitis/otitis, anesthesia (spinal, ventilation, nitric oxide induced), and tumors. Accumulation of trapped air in subdural and interhemispheric space bilaterally, is seen as hypodense collections causing compression and separation of the frontal lobes (Mount Fuji sign). Emergency management is by decompression, usually by opening up previous burr hole (if present) or making a new one. Definitive management will involve identifying the site of air entry and intracranial or extracranial repair.

Image from Jakherea, SG, Yadava DA, Jaina, DG, Balasubramaniamb, S; Does the Mount Fuji Sign always signify "tension" pneumocephalus? An exception and a reappraisal, European Journal of Radiology Extra, 2011;78(1): e5-e7.

14. **c**—Compression or loss of visualization of the temporal horns

The clinical scenario suggests a Cushing's reflex secondary to an expanding right sided posterior fossa extradural hematoma, most probably due to transverse sinus laceration, and evidence of 4th ventricular effacement and obstructive hydrocephalus. Upward herniation of cerebellar vermis through the tentorial incisura is also seen. Indications for surgery include neurological dysfunction or deterioration referable to the lesion, or presence of mass effect: distortion, dislocation, or obliteration of the fourth ventricle; compression or loss of visualization of the basal cisterns, or the presence of obstructive hydrocephalus. Evacuation via suboccipital craniectomy should be performed as soon as possible because these patients can deteriorate rapidly, thus, worsening their prognosis. Patients with lesions and no significant mass effect on CT scan and without signs of neurological dysfunction may be managed by close observation and serial imaging.

Image from Naidich T, Castillo M, Cha S. Smirniotopoulos J, Imaging of the Brain, Elsevier, Saunders, 2013.

FURTHER READING

Bullock MR, Chesnut R, Ghajar, J et al. Surgical management of posterior fossa mass lesions. Neurosurgery. 2006;58(3 Suppl):S47-S55; discussion Si-Siv. Review.

15. **b**—Diffuse axonal injury

Diffuse axonal injury is the most common cause of coma in the head-injured patient without an intracranial mass lesion. It is characterized pathologically by diffusely spread axonal swellings affecting the white matter, corpus callosum, and upper brainstem. These foci are usually hemorrhagic. The etiology is thought to be due to shearing forces on axons in certain susceptible regions of the brain, notably those that are particularly vulnerable to rotational forces, such as the subcortical white matter, corpus callosum, and upper brainstem. On MRI the spots will appear as T2 bright lesions and appear dark on GRE. Classically, DAI has been considered to be a major neuropathological feature of severe TBI, but most experts now agree that almost all TBI is usually accompanied by some degree of DAI and brain volume loss. There have been no evidence-based effective treatments specifically for DAI, hence avoidance of secondary brain injury, and medial and/or surgical management of ICP are the mainstay.

Image from Haaga JR, et al. (Eds). CT and MRI of the Whole Body, 5th ed., Elsevier, Mosby, 2009.

16. **e**—They are more common in females than males at all ages

A chronic subdural hematoma (CSDH) is a collection of blood breakdown products in the subdural space. Estimates of the incidence of CSDH range from 8.2 to 14.0 per 100,000 person-years. Presentation is predominantly in the seventh decade onwards and is more frequent in males (approximately 3:1 male to female ratio across all age groups). CSDH arises at the dural border cell layer (between the dura mater and arachnoid mater) which is prone to separation creating a "subdural space," particularly in those with cerebral atrophy (e.g. elderly, alcoholics). Minor precipitant trauma can generate CSDH either from the incomplete breakdown/reabsorption of ASDH or recurrent microhemorrhage into subdural hygromas. ASDH may occur due to tearing of the bridging veins that traverse the dural border cell layer or, less commonly, tearing of cortical arteries or veins. In contrast, a subdural hygroma (CSF collection), is caused by splitting of the dural border cell layer at points of tension between the dura mater and arachnoid mater. Neovascularization occurs in the newly formed subdural space and hemorrhage from these new vessels leads to the formation of a CSDH. In both cases, the opening of the dural border cell layer into a subdural space triggers a reparatory response which either causes hematoma/hygroma resolution or hematoma enlargement. The latter is thought to be due to a localized inflammatory reaction, which results in hyperfibrinolysis of the clot and production of angiogenic factors that promote neovascularization and further bleeding from fragile capillaries. Formation of neomembranes is one of the main features of CSDH—the inner (visceral) membrane is less vascular and usually thinner than the outer (parietal) membrane. Risk factors for CSDH include advancing age, a history of falls, minor head injury, use of anticoagulants or antiplatelet drugs, bleeding diatheses, alcohol (contributing to globalized brain atrophy, increased risk of falls, and hepatogenic coagulopathy), epilepsy, intracranial hypotension, and hemodialysis.

FURTHER READING

Kolias AG, Chari A, Santarius T, Hutchinson PJ. Chronic subdural haematoma: modern management and emerging therapies, Nat Rev Neurol. 2014;10(10):570-578.

17. **b**—Single burr hole with subdural drain

Medical management of Subacute SDH or CSDH generally involves correction of bleeding disorders/anticoagulation and any interventions required to improve anesthetic fitness (e.g. treat infections, optimize gas exchange, etc.). Steroids may be useful as adjunctive therapy preoperatively or postoperatively, or as monotherapy as an alternative to surgical intervention (in small, mildly symptomatic CSDH), but their role remains ill-defined in the absence of level I evidence. Preoperative antiepileptic prophylaxis has been shown to affect postoperative seizure rate but not discharge outcome, hence is not particularly advocated. In patients with mild or no symptoms and relatively small collections, or moribund patients with poor baseline function may both be managed non-operatively. However, surgical treatment of symptomatic CSDH results in rapid improvement of symptoms, and produces a favorable outcome in over 80% of patients. Coupled with relatively low surgical risk, surgical evacuation is currently the mainstay of management for symptomatic patients. Three primary surgical techniques are used: twist drill craniostomy (TDC) involving small openings (<10 mm) made using a twist drill, burr hole craniostomy (BHC; most popular) involving openings of 10-30 mm, and craniotomy involving larger openings. The BHC technique involves the drilling of burr holes over the cerebral convexity followed by durotomy, usually under general anesthetic. Insertion of a subdural drain in the anterior hole connected to a closed drainage system for approximately 48 h decreased CSDH recurrence after BHC from 24.3% to 9.3% ($P=0.003$) and 6-month mortality from 18.1% to 9.6% ($P=0.042$). Twist drill craniostomy can be performed under local anesthesia either at the bedside or in the operating theatre, making it an attractive option for the elderly patient with multiple comorbidities. A recent modification to the original technique involves the insertion of a hollow screw to set up a closed drainage system. This technique, unlike the traditional TDC technique, does not require the blind insertion of a catheter in the subdural space, thereby minimizing the risks of brain laceration and bleeding from cortical vessels. Craniotomy involves general anesthesia and is commonly reserved for recurrent CSDH with extensive organization and membrane formation (preventing brain re-expansion) or primary evacuation of a CSDH that has a substantial acute component. Systematic reviews comparing the three techniques have generally found either no difference between TDC and BHC, or lower recurrence rates with BHC and craniotomy, higher morbidity with craniotomy (and in one review BHC), and a higher mortality with craniotomy.

Image with permission from Takemotoa, Y, Hashiguchib, A, Morokib, K et al. Chronic subdural hematoma with persistent hiccups: A case report, Interdisciplinary Neurosurgery, 2016;3:1-2.

FURTHER READING

Kolias AG, Chari A, Santarius T, Hutchinson PJ. Chronic subdural haematoma: modern management and emerging therapies, Nat Rev Neurol. 2014;10(10):570-578.

Santarius T et al. Use of drain versus no drains after burr hole evacuation of chronic subdural haematoma: a randomised controlled trial. Lancet. 2009;364:1067-1073.

18. **b**—Unilateral uncal herniation

Subfalcine herniation is the commonest type of herniation patter as it is measured by midline shift of the septum pellucidum, and reflects cingulate gyrus, anterior cerebral artery, internal cerebral vein and lateral ventricle compression. Complications of subfalcine herniation are contralateral lateral ventricle hydrocephalus due to obstruction of the foramen of Monro, and ipsilateral ACA compression against the falx resulting in infarction and contralateral leg weakness. Following subfalcine herniation, descending transtentorial herniation is the second most common type of herniation syndrome and may occur unilaterally or bilaterally. With increasing supratentorial mass effect, the uncus of the anteromedial temporal lobe is driven medially to efface the suprasellar cistern (uncal herniation). Medial shift of the hippocampus and parahippocampal gyrus then follows with subsequent effacement of the mesencephalic and quadrigeminal cisterns and compression of the midbrain. Kernohan's notch phenomenon is an uncommon but important scenario described by this case where a unilateral hemispheric expanding mass lesion causing ipsilateral uncal herniation (descending transtentorial herniation; associated with 3rd nerve palsy) results in compression of the contralateral cerebral peduncle against the tentorium cerebelli creating a "notch" in it. This leads to the confusing picture of hemiparesis on the same side as the mass lesion (false localizing sign). By contrast, diffuse brain swelling (e.g. hypoxic brain injury) is likely to cause a more symmetrical uncal herniation without this phenomenon. With midbrain caudal compression, there is progressive narrowing of the normal angle ($\sim$90°) between the ventral midbrain and pons with subsequent compression of basilar artery perforators and potentiation for secondary midbrain hemorrhagic infarct—Duret hemorrhage. Ascending transtentorial cerebellar herniation through the tentorial notch due to a mass lesion in the posterior fossa causes rapid loss of consciousness, noncommunicating hydrocephalus and PCA/SCA territory infarction. Descending transalar herniation occurs as a result of frontal lobe mass effect with posterior and inferior displacement of the posterior aspect of the frontal lobe orbital surface over the sphenoid wing and MCA compression. Ascending transalar herniation is produced by middle cranial fossa or temporal lobemass effect resulting in displacement of the temporal lobe superiorly and anteriorly across the sphenoid ridge causing compression of the ICA. Tonsillar cerebellar herniation though the foramen magnum may be chronic/congenital (e.g. Chiari I malformation), due to primary posterior fossa mass lesions or secondary to descending transtentorial herniation from a supratentorial mass lesion; compression of the brainstem against the clivus results in compression of respiratory and cardiac centers.

19. **c**—GCS score less than 9, with or without ICP >20 mmHg

Acute SDH complicates 11% of all TBI, and 10-30% of severe TBI. Most SDH are caused by motor vehicle-related accidents (MVA), falls, and assaults. The elderly population is particularly susceptible due to increased fragility of vessel walls, falls and greater use of antithrombotic and anticoagulants agents. Between 37% and 80% of patients with acute SDH present with initial GCS scores of 8 or less. A lucid interval has been described in 12-38% of patients before admission but there is no conclusive evidence that this correlates with outcome. The definition of lucid interval is vague. Authors interpret the lucid interval differently and analysis of its frequency requires documentation during the prehospital phase. Pupillary abnormalities are observed in 30-50% of patients on admission or before surgery. Compared with EDH, the degree of underlying brain damage associated with ASDH is more severe, and mortality rates are greater especially in older patients with poor initial

GCS, and other associated brain or systemic injuries. Studies looking at patients from all age groups with GCS scores between 3 and 15 with SDH requiring surgery quote mortality rates between 40 and 60%. Mortality among patients presenting to the hospital in coma with subsequent surgical evacuation is between 57% and 68%. Only 30-40% of SDH requiring surgery are isolated lesions. In the majority of cases, the SDH is associated with other intracranial and extracranial injuries. An acute subdural hematoma (SDH) with a thickness greater than 10 mm or a midline shift greater than 5 mm on computed tomographic (CT) scan should be surgically evacuated, regardless of the patient's Glasgow Coma Scale (GCS) score. All patients with acute SDH in coma (GCS score less than 9) should undergo intracranial pressure (ICP) monitoring. A comatose patient (GCS score less than 9) with an SDH less than 10 mm thick and a midline shift less than 5 mm should undergo surgical evacuation of the lesion if the GCS score decreased between the time of injury and hospital admission by 2 or more points on the GCS and/or the patient presents with asymmetric or fixed and dilated pupils and/or the ICP exceeds 20 mmHg. In patients with acute SDH and indications for surgery, surgical evacuation should be performed as soon as possible, with or without bone flap removal and duraplasty. Patients with less severe ASDH can be monitored clinically; after 7-10 days an ASDH may liquefy, to become drainable with burr holes, thus avoiding the major morbidity of craniotomy.

Image from Fujimoto K, Otsuka T, Yoshizato K, Kuratsu J. Predictors of rapid spontaneous resolution of acute subdural hematoma, Clin Neurol Neurosurg. 2014;118:94-97.

FURTHER READING

Bullock MR, et al. Surgical management of acute subdural hematomas. Neurosurgery. 2006;58(3 Suppl):S16-S24; discussion Si-Siv. Review.

20. **b**—5%

Post-traumatic seizures are classified into early (<1 week post-injury) and late (>1 week post-injury). Generally children are more likely to develop early seizures, whereas adults are more likely to develop post-traumatic epilepsy. Overall, the rate of post-traumatic epilepsy after TBI is approximately 2% over the subsequent 10 years. However, frequency increases with severity of TBI: the risk is only marginally higher than the general population in mild TBI, less than 5% in moderate TBI and affects 10-15% of patients after severe TBI. Short-term anti-epileptic prophylaxis for high-risk cases (e.g. cortical contusion, depressed skull fracture) as it has been shown to reduce the incidence of early seizures; however, there is no evidence supporting the use of long-term prophylaxis to prevent post-traumatic epilepsy.

21. **c**—Associated with ascending transalar herniation

Bifrontal contusions are present in about 20% of cases of moderate TBI with cerebral contusion and are due to acceleration/deceleration forces pushing the inferior frontal lobes and temporal pole against the irregular skull base. Hemorrhagic swelling of these contusions may disrupt the median forebrain bundle, gyrus rectus, and anterior hypothalamic nuclei. These structures are involved in behavior control and are associated with changes in personality, volition, motivation, judgment, and social interactions. When these contusions swell, the brain is displaced posteriorly (descending transalar herniation) and abrupt deterioration because of descent of the brain stem into the posterior fossa with stretching and deformity of the small perforating blood vessels of the basilar artery with risk of death due to respiratory arrest, sudden coma, and autonomic changes. These lesions are also very often associated with disturbances of sodium and water metabolism (e.g. diabetes insipidus or SIADH). Aggressive surgical resection of these contusions may worsen the late neurological deficit and neuropsychological consequences. Surgical decompression requires bifrontal decompressive craniotomy and cutting of the falx and sagittal sinus on the frontal cranial fossa. This is a major procedure, caries hemorrhage risk, and requires delayed cranioplasty 2-3 months later. The risk of this surgical procedure must, therefore, be balanced against risk of death due to herniation. The timing of deterioration is variable, but brain edema will usually peak around the 5th to the 10th day, with resolution of the swelling after this time hence observation for up to 2 weeks with serial CT scanning every 2-3 days is necessary to exclude progression of the lesions. When the patients are unable to obey commands, are very restless, or deteriorate, ICP monitoring with titrated osmotherapy may be an option with decompression the next stage. Particular problems are posed by the patient with progressive swelling, especially posterior shift of the third ventricle, but preserved capacity to obey commands. For these patients, prophylactic decompressive bifrontal craniectomy is usually preferable to the risk of sudden death or permanent disability that can result from rapid herniation.

Image from Vincent JL, et al. (Eds.), Textbook of Critical Care, 6th ed., Elsevier, Saunders, 2011.

FURTHER READING

Kolias AG, Guilfoyle MR, Helmy A. Traumatic brain injury in adults, Pract Neurol. 2013;13(4):228-235.

Godoy DA, Rubiano A, Rabinstein AA, et al. Moderate Traumatic Brain Injury: The Grey Zone of Neurotrauma, Neurocrit Care. 2016 Feb 29.

22. **b**—12 cm

Unilateral DC (also termed hemicraniectomy) is usually performed in cases with predominantly unilateral hemispheric edema—a feature that is evident on brain imaging as a midline shift to the contralateral side. Bifrontal DC, which extends from the floor of the anterior cranial fossa anteriorly to the coronal suture posteriorly and to the pterion laterally, is usually performed in patients with diffuse brain edema. Removal of the inferior part of the temporal bone to the floor of the middle cranial fossa is an important maneuver for both types of DC, especially in the presence of temporal pole lesions or edema causing brainstem compression. It is now well recognized that, during DC, the dura mater has to be widely opened as bony decompression alone cannot sufficiently accommodate severe brain swelling. Leaving the dura open while covering the brain with a sheet of hemostatic material (such as Surgicel®, Ethicon Inc., Somerville, NJ) is our preferred option as it allows for faster closure with a low chance of complications. If a duraplasty is performed, it should be wide enough to accommodate further brain expansion. A decompressive hemicraniectomy diameter of 12 cm has been postulated to represent the minimum size for effective decompression, as the incidence of hemicraniectomy-associated lesions increases sharply with defects of smaller size. Cerebral herniation, shear stress along a bony ridge due to steep pressure gradients as well as compression of cortical veins and aggravated swelling are examples of the mechanisms thought to contribute to new postoperative contusions, hemorrhage and ischemia. As a consequence, a minimum diameter exceeding 12 cm is commonly pursued, with adequate decompression to the floor of the middle cranial fossa being crucial to prohibit uncal herniation. In a recent study where all patients had ICP control and all decompressions were >12 cm in AP diameter, no significant difference in outcome or complication rate was seen in those <18 cm versus those >18 cm in AP diameter, craniectomies of 12-15 or 18 cm, though commonly perceived to be somewhat faster and less invasive and traumatic, were not associated with a more favorable procedural risk profile, i.e. shorter operating time, a lower incidence of structural laceration or transfusion requirements. Equally, an additional benefit for an exposure that exceeds 15 or 18 cm could not be found. A small proportion of craniectomies extended over the sagittal midline and did not result in a statistically significant increase in structural laceration or development of hygroma, but were associated with significantly more contusions/hemorrhages, higher rate of meningitis and shunt-dependency, but also with better GOS outcome.

FURTHER READING

Wagner S, Schnippering H, Aschoff A, et al. Suboptimum hemicraniectomy as a cause of additional cerebral lesions in patients with malignant infarction of the middle cerebral artery, J Neurosurg. 2001;94(5):693-696.

Tanrikulu L, Oez-Tanrikulu A2, Weiss C, et al. The bigger, the better? About the size of decompressive hemicraniectomies, Clin Neurol Neurosurg. 2015;135:15-21.

23. **a**—DECRA trial has shown the utility of early decompressive craniectomy in neuroprotection

In the modern era of TBI management, DC can be grouped into two major categories: primary or secondary. Primary decompressive craniectomy is usually performed during evacuation of an acute subdural hematoma (ASDH), either because the brain is swollen beyond the confines of the skull or because the patient is thought to be at high risk of worsening of brain swelling within the ensuing few days. Secondary decompressive craniectomy is usually undertaken as a last-tier (life-saving) therapy when a patient has intracranial hypertension that is sustained at 20-35 mmHg and refractory to medical management. However, secondary DC can also be undertaken earlier (that is, before the stages of last-tier therapy) and in individuals with less-sustained periods of intracranial hypertension. In such cases, secondary DC can be regarded as a neuroprotective measure. This was examined in the DECRA study where 155 adults aged <60 with diffuse TBI, <72 h post injury and moderate intracranial hypertension (ICP exceeded 20 mmHg for more than 15 min within a 1-h period, and if they did not respond to optimized first-tier interventions) were randomly assigned to receive either standard medical management alone or medical management plus bifrontal DC. At 6-month follow-up, the investigators observed a higher rate of unfavorable outcomes in the DC group than in the control group (70% vs. 51%). However, 27% of patients in the surgical arm had bilaterally unreactive pupils compared with only 12% in the control arm. As pupil reactivity is known to be a major prognostic indicator of outcome following TBI, the investigators performed a post-hoc adjustment for pupil reactivity at baseline, which revealed that the between-group difference in terms of unfavorable outcome was not significant. In contrast to the DECRA study of early DC for intracranial hypertension, the RESCUEicp trial is examining the effectiveness of DC as a last-tier therapy for patients with refractory intracranial hypertension. The RESCUEicp study differs from DECRA in a number of features: sample size (400 patients in RESCUEicp vs. 155 patients in DECRA); surgical technique (bifrontal DC or hemicraniectomy versus bifrontal DC alone); threshold for ICP (25 mmHg vs. 20 mmHg); duration of refractory intracranial hypertension (at least 1 h vs. 15 min); timing of randomization (any time when inclusion criteria are met versus within 72 h post-injury); and follow-up period (2 years vs. 6 months).

FURTHER READING

Kolias AG, Guilfoyle MR, Helmy A. Traumatic brain injury in adults, Pract Neurol. 2013;13(4):228-235.

ANSWERS 24–33

Additional answers 24–33 available on ExpertConsult.com

EMI ANSWERS

34. 1—k, Thiopentone, 2—c, External ventricular drain and/or hematoma evacuation, 3—b, Decompressive craniectomy

Raised ICP after head injury increases in cerebral blood volume due to reduced venous outflow (mechanical obstruction of intracranial or extracranial venous structures, head-down position, obstructed ventilation, high positive end-expiratory pressure [PEEP], tight neck collar, etc.) or increased CBF (loss of vascular autoregulation at low or high CPP, increase in $PaCO_2$, hypoxia, acidosis, coupling to increased metabolism). Many current clinical strategies aimed at reducing ICP are based on the described pathophysiologic mechanisms, for example, correction of hypoxia and hypotension (prevention of cellular brain edema), hyperosmolar agents (reflex vasoconstriction to reduce CBF), head elevation (increase in venous outflow), low-end normocapnia (reduction in CBF and therefore CBV via decreased $PaCO_2$), sedation and muscle paralysis, normothermia (reduction in metabolism with a coupled reduction in CBF/CBV), optimization of CPP (improvement in O_2 delivery without increasing vasogenic edema), ventriculostomy (CSF diversion) and/or removal of mass lesions, and decompressive craniectomy (mechanical increase in intracranial volume). Regarding the role of hypothermia, evidence to date suggests that early institution (i.e. at tier 2 in patients with TBI in last 10 days recently admitted to intensive care setting in Eurotherm trial to treat ICP, or within 2.5 h of injury in NABIS:HII as a neuroprotectant) does not improve outcome.

FURTHER READING

Gupta K, Gelb AW (Eds.), Essentials of Neuroanesthesia and Neurointensive Care, Elsevier, Saunders, 2008.

35. 1—j, Near-infrared spectroscopy, 2—f, Glycerol, 3—i, Lactate/pyruvate ratio, 4—c, External ventricular drain ICP, 5—l, Pressure reactivity index

Multi-Modality Monitoring in Traumatic Brain Injury

Modality	Description
ICP monitor	Single measurements not clinically as relevant as its long-term average, variability in time, presence of waveforms, and correlation with other variables in brain monitoring. ICP also provides information regarding autoregulation of cerebral blood flow, pressure reactivity, and compliance of the cerebrospinal system. Intraparenchymal systems may be inserted through an airtight support bolt (e.g. Codman or Camino systems) or tunneled subcutaneously from a bur hole either at the bedside or after craniotomy (Codman system). With the most common intraparenchymal arrangement, the measured pressure may be local and not necessarily representative of CSF pressure, and cannot generally be recalibrated after insertion, and zero drift may occur with long-term monitoring

Continued

Modality	Description
Cerebral microdialysis	
Glycerol	Release from phospholipids cell membrane degradation after cell injury. Systemic lipolysis or the administration of glycerol-containing drugs may affect its cerebral levels
Glucose	Reduced CBF (ischemia) or increased consumption of glucose may lead to a decrease in its extracellular concentration. Low extracellular glucose levels are associated with poor outcome after traumatic brain injury (TBI)
Lactate/glucose ratio	Marker of ischemia or increased glycolysis
Lactate/pyruvate ratio	Under normal conditions glucose is metabolized to pyruvate and lactate, and the former is used as substrate for the citric acid cycle to generate ATP. There is normally a relative balance between glucose, lactate, and pyruvate concentrations in ECF. Ischemia and increased anaerobic respiration increases the L/P ratio and relates to poorer neurologic outcome
Glutamate	Cerebral extracellular glutamate levels increase in tissue ischemia and hypoxia
Near-infra red spectroscopy	Differential absorption and scatter of near-infrared light allow assessment of changes in the chromophores oxyhemoglobin (HbO_2), deoxyhemoglobin (Hb), and cytochrome oxidase. Provides regional cerebral hemoglobin oxygen saturation, cerebral blood volume (CBV), and cerebrovascular responses to therapeutic interventions
Jugular bulb venous oximetry (Sjv O_2)	A method of estimating global cerebral oxygenation and metabolism. Although Sjv O_2 does not give quantitative information about either cerebral blood flow (CBF) or the cerebral metabolic rate of oxygen ($CMRO_2$), it does reflect any mismatch between them. Low Sjv O_2 values indicate either low oxygen delivery to the brain (low CBF or arterial O_2 content) or high $CMRO_2$ and increased oxygen extraction. High Sjv O_2 values reflect high oxygen delivery (hyperemia, arteriovenous mixing) or low $CMRO_2$. The two most common causes of jugular bulb desaturation (Sjv O_2 <55%) are decreased CPP (raised ICP or reduced MAP) or hypocapnia. In head-injured patients, Sjv O_2 values less than 50% have been shown to increase mortality. samples may be contaminated by extracranial venous blood
PbO_2 (LICOX)	Brain tissue oxygen tension (PbO_2) is the partial pressure of oxygen in the extracellular fluid of the brain and reflects the availability of oxygen for oxidative energy metabolism. It represents the balance between oxygen delivery and consumption. Exact localization of the sensor tips on CT after insertion is essential for accurate interpretation and use. To exclude insertion-related microhemorrhage or sensor damage, FiO_2 can be increased transiently to confirm appropriate corresponding increases in PbO_2. An equilibration time of about half an hour after insertion is required before readings are stable
EVD ICP	Still considered the "gold standard" for measurement of ICP due to ability to recalibrate and drain CSF, but may be impossible in patients with advanced brain swelling
CPP	Calculated by subtracting mean ICP from mean arterial blood pressure (CPP = MAP − ICP)
Pressure reactivity index (PRx)	The correlation between spontaneous waves in ABP and ICP is dependent on the ability of cerebral vessels to autoregulate. With intact autoregulation, a rise in ABP produces vasoconstriction, a decrease in cerebral blood volume, and a fall in ICP. With disturbed autoregulation, changes in ABP are transmitted to the intracranial compartment and result in a passive pressure effect. The correlation coefficient between slow changes in mean ABP and ICP is negative when cerebral vessels are pressure reactive (i.e. intact autoregulation). A positive correlation coefficient indicates disturbed cerebrovascular pressure reactivity. This index may fluctuate with time as ICP and CPP vary, but on average it expresses most of the phenomena related to cerebral hemodynamics and volume expansion processes
Non-invasive ICP	Options under investigation include transcranial Doppler examination, tympanic membrane displacement, and ultrasound "time-of-flight" techniques have been suggested

36. 1—h, Hemorrhagic progression of contusion, 2—n, Subdural hygroma, 3—a, Aseptic bone flap resorption

General frequency of complications related to decompressive craniectomy (TBI specific where available):

New ipsilateral hematoma 12.9%, New contralateral/remote hematoma 8.6%, Hemorrhagic progression of contusion 12.6%, Meningitis/ventriculitis 6.1%, deep complications in total (meningitis, ventriculitis, cerebral abscess, extradural/subdural empyema) 5.1%, Hydrocephalus 14.8%, CSF leak 6.7%, Syndrome of the trephined 10%, superficial complications 8.1% (wound necrosis/poor healing, wound infection, subgaleal infection), Subdural hygroma 27.4%. Specific frequencies not available for paradoxical herniation or falls onto unprotected cranium.

General frequency of complications related to cranioplasty following decompressive craniectomy (TBI specific where available):

New ipsilateral hematoma 5.4%, meningitis/ventriculitis 4.5%, deep complications in total (meningitis, ventriculitis, cerebral abscess, extradural/subdural empyema) 4.8%, Hydrocephalus 6.2%, CSF leak 6.8%, superficial complications 5.4% (wound necrosis/poor healing, wound infection, subgaleal infection), Subdural hygroma 6.5%, bone flap/prosthesis infection 5.4%, aseptic bone flap reabsorption 13.5% adults and 39.2% children, bone flap depression/cosmetic defect 3.1%.

Cranioplasty is mainly performed following craniectomy for traumatic injuries. For all age groups, tumor removal or decompressive craniectomies are the main reasons for cranioplasty. Contraindications for cranioplasty include infection, hydrocephalus, and brain swelling. Delaying cranioplasty could prevent devitalized autograft or allograft infections. The ideal material used for cranioplasty would be radiolucent, resistant to infections, not conductive of heat or cold, resistant to biomechanical processes, malleable to fit defects with complete closure, inexpensive, and ready to use. Replacement of the original bone removed during craniectomy is optimal as no other graft or foreign materials are introduced. In pediatric patients, this is preferable as the child's original skull material will become reintegrated as he or she matures. Moreover, autologous cranial bone grafts can be harvested with ease and have an enhanced survival time relative to other types of bone. When the cranial bone grafts are split, reconstruction of the donor site is greatly simplified, which reduces donor site morbidity. Autologous split-thickness bone grafts have become the graft of choice in craniofacial reconstructions in children. Autologous bone can be preserved either by cryopreservation or by placement in a subcutaneous abdominal pocket. Both of these methods may be equally efficacious for storage in a non-traumatic brain injury setting. However, in a traumatic brain injury setting, the subcutaneous pocket may be the preferred method of storage because cryopreservation may have a higher surgical site infection rate. Many studies have validated the efficacy, low infection rate, and low cost of storing a cranioplasty flap in the subcutaneous pouch of the abdominal wall. Furthermore, in a battlefield setting where injured soldiers are often transported off the battlefield, storage of cranioplasty flaps in the subcutaneous abdominal wall ensures that the flap will not be lost in transport. Although preferred, autologous bone transplants are not without risks. A common complication in pediatric patients is bone flap resorption, which results in structural breakdown. This necessitates reoperation and replacement with plastic, metal, or other materials. Cranioplasty depends on osteoconduction, whereby the bone graft provides the structure to allow osteoprogenitor cells to enter and take root. This requires a matrix, which could potentially be destroyed when the flap is frozen or autoclaved. This explains the higher resorption rate of autologous bone grafts. autologous bone grafts had the highest rates of infection than polymethylmethacrylate (PMMA), alumina ceramics, and titanium mesh. Synthetic materials are largely being considered as an alternative to prevent the complications of bone resorption, infection, donor site morbidity, and reduced strength and malleability for esthetic contour.

FURTHER READING

Kurland DB, et al. Complications Associated with Decompressive Craniectomy: A Systematic Review. Neurocrit Care. 2015;23(2):292-304.

37. 1—b, Chronic subdural hematoma, 2—a, Carotid-cavernous fistula (high flow)
Complications after TBI may include:

Complications of Traumatic Brain Injury

Bony/Dural/CSF	Vascular	Parenchymal
Air sinus injury	Traumatic SAH	Contusion
Mucocele	EDH	Hypopituitarism
Ossicular disruption	ADH	GH deficiency
CSF fistula	Dissection	Hypogonadotrophic hypogonadism
Hydrocephalus	Carotid-cavernous fistula	Hypothyroidism
Meningitis	Traumatic aneurysm	Secondary adrenal insufficiency
Pneumocephalus		Diabetes insipidus
Subdural hygroma		Seizures
Cranial nerve injury		

CHAPTER 22A

CRANIAL VASCULAR NEUROSURGERY I: ANEURYSMS AND AVMs

SINGLE BEST ANSWER (SBA) QUESTIONS

1. Which one of the following pathologies is most likely to give the appearances shown?

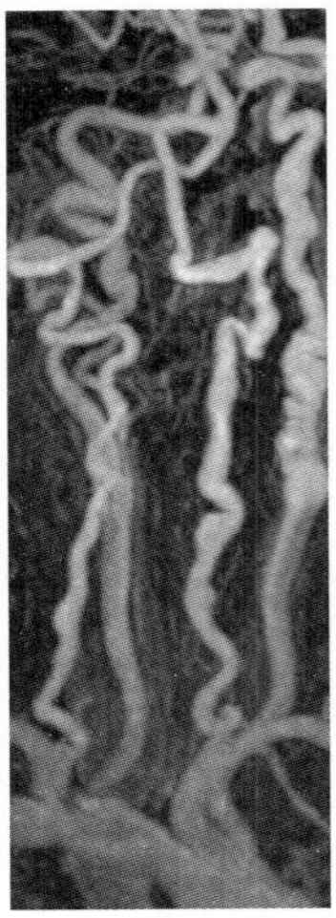

a. Atrial myxoma
b. Ehlers-Danlos syndrome
c. Fibromuscular dysplasia
d. Marfan syndrome
e. Polycystic kidney disease

2. Which one of the following pathologies is most likely to give the appearances shown?

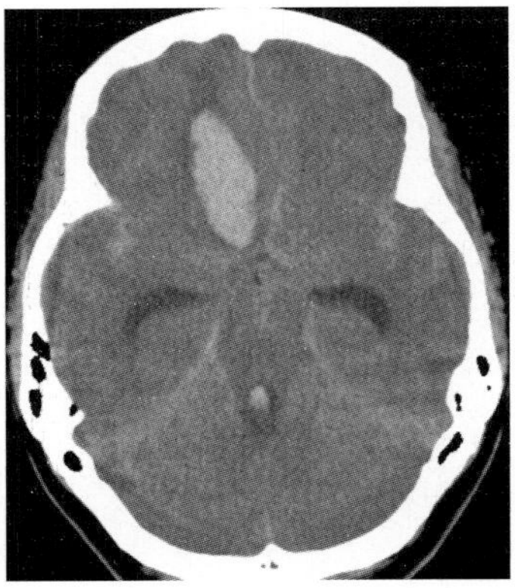

a. Anterior communicating artery aneurysm
b. Basilar tip aneurysm
c. Posterior communicating artery aneurysm
d. Posterior inferior cerebellar artery aneurysm
e. Middle cerebral artery aneurysm

3. A 33-year-old man presents with spontaneous tinnitus and nausea. Which one of the following is most likely based on the imaging shown?

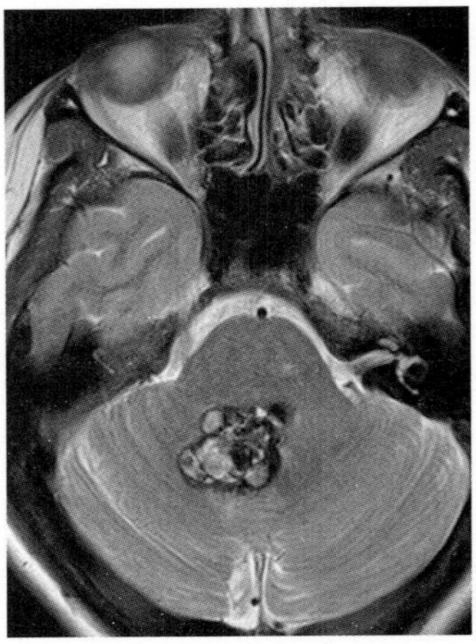

a. Arteriovenous malformation
b. Cavernous angioma
c. Hemangioblastoma
d. Intracerebral hemorrhage
e. Medulloblastoma

4. A 49-year-old man attends the Emergency department complaining of headache and vomiting for the last 2 days and now he has clumsiness of his left hand. There is no history of trauma. His GCS is 15/15. CT head shows there is a right sided acute subdural hematoma with midline shift of 5 mm. Which one of the following would you perform next?
a. CT intracranial angiogram
b. CT head with contrast
c. CT perfusion scan
d. MRI head with diffusion weighted sequences
e. Transcranial Doppler

5. Which one of the following is most likely given the image below?

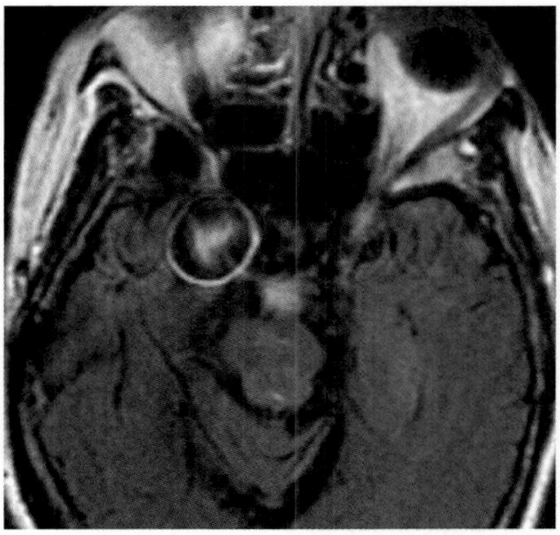

a. Arachnoid cyst
b. Cavernous sinus meningioma
c. Craniopharyngioma
d. Giant MCA aneurysm
e. Pituitary macroadenoma

6. A 46-year-old female presents with sudden onset right facial numbness, hearing loss, and diplopia. CT head was unremarkable. Which one of the following therapies may be most appropriate based on the subsequent imaging shown?

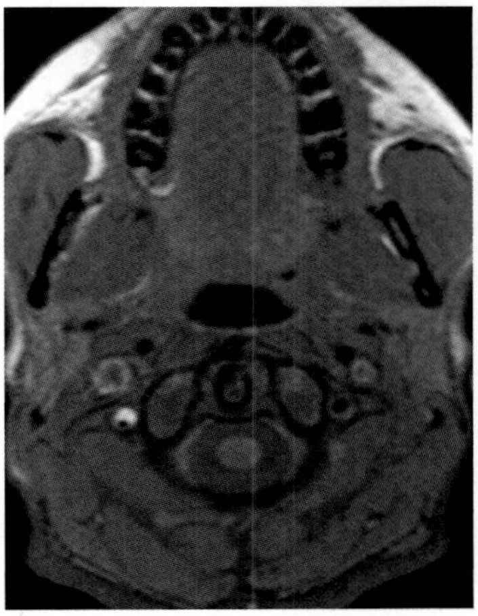

a. Anticoagulant therapy
b. Balloon Angioplasty
c. Intra-arterial nimodipine
d. Surgical clipping
e. Thrombolytic therapy

7. A 37-year-old man presents with seizures. Which one of the following is NOT thought to increase risk of hemorrhage in this type of lesion?

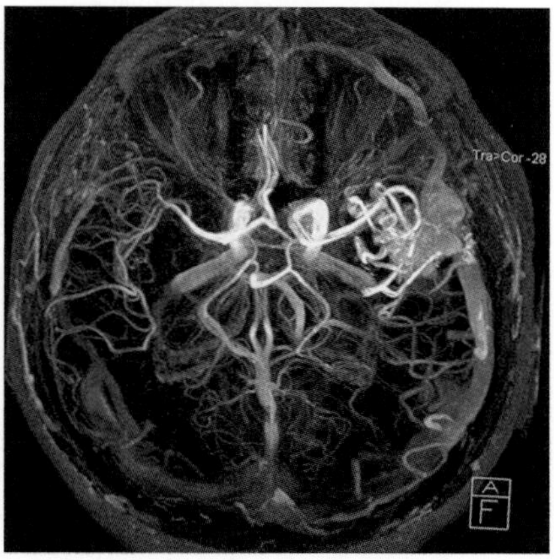

a. Deep venous drainage
b. Intranidal aneurysm
c. Prior hemorrhage
d. Single draining vein
e. Smoking

8. A 54-year-old woman presents with sudden onset severe headache. Her GCS is 15/15 with no neurological deficit on examination. Rupture of a vertebrobasilar aneurysm is thought to be responsible for the imaging appearances shown in what proportion of cases?

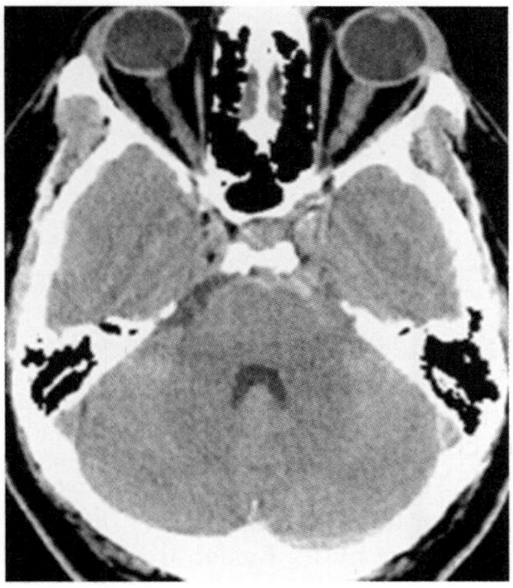

a. 2%
b. 4%
c. 6%
d. 8%
e. 10%

9. Which one of the following supraclinoid internal carotid artery aneurysm locations is most frequent?
   a. Anterior choroidal artery aneurysm
   b. Carotid bifurcation aneurysm
   c. Hypophyseal artery aneurysm
   d. Posterior communicating artery aneurysm
   e. Supraopthalmic aneurysm

10. Which one of the following pathologies is most likely demonstrated by the angiogram?

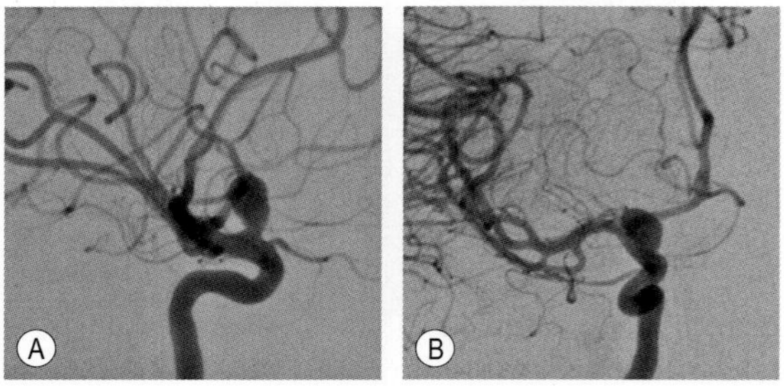

   a. Anterior choroidal artery aneurysm
   b. Basilar tip aneurysm
   c. MCA bifurcation
   d. PCA aneurysm
   e. Supraopthalmic aneurysm

11. Which one of the following is most likely based on this AP view of a right ICA injection?

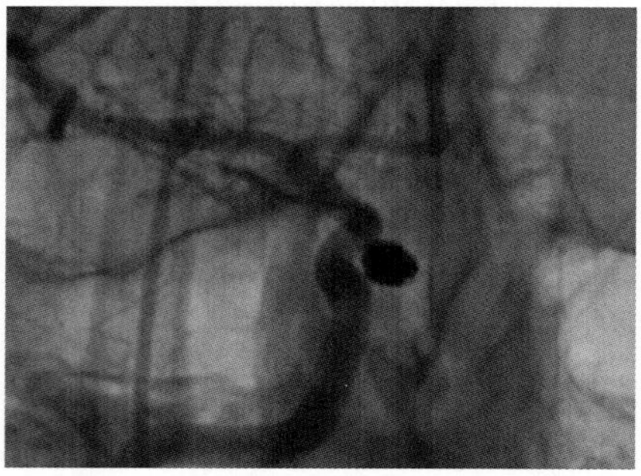

   a. A1 branch of ACA
   b. Acomm artery
   c. MCA bifurcation
   d. M3 branch of MCA
   e. Superior hypophysial artery

12. Which one of the following clinical findings would you look for in this patient?

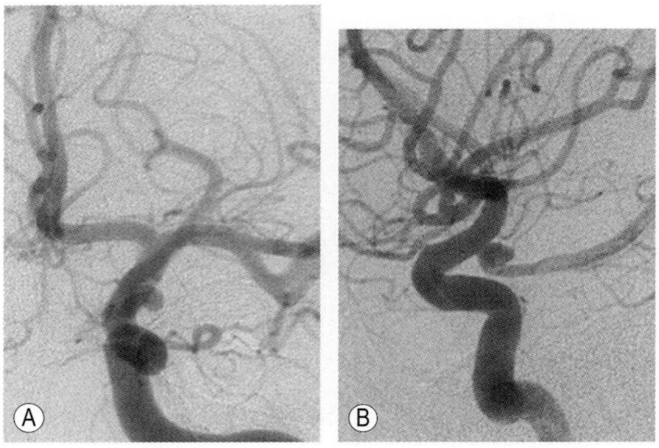

   a. Abducens palsy
   b. Absent corneal reflex
   c. Bitemporal hemianopia
   d. Oculomotor palsy
   e. Pituitary dysfunction

13. Which one of the following pathologies is most likely demonstrated by the angiogram?

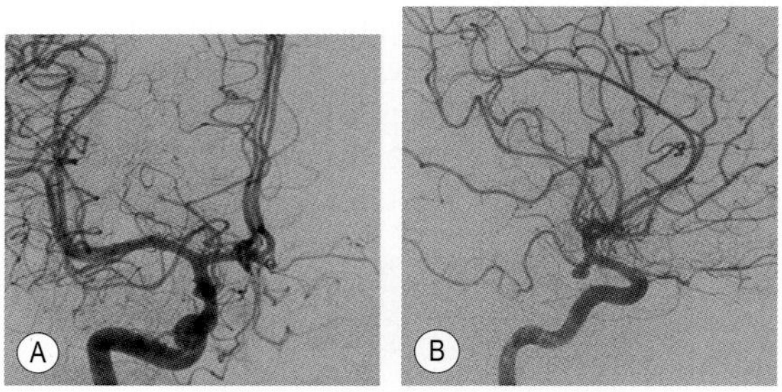

   a. Anterior choroidal artery aneurysm
   b. Anterior communicating artery aneurysm
   c. Pericallosal aneurysm
   d. Supraopthalmic aneurysm
   e. Trigeminal artery aneurysm

14. The aneurysm type shown below constitutes which one of the following proportions of all intracranial aneurysms?

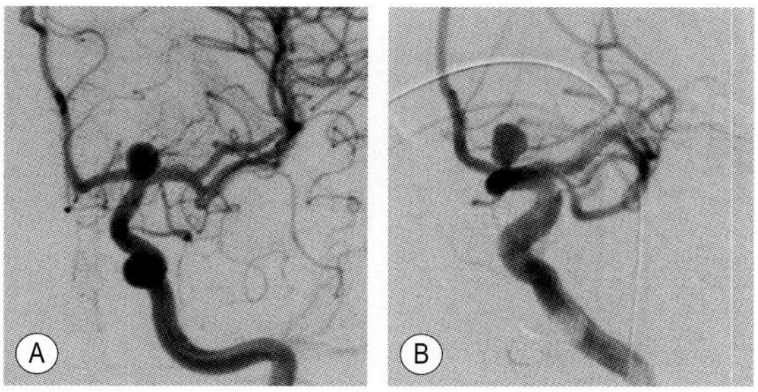

a. 1%
b. 5%
c. 15%
d. 25%
e. 35%

15. Which one of the following pathologies is most likely demonstrated by the angiogram?

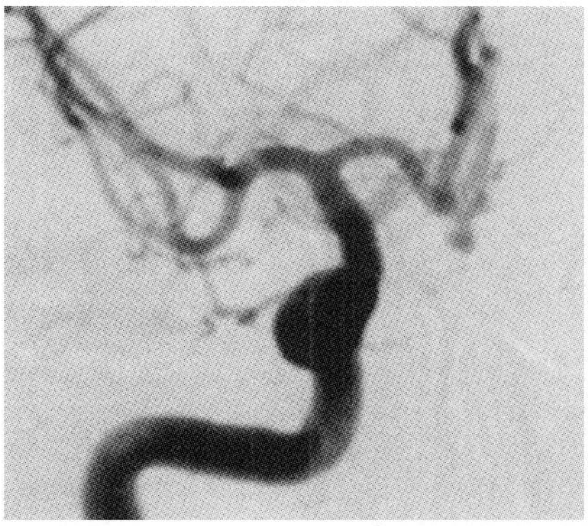

a. Anterior communicating artery aneurysm
b. Basilar artery aneurysm
c. Basilar invagination
d. Left PCA artery aneurysm
e. Superior hypophyseal artery aneurysm

16. The following appearances are seen during endovascular treatment of an anterior communicating artery aneurysm. What is the next appropriate management step?

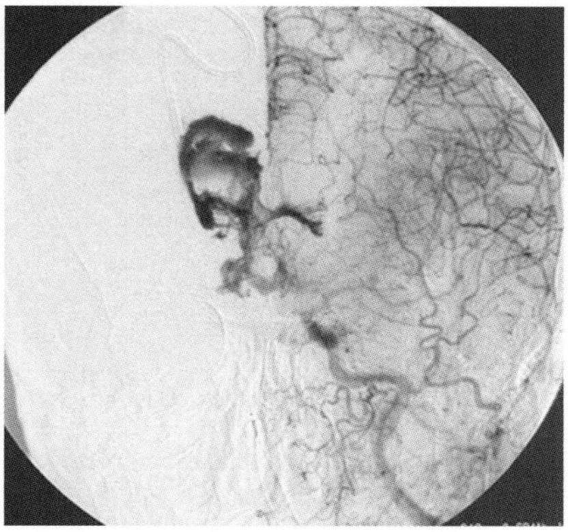

a. Ask the anesthetist to reduce systolic blood pressure to 100 mmHg
b. Check pupillary reflexes and perform CT head
c. Continue with endovascular treatment
d. ICP monitoring
e. Insertion of external ventricular drain

17. Which one of the following pathologies is most likely demonstrated by the angiogram?

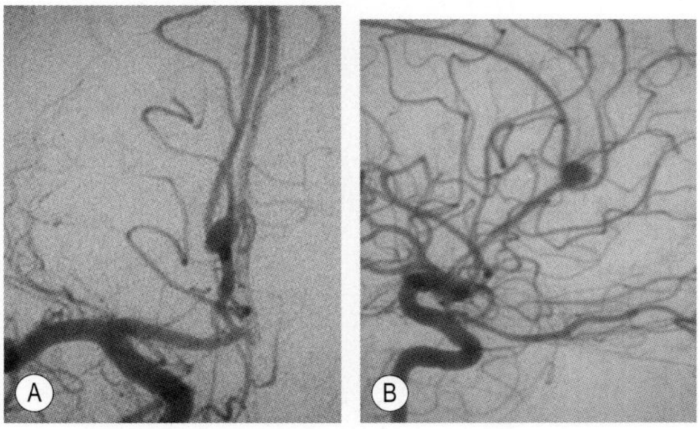

a. A1 branch of ACA aneurysm
b. Corpocallosal AVM
c. MCA bifurcation aneurysm
d. Pericallosal aneurysm
e. Posterior communicating artery aneurysm

18. Which one of the following is most likely demonstrated by the angiogram?

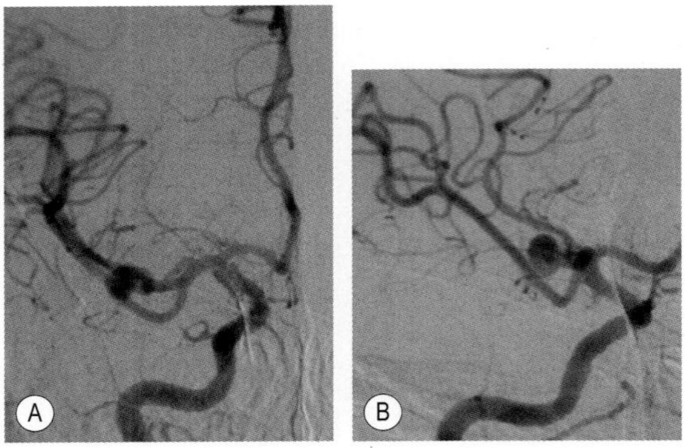

a. Anterior communicating artery
b. MCA bifurcation aneurysm
c. Pericallosal aneurysm
d. Posterior communicating artery
e. Terminal ICA aneurysm

19. Which one of the following pathologies is most likely demonstrated by the angiogram?

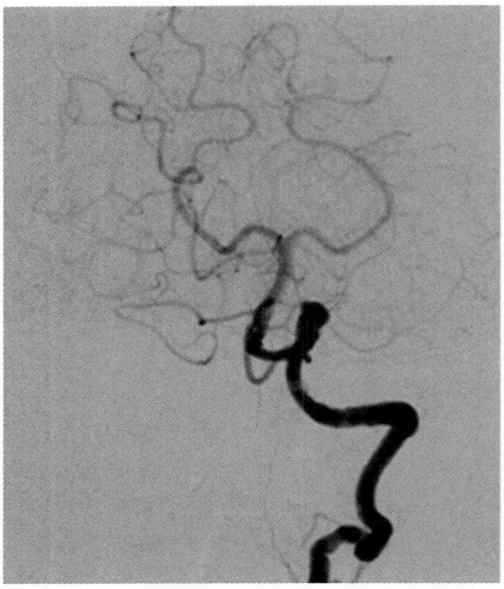

a. Anterior inferior cerebellar artery aneurysm
b. Basilar tip aneurysm
c. Posterior cerebral artery aneurysm
d. Posterior inferior cerebellar artery aneurysm
e. Superior cerebellar artery aneurysm

20. Which one of the following pathologies is most likely demonstrated by the angiogram?

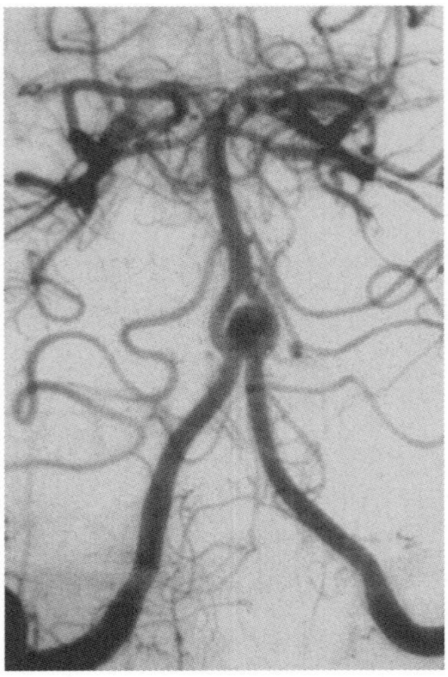

a. Asymmetric fusion of caudal divisions of fetal ICA
b. Basilar fenestration
c. Basilar invagination
d. Fetal origin of PCA
e. Hypoplastic posterior communicating artery

21. Which one of the following clinical findings would you look for in this patient?

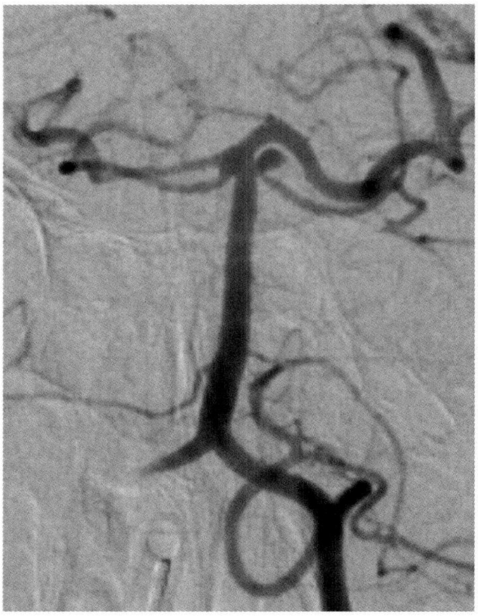

a. Abducens palsy
b. Internuclear opthalmoplegia
c. Occulomotor palsy
d. Parinaud's syndrome
e. Trochlear palsy

22. Which one of the following pathologies is most likely demonstrated by the angiogram?

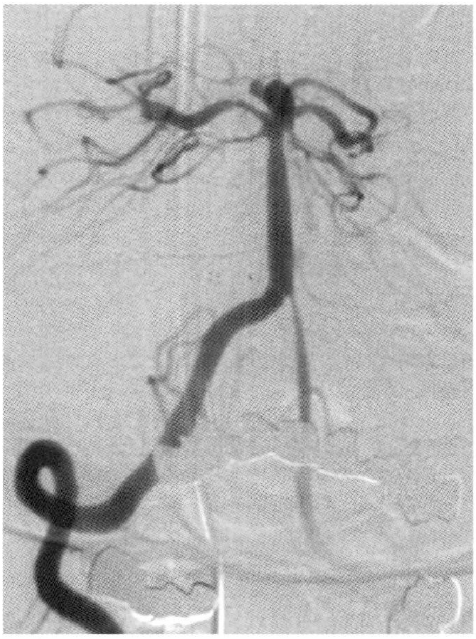

a. Basilar fenestration
b. Basilar tip aneurysm
c. Persistent trigeminal artery
d. Persistent otic artery
e. Vertebral artery occlusion

23. Which one of the following mechanisms is most likely responsible for the finding in the angiogram?

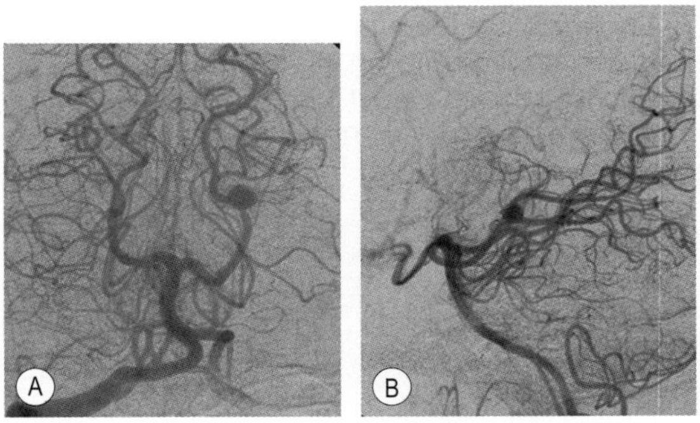

a. Connective tissue disorder
b. Infection
c. Traumatic dissection
d. Neoplasia
e. Toxin

QUESTIONS 24–32

Additional questions 24–32 available on ExpertConsult.com

EXTENDED MATCHING ITEM (EMI) QUESTIONS

33. **Posterior circulation stroke syndromes:**
a. Anton syndrome
b. Babinski-Nageotte syndrome
c. Balint syndrome
d. Benedikt syndrome
e. Claude syndrome
f. Dejerine syndrome
g. Dejerine-Roussy syndrome
h. Foville syndrome
i. Locked-in syndrome
j. Marie-Foix syndrome
k. Millard-Gubler syndrome
l. Raymond syndrome
m. Top of basilar syndrome
n. Wallenberg syndrome
o. Weber syndrome

For each of the following descriptions, select the most appropriate answers from the list above. Each answer may be used once, more than once or not at all:
1. Contralateral hemisensory loss and contralateral hemibody pain
2. Visual deficit without recognition of blindness
3. Ipsilateral loss of facial sensation/pain, ipsilateral Horner's syndrome, ipsilateral ataxia, loss of gag reflex, and contralateral hemibody loss of pain and temperature
4. Ipsilateral oculomotor palsy and contralateral temor and ataxia

34. **Arterial supply:**
a. Anterior choroidal artery
b. Anterior inferior cerebellar artery
c. Anterior temporal artery
d. Anterior thalamoperforating arteries
e. Calcarine artery
f. Inferolateral trunk of ICA (C4)
g. Labyrinthine artery
h. Lateral posterior choroidal artery
i. Medial and lateral lenticulostriate arteries
j. Medial posterior choroidal artery
k. Ophthalmic artery
l. Posterior inferior cerebellar artery
m. Recurrent artery of Heubner
n. Thalamogeniculate arteries

For each of the following descriptions, select the most appropriate answers from the list above. Each answer may be used once, more than once or not at all:
1. Supplies visual cortex
2. Arises from P2 segment to supply pulvinar and superior colliculus

35. **Venous drainage:**
   a. Thalamostriate veins
   b. Superior anastomotic vein of Trolard
   c. Inferior anastamostic vein of Labbe
   d. Internal cerebral vein
   e. Great cerebral vein of Galen
   f. Superficial middle cerebral (Sylvian) vein
   g. Basal vein of Rosenthal
   h. Anterior cerebral vein
   i. Deep middle cerebral vein
   j. Straight sinus
   k. Transverse sinus
   l. Occipital sinus
   m. Inferior petrosal sinus
   n. Superior petrosal sinus
   o. Cavernous sinus
   p. Superior saggital sinus
   q. Inferior saggital sinus

For each of the following descriptions, select the most appropriate answers from the list above. Each answer may be used once, more than once or not at all:

1. Drains from the Sylvian fissure to the superior saggital sinus
2. Drains from the Sylvian fissure to the transverse sinus
3. Drains into the cavernous sinus, vein of Trolard, and vein of Labbe

36. **Trials in Vascular Neurosurgery:**
   a. ARUBA
   b. BRANT
   c. BRAT
   d. ISAT
   e. ISUIA
   f. JAM
   g. NASCET
   h. STASH
   i. STICH
   j. ESCAPE/EXTEND-IA/SWIFT-PRIME

For each of the following descriptions, select the most appropriate answers from the list above. Each answer may be used once, more than once or not at all:

1. Prospective study of natural history of unruptured intracranial aneurysms
2. Randomized trial showing superiority of mechanical thrombectomy over thrombolysis in acute ischemic stroke
3. Randomized trial showing reduction in cerebral ischemic events in subarachnoid hemorrhage in patients taking oral nimodipine
4. Randomized trial showing no difference in favorable outcome when simvastatin given in aneurysmal subarachnoid hemorrhage

37. **Triangle of cavernous sinus and middle fossa:**
   a. Anteromedial triangle
   b. Medial (Hakuba's) triangle
   c. Paramedian triangle
   d. Parkinson's triangle
   e. Anterolateral (Mullan's) triangle
   f. Lateral triangle
   g. Posterolateral (Glasscock's) triangle
   h. Posteromedial (Kawase's) triangle
   i. Inferomedial triangle
   j. Inferolateral triangle

For each of the following descriptions, select the most appropriate answers from the list above. Each answer may be used once, more than once or not at all:

1. Access to entire intracavernous ICA
2. Access to petroclival area, anterolateral brainstem, and vertebrobasilar junction
3. Access horizontal intrapetrosal ICA for proximal control or bypass graft

SBA ANSWERS

1. **c**—Fibromuscular dysplasia. FMD occurs predominantly in middle-aged women and most often affects the cervical ICA (75%). The vertebral (12%) and external carotid arteries may also be involved. Disease is bilateral in 60% of cases. Angiographic images, almost always with non-invasive techniques, demonstrate alternating luminal narrowing and dilatation, the resulting appearance often described as a "string of beads." This "corrugation" typically affects the mid ICA, usually 2 cm distal to bulb. Uni- or multifocal tubular stenoses are less common, and where observed, the degree of stenosis is usually modest (less than 40%). FMD can occasionally be observed intracranially and is associated with aneurysms.

Image with permission from Adam A, et al. (Eds.). Grainger & Allison's Diagnostic Radiology, 6th ed., Elsevier, Churchill Livingstone, 2014.

2. **a**—Anterior communicating artery aneurysm. The classical flame shaped hemorrhage associated with acute rupture of these aneurysms is depicted.

Image with permission from Adam A, et al. (Eds.). Grainger & Allison's Diagnostic Radiology, 6th ed., Elsevier, Churchill Livingstone, 2014.

3. **b**—Cavernous angiomas are mulberry-like lesions consisting of vascular spaces with little intervening tissue and hemorrhage of different ages. The incidence of clinically symptomatic hemorrhage remains uncertain, but is less frequent than with cerebral AVMs or dural fistulae. A previous bleed and infratentorial location are the main prognostic factors for recurrent hemorrhage. Lesions in or close to the cerebral cortex may cause epilepsy. They are occasionally intraventricular or arise on a cranial nerve. They appear as relatively well-defined, dense, or calcified lesions on CT, which may show patchy contrast enhancement. On MRI they appear multilobular with mixed but predominantly elevated T2 signal intensity centrally surrounded by a dark hemosiderin rim. Not surprisingly, susceptibility-based sequences are the most sensitive. They may be multiple, particularly in familial cases. In many clinical situations the discovery of a cavernoma represents an incidental finding.

Image with permission from Adam A, et al. (Eds.). Grainger & Allison's Diagnostic Radiology, 6th ed., Elsevier, Churchill Livingstone, 2014.

4. **a**—CT intracranial angiogram

Occasionally, rupture of a cerebral aneurysm may cause an acute subdural hematoma, most frequently a posterior communicating artery aneurysm lying next to the free edge of the tentorium cerebelli. A dural arteriovenous fistula may also bleed into the subdural space. Angiography is therefore indicated following a spontaneous acute subdural hematoma, particularly in a young patient prior to craniotomy and evacuation of the clot.

5. **d**—Giant MCA aneurysm

On MRI imaging, giant aneurysms have a characteristic appearance, as in this case. Findings include signal void consistent with flow in the patent lumen; phase artifact related to flow, as is seen in this case; and heterogeneous signal intensity representing thrombi of varying ages.

Image with permission from Loevner L. Brain Imaging: Case Review Series, 2nd ed., Elsevier, Mosby, 2009.

6. **a**—Anticoagulation. The MRI shows a spontaneous right vertebral artery dissection—the main treatment for which is anticoagulation or antiplatelet therapy once subarachnoid hemorrhage has been excluded. Intra-arterial thrombolytics have only been used in selected cases.

Image with permission from Loevner L. Brain Imaging: Case Review Series, 2nd ed., Elsevier, Mosby, 2009.

7. **e**—Smoking. Brain arteriovenous malformations (AVMs) are abnormal vascular anomalies within the brain, presumably congenital in nature, but tend to present later in life (20-40 years). There are several subgroups, including the glomerular (most common) and fistulous (less common) types of AVMs. AVMs, often pial-based, are defined by presence of arteriovenous shunting through a nidus of coiled and tortuous vascular connections that connect feeding arteries to draining veins, without a capillary bed. Most (approximately 60-70%) of AVMs are located in the cerebral hemispheres, 11-18% within the cerebellum, and 13-16% in the brainstem; 8-9% are deep-seated. Factors that increase risk of hemorrhage from an AVM include history of hypertension or previous hemorrhage, flow-related aneurysm, intranidal aneurysm, deep venous drainage, deep (periventricular) location, small nidus size (<3 cm), high feeding artery pressure, slow arterial filling, and venous stenosis. Presence of intracranial hemorrhage indicates a poorer prognosis and is associated with an increasing morbidity and mortality. Presence of AVMs can lead to arterial steal phenomenon, venous congestion, gliosis, or hydrocephalus.

Image with permission from Fatterpekar GM, Naidich TP, Som PM. The Teaching Files: Brain and Spine, Elsevier, Saunders, 2012.

8. **b**—4%—Nontraumatic, nonaneurysmal perimesencephalic hemorrhage (PMH), presumably of venous origin, accounts for 96% of all perimesencephalic hemorrhage. The remaining 4% have been reported to result from rupture of vertebrobasilar aneurysm. Nontraumatic, nonaneurysmal perimesencephalic hemorrhage is characterized by relatively mild symptoms at onset, confinement of the extravasated blood in the perimesencephalic cisterns, and absence of aneurysm. It has a benign clinical course and excellent prognosis.

Image with permission from Loevner L. Brain Imaging: Case Review Series, 2nd ed., Elsevier, Mosby, 2009.

9. **d**—Posterior communicating artery aneurysm

Thirty-five percent of all intracranial aneurysms arise at one of the following five sites along the supraclinoid ICA

Type	Site	Frequency of all IC aneurysms (%)
supraopthalmic aneurysm	Upper surface of ICA at the origin of the ophthalmic artery	5
Hypophyseal artery aneurysm	Medial wall of ICA at the origin of the superior hypophyseal artery	1
Posterior communicating artery aneurysm	Posterior wall of ICA immediately superolateral to the origin of the PcommA	25
Carotid bifurcation aneurysm	Apex of the terminal ICA bifurcation into ACA and MCA	5
Anterior choroidal artery aneurysm	Posterior wall of the ICA immediately superior to the origin for the anterior choroidal artery	5

10. **e**—Supraopthalmic aneurysm. These typically arise from the superior wall of the carotid artery at the distal edge of the origin of the ophthalmic artery close to the roof of the cavernous sinus. At this point, the ICA changes direction from superior toward posterior, so the maximal hemodynamic force is directed toward the superior wall of the carotid artery just distal to the ophthalmic artery. Therefore, these aneurysms project upward toward the optic nerve and are often large with complex, multi-lobulated shape. Surgical exposure may be difficult as the ophthalmic artery has a variable origin and course and because multiple folds of the dura enclose the region of the optic foramen and clinoid process. Many are wide-necked aneurysms that may require remodeling techniques. Unruptured aneurysms may become symptomatic due to headaches or compression of cranial nerves.

Images with permission from Naidich T, Castillo M, Cha S, Smirniotopoulos J. Imaging of the Brain, Elsevier, Saunders, 2013.

11. **e**—Superior hypophysial artery aneurysms arise just distal to the origin of the superior hypophysial artery from the medial or posterior wall of the ICA where the curvature of the ICA is convex medially. In this location they lie lateral to the pituitary stalk and point medially under the optic chiasm. Medial expansion of the aneurysm may compromise the perforating arteries to the floor of the third ventricle, the optic nerves, the chiasm, the pituitary stalk, and the hypophysial vascular supply.

Image with permission from Naidich T, Castillo M, Cha S, Smirniotopoulos J. Imaging of the Brain, Elsevier, Saunders, 2013.

12. **d**—Oculomotor palsy

The posterior communicating artery arises from the posterior wall of the ICA where it forms a posteriorly convex curve as it ascends to its terminal bifurcation under the anterior perforated substance. These aneurysms arise near the apex of the posteriorly convex turn, immediately superior to the distal edge of the origin of the posterior communicating artery. They point downward and posteriorly toward the oculomotor nerve, so the posterior communicating artery is usually found inferomedial to the neck of the aneurysm (the anterior choroidal artery is found superior or superolateral to the neck of the aneurysm). The oculomotor nerve enters the dural roof of the cavernous sinus lateral to the posterior clinoid process and medial to a dural band that runs between the tentorium cerebelli and the anterior clinoid process. Posterior communicating artery aneurysms larger than 4-5 mm may compress the oculomotor nerve at its entrance into the dural roof, causing opthalmoplegia.

Images with permission from Naidich T, Castillo M, Cha S, Smirniotopoulos J. Imaging of the Brain, Elsevier, Saunders, 2013.

13. **a**—Anterior choroidal artery aneurysm

Should the posteriorly convex curve of the supraclinoid ICA form its apex at the level of the anterior choroidal artery the hemodynamic force is shifted distally from the origin of the posterior communicating artery to the origin of the anterior choroidal artery. The anterior choroidal aneurysms form just distal, superior, or superolateral to the origin of the anterior choroidal artery. They also point posterior or posterolaterally but are usually well above the oculomotor nerve. Aneurysms arising from the choroidal segment commonly have more perforating branches stretched around their neck than those arising from the communicating or ophthalmic segment, because the choroidal segment has a greater number of perforating branches arising from it and the majority arise from the posterior wall, where the neck of the aneurysm is situated.

Images with permission from Naidich T, Castillo M, Cha S, Smirniotopoulos J. Imaging of the Brain, Elsevier, Saunders, 2013.

14. **b**—5%

Aneurysms arise at the apex of the T-shaped carotid bifurcation and point superiorly in the direction of the long axis of the pre-bifurcation segment of the artery. As they grow, they lie lateral to the optic chiasm and may indent the undersurface of the anterior perforated substance. The perforating branches arising from the choroidal segment of the internal carotid and the proximal segments of the anterior and middle cerebral arteries are stretched around the posterior aspect of the neck and wall of the aneurysm.

Images with permission from Naidich T, Castillo M, Cha S, Smirniotopoulos J. Imaging of the Brain, Elsevier, Saunders, 2013.

15. **a**—Anterior communicating artery aneurysm

Aneurysms of the ACA typically form close to the anterior communicating artery complex. They constitute about 30% of all intracranial aneurysms and are considered one of the most common types of aneurysm. They are frequently associated with anatomical variants. Aneurysms often occur when one A1 segment is hypoplastic and the dominant A1 gives rise to both A2s. In such case, the aneurysm arises at the level of the anterior communicating artery at the point where the dominant A1 segment bifurcates to give rise to both the left and right A2 segments. The direction in which the dome of the aneurysm points is determined by the course of the dominant A1 segment proximal to its junction with the anterior communicating artery. Thus, these aneurysms usually point away from the dominant segment toward the opposite side. Approaches to anterior communicating artery aneurysms must ensure that the anterior communicating artery and the adjacent recurrent artery of Heubner remain patent. The AcomA gives rise to small perforating branches for the dorsal surface of the optic chiasm and suprachiasmatic area that perfuse the fornix, corpus callosum, and septal region. Occlusion of the anterior communicating artery may lead to personality disorders, even if both A2 segments are perfused from their respective A1 segments. The recurrent artery of Heubner arises, variably, from the distal A1, the proximal A2, or the frontopolar branch of the ACA before looping forward on the gyrus rectus or the posterior part of the orbital surface of the frontal lobe and then passing back over the carotid bifurcation to accompany the MCA and enter the anterior perforating substance. Occlusion of the recurrent artery of Heubner may cause hemiparesis or aphasia.

Image with permission from Naidich T, Castillo M, Cha S, Smirniotopoulos J. Imaging of the Brain, Elsevier, Saunders, 2013.

16. **b**—Check pupillary reflexes and perform CT head. This angiogram shows active extravasation of contrast material into the subarachnoid spaces, suggesting acute rupture of this aneurysm necessitating clinical reassessment and surgical intervention if appropriate.

Image with permission from Naidich T, Castillo M, Cha S, Smirniotopoulos J. Imaging of the Brain, Elsevier, Saunders, 2013.

17. **d**—Pericallosal aneurysm

The second most common aneurysm of the ACA is the so-called pericallosal aneurysm, which arises at the origin of the callosomarginal artery from the pericallosal artery, usually in close proximity to the anterior portion of the corpus callosum, near the point where the genu of the ACA has its greatest angulation. Pericallosal aneurysms account for approximately 3% of all intracranial aneurysms. They point distally into the window between the junction of the pericallosal and callosomarginal arteries.

Images with permission from Naidich T, Castillo M, Cha S, Smirniotopoulos J. Imaging of the Brain, Elsevier, Saunders, 2013.

18. **b**—MCA bifurcation aneurysm

Approximately 15% of all saccular aneurysms arise from the MCA. Typically they originate at the level of the first major bifurcation or trifurcation of the artery and point laterally in the direction of the long axis of the pre-bifurcation segment of the MCA. The more proximal the bifurcation, the greater the number of lenticulostriate branches arising distal to the bifurcation that may be stretched around the neck of the MCA aneurysm. When unruptured, these aneurysms are typically clinically silent. Proximal M1 segment aneurysms at origins of lenticulostriate arteries are exceedingly rare but when present tend to point upward toward the anterior perforated substance. MCA aneurysms may also arise from the temporopolar branch of the M1 segment. When present, these tend to point inferiorly. Aneurysms distal to the MCA bifurcation are rare and are typically encountered in the setting of infectious diseases.

Images with permission from Naidich T, Castillo M, Cha S, Smirniotopoulos J. Imaging of the Brain, Elsevier, Saunders, 2013.

19. **d**—Posterior inferior cerebellar artery aneurysm

Most aneurysms of the vertebral artery take origin at the posterior inferior cerebellar artery (PICA), especially when the origin of the PICA falls at the apex of a superiorly directed curve of the vertebral artery. These aneurysms almost invariably point upward and usually communicate widely with the PICA. The size of the territory supplied by the PICA varies widely, and will influence the best approach to aneurysm therapy. Common anatomic variants associated with the vertebral artery include unilateral agenesis/hypoplasia, double (duplicated, fenestrated) origin, and extracranial or epidural origin. There are close reciprocal inverse relationships among the sizes of the hemispheric territories supplied by the PICA, AICA, and SCA. Any one may annex (part of) the territory of the adjacent vessel, commonly leading to variations such as the AICA-PICA trunk. PICA supply to both cerebellar hemispheres is very uncommon but does occur and must be considered prior to endovascular procedures.

Image with permission from Naidich T, Castillo M, Cha S, Smirniotopoulos J. Imaging of the Brain, Elsevier, Saunders, 2013.

20. **b**—Basilar fenestration

The incidence of basilar artery aneurysms increases when the basilar system shows anomalous or variant architecture, including basilar nonfusion (fenestration), asymmetric or caudal fusion of the caudal divisions of the fetal ICA, hypoplastic communicating artery, or fetal (persistent carotid) origin of the posterior cerebral artery. Proximal non-dissecting basilar artery aneurysms are rare and typically arise in patients with failure to form a single basilar artery during embryologic development. The single basilar artery normally develops by union of paired longitudinal neural arteries that fuse together by about the fifth fetal week (when the embryo is 9 mm long). Each of the longitudinal neural arteries gives rise to the perforating arteries for its own side of the brain stem. Failed fusion of the neural arteries is often associated with aneurysms at the proximal portion of the nonfused artery. The lateral walls of the unfused arteries have normal intrinsic architecture. At the base of the medial wall, however, the media is absent, the elastic is discontinuous, and the subendothelium is thinned. These segments are more likely to develop arterial aneurysms when subject to secondary "offensive" triggers such as hemodynamic stress. The surgical treatment of these aneurysms is difficult due to their relationship to the cranium, lower cranial nerves, and the complex surgical approaches to this region. Endovascular embolization of aneurysms at an unfused basilar artery is an alternative to surgery. However, it must be recognized that both limbs of the unfused basilar artery have to be preserved, that the neck of such aneurysms is often broad, and that the aneurysm may regrow due to the unfavorable hemodynamics at the site of an unfused segment.

Image with permission from Naidich T, Castillo M, Cha S, Smirniotopoulos J. Imaging of the Brain, Elsevier, Saunders, 2013.

21. **c**—Oculomotor palsy

Basilar artery aneurysms at the level of the SCA often arise where the upper basilar artery curves and tilts, so the hemodynamic thrust created by flow along the basilar artery impacts just above the origin of the SCA rather than at the basilar apex. SCA aneurysms often have a broad connection with the SCA, a rather large neck, and a neck-to-dome ratio that makes endovascular therapy demanding. Endovascular therapy must attempt to preserve this artery, because this is the major vessel to supply the deep nuclei of the cerebellum. Large SCA aneurysms may cause oculomotor nerve palsies by direct impression on the oculomotor nerve as it courses through the interpeduncular cistern just cranial to the SCA.

Image with permission from Naidich T, Castillo M, Cha S, Smirniotopoulos J. Imaging of the Brain, Elsevier, Saunders, 2013.

22. **b**—Basilar tip aneurysm

About 15% of saccular aneurysms occur in the vertebrobasilar system and of these 60% arise at the basilar bifurcation where the posterior cerebral arteries branch off from the tip of the basilar artery. At the aneurysm site the blood flow changes from vertical to nearly horizontal, so these aneurysms project upward in the direction of the long axis of the basilar artery. The largest and most important perforators to arise from the basilar tip are the posterior thalamoperforate arteries (retromammillary arteries). These originate from the basilar tip and P1, enter the brain through the posterior perforated substance in the interpeduncular fossa medial to the cerebral peduncles, and ascend through the midbrain to the thalamus. The risks from occlusion of these vital perforating vessels include visual loss, paralysis, sensory disturbances, weakness, memory deficits, autonomic and endocrine imbalance, abnormal movements, diplopia, and depression of consciousness. Endovascular approaches have been widely adopted to treat basilar apex aneurysms, because the surgical approach is associated with a higher morbidity. This is especially true for the more posterior basilar tip aneurysms, because greater numbers of vital thalamoperforators are affected as the aneurysm enlarges and projects more deeply into the interpeduncular fossa.

Image with permission from Naidich T, Castillo M, Cha S, Smirniotopoulos J. Imaging of the Brain, Elsevier, Saunders, 2013.

23. **c**—Microtrauma

Intradural traumatic aneurysms most commonly involve the internal carotid and vertebral arteries at their transdural portions. Traumatic aneurysms may result from penetrating injuries such as a stabbing accident, a high-velocity gunshot wound, or iatrogenic trauma (e.g., third ventriculostomy). Similarly, traumatic arterial aneurysms have been described as involving the ACA along the falx and the tentorium, either following major head injuries or as part of the shaken baby syndrome. Distal posterior cerebral artery aneurysm are most likely dissecting in nature. They typically appear at the junction between the P2 and P3 segments, where the PCA crosses the tentorium resulting in microtrauma. Angiographic criteria for spontaneous dissections are the stagnation of the contrast medium in an aneurysmal pouch, the presence of stenotic segments proximal and/or distal to the ectasia, and a fusiform appearance of the aneurysm. Spontaneous hemorrhagic intracranial dissection is an uncommon disease but has been increasingly recognized as a cause for SAH with an unfavorable prognosis and a high rebleeding rate. One percent to 10% of all intracranial nontraumatic SAH is thought to result from ruptured intracranial dissections. This rate may rise to 5-20% in young patients. The choice of treatment and its timing continue to be controversial. Acutely ruptured dissections are unstable. Up to 70% of cases rebleed, often soon after the initial hemorrhage, with a mortality rate from rebleeding as high as 50%. After SAH, 70% of rebleeding occurs within the first 24 h, with 80% occurring within the first week. The rebleeding rate decreases considerably beyond the first week after initial hemorrhage, and only 10% of rebleeding occurs more than 1 month after the initial hemorrhage. The dissection may lead to an extensive mural hematoma that may compress perforating arteries close to the site of dissection. Treatment should be targeted at excluding the damaged vessel wall segment from the circulation, either endovascularly or via surgical approaches.

Image with permission from Naidich T, Castillo M, Cha S, Smirniotopoulos J. Imaging of the Brain, Elsevier, Saunders, 2013.

ANSWERS 24–32

Additional answers 24–32 available on ExpertConsult.com

EMI ANSWERS

33. 1—g, Dejerine-Roussy syndrome; 2—a, Anton syndrome; 3—n, Wallenberg's syndrome; 4—d, Benedikt's syndrome

Name	Features	Localization	Supply
Claude syndrome	Ipsilateral CNIII palsy contralateral ataxia and tremor Contralateral hemiparesis Contralateral hemiplegia of lower facial muscles/tongue/shoulder	Red nucleus, III nucleus, superior cerebral peduncle Corticospinal tract Corticobulbar tract	P1 PCA
Weber syndrome	Ipsilateral CNIII palsy Contralateral hemiplegia	Medial midbrain/cerebral peduncle	P1 PCA
Benedikt's syndrome	Ipsilateral CNIII palsy Contralateral ataxia and tremor	III nucleus Red nucleus	P1 PCA
Dejerine-Roussy syndrome (thalamic pain syndrome)	Contralateral hemisensory loss Contralateral hemibody pain	Thalamus	P1 PCA

Continued on following page

Name	Features	Localization	Supply
STN	Contralateral hemiballismus	STN	P1 PCA
Anton syndrome (cortical blindness)	Visual agnosia (deficit without recognition of blindness)	Bilateral occipital lobe	Bilateral P2 PCA/top of basilar
Balint syndrome	Bilateral loss of voluntary but not reflex eye movements Bilateral optic ataxia Asimultagnosia	Bilateral parieto-occipital lobe	Bilateral P2 PCA
Top of Basilar syndrome	Opthalmoplegia Behavioral abnormalities Somnolence/hallucinations Usually no motor deficit	Bilateral rostal midbrain and posterior thalamus	Basilar
Wallenberg's syndrome (lateral medullary)	Ipsilateral loss facial pain and sensation Ipsilateral Horner's syndrome Ipsilateral ataxia Dysarthria/dysphagia/loss of gag reflex Vertigo/nystagmus Loss of taste Contralateral body pain and temperature loss Ipsilateral numbness	Trigeminal nucleus Cerebellar peduncle Nucleus ambiguus Vestibular nucleus Solitary nucleus Spinothalamic tract Cuneate/gracile nuclei	PICA or VA
Dejerine syndrome (medial medullary)	Contralateral hemiparesis Contralateral hemisensory loss Ipsilateral CNXII palsy		VA/BA/ASA
Babinski-Nageotte syndrome	Combination of Wallenberg's and Dejerine syndromes	Hemimedullary infarct	VA (proximal to PICA and spinal artery)
Marie-Foix syndrome	Ipsilateral ataxia Contralateral hemiparesis Contralateral hemisensory loss	Lateral inferior pons	AICA
Locked-in syndrome	Quadriplegia Bilateral VI/VII weakness Aphonia (lower CN) Intact upgaze and blinking	Bilateral ventral pons	Basilar perforators
Foville syndrome	Ipsilateral facial palsy Ipsilateral lateral gaze palsy Contralateral hemiparesis	Inferior medial pons PPRF/CN VI	Basilar perforators
Millard-Gubler syndrome	Ipsilateral abducens palsy Ipsilateral facial palsy Contralateral hemiparesis	Ventral pons	Basilar perforators
Raymond syndrome	Ipsilateral abducens palsy Contralateral hemiparesis	CNVI nucleus Corticospinal tracts	Basilar perforators

34. 1—e, Calcarine artery; 2—n, Thalamogeniculate arteries

35. 1—b, Superior anastomotic vein of Trolard; 2—c, Inferior anastamostic vein of Labbe; 3—f, Superficial middle cerebral (Sylvian) vein

36. 1—e, ISUIA; 2—j, ESCAPE/EXTEND-IA/SWIFT-PRIME; 3—b, BRANT; 4—h, STASH

STASH	Simvastatin in aneurysmal subarachnoid hemorrhage	In the STASH trial, within 96 h of ictus patients were randomized in a 1:1 fashion to a 21 day course of either 40 mg simvastatin or placebo. The analysis of mRS at 6 months follow-up (primary outcome) showed no difference between favorable outcome. Fewer patients receiving simvastatin required extended hypervolemic therapy (21% vs. 29%, respectively; $p=0.009$), but there was no significant difference in the rates of DIND or mortality between the two groups
STICH	Early surgery versus initial conservative treatment in patients with spontaneous supratentorial intracerebral hematomas in the International Surgical Trial in Intracerebral Hemorrhage (STICH)	Patients with spontaneous supratentorial intracerebral hemorrhage in neurosurgical units show no overall benefit from early surgery (<24 h after randomization) when compared with initial conservative treatment (with delayed surgery if judged necessary)
STICH II	Early surgery versus initial conservative treatment in patients with spontaneous supratentorial lobar intracerebral hematomas (STICH II)	In conscious patients with spontaneous superficial (<1 cm from cortical surface; volume 10-100 ml) intracerebral hemorrhage without intraventricular hemorrhage early surgery (<12 h after randomization) does not increase the rate of death or disability at 6 months compared to initial conservative management (with delayed surgery if judged necessary). Patients in the STICH II trial with a poor prognosis did better with early surgery, whereas those with a good prognosis did not
ISAT	International Subarachnoid Aneurysm Trial	In contrast to the statistically significant difference in death or dependence [modified Rankin Scale (mRS) 3-6] at 1 year after ruptured aneurysm coiling as compared to clipping (23.5% vs. 30.9%, respectively; $p=0.0001$), at 5-year follow-up no statistically significant difference in independence was seen. However, the risk of death remained significantly lower in the endovascular cohort at 5-year follow-up [relative risk (RR) 0.77; 95% CI 0.61-0.98]. At 10-year follow-up, rates of independence still did not differ between the two groups, however, the probability of being alive and independent was more likely in the endovascular cohort (OR 1.34; 95% CI 1.07-1.67). The risk of rebleeding was higher in the endovascular group than the clipping group (1.56 bleeds per 1000 patient years vs. 0.49 bleeds per 1000 patient years, respectively)
ISUIA (1998, 2003)	International Study of Unruptured Intracranial Aneurysms	Risk of rupture 0.05% per year if <10 mm and no previous SAH from different aneurysm Risk of rupture 0.5% per year if <10 mm but previous SAH from different aneurysm Risk of rupture 1% per year if >10 mm (with or without previous SAH) Ninety percent of unruptured aneurysms in anterior circulation Criticism: Selection bias, retrospective, 7.5 years follow up and Pcomm aneurysms included in posterior circulation
ARUBA	A Randomized trial of Unruptured Brain AVMs	Comparing no treatment and any treatment modality (embolization, radiosurgery, microsurgery, alone or in combination) in the management of unruptured brain AVMs. The primary end point was death or symptomatic stroke. After a mean follow-up of 33.3 months, the primary end point was observed in 10.1% of the patients receiving no treatment and in 30.7% of patients assigned to treatment (RR 0.33; 95% CI 0.18-0.61). Main criticism is expected benefit from radiosurgery would not be seen within such short follow-up times (used in

Continued on following page

		alone or in combination in more than half of patients assigned to treatment in this study). Higher rate of hemorrhage could not be attributed to radiosurgery or surgical treatment and therefore likely underscores a prohibitively high rate of overzealous and/or partial embolization employed in the study. This highly unusual practice has poor external validity to high volume centers that treat AVMs. Although 68% of patients in the treatment arm were designated Spetzler-Martin Grade I or II (93% Grades I-III), only five patients (4.3%) were treated with microsurgery alone
BRAT	Barrow Ruptured Aneurysm Trial	At 1 year intention to treat analysis a poor outcome (mRS score >2) was observed in 33.7% of the patients assigned to aneurysm clipping and in 23.2% of the patients assigned to coil embolization (OR 1.68, 95% CI 1.08-2.61; $p=0.02$) At 3 years analysis was based on received treatment (rather than ITT) which showed the risk of a poor outcome in patients assigned to clipping compared with those assigned to coiling (35.8% vs. 30%) was no longer significant (OR 1.30, 95% CI 0.83-2.04, $p=0.25$). In addition, the degree of aneurysm obliteration ($p=0.0001$), rate of aneurysm recurrence ($p=0.01$), and rate of retreatment ($p=0.01$) were significantly better in the group treated with clipping compared with the group treated with coiling Criticisms: 38% crossed over to clipping, no intention to treat analysis in 3-year data
BRANT	British Aneurysm Nimodipine Trial	At 3 months after subarachnoid hemorrhage in patients given nimodipine the incidence of cerebral infarction was 22% (61/278) compared with 33% (92/276) in those given placebo, a significant reduction of 34% (95% confidence interval 13-50%). Poor outcomes (death, vegetative state, severe disability) were also significantly reduced by 40% (95% confidence interval 20-55%) with nimodipine [20% (55/278) in patients given nimodipine vs. 33% (91/278) in those given placebo]
JAM	Japanese Adult Moyamoya trial	Compared medical management and EC-IC bypass for prevention of rebleeding in Japanese adults with hemorrhagic Moyamoya disease over a 5-year period. Forty-two were randomized to surgery and 38 to conservative management. The primary outcome was defined as adverse events (stroke, transient ischemic attack, or recurrent hemorrhage) and it occurred in 14.3% of patients in the surgical group and 34.2% in the conservative care group ($p=0.048$). The secondary outcome, rebleeding, was observed in 11.9% of patients in the surgical group and 31.6% in the conservative care group ($p=0.042$)
ESCAPE/ EXTEND-IA/SWIFT-PRIME	Endovascular treatment for Small Core and Anterior circulation Proximal occlusion with Emphasis on minimizing CT to recanalization times Extending the time for Thrombolysis in Emergency Neurological Deficits with Intra-Arterial therapy Solitaire™ With the Intention For Thrombectomy as PRIMary treatment for acute ischemic stroke	All three of these trials aiming to validate mechanical thrombectomy for acute ischemic stroke were prematurely halted due to positive interim analyses compared to intravenous thrombolysis

37. 1—d, Parkinson's triangle; 2—h, Kawase's triangle; 3—g, Glasscock's triangle

Triangle	Borders	Access to
Anteromedial triangle	Medial IIIrd, lateral optic nerve, tentorial edge between IIIrd and optic nerve entry to optic canal	Clinoid ICA
Medial (Hakuba's) triangle	Connect points: Lateral margin supraclinoid ICA, dural entrance of IIIrd, anterolateral posterior clinoid process	Horizontal portion of cavernous ICA
Paramedian triangle	Lateral edge IIIrd, medial IVth, tentorial edge between entry points of III and IV	Medial loop of intracavernous ICA and meningohypophyseal trunk
Parkinson's triangle	Lateral aspect of IV, medial aspect of V1, dural edge between entry points of IV and V1	Entire intracavernous ICA (lateral to proximal ring) Entire intracavernous course VI (Dorello's canal to SOF)
Anterolateral (Mullan's) triangle	Between V1, V2 and bone between foramen rotundum (V2 exit) and SOF	Superior orbital vein, CN VI, carotid-cavernous fistulae
Lateral triangle	Between V2, V3 and bone between foramen rotundum (V2 exit) and foramen ovale (V3 exit)	Sphenoidal emissary vein (between cavernous sinus and pterygoid venous plexus), masses extending laterally in the cavernous sinus
Posterolateral (Glasscock's) triangle	Greater superficial petrosal nerve, posterior aspect of V3, and line between foramen spinosum and arcuate eminence of petrous bone	Identifies the triangular area of bone that must be removed to access horizontal intrapetrosal ICA for proximal control or bypass graft
Posteromedial (Kawase's) triangle	Quadrangular space. Posterior border of V3, arcuate eminence, greater superficial petrosal nerve, petrous ridge/superficial petrosal sinus	Removal of bone here gives access to petroclival area, anterolateral brainstem, and vertebrobasilar junction. Corridor between V and VII/VIII
Inferomedial triangle	Posterior clinoid process, VI at Dorello's canal, IV at edge of tentorium, petrous apex	Dural opening to Dorello's canal (Gruber's ligament forms lateral wall)
Inferolateral triangle	Lateral to inferomedial triangle. VI at Dorello's canal, IV at edge of tentorium, petrosal vein at superior petrosal sinus, petrous apex at base	Dural opening into Meckel's cave

CHAPTER 22B

Cranial Vascular Neurosurgery II: Cerebral Revascularization and Stroke

SINGLE BEST ANSWER (SBA) QUESTIONS

1. A 75-year-old man with a history of recent memory impairment is admitted with headache, confusion, and a left homonymous hemianopsia. There is no history of hypertension or malignancy. Non-contrast CT scan and GRE MRI are shown. Which one of the following is the most likely cause of this patient's symptoms and signs?

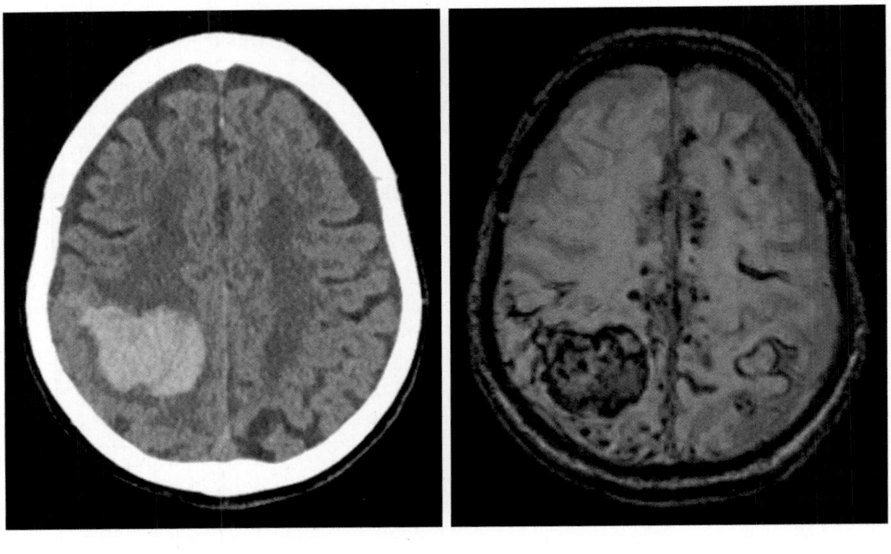

a. Multi-infarct dementia
b. Mycotic aneurysm
c. Amyloid angiopathy
d. Undiagnosed hypertension
e. Gliomatosis cerebri

2. A 71-year-old presents with sudden headache and confusion. CT is shown. Which one of the following is most likely cause?

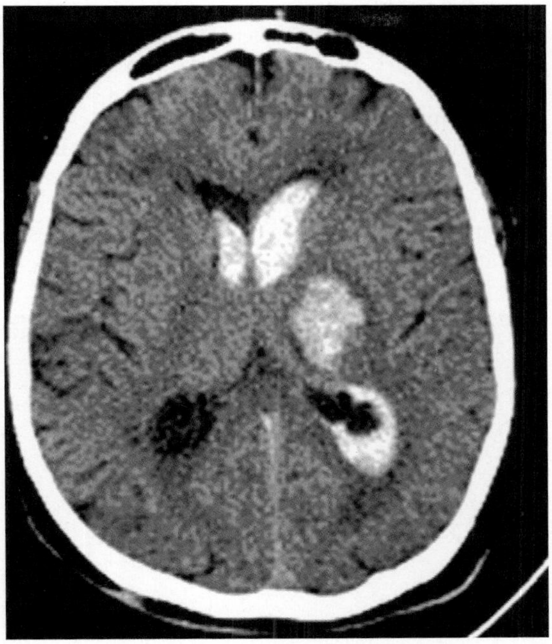

a. Vasculitis
b. Mycotic aneurysm
c. Amyloid angiopathy
d. Undiagnosed hypertension
e. Gliomatosis cerebri

3. Which one of the following statements regarding the World Federation of Neurological Surgeons (WFNS) subarachnoid grading scale is most accurate?
a. It was derived from statistical analysis of a large cohort of consecutive SAH patients from a single center
b. It was derived from statistical analysis of a large cohort of consecutive SAH patients from multiple centers
c. It was created based on expert opinion using the results of the International Cooperative Aneurysm Study
d. It is inferior to the Hunt & Hess grading scale in terms of predicting outcome at 3 months
e. It is superior to the modified Fisher score in predicting risk of vasospasm

4. Which one of the following statements regarding the Hunt & Hess subarachnoid hemorrhage grading scale is most accurate?
a. Based on a prospective study of 275 patients with aneurysmal subarachnoid hemorrhage treated in a single center
b. Assesses risk of vasospasm on initial diagnostic cerebral angiography
c. Intended to guide timing of aneurysm clipping based on grades of surgical risk
d. Meningeal reaction alone does not increase surgical hazard
e. Suggests that in the absence of ICH, grade III patients should be operated on early

5. Which one of the following statements regarding the Fisher and Modified Fisher scales is LEAST accurate?
a. Fisher Scale (1980) was proposed to predict cerebral vasospasm after aneurysmal SAH and retrospectively validated in 47 patients
b. Fisher scale (1980) utilized blood clot thickness measurements still calculable from modern CT scans
c. Fisher scale (1980) grade 4 SAH is characterized by localised clot and/or vertical layer within the subarachnoid space >1 mm thick
d. After adjusting for early angiographic vasospasm, history of hypertension, neurological grade, and elevated admission mean arterial pressure, the Fisher scale (1980) remains a significant predictor of vasospasm
e. Odds ratio of symptomatic vasospasm in Modified Fisher grade 4 SAH is two-fold higher than those with Grade 0-1 SAH

6. Which one of the following statemen regarding moyamoya disease is LEAS accurate?
a. Incidence is higher in Japan compare Western countries
b. More prevalent in females
c. Adults usually present with prog cerebral ischemia
d. Progression of disease is more co seen in children
e. Ischemic symptoms can be tri crying in children with moyam

7. Which one of the following regarding moyamoya in pregr is LEAST accurate?
a. Contraception increases graft thrombosis
b. Blood donation may in TIA/stroke in moyamo
c. Cesarean section is adv Suzuki stage 3 moyan
d. Aspirin should be cc pregnancy

e. Good cerebral circulation on SPECT or absence of frequent symptoms due to moyamoya disease within 1 year before pregnancy may reduce complications associated with vaginal delivery

8. Which one of the following statements regarding diagnosis of moyamoya disease is most accurate?
   a. Unilateral moyamoya disease can be diagnosed with MRI and MRA
   b. Suzuki stage 1 shows first evidence of developing moyamoya vessels at the base of the brain
   c. Diagnosis does not requires exclusion of causes of secondary “moyamoya syndrome”
   d. Bilateral stenosis at the terminal portion of the ICA and abnormal vascular networks in the vicinity of the stenotic lesion in the arterial phase on angiography and no secondary cause for this appearance would be sufficient to diagnose moyamoya disease
   e. Suzuki stage 6 is characterized solely by the complete absence of moyamoya vessels

9. Which one of the following is the most appropriate indications of cerebral revascularization surgery in moyamoya disease?
   a. Suzuki stage 3 moyamoya disease on cerebral angiography
   b. Intracranial hemorrhage
   c. Recurrent ischemic episodes in a child triggered by crying
   d. Asymptomatic moyamoya
   e. Planned pregnancy

10. Which one of the following statements regarding complications of cerebral bypass surgery for moyamoya disease is LEAST accurate?
   a. Cerebral hyperperfusion syndrome generally occurs 2-6 days after STA-MCA bypass
   b. Cerebral hyperperfusion can result in hemorrhagic conversion of moyamoya disease
   c. Watershed shift phenomenon is commoner in adults than children
   d. Watershed shift phenomenon describes retrograde blood supply from STA-MCA bypass may interfere with the anterograde blood flow from the proximal MCA
   e. Mechanical compression by swollen temporal muscle flap can result in cerebral edema

11. A 73-year-old patient has sudden onset left facial droop left hemiparesis 3/5 and slurred speech, left facial droop developing 90 min ago. CT head scan does not show any large infarct of hemorrhage. ASPECT score is 10. CT angiography is performed and shown below. CT perfusion shows elevated mean transit time, reduced cerebral blood flow, and preserved cerebral blood volume in the right MCA territory. There is no past medical history and he has not had any recent surgery. BP is 179/95, HR 102. Which one of the following evidence-based strategies is appropriate?

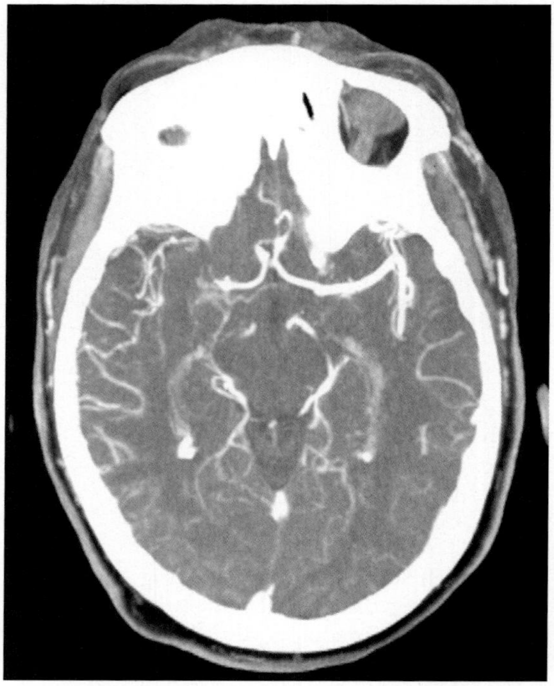

   a. Intravenous thrombolysis, if unsuccessful in 30 min proceed to mechanical thrombectomy
   b. Mechanical thrombectomy without thrombolysis
   c. Intravenous thrombolysis followed by heparin infusion
   d. Aspirin 300 mg
   e. Warfarinization

12. Which one of the following statements regarding stroke imaging is LEAST accurate?

a. ASPECT score of >7 is associated with unfavorable outcome with thrombolysis
b. Acute infarction is visible earlier on diffusion weighted imaging
c. MRI gradient echo (GRE) is useful for demonstrating microbleeds
d. CT/MR angiography can assess tissue perfusion
e. Prenumbra shows a normal or elevated regional cerebral blood volume, whereas this is reduced in infarcted tissue.

13. Which one of the following statements regarding randomized clinical trials comparing carotid endarterectomy to best medical therapy is LEAST accurate?
a. NASCET and ECST showed that the degree of benefit individual symptomatic patients gained from carotid endarterectomy was directly proportional to the risk they faced without surgery
b. Symptomatic male patients and those >70 years old benefit from CEA more
c. Risk of stroke recurrence at 30 days is 3% after first ever stroke
d. Patients with carotid "near-occlusion" benefitted most from surgery
e. Carotid endarterectomy is 70-99% carotid stenosis

14. A 59-year-old man with a background of diabetes mellitus, hyperlipidemia, and hypertension presented with sudden left hemiparesis, hemisensory loss, and dysarthria due to right MCA infarct. He was treated with systemic thrombolysis and made some recovery. A carotid duplex ultrasound and CT angiogram of the carotid arteries confirmed a severe (70-99%) stenosis in the right internal carotid artery (ICA) secondary to a 23-mm-long atherosclerotic plaque extending from the carotid bifurcation to the level of C3 vertebral body with evidence of intraluminal thrombus. The left ICA showed moderate (50-69%) stenosis. Which one of the following is most appropriate?
a. Carotid endarterectomy
b. Carotid stent
c. Carotid angioplasty
d. Best medical therapy
e. EC-IC bypass

15. Which one of the following randomized clinical trials comparing carotid endarterectomy and carotid artery stenting showed non-inferiority of carotid artery stenting to endarterectomy in high-risk patients?
a. SAPPHIRE
b. EVA-3S
c. SPACE
d. ICSS
e. CREST

16. Which of the following trials demonstrated 2-year stroke reduction benefit for symptomatic intracranial atherosclerotic disease patients with baseline hemodynamic insufficiency as defined by decreased cerebral blood flow and cerebrovascular reactivity on acetazolamide challenge as measured on SPECT who underwent STA-MCA bypass?
a. EC-IC Bypass Study (1985)
b. Japanese EC-IC Bypass Trial (JET)
c. Carotid Occulsion Surgery Study
d. SAMMPRIS
e. St. Louis Carotid Occlusion Study

17. In the modern era, which one of the following is the commonest indication for cerebral bypass surgery?
a. Moyamoya disease
b. Complex intracranial aneurysm
c. Skull base tumor causing carotid compression
d. Traumatic ICA dissection
e. Extracranial carotid occlusion

18. Which one of the following statements regarding cerebral bypass grafts is LEAST accurate?
a. STA graft patency is >95% at 2 years
b. STA is a medium-high flow graft (initially 40-80 ml/min)
c. Saphenous vein graft patency is 82% at 5 years
d. Initial flow through saphenous vein graft is 70-140 ml/min
e. High risk of vasospasm with radial artery interposition graft

19. Which one of the following statemen[t]
regarding management of complex intrac[ra]
nial aneurysms not amenable to clip rec[on]
struction or coiling is LEAST accurate[?]
a. Flow-diverting stents can be us[ed to]
reconstruct the parent artery [...]
deployed across the neck of the
mal segment
b. Flow-diverting stents become
lized over time
c. Intracranial-intracranial by
required distal to complex
d. A radial interposition gra[ft]
short segment IC-IC by
e. Flow diverting stents
conjunction with deta
necked aneurysms

SBA ANSWER

1. **c**—Amyloid angiopathy

Cerebral amyloid angiopathy (CAA) as a cause of ICH has been implicated in as many as 15% patients older than 60 years of age and almost 20% of patients 70 years of age and older. Deposition of β-amyloid protein in the vessel walls of small and medium sized arteries within the aging brain predisposes to both ICH and dementia. The locations of the bleeds are lobar or cortical-subcortical as opposed to the basal ganglia location in hypertensive IPH. Most commonly, bleeds are seen in the frontal lobe, followed by the parietal, occipital, and temporal lobes. Hemorrhage into the deep gray matter or cerebellum is uncommon and there may be evidence of prior macrohemorrhages or microhemorrhages. Patients with CAA are at substantial increased risk for recurrent hemorrhage, estimated at approximately 10% annually. On CT it is common to see multiple microhemorrhages and hematomas of varying ages. Magnetic resonance imaging including GRE and/or susceptibility-weighted imaging (SWI) is recommended as a further step in evaluation of patients suspected of CAA. MRI including MRA/MRV is reasonably sensitive at identifying secondary causes of hemorrhage. A catheter angiogram may be considered if clinical suspicion is high or noninvasive studies are suggestive of an underlying vascular cause. On GRE sequences microbleeds are round, punctate, hypointense foci less than 5-10 mm in size in brain parenchyma seen in 80% of patients with primary ICH (hypertension and amyloid angiopathy), 25% of patients with ischemic stroke, and 8% of elderly people. They correspond to hemosiderin-laden macrophages lying adjacent to the vessels and indicate prior extravasation of blood. Microbleeds have been suggested to be predictors of bleeding-prone angiopathy. Some studies have shown that patients with microbleeds may be at increased risk for ICH after anticoagulation or thrombolytic treatment; however, this is controversial and not confirmed in all studies. The STICH trial randomized patients with spontaneous supratentorial ICH (<72 h; unlikely due to vascular malformation/aneurysm/tumor), hematoma >2 cm, and GCS 5 or more where there was clinical equipoise about hematoma evacuation to either early surgery or initial conservative management with possibility of ICH evacuation if deemed appropriate by the treating physicians. They found that except for possibly those with superficial ICHs, craniotomy 1 day or longer after onset is not better than initial conservative medical treatment with or without later craniotomy for patients who have deterioration. STICH II trial focused on those with spontaneous, superficial lobar ICH (<1 cm from cortical surface; volume 10-100 ml) without intraventricular hemorrhage in conscious patients and found that early surgery (<12 h after randomization) does not increase the rate of death or disability at 6 months compared to initial conservative management (with delayed surgery if judged necessary). Patients in the STICH II trial with a poor prognosis (GCS 9-12) did better with early surgery, whereas those with a good prognosis did not (as the ability to observe and operate on only those who deteriorate is more beneficial overall for this group).

Image with permission from Mirvis SE, et al., editors. Problem Solving in Emergency Radiology, Saunders, Elsevier, 2015.

FURTHER READING

Mendelow AD, Gregson BA, Rowan EN, Murray GD, Gholkar A, Mitchell PM. STICH II Investigators. Early surgery versus initial conservative treatment in patients with spontaneous supratentorial lobar intracerebral haematomas (STICH II): a randomised trial. Lancet 2013 Aug 3;382 (9890):397-408. doi: 10.1016/S0140-6736(13)60986-1. Epub 2013 May 29. Erratum in: Lancet. 2013 Aug 3;382 (9890):396. PubMed PMID: 23726393; PubMed Central PMCID: PMC3906609.

Mendelow AD, Gregson BA, Fernandes HM, Murray GD, Teasdale GM, Hope DT, Karimi A, Shaw MD, Barer DH. STICH investigators. Early surgery versus initial conservative treatment in patients with spontaneous supratentorial intracerebral haematomas in the International Surgical Trial in Intracerebral Haemorrhage (STICH): a randomised trial. Lancet 2005 Jan 29-Feb 4;365(9457):387-97. PubMed PMID: 15680453.

2. **d**—Undiagnosed hypertension

Hypertensive ICH accounts for over 50% of cases. Hemorrhage occurs most commonly in the basal ganglia /thalamus (80%), pons (5-10%) and the cerebellar hemispheres (5-10%). Over 90% of the patients are older than 45 years of age. The bleeding results from the rupture of small penetrating arteries. In 1868 Charcot and Bouchard described the cause of the bleeding as rupture of Charcot-Bouchard microaneurysms in the walls of small penetrating arterioles (microaneurysms). Intraparenchymal hemorrhage may result from a large and heterogeneous group of causes, including primary causes such as hypertension and amyloid angiopathy or secondary causes such as AVM, intracranial aneurysms, cavernous angiomas, dural venous sinus thrombosis, intracranial neoplasms, coagulopathy, vasculitis, drug use, and hemorrhagic ischemic stroke. Underlying vascular abnormalities must always be considered and excluded if suspected due to the high risk for recurrent hemorrhage and the availability of treatment options. Clinical symptoms suggesting a secondary cause include prodrome of headache or neurologic deficits before the onset of the accident or other clinical findings that suggest an underlying disease. Imaging findings suggestive of secondary causes include the presence of SAH and ICH at the same time, unusual shape of the hematoma, increased edema compared to the size of the hematoma, and visualization of a masslike lesion or abnormal vessels. Hematoma expansion occurs in approximately one third of acute primary IPH cases and is associated with high mortality, disability, and functional deterioration. The CT shown demonstrates basal ganglia hemorrhage with intraventricular extension and surgical management will be directed towards developing hydrocephalus via external ventricular drainage.

Image with permission from Hernalsteen D, Dignac A, Oppenheim C, et al. Hyperacute intraventricular hemorrhage: detection and characterization, a comparison between 5 MRI sequences, J Neuroradiol 2007 Mar;34(1):42-8.

3. **c**—It was created based on expert opinion using the results of the International Cooperative Aneurysm Study

In 1988, an expert opinion committee proposed the WFNS Scale based on the committee members' opinions that a SAH scale should (a) include five grades, (b) be based on the GCS, and (c) acknowledge the presence of a focal neurological deficit. They considered data from the International Cooperative Aneurysm Study that assessed the prognostic importance of headache, stiff neck, and major focal neurological deficits. The analysis showed that Hunt and Hess grades 1 and 2 were prognostically the same because, as long as consciousness was normal, headache and/or stiff neck had no significant effect on outcome. Secondly, the most important predictor of mortality and disability was level of consciousness, and lastly the most important predictor of disability (but not mortality) was hemiparesis and/or aphasia. The WFNS Scale compresses the GCS into five grades, with the addition of a fourth axis (focal neurological deficit) to differentiate grades 2 and 3. In a series of approximately 3500 patients with SAH who were graded prospectively and assessed for outcome on the GOS 3 months after aneurysmal clipping (favorable outcome was good recovery or moderate disability [GOS 4-5] and an unfavorable outcome was severe disability, a vegetative state, or death [GOS 1-3]) admission WFNS was shown to be predictive of outcome ($p < 0.0001$).

WFNS	Description	Unfavorable Outcome (GOS1-3) at 3 months
I	GCS 15 without motor deficit	13%
II	GCS 13-14 without motor deficit	24%
III	GCS 13-14 with motor deficit	48%
IV	GCS 7-12 with or without motor deficit	55%
V	GCS 3-6 with or without motor deficit	66%

FURTHER READING

Report of World Federation of Neurological Surgeons Committee on a Universal Subarachnoid Hemorrhage Grading Scale. J Neurosurg 1988;68:985.

Rosen DS, Macdonald RL. Grading of subarachnoid hemorrhage: modification of the World Federation of Neurosurgical Societies scale on the basis of data for a large series of patients. Neurosurgery 2004;54:566-75.

Rosen DS, Macdonald RL. Subarachnoid hemorrhage grading scales: a systematic review. Neurocrit Care 2005;2 (2):110-18.

4. **c**—Intended to guide timing of aneurysm clipping based on grades of surgical risk

The Hunt and Hess scale (1968) aimed to retrospectively create an index of surgical risk and to aid neurosurgeons in deciding on the appropriate time after SAH at which the neurosurgeon should operate. Surgical risk was felt to be best estimated by the intensity of meningeal inflammatory reaction, the severity of neurological deficit/level of arousal (indicating arterial spasm, ischemia, and brain edema and thus greater vulnerability to manipulation), and the presence of associated disease. Their practice at that time was to take grade I and II to surgery as soon as a diagnosis could be made (ideally <24 h admission), while graded III-V treated conservatively until they improved to Grade I or II (except in the case of multiple rebleeds or life-threatening ICH). After retrospective review of 275 cases, they concluded that aneurysm clipping can be accomplished with an extremely low mortality rate in the absence of severe meningeal reaction, neurological deficit, or serious associated disease (preop Grade I 1.4% versus Grade II 22% versus Grade III-IV approx. 40%) and that meningeal reaction alone (Grade II) increases surgical hazard. Thus they suggested prompt surgical intervention is important for patients admitted in good condition, while for the more seriously ill conservative therapy should be utilized until their condition improves. In 1974, Hunt and Kosnik proposed a modification of their SAH scale by adding a zero grade for unruptured aneurysms and 1a grade for a fixed neurological deficit in the absence of other signs of SAH. Although the Hunt and Hess scale is easy to administer, the classifications are arbitrary, some of the terms are vague (e.g. drowsy, stupor, and deep coma) and some patients may present with initial features that defy placement within a single grade. In one study which compared Hunt and Hess Scale with GCS, and WFNS Scale in a series of 185 patients with aneurysmal SAH showed that it had the strongest predictive power for GOS at 6 months, though half of poor-grade patients achieved good recoveries suggesting that current admission grading scales are not accurate enough to be the sole basis for treatment decisions. They also found that scores on the day of operation were of more prognostic value than values observed immediately after hospitalization. Furthermore other studies have struggled to find outcome differences between the individual grades, but did when lower grades were merged suggesting the possibility of an oversplitting error weakening the prognostic power of the scale.

Hunt and Hess SAH Scale (1968)

Grade	Description NOTE: Grade must be increased by one level in the presence of serious systemic disease (hypertension, diabetes, severe arteriosclerosis, COPD) or severe vasospasm on angiography.
I	Asymptomatic or minimal headache and slight nuchal rigidity
II	Moderate to severe headache, nuchal rigidity, cranial nerve palsy (but no other neurological deficit)
III	Drowsy, confusion, or mild focal deficit
IV	Stupor, moderate-to-severe hemiparesis, possibly early decerebrate rigidity, and vegetative disturbances
V	Deep coma, decerebrate rigidity, moribund appearance

FURTHER READING

Hunt W, Hess R. Surgical risk as related to time of intervention in the repair of intracranial aneurysms. J Neurosurg 1968;28:14.

Rosen DS, Macdonald RL. Subarachnoid hemorrhage grading scales: a systematic review. Neurocrit Care 2005;2 (2):110-18.

5. **e**—Odds ratio of symptomatic vasospasm for Modified Fisher grade 4 SAH is two-fold higher than those with Grade 0-1 SAH

The Fisher Scale (1980) was proposed to predict cerebral vasospasm after aneurysmal SAH and prospectively validated in 47 patients: slight to severe vasospasm was seen in 4/11 (36%) grade 1, 3/7 (43%) grade 2, 24/24 (100%) of grade 3, and 2/3 (67%) of grade 4 patients. Limitations of this original scale include: (i) poor resolution compared to current CT scans, (ii) blood thickness measurements used were actual measurements on printed CT scan images and had no relationship to the real clot thickness, (iii) No SAH and SAH <1 mm in true thickness (Grades 1 and 2) are both uncommon, and (iv) it does not account for patients with thick SAH with ICH/IVH or those with ICH/IVH alone. More recent evidence that the Fisher scale may not correlate with risk of vasospasm resulted in the Fisher scale being compared to the Modified Fisher scale (2006) in 1355 patients with SAH (in placebo arm of RCT for tirilazad), of whom 33% developed vasospasm. Early angiographic vasospasm, history of hypertension, neurological grade, and elevated admission mean arterial pressure were identified as risk factors for symptomatic vasospasm. After adjusting for these variables, the modified Fisher scale remained a significant predictor of symptomatic vasospasm (adjusted OR 1.28, $p = 0.01$) while the original Fisher scale was not (adjusted OR 1.1, $p = 0.488$).

Risk of Vasospasm Based on Fisher and Modified Fisher Scales

Grade	Fisher Scale	Vasospasm OR	Modified Fisher Scale	Vasospasm OR
0			No SAH or IVH	-
1	No subarachnoid hemorrhage	-	Focal or diffuse thin SAH, no IVH	-
2	Diffuse or vertical layer of subarachnoid blood <1 mm thick (Diffuse thin SAH)	1.3	Focal or diffuse thin SAH, with IVH	1.6
3	Localized clot and/or vertical layer within the subarachnoid space >1 mm thick (focal or diffuse thick SAH)	2.2	Focal or diffuse thick SAH, no IVH	1.6
4	Diffuse thin SAH or no SAH, with ICH or IVH	1.7	Focal or diffuse thick SAH, with IVH	2.2

FURTHER READING

Fisher CM, Kistler JP, Davis JM. Relation of cerebral vasospasm to subarachnoid hemorrhage visualized by computerized tomographic scanning. Neurosurgery 1980;6:1-9.

Frontera JA, Claasen J, Schmidt JM, Wartenberg KE, Temes R, Connolly ES, Loch Macdonald R, Mayer SA. Prediction of symptomatic vasospasm after subarachnoid haemorrhage: the modified Fisher scale. Neurosurgery 2006;58(7):21-27.

Rosen DS, Macdonald RL. Subarachnoid hemorrhage grading scales: a systematic review. Neurocrit Care 2005;2 (2):110-18.

6. **c**—Adults usually present with progressive cerebral ischemia

Moyamoya disease is characterized by bilateral stenosis or occlusion of the terminal portion of the ICAs and/or the proximal portions of the ACAs and MCAs. Moyamoya disease is also characterized by irregular perforating vascular networks, called moyamoya vessels, near the occluded or stenotic regions corresponding to the lenticulostriate and thalamoperforate arteries. The associated tuft of collateral vessels that forms at the base of the skull gives the angiographic appearance of a hazy "puff of smoke," or "moyamoya" in Japanese. Incidence rate in Japan is 0.5-1 per 100,000 people, with a prevalence of 10.5 patients per 100,000. Improved diagnostic measures and prognosis for these patients may have contributed to the increase in the incidence and prevalence of the disease. MMD cases in the US show a lack of bimodal age of onset, prevalence of the ischemic type at all ages, more benign symptoms at presentation, and better response to surgical treatment. The incidence of MMD in California was only 0.087 per 100,000 from 1987 to 1998, even with a higher Asian population. It is more prevalent among women. Genome-wide association study identified the RNF213 gene in the 17q25 region as a susceptibility gene for moyamoya disease among East Asians. Secondary causes of "moyamoya syndrome" include infection, autoimmunity, other inflammatory conditions, and cranial irradiation. Presentation may be: ischemic 63.4%, hemorrhagic 21.6%, epileptic 7.6%, and "other" 7.5%. The ischemic type of MMD predominates in childhood, making up 69% of cases in patients under 10 years old and Ischemic symptoms are often instigated by hyperventilation (e.g. crying). The symptoms may present repetitively and can result in motor aphasia, cortical blindness, mental retardation, and low IQ over the long term. The hemorrhagic type of MMD occurs in 66% of adult cases exhibit hemorrhages with a higher occurrence in females. Progression of occlusion is more common in children than adults. Due to a poor response to medical therapy, direct and indirect cerebral bypass techniques have been devised with the goals of promoting neoangiogenesis, inducing collateral vessel formation, and restoring perfusion to oxygen-deprived areas of the brain. The direct techniques can immediately augment the blood supply as well as promote neoangiogenesis. surgical intervention improves the outcomes of patients with symptomatic MMD. Direct revascularization is the treatment of choice and may lead to immediate improvement of symptoms, but is technically challenging and is associated with risks such as hemorrhage and cerebral hyperperfusion syndrome. The pediatric population is typically treated with indirect revascularization because (i) the likelihood of angiogenesis is higher in children than in adults and (ii) direct bypass is technically challenging and more prone to thrombosis in children. Disadvantages of indirect revascularization relate to longer time for collateral formation and angiogenesis and that it may preclude the option of subsequent direct bypass in symptomatic children if the STA is used or compromised.

FURTHER READING

Burke GM, et al. Moyamoya disease: a summary. Neurosurg Focus 2009;26(4):E11.

Baaj AA, et al. Surgical management of Moyamoya disease: a review. Neurosurg Focus 2009;26(4):E7.

7. **c**—Cesarean section is advisable in those with Suzuki stage 3 moyamoya

General lifestyle advice for pre- or post-bypass moyamoya patients includes: (i) avoid oral contraceptives or hormone replacement therapy due to the risk of cerebral thrombosis (especially through bypass graft), (ii) lifelong aspirin, (iii) ensure headgear/helmets do not constrict blood supply to the bypass, (iv) avoid donating blood due to risk of TIA/stroke from loss of intravascular volume, (v) normal pregnancy and vaginal delivery is possible under specialist joint care. Cerebral infarction and intracranial hemorrhage are the major concerns in pregnancies with moyamoya disease because these conditions greatly influence the prognoses of the mother and newborn infant. Intrapartum, cerebral blood flow decreases due to hyperventilation and increases due to elevation of blood pressure caused by pain and uterine contractions. These increases and decreases of cerebral blood flow cause cerebral ischemia and hemorrhage. However, vaginal delivery is possible if cerebral blood flow can be controlled, and this may be achieved by controlling blood flow to the brain with epidural anesthesia. When vaginal delivery is selected, there is evidence to suggest that good cerebral circulation on SPECT or absence of frequent symptoms due to moyamoya disease within 1 year before pregnancy is important for avoiding complications.

FURTHER READING

Stanford Medicine (Neurosurgery): http://med.stanford.edu/neurosurgery/moyamoya/faq.html

Tanaka H, Katsuragi S, Tanaka K, et al. Vaginal delivery in pregnancy with Moyamoya disease: experience at a single institute. J Obstet Gynaecol Res 2015;41:517-22.

8. **d**—Bilateral stenosis at the terminal portion of the ICA and abnormal vascular networks in the vicinity of the stenotic lesion in the arterial phase on angiography and no secondary cause for this appearance would be sufficient to diagnose moyamoya disease

Clinical diagnosis of moyamoya disease is based on (A) cerebral angiography (gold standard) and/or (B) MRI/MRA, and (C) exclusion of secondary moyamoya syndrome (arteriosclerosis, autoimmune, meningitis, brain tumor, Down's syndrome, NF-1, head trauma, cranial irradiation, sickle cell disease, and others). Historically, only bilateral cases could be diagnosed definitively while unilateral cases with appropriate criteria could be termed probable moyamoya disease. However, the most recent Japanese diagnostic criteria state that definitive diagnosis of moyamoya disease requires catheter angiography in unilateral cases while bilateral cases could be promptly diagnosed by either catheter angiography or magnetic resonance (MR) imaging/angiography. Cerebral angiography should show (i) stenosis or occlusion at the terminal portion of the ICA and/or at the proximal portion of the ACAs and/or the MCAs and (ii) abnormal vascular networks in the vicinity of the occlusive or stenotic lesions in the arterial phase. Cerebral angiography is not mandatory when MR imaging and MR angiography clearly demonstrate: (i) bilateral stenosis or occlusion at the terminal portion of the ICA and at the proximal portion of the ACAs and MCAs on MR angiography, and (ii) bilateral abnormal vascular network in the basal ganglia on MR angiography (>2 apparent flow voids are observed in 1 side of the basal ganglia on MR imaging). Cerebral angiography serves for diagnosis, surgical planning, and monitoring progression via Suzuki staging. The utility of Suzuki staging may be mostly in children (as many adults remain within the same stage), and even then most cases belong to stages 3-5, and stages are not strongly related to clinical symptoms.

Suzuki Angiographic Staging of Moyamoya Disease

Suzuki Stage	Angiographic Findings
1	Stenosis of suprasellar ICA, usually bilateral
2	Development of moyamoya vessels at base of brain
3	Increasing ICA stenosis and prominence of moyamoya vessels (most cases diagnosed at this stage)
4	Entire circle of Willis and PCAs occluded, extracranial collaterals start to appear, moyamoya vessels begin to diminish
5	Further progression of Stage 4
6	Complete absence of moyamoya vessels and major cerebral arteries

FURTHER READING

Suzuki J, Takaku A. Cerebrovascular "moyamoya" disease. Disease showing abnormal net-like vessels in base of brain. Arch Neurol 1969;20:288-99.

Research Committee on the Pathology and Treatment of Spontaneous Occlusion of the Circle of Willis; Health Labour.

Sciences Research Grant for Research on Measures for Intractable Diseases (2012) Guidelines for diagnosis and treatment of moyamoya disease (spontaneous occlusion of the circle of willis). Neurol Med Chir (Tokyo) 2012;52:245-66.

9. **c**—Recurrent ischemic episodes in a child triggered by crying

Direct revascularization surgery such as STA-MCA anastomosis, as well as indirect revascularization, is established as an effective procedure for the moyamoya disease patients with ischemic symptoms. However, the recently published results of the Japanese Adult Moyamoya trial have provided us with level I evidence for the potential benefit of direct cerebral revascularization for preventing recurrent bleeds in adults with hemorrhagic moyamoya disease. In summary, 80 adult patients with a recent history (<12 months) of cerebral hemorrhage were randomly assigned to either direct extracranial-to-intracranial (EC-IC) bypass or medical management and followed for 5 years. Significant morbidity was seen in 34% of the patients managed conservatively compared with 14.3% of the patients in the surgical group. Similarly, patients in the nonsurgical arm were approximately 3 times more likely to experience a recurrent bleed than patients who underwent surgery (31.6% vs. 11.9%) suggesting a preventive effect of direct bypass against rebleeding. JAM trial strongly encourages direct revascularization surgery for reducing the risk for rebleeding in adult moyamoya disease patients presenting with intracranial hemorrhage, although the statistical significance was marginal. Finally, revascularization surgery for asymptomatic moyamoya disease patients is not recommended due to the uncertainty of the natural history of this patient population.

FURTHER READING

Howard BM, Barrow DL. Cerebral revascularization: which patients should be bypassed and which patients should be passed by? World Neurosurg 2015 Mar;83(3):288-90.

Fujimura M, et al. Current status of revascularization surgery for moyamoya disease: special consideration for its "internal carotid-external carotid (IC-EC) conversion" as the physiological reorganization system. Tohoku J Exp Med 2015;236:45-53.

10. **d**—Watershed shift phenomenon is more common in adults than children

Surgical complications of moyamoya disease include both neurological and non-neurological complications, and neurological complications include perioperative cerebral infarction and cerebral hyperperfusion syndrome. Mechanisms for ischemia include "watershed shift phenomenon" where retrograde blood supply from STA-MCA bypass may interfere with the anterograde blood flow from the proximal MCA, and thus result in the temporary decrease in CBF at the cortex supplied by the adjacent branch of MCA—particularly in pediatric moyamoya disease. Secondly, thrombo-embolic complications related to the anastomosed site and the mechanical compression by swollen temporal muscle flap could also cause cerebral ischemia in the acute stage. STA-MCA bypass may temporarily lead to heterogeneous hemodynamic condition even within the hemisphere operated on. Cerebral hyperperfusion syndrome is one of the most serious complications and may occur in nearly 40% of adult patients with moyamoya disease 2-6 days after STA-MCA bypass. Rapid focal increase in CBF (hyperemia) at the site of the anastomosis could result in vasogenic edema and/or hemorrhagic conversion in moyamoya disease. Focal cerebral hyperperfusion can cause temporary focal neurological deficit such as aphasia, hemiparesis, and dysarthria in a blood pressure dependent manner. In general, good perioperative hydration, hemoglobin control, and routine use of anti-platelet agent are essential to avoid ischemic complications.

FURTHER READING

Fujimura M, et al. Current status of revascularization surgery for moyamoya disease: special consideration for its "internal carotid-external carotid (IC-EC) conversion" as the physiological reorganization system. Tohoku J Exp Med 2015;236:45-53.

11. **a**—Intravenous thrombolysis, if unsuccessful in 30 minutes proceed immediately to mechanical thrombectomy

In 1995 with the validation of intravenous recombinant tissue plasminogen activator (IV rtPA) in studies demonstrating improved clinical outcomes in patients treated within 3 h of stroke ictus dramatically improved stroke therapy. Despite the clinical benefits of IV rtPA, disappointments remained concerning modest recanalization rates, ranging between 4.4% for distal internal carotid artery occlusion, 4% for basilar artery occlusions and 30% for middle cerebral artery (MCA) M1 and M2 segment occlusions. Initial trials of endovascular therapy versus IV rtPA alone (e.g. MERCI, IMS III, SYNTHESIS Expansion, MR RESCUE trials) failed to definitively demonstrate superiority of mechanical embolectomy—possibly due to use of first generation stent retrievers with poor recanalization rates, and limited availability of advanced imaging to confirm vessel occlusion and identify prenumbral pattern/infarct core. Recently, however, 5 published randomized controlled studies (ESCAPE, MR CLEAN, SWIFT Prime, EXTEND IA, REVASCAT) using new generation devices with recanalization rates 58-88% and advanced CT/MR imaging for patient selection (assessing collateral circulation, mismatch ratio and ischemic core volume) have provided overwhelming evidence in support of IV rtPA plus mechanical thrombectomy for acute ischemic stroke in patients with proximal large artery (ICA/MCA) compared to IV rtPA alone. In the studies, the odds of a favorable outcome (mRS 2 or less at 90 days) in the endovascular group were at least twice that in controls, without any difference in 30-day mortality or symptomatic ICH between groups. Furthermore, the benefit was maintained in old age (>80) and those with severe stroke (based on NIHSS). Further studies underway to assess its role in those with wake up strokes and those outside treatment timeframe as stratified by advanced imaging.

Image with permission from Quiñones-Hinojosa A. Schmidek and Sweet's Operative Neurosurgical Techniques, 6th ed. Saunders, Elsevier, 2012.

FURTHER READING

Palaniswami and Yan: Mechanical Thrombectomy Is Now the Gold Standard for Acute Ischemic Stroke: Implications for Routine Clinical Practice. Intervent Neurol 2015;4:18-29.

12. **d**—CT/MR angiography can assess tissue perfusion

Advance imaging in stroke has and increasing role in patient selection, and may be crucial in future to discriminate where endovascular therapy may be of benefit in those outside of established treatment windows or with wakeup strokes. Alberta Stroke Program Early Computed Tomography Score (ASPECTS) is a 10 point score used in MCA infarcts whereby 1 point is deducted for every vascular region involved. An ASPECT score of 7 or below is associated with a worse functional outcome at 3 months, higher risk of symptomatic hemorrhage and unfavorable outcome with thrombolysis. CT and MR angiography can demonstrate occlusion and length of clot and recanalization post-thrombolysis. MR gradient echo can demonstrate hemorrhage (and microhemorrhage), while DWI can demonstrate acute infarction very early on (e.g. 10 min in animal models). CT and MR perfusion imaging can be used to assess the proportion of salvageable (prenumbra) and non-salvageable (infarcted) tissue before deciding on endovascular therapy utilizing parameters shown below (TTP, MTT, CBF, CBV).

	rTTP	MTT	rCBF	rCBV
Tissue at risk (prenumbra)	Increased	Increased	Reduced	Normal or elevated
Infarct/dead	Significantly increased	Increased	Reduced	Reduced

TTP, time to peak; MMT, mean transit time, CBF, cerebral blood flow, CBV, cerebral blood volume (area under the curve).

13. **d**—Patients with carotid "near-occlusion" benefitted most from surgery

The estimated 30-day risk of stroke recurrence after first stroke is ~3% at 30 days and 26% at 5 years. The NASCET investigators stratified patients into groups with "low moderate" (<50%), "high moderate" (50-69%) and "severe" (70-99%) carotid stenosis. For the severe stenosis, the risk of any major stroke or death was 32.3% in the medical group and 15.8% in the surgical group at two years and statistically significant. Furthermore, the degree of benefit individual symptomatic patients gained from carotid endarterectomy was directly proportional to the risk they faced without surgery: patients with 50-69% stenosis had attenuated benefit, therefore would be expected to face a lower risk without surgery. Patients with <50% stenosis did not achieve a significant reduction in the risk of ipsilateral stroke. In ECST, the method of measurement of carotid stenosis differed, but when the trial results were reanalyzed using the NASCET method, similar benefit for CEA was demonstrated. The five-year risk reduction of "stroke or surgical death" in ECST patients with 70-99% stenosis randomized to CEA rather than medical treatment was 21.2%. In patients with 50-69% stenosis, the risk reduction was 5.7%. As expected, patients with a lesser degree of stenosis did not benefit from surgery. However, an additional important finding is that patients with "near-occlusion"—those with evidence of collapse of the distal vessel indicating poor run-off flow in the carotid—did not benefit significantly from surgery. Indeed, many patients with near-occlusion will progress to complete occlusion of the artery, which precludes intervention. The risk/benefit ratio most favors surgery over medical treatment in men and in the elderly. In addition, the overall benefit of surgery is diminished as the time between symptoms and surgery increases, strongly arguing for intervention in the stable patient within two weeks of last symptoms. The rate of ipsilateral stroke in patients with asymptomatic carotid stenosis is much lower: possibly <0.5% per year in patients with ≥50% stenosis treated with best medical therapy. Two large randomized trials provide much of the data available to address the question of whether prophylactic CEA in the asymptomatic patient prevents stroke. The Asymptomatic Carotid Atherosclerosis Study (ACAS) randomized 1662 patients with an asymptomatic carotid stenosis of 60% or greater (measured using NASCET criteria) as detected on cerebral angiography or computerized tomography angiogram (CTA) either to daily aspirin with risk factor management (BMT) or to CEA plus BMT. CEA reduced the rate of rate of ipsilateral stroke or any perioperative stroke or death from 11.0% to 5.1%. The Asymptomatic Carotid Surgery Trial (ACST) randomized 3,120 patients with 60-99% carotid stenosis on Doppler ultrasound to either "immediate" endarterectomy (with half of patients being operated on within one month after randomization) or deferral of CEA until a clinician considered there to be a clear indication for surgery. When perioperative adverse events were combined with subsequent strokes over a five-year period, CEA reduced the rate of events from 11.8% to 6.4% ($p < 0.0001$) and subsequently maintained at 10 year follow up in those operated <75. The results of these two trials, when combined in meta-analysis with the asymptomatic patients of the Veterans Affairs Cooperative Studies, appear to support the practice of endarterectomy for asymptomatic carotid stenosis to reduce the risk of ipsilateral stroke over three years but this risk reduction was marginal (6% reduction over 10 years) compared to that in symptomatic patients, and that to be worthwhile the surgical risk (MI, stroke, death) must be low and patient must also be prepared to incur an early risk of perioperative stroke to reduce the risk of a stroke that might not happen for many years. In subgroup analyses, surgical intervention appeared to benefit men more than women and younger patients more than older.

FURTHER READING

Doig D, Brown M. Carotid stenting versus endarterectomy. Annu Rev Med 2012;63:259-76.

North American Symptomatic Carotid Endarterectomy Trial Collaborators. Beneficial effect of carotid endarterectomy in symptomatic patients with high-grade carotid stenosis. N Engl J Med 1991;325:445-453.

Barnett HJ, Taylor DW, Eliasziw M, Fox AJ, Ferguson GG, Haynes RB, Rankin RN, Clagett GP, Hachinski VC, Sackett DL, Thorpe KE, Meldrum HE, Spence JD. Benefit of carotid endarterectomy in patients with symptomatic moderate or severe stenosis. North American Symptomatic Carotid Endarterectomy Trial Collaborators. N Engl J Med 1998;339:1415-1425.

Randomized trial of endarterectomy for recently symptomatic carotid stenosis: final results of the MRC European Carotid Surgery Trial (ECST). Lancet 1998;351:1379-1387.

Endarterectomy for asymptomatic patients with high-grade stenosis. Executive Committee for the Asymptomatic Carotid Atherosclerosis Study. JAMA 1995;273:1421-1428.

Halliday A, Mansfield A, Marro J, Peto C, Peto R, Potter J, Thomas D. MRC Asymptomatic Carotid Surgery Trial (ACST) Collaborative Group. Prevention of disabling and fatal strokes by successful carotid endarterectomy in patients without recent neurological symptoms: randomised controlled trial. Lancet 2004;363:1491-1502.

14. **a**—Carotid endarterectomy

Best medical therapy (BMT) alone may be preferred for asymptomatic carotid occlusion if (i) patient life expectancy is less than the time to achieve stroke reduction benefit from revascularization (i.e. 2-3 years for CEA, and 5 years for CAS), or (ii) if established periprocedure risk of death/stroke is small enough (<3%) and/or high future stroke risk factors (e.g. plaque ulceration, contralateral ICA occlusion, male, intraluminal thrombus, young age) to ensure benefit despite small absolute risk reduction seen in studies (6% at 5 years in ACAS). In contrast, symptomatic patients benefit almost immediately from CEA due to their higher short-term stroke risk. However, even symptomatic patients with dense hemispheric neurological deficits, significant dementia, or severely limited functional status attributable to poor cardiac, renal, or pulmonary reserve are unlikely to benefit from any form of carotid revascularization. Factors outlining the decision between CEA and CAS in appropriate individuals with symptomatic carotid stenosis are shown below, although patient preference and operator experience/center specific outcomes are just as important.

Patient Selection in Carotid Endarterectomy Versus Stenting

Factors	Carotid Endarterectomy (CEA) plus BMT	Carotid Artery Stent (CAS) plus BMT
Age	Safer than CAS in patients ≥70 years of age.	Significantly increased risk of periprocedural stroke or death in CAS-treated patients ≥70 years of age.
Life expectancy to see stroke reduction relative to BMT alone	At least 3 years	At least 5 years
Stroke risk factors present	Ipsilateral neurology in last 6 months High grade (70-99%) stenosis High risk plaque (ulcer, hemorrhage etc.) Contralateral carotid occlusion increases risk of CEA (inadequate collateral circulation)	Not suitable for lesions at high risk of periprocedural embolization (e.g. intraluminal thrombus)
Neck anatomy	Challenging if hostile neck anatomy Unclear if preferable to CAS for recurrent carotid artery stenosis	Preferred for patients with hostile neck (previous neck surgery/radiotherapy, contralateral laryngeal nerve palsy, tracheostomy)
Carotid/aortic arch anatomy	Better outcomes than CAS if: ICA-CCA angulation >60 deg., ICA lesion >10-15 mm long, ostial involvement of lesion, excessive calcification	Preferred if hostile carotid: lesion distal to C2 vertebral body or proximal to clavicle Increased risk of periprocedural stroke if aortic arch challenging configuration, tortuous, calcified.
Stroke risk reduction and outcome	16% absolute risk reduction at 2 years compared to BMT alone in symptomatic patients in NASCET (overall 10% risk reduction once 6% perioperative risk considered)	Conflicting evidence as to whether non-inferior to CEA. Worse outcomes in symptomatic patient and >70. Non-inferior to CEA in high risk patients
Complications	Greater risk of MI and cranial nerve injury compared to CAS Lower risk of periprocedure stroke risk than CAS	Higher stroke risk and death Lower risk of MI

15. **a**—SAPPHIRE

Several large trials have shown the superiority of carotid endarterectomy to best medical management in patients with significant carotid stenosis (>70-99%) in terms of reducing risk of recurrent stroke. Many head to head trials of carotid end-arterectomy (e.g. EVA-3S, SPACE, ICSS) have failed to prove non-inferiority of CAS compared to CEA in standard risk patients. The CREST trial found CAS to be non-inferior to CEA in symptomatic or asymptomatic standard risk patients, with no difference in rates of death, stroke or MI at 4 years (but did find a statistically higher 30-day risk of stroke for CAS and MI for CEA). The Stenting and Angioplasty with Protection in Patients at High Risk for Endarterectomy (SAPPHIRE) trial, showed non-inferiority of CAS in high-risk patients at 3 years (e.g. clinically significant cardiac disease [congestive heart failure, abnormal stress test, or need for open-heart surgery], contralateral carotid disease, severe pulmonary disease). These results, have meant that in symptomatic patients CAS is a viable option in high risk patients, those with stenosis distal to C2 vertebral body (difficult to treat with CEA), or if being performed by an experienced operator with established outcomes equivalent to CEA. Due to fewer trials demonstrating non-inferiority of CAS for asymptomatic patients, it should at present only be considered if being performed by an experienced operator with established outcomes equivalent to CEA.

FURTHER READING

Hussain MA, et al. Carotid artery revascularization: what's the best strategy? Circulation 2015;131:2226-31.

16. **b**—Japanese EC-IC Bypass Trial (JET)

Symptomatic ICAD portends a high rate of recurrent, disabling ischemic strokes. In fact, several large clinical trials have documented recurrence rates of 14% -19% over 2 years, with the majority of events occurring in the 1st year. In the Warfarin-Aspirin Symptomatic Intracranial

Disease (WASID) study –a retrospective, multicenter trial that compared the efficacy of warfarin with aspirin for the prevention of major vascular events –73% of patients with recurrent strokes had ischemic lesions in the territory of the symptomatic artery. One recent clinical trial –Stenting versus Aggressive Medical Management for Preventing Recurrent stroke in Intracranial Stenosis (SAMMPRIS) –also demonstrated that in patients with symptomatic ICAD, best medical therapy was superior to angioplasty and stenting. 451 patients with symptomatic major intracranial artery stenosis of 70% -99% were randomized to stenting with the Wingspan system or "aggressive medical therapy" alone. Both groups received aspirin, clopidogrel, and management of cardiovascular risk factors including blood pressure and cholesterol. The trial included 94 patients with intracranial carotid stenosis. The overall 30-day rate of stroke or death for all trial patients was 14.7% in the stenting group and 5.8% in the medical management group, a significant difference that prompted the trial's data and safety monitoring board to recommend termination of enrollment. In the medical management group, 12.2% of patients reached the primary endpoint (stroke or death within 30 days after enrollment or after a revascularization procedure for the qualifying lesion, or ischemic stroke in the territory of the qualifying artery after day 31) at one year, a lower figure than that reported in the medical management arms of the trials of CEA for carotid stenosis. Although these cohorts might not be directly comparable, this lower rate of stroke may again reflect advances in medical therapy in recent decades. The EC-IC Bypass Study (1985) was the first prospective, multicenter international study comprising 1377 patients with symptomatic intracranial ICA stenosis who were randomly assigned to best medical care and EC-IC bypass (superficial temporal or occipital artery to MCA). Despite a bypass patency rate of 96%, 30-day surgical mortality and major stroke morbidity rates were 0.6% and 2.5%, respectively. The study was highly criticized because the authors were unable to identify a subgroup of patients for whom EC/IC bypass may yield benefit. However, in light of the high bypass patency rate, hope remained that if an appropriate cohort could be identified, patients with symptomatic cerebral ischemia could still benefit from surgical revascularization. The St. Louis Carotid Occlusion Study, which showed that patients with cerebral hemodynamic insufficiency demonstrated by increased oxygen extraction fraction (OEF) on PET were at the greatest risk of stroke after medical management for atherosclerotic carotid occlusion. Based on this finding, the Carotid Occlusion Surgery Study (COSS; 2011) was a prospective, randomized, open-label, blinded-adjudication trial that randomly assigned 195 patients with i) angiographically demonstrated complete occlusion of the ICA causing either TIA/ischemic stroke within 120 days and ii) hemodynamic cerebral ischemia indicated by an increased OEF on PET imaging to either STA-MCA bypass or medical management. The STA-MCA arterial bypass patency rate was 98% at the 30-day postoperative visit and 96% at the last follow-up examination. The STA-MCA arterial bypass markedly improved, although it did not normalize, the level of elevated OEF in the symptomatic cerebral hemisphere. However, STA-MCA bypass failed to afford patients in the surgical arm any benefit over patients in the medical group, primarily because of better than expected stroke reduction in the non-operative arm. COSS trial design has been criticised for counting severe, disabling stroke as an endpoint and not giving equal weight to the effects of living with chronic hypoperfusion or continuous TIA events. These trials also do not address `hot patients' such as those with postural hypoperfusion, crescendo TIAs and recurrent stroke. In contrast, the Japanese EC/IC Bypass Trial (JET) demonstrated 2-year stroke reduction benefit for patients with baseline hemodynamic insufficiency as defined by decreased cerebral blood flow and cerebrovascular reactivity on acetazolamide challenge as measured on SPECT who underwent STA-MCA bypass, suggesting that better patient selection using SPECT and PET may be required to determine those likely to benefit. Patients with known carotid occlusive disease were screened for hemodynamic insufficiency by measuring cerebral blood flow and cerebrovascular reactivity on SPECT as well as OEF on positron emission tomography. The study prospectively enrolled 49 patients, and STA-MCA statistically reduced strokes compared with medical therapy (0.7% vs. 6.5%) for patients with reduced cerebral blood flow and cerebrovascular reactivity and increased OEF.

FURTHER READING

Powers WJ, Clarke WR, Grubb RL Jr, Videen TO, Adams HP Jr, Derdeyn CP; COSS Investigators. Extracranial-intracranial bypass surgery for stroke prevention in hemodynamic cerebral ischemia: the Carotid Occlusion Surgery Study randomized trial. JAMA. 2011 Nov 9;306 (18):1983-92.

Bauer AM, Bain MD, Rasmussen PA. Chronic Cerebral Ischemia: Where "Evidence-Based Medicine" Fails Patients. World Neurosurg. 2015 Sep;84(3):714-8.

Howard BM, Barrow DL. Cerebral revascularization: which patients should be bypassed and which patients should be passed by? World Neurosurg. 2015 Mar;83(3):288-90. doi: 10.1016/j.wneu.2014.12.045. Epub 2015 Jan 14. PubMed PMID: 25596433.

17. **a**—Moyamoya disease

Yasargil first described intracranial arterial bypass, and indications for surgery quickly expanded to include treatment of complex aneurysms, moyamoya disease, extensive skull base neoplasms, and occlusive vasculopathy. However, the rates of bypass are falling for all of these indications due to advances in (medical, endovascular and radiotherapy) and well as better evidence showing absence of long term benefit (except in highly selected patients). Innovations and increased experience in endovascular techniques (e.g. flow-diverting stents) have limited the number of complex aneurysms that require open surgical trapping and bypass. Similarly, skull base tumors, previously treated by resection and bypass, are often managed with less invasive surgery combined with newer, more effective chemotherapy and radiosurgery regimens. Microsurgical bypass in most centers following publication of the EC/IC Bypass Study and the Carotid Occlusion Surgery Study (COSS). Although extracranial/intracranial (EC/IC) bypass remains a viable treatment for moyamoya angiopathy, particularly in adults, patients are increasingly being treated with various indirect revascularization procedures, such as encephaloduroarteriosynangiosis (EDAS).

FURTHER READING

Howard BM, Barrow DL. Cerebral revascularisation: which patients should be bypassed and which patients should be passed by? World Neurosurg 2015;83(3):288-90.

18. **b**—STA is a medium-high flow graft (initially 40-80 ml/min)

Intravascular thrombosis is more likely when grasping the intima, if there is vessel stenosis at the anastomotic line (ideally fish mouthing required) or if the vessel is overly stretched. Maintaining patency is favored by fish mouthing the anastomosis in end to side grafts, using interrupted sutures to allow maximum expansion, and other factors such as flow demand through the bypass and length of the donor graft used in the bypass. Properties of common grafts are shown above.

Type	Comments	Demand	Initial Flow	Patency
Superficial temporal artery	Pedicle vessel	Low flow	15-25 ml/min (may increase with time)	>95% (e.g. EC-IC bypass trial, COSS)
Radial Artery interposition graft	Same size as M2 branch. Risk of vasospasm.	Moderate-High flow	40-80 ml/min	>90% at 5 years
Saphenous vein graft	Greater length but has valves	High flow	70-140 ml/min	82% patency at 5 years

FURTHER READING

Regli L, Piepgras DG, Hansen KK. Late patency of long saphenous vein bypass grafts to the anterior and posterior cerebral circulation. J Neurosurg 1995;83:806-11.

Houkin K, Kamiyama H, Kuroda S, et al. Long-term patency of radial artery graft bypass for reconstruction of the internal carotid artery. J Neurosurg 1999;90:786-90.

19. **e**—Flow diverting stents are usually used in conjunction with detachable coils for wide necked aneurysms

Complex aneurysms (e.g. dolichoectactic and thrombosed aneurysms) not amenable to coiling, direct clipping or clip reconstruction in the modern era can be managed with cerebral bypass, or increasingly with flow diverting stents like the Pipeline Embolization Device (ev3, Irvine, California, USA) for large, giant, wide-necked, failed treatment and fusiform aneurysms by reconstructing the parent artery. During a flow-diversion/Pipeline™ procedure, a microcatheter is navigated past the aneurysm (without entering it) then, the flow-diverting stent is deployed across the neck of the aneurysm in the parent blood vessel, immediately reducing blood flow to the aneurysm and inducing thrombosis within it. The device becomes endothelialized, forming a permanent biological seal across the diseased (aneurysmal) segment of the parent artery. The recently published results of the International Retrospective Study of the Pipeline Embolization Device demonstrated an overall combined neurologic morbidity and mortality rate of 8.4%. The combined morbidity and mortality rate in patients with ICA aneurysms 10 mm was 9.5% and in patients with posterior circulation aneurysms was 16.4%. Since the introduction of the EC/IC bypass, several intracranial/intracranial (IC-IC) bypass methods, which represent an elegant solution to otherwise untreatable aneurysms, have been described. The in situ bypass requires 2 parallel arteries (e.g. ACA, PCA, SCA, distal PICA, MCA branches) which are anastomosed side-to-side distal to the aneurysm. Alternatively, reanastomosis of the parent artery or branches there of proximal and distal to the aneurysm after complete resection of the diseased portion of the vessel is an attractive technique in places where the parent artery has sufficient slack. Short segment intracranial/intracranial bypass with a radial artery interposition graft is often a good alternative to EC/IC bypass, due to graft artery diameter being similar to intracranial vessels. Finally, the ability to reimplant an important arterial branch that originates from the aneurysm itself is an advantage of bypass when endovascular therapy would risk occluding the perforating branch or clip reconstruction would risk incomplete neck occlusion and aneurysm recurrence.

FURTHER READING

Kallmes DF, et al. International retrospective study of the pipeline embolization device: a multicenter aneurysm treatment study. AJNR Am J Neuroradiol 2015 Jan;36(1):108-15 (Erratum in: AJNR Am J Neuroradiol 2015 May;36(5)).

Howard BM, Barrow DL. Cerebral revascularization: which patients should be bypassed and which patients should be passed by? World Neurosurg 2015 Mar;83(3):288-90.

CHAPTER 23

CRANIAL ONCOLOGY

SINGLE BEST ANSWER (SBA) QUESTIONS

1. In the UK, which one of the following statements regarding driving restrictions due to neurological disorders is LEAST accurate?
   a. Driving can be reconsidered 6 months after craniotomy for a benign meningioma if there is no seizure history
   b. Driving can be considered after 12 months for most craniotomies
   c. Driving can be considered whenever there is no residual impairment likely to affect driving after trans-sphenoidal pituitary surgery
   d. Driving can be considered after 6 months for after craniotomy for a benign brainstem tumor if asymptomatic
   e. Driving can be considered 3 years after craniotomy for high-grade glioma if safe to do so and no evidence of tumor progression

2. Which one of the following lists of primary brain tumors is in order of frequency (highest to lowest)?
   a. Glioblastoma multiforme, meningioma, nerve sheath tumors, diffuse astrocytoma, pituitary tumors
   b. Meningioma, glioblastoma multiforme, diffuse astrocytoma, pituitary tumors, nerve sheath tumors
   c. Meningioma, glioblastoma multiforme, pituitary tumors, nerve sheath tumors, diffuse astrocytoma
   d. Meningioma, pituitary tumors, glioblastoma multiforme, nerve sheath tumors, diffuse astrocytoma
   e. Pituitary tumors, meningioma, glioblastoma multiforme, nerve sheath tumors, diffuse astrocytoma

3. Which one of the following statements regarding brain metastases in adults is LEAST accurate?
   a. Brain metastases are over twice as common in small cell lung cancer than non-small cell lung cancer
   b. Distribution of brain metastases in the CNS is proportional to amount of arterial blood supplied
   c. Colorectal cancer has a higher propensity for brain metastases than breast cancer
   d. Melanoma is the third most commonly diagnosed type of brain metastases
   e. Prostate cancer is the most frequent cancer of males but has a low propensity to metastasize to the brain

4. A 67-year-old patient presents with left hemisensory change. Postcontrast MRI is shown below, and diffusion weighted imaging shows the lesion to be dark on DWI and bright on ADC map. Which one of the following options is most appropriate next?

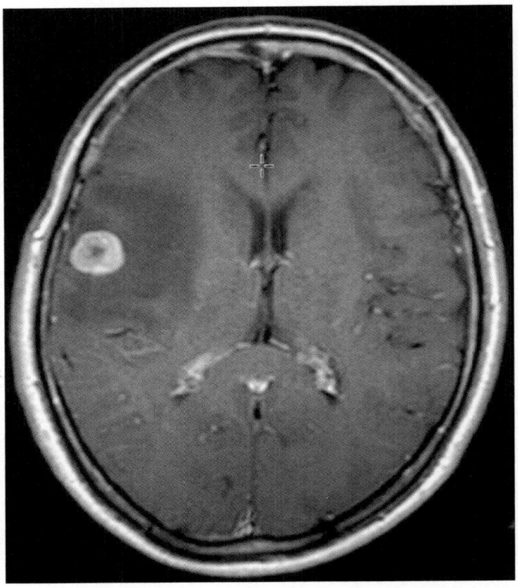

   a. Urgent image-guided drainage of lesion
   b. CT of chest, abdomen and pelvis with contrast
   c. Imaging surveillance
   d. Intravenous antibiotics
   e. Lumbar puncture

5. Which one of the following indications for stereotactic biopsy of a brain lesion is LEAST appropriate?
   a. Deep seated lesions
   b. Infiltrative lesion
   c. Lesions in eloquent cortex
   d. Lesions not curable by surgical excision (e.g. brainstem tumors)
   e. Suspected frontal renal cell carcinoma brain metastasis

6. Which one of the following statements regarding biopsy of brainstem lesions is LEAST accurate?
   a. Contralateral extraventricular transfrontal approach is suited to more lateral pontine lesions
   b. Ipsilateral transfrontal approach may have a higher risk of intraventricular hemorrhage
   c. Is more commonly used in adults compared to children
   d. Occipital transtentorial approach is routinely used
   e. Suboccipital, transcerebellar approach is associated with greater postoperative pain

7. Which one of the following statements regarding average prognosis of patients presenting with Karnofsky of score less than 70 is most accurate?
   a. A Karnofsky performance score less than 70 is associated with a median survival of 2 months
   b. A Karnofsky performance score less than 70 is associated with a median survival of 4 months
   c. A Karnofsky performance score less than 70 is associated with a median survival of 6 months
   d. A Karnofsky performance score less than 70 is associated with a median survival of 8 months
   e. A Karnofsky performance score less than 70 is associated with a median survival of 12 months

8. Which one of the following statements regarding management of brain metastases is LEAST accurate?
   a. Chemotherapy/biologics should be considered alone when asymptomatic brain metastasis is found on screening before planned systemic therapy
   b. Whole brain radiotherapy should be considered in the setting of multiple brain metastasis (4-10) especially if primary tumor is known to be radiotherapy sensitive
   c. SRS could be considered in multiple brain metastases (4-10) when the primary tumor is known to be radiotherapy resistant
   d. Surgical resection should be considered in the setting of a dominant hemisphere metastasis in a critical location
   e. SRS could be considered in oligometastases if they are greater than 4 cm in diameter

9. A 55-year-old right handed male presents with headache and cognitive slowing. There is no significant past medical history. MRI is shown. Which one of the following management strategies is most appropriate?

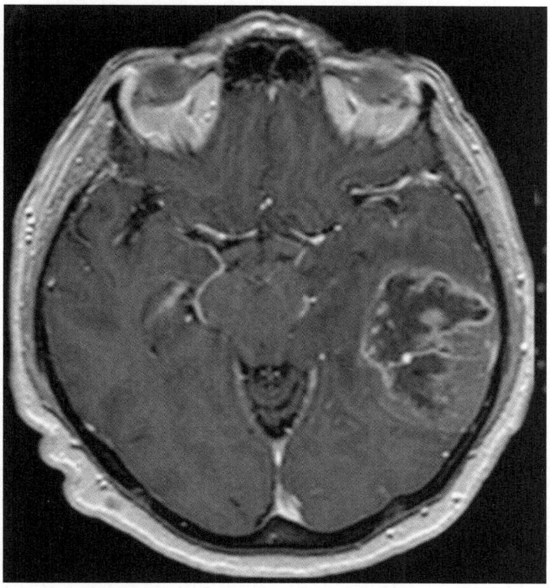

   a. Surveillance imaging
   b. Awake craniotomy with goal of maximal safe resection
   c. Cerebral angiogram
   d. Gross total resection under general anesthetic
   e. Stereotactic biopsy for molecular classification

10. A 44-year-old patient with a known history of relapsing remitting multiple sclerosis presents with worsening memory. MRI is shown below. MRI spectroscopy shows reduced NAA and myoinositol, increased choline and lipid, lactate peaks. Perfusion weighted MR shows markedly elevated cerebral blood flow in the rim of the necrotic mass. Which one of the following best explains his new deterioration?

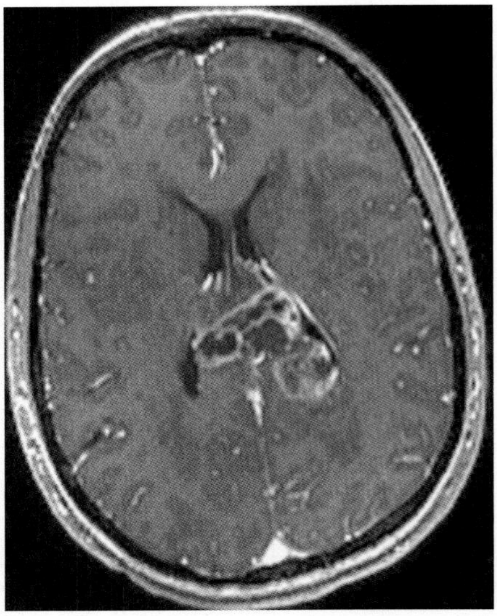

a. Tumefactive multiple sclerosis
b. Glioblastoma
c. Lymphoma
d. Oligodendroglioma
e. Choroid plexus carcinoma

11. Which one of the following factors is most important in improving length of survival in gliomas?
a. 1p19q codeletion
b. ATRX mutation
d. EGFR mutation
e. IDH1/2 mutations
c. TERT mutation

12. Median survival advantage in glioblastoma multiforme patients undergoing 5-ALA fluorescence assisted tumor resection versus conventional surgery in the randomized controlled trial by Stummer and colleagues (2006) was which one of the following?
a. No advantage
b. 1 month advantage
c. 3 month advantage
d. 5 month advantage
e. 7 month advantage

13. Two-year survival in glioblastoma multiforme patients receiving post-surgery temozolomide and radiotherapy verus in the randomized controlled trial by Stupp and colleagues (2005) is which one of the following?
a. 16.5%
b. 26.5%
c. 36.5%
d. 46.5%
e. 56.5%

14. Which one of the following statements regarding radiological phenomena following modern treatment of high-grade gliomas is most accurate?
a. Tumor recurrence has a lower FDG PET uptake than radiation necrosis
b. Radiation necrosis typically occurs 2-3 months after radiotherapy
c. Pseudoprogression is associated with anti-VEGF pharmacotherapy
d. Pseudoresponse typically occurs 6-12 months after temozolomide chemoradiotherapy
e. Recurrent tumors usually show a lower ADC than radiation necrosis on diffusion weighted MRI

15. Which one of the following statements regarding advanced imaging in gliomas is LEAST accurate?
a. Anaplastic astrocytoma
b. Oligodendrogliomas commonly show calcification (central, peripheral or ribbon like)
c. FDG-PET imaging of WHO grade III gliomas shows an uptake greater than white matter but lower than gray matter, whereas grade II gliomas have an uptake similar to white matter
d. MR perfusion imaging shows elevated regional cerebral blood flow in grade III oligodendrogliomas compared to grade II oligodendrogliomas
e. Glioblastomas show reduced NAA and myoinositol peaks and increased choline, lipid and lactate peaks on MR spectroscopy

16. Which one of the following PET tracers is LEAST appropriate for detection of de novo low-grade glioma?
a. ^{18}F-FET
b. ^{18}F-FDG
c. ^{18}F-DOPA
d. ^{11}C-MET
e. ^{18}F-DOPA

17. A 34-year-old male presents with seizures. He has no significant past medical history. MRI is shown (FLAIR) and T1 postcontrast imaging does not show any enhancement. Which one of the following management strategies is most appropriate?

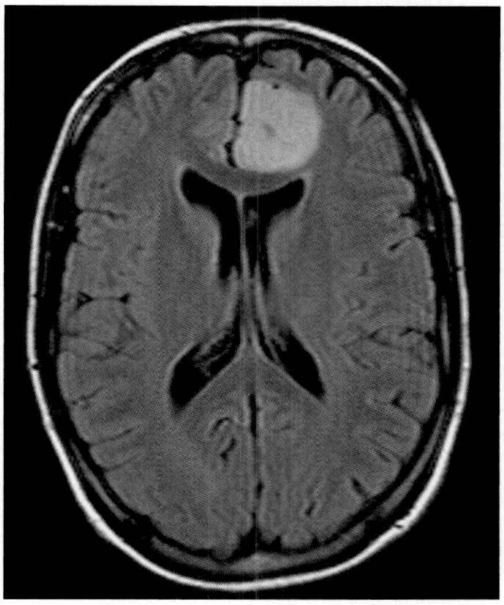

a. Imaging surveillance until starts to show focal enhancement
b. Gamma knife surgery
c. Methotrexate chemotherapy
d. Dexamethasone
e. Maximal safe resection

18. A 27-year-old presents with a generalized tonic-clonic seizure. On examination there is no residual neurological deficit or speech disturbance. Some spots of calcification are seen on CT therefore MRI is performed. Which one of the following statements regarding this type of tumor is LEAST accurate?

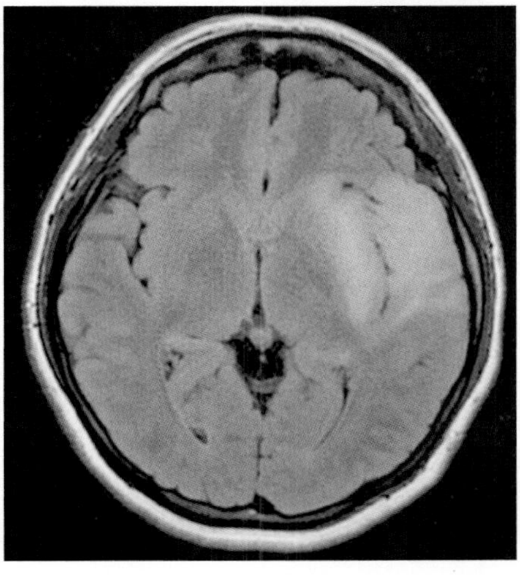

a. Functional mapping is a perquisite for resection
b. MRS findings may include increased 2-hydroxyglutarate
c. Prognosis is related to extent of resection
d. The majority of patients with dominant hemisphere lesions of this type present with seizures
e. Tumor margins are usually seen best on T1 + gad MRI sequences

19. Which one of the following statements regarding surgical management of low grade glioma (LGG) is LEAST accurate?
a. Gross total resection involves taking the tumor until its border as visualized on T2/FLAIR MRI sequences
b. Craniotomy under GA with functional mapping is the standard of care for low-grade gliomas in eloquent cortex
c. Biopsy of low-grade gliomas are prone to histological undergrading as they may miss anaplastic foci
d. Extent of resection correlated with survival
e. PET imaging can facilitate biopsy targets in low-grade glioma

20. Which one of the following statements regarding brain mapping is LEAST accurate?
a. Connectome refers to the organization of the CNS into parallel networks, which are dynamic, interactive and able to compensate for each other
b. Hodotopy suggests individual functions of the brain are supported by extensive circuits comprising both the cortical nodes and connections between them created by associating bundles of white matter
c. Cortical map reorganization for a given function can occur as long as the subcortical white matter tracts subserving it are preserved
d. Brodmann areas represent a connectionist model of brain function
e. Neuroplasticity is seen in slow growing low-grade gliomas more than in acute insults such as stroke

21. Which one of the following chemotherapy options is most likely to be utilized in the context of anaplastic oligodendroglioma?
a. Anti-VEGF
b. Cyclophosphamide
c. Etoposide
d. PCV
e. Temozolomide

22. Which one of the following statements regarding O(6)-Methylguanine-DNA Methyl Transferase (MGMT) promoter methylation status is LEAST accurate?
   a. MGMT is a DNA repair enzyme that reverts the naturally occurring mutagenic O6-methylguanine back to guanine, preventing errors during DNA replication
   b. Functional MGMT increases the effectiveness of cancer chemotherapy
   c. Hypermethylation of the MGMT promoter results in less DNA repair activity of MGMT
   d. Temozolomide chemotherapy is more effective in glioblastoma multiforme cells with a hypermethylated MGMT promoter
   e. MGMT promoter-unmethylated tumors have no survival benefit from temozolomide chemotherapy

23. Which one of the following statements regarding telomerase reverse transcriptase (TERT) promotor mutations in gliomas is LEAST accurate?
   a. Overexpression of TERT in cells results in an increase in the number of times a cell can successfully divide
   b. TERT normally prevents telomerase repair ensuring that cells become replicatively senescent
   c. TERT promoter mutations were also strongly associated with 1p/19q codeletion and co-occur with IDH1/2 in oligodendrogliomas
   d. TERT and IDH1/2 mutations are largely mutually exclusive in GBM and astrocytomas
   e. Gliomas with TERT promoter mutations but no IDH1/2 mutation have been shown to have poor overall survival

24. Which one of the following statements regarding isocitrate dehydrogenase 1 or 2 (IDH1/2) gene mutations in gliomas is LEAST accurate?
   a. The most common mutation (~90%) in glial brain tumors causes a substitution of the amino acid Arginine to Histidine at codon 132 of the IDH1 gene
   b. IDH1 and 2 are homologous enzymes decarboxylate isocitrate to α-ketoglutarate (αKG)
   c. IDH1/2 mutations result in accumulation of 2-hydroxyglutarate to high levels in glioma tissues possibly promoting oncogenic transformation through epigenetic mechanisms
   d. Mutant IDH is the molecular basis of the CpG island methylator phenotype (CIMP) in gliomas, leading to global dysregulation of gene expression
   e. IDH1/2 mutations co-segregate with 1p/19q codeletion in oligodendrogliomas
   f. IDH1/2 mutation is associated with an improved prognosis in grade II astrocytomas

QUESTIONS 25–40

Additional questions 25–40 available on ExpertConsult.com

EXTENDED MATCHING ITEM (EMI) QUESTIONS

41. **Supratentorial lesions:**
   a. Anaplastic oligodendroglioma
   b. Central neurocytoma
   c. Diffuse astrocytoma
   d. DNET
   e. Germinoma
   f. Glioblastoma multiforme
   g. Metastatic melanoma
   h. Non-germinomatous germ cell tumor
   i. Oligodendroglioma
   j. Pineoblastoma
   k. Primary CNS lymphoma
   l. Subependymal giant cell astrocytoma

For each of the following descriptions, select the most appropriate answers from the list above. Each answer may be used once, more than once or not at all.

1. A 30-year-old man with AIDS develops headaches and left hemiparesis and is found to have a right frontal white matter homogeneously enhancing lesion. The lesion shows increased uptake on Thallium SPECT
2. A 13-year-old presents with diabetes insipidus
3. A 17-year-old presents with Parinaud syndrome. Blood tests show a markedly raised HCG, but normal AFP

42. **Posterior fossa lesions:**
   a. Brainstem glioma
   b. Choroid plexus papilloma
   c. Dysplastic cerebellar gangliocytoma
   d. Ependymoma

e. Epidermoid
f. Hemangioblastoma
g. Medulloblastoma
h. Meningioma
i. Pilocytic astrocytoma
j. Vestibular schwannoma

For each of the following descriptions, select the most appropriate answers from the list above. Each answer may be used once, more than once or not at all.

1. Commonest posterior fossa primary brain tumor in adults
2. Commonest posterior fossa primary brain tumor in children
3. Associated with mutation in PTEN tumor suppressor gene

43. **Molecular classification of brain tumors:**
   a. TERT
   b. TP53
   c. IDH1/2 mutation
   d. MGMT promoter methylation
   e. 1p19q co-deletion
   f. EGFRvIII
   g. Histone H3
   h. ATRX
   i. BRAF
   j. 10q loss

For each of the following descriptions, select the most appropriate answers from the list above. Each answer may be used once, more than once or not at all.

1. A mutation which gives patients with IDH wild type, ATRX mutant (negative) astrocytoma a similar prognosis to glioblastoma multiforme
2. Highly prevalent in all gliomas except primary glioblastoma multiforme
3. Improves prognosis in oligodendrogliomas, irrespective of IDH1/2 status
4. Target for glioblastoma vaccine trials
5. Predictive of benefit from temozolomide in primary GBM

SBA ANSWERS

1. **e**—Driving can be considered 3 years after craniotomy for high-grade glioma if safe to do so and no evidence of tumor progression

The guidelines below relate to car/motorcycle use (not heavy goods vehicles) and will vary based on individual risk assessment:

- First seizure: 6 months off driving if the license holder has undergone assessment by an appropriate specialist and no relevant abnormality has been identified on investigation, for example, EEG and brain scan where indicated. For patients with established epilepsy they must be fit free for 12 months before being able to drive
- Stroke or TIA: 1 month off driving, multiple TIAs over a short period of time: 3 months off driving
- Craniotomy for low-grade tumor: 1 year off driving (if the tumor is a benign meningioma and there is no seizure history, license can be reconsidered 6 months after surgery if remains seizure free)
- Craniotomy for high-grade tumor: 2 years off driving, and no evidence of tumor progression before
- Pituitary tumor surgery: driving can resume when safe after trans-sphenoidal surgery but if a craniotomy is required 6 months off driving
- Chronic neurological disorders (e.g. multiple sclerosis, motor neuron disease, Alzheimer's) DVLA should be informed, complete application for driving license holders state of health
- Syncope: simple faint: no restriction, single episode, explained and treated: 4 weeks off, single episode, unexplained: 6 months off, two or more episodes: 12 months off.
- Stereotactic radiosurgery: Do not drive for 1 month after treatment
- Benign brainstem/posterior fossa tumor: can return to driving as soon as recovered from surgery but let DVLA know (you do not need to tell DVLA about acoustic neuromas unless you have dizziness).

2. **d**—Meningioma, pituitary tumors, glioblastoma multiforme, nerve sheath tumors, diffuse astrocytoma

The commonest intracranial tumors are brain metastases (just over 50%). Incidence of primary brain tumors is approximately 20-30 per 100,000 in adults and 5 per 100,000 children. Approximately one third of primary brain tumors in adults are malignant whereas they account for two thirds in childhood. Frequency of WHO subgroups and specific tumors is given:

Brain Tumour Frequency

Commonest Primary Brain Tumors by WHO Group	Commonest Primary Brain Tumors by Subtype
Meninges (37.6%) Neuroepithelial tissue (29.9%) Sellar region (16.3%) Cranial and spinal nerves (8.1%) Unclassified (5.6%) Lymphoma and hematopoietic (2.1%) Germ cell tumors and cysts (0.4%)	Meningioma (36%) Pituitary tumors (15.5%) Glioblastoma multiforme (15.1%) Nerve sheath tumors (8.1%) Diffuse astrocytoma (2.3%) Primary CNS lymphoma (2%) Ependymal (1.9%) Anaplastic astrocytoma (1.7%) Pilocytic astrocytoma (1.4%) Neuronal and neuronal-mixed (1.2%) Oligodendroglioma (1.1%) Oligoastrocytoma (0.9%) Craniopharyngioma (0.8%) Anaplastic oligodendroglioma (0.5%)

Ostrom QT, Gittleman H, Fulop J, et al. CBTRUS Statistical Report: Primary Brain and Central Nervous System Tumors Diagnosed in the United States in 2008-2012. Neuro Oncol 2015;17 Suppl 4:iv1.

3. **c**—Colorectal cancer has a higher propensity for brain metastases than breast cancer

The majority of brain metastases diagnosed originate from lung, breast, melanoma, renal and colorectal primary tumors—reflecting how common those primary cancers are, but not necessarily their respective propensity for metastasizing to the brain. Propensity for spread to brain parenchyma is high in melanoma, small cell lung cancer, choriocarcinoma, and other germ cell tumors; intermediate in breast cancer, non-small cell lung cancer (adenocarcinoma > squamous cell), and renal cell carcinoma; low in prostate, colorectal, ovarian carcinoma, thyroid cancer and sarcomas. Metastases spread via the circulation and seed at the gray-white matter junction, and particularly watershed areas (most obviously PCA vs. MCA border) in a distribution proportional to amount of arterial blood supplied: 80% occur in cerebral hemispheres, 15% in posterior fossa and 5% in the brainstem. The frequency of metastases found at autopsy is much higher than that detected during the illness.

FURTHER READING

Schouten LJ, Rutten J, Huveneers HA, Twijnstra A. Incidence of brain metastases in a cohort of patients with carcinoma of the breast, colon, kidney, and lung and melanoma. Cancer. 2002;94(10):269.

Barnholtz-Sloan JS, et al. Incidence proportions of brain metastases in patients diagnosed (1973-2001) in the Metropolitan Detroit Cancer Surveillance System. J Clin Oncol. 2004;22(14):2865.

Cancer Research UK, http://www.cancerresearchuk.org/health-professional/cancer-statistics/incidence/common-cancers-compared, Accessed February 2016.

Brain Metastases. In: Oncology of CNS tumours. Springer Verlag, Berlin 2010 pp.345-346.

Frequency of Metastatic Cancer and Relationship to Occurence of Brain Metastases

Cancer in Order of Frequency (Overall)	Cancer in Order of Frequency (Males)	Cancer in Order of Frequency (Females)	Propensity for Radiological Brain Metastases at 5 Years Follow Up (Descending Frequency)	Contribution to Total Brain Metastases Diagnosed (in Descending Frequency)
(1) Breast (2) Prostate (3) Lung (4) Colorectal (5) Uterus (6) Malignant melanoma	(1) Prostate (26%) (2) Lung (14%) (3) Colorectal (13%) (4) Bladder (4%) (5) Kidney (4%) (6) NHL (4%) (7) Malignant melanoma (4%)	(1) Breast (31%) (2) Lung (12%) (3) Colorectal (11%) (4) Uterus (5%) (5) Malignant melanoma (4%) (6) Ovarian (4%)	(1) Lung (16-20%; SCLC 29% vs. NSCLC 12%) (2) Melanoma (7%) (3) Renal cell carcinoma (7-10%) (4) Breast (5%) (5) Colorectal (1%)	(1) Lung (2) Breast (3) Melanoma (4) Colon (5) Prostate (6) Liver/pancreas

4. **b**—CT of chest, abdomen and pelvis with contrast

MRI shows a peripherally enhancing, centrally necrotic lesion in the right thalamus, with DWI pattern consistent with a relatively unrestricted diffusion in the center of the mass hence this is most likely a metastasis (given previous history of breast cancer) or a primary tumor. As such, initial management in a patient should consist of a search for the primary tumor based on a full clinical examination and staging CT of the body, followed by discussion in the primary tumor site multidisciplinary meeting to decide on options for tissue diagnosis and further management, as well as the neuro-oncology MDT. The primary neoplasms that most commonly metastasize to the brain are carcinoma of the lung, breast, malignant melanoma, renal cell carcinoma, and GI cancers (e.g. colorectal). Generally, metastases appear as multiple rounded lesions with a tendency to seed peripherally in the cerebral substance, at the gray/white matter junction. They can, however, occur anywhere in the cerebrum, brainstem or cerebellum, and can also spread to the meninges. Metastases are characterized by edema in the surrounding white matter which is often disproportionate to the size of the tumor itself. On T2 images, the neoplastic nodule may blend with the surrounding edema, giving a picture of widespread vasogenic edema and obscuring the diagnosis. Most metastases enhance strongly with IV contrast medium, either uniformly, or ring-like if the metastasis has outgrown its blood supply. Most metastases from lung and breast are similar in density to normal brain parenchyma on CT, but some types are spontaneously dense, particularly deposits from malignant melanoma. Hemorrhage occurs in about 10% of metastases, resulting in high signal on T1 images and high or low signal on T2 images. Similar signal characteristics can also occur in non-hemorrhagic metastases from melanoma, due to the paramagnetic properties of melanin. Small metastases and those that are not made conspicuous by surrounding edema are often only detected on contrast-enhanced studies. Increasing the contrast dose or relaxivity of gadolinium compounds can improve the sensitivity for detection of metastases on MRI.

Image with permission from Kang TW, Kim ST, Byun HS, et al. Morphological and functional MRI, MRS, perfusion and diffusion changes after radiosurgery of brain metastasis, Eur J Radiol. 2009;72(3):370-380.

5. **e**—Suspected frontal renal cell carcinoma brain metastasis

The significant development of intracranial imaging over the past few decades has allowed much earlier diagnosis of brain tumors. Although some tumors have a characteristic appearance on imaging, no imaging modality is yet able to provide sufficient diagnostic information to direct subsequent aggressive therapy. The goal of biopsy is to provide a representative sample for pathologic diagnosis to guide subsequent treatment, which can include cytoreductive surgery, radiotherapy, or chemotherapy. The main stimulus for the adoption of stereotactic biopsy over an open operative procedure is to achieve a higher rate of diagnostic accuracy while minimizing potential adverse effects. Diagnostic accuracy is important for dictating appropriate adjuvant therapy. Particular characteristics of the tumor that favor the use of stereotactic biopsy over open biopsy include (1) lesions not requiring emergent surgery or that are not curable by surgical excision, such as metastases or malignant intrinsic brain tumors; (2) deep-seated lesions or those occupying space in eloquent cortex or deep nuclei (i.e. basal ganglia, thalamus), where open resection would lead to unacceptable morbidity/mortality; and (3) infiltrative lesions (i.e. gliomatosis cerebri) that do not have a clear brain-tumor margin and are unlikely to be excised completely without significant loss of normal brain parenchyma. Moreover, if the lesion's appearance on imaging or the course of the disease suggests an alternative cause such as an infectious or demyelinating process rather than a neoplastic one, stereotactic biopsy is a more appropriate first step than a large open procedure. Relative contraindications include vascular tumors (e.g. metastatic renal cell carcinoma, choriocarcinoma, or metastatic melanoma) where diagnosis and biopsy the primary neoplasm instead is generally recommended, close proximity to a major blood vessel/sylvian fissure/cavernous sinus/brain-pial border all increase the risk of hemorrhage.

6. **d**—Occipital transtentorial approach is routinely used

Lesions within the brainstem have long been considered challenging to diagnose and treat. Although brainstem tumors represent only about 2% of all intracranial tumors in adults as compared with about 10-15% in the pediatric population, radiologic diagnosis of brainstem lesions in adults is inaccurate 10-20% of the time whereas in children the majority are gliomas (diagnosable on MRI). In general, because most adult brainstem tumors are not amenable to surgical excision, stereotactic biopsy is important for obtaining a pathologic diagnosis enabling replacement of empirical treatment modalities with more specific therapies, as well as determination of a more accurate prognosis. Equally, given the great diversity of

Approaches for Brainstem Biopsy

Brainstem Biopsy Approach	Comments
Occipital, transtentorial	Uncommon as crosses the pia superior and inferior to the tentorium and places vital vasculature and cranial nerves at risk
Suboccipital, transcerebellar	For lesions of the lower midbrain, pons, and rostral medulla projects through the ipsilateral middle cerebellar peduncle, pain associated with muscle dissection before making the twist drill hole in the skull. A more decisive contraindication to this approach is the risk for posterior fossa subdural hematomas caused by blind puncture of the cerebellar cortex
Ipsilateral transfrontal	Midbrain, upper pons, and medulla. For lower pons or medulla biopsies, an ipsilateral transfrontal approach necessitates a trajectory traversing the lateral ventricle before entering the anterior thalamus, cerebral peduncle, and then the brainstem. Lateral midbrain, a trajectory lateral to the ventricle suffices. approaching the pons and medulla with this method often requires entering the frontal horn of the lateral ventricle, which violates two ependymal surfaces and places the patient at risk for intraventricular hemorrhage. Second, ventriculostomy may lead to intraoperative loss of cerebrospinal fluid, which may contribute to postoperative headache and shifting of intracranial contents, thereby possibly altering the location of the target. Third, this route is limited to midline regions of the pons and midbrain by the tentorial incisura
Contralateral extraventricular transfrontal	Lesions below lower pons, and lateral pontine lesions. An intraparenchymal trajectory is projected to avoid the lateral ventricle, the tentorium, major vessels, and the cerebral aqueduct

brainstem lesions, patients most likely to benefit from stereotactic biopsy are those who are given a better prognosis based on biopsy results or who are spared a course of debilitating therapy. Such patients include those with radiation necrosis, chemotherapy-sensitive metastasis, a lymphoma, or an abscess rather than a malignant glioma. In terms of complications, 6.6% have transient or mild symptoms and 1.8% have permanent deficits.

7. **a**—A Karnofsky performance score less than 70 is associated with a median survival of 2 months

The median survival of patients who receive supportive care with brain metastases and are treated only with corticosteroids is approximately 1-2 months. The use of whole brain radiation therapy in large series increased the average survival to 3-6 months, and larger gains were seen in carefully selected subsets. The key parameters that determine survival after the diagnosis of brain metastases are performance status, the extent of extracranial disease, and age, as well as the primary diagnosis. Recursive partitioning analysis (RPA) system was based upon an analysis of prognostic factors in 1200 patients from three Radiation Therapy Oncology Group (RTOG) brain metastases trials and resulted in three groups being identified:

Class 1 (20%)—Patients who had a Karnofsky performance score 70 or higher, were less than 65 years of age, and had a controlled primary tumor without extracranial metastases had a favorable prognosis (median survival was 6-7 months).

Class 2 (65%)—Patients with a Karnofsky performance score 70 or higher, but with other unfavorable characteristics (e.g. uncontrolled primary tumor, other extracranial metastases, age >65 years) had an intermediate prognosis (median survival 4 months). From a further management point of view, they are treated as either RPA Class 1 or RPA Class 3, depending largely upon the likelihood of controlling systemic disease.

Class 3 (15%)—Patients with a Karnofsky performance score less than 70 have a poor prognosis (median survival of 2 months).

FURTHER READING

Uptodate. Overview of the clinical manifestations, diagnosis, and management of patients with brain metastases. Topic 5217 Version 16.0.

8. **e**—SRS could be considered in oligometastases if they are greater than 4 cm in diameter

Brain Metastases: Indications for Different Treatment Modalities
Consider chemotherapy/biologics in brain metastasis: • From highly chemotherapy-sensitive primary tumor • Asymptomatic/found on screening MRI with planned systemic therapy • Primary tumor with identified molecular alteration amenable to targeted therapy • Other options exhausted and there is a reasonable drug available
Consider WBRT in brain metastasis when: • CNS and systemic progression of disease, with few systemic treatment options and poor performance status • Multiple (4-10) brain metastasis especially if primary tumor known to be radiotherapy sensitive (NB current data support SRS use in up to 3 metastasis but there is a growing trend to use it in up to 10). • Large (>4 cm) brain metastasis not amenable to SRS • Postsurgical resection of a dominant hemisphere brain metastasis with multiple (4-10) remaining BMs • Salvage therapy for recurrent BM after SRS or WBRT failure
Consider SRS when: • Oligometastases (1-3) or multiple (4-10) metastases especially if primary tumor is known to be radiotherapy resistant • Postsurgical resection of a single BM, especially if 3 cm or bigger and in the posterior fossa • Local relapse after surgical resection of a single brain metastasis • Salvage therapy for recurrent oligometastases (1-3) after WBRT
Consider surgical resection when: • Uncertain diagnosis of CNS lesion(s) • 1-2 BMs, especially when associated with extensive cerebral edema • Dominant BM in a critical location
No treatment is reasonable when: • Systemic progression of disease with few treatment options and poor performance status

Table with permission from Lin X, DeAngelis LM. Treatment of Brain Metastases. J Clin Oncol. 2015;33(30):3475-3484.

FURTHER READING

Lin X, DeAngelis LM. Treatment of Brain Metastases. J Clin Oncol. 2015;33(30):3475-3484.

9. **b**—Awake craniotomy with goal of maximal safe resection

Glioblastoma (WHO grade IV) is the commonest primary intracranial neoplasm in adults (fourth commonest intracranial tumor after metastases, meningioma and pituitary tumors). About 90% of glioblastomas arise de novo (primary glioblastoma) and 10% are from malignant transformation of lower-grade astrocytomas (secondary glioblastoma). The two groups have different genetic characteristics: primary glioblastomas, which occurs in a slightly older age group, show EGFR overexpression and secondary glioblastomas show IDH mutations like the lower-grade gliomas from which they arise. Methylation of the DNA repair gene MGMT is associated with a better response to temozolomide and better prognosis in glioblastomas. The MRI appearances of glioblastomas are heterogeneous, showing a mixture of solid tumor portions, central necrosis and surrounding edema. The solid portion is usually T1 hypointense, but T2/FLAIR hyperintensity is to a lesser degree than areas of central necrosis and surrounding edema, which are similar to CSF. The solid portion of the glioblastomas may show complete or partial or enhancement with contrast. The standard treatment for glioblastoma (GBM) consists of surgery (with a variable extent of resection depending on tumor location and the patient's clinical status), followed by a combination of radiotherapy and chemotherapy with temozolomide.

Image with permission from Zikou AK, Alexiou GA, Kosta P, et al. Diffusion tensor and dynamic susceptibility contrast MRI in glioblastoma, Clin Neurol Neurosurg. 2012;114(6):607-612.

10. **b**—Glioblastoma

Tumefactive multiple sclerosis, high-grade glioma (GBM), PCNSL and occasionally an abscess can appear similar on imaging. Tumefactive MS refers to patients with known MS developing large tumefactive demyelinating plaques (as opposed to patients presenting with tumefactive demyelinating lesions who rarely go on to develop MS).

Image with permission from Loevner, L, Brain Imaging: Case Review Series, 2nd ed., 2009, Elsevier, Mosby.

Advanced MRI for Heterogenously Enhancing Lesions (Non-infective)

	MRI	MR Spectroscopy	MR Perfusion
Tumefactive demyelination	50% show enhancement, usually an open ring with incomplete portion facing grey matter Mildly increased diffusion (unlike abscess)	Elevation glutamate/ glutamine peaks Red NAA Inc cho, lipid, lactate	No elevation in rCBV
High-grade glioma	Peripheral, heterogeneous enhancement with nodules and necrosis Can be ring enhancing Solid parts have diffusion similar to normal white matter, but appears markedly elevated relative to facilitated diffusion in edema/necrotic/cyst	Reduced NAA Reduce Myoinositol Inc lipids, choline and lactate	Marked elevation rCBV
Primary CNS Lymphoma	Homogeneous enhancement common Ring enhancing in HIV/immunocompromise Restricted diffusion (lower ADC than metastasis or HGG)	Large choline peak Reversed Cho/Cr ratio Markedly reduced NAA Lactate peak possible	Modest elevation rCBV

11. **b**—ATRX mutation

FURTHER READING

Almeida JP, Chaichana KL, Rincon-Torroella J, Quinones-Hinojosa A. The value of extent of resection of glioblastomas: clinical evidence and current approach. Curr Neurol Neurosci Rep. 2015;15(2):517.

12. **d**—5 month advantage (16.8 months vs. 11.8 months)

FURTHER READING

Stummer W, Pichlmeier U, Meinel T, Wiestler OD, Zanella F, Reulen HJ; ALA-Glioma Study Group. Fluorescence-guided surgery with 5-aminolevulinic acid for resection of malignant glioma: a randomised controlled multicentre phase III trial. Lancet Oncol. 2006;7(5):392-401. PubMed PMID:16648043.

13. **b**—26.5%

FURTHER READING

Hegi ME, et al. MGMT gene silencing and benefit from temozolomide in glioblastoma. N Engl J Med. 2005;352 (10):997-1003.

Stupp R, et al. Radiotherapy plus concomitant and adjuvant temozolomide for glioblastoma. N Engl J Med. 2005;352 (10):987-996.

14. **e**—Recurrent tumors usually show a lower ADC than radiation necrosis on diffusion weighted MRI

Radiation necrosis is a late complication of radiotherapy or gamma knife surgery, and can present as an enhancing mass lesion 6-12 months after radiotherapy, difficult to distinguish from recurrent tumor on conventional imaging. FDG-PET, PWI and DWI may help to distinguish between radiation necrosis and tumor recurrence. In radiation necrosis the enhancing lesion has a low glucose metabolism (FDG uptake) and low rCBV, both of which tend to be high in tumor recurrence. On DCE perfusion imaging, recurrent tumors show a much higher maximum slope of enhancement than radiation necrosis. ADC measurements of the enhancing components in recurrent tumor are significantly lower than in radiation necrosis, mirroring the higher cellular density in recurrent neoplasms. The assessment of tumor response and progression in GBM had traditionally been based on measurements of enhancing tumor portions known as Macdonald criteria. With the advent of combined chemoradiation as standard therapy and antiangiogenic drugs as second-line treatment, new phenomena such a pseudoprogression and pseudoresponse have to be taken into account and have made an assessment solely based on assessment of enhancing tumor portion unreliable. Pseudoprogression (therapy induced necrosis) is due to an inflammatory reaction, which results in a temporary increase of contrast enhancement and edema in 20% of patient, usually within 12 weeks of temozolomide chemoradiotherapy, and subsides subsequently without additional treatment. Pseudoprogression is more frequently observed in patients with methylation of the DNA repair gene MGMT, and is associated with a better prognosis (longer overall survival). Advanced MR imaging such as DSC and DCE perfusion imaging shows promise in differentiating these two conditions from true tumor progression. Pseudoresponse is characterized by a decrease of enhancement and edema following the administration of antiangiogenic drugs without improved survival. In pseudoresponse the tumor progresses by infiltrative patterns without neoangiogenesis, resulting in an increase of non-enhancing T2/FLAIR hyperintense tumor portions

FURTHER READING

Hygino da Cruz Jr LC, et al. Pseudoprogression and pseudoresponse: imaging challenges in the assessment of posttreatment glioma. AJNR 2011;32:197801985.

15. **d**—MR perfusion imaging shows elevated regional cerebral blood flow in grade III oligodendrogliomas compared to grade II oligodendrogliomas

With recent advances in our understanding of prognostic and predictive factors of gliomas and within current paradigms of care, glioma grade and molecular genetic features frequently guide our management approach. In general, high-grade gliomas are treated aggressively with upfront surgical resection followed by radiotherapy with or without chemotherapy. In contrast, the management of LGG is often more conservative, even with an initial period of close observation, with serial imaging being considered in some cases. Common molecular and genetic features that are considered in the overall management approach for gliomas include 1p/19q deletion status and isocitrate dehydrogenase (IDH) mutation status. With advances in MRI and positron emission tomography (PET) imaging, there have been developments to better characterize tumors noninvasively with respect to grade, known molecular, and genetic factors such as 1p/19q deletion status and additional physiological features including tumor vascularity and metabolism. In the future, the use of multiparametric/multimodality imaging more routinely may make preoperative distinction between grade II and grade III gliomas more sensitive.

Differential Appearances of Glioma Subtypes on Multi-modal Imaging

Glioma	CT	MRI	MRS/Perfusion	PET
Diffuse (infiltrative) astrocytoma (WHO grade II)	Hyperdense No enhancement (possibly wispy in gemistocytic) May be cystic	T1 iso-hypointense, T2/FLAIR hyperintense white matter lesion expanding cortex No enhancement	No restricted diffusion (unlike infarct) Elevated choline, low NAA, elevated Ch/Cr ratio, myoinositol and ml/Cr ratio Increased 2-hydroxyglutarate in LGG if mutant IDH1/2	FDG uptake similar to while matter Most hypermetabolic area on FDG, 18F-Chlorine and 11C-Chlorine PET useful for biopsy
Anaplastic astrocytoma (WHO grade III)	Heterogeneous low density Intense and heterogeneous enhancement	Heterogeneous signal intensities—predominantly T1 isointense, T2 hyperintense, ring-like enhancement, mass effect	Reduce NAA, reduced creatinine Increasing choline, lipids and lactate Increased rCBV	FDG uptake greater than white matter
Oligodendroglioma (WHO grade II)	Hypodense Calcification (central, peripheral or ribbon like) No enhancement in 50%, rest variable Cysts uncommon	Hypointense T1 Hyperintense T2/FLAIR Minimal/no edema None or dot-like lacy enhancement	Increased regional TBV (?only if 1p19q loss) Elevated rCBV compared to anaplastic oligodendroglioma (due to chicken wire capillaries) Increased 2-hydroxyglutarate in LGG if mutant IDH1/2	FDG uptake similar to normal *white* matter 11C-Methionine studies can be used to differentiate ODs from anaplastic oligodendrogliomas
Anaplastic oligodendroglioma (WHO grade III)	Similar to grade II oligodendroglioma	Similar to grade II oligodendroglioma	More diffusion restriction (low ADC) than grade II oligo Lower rCBV compared to grade II oligodendroglioma	FDG uptake similar to normal *grey* matter 11C-Methionine studies can be used to differentiate ODs from anaplastic oligodendrogliomas

Continued on following page

Differential Appearances of Glioma Subtypes on Multi-modal Imaging (Continued)

Glioma	CT	MRI	MRS/Perfusion	PET
Primary or secondary glioblastoma multiforme (WHO grade IV)	Iso to hyperdense (cellularity) ± hypodense (necrotic) center. Marked edema and mass effect. Intense, irregular, heterogeneous enhancement of margins	Within white matter, T1 hypo-isointense with heterogeneous center (bleed, necrosis). T2/FLAIR hyperintense, edema, flow voids. Enhancement present but heterogeneous, ring-like but nodules.	GRE/SWI may show blood products inside necrotic pockets. Heterogeneous DWI pattern—restricted in solid component, facilitated in edematous and cystic. Low ADC = GBM, high ADC = low grade. Elevated rCBV. NAA and myoinositol decreased, increased choline/lipid/lactate	FDG uptake similar or higher than normal *grey* matter

FURTHER READING

Chung C, Metser U, Ménard C. Advances in Magnetic Resonance Imaging and Positron Emission Tomography Imaging for Grading and Molecular Characterization of Glioma. Semin Radiat Oncol. 2015 Jul;25(3):164-171. doi: 10.1016/j.semradonc.2015.02.002. Epub 2015. Review. PubMed PMID:26050586.

Law M, Yang S, Wang H, et al. Glioma grading: sensitivity, specificity, and predictive values of perfusion MR imaging and proton MR spectroscopic imaging compared with conventional MR imaging. AJNR Am J Neuroradiol. 24(10):1989-1998.

16. **b**—^{18}F-FDG

F-FDG PET was the first tracer used for assessment of brain tumors; however, it has a low tumor-to-background ratio in brain, limiting its utility. ^{18}F-FDG uptake correlates with tumor grade, with high-grade gliomas (grades III and IV) showing higher uptake than low-grade gliomas. Therefore, in spite of its limitations, ^{18}F-FDG PET-CT is used for imaging of high-grade glioma. Amino acid PET radiotracers including ^{18}F-FDOPA display superior contrast to ^{18}F-FDG because of low uptake of amino acids in normal brain tissue. They have particularly special value in the detection of low-grade gliomas. However, ^{18}F-FDOPA tumor uptake cannot provide reasonable predictions about tumor grade and proliferation in recurrent tumors that have undergone treatments. Also, their difficult synthesis or need for an on-site cyclotron limits their widespread use. The present case shows the utility of ^{18}F-FDOPA PET-CT in detection of a recurrent high-grade AA that was missed by ^{18}F-FDG PET-CT. It highlights that ^{18}F-FDG PET-CT can be falsely negative, even in high-grade recurrent gliomas and, therefore, in cases with strong clinical suspicion ^{18}F-FDOPA PET-CT can be an alternative imaging modality to rule out recurrence even when ^{18}F-FDG PET-CT is negative. In general, practical and experimental roles of PET imaging in glioma management include: (1) Grading tumors and estimating prognosis; (2) Localizing the optimum biopsy site, (3) Defining target volumes for radiotherapy (RT), (4) Assessing response to therapy, and (5) Detecting tumor recurrence and distinguishing it from radionecrosis.

FURTHER READING

Chung C, Metser U, Ménard C. Advances in Magnetic Resonance Imaging and Positron Emission Tomography Imaging for Grading and Molecular Characterization of Glioma. Semin Radiat Oncol. 2015;25(3):164-171. doi: 10.1016/j.semradonc.2015.02.002. Epub 2015. Review. PubMed PMID:26050586.

17. **e**—Maximal safe resection

Diffused astrocytomas are WHO grade II (low-grade) gliomas. Infiltrating low-grade tumors which occur typically in the cerebral hemispheres of young adults, involving cortex and white matter with less well-defined borders than pilocytic astrocytomas. They frequently show IDH1 and IDH2 mutations, which have a favorable impact on overall survival. WHO grade II astrocytomas appear iso- or hypodense on CT and show areas of calcification in up to 20%. MRI is better in defining the extent of the low-grade gliomas. They are hyperintense on T2 images and FLAIR images and hypo/isointense on T1 images and show no contrast enhancement as opposed to pilocytic (WHO grade I) and anaplastic (WHO grade III) astrocytomas. All diffuse astrocytomas (as well as other low-grade gliomas such as grade II oligodendrogliomas and oligoastrocytoma have) will inevitably transform into a higher high-grade glioma usually within 3-10 years. As such, from a surgical management perspective they are considered collectively. Current standard of care for low-grade gliomas is maximal safe anatomical resection based on tumor borders as seen on FLAIR MRI, with or without early radiotherapy to the tumor bed (especially if residual) or late radiotherapy at the time of tumor progression on imaging. More recently, some have argued that since tumor cells are likely to have spread significantly further along white matter than visualized on FLAIR MRI the limit of tumor resection should instead be based on functional limits identified by continuous intraoperative functional mapping/testing during surgery. Adjuvant treatment with stereotactic radiosurgery is under investigation.

Image with permission from Senft C, Franz K, Ulrich CT, et al. Low field intraoperative MRI-guided surgery of gliomas: a single center experience. Clin Neurol Neurosurg. 2010;112(3):237-243.

18. **e**—Tumor margins are usually seen best on T1 + gad MRI sequences

Oligodendrogliomas account for 10-15% of all gliomas and occur predominantly in adults. They are diffusely infiltrating neoplasms, which are found almost exclusively in the cerebral hemispheres, most commonly in the frontal or temporo-frontal region, and typically involving subcortical white matter and cortex. The WHO classification distinguishes between WHO grade II (well-differentiated low-grade) and WHO grade III (anaplastic high-grade) oligodendrogliomas. The former are slowly growing tumors with rounded homogeneous nuclei; the latter have increased tumor cell density, mitotic activity, microvascular proliferation and necrosis. Both low- and high-grade oligodendral tumors express proangiogenic mitogens and may contain regions of increased vascular density with finely branching capillaries that have a "chicken wire" appearance. This contributes to their appearance on contrast-enhanced MRI and MR perfusion. Up to 90% of oligodendrogliomas contain visible calcification on CT, which can be central, peripheral or ribbon-like. On MRI, intratumoral calcification appears typically T2 hypo- and T1 hyperintense and causes marked signal loss on T2* or SWI images. Contrast enhancement is variable and often heterogeneous. Unlike in astrocytomas, contrast enhancement is not a reliable indicator of tumor grade in oligodendrogliomas: it occurs in about 20% of WHO grade II tumors and in over 70% of WHO grade III oligodendrogliomas. Low-grade oligodendrogliomas may also have an elevated rCBV on PWI. Despite commonly being located in functional "eloquent" areas of cortex and corresponding white matter, their slow growth and tumor-induced plasticity means that seizures rather than functional deficits are by far the most common presenting features. As with astrocytomas, standard of care is maximal safe resection to the FLAIR border, often requiring awake intraoperative functional mapping for eloquent area tumors due to distortion of cortical functional maps by the tumor.

Image with permission from Kaye, AH, Brain Tumors an Encyclopedic Approach, 3rd ed., 2012, Elsevier.

19. **b**—Craniotomy under GA with functional mapping is the standard of care for low-grade gliomas in eloquent cortex

The primary goal in the initial treatment of LGG is maximum safe resection in the majority of patients. The goal of achieving more extensive resection (over biopsy alone) is often favored because, in retrospective analyses, it is associated with prolonged survival, greater seizure control and reduced risk of transformation to a higher grade. However, surgical treatment of suspected LGGs poses a special challenge for the neurosurgeon for the following reasons: (1) Gross total resection is difficult as their diffusely infiltrative growth pattern means that intraoperative identification of the exact tumor border in an LGG is frequently not possible with certainty, hence image guidance based on tumor limits on FLAIR MRI is key. (2) Histopathological undergrading is common with biopsy as LGG generally exhibits focal areas of malignant transformation (anaplastic foci) therefore the surgical goal is to perform precise tissue sampling from a potential anaplastic focus to avoid this and reduce subsequent treatment failure. (3) "Eloquent" tumor localization and infiltrative growth pattern means that awake surgery and/or functional mapping are generally employed to avoid new postoperative neurological deficits. (4) precise localization of the tumor and its relation to cortical surface anatomy and vasculature in the preoperative planning phase as well as during the operative approach is required to avoid morbidity (e.g. insular gliomas).

20. **d**—Brodmann areas represent a connectionist model of brain function

The locationist view that each region of the brain corresponds to a given function (e.g. Brodmann areas) producing a topographical map has been used for over a century, and implies that brain injury in an "eloquent" area will result in a massive and permanent neurological deficit. However, it is unable to explain the many observations of recovery after brain damage, even in eloquent regions as well as fMRI and intraoperative mapping evidence of pre- and postoperative cortical topographic map reorganization in diffuse low-grade glioma patients with "eloquent" lesions. More recently, the idea of a brain connectome where the CNS is organized into parallel networks, which are dynamic, interactive and able to compensate for each other (at least to a certain extent) has gained favor. This is underpinned by the hodotopic principle where functions of the brain are supported by extensive circuits comprising both the cortical nodes (topos) and connections between them created by associating bundles of white matter (hodos). Neurological function arises from the synchronization between different nodes, working in phase during a given task, and the same node may take part in several functions depending on the other cortical areas with which it is temporarily connected at any one time. Functional maps may be reorganized within remote networks over time, making neuroplasticity mechanisms possible. Modest redistribution of neurosynaptic networks occurs in acute injuries (e.g. stroke) explaining the limited recovery, whereas massive redistribution of function can occur in chronic slowly progressive injuries (e.g. DLGG) so that an "eloquent" location generally does not result in functional deficit. Cortical map reorganization mechanisms involve recruitment of areas around the lesion and/or within the hemisphere remote to the glioma and/or contralateral to the lesion. However, the plasticity index is high for cortical reorganization but very limited for subcortical connectivity hence it is crucial to preserve functionally important subcortical white matter (determined by intraoperative white matter functional mapping), allowing post injury/operative cortical map reorganization and avoidance of permanent neurological deficit. In this way, supratotal resection of diffuse low-grade gliomas (i.e. to the functional limit defined by intraoperative white matter mapping, rather than to the tumor limit defined by FLAIR MRI) has been supported by some. While this approach may tackle microscopic tumor spread, all cases must be done awake with functional mapping, requires a large craniotomy, and is seen as too aggressive by many at present.

FURTHER READING

Duffau H. Nat Rev Neurol 2015;11:255-265.

21. **d**—PCV

LGG management involves surgery, radiotherapy, chemotherapy, or a combination of these modalities. Surgery is first-line therapy whose chief role is to provide tissue to confirm the diagnosis. The next most common step in management is radiotherapy: either early radiotherapy (within a few weeks of surgery) or delayed radiotherapy (at time of clinical or imaging progression). Controversy exists on its optimal timing, particularly due to the long term neurocognitive side effects in LGG patients who are mostly young adults. Early adverse effects of radiation include headache, dizziness, ear inflammation, nausea, vomiting, seizure, altered level of consciousness, alopecia, dermatitis, urinary incontinence, and personality change. Late clinical consequences of brain irradiation include leukoencephalopathy, neurocognitive decline, reduced quality of life, and tissue necrosis that may mimic tumor progression. The toxic effects of radiotherapy must be carefully weighed against the benefits for tumor control, including an improvement of seizures. SRS can produce long-term control with an acceptable toxicity profile, and is generally reserved for inoperable tumors in close proximity to critical structures. Similarly, chemotherapy has potential either as a concurrent treatment or substitute for radiotherapy and can also improve seizure control. Studies have focused primarily on a three-drug regimen of procarbazine, lomustine, and vincristine (PCV) or single agent temozolomide (temozolomide response may be predicted by IDH1/2 mutation). Ongoing randomized controlled trials are evaluating whether temozolomide can substitute for radiotherapy, or whether concurrent temozolomide and radiotherapy is superior to radiotherapy alone for postoperative tumor control.

22. **b**—Functional MGMT increases the effectiveness of cancer chemotherapy

The O(6)-Methylguanine-DNA Methyl Transferase (MGMT) is a DNA repair enzyme that reverts the naturally occurring mutagenic O6-methylguanine back to guanine. This prevents errors during DNA replication. In the context of chemotherapy with alkylating agents (e.g. temozolomide) it removes a cytotoxic lesion, thus counteracting the chemotherapeutic effects of the drug. Aberrant, cancer related methylation of the MGMT promoter region leads to its silencing, a reduction of the MGMT enzyme expression and subsequently to less repair activity of DNA damage, including that induced by temozolomide (TMZ). MGMT promoter methylation in GBM is a prognostic and predictive biomarker indicating response to chemoradiation. It has no diagnostic value. This was demonstrated in the EORTC NCIC registration trial for TMZ in newly diagnosed GBM where patients with MGMT promoter methylated tumors derived most benefit when treated with TMZ. Patients with tumors with methylated MGMT promoter had a survival benefit when treated with TMZ and radiotherapy, compared with those who received radiotherapy only, whereas absence of MGMT promoter methylation resulted in a smaller and statistically insignificant difference in survival between the treatment groups. Further studies showed that patients with MGMT promoter-unmethylated tumors had no survival benefit from chemotherapy, regardless of whether given at diagnosis together with RT or as a salvage treatment. Prospective randomized trials (NOA-08), the Nordic trial and RTOG 0525 concluded that MGMT promoter methylation is a useful predictive biomarker to stratify elderly (>70 years of age; the Stupp protocol was studied in GBM patients under 70) GBM patients for RT versus alkylating agent chemotherapy and should be tested for.

FURTHER READING

Brandner S, et al. Invited review: diagnostic, prognostic and predictive relevance of molecular markers in gliomas. Neuropathology and Applied Neurobiology 2015;41:694-720.

23. **b**—TERT normally prevents telomerase repair ensuring that cells become replicatively senescent

Telomere (repetitive nucleotide sequences at the ends of chromosomes) length shortens with each cell division, normally leading to replicative senescence and thus a limit to the number of times a cell can divide. Cancer cells bypass this limit in various ways, including an increased ability to maintain telomere length. The enzyme telomerase reverse transcriptase (TERT) plays a critical role in extending the telomeres in normal cells and mutations in the TERT promoter, resulting in overexpression of TERT is a feature of most human cancers including gliomas. It has been suggested that tumors derived from cell populations with low self-renewal capacity generally rely on alterations that restore/gain telomerase activity, while epigenetic mechanisms maintain/prevent loss of telomerase activity in tumor types derived from self-renewing stem cells. In contrast, ATRX or DAXX mutations have been shown to underlie a telomere maintenance mechanism not involving telomerase ("alternative lengthening of telomeres;" ALT). TERT is essential in maintaining telomere length and its activity is pathologically increased in a number of human cancers, including GBM. Analysis of TERT promoter mutations in 1515 CNS tumors showed 327 mutations, predominantly in adult patients, with a strong association with older age. Mutations were seen in gliosarcomas (81%), oligodendrogliomas (78%), oligoastrocytomas (58%) and primary GBMs (54%). TERT promoter mutations were also strongly associated with 1p/19q codeletion and inversely associated with loss of ATRX expression and IDH1/IDH2 mutations. In general, TERT and IDH mutations are largely mutually exclusive in GBM and astrocytomas but co-occur in most oligodendrogliomas. In a study of 400 gliomas patients with TERT promoter mutations alone (i.e. no IDH mutation) had the poorest overall survival (median 11.3 months), patients with tumors without TERT or IDH1/2 mutations had a slightly better survival (median 16.6 months), whereas patients with IDH-only mutant GBM had the best survival (median 42.3 months). Although an earlier study with 358 patients found no significant difference in overall survival between TERT mutant and TERT wild-type (IDH wt) GBM, the role of TERT mutations may in the future provide a tool to identify non-IDH1/2 mutant GBMs and suggests that combined IDH1/2 and TERT promoter genotyping will be useful for patient management.

FURTHER READING

Brandner S, et al. Invited review: diagnostic, prognostic and predictive relevance of molecular markers in gliomas. Neuropathology and applied neurobiology 2015;41:694-720.

24. **f**—IDH1/2 mutation is associated with an improved prognosis in grade II astrocytomas

Pathogenic mutations in the isocitrate dehydrogenase genes 1 (IDH1; chromosome 2q) or 2 (IDH2; chromosome 15q) were discovered in next-generation sequencing studies of 22 GBM, including in secondary GBM. Likely to be a tumor initiating or driver mutation in astrocytomas and oligodendrogliomas, even in the presence of a pre-existing mutation of the tumor suppressor p53 (TP53) gene. The most common mutation (~90%) in glial brain tumors causes a substitution of the amino acid Arginine to Histidine at codon 132 of the IDH1 gene (IDH1 R132H); alternatively, a mutually exclusive mutation in codon 172 of the mitochondrial IDH2 gene can occur. These homologous enzymes decarboxylate isocitrate to α-ketoglutarate (αKG) and this "neomorphic" mutation renders the IDH enzyme to reduce αKG into 2-hydroxyglutarate (2-HG) in an NADPH dependent manner. Accumulation of 2-HG to high levels in glioma tissues may cause epigenetic alterations in both, DNA and histones, altering gene expression and promoting oncogenic transformation. Reorganization of the methylome due to mutant IDH is the molecular basis of the CpG island methylator phenotype (CIMP) in gliomas, leading to global dysregulation of gene expression.

IDH1 mutations occur early, with a high frequency, in WHO grade II and III astrocytic and oligodendroglial tumors and in secondary GBMs, which develop from astrocytomas. IDH mutations in gliomas are early events in their pathogenesis, and are associated with several clinically relevant parameters including patient age, histopathological diagnosis, combined 1p/19q deletion (co-segregate in oligodendrogliomas), TP53 mutation, MGMT promoter hypermethylation and patient survival. Diagnostically it serves 2 roles when used with ATRX and 1p19q status: (1) differentiate grade II/III oligodendrogliomas from other lesions with potentially similar histological appearance or "oligodendroglial-like differentiation" (e.g. primary GBM, clear cell ependymomas, neurocytomas or pilocytic astrocytomas), and (2) high-grade astrocytomas or oligodendrogliomas from "primary GBMs with oligodendroglial differentiation." The association between IDH1/2 mutation and a favorable prognosis is better established in high-grade gliomas. The majority of studies reporting mutant IDH1 as a favorable factor in WHO grade II tumors often include oligodendroglial tumors (which will also have 1p19q loss hence better chemotherapy response) and studies comprising low-grade astrocytomas only showed no prognostic value of mutant IDH1/2. The NOA4 trial identified that MGMT promoter methylation is prognostic for patients with IDH1/2-mutant WHO grade III gliomas, but in patients with IDH-wild-type tumors it was predictive for benefit from alkylating chemotherapy.

FURTHER READING

Brandner S, et al. Invited review: diagnostic, prognostic and predictive relevance of molecular markers in gliomas. Neuropathology and applied neurobiology 2015;41:694-720.

ANSWERS 25–40

Additional answers 25–40 available on ExpertConsult.com

EMI ANSWERS

41. 1—k, Primary CNS lymphoma; 2—e, Germinoma; 3—h, Non-germinomatous germ cell tumor (most likely choriocarcinoma given markedly raised HCG)

42. 1—f, Hemangioblastoma; 2—i, Pilocytic astrocytoma; 3—c, Dysplastic cerebellar gangliocytoma (Lhermitte-Duclos disease)

43. 1—f, Histone H3; 2—g, IDH1/2 mutation; 3—a, 1p19q co-deletion; 4—e, EGFRvIII; 5—h, MGMT methylation

BRAF gene mutations are diagnostically useful in differentiating low-grade glial and glioneuronal (pilocytic astrocytoma, PXA, ganglioglioma, SEGA) from diffuse astrocytomas, but not prognostically relevant. The table below reflects commonest patterns of molecular status according to histological grades.

Molecular Classification of Gliomas

WHO Grade	1p19q Status	IDH1/2 Status	ATRX Status	MGMT Promoter Methylation	Other Molecular Markers
Astrocytoma (grade II)	Preserved 19q loss only exceptionally	Mutant IDH in majority	ARTX loss in IDH mutants		
Oligodendroglioma (grade II)	Codeleted in vast majority	Mutant IDH in majority	ARTX loss in 25%, but rare if 1p19q loss		TERT promoter methylation (co-occurs with IDH mutation unlike in GBM)
Anaplastic astrocytoma (Grade III)	Preserved 19q loss only in minority.	Mutant IDH in majority, confers better prognosis than wild type	ATRX loss in IDH1/2 mutants = favorable prognosis	Associated with better prognosis in IDH mutants Predictive for benefit from temozolomide in IDH wild type	H3 Histone mutation predicts worse prognosis (similar to GBM)
Anaplastic oligodendroglioma (Grade III)	Codeleted in vast majority, better prognosis and 1p loss confers response to TMZ/PCV	Mutant IDH in majority, confers better prognosis than wild type IDH	ARTX loss in 7%, but rare if 1p19q loss	Associated with better prognosis in IDH mutants Predictive for benefit from temozolomide in IDH wild type	TERT promoter methylation

Continued

WHO Grade	1p19q Status	IDH1/2 Status	ATRX Status	MGMT Promoter Methylation	Other Molecular Markers
Primary GBM	Preserved 19q loss only in a small minority	Wild type IDH in all adult primary GBM If IDH mutant present likely represents secondary GBM	ARTX loss rare in primary GBM ATRX loss seen in IDH mutant secondary GBM and pediatric GBM	Predictive for benefit from temozolomide	7p gain; 10q loss; TERT promoter methylation; EGFR amplification; Histone H3 mutation in younger patients

FURTHER READING

Brandner S, et al. Invited review: diagnostic, prognostic and predictive relevance of molecular markers in gliomas. Neuropathology and Applied Neurobiology 2015;41:694-720.

Louis DN, Perry A, Reifenberger G, von Deimling A, et al. The 2016 World Health Organization Classification of Tumors of the Central Nervous System: a summary. Acta Neuropathol. 2016 Jun; 131(6):803-20.

CHAPTER 24

SKULL BASE AND PITUITARY SURGERY

SINGLE BEST ANSWER (SBA) QUESTIONS

PITUITARY

1. A 45-year-old man presents with sudden onsent headache, nausea, vomiting and visual disturbance. On examination he is apyrexial, hypotensive, and tachycardic but does not have neck stiffness or photophobia. Visual fields appear to be constricted on confrontation. CT head is abnormal therefore MRI is done. Which one of the following is appropriate acute management?

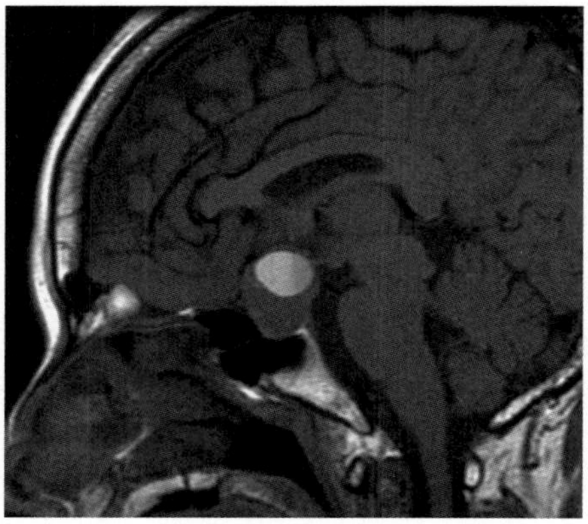

   a. Dexamethasone
   b. Formal visual field tests
   c. Pituitary profile and start empirical intravenous hydrocortisone
   d. Lumbar puncture
   e. Transsphenoidal surgery

2. A 64-year-old male presented with severe headache and visual disturbance. Plain CT imaging revealed a sellar mass but no other acute abnormality. Contrast imaging was performed (below). Which one of the following is the most important next management step?

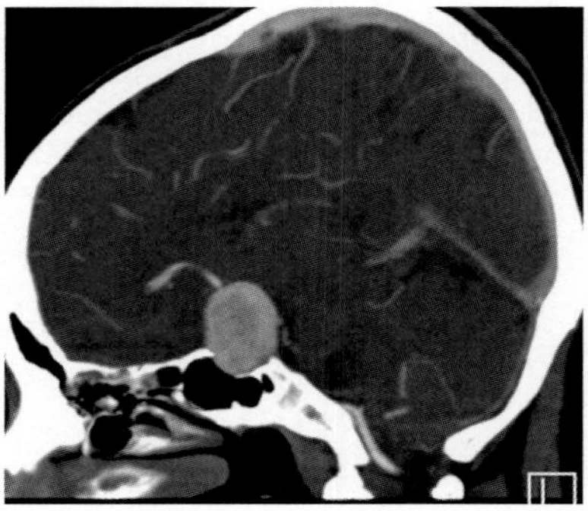

   a. Pituitary profile
   b. Formal visual field assessment
   c. Image guided biopsy
   d. Lumbar puncture
   e. ICP monitoring

3. A 57-year-old undergoes elective transsphenoidal surgery for a non-functioning macroadenoma compressing the optic chiasm. Recovery was uneventful and routine bloods on postoperative day 1 were normal, and endocrine profile showed FT4 12 pmol/L (11.5-22), TSH 0.9 mU/L (0.35-5.5) and 9 am cortisol 154 nmol/L. Which one of the following statements regarding further management is LEAST accurate?
   a. If thyroid function tests are normal on day 3 or 4 a further assessment should take place at 4-8 weeks
   b. Evening steroid dose should not be omitted if checking 9 am cortisol
   c. If day 2 postoperative 9 am cortisol >550 nmol/L does not require steroid replacement
   d. If day 2 postoperative 9 am cortisol 400-550 nmol/L requires hydrocortisone only during severe illness

e. If day 2 postoperative 9 am cortisol <400 nmol/L does requires regular oral hydrocortisone

4. A 65-year-old man undergoes transsphenoidal surgery for a non-functioning macroadenoma. Postoperatively on day 1 the nurses notice he is passing large volumes of dilute urine via his catheter. Which one of the following criteria is LEAST suggestive of diabetes insipidus?
   a. Urine specific gravity <1.003 or osmolality <200 mOsmol/kg
   b. Urine output >250 ml/h for 2 consecutive hours
   c. Serum sodium normal or raised
   d. Primary adrenal insufficiency
   e. Inability to concentrate urine to >300 mOsmol/L in the presence of clinical dehydration

5. A 17-year-old female presents with an 8 month history of secondary amenorrhea. More recently she has noticed that she is more thirsty and is passing large volumes of urine. Her examination is otherwise unremarkable. Routine blood tests are normal and endocrine profile shows: FSH 5.5 U/L (follicular 0.5-5, mid-cycle 8-33, luteal 2-8), LH 2.8 U/L (follicular 3-12, mid-cycle 20-80, luteal 3-16), estradiol 32 pmol/L (follicular 17-260, luteal 180-1100), prolactin 990 mU/L (60-620), 9 am cortisol 400 nmol/L, fasting blood glucose 5.5 mmol/L, serum calcium 2.35 mmol/L (2.2-2.6). Water deprivation test: serum osmolality 300 mOsmol/kg, urine 200 mOsmol/kg at 6 h, post-DDAVP urine osmolality 800 mOsmol/kg. MRI head is shown. Which one of the following would you perform next?

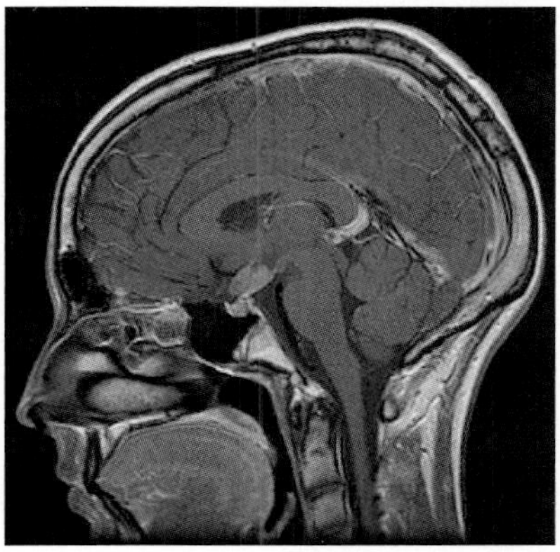

   a. Serum and CSF HCG and AFP
   b. Ultrasound pelvis/ovaries
   c. Insulin tolerance test
   d. Short synacthen test
   e. Visual field tests

6. A 33-year-old female who presents with a several week history of headache, extreme fatigue and malaise. She gave birth to her first child 2 months ago via vaginal delivery. Examination was unremarkable. Routine bloods were normal, and endocrine profile showed: Prolactin 801 mU/L (100-550), FT4 10 pmol/L (11.5-22), TSH 0.1 mU/L (0.35-5.5). Short synacthen test: 0 h cortisol 55 nmol/L, 30 min cortisol 155 nmol/L. MRI is shown. Which one of the following is most likely?

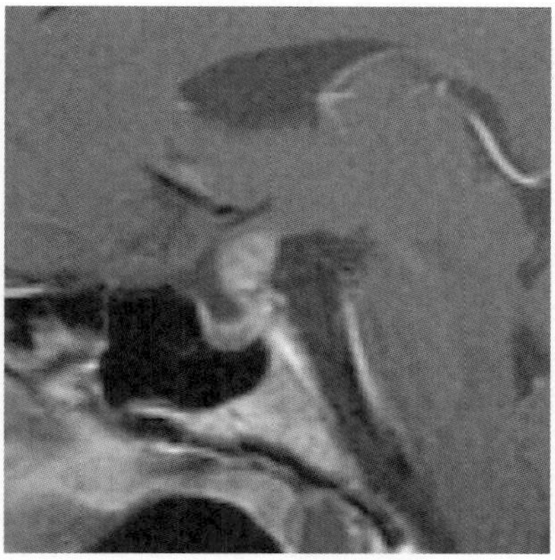

   a. Lymphocytic hypophysitis
   b. Sheehan's syndrome
   c. Non-functioning adenoma
   d. Langerhans cell histiocytosis
   e. Sarcoidosis

7. A 48-year-old male presents with low mood, malaise and reduced exercise tolerance. He has a past history of IHD and a non-functioning pituitary adenoma resected 5 years ago resulting in partial anterior hypopituitarism. He is normally on thyroxine and hydrocortisone replacement therapy. On examination his BMI is 39 kg/m^2 and shows central adiposity. His endocrine tests show 9 am cortisol 410 nmol/L, IGF-1 8 nmol/L (16-118), FT4 16 pmol/L (11.5-22) and TSH 0.03 mU/L

(0.35-5.5). Which one of the following is most appropriate to confirm the diagnosis?
a. Growth hormone levels
b. GHRH-arginine stimulation test
c. IGF-binding protein 3 measurement
d. Insulin tolerance test
e. Water deprivation test

8. A 56-year-old presents with a 2-month history of headache and visual disturbance. Confrontation testing revealed a bitemporal hemianopia. Routine bloods were normal and endocrine profile is: FT4 pmol/L 8.5 (11.5-22), TSH 0.5 mU/L (0.35-5.5), FSH 1.0 U/L (1.4-18.1), LH 2.5 U/L (3-8), prolactin 900 mU/L (45-375), testosterone 3.5 nmol/L (8.4-28.7), 9 am cortisol 405 nmol/L. MRI is shown. Which one of the following is most likely?

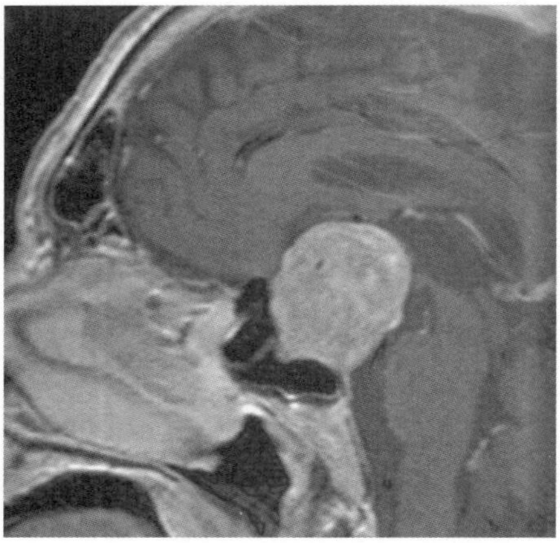

a. Non-functioning adenoma
b. Thyrotropinoma
c. GH-secreting pituitary adenoma
d. Prolactinoma
e. Cushing's disease

9. A 50-year-old male presents with a 12 month history of reduced libido and lethargy. On examination there were mild left sided 3rd and 6th nerve palsies. Routine bloods were normal and endocrine profile showed: FT4 8 pmol/L (11.5-22), TSH 0.4 mU/L (0.35-5.5), FSH 2.2 U/L (1.4-18.1), LH 3.5 U/L (3-8), testosterone 6.8 nmol/L (8.4-28.7), IGF-1 35 nmol/L (16-118), prolactin 880 mU/L (45-375). MRI is shown. Which one of the following is most appropriate next?

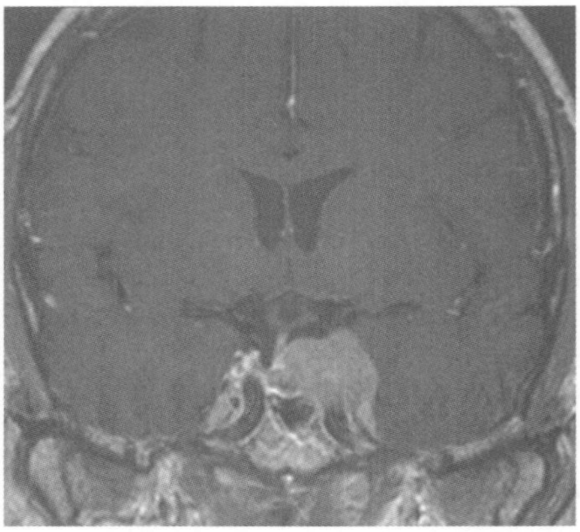

a. Stereotactic radiosurgery
b. Transsphenoidal debulking followed by stereotactic radiosurgery
c. Cabergoline
d. Somatostatin
e. Petrous sinus sampling

10. Which one of the following statements regarding diagnosis and management of prolactinomas is LEAST accurate?
a. Prolactinomas are managed medically with dopamine receptor agonists
b. Hook effect describes spuriously high prolactin levels due to macroprolactin complexes
c. Compression of the pituitary stalk can cause a mildly raised prolactin
d. Prolactin levels in a prolactinoma are usually >2000 mU/L
e. Hypothyroidism may result in hyperprolactinemia

11. Which one of the following statements regarding management of incidentally found pituitary adenomas (except prolactinomas) is most accurate?
a. Anterior pituitary hormone profile should only be performed if the patient is symptomatic
b. MRI surveillance for lesions <10 mm and >10 mm is the same
c. Indications for surgery include secreting tumours
d. Macroincidentalomas should be reimaged at 12 months
e. Formal visual field testing should be performed as a baseline

12. Which one of the following statements regarding medical management of secreting pituitary adenomas is LEAST accurate?
   a. Octreotide used in patients with acromegaly
   b. Cabergoline is a dopamine receptor antagonist
   c. Bromocriptine is used in the treatment of prolactinoma
   d. Pegvisomant is a GH receptor blocker and useful if somatostatin fails in acromegaly
   e. Mitotane used for Cushing's disease

13. A 36-year-old patient with Cushing's syndrome but normal ACTH levels is referred. There is no visual compromise. Pituitary MRI shows a 3 mm hypodense area in the lateral aspect of the pituitary gland. Which one of the following is the next appropriate management?
   a. Laparoscopic adrenalectomy
   b. Transsphenoidal surgery
   c. Inferior petrosal sinus sampling
   d. High-dose dexamethasone test
   e. Start octreotide

14. Which one of the following statements regarding Cushing's disease is most accurate?
   a. It is often due to ACTH-secreting pituitary adenoma
   b. Primary management is surgical resection of the tumor
   c. High-dose dexamethasone suppression test is able to lateralize the side of ACTH-secreting microadenoma within the pituitary gland
   d. It may be caused by ectopic ACTH producing tumors
   e. Can cause amenorrhea in females and infertility in males

15. Which one of the following would be most appropriate treatment following failure of transsphenoidal surgery to treat Cushing's disease?
   a. Surveillance imaging
   b. Repeat transsphenoidal surgery
   c. Cabergoline
   d. Octreotide
   e. Bilateral adrenalectomy

16. A 43-year-old female presents with coarse facial appearance, macroglossia and large hands and feet. She has also been experiencing worse glycemic control on a background of type II diabetes mellitus. Routine bloods are normal and endocrine profile shows: IGF-1 102 nmol/L (16-118), prolactin 610 mU/L (45-375), FT4 12.5 pmol/L (11.5-22), and TSH 1.5 mU/L (0.35-4.5). Which one of the following would you perform to confirm your biochemical diagnosis?
   a. Oral glucose tolerance test
   b. Insulin tolerance test
   c. Short synacthen test
   d. Dexamethasone suppression test
   e. Domperidone test

17. Endoscopic view from within sphenoid sinus. Which one of the following labels appropriately identifies the opticocarotid recess?

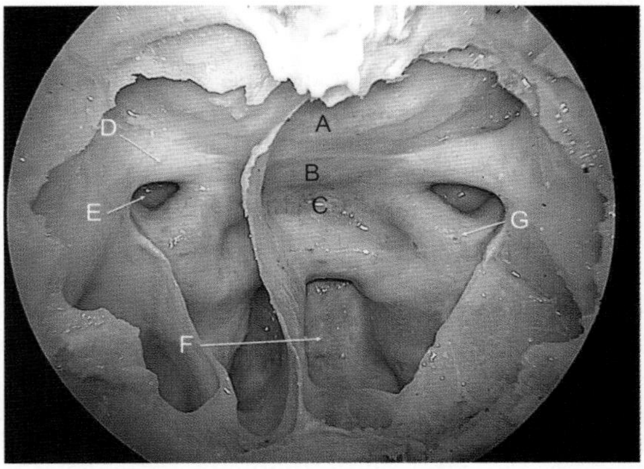

18. A patient presents 7 days after transsphenoidal resection of pituitary adenoma with headache, neck stiffness, fever and clear fluid discharge from his nose. Which one of the following is the most appropriate management?
   a. Endoscopic repair
   b. External ventricular drain
   c. Bed rest and lumbar puncture
   d. Lumbar drain
   e. Empirical antibiotics and CT head

QUESTIONS 19–37

Additional questions 19–37 available on ExpertConsult.com

EXTENDED MATCHING ITEM (EMI) QUESTIONS

38. **Sellar and parasellar lesions:**
    a. ACTH-secreting pituitary adenoma
    b. Arachnoid cyst
    c. Craniopharyngioma
    d. Germinoma
    e. GH-secreting pituitary adenoma
    f. Gonadotropin-secreting adenoma
    g. Hypothalamic hamartoma
    h. Langerhans cell histiocytosis
    i. Lymphocytic hypophysitis
    j. Non-functioning pituitary adenoma
    k. Optic pathway glioma
    l. Prolactin-secreting pituitary adenoma
    m. Thyrotropinoma

For each of the following descriptions, select the most appropriate answers from the list above. Each answer may be used once, more than once or not at all.

1. A 24-year-old female presents with a 3 year history of menstrual irregularities. Prior to this she had regular menstrual cycles. Examination was unremarkable. Routine bloods were normal, and endocrine profile showed: FSH 45 U/L (follicular 0.5-5, mid-cycle 8-33, luteal 2-8), LH 2.5 U/L (follicular 3-12, mid-cycle 20-80, luteal 3-15), estradiol 1332 pmol/L (follicular 17-260, luteal 180-1100), prolactin 604 mU/L (45-375). Ultrasound of pelvis shows bilateral enlarged and cystic ovaries. MRI shows a pituitary tumor without optic chiasm compression.
2. A 49-year-old female presents with a 6 month history of palpitations, weight loss, increased sweating and shortness of breath. Her examination was unremarkable except for sinus tachycardia. Routine bloods were normal and TFTs showed: FT4 27 pmol/L (9-19), FT3 pmol/L (8 (2.6-5.7), TSH 7 (0.35-5.5). Further tests show alpha-subunit to TSH ratio >1.
3. A 9-year-old girl presents with bitemporal hemianopia and café-au-lait spots. Autoantibody screen in normal. MRI shows a lesion involving the chiasm and hypothalamus.

39. **Pituitary dysfunction:**
    a. Acromegaly
    b. Conn's syndrome
    c. Cushing's disease
    d. Diabetes insipidus
    e. Hyperprolactinemia
    f. Hyperthyroidism
    g. Hypothyroidism
    h. Nelson's syndrome
    i. Panhypopituitarism
    j. Pituitary apoplexy
    k. Primary adrenal insufficiency (Addison's disease)
    l. Secondary adrenal insufficiency
    m. Syndrome of inappropriate ADH secretion

For each of the following descriptions, select the most appropriate answers from the list above. Each answer may be used once, more than once or not at all.

1. A 37-year-old male presents with abdominal pain, fatigue, hypotension and skin hyperpigmentation. Neither short or long synacthen tests show cortisol response.
2. A 57-year-old male undergoes transsphenoidal surgery for non-functioning adenoma. On day 2 postoperatively his serum sodium rises to 149 mmol/L and urine output is 300 ml/h for greater than 2 h despite previously normal fluid balance. Serum osmolality is 295 mOsmol/kg and urine osmolality is 105 mOsmol/kg.
3. A 44-year-old on pituitary hormone replacement with bitemporal hemianopia and right ocular paresis. She was diagnosed with a brain tumor but had an operation on her abdomen to stop it causing symptoms.

40. **Skull base foramina:**

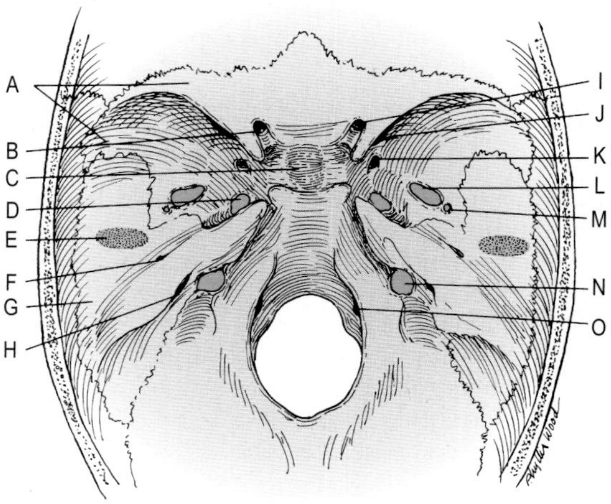

For each of the following descriptions, select the most appropriate answers from the image above.

Each answer may be used once, more than once or not at all.

1. Contains maxillary nerve (CNV2)
2. Contains greater petrosal nerve (VII) which joins with deep petrosal nerve to form vidian nerve (of the pterygoid canal).
3. Contains facial nerve (VII), vestibulocochlear (VIII)

41. **Skull base approaches:**
   a. Anterior clinoidectomy
   b. Anterior petrosectomy
   c. Combined transpetrosal approach
   d. Frontotemporal orbitozygomatic approach
   e. Middle cranial fossa approach
   f. Retrolabyrinthine
   g. Retrosigmoid
   h. Transcochlear
   i. Transcondylar and far lateral approach
   j. Translabyrinthine
   k. Transotic
   l. Transpetrous

For each of the following descriptions, select the most appropriate answers from the list above. Each answer may be used once, more than once or not at all.

1. Presigmoid approach that uses a mastoidectomy and skeletonization of the sigmoid sinus
2. Includes drilling the posterior and superior external auditory canal and sacrificing middle ear structures and inner ear (cochlea), and rerouting the facial nerve to provide access to the anterior cerebellopontine angle, petrous apex, and ventral brainstem.

SBA ANSWERS

1. **c**—Pituitary profile and start empirical intravenous hydrocortisone

Pituitary apoplexy is characterized by sudden onset headache, nausea, vomiting, with or without acute visual disturbance and cranial nerve palsy (2nd, 3rd, 4th, 6th) due to pituitary hemorrhage and/or infarction. Precipitating factors in those with or without an underlying pituitary tumor include hypertension, major surgery, dynamic testing of pituitary function, anticoagulation/coagulopathy, estrogen therapy, dopamine receptor agonist initiation/withdrawal, radiotherapy, pregnancy and head trauma. Assessment should focus on history and examination findings consistent with preexisting pituitary dysfunction. Anterior pituitary function tests (FT4, TSH, IGF-1, random cortisol, prolactin, growth hormone, FSH/LH, and testosterone in men or estradiol in women) should be checked urgently but those with hemodynamic instability (i.e. Addisonian crisis) should be started on empirical hydrocortisone. Indications for empirical steroid therapy in patients with pituitary apoplexy are hemodynamic instability, altered consciousness level, reduced visual acuity and severe visual field defects. Patients who do not fulfill the criteria for urgent empirical steroid therapy should be considered for treatment with steroids, if their 09·00 serum cortisol is less than 550 nmol/L; The majority of the patients (nearly 80%) will have deficiency of one or more anterior pituitary hormones at presentation. As most of the patients have underlying macroadenomas, partial hypopituitarism would be expected to have been present in the majority even before the apoplectic episode. Clinically, the most crucial deficit is that of adrenocorticotroph hormone (ACTH) in up to 70% of the patients. Thyrotrophin and gonadotrophin deficiencies are observed in 50% and 75% of the patients, respectively. Hyponatremia has been reported in up to 40% of the patients because of either the syndrome of inappropriate antidiuretic hormone secretion or hypocortisolism. Patients with pituitary apoplexy who have low serum prolactin (PRL) levels at presentation have the highest intrasellar pressure and are the least likely to recover from hypopituitarism after decompressive surgery. Formal visual fields assessment, using Humphrey visual field analyzer or Goldmann perimeter must be undertaken when the patient is clinically stable, preferably within 24 h of the suspected diagnosis. MRI of the pituitary is required to confirm the diagnosis. Hemorrhage appears hyperintense on non-enhanced T1W images and, in the acute stage, hyperdense on CT and may rarely contain a fluid level (as in this case) with evidence of optic chiasm being stretched across the top of the mass. Patients with pituitary apoplexy who are without any neuro-ophthalmic signs or mild and stable signs can be considered for conservative management with careful monitoring. In patients with reduced visual acuity or defective visual fields, formal assessment of visual fields and acuity should be performed every day until a clear trend of improvement is observed. Indications for urgent neurosurgical decompression include deteriorating level of consciousness, severely reduced visual acuity, severe/persistent/

worsening visual field defect. Ocular paresis because of involvement of III, IV or VI cranial nerves in cavernous sinus in the absence of visual field defects or reduced visual acuity is not in itself an indication for immediate surgery. Resolution will typically occur within days or weeks with conservative management. Surgery should be performed preferably within the first 7 days of onset of symptoms by an experienced pituitary surgeon.

Image with permission from Adam A, et al. (Eds.), Grainger & Allison's Diagnostic Radiology, 6th ed. Elsevier, Churchill Livingstone, 2014.

FURTHER READING

Rajasekaran S, Vanderpump M, Baldeweg S, Drake W, Reddy N, Lanyon M, Markey A, Plant G, Powell M, Sinha S, Wass J. UK guidelines for the management of pituitary apoplexy. Clin Endocrinol (Oxf) 2011;74(1):9-20.

2. **d**—Lumbar puncture

Imaging above is a CT angiogram demonstrating a giant ICA aneurysm expanding the sella. The most important next step is to clarify the likelihood that it has ruptured, and if so the patient will need to be started on subarachnoid hemorrhage treatment and the aneurysm secured. Options include lumbar puncture (though many would avoid this given the risk of aneurysm rupture) or assessing hemosiderin on MRI. Others may argue that given the history and the size of the aneurysm, treatment should be performed expediently as in aneurysmal subarachnoid hemorrhage patients.

Image with permission from Adam A, et al. (Eds.), Grainger & Allison's Diagnostic Radiology, 6th ed. Elsevier, Churchill Livingstone, 2014.

3. **b**—Evening steroid dose should not be omitted if checking 9 am cortisol

If preoperative steroid reserve adequate or unknown:

- Check 9 am serum cortisol on day 2 and on day 3 after surgery, in patients with no evidence of cortisol deficiency before operation. If already on hydrocortisone replacement, omit the evening dose for the previous day before checking.

In patients without Cushing's disease (9 am cortisol: >550 nmol/L no requirement for hydrocortisone, 400-550 nmol/L hydrocortisone only during severe illness or stress, <400 nmol/L start regular oral hydrocortisone).

If preoperative steroid reserve deficient:

- In patients with proven cortisol deficiency before surgery, continue hydrocortisone and consider changing over to maintenance dosage when stable. These patients will need further assessment at 4-8 weeks with anterior hormone profile and short synacthen test to determine whether they will need long-term steroids;
- FT4 and TSH should be assessed on day 3 or day 4 and thyroid hormone replacement should be considered if deficient.
- If FT4 and TSH normal further assessment should take place at 4-8 weeks.

FURTHER READING

Rajasekaran S, Vanderpump M, Baldeweg S, Drake W, Reddy N, Lanyon M, Markey A, Plant G, Powell M, Sinha S, Wass J. UK guidelines for the management of pituitary apoplexy. Clin Endocrinol (Oxf) 2011;74(1):9-20.

4. **d**—Primary adrenal insufficiency

Diabetes insipidus cannot occur in primary adrenal insufficiency (hypocortisolism/hypoaldosteronism) because mineralocorticoid activity is required for kidneys to produce free water.

5. **a**—Serum and CSF HCG and AFP

Water deprivation test involves serial 2 hourly measurement of serum and urine osmolality (and body weight) over a water deprivation period of 6-8 h—if serum osmolality >290 and urine <300 by the end it is suggestive of DI and DDAVP is given. If kidneys are functioning normally, DDAVP should cause a rise in urine osmolality to >750 suggesting a cranial (failure of posterior pituitary vasopressin secretion, as in this case) cause for the DI. This case describes an adolescent presenting with a hypopituitarism including cranial diabetes insipidus, with an homogeneously enhancing suprasellar mass and smaller enhancing pineal cyst. The main concern is of a germinoma (synchronous suprasellar and pineal) given her age and imaging, rather than lymphocytic hypophysitis which presents later although the two may be difficult to distinguish. MRI of the whole spine with contrast should also be performed given these findings. In a small proportion of germinomas, there may be non-germinomatous elements secreting BHCG or AFP hence serum and CSF should be checked urgently. If these are both negative biopsy should be performed to confirm a diagnosis of germinoma and start radiotherapy with or without chemotherapy.

Image with permission from Jensen AW, Laack NN, Buckner JC. Long-term follow-up of dose-adapted and reduced-field radiotherapy with or without chemotherapy for central nervous system germinoma. Int J Radiat Oncol Biol Phys 2010;77(5):1449-56.

Water Deprivation Test Interpretation			
Post-Dehydration Serum Osmolality	**Post-Dehydration Urine Osmolality**	**Post-DDAVP Urine Osmolality**	**Diagnosis**
280-90	>750	Do not give DDAVP	Normal
>290-300<	<300	<300	Nephrogenic DI
>290-300<	<300	>750	Cranial DI
>290-300<	300-750	>750	Partial cranial DI
<290	300-750	300-750	Partial nephrogenic DI, chronic psychogenic polydipsia
<290	300-750	>750	Psychogenic polydipsia

6. **a**—Lymphocytic hypophysitis

The clinical picture is that of anterior pituitary pathology with early involvement/impairment of corticotrophs (short synacthen test suggesting adrenal insufficiency; normally increase should be >200 nmol/L and 30 min value >600 nmol/L) and thyrotrophs (low TSH). This is in contrast to non-functioning pituitary adenomas where there is usually early involvement of gonadotrophs. Lymphocytic hypophysitis is most commonly seen during pregnancy or postpartum period and represents an inflammatory/autoimmune process affecting the pituitary gland and the pituitary stalk (infundibulum). Presentation is with pituitary failure such as lethargy, amenorrhea, diabetes insipidus and visual disturbance (if there is optic chiasm compression). MRI may show a homogeneously enhancing sellar/infundibular mass and T1WI may even show loss of posterior pituitary bright spot (normally present due to vasopressin storage) in cranial diabetes insipidus. Where there is a high clinical suspicion (e.g. postpartum, other autoimmune conditions, ipilimumab use, absence of serum markers for sarcoidosis) treatment with steroids and supportive therapy can be initiated. However, if the picture is uncertain or no response to steroids biopsy should be performed as it is the only way to make the diagnosis.

Image with permission from Hess CP, Dillon WP. Imaging the pituitary and parasellar region. Neurosurg Clin N Am 2012;23(4):529-42.

7. **b**—GHRH-arginine stimulation test

The clinical features of growth hormone deficiency are nonspecific and include lethargy, low mood, poor quality of life, loss of muscle mass and central adiposity. GH is normally secreted in a pulsatile fashion (5 per 24 h) hence random measurement of levels is not helpful. A low IGF-1 level may be present in 60-70% of patients with GH deficiency, and may suggest the need for dynamic tests of GH secretion. Equally, a low IGF-1 in the presence of 3 or more other anterior pituitary hormone deficiencies in an otherwise healthy individual is a strong predictor of GH deficiency and treatment should be considered without dynamic testing. Contraindications to GH therapy is active malignancy (other than pituitary). If dynamic testing is required, the gold standard is insulin tolerance test (ITT) where insulin administration should provoke a rise in GH (peak level <10 mU/L or <3 μg/L is suggestive of severe GH deficiency). However, ITT is contraindicated in those with IHD and epilepsy due to the risks associated with hypoglycemia and may give a false result in obese patients. In this situation, other dynamic tests include GNRH-arginine stimulation and glucagon stimulation test which have a higher sensitivity than IGFBP-3 levels.

8. **a**—Non-functioning adenoma

Pituitary adenomas are the most common neoplasms in the sellar region and comprise 10-15% of all primary brain tumors. They are classified as microadenomas (<10 mm) and macroadenomas (>10 mm). Furthermore, they may be non-functional pituitary adenomas (clinically not hormonally active) or functional (clinically showing signs of hormone excess). Non-functional adenomas account for 15-30% of pituitary adenomas and show gonadotroph (FSH, LH) deficiency in 80%, followed by somatotrophy (GH secretion) deficiency, and later thyrotrophs (TSH) and corticotrophs (ACTH) deficiency in 20-50%. Gonadotrophs are the commonest primary cell type involved in NFPA. As such, patients tend to present with hypogonadotrophic hypogonadism early, and features of GH deficiency, secondary hypothyroidism and secondary adrenal insufficiency later on. Hypogonadotrophic hypogonadism is characterized by Large NFSs compress the pituitary stalk, causing impairment of dopamine transport to the lactotrophs and a slight rise in prolactin secretions above normal (but prolactinoma is usually associated with levels >200 mU/L). Macroadenomas of either type (functional or non-functional) may present with mass effect on adjacent structures (e.g. chiasmal compression) or pituitary apoplexy. MRI with and without contrast is the imaging modality of choice. Management of nonfunctioning pituitary adenoma is with elective transsphenoidal surgery if there is evidence of optic chiasm compression (as in this case with suprasellar extension)—otherwise endocrine, ophthalmologic and imaging surveillance is appropriate.

Image with permission from Roser F, Honegger J, Schuhmann MU, Tatagiba MS. Meningiomas, nerve sheath tumors, and pituitary tumors: diagnosis and treatment. Hematol Oncol Clin North Am 2012;26 (4):855-79.

9. **b**—Transsphenoidal debulking followed by stereotactic radiosurgery

There is extensive cavernous sinus involvement hence transsphenoidal surgery alone is unlikely to be sufficient (but will decompress/separate tumour mass from optic nerve), and given the features of a non-functional pituitary adenoma stereotactic radiosurgery is the appropriate next action as medical therapy is unlikely to be of benefit.

Image with permission from Loevner L. Brain Imaging: Case Review Series, 2nd ed. Elsevier, Mosby, 2009.

10. **b**—Hook effect describes spuriously high prolactin levels due to macroprolactin complexes

Prolactinomas are the most common secreting pituitary adenomas and tend to arise laterally within the anterior lobe of the pituitary gland. They may depress the floor of the sella turcica or expand one side of the gland, causing a subtle upwardly convex bulge and contralateral displacement of the infundibulum. Hyperprolactinemia in men interferes with sperm production (infertility) and testosterone production (lethargy, reduced libido, reduced muscle mass), galactorrhea, loss of pubic/axillary hair, and erectile dysfunction (and small gonads in prepubertal boys). In females, hypeprolactinemia reduces estradiol production and this causes irregular menstrual cycles, amenorrhea, galactorrhea and premature menopausal symptoms (does not cause similar symptoms in postmenopausal women). Blood tests show prolactin levels >2000 mU/L (note that hypothyroidism may also cause hyperprolactinemia). Macroprolactin with its longer half-life and biological inert nature needs to be measured, and may cause a spuriously high prolactin level. Equally, depending on the assay used, if prolactin levels are truly very high they may saturate the assay giving a near-normal result (Hook effect). Estrogen containing oral contraceptives can stimulate lactotrophs and cause hyperprolactinemia. The primary treatment of prolactin-secreting microadenomas is medical and the role of imaging in cases of hyperprolactinemia is to assess size and any chiasmal compression. Bromocriptine and cabergoline are both safe options for females in the reproductive age group presenting with a microprolactinoma if they are planning a pregnancy in the near future, and have not been associated with fetal malformation. The therapy can be stopped once pregnancy is confirmed. Dopamine agonists reduce prolactin levels and induce ovulation, hence females started on them are possibly at higher risk of pregnancy and should be given advice regarding contraception at initiation if they do not wish to become pregnant. Management of prolactinomas during pregnancy is challenging as prolactin measurements are unreliable. There is <5% chance of microprolactinoma regrowth and 15-40% chance of macroprolactinoma regrowth during pregnancy. As such, patients need to be kept under close surveillance with periodic formal visual field assessments. Imaging in other secreting pituitary adenomas (TSH, GH, ACTH) is also important to localize the exact position of the tumor for surgical treatment. In particular, given the high morbidity of Cushing's disease if no lesion is found on MRI then inferior petrosal and/or cavernous sinus venous sampling may be necessary to grossly lateralize an adenoma for surgery.

11. **c**—Indications for surgery include a secreting tumor

Due to improvements in imaging there has been a rise in the number of incidental pituitary adenomas discovered on cranial imaging with rates of 5-30% for those <10 mm (microincidentaloma) and 0.1-0.25% for those >10 mm in size (macroincidentaloma). They should be investigated for subclinical disease even if asymptomatic including endocrinological history and examination, anterior pituitary profile, MRI pituitary (if lesion found on CT) and, if clinical visual field defect or evidence of chiasmal compression on imaging, formal visual field testing. If all results are normal, microincidentalomas should be rescanned at

1 year then every 1-2 years for the first 3 years then less frequently after that. Macroincidentalomas should be rescanned at 6 months then at least yearly for the first 3 years. Repeat anterior pituitary hormone profile should only be performed if symptomatic or MRI changes are seen. Indications for surgery include visual field deficit, optic nerve/chiasm compression, ophthalmoplegia, pituitary apoplexy with severely reduced visual acuity or field defect, and evidence of secreting tumor (e.g. Acromegaly, Cushing's disease).

FURTHER READING

Freda PU, Beckers AM, Katznelson L. Pituitary incidentaloma: an endocrine society clinical practice guideline. J Clin Endocrinol Metab 2011;96(4):894-904.

12. **b**—Cabergoline is a dopamine receptor antagonist

Dopamine receptor agonists (e.g. bromocriptine, cabergoline) augment physiological inhibition of prolactin secretion. Octreotide is a somatostain analog used in the treatment of acromegaly is associated with the development of gallstones and reduced gall bladder contractility, but causes >2% tumor reduction in 75% of patients treated. GI side effects are common, and glycemic control also.

13. **c**—Inferior petrosal sinus sampling

This finding is nonspecific and occurs in up to 10% of healthy people. It may or may not be related to Cushing syndrome. The odds are good that the patient has a pituitary tumor, but the MRI findings do not prove this. The MRI is diagnostic only if it shows a large tumor. One option is to proceed directly to pituitary surgery because a patient with abnormal MRI findings has a 90% chance of having an ACTH-secreting pituitary tumor. To achieve more diagnostic certainty, one has to perform bilateral simultaneous inferior petrosal sinus sampling (IPSS) for ACTH levels. Catheters are advanced through the femoral veins into the inferior petrosal sinuses, which drain the pituitary gland, and blood samples are obtained for ACTH levels. If ACTH levels in the petrosal sinuses are significantly higher than those in peripheral samples, the pituitary gland is the source of excessive ACTH. If there is no gradient between petrosal sinus and peripheral levels of ACTH, the patient probably has a carcinoid tumor somewhere. The accuracy of the test is further increased if ACTH responses to injection of exogenous CRH are measured. If sinus sampling is positive for a gradient transsphenoidal surgery (TSS) should be scheduled with an experienced neurosurgeon who is comfortable examining the pituitary for small adenomas. ACTH levels from the right and left petrosal sinuses obtained during the sampling study may tell the neurosurgeon in which side of the pituitary gland the tumor is likely to be found, but this information is not 100% accurate. If IPSS shows no gradient in ACTH levels, start the search for a carcinoid tumor (e.g. lung, adrenal, GI) and treatment as appropriate.

FURTHER READING

Samuels MH. Cushing syndrome. In: McDermott MT (Ed.), Endocrine secrets. Saunders, Elsevier, 2013.

14. **e**—Can cause amenorrhea in females and infertility in males

Cushing's syndrome (hypercortisolism) can present in children and young adults with an increase in body weight, central obesity and growth retardation. In adults, it is associated with mood facies, proximal myopathy, bruising, abdominal striae, oligomenorrhea/amenorrhea in females, impotence in males, infertility, hirsutism, hypertension and diabetes. Adrenal tumors are commoner in children under 10 (neuroblastoma) causing ACTH-independent Cushing's syndrome with signs of virilization. Cushing's disease due to ACTH-secreting pituitary tumor is commoner in older children and adults. In adults, ectopic ACTH production due to lung cancer or carcinoid/neuroendocrine tumor can also occur. Initial screening tests such as 24 h urinary cortisol collection, 9 am and midnight cortisol (loss of diurnal variation; remains high), and overnight (low-dose) dexamethasone suppression test help confirm the diagnosis of hypercortisolism. Second line localization tests aim to differentiate hypercortisolism based on whether it is secondary to increased ACTH secretion (e.g. ACTH-secreting pituitary tumor or ectopic/carcinoid tumor) or not (e.g. adrenal tumor). Third line tests aim to differentiate location of ACTH-dependent hypercortisolism as pituitary (reduces ACTH/cortisol production in response to high-dose dexamethasone; gradient on petrosal sinus sampling) or ectopic tumor (no reduction in ACTH/cortisol secretion in response to high-dose dexamethasone; cortisol rise if CRH stimulation test; no cortisol rise on CRH stimulation; no gradient on petrosal sinus sampling).

15. **b**—Repeat transsphenoidal surgery

Patients with inadequately treated Cushing's syndrome have a markedly increased mortality rate (four- to fivefold above the normal rate), usually from cardiovascular disease or infections. Hypertension, impaired glucose tolerance, dyslipidemia, and visceral obesity all contribute to the excess risk for cardiovascular mortality. This excess mortality normalizes with adequate therapy. If TSS does not cure a patient with Cushing's disease, alternative therapies must be tried because patients with inadequately treated hypercortisolism have increased morbidity and mortality rates. Of the various options after failed surgery, none is ideal. Patients may require repeat pituitary surgery, radiation therapy, medical therapy to block adrenal cortisol secretion (e.g. ketoconazole, metyrapone, mitotane, or etomidate), centrally acting agents that suppress ACTH secretion, and glucocorticoid receptor blocker (mifepristone). Bilateral adrenalectomy can be safely performed via a laparoscopic approach, with low morbidity in experienced hands. However, this procedure leads to lifelong adrenal insufficiency and dependence on exogenous glucocorticoids and mineralocorticoids. The other main drawback is the development of Nelson syndrome in up to 30% of patients after adrenalectomy. Nelson syndrome is the appearance, sometimes years after adrenalectomy, of an aggressive corticotroph pituitary tumor.

16. **a**—Oral glucose tolerance test

Acromegaly is due to excess secretion of GH/IGF-1 and results in coarsening of facial features, increased ring/shoe size, prognathism, macroglossia, widely spaced teeth, enlargement of the extremities and increased sweating. Due to pulsatile release of GH, serum GH levels are rarely helpful—the main test should be random IGF-1 serum level which is useful in diagnosis and monitoring of subsequent treatment. However, a normal IGF-1 level does not exclude acromegaly and an oral glucose tolerance test (OGTT) with measurements of GH remains the gold standard. Failure of oral glucose administration to suppress GH level below 1 ng/mL (or higher sensitivity if <0.4 ng/mL cutoff) is supportive of a diagnosis of acromegaly. In those suspected to have acromegaly, MRI pituitary should be performed.

17. **E**—Opticocarotid recess.

A—planum sphenoidale, B—chiasmatic groove (CG), C—tuberculum sellae, D—optic nerve prominence, E—opticocarotid recess, F—clival recess, G—prominence of the internal carotid artery

The panoramic view provided by the endoscope of the bony prominences and depressions inside the sphenoid sinus allows one to see a sort of "fetal face," where the forehead corresponds to the planum sphenoidale, the eyes to the two opticocarotid recesses, the eyebrows to the two bony protuberances covering the optic nerves, the nose to the sellar floor, and the mouth to the clival indentation, laterally limited by the two paraclival carotid arteries, representing the cheeks.

Image with permission from Laws ER, Lanzino G (Eds.), Transsphenoidal Surgery, Saunders, Elsevier, 2010.

18. **e**—Empirical antibiotics and CT head

CT head should be done initially to exclude development of postoperative hydrocephalus and exclude subdural hematoma formation from intracranial hypotension due to CSF leak. In patients who have a traumatic leak and normal CSF pressure, conservative treatment consists of bed rest with head of bed elevation and lumbar drainage of CSF for 5-10 days. With conservative management, there is a reported risk ranging from 7% to 30% of ascending meningitis. The incidence of spontaneous resolution with conservative management is reported to be 70%. The general consensus among practicing otolaryngologist is that antibiotics should not be used for conservative management unless there is a very large defect with comminuted bone of the skull base as a simple CSF leak carries a 7% infection rate (meningitis, intracranial abscess, cellulitis/abscess, and osteomyelitis) and prophylactic antibiotics have not been shown to decrease the risk of infection. After endoscopic repair, antibiotics are generally recommended for 24-48 h. This is done to cover possible contamination at the time of surgery in a non-sterile field with concomitant sealing of the sterile to non-sterile flushing of an active leak. A reconstructive ladder should be used to help determine the type of repair performed. For simple, small (less than 1 cm) defects, a fat plug harvested from the earlobe or abdomen can be used to plug the defect. The next option includes a simple overlay graft harvested from the nasal floor mucosa, turbinate mucosa, or nasal septum. If a more complex, larger reconstruction is in order, a composite (underlay and overlay) graft can be used consisting of an intracranial underlay of bone or cartilage from nasal septum, auricular cartilage or turbinate bone, and an overlay graft of mucosa (free or pedicled) as above. Local pedicled flaps should include the nasoseptal flap, which is supplied by the posterior nasal septal artery, a terminal branch of the sphenopalatine artery. Additional grafts that can be useful in larger defects include temporal fascia or tensor fascia lata grafts. These grafts are often bolstered in the sinonasal cavity with abdominal fat, a nasoseptal flap or both. In complex situations of extensive defects or poor local tissue, such as in chemoradiated patients, a craniotomy with pericranial flap or free flap reconstruction of the skull base may be necessary. A multitude of studies over the past 20 years have shown high success rates of primary repair around 90%, and secondary repair around 97%. These success rates compare favorably to traditional craniotomy approaches with reported success rates between 70% and 80% that carry a higher morbidity profile.

FURTHER READING

Scholes MA. ENT Secrets, 4th ed. Elsevier, 2016.

ANSWERS 19–37

Additional answers 19–37 available on ExpertConsult.com

EMI ANSWERS

38. 1—f, Gonadotropin-secreting adenoma. This a rare tumor presenting with ovarian cysts and menstrual abnormalities, high or normal estradiol and usually suppressed LH due to secretion of FSH by the pituitary adenoma. Treatment is surgery. 2—m, TSH-secreting tumor (thyrotropinoma, TSHoma). Inappropriately high or normal TSH in the presence of high free T3 and T4 levels is suggestive of either TSH-secreting tumor or thyroid hormone resistance syndromes. TSH-secreting tumors represent 0.5-1% of pituitary adenomas and present with features of thyrotoxicosis and goiter, and is distinguished from hormone resistance by its alpha-subunit to TSH ratio >1 (if >5.7 is diagnostic), presence of pituitary adenoma on MRI, lack of TSH response to TRH stimulation testing and lack of a family history of thyroid problems. Surgery is the treatment of choice, but octreotide may be used in non-surgical candidates or surgical failure. 3—k, Optic pathway glioma. Increased association with NF-1.

39. 1—k, Primary adrenal insufficiency (Addison's disease). Short synacthen tests can demonstrate adrenal insufficiency (lack of cortisol production in response to synthetic ACTH). Long synacthen tests differentiate between primary causes (e.g. adrenal infarction) which fail to respond even after several doses, compared to secondary causes (e.g. non-functioning adenoma causing reduced ACTH release) which start to produce cortisol after several doses. 2—d, Diabetes insipidus. 3—h, Nelson-Salassi syndrome. When bilateral adrenalectomy is performed for ACTH-secreting pituitary adenoma (Cushing's disease) to treat the associated hypercortisolism, loss of negative cortisol feedback to hypothalamus causes increased secretion of corticotropin releasing hormone and growth of pituitary tumors. This was seen before the advent of transsphenoidal surgery and radiotherapy, when adrenalectomy was more commonly performed.

40. 1—k, Foramen rotundum; 2—d, Foramen lacerum, 2—h, Internal auditory meatus

a—Lesser, greater wings of sphenoid bone, b—Carotid groove, c—Pituitary fossa, d—Foramen lacerum, e—Condylar fossa (mandibular), f—Facial hiatus, g—Temporal bone, h—Internal auditory meatus, i—Optic canal, j—Superior orbital Fissure, k—Foramen rotundum, l—Foramen ovale, m—Foramen spinosum, n—Foramen jugulare, o—Hypoglossal Canal.

Image with permission from Flint PW (Eds.), Cummings Otolaryngology, 6th ed. Saunders, Elsevier, 2015.

Contents of Skull Base Foramina

Skull Base Foramina	Contents
Cribiform plate	CN I, anterior ethmoidal artery (branch of ophthalmic artery)
Opitc canal	CN II, ophthalmic artery (branch of ICA), meninges, optic nerve sheath
Superior orbital fissure	Middle part: nasociliary nerve (CN V1 branch), oculomotor nerve (III), abducens nerve (CN VI) Lateral part: Trochlear nerve (CN IV), frontal nerve (V1), lacrimal nerve (V1), orbital branch of medial meningeal artery, superior ophthalmic vein

Continued on following page

Contents of Skull Base Foramina (Continued)

Skull Base Foramina	Contents
Foramen rotundum	Maxillary nerve (CNV2)
Foramen ovale	Mandibular nerve (CNV3), emissary vein (cavernous sinus to pterygoid plexus)
Foramen lacerum	Connective tissue, meningeal branches of ascending pharyngeal artery, and emissary vein (cavernous sinus to pterygoid plexus). Greater petrosal nerve (VII) joins with deep petrosal nerve to form vidian nerve (of the pterygoid canal). Lacerum segment of ICA courses above as it exits the carotid canal.
Foramen spinosum	Meningeal branch of CN V3, medial meningeal artery (branch of maxillary artery)
Carotid canal	Petrous ICA, internal carotid venous and sympathetic plexus
Internal acoustic meatus	Facial nerve (VII), vestibulocochlear (VIII): superior vestibular, inferior vestibular, cochlear nerve, labyrinthine artery (branch of basilar artery), labyrinthine veins
Jugular foramen	Rostromedial: Inferior petrosal sinus, meningeal branch of ascending pharyngeal artery Middle part: Cranial nerves IX, X, XI Caudolateral: Internal jugular vein, meningeal branch of occipital artery, meningeal branch of X
Hypoglossal canal	Hypoglossal nerve (XII) and venous plexus
Foramen magnum	Meninges, marginal sinus, vertebral arteries, anterior spinal artery, medulla oblongata/ spinal cord, spinal accessory nerve (XI)

41. 1—f, Retrolabyrinthine; 2—h, Transcochlear

Serviceable hearing includes a pure tone average threshold better than 50 dB and/or speech discrimination greater than 50% (50/50 rule), and may favor the use of hearing-sparing approaches depending on tumor size and location (e.g. middle fossa, retrosigmoid, retrolabyrinthine). Use of other approaches sacrifices hearing, hence other criteria such as surgical exposure gained and risk of facial nerve injury become prime considerations.

Surgical Approaches to the Cerebellopontine Angle (CPA)

Approach	Rationale	Indications	Contraindications
Retrosigmoid craniotomy	Easy and rapid access to the CPA. Extended retrosigmoid approach permits access ventral to the brainstem and near the tentorium (safe alternative to more radical cranial base approaches).	Extra-axial lesions in the CPA and intra-axial lesions arising along the petrosal surface of the cerebellum, cerebellar peduncles, or brainstem.	Patients must have patent contralateral transverse and sigmoid sinuses before manipulation of the sinuses ipsilateral to the approach.
Translabyrinthine	Sacrificing the labyrinth (i.e. hearing) to give direct access to the internal auditory canal (IAC) and cerebellopontine angle without cerebellar retraction Exposure of the posterior fossa and 320-degree exposure of the IAC circumference.	Indications include removal of CPA lesions with preoperative unserviceable hearing, regardless of lesion size.	Lesions extending anteriorly to prepontine cistern Ipsilateral chronic otitis media (relative) Only hearing ear

Continued

Surgical Approaches to the Cerebellopontine Angle (CPA) (Continued)

Approach	Rationale	Indications	Contraindications
Transcochlear	Extension of the translabyrinthine approach anteriorly, which includes drilling the posterior and superior external auditory canal and sacrificing middle ear structures and inner ear (cochlea), and rerouting the facial nerve to provide access to the anterior cerebellopontine angle, petrous apex, and ventral brainstem.	CPA tumors with anterior extension and unserviceable hearing. Extensive petrous apex lesions with inner ear compromise (e.g. petrous apex cholesteatomas). Petroclival lesion with extension ventral to the brainstem. Temporal bone and clival lesions with extension to the posterior fossa (e.g. chordomas)	Ipsilateral chronic otitis media (relative) Only hearing ear (relative)
Retrolabyrinthine approach	The retrolabyrinthine approach is a hearing-preserving presigmoid approach that uses a mastoidectomy and skeletonization of the sigmoid sinus to expose the presigmoid dura between the labyrinth (semicircular canals) and sigmoid sinus.	Expose widely the posterior petrous face and cisternal portions of cranial nerves VII and VIII with a minimal degree of cerebellar retraction identify and expose the superior petrosal sinus, as a first step for division of the tentorium	This approach is unable to access the internal auditory canal or petrous apex directly because of the interposition of the labyrinthine and cochlear structures between the surgeon and these regions.
Transotic approach	The objective of this approach is to obtain a direct lateral exposure and the widest possible access to the CPA through the medial wall of the temporal bone, from the superior petrosal sinus to the jugular bulb, and from the internal carotid artery to the sigmoid sinus. The tympanic and mastoid portions of the fallopian canal are left in situ. This transtemporal access is achieved at the expense of bony exenteration, rather than cerebellar retraction.	CPA or the temporal bone lesions with invasion of the IAC or the otic capsule in patients with *no* serviceable hearing. In this clinical setting, the transotic approach offers the best possible exposure for tumor extirpation and preservation of facial nerve with minimal morbidity.	
Middle cranial fossa approach	a largely extradural approach to the bony structures that make up the floor of the middle fossa.	Convex floor of the middle fossa is the most straightforward region to access with this approach, this approach is commonly the starting point for anterior transpetrosal approaches to the internal auditory canal (IAC) or petroclival junction.	Tumors with significant posterior fossa extension Tumors caudal to the IAC

CHAPTER 25

CRANIAL INFECTION

SINGLE BEST ANSWER (SBA) QUESTIONS

1. A 35-year-old transplant patient develops headache, neck stiffness, photophobia and fever. Cerebrospinal fluid (CSF) testing with India ink stain reveals a fungal infection. Which one of the following is the cause of this patient's fungal meningitis?
   a. *Aspergillus*
   b. *Blastomyces*
   c. *Candida*
   d. *Cryptococcus*
   e. *Mucor*

2. An 82-year-old previously healthy female with a recent history of upper respiratory tract infection presents with generalized weakness, headache, and blurry vision. Other symptoms include fever, vomiting and eye pain on movement with mild photosensitivity. She has no drug allergies. Examination findings include temperature of 102.5 °F (39.1 °C), nuchal rigidity, and drowsiness GCS is E3V4M5. Her blood pressure is 82/56 and she is tachycardic, with only a transient response to fluid challenge. Which one of the following is the next most appropriate action in this case?
   a. Cranial imaging then perform a lumbar puncture
   b. Give the patient a prescription for oral co-amoxiclav (Augmentin)
   c. Immediately start intravenous antibiotics
   d. Immediately start oral dexamethasone
   e. Obtain CSF and blood cultures and observe the patient in high dependency unit the results come back

3. A 9-year-old is brought into the emergency room lethargic with a stiff neck and fever. Despite aggressive therapy in the ITU the child dies. Postmortem evaluation reveals that the child had primary amoebic meningoencephalitis. This condition is usually acquired through which one of the following means?
   a. Animal bites
   b. Drinking contaminated water
   c. Eating contaminated meat
   d. Freshwater swimming
   e. IV drug abuse

4. A 27-year-old man presents to his primary care doctor with a low-grade fever, headache, and neck stiffness, which have become more bothersome over the past 1-2 weeks. Serum is positive for *Borrelia burgdorferi* IgM. CSF polymerase chain reaction (PCR) is also positive for this organism. The cranial nerve most commonly affected in this disease is most likely?
   a. Abducens nerve
   b. Facial nerve
   c. Glossopharyngeal nerve
   d. Oculomotor nerve
   e. Trigeminal nerve

5. An 11-year-old girl is bitten on her upper arm by a stray dog while on holiday in South America. Two weeks later she develops throat spasms and confusion. Which one of the following is most accurate regarding the causative virus?
   a. Cause of death is usually dehydration
   b. Commonly causes progression to quadriplegia in 80%
   c. Inducing an artificial coma obviates the need for post-exposure prophylaxis
   d. Post-exposure prophylaxis consists of a vaccine
   e. Spreads retrogradely in peripheral nerves

6. A 64-year-old female presents with progressive cognitive impairment, tremors, gait ataxia, and myoclonic jerks over the course of 6 months. There is no relevant family history. MRI of the head reveals a subtle increase in T2 signal in the basal ganglia bilaterally. EEG reveals disorganized background activity with periodic sharp-wave discharges that occur repetitively at 1-s intervals and extend over both sides of the head. There was also evidence of diffuse slowing and triphasic waves. The clinical picture is most consistent with which one of the following?
   a. Alzheimer's dementia
   b. Friedreich's ataxia
   c. Multi-infarct dementia
   d. Parkinson's disease
   e. Spongiform encephalopathy

7. An 85-year-old woman has 3 days of gradually worsening fever and headache. She then develops blurry vision and a stiff neck. MRI with contrast has an enhancement pattern suggesting rhombencephalitis. CSF shows a mild pleocytosis with no organisms. All blood and CSF cultures are negative. Which one of the following is the most likely organism responsible for the patient's condition?
   a. *Borrelia burgdorferi*
   b. *E. coli*
   c. HTLV-1
   d. *Listeria monocytogenes*
   e. MRSA

8. A 75-year-old left-handed woman presented to the emergency room with what at first was thought to be a stroke. There is no clear history of recent infection. MRI head was performed and T1+gadolinium, DWI and ADC map are shown. Which one of the following is the most appropriate next step?

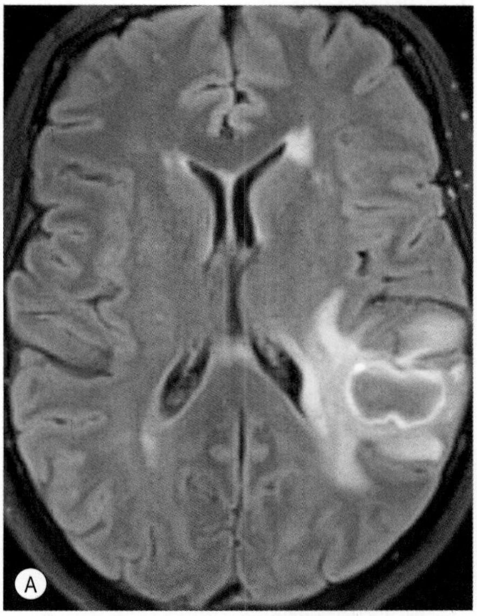

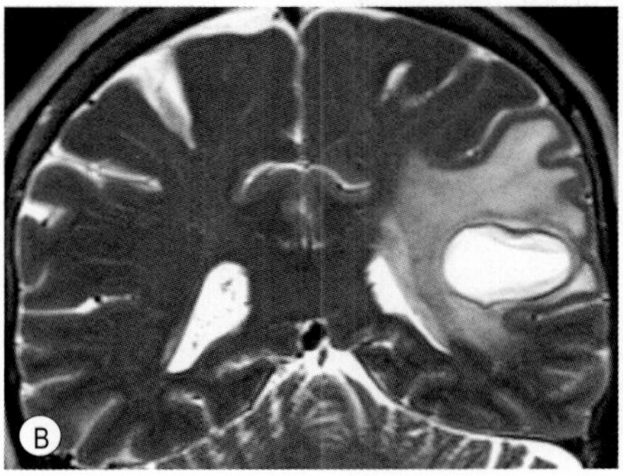

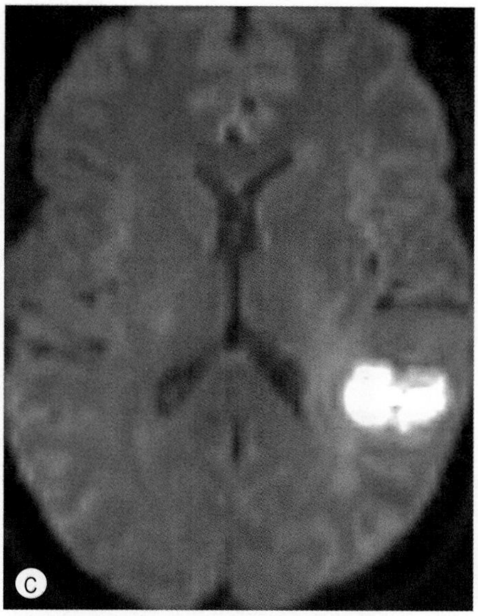

   a. Cerebral angiogram
   b. Image guided attempted gross total resection
   c. Lumbar puncture and oligoclonal bands
   d. Stereotactic biopsy
   e. Stereotactic needle aspiration

9. During formation of an abscess capsule, when does necrosis begin?
   a. Days 1-3
   b. Days 4-9
   c. Days 10-13
   d. Days 14-20
   e. Day 21 onwards

10. A 40-year-old ex-IV drug abuser presents to the emergency room with a seizure. CT head with contrast shows 3 cm diameter ring enhancing lesion periventricular location. MRI is performed and the lesion is bright on DWI and dark on ADC map. Which one of the following would be the appropriate next step in management?
   a. Blood cultures and external ventricular drain then start intravenous antibiotics
   b. Craniotomy and excision of abscess then start intravenous antibiotics
   c. Image-guided aspiration of abscess then start intravenous antibiotics
   d. Endoscopic aspiration and irrigation
   e. Real-time ultrasound-guided excision of abscess and start intravenous antibiotics

11. A 37-year-old HIV positive male presents with headache, confusion, new right-sided weakness progressing over the previous week. He has been on highly active retroviral therapy for the last 10 years and not had any problems. On examination, his responses are slow and he has some difficulty sustaining attention. He has a right hemiparesis with increased reflexes on the right. FBC, U+E and CRP are normal. T1 contrast MRI is shown. Which one of the following organisms is the most likely cause?

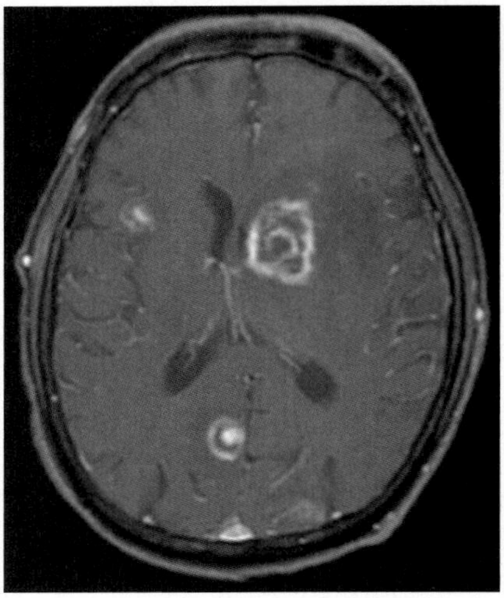

a. *Cryptococcus neoformans*
b. *Herpes zoster*
c. *Pneumocystic jerovecii*
d. *Toxoplasma gondii*
e. *Tuberculosis*

12. A 45-year-old renal transplant patient presents with a 3-week history of worsening right headache, ear pain, and pyrexia. His medications include tacrolimus and cyclosporin. He is diagnosed with malignant fungal otitis externa and secondary osteomyelitis of the skull base. Which one of the following organisms is most likely?
a. *Actinomyces*
b. *Aspergillus*
c. *Candida*
d. *Cryptococcus neoformans*
e. *Naegleria fowleri*

13. A 67-year-old with chronic sinusitis presents with severe frontal headache and change in smell. T1-gadolinium enhanced MRI head is shown. Which one of the following is most likely?

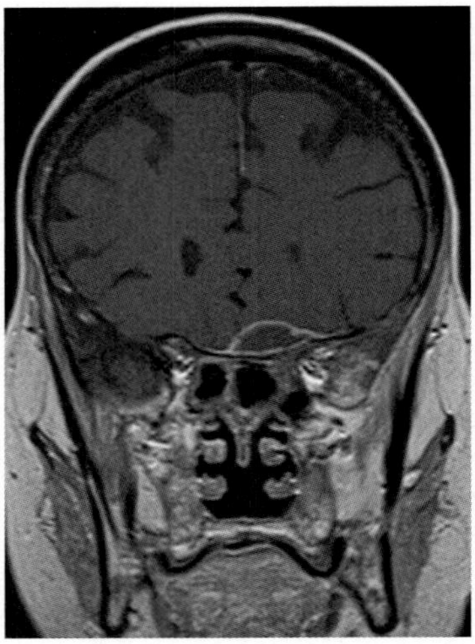

a. *Basal meningitis*
b. *Cerebral abscess*
c. *Epidural abscess*
d. Resolving hematoma
e. *Subdural abscess*

14. A 29-year-old ex-IVDU who previously underwent aspiration of a brain abscess and prolonged inpatient antibiotic course re-presents after several generalized tonic-clonic seizures progressing into status epilepticus. Contrast CT head is shown. What is the next appropriate action?

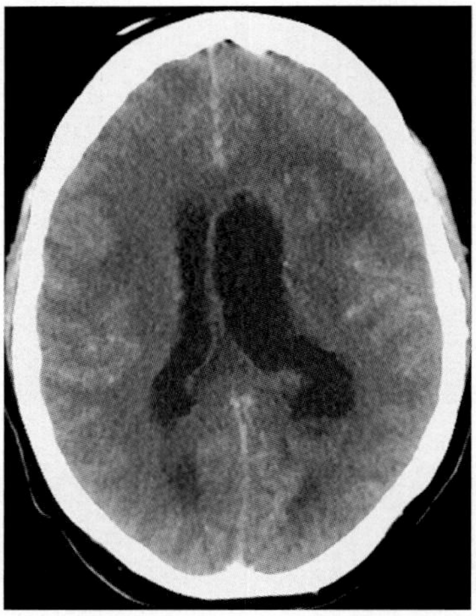

a. Cerebral angiogram
b. Decompressive craniectomy
c. External ventricular drain
d. Lumbar drain
e. Palliative care

15. A 27-year-old immigrant from South America presents with a generalized seizure. After awakening, he relates that he has had two or three episodes of unexplained loss of consciousness in the past 2 years. He has otherwise been healthy and worked as a farmer. His examination is normal. MRI head was performed and T2 and T1+GAD images are shown. What is the most likely organism?

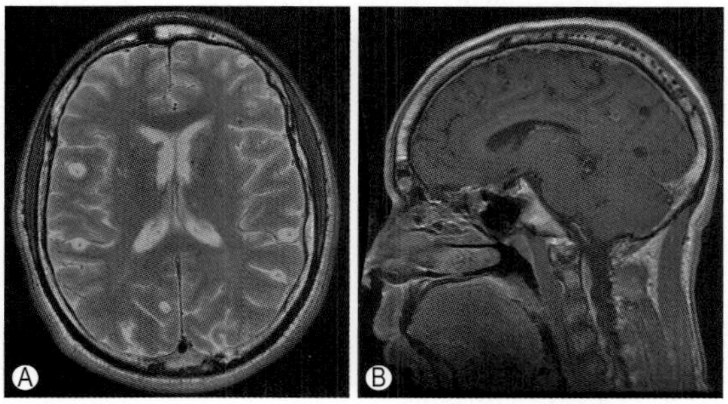

a. Histoplasma
b. *Mucor*
c. *Shistosoma mansonii*
d. *Taenia solium*
e. *Toxoplasma gondii*

16. A 35-year-old woman has progressive numbness of the right arm and difficulty seeing objects in the right visual field. She is known to be HIV positive, but has not consistently taken medications in the past. On examination, she appears healthy, but has a right homonymous hemianopsia and decreased sensory perception in her right upper extremity and face. Her CD4 count is 75 cells per μL, and her MRI is consistent with a demyelinating lesion of the left parieto-occipital area. CSF PCR for JC virus is positive. Which one of the following is the most appropriate treatment in this case?

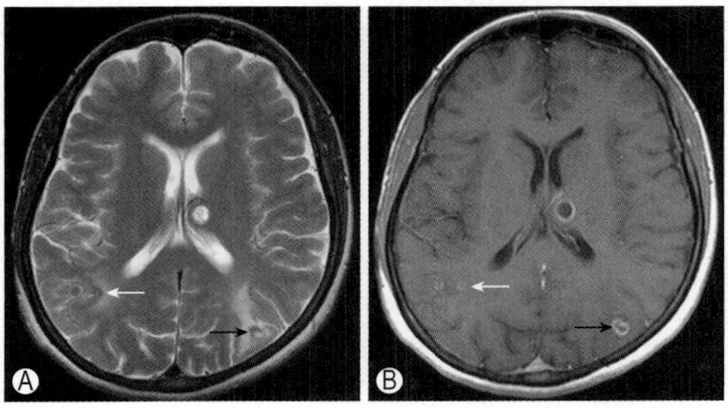

a. Amphotericin B
b. Fluconazole
c. Highly active antiretroviral therapy (HAART)
d. Intravenous acyclovir
e. Intravenous rifampicin

17. A 52-year-old woman with acquired immune deficiency syndrome (AIDS) presents to the emergency room with mild left hemiparesis and altered mental status. A CT scan reveals several ring-enhancing lesions with minimal mass effect. Which one of the following is the best next step in management?
a. Get a cerebral angiogram
b. Order a ventricular CSF aspiration
c. Perform a lumbar puncture and include CSF for Epstein-Barr virus (EBV) PCR in tests ordered
d. Stop all antiretroviral therapy
e. Treat with intravenous acyclovir

18. A 12-year-old boy has left body weakness. A brain magnetic resonance imaging (MRI) scan reveals a polycystic lesion. Which one of the following is most likely?

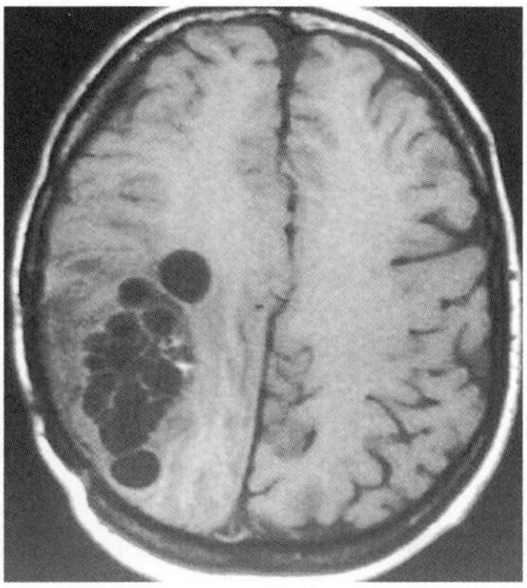

a. *Diphyllobothrium latum*
b. *Echinococcus*
c. *Schistosoma hematobium*
d. *Schistosoma japonicum*
e. *Taenia solium*

QUESTIONS 19–22

Additional questions 19–22 available on ExpertConsult.com

EXTENDED MATCHING ITEM (EMI) QUESTIONS

23. **Intracerebral abscess:**
    a. *Actinomyces*
    b. *Aspergillus*
    c. *Bacillus*
    d. *Candida*
    e. *E. coli*
    f. *Klebsiella*
    g. *Listeria monocytogenes*
    h. *Nocardia*
    i. *Pseudomonas*
    j. *Propionibacterium*
    k. *Staphylococcus aureus*
    l. *Toxoplasma gondii*
    m. *Viridans streptococci*

For each of the following descriptions, select the most appropriate answers from the list above. Each answer may be used once, more than once or not at all.

1. Commonest cause of brain abscess post-neurosurgery
2. Brain abscess secondary to otitis externa
3. Commonest cause of pyogenic brain abscesses

24. **Viral encephalitis:**
    a. *Cytomegalovirus*
    b. Enterovirus
    c. Epstein Barr Virus
    d. Herpes simplex virus
    e. HIV
    f. Human herpes virus 6
    g. JC virus
    h. Measles
    i. Mumps
    j. Rabies virus
    k. Varicella zoster virus

For each of the following descriptions, select the most appropriate answers from the list above. Each answer may be used once, more than once or not at all.

1. A 35-year-old intravenous drug abuser presents with inability to control his left hand. He reports that at times he will button his shirt with his right hand, only to find that his left hand is unbuttoning the shirt against his control. He has a history of thrush. He is alert and oriented. MRI shows an increased T2 signal affecting the subcortical white matter of the right parietal lobe without enhancement.
2. A 21-year-old male presents with 3 days of headaches and fever, followed by hallucinations, speech disturbance, and lethargy. On examination, he has mild left hemiparesis. MRI shows abnormal signal, with enhancement, in the right anterior temporal lobe.
3. An 8-year-old girl shows rapidly deteriorating school performance and personality change over several weeks, then experiences a generalized tonic-clonic seizure. A neurologist examining the child discovers chorioretinitis, ataxia, and bilateral upper motor neuron signs. Her EEG exhibits periodic bursts of high-voltage slow waves, followed by recurrent periods of burst suppression. CSF shows an increased γ-globulin fraction.

25. **Infections affecting the CNS:**
    a. Amoebiasis
    b. Aspegillosus
    c. Bartonella hensae
    d. Candidiasis
    e. Cryptococcosis
    f. Echinococcosis
    g. Leptospirosis
    h. Neurocystercercosis
    i. Tabes dorsalis
    j. Toxoplasma
    k. Whipple disease

For each of the following descriptions, select the most appropriate answers from the list above. Each answer may be used once, more than once or not at all.

1. A 50-year-old presents with a several-month history of difficulty with bladder control, an unsteady gait, and pain in his legs. The pain in his legs is sharp, stabbing, and paroxysmal. He has no history or tests suggestive of diabetes. He has absent deep tendon reflexes in his legs, markedly impaired vibration sense in his feet, and a positive Romberg sign. He has no cerebellar signs or weakness.
2. A 29-year-old HIV positive female pet store worker presents with 2 days of confusion and seizures, which progressed to status epilepticus. General examination discloses epitrochlear lymphadenopathy. CSF analysis is normal. MRI brain is unremarkable.
3. A 54-year-old woman presents with 6 months of progressive memory loss. She has limited vertical eye movements, and on examination, she has rhythmic, synchronous grimacing and eye closure movements. Jejunal biopsy reveals periodic acid-Schiff (PAS)-positive cells.

SBA ANSWERS

1. **d**—*Cryptococcus*

Cryptococcosis is usually acquired through the lungs and spreads to the CNS through the bloodstream. In the CNS, it may produce either a meningitis or a meningoencephalitis. Other examples include histoplasma, and candida (very rare and usually in premature babies). Fungal CNS infections occur in immunodeficiency states (e.g. AIDS, or immunosuppressive drugs, lymphoproliferative disorders). *Aspergillus*, *Candida*, *Mucor*, and *Rhizopus* can also cause CNS fungal infections, but rarely meningitis. *Aspergillus* tends to cause abscesses in immunocompromised individuals, and *Mucor* affects mostly diabetics.

2. **c**—Immediately start intravenous antibiotics

This patient has presented with probable meningitis, but with evidence of septic shock hence antibiotics should be administered at the resuscitation stage after taking blood cultures. Cranial imaging should be performed before a lumbar puncture (at least when no previous imaging is available), but delaying antibiotics until this has all been done could be catastrophic.

3. **d**—Freshwater swimming

Primary amoebic meningoencephalitis (PAM) is caused by *Naegleria fowleri* found in warm bodies of freshwater, and although rare is nearly always fatal. The parasites enter the nervous system through the cribriform plate at the perforations for the olfactory nerves.

4. **b**—Facial nerve

Facial weakness may be the only neurological sign of Lyme disease, and may be bilateral. The neurological deficits usually appear weeks after the initial rash. The facial palsy or optic neuritis that develops with CNS disease is characteristically associated with meningitis. *B. burgdorferi* is a spirochete usually transmitted to humans through tick bites. Another feature is erythema chronicum migrans, an expanding reddish discoloration of the skin that spreads away from the site of the bite as a ring of erythema; evolving over 3-4 weeks then spontaneously clearing. If there is meningeal involvement, high-dose intravenous antibiotics is given for 10-14 days.

5. **e**—Spreads retrogradely in peripheral nerves

Rabies virus is usually spread through the saliva of an infected animal (e.g. dogs, bats, skunks, foxes, and raccoons). After introduction of the virus, the incubation period until fulminant infection appears extends from a few days to over 1 year, but usually ranges from 1 to 2 months. Bites of the head and face carry the greatest risk of causing fatal disease. Early after exposure, the patient will often complain of pain or paresthesias at the site of the animal bite. Animals transmitting the virus include. Furious form (80%) is commonly associated with hydrophobia, where viral multiplication in the salivary glands results in painful spasms of throat/larynx, especially when saliva production is increased associated with drinking or the thought of it. Dehydration is no longer likely because intravenous fluids can be given to completely replace what the hydrophobic patient cannot consume by mouth. Other complications of rabies include a paralytic form of the disease that progresses to quadriplegia (dumb rabies) in 20% of patients. With the classic form of the disease, the patient will also exhibit intermittent hyperactivity. Post-exposure prophylaxis consists of a single dose of rabies immunoglobulin and 3-4 doses of rabies vaccine. Patients have also been treated by inducing a coma (Milwalkee protocol) with some success even without post-exposure prophylaxis.

6. **e**—Spongiform encephalopathy

The clinical, EEG and MRI findings are typical of a spongiform encephalopathy most probably due to Creutzfeldt-Jakob disease. This prion disease can be transmitted via infected nervous system tissue, including dura mater grafts, and occasionally via growth hormone preparations acquired from cadaver pituitary glands. CSF is usually normal, but may show slightly elevated protein, increased IgG, oligoclonal bands, and may contain a specific protein (14-3-3 proteinase inhibitor). Vascular causes are unlikely given the gradual deterioration and imaging findings. Friedreich disease may produce some dementia, but it is not a prominent part of the clinical deterioration and usually affects younger patients.

7. **d**—Listeria monocytogenes

The presentation is highly suggestive of *Listeria monocytogenes* meningitis. This infection commonly develops in renal transplant recipients, patients with chronic renal disease, immunosuppressed persons, and occasionally in otherwise unimpaired persons. It may also affect neonates. This type of meningitis is not usually seen in older children. It may on occasion lead to intracerebral abscess formation. Third-generation cephalosporins are inactive against *Listeria*, and ampicillin and gentamicin are recommended therapy. Neither ampicillin nor penicillin alone is bactericidal.

8. **e**—Stereotactic needle aspiration

Brain abscess are commonly due to hematological (e.g. pneumonia, endocarditis, dental work) or direct local spread of infection (e.g. mastoiditis, chronic otitis). They usually start from a microscopic focus of infection at the gray-white matter junction and takes the following course: early cerebritis 1-3 days, late cerebritis 4-9 days, early capsule 10-13 days, late capsule >14 days. As the infection develops, a cerebritis appears, and subsequently this focus of infection becomes necrotic and liquefies. Around the enlarging abscess, there is usually a disproportionately large area of edema. Mature abscess collagen capsule thinner on ventricular side, presence of dimple or small evagination for ring enhancing lesion should suspect abscess but this is not always distinguishable. Patient commonly present with headache, seizures, and focal neurological deficit. Streptococcal bacteria occur in more than half of all brain abscesses; *Staphylococcus aureus* most often occurs in patients who have had penetrating head wounds or have undergone neurosurgical procedures. Enteric bacteria (eg, *Escherichia coli*, *Proteus*, and *Pseudomonas*) account for twice as many abscesses as *S. aureus*. The important differentials of a ring enhancing brain lesion include primary tumor, metastasis, and abscess (although other causes are demyelination, maturing hematoma, and radiation necrosis). Due to the high mortality associated with intraventricular rupture of a brain abscess, emergency MRI should be performed to determine if the lesion is diffusion restricting (bright on DWI, dark on ADC) and thus likely to require emergency neurosurgical drainage. Although uncommon, diffusion restriction has been reported in metastases and glioblastomas and other modalities such as dynamic contrast-enhanced perfusion MRI may help distinguish between brain abscess and tumor; abscesses have a lower relative cerebral blood volume in their enhancing rim than gliomas.

Image with permission from Adam A, et al. (Eds.), Grainger & Allison's Diagnostic Radiology, 6th ed., Elsevier, Churchill Livingstone, 2014.

9. **b**—Days 4-9

Early cerebritis (days 1-3) is a poorly circumscribed lesion characterized by acute inflammation and cerebral edema associated with bacterial invasion. Later (days 4-9), the zone of cerebritis expands, and necrosis develops, with pus forming at the center of the lesion. CT scanning reveals some ring enhancement with diffusion of contrast material into the necrotic center. The early capsule stage (days 10-13) demonstrates the establishment and maturation of a well-formed collagenous capsule associated with a reduction in the degree of cerebritis and some regression in the local edema. At the late capsule stage (day 14 and beyond), there is continued maturation of a thick capsule with extracapsular gliosis and dense ring enhancement with little contrast diffusion on CT scan. Capsule formation and ring enhancement on imaging studies are generally thinner and less complete on the ventricular side of the abscess. This situation is probably related to the relatively poor vascularity of the deep white matter and reduced migration of fibroblasts into the area. This thinner area of capsule predisposes to ventricular rupture of the abscess.

10. **c**—Image-guided aspiration of abscess then start intravenous antibiotics

Image-guided craniotomy for excision of brain abscess with its capsule has a lower recurrence rate compared to aspiration methods. Excision of brain abscesses is useful in: large (more than 2.5 cm) superficial abscesses, multi-loculated abscesses, failure of resolution after several aspirations; some posterior fossa lesions; some fungal abscesses; post-traumatic abscesses with retained bone fragments or foreign bodies; and gas-containing abscesses, usually signifying the presence of an associated CSF fistula. For surgical excision of a brain abscess that has failed to respond to aspiration and antimicrobial therapy or is in a particularly dangerous location, such as a posterior fossa abscess associated with edema, mass effect, and impending or actual obstructive hydrocephalus, image-guided craniotomy is favored to excise the lesion, relieve the mass effect on the brain stem, and reduce the chances of recurrence. Excision is not the procedure of choice in the cerebritis stage or in deep-seated brain abscesses, especially in eloquent areas. During the stage of cerebritis, antimicrobials are used with serial neurologic examinations and imaging studies to guide therapy. In most other settings, however, surgical intervention is undertaken. In the obtunded patient with a severe neurologic deficit and an encapsulated lesion, surgery for diagnosis and decompression is carried out emergently. If multiple lesions are discovered, those greater than 2.5 cm in diameter should be aspirated. If all lesions are less than 2.5 cm and do not exert mass effect, the largest or most accessible one should be aspirated for culture.

11. **d**—*Toxoplasma gondii*

The timing of this presentation suggests that he has now developed AIDS. While fungal abscesses develop with unusual frequency in patients with AIDS, *T. gondii* is considerably more common than fungi as the cause of abscess formation. Cerebral toxoplasmosis usually presents as multiple ring-enhancing lesions in the basal ganglia, thalamus, or corticomedullary junction. Note the "eccentric target sign," which is shown best in the right parahippocampal lesion. Although this sign is not sensitive, it is fairly specific for toxoplasmosis. The combination of sulfadiazine and pyrimethamine is proper treatment for *T. gondii* infection. Neurosurgical drainage of the lesions is usually not indicated. The fungi that do produce abscesses in persons with AIDS are most often *Cryptococcus*, *Candida*, *Mucor*, and *Aspergillus*. *Tuberculosis meningitis* and abscesses are also common in immunocompromised individuals.

Image with permission from Aiken AH. Central nervous system infection. Neuroimaging Clin N Am 2010;20 (4):557-80.

12. **b**—*Aspergillus*

Fungal otitis exerna is usually caused by *Aspergillus* (black exudate), followed by *Candida* (cheesy white exudate) and *Actinomyces*. Although *Aspergillus* is the most common cause of fungal abscesses, it is a relatively uncommon cause of fungal meningitis or meningoencephalitis.

13. **c**—Epidural abscess

There is left subfrontal epidural fluid collection surrounded by an enhancing rim of thickened dura, which differentiates cranial epidural abscess from a sterile collection. They arise between the skull and the dura, usually in the frontal region, as a result of contiguous spread of infections from adjacent structures, such as the paranasal sinuses or the mastoid cells. It is associated with paranasal sinusitis, cranial osteomyelitis, or head trauma or occurs post-surgery. Risk factors for intracranial epidural abscess include prior craniotomy, head injury, sinusitis, otitis media, and mastoiditis. The bacteriology of these lesions is analogous to that of brain abscess. Generally, the epidural abscess is an indolent lesion when compared to subdural empyema. Neurologic symptoms and complications are rare, because the dura mater protects the brain parenchyma, and the tight adherence of the dura to the skull limits the spread. The most common presenting symptoms are fever, headache, and neurologic signs. Untreated, this parameningeal focus can extend intracranially and involve the dural venous sinuses, resulting in septic thrombophlebitis. The treatment consists of antibiotic therapy, usually in combination with surgical drainage to prevent progression to subdural empyema. Drainage of the epidural abscess can be done either by a minimally invasive approach or by a craniotomy with removal of infected bone. A higher rate of recurrence was reported after burr hole drainage. In preceding sinusitis, a combination of neurosurgical and ENT approaches are needed.

Image with permission from Adam A, et al. (Eds.), Grainger & Allison's Diagnostic Radiology, 6th ed., Elsevier, Churchill Livingstone, 2014.

14. **c**—External ventricular drain

Axial CT shows dilated lateral ventricles that contain intermediate attenuation debris suggestive of pyogenic ventriculitis, with a rim of low-attenuation interstitial edema surrounding the ventricles. The intraventricular rupture of a brain abscess occurs with progressive growth of the lesion. As the pus increases, the abscess expands toward the ventricle and may rupture, resulting in the sudden, catastrophic deterioration of the patient. The diagnosis is confirmed by the presence of hydrocephalus and enhancement of the ventricular walls. Immediate ventricular drainage, intraventricular instillation of antibiotics, evacuation of the remaining abscess, and systemic antibiotic therapy are still associated with a management mortality rate of greater than 80%

Image with permission from Adam A, et al. (Eds.), Grainger & Allison's Diagnostic Radiology, 6th ed., Elsevier, Churchill Livingstone, 2014.

15. **d**—*Taenia solium*

MRI shows extensive parenchymal and subarachnoid cysticercosis. Most of the lesions are in the vesicular stage showing thin-walled cysts with little or no enhancement and a scolex (worm head) in the center of the cyst. Cysticercosis is produced by the larval form (cysticercus) of the pork tapeworm, *Taenia solium*. This is the most common neurological infection throughout the world, occurring most commonly in South America, Southeast Asia, and Africa. It is transmitted by fecal-oral contact; tapeworm eggs hatch in the human GI tract, invade the bowel mucosa, and migrate throughout the body, particularly into CNS, muscle, eye, and subcutaneous tissues. Cysticercal infection of muscles produces a nonspecific myositis. Brain involvement may lead to seizures. The lesions in the brain may calcify and often appear as multiple small cysts spread throughout the cerebrum. Treatment of neurocysticercosis depends on whether the cyst is dead (antiseizure medication) or viable. Viable cysts in the presence of vasculitis/arachnoiditis/encephalitis, immunosuppressant therapy is usually given before anticystercal drugs (albendazole and praziquantel). Neurosurgical management may be indicated when intraventricular or racemose cysts cause hydrocephalus.

Image with permission from Adam A, et al. (Eds.), Grainger & Allison's Diagnostic Radiology, 6th ed., Elsevier, Churchill Livingstone, 2014.

16. **c**—Highly active antiretroviral therapy (HAART)

Progressive multifocal leukoencephalopathy is caused by the JC virus, which is a double-stranded DNA virus transmitted via respiratory droplets. MRI demonstrates widespread hyperintense signal change in the left corona radiate with typical involvement of the subcortical U fibers, and DWI shows a hyperintense edge of the lesion medially reflecting zones of active demyelination. The prognosis is poor, but HAART has been known to be effective in improving survival.

Image with permission from Adam A, et al. (Eds.), Grainger & Allison's Diagnostic Radiology, 6th ed., Elsevier, Churchill Livingstone, 2014.

17. **c**—Perform a lumbar puncture and include CSF for Epstein-Barr virus (EBV) PCR in tests ordered.

The most common etiologies of rim-enhancing brain lesions in AIDS patients are primary CNS lymphoma and *Toxoplasma gondii* infection. Other etiologies such as bacterial or fungal abscess are also possible. CSF EBV PCR test is highly sensitive and specific for primary CNS lymphoma. Because there is no mass effect, it is safe to do a lumbar puncture, so a ventricular CSF aspiration is not necessary. A cerebral angiogram should be done if you suspect an aneurysm or vascular malformation. These are unlikely in this case. There is no reason to stop all antiretroviral therapy. Intravenous acyclovir is used to treat herpes encephalitis, which is unlikely in this case.

18. **b**—*Echinococcus*

Echinococcosis is usually acquired by ingesting material contaminated with fecal matter from sheep or dogs. Children are more likely to develop cerebral lesions than adults, but people at any age may develop this encephalic hydatidosis, which entails the development of a major cyst with multiple compartments in which smaller cysts are evident. This hydatid cyst of the brain behaves like a tumor and may become massive enough to cause focal deficits.

Image with permission from Adam A, et al. (Eds.), Grainger & Allison's Diagnostic Radiology, 6th ed., Elsevier, Churchill Livingstone, 2014.

ANSWERS 19–22

Additional answers 19–22 available on ExpertConsult.com

EMI ANSWERS

23. 1—k, *Staphylococcus aureus*; 2—i, *Pseudomonas*; 3—m, *Viridans streptococci*

24. 1—g, JC Virus. Progressive multifocal leukoencephalopathy is a progressive leukoencephalopathy seen in immunocompromised patients, most notably those with AIDS. Lesions in the occipital or parietal regions can result in visual complaints or "alien hand syndrome." 2—d, Herpes simplex virus. Herpes simplex virus (HSV) encephalitis is the most common form of sporadic encephalitis in the United States. Patients may present with acute onset of seizures or with a subacute course characterized by deficits referable to temporal lobe structures, such as amnesia, aphasia, or psychosis. Motor deficits also often occur. 3—h, Measles virus. Subacute sclerosing panencephalitis (SSPE) usually develops in children and is rarely seen after the age of 18. Most affected children have had a bout of measles (rubeola) that occurred before they were 2 years old. SSPE may not appear for as long as 6-8 years after the episode of measles. Death usually occurs within 1-3 years after the onset of symptoms. SSPE produces a CSF pattern similar to that seen with multiple sclerosis, whose features include an increase in the γ-globulin fraction and the presence of oligoclonal bands. The measles virus appears to be directly responsible for this demyelinating disease, and the oligoclonal bands that appear in the CSF include a substantial proportion of measles-specific antibody.

25. 1—i, Tabes dorsalis. *Treponema pallidum* causes syphilis, and neurosyphilis may take the form of general paresis (dementia, personality change, myoclonus, rhombencephalitis) or tabes dorsalis (leptomeningitis). The posterior columns of the spinal cord

and the dorsal root ganglia are hit especially hard by degenerative changes associated with this form of neurosyphilis. The bladder is usually hypotonic (flaccid), and megacolon may develop. Patients with tabes dorsalis routinely exhibit abnormal (Argyll Robertson) pupils and optic atrophy. 2—c, Bartonella hensae. Cat-scratch disease produces a regional adenitis, frequently involving epitrochlear nodes caused by scratches on the patient's arm from an animal infected with Bartonella hensae. CNS involvement occurs in only 5% of cases. In immunocompetent hosts, it may produce a self-limited aseptic meningitis. In HIV-infected individuals, it may produce a more virulent encephalitis associated with status epilepticus. 3—k, Whipple disease. Treponema whippeli can cause a rare multisystem disorder with symptoms of bowel and CNS infection. Central nervous system (CNS) infection may produce seizures, myoclonus, ataxia, supra-nuclear gaze disturbances, hypothalamic dysfunction, and dementia. Oculomasticatory myorhythmia (pendular convergence movements of the eyes in association with contractions of the masticatory muscles) may occur and is considered pathognomonic.

PART IV
SPINAL NEUROSURGERY

CHAPTER 26

SPINE: GENERAL PRINCIPLES

SINGLE BEST ANSWER (SBA) QUESTIONS

1. The attachments of the ligamentum flavum are best described as:
   a. The body of the axis to the sacrum binding the anterior aspect of the vertebral bodies and intervertebral discs together
   b. Extending from the axis to the sacrum
   c. The ventral aspect of the superior lamina and the dorsal aspect of the inferior lamina
   d. The spinous processes of adjacent vertebrae
   e. Dorsal to the spinous process and in continuity with the ligamentum nuchae

2. The transverse sinus is located in close proximity to which one of the landmarks below?

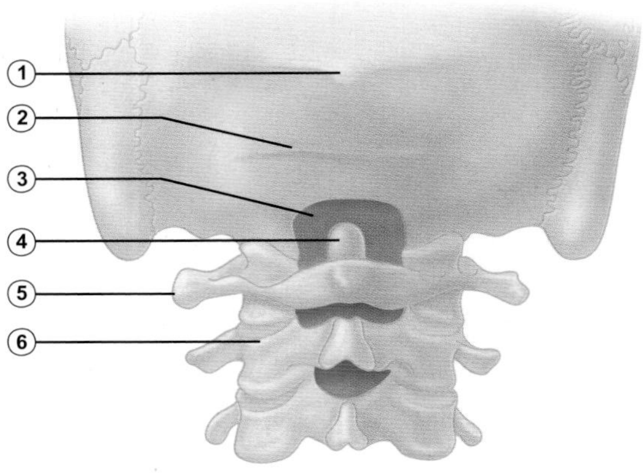

3. Which one of the following statements is most accurate regarding the C1 vertebra?
   a. Possesses a groove for the vertebral artery on its anterior-superior aspect
   b. It is weakest where the anterior and posterior arches connect to the lateral masses
   c. Load bearing occurs through the anterior tubercle
   d. Vertebral artery passes through C1 foramen transversarium
   e. Possesses concave superior facets and convex inferior facets

4. Which one of the following statements is most accurate regarding the C2 vertebra (axis)?
   a. Atlantodens interval is normally <11 mm in children
   b. Superior articular facet is located posterolaterally to the spinal canal
   c. Inferior articular facet is located anterolaterally to the spinal canal
   d. Atlantodens interval is normally >3 mm in adults
   e. Pars interarticularis may fracture in hyperflexion or hyperextension

5. Which one of the following best describes the uncovertebral (Lushka's) joints in subaxial cervical spine?
   a. Between superior and inferior articular facets
   b. Between vertebra below and inferolateral uncinate processes of the vertebra above
   c. Between vertebra above and the superolateral uncinate processes of the vertebral body below
   d. Between transverse processes of adjacent vertebrae
   e. Between spinous processes of adjacent vertebrae

6. Which one of the following is NOT a unique anatomic feature of the C7 vertebra?
   a. Inferior articular process of C7 is oriented in a relatively perpendicular direction
   b. It has the thinnest lateral mass in the cervical spine
   c. Its transverse process only possesses a posterior tubercle

d. Its foramen transversarium is the entry point for the vertebral artery
e. It has a long, non-bifid spinous process

7. Orientation of facet joint planes in the subaxial cervical spine are which one of the following?
a. 75° in the sagittal plane and 30° in the coronal plane
b. 60° in the sagittal plane and 15° in the coronal plane
c. 45° in the sagittal plane and 0° in the coronal plane
d. 30° in the sagittal plane and 15° in the coronal plane
e. 15° in the sagittal plane and 30° in the coronal plane

8. Which one of the following best describes the constituents of the intervertebral disc?
a. Annulus fibrosus type I collagen, nucleus pulposus type IV collagen
b. Annulus fibrosus type I collagen, nucleus pulposus type II collagen
c. Annulus fibrosus type II collagen, nucleus pulposus type II collagen
d. Annulus fibrosus type IV collagen, nucleus pulposus type II collagen
e. Annulus fibrosus type IV collagen, nucleus pulposus type III collagen

9. Site of entry for thoracic pedicle screw is best described as which one of the following?
a. Where the facet joint and transverse process intersect
b. Where the pars interarticularis and lamina intersect
c. Where the superior facet and lamina intersect
d. Where the inferior facet and lamina intersect
e. Where the transverse process and lamina intersect

10. Which one of the following labels denotes the pedicle in this lumbar vertebra?

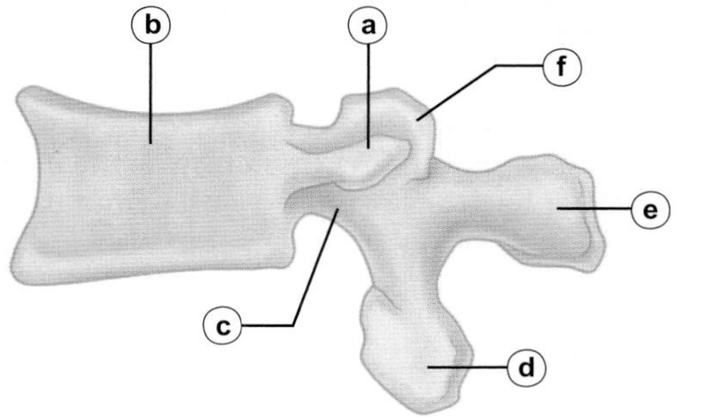

11. Which one of the following best describes Batson's plexus?
a. System of valveless veins located within the vertebral canal and body
b. Sympathetic plexus located along the anterior prevertebral tissues in the region of L5 vertebral body and L5/S1 disc
c. Paired segmental arteries from L1 to L4 vertebrae arising from the aorta
d. Parasympathetic plexus located along the anterior prevertebral tissues in the region of L4 vertebral body and L3/L4 disc
e. Nervous supply to the bladder

12. Vertebral artery V2 segment is best described as which one of the following?
a. Runs from transverse foramen of C6 to transverse foramen of C2
b. Curves around the C1 lateral mass
c. Runs from transverse foramen of C2 to the dura
d. Ascends anterior to the roots of the hypoglossal nerve
e. Runs from the posterior atlanto-occipital membrane to the origin of PICA

13. Panjabi & White's definition of spinal stability is most accurately described by which one of the following?
a. The loss of the ability of the spine under physiological loads to maintain relationships between vertebrae to prevent pain or deformity
b. The loss of the ability of the spine under physiological loads to maintain relationships between vertebrae to prevent pain
c. The loss of the ability of the spine under physiological loads to maintain relationships between vertebrae to prevent pain, deformity or neurological injury
d. The loss of the ability of the spine under physiological loads to maintain relationships between vertebrae to prevent neurological injury
e. The loss of the ability of the spine under physiological loads to maintain relationships between vertebrae to prevent pain or neurological injury

14. Load-sharing concept of spinal biomechanics holds that in the normal lumbar spine:
a. Approximately 80% of axial load is carried by the anterior spinal column and the remaining 20% is transmitted through the posterior spinal column

b. Approximately 70% of axial load is carried by the anterior spinal column and the remaining 30% is transmitted through the posterior spinal column
c. Approximately 60% of axial load is carried by the anterior spinal column and the remaining 40% is transmitted through the posterior spinal column
d. Approximately 50% of axial load is carried by the anterior spinal column and the remaining 50% is transmitted through the posterior spinal column
e. Approximately 40% of axial load is carried by the anterior spinal column and the remaining 60% is transmitted through the posterior spinal column

15. Placement of lumbar pedicle screws at L3 and L4 level should use which one of the following entry point?
a. The site where the transverse process joins the superior articular process just lateral to the pars interarticularis
b. The site where the lamina joins the superior articular process just lateral to the pars interarticularis
c. The site where the transverse process joins the inferior articular process just lateral to the pars interarticularis
d. The site where the lamina joins the inferior articular process just lateral to the pars interarticularis
e. The pars interarticularis

16. Which one of the following is most accurate regarding placement of thoracic pedicle screws?
a. Varies widely depending on level
b. Straight-head screw trajectory is parallel to the facet joint
c. Anatomic screw trajectory is along the long axis of the pedicle
d. Entry point is where the transverse process joins the superior articular process just medial to the pars interarticularis
e. The pars interarticularis is the LEAST useful landmark

17. The primary goal of dynamic stabilization techniques in the spine is best described as which one of the following?
a. Produce less stress on adjacent vertebral segments
b. Reduce implant failure
c. Reduce motion between segments compared to currently available constructs
d. Increase the rate of spinal arthrodesis
e. Avoid the need for pedicle screw placement

18. The spinal construct shown below would most likely have been used for which one of the following

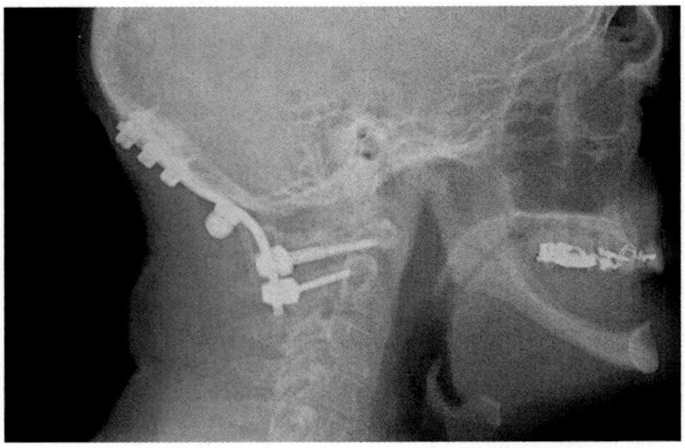

a. Basilar invagination in rheumatoid arthritis
b. C3 vertebral body metastasis
c. Hangman fracture
d. Jefferson fracture
e. Type II odontoid peg fracture

19. The normal anatomical variant ponticulus posticus may increase the risk of vertebral artery injury during which one of the following?
a. C1 lateral mass screw placement
b. C2 pars screw placement
c. C2 pedicle screw placement
d. C2 translaminar screw placement
e. C1-C2 transarticular screws

QUESTIONS 20–28

Additional questions 20–28 available on ExpertConsult.com

EXTENDED MATCHING ITEM (EMI) QUESTIONS

29. For each of the following descriptions, select the most appropriate answers from the image below. Each answer may be used once, more than once or not at all:

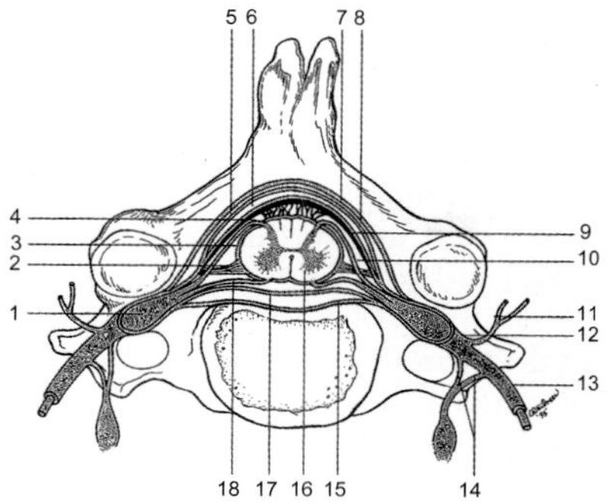

1. Dentate ligament
2. Dorsal root ganglion
3. Ramus communicans
4. Dorsal ramus
5. Ventral root of spinal nerve

30. For each of the following descriptions, select the most appropriate answers from the image below. Each answer may be used once, more than once or not at all:

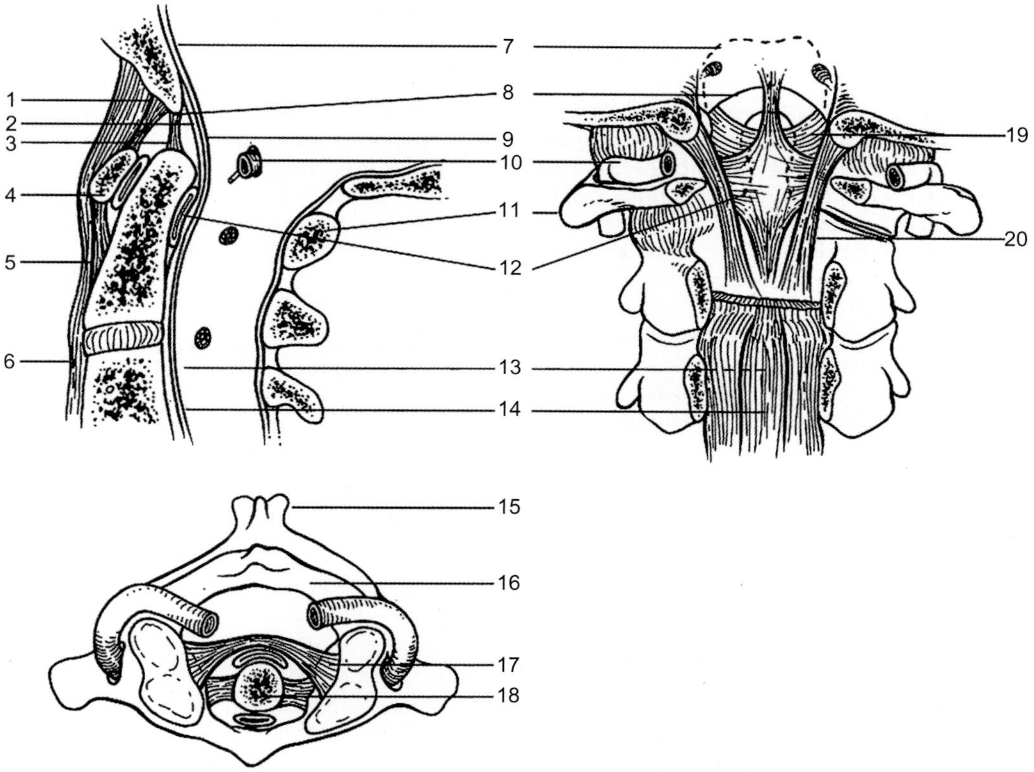

1. Apical ligament
2. Tectorial membrane
3. Transverse ligament
4. Anterior atlanto-occipital membrane
5. Alar ligament

31. **Descending tracts:**
   a. Anterior Corticospinal
   b. Rubrospinal
   c. Tectospinal
   d. Medial Reticulospinal
   e. Lateral reticulospinal
   f. Vestibulospinal tract
   g. Lateral corticospinal
   h. Septomarginal fasciculus
   i. Tract of Lissauer

For each of the following descriptions, select the most appropriate answers from the list above. Each answer may be used once, more than once or not at all:

1. Fine skilled movements in hand, foot, and lower limb.

2. Controlling movements of the hands and digits by facilitating flexor muscles and inhibiting extensors in the upper limb.
3. Head and neck movements while maintaining gaze fixation on an object.

32. **Ascending tracts:**
   a. Cuneocerebellar tract
   b. Dorsal spinocerebellar tract
   c. Fasciculus cuneatus
   d. Fasciculus gracilis
   e. Rostral spinocerebellar tract
   f. Spinohypothalamic tract
   g. Spinomesencephalic tract
   h. Spinoreticular tract
   i. Spinotectal tract
   j. Spinothalamic tract
   k. Ventral spinocerebellar tract

For each of the following descriptions, select the most appropriate answers from the list above. Each answer may be used once, more than once or not at all:

1. First-order neurons synapse in nucleus dorsalis (Clarke's column) and second-order neurons ascend ipsilaterally to the inferior cerebellar peduncle (restiform body), where third-order mossy fibers project to cerebellar vermis. Relays touch, pressure and proprioception from ipsilateral lower trunk and lower limb.
2. First-order neurons ascend synapse in the accessory cuneate nucleus and second-order neurons ascend ipsilaterally to the inferior cerebellar peduncle (restiform body), where third-order mossy fibers project to ipsilateral anterior lobe of the cerebellum. Relay touch, pressure and proprioception from ipsilateral upper trunk and upper limb.
3. Reflex movement of eyes, head, and upper body towards painful stimulus.
4. Autonomic and reflex responses (cardiac, endocrine) to pain.

33. **Spinal laminae and nuclei:**
   a. Lamina I
   b. Lamina II/III
   c. Lamina III/IV/V
   d. Lamina VI
   e. Lamina VII
   f. Lamina VIII
   g. Lamina IX
   h. Lamina X

For each of the following descriptions, select the most appropriate answers from the list above. Each answer may be used once, more than once or not at all:

1. Contains Onuf's nucleus in sacral region
2. Contains sympathetic outflow and Clarke's column (nucleus dorsalis)
3. Substantia gelatinosa

QUESTIONS 34–35

Additional questions 34–35 available on ExpertConsult.com

SBA ANSWERS

1. **c**—The ventral aspect of the superior lamina and the dorsal aspect of the inferior lamina

Ligament	Comments
Anterior longitudinal ligament (ALL)	Runs from body of the axis (C2) to the sacrum binding the anterior aspect of the vertebral bodies and intervertebral discs together
Posterior longitudinal ligament (PLL)	Extends from the axis to the sacrum binding the posterior aspect of the vertebral bodies and intervertebral discs together
Ligamentum flavum	Attaches to the ventral aspect of the superior lamina and the dorsal aspect of the inferior lamina—segments run from C2 to first segment of the sacrum. Laterally, the ligamentum flavum is in continuity with the facet capsules
Interspinous ligament	Lies between spinous processes
Supraspinous ligament	Lies dorsal to spinous process and is in continuity with the ligamentum nuchae

2. **a**—1: inion (external occipital protuberance)

The transverse sinus is located in close proximity to the inion, and below the superficial nuchal lines extending laterally. The occipital area in the midline below the inion is the ideal location for screw insertion for occipitocervical fixation as it is the thickest portion of the occiput and below the transverse sinus.

1	Inion (external occipital protuberance) with superior nuchal lines extending laterally
2	C1 transverse process
3	C2 Odontoid peg
4	Foramen magnum: posterior border (opisthion), anterior border (basion/clivus; not shown)
5	Inferior nuchal line
6	C3 lateral mass

Image adapted with permission from Devlin VJ. Spine Secrets Plus, 2nd ed., Elsevier, Mosby, 2012.

3. **b**—Weakest where the lateral mass connects to anterior and posterior arches

The ring-like atlas (C1) is unique because during development its body fuses with the axis (C2) to form the odontoid process. Thus, it is composed of two thick, load-bearing lateral masses, with concave superior and inferior articular facets. There is a short anterior arch with a tubercle and articular facet on its posterior aspect for articulation with the dens (odontoid process). The posterior arch is longer and curved, and has a grove on its posterior-superior surface for the vertebral artery. The transverse process of the atlas has a single tubercle, which protrudes laterally and can be palpated in the space between the tip of the mastoid process and the ramus of the mandible. It is weakest at the junction of the anterior and posterior arches with the lateral masses explaining the nature of Jefferson (burst) fracture of C1.

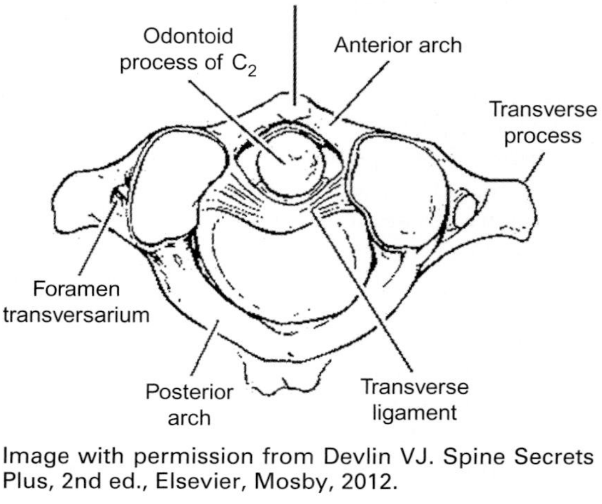

Image with permission from Devlin VJ. Spine Secrets Plus, 2nd ed., Elsevier, Mosby, 2012.

4. **e**—Pars interarticularis may fracture in hyperflexion or hyperextension

The axis (C2) receives its name from its odontoid process (dens), which forms the axis of rotation in the atlantoaxial joint. The dens has an anterior hyaline articular surface for the anterior arch of C1, and a posterior articular surface articulates for the transverse ligament. Relative to the spinal canal, the superior articular processes are located anterolaterally while the inferior articular processes are located posterolaterally—they are connected by the pars interarticularis. Hyperflexion or hyperextension injuries may subject C2 to shear stresses, resulting in a fracture through the pars region (*hangman's fracture*). The C2 pedicle is a narrow area between the vertebral body and the pars. The atlantodens interval (ADI) is the space between the hyaline cartilage surfaces of the anterior tubercle of the C1 and the anterior dens; it is <3 mm adults and 5 mm children.

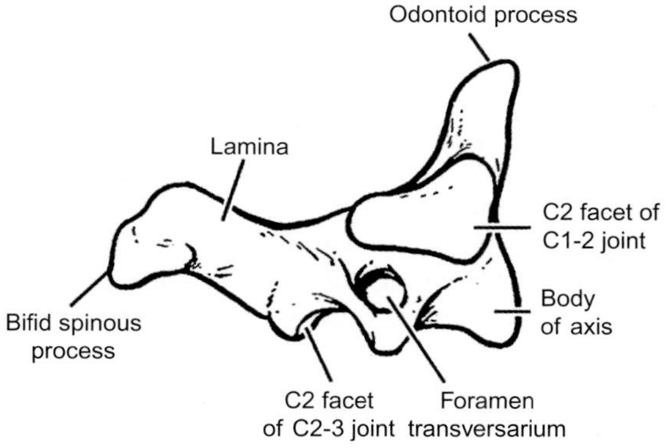

Image with permission from Devlin VJ. Spine Secrets Plus, 2nd ed., Elsevier, Mosby, 2012.

5. **c**—Between vertebra above and the superolateral uncinate processes of the vertebral body below

Typical cervical vertebra (C3-C6) have an anterior body and a posterior arch formed by lamina and pedicles. The lamina blends into the lateral masses, which comprises the bony region between the superior and inferior articular facets/processes. The uncovertebral (Lushka's) joints are formed by uncinate processes that extend upward from the lateral margin of the superior surface of the vertebral body and limit lateral flexion/guide flexion-extension. Spinal nerves exit via the intervertebral foramina formed between adjacent pedicles, facet joint and posterior aspect of the vertebral body. The transverse processes of the lower cervical spine are directed anterolaterally and composed of an anterior costal element and a posterior transverse element. The transverse foramen, located at the base of the transverse process, permits passage of the vertebral artery. The spinous process originates in the midsagittal plane at the junction of the lamina and is bifid between C2 and C6.

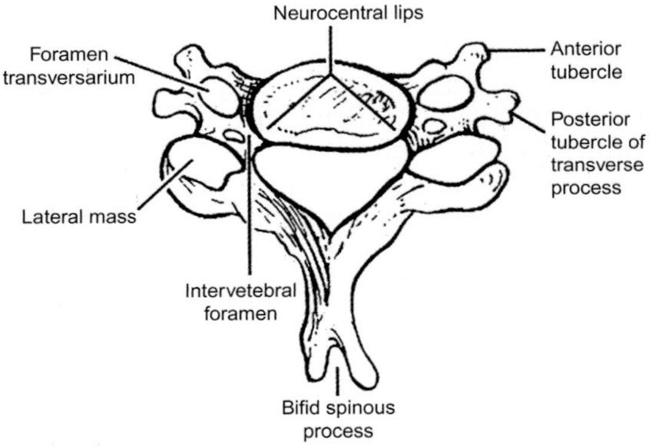

Image with permission from Devlin VJ. Spine Secrets Plus, 2nd ed., Elsevier, Mosby, 2012.

6. **d**—Its foramen transversarium is the entry point for the vertebral artery

The unique anatomic features of the C7 vertebra reflect its location as the transitional vertebra at the cervicothoracic junction:

- Long non-bifid spinous process
- Its foramen transversarium usually contains vertebral veins only (vertebral artery enters at the C6 level)
- The C7 transverse process is large in size and possesses only a posterior tubercle
- The C7 lateral mass is the thinnest lateral mass in the cervical spine
- The inferior articular process of C7 is oriented in a relatively perpendicular direction (like a thoracic facet joint)

7. **c**—45° in the sagittal plane and 0° in the coronal plane

The orientation of the facet joints is a major factor in the range of motion of the cervical spine. Approximately 50% of cervical flexion-extension occurs at the occiput-C1 level. Approximately 50% of cervical rotation occurs at the C1-C2 level. Lesser amounts of flexion-extension, rotation, and lateral bending occur segmentally between C2 and C7 where facet joints are oriented 45° in the sagittal plane and 0° in the coronal plane. These are the most horizontally oriented regional facet joints in the spinal column. The orientation of these facets allows flexion-extension (greatest at the C5-C6 and C6-C7), lateral flexion, and rotation of the lower cervical spine. Laxity of the joint capsule permits sliding motion to occur and explains why unilateral or bilateral dislocation without fracture may occur.

8. **b**—Annulus fibrosus type I collagen, nucleus pulposus type II collagen

Each intervertebral disc is composed of a central gel-like nucleus pulposus surrounded by a peripheral fibrocartilaginous annulus fibrosus. The annulus fibrosus (type I collagen) attaches to the cartilaginous endplates via collagen fibers, which run obliquely at a 30° angle to the surface of the vertebral body and in a direction opposite to the annular fibers of the adjacent layer. The nucleus pulposus (glycosaminoglycans and type II collagen) can bind large amounts of water. In a normal healthy disc, loads acting on the disc are transferred to the annulus by intradiscal pressure generated by the nucleus. With aging, then nucleus binds less water and becomes dehydrated resulting in increased loading of the annulus. Fissuring and disruption of the annulus predisposes to herniation of nuclear material through it.

9. **a**—Where the facet joint and transverse process intersect

The paired pedicles arise from the posterior-superior aspect of the vertebral bodies. The superior-inferior pedicle diameter is consistently larger than the medial-lateral pedicle diameter. Pedicle widths are narrowest at the T4-T6 levels, with medial-lateral pedicle diameter increasing both above (T1-T3) and below this region. The medial pedicle wall is two to three times thicker than the lateral pedicle wall across all levels of the thoracic spine. The medial angulation of the pedicle axis decreases from T1 to T12. The site for entry into the thoracic pedicle from a posterior spinal approach is in the region where the facet joint and transverse process intersect and varies slightly, depending on the specific thoracic level.

10. **c**—C

Lumbar vertebral bodies are kidney-shaped with the transverse diameter exceeding the antero-posterior diameter. An imaginary line passing beneath the pedicles divides it into upper and lower halves, with three posterior elements aligned above (superior facet, transverse process, pedicle) and three below (lamina, inferior facet, spinous process). The pars interarticularis (concave lateral part of the lamina that connects the superior and inferior articular facets) is located along this imaginary dividing line (fracture here is termed spondylolysis).

1. Vertebral bodies increase in size from L1 to L5
2. Pedicle width 6 mm at L1 and 18 mm at L5, and become more medially inclinated (12° at L1 and 30° at L5).
3. Lateral border of pars aligns with medial border of pedicle at L1-L4, but middle of the pedicle at L5.
4. The inferior articular facet of the vertebra above is located posteromedially to the superior articular facet of the vertebrae below; facets are oriented in sagittal plane (allowing flexion-extension only) except at L5/S1 facet oriented coronal plane (allowing rotation only).
5. The transverse processes are long and thin except at L5, where they are thick and broad and possess ligamentous attachments to the pelvis.

Image adapted with permission from Devlin VJ. Spine Secrets Plus, 2nd ed., Elsevier, Mosby, 2012.

11. **a**—Batson's plexus is a system of valveless veins located within the spinal canal and around the vertebral body. It is an alternate route for venous drainage to the inferior vena cava system. Because it is a valveless system, any increase in abdominal pressure (e.g. prone positioning) can cause blood to flow preferentially toward the spinal canal and surrounding bony structures. Batson's plexus also serves as a preferential pathway for metastatic tumor and infection spread to the lumbar spine.

12. **a**—Runs from transverse foramen of C6 to transverse foramen of C2

The vertebral artery is the first branch off the subclavian artery and provides the major blood supply to the cervical spinal cord, nerve roots, and vertebrae. It can be divided into four segments.

Segment	Course
V1	Passes from the subclavian artery anterior to C7 to enter the C6 transverse foramen
V2	Enters the transverse foramina at C6 and continues to the level of the atlas; lies lateral to the vertebral body and in front of the lateral mass; gradually shifts to an anterior and medial position, thereby placing the artery at greater risk of injury during anterior decompressive procedures at the upper cervical levels
V3	Exits C2 transverse foramen laterally, travels vertically to enter C1 transverse foramen then exits horizontally to curve around the C1 lateral mass, running medially along the cranial surface of the posterior arch of C1 in its sulcus, before passing through the atlanto-occipital membrane and entering the foramen magnum. The artery stays at least 12 mm lateral from midline of C1, making this a safe zone for dissection
V4	Intradural segment ascending anterior to roots of XII, joining contralateral V4 to form basilar artery at lower boder of pons. Gives off PICA and spinal arteries

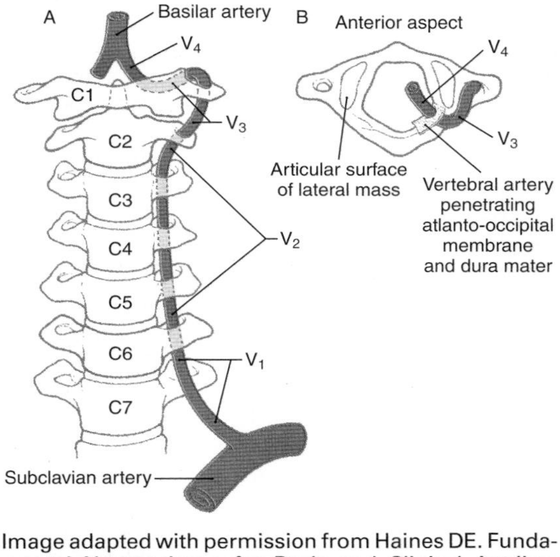

Image adapted with permission from Haines DE. Fundamental Neuroscience for Basic and Clinical Applications, 4th ed., Saunders, Elsevier, 2013.

13. **c**—The loss of the ability of the spine under physiological loads to maintain relationships between vertebrae to prevent pain, deformity or neurological injury.

Stabilization of the spine can be provided by spinal implants in the short-term, but long-term stabilization occurs only if vertebral bony fusion is successful. Non-fusion will ultimately result in spinal implant failure. The surgical factors include fusion technique, appropriate location (anterior, posterior, or combined anterior and posterior column fusion), and use of appropriate spinal implants to adequately support the spine during bony fusion. Spinal implants:

1. Immobilize spinal segments during the fusion process to increase the rate of successful arthrodesis
2. Restore spinal stability lost due to pathologic processes (e.g. tumor, infection, fracture)
3. Correct spinal deformities (e.g. scoliosis, kyphosis, spondylolisthesis)
4. Maintain stability/prevent post-surgical spinal deformity when extensive decompression of the neural elements is required (e.g. spinal stenosis).

FURTHER READING

White AA, Panjabi MM. Clinical biomechanics of spine. Abnormal flexion-extension mobility—Paradoxical motion. Kinematics of Spine Chap. 2; 89., Philadelphia, JB Lippincott, 1990.

14. **a**—Approximately 80% of axial load is carried by the anterior spinal column and the remaining 20% is transmitted through the posterior spinal column

This 80/20 relationship between anterior and posterior columns is termed the load-sharing concept, and it becomes clear that any anterior column incompetence would require the entire axial load to pass through the posterior column (exceeding the strength of any posterior spinal implant). In this situation, posterior spinal implants will fail by fatigue, permanent deformation, or implant migration through bone if used alone—hence it is critical to assess the need to reconstruct an incompetent anterior spinal column.

15. **a**—The site where the transverse process joins the superior articular process just lateral to the pars interarticularis

In the lumbar region, the entry site for screw placement is located at the upslope where the transverse process joins the superior articular process just lateral to the pars interarticularis. This site can be approximated by making a line along the midpoint of the transverse process and a second line along the lateral border of the superior articular process. The crossing point of these two lines defines the entry site to the pedicle. Advantages of pedicle screws include secure fixation, the ability to apply forces to both the anterior and posterior columns of the spine from a posterior approach, and the capability to achieve fixation when lamina are deficient. The disadvantages of pedicle screws include technical challenges related to screw placement and the potential for neurologic, vascular, and visceral injury due to misplaced screws. Pedicle screws may be: fixed head (monoaxial), mobile head (polyaxial), or bolts (require a separate connector for attachment to the longitudinal member).

16. **c**—Anatomic screw trajectory is along the long axis of the pedicle

In the thoracic region, screw placement is initiated at the lateral aspect of the pedicle. The pedicle entry site is determined by referencing the transverse process, the superior articular process, and the pars interarticularis. Exact position of the entry site is adjusted depending on the specific level of the thoracic spine and whether the screw trajectory is straight-ahead (perpendicular to vertebral body) or anatomic (along true axis of pedicle; angulated relative to vertebral body).

17. **a**—Produce less stress on adjacent vertebral segments

Dynamic stabilization is a concept of placing anchors (generally pedicle screws) into the spine and connecting these anchors with a flexible longitudinal member (e.g. rod, cable, spring). The goal of this type of implant is to constrain but not eliminate motion. Proponents of this concept believe this type of implant will produce less stress on the adjacent spinal segments and may prevent some of the complications observed following spinal fusion (e.g. adjacent-level degenerative changes). Opponents worry that without concurrent spinal arthrodesis, these implants may loosen or fail prematurely and require revision surgery. Currently, there are limited data to prove or disprove the scientific utility of this concept.

18. **a**—Basilar invagination in rheumatoid arthritis

Image with permission from Devlin VJ. Spine Secrets Plus, 2nd ed., Elsevier, Mosby, 2012.

19. **a**—C1 lateral mass screw placement

A bony bridge, the arcuate foramen (ponticulus posticus) may overlie the vertebral artery due to calcification of the oblique atlanto-occipital ligaments and may be mistaken for the C1 lateral mass. The entry point for C1 lateral mass screws is at the junction of the C1 lateral mass with the undersurface of the C1 posterior arch. The extensive venous plexus in this region makes dissection challenging and the C2 nerve root is in close proximity to the screw entry point and must be retracted distally. Screws are directed with 5-10° of convergence and parallel to the C1 arch. Alternatively, C1 pedicle screw placement has an entry point on the dorsal aspect of the posterior arch into the lateral mass. With either technique, excessive superior C1 screw angulation will violate the occiput-C1 joint. An excessively long C1 screw may potentially compromise the internal carotid artery or hypoglossal nerve.

ANSWERS 20–28

Additional answers 20–28 available on ExpertConsult.com

EMI ANSWERS

29. 1—2, 2—1, 3—14, 4—11, 5—18

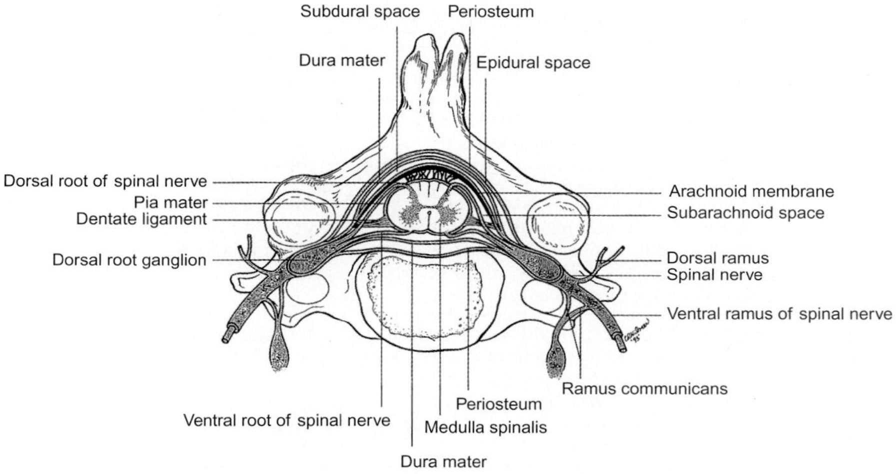

Image adapted with permission from Devlin VJ. Spine Secrets Plus, 2nd ed., Elsevier, Mosby, 2012.

30. 1—3, 2—9, 3—12, 4—1, 5—19

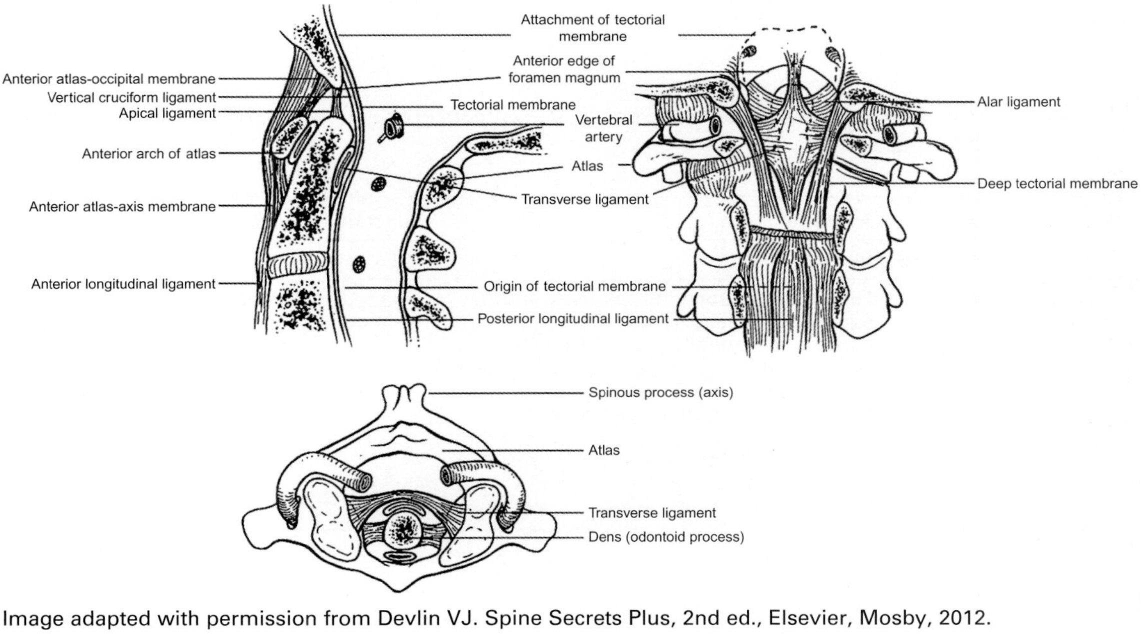

Image adapted with permission from Devlin VJ. Spine Secrets Plus, 2nd ed., Elsevier, Mosby, 2012.

31. 1—g, Lateral corticospinal tract, 2—b, Rubrospinal tract, 3—f, Medial vestibulospinal tract

	Anatomy	Function
Direct (pyramidal) tracts Fibers from primary motor cortex, secondary motor cortex (PMA, SMA), and somatosensory cortex Cortex > Corona radiate > Genu/posterior limb of internal capsule > Midbrain crus (basis pedunculi) > Pons > Medullary pyramids and decussation		
Lateral corticospinal	Formed by decussating fibers (85%)	Fine skilled movements hand, foot and lower limb Sensory input modulation
Ventral corticospinal	Formed by non-decussating (15%) fibers	Control of axial and proximal upper limb muscles
Corticonuclear	Diverges from corticospinal tract at multiple levels in brainstem to bilaterally innervate cranial nerve somatic motor or branchiomotor nuclei (but not directly to III, IV, VI)	Cranial nerve function
Indirect (extrapyramidal) tracts		
Rubrospinal	Leave red nucleus, decussate in anterior midbrain tegmentum, descends to terminate in anterior horn motor neurons	Controlling movements of the hands and digits by facilitating flexor muscles and inhibiting extensors in the upper limb
Tectospinal	Superior colliculus, decussate at level of red nucleus, descends through medulla in medial longitudinal fasciculus and continues in spinal cord to interneurons in cervical/upper thoracic segments	Important in reflexive movements of the eyes, head, neck and upper trunk in response to visual, auditory and vestibular stimuli
Medial (pontine) Reticulospinal Lateral (medullary) reticulospinal	From pontine reticular nuclei descending ipsilaterally to all levels of cord synapsing with interneurons/motor neurons From medullary reticular nucleus descending bilaterally to intermediate zone grey matter	Excitatory to trunk/proximal limb extensor muscles and inhibit flexors. Acts in concert with the vestibulospinal tracts Excitatory to trunk/proximal limb flexors and inhibit extensors Autonomic system output
Medial Vestibulospinal tract	From medial vestibular nucleus, descending ipsilaterally in MLF then continues in SC to cervical and upper thoracic interneurons or alpha motor neurons	Head and neck movements while maintaining gaze fixation on an object
Lateral vestibulospinal tract	From lateral vestibular nucleus, descend ipsilaterally to all cord levels terminating on excitatory interneurons	Maintenance of posture and balance by facilitating limb extensor (antigravity) muscles and inhibiting limb flexors

32. 1—Posterior (dorsal) spinocerebellar tract, 2—Cuneocerebellar tract, 3—Spinotectal tract, 4—Spinohypothalamic tract

Ascending tract	Anatomy	Function
Dorsal column-Medial lemniscal		
Fasciculus cuneatus* (only present above T6)	First-order neuron with cell body in DRG supplying spinal cord level T6 and higher ascends ipsilaterally to synapse with second-order neurons in nucleus cuneatus (medulla) which decussate (internal arcuate fibers) then ascend as medial lemniscus. They synapse with third-order neurons in VPL thalamus which ascend in posterior limb of internal capsule to terminate in somatosensory cortex	Fine touch, pressure, proprioception from upper trunk, upper limbs and neck

Continued

Ascending tract	Anatomy	Function
Fasciculus gracilis*	First-order neuron with cell body in DRG supplying spinal cord levels below T6 ascends ipsilaterally to synapse with second-order neurons in nucleus gracilis (medulla) which decussate (internal arcuate fibers) then ascend as medial lemniscus. They synapse with third-order neurons in VPL thalamus which ascend in posterior limb of internal capsule to terminate in somatosensory cortex	Fine touch, pressure, proprioception from lower limbs and inferior trunk
Somatosensory to cerebellum (subconscious)		
Posterior (dorsal) spinocerebellar tract	First-order neurons synapse in nucleus dorsalis (Clarke's column) and second-order neurons ascend ipsilaterally to the inferior cerebellar peduncle (restiform body), where third-order mossy fibers project to cerebellar vermis	Relay touch, pressure and proprioception from ipsilateral lower trunk and lower limb. Posture and coordination of lower limb movement
Cuneocerebellar tract	First-order neurons ascend in fasciculus cuneatus to synapse in the accessory cuneate nucleus and second-order neurons ascend ipsilaterally to the inferior cerebellar peduncle (restiform body), where third-order mossy fibers project to ipsilateral anterior lobe of the cerebellum	Relay touch, pressure and proprioception from ipsilateral upper trunk and upper limb. Coordinated movement of head and upper limb
Anterior (ventral) spinocerebellar tract	First-order neurons synapse in laminae V-VII and second-order neurons decussated and ascend to the superior cerebellar peduncle where third-order mossy fibers project to cerebellar vermis and decussate again to side of origin	Relays proprioception. Posture and coordination of lower limb movement
Rostral spinocerebellar tract	First-order neurons synapse in laminae VII and second-order neurons ascend ipsilaterally to inferior cerebellar peduncle where third-order mossy fibers project to cerebellum	Movement of head and upper limb
Anterolateral		
Anterior spinothalamic tract*	Second-order neuron from dorsal horn decussates to synapse with third-order neuron in thalamus which terminates in somatosensory cortex	Light touch
Lateral spinothalamic tract*	Second-order neuron from dorsal horn decussates to synapse with third-order neuron in thalamus which terminates in somatosensory cortex	Pain and temperature
Spinoreticular tract	Second-order neurons remain ipsilateral (majority) or decussate (minority) and ascend bilaterally to reticular formation where they synapse on reticulothalamic fibers	Increased arousal following nociceptive, thermal, non-discriminatory (crude) touch
Spinomesencephalic tract	Terminate in periaqueductal grey and midbrain raphe nuclei Terminate in parabranchial nucleus (then amygdala)	Descending pain inhibiting system Emotional component of pain
Spinotectal tract	Terminate in superior colliculus	Reflex movement of eyes, head, and upper body towards painful stimulus
Spinohypothalamic	Terminate in hypothalamus where synapse with neurons that give rise to hypothalamospinal tract	Autonomic and reflex responses (e.g. cardiac, endocrine) to pain

*Pathways transmitting consciously perceived stimuli.

33. 1—g, Lamina IX, 2—e, Lamina VII, 3—b, Lamina II/III

Rexed Lamina	Description
Lamina I	Substantia marginalis (marginal nucleus; receives/relays pain and temperature from Lissauer's tract)
Lamina II/III	Substantia gelatinosa (first-order neurons of spinothalamic tract synapse)
Lamina III/IV/V	Nucleus proprius (first-order neurons of spinothalamic tract synapse)
Lamina VI	Base of the dorsal horn
Lamina VII	Intermediolateral nucleus (T1-L2; sympathetic output) and nucleus dorsalis (Clarke's column; proprioception via spinocerebellar tract)
Lamina VIII	Motor interneurons
Lamina IX	Lateral and medial motor neurons; cervical phrenic and spinal accessory nuclei; sacral Onuf's nucleus (S2 level; pudendal nerve origin; micturition, defecation)
Lamina X	Substantia gelatinosa centralis

ANSWERS 34–35

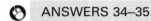

Additional answers 34–35 available on ExpertConsult.com

CHAPTER 27

Scoliosis and Spinal Deformity

SINGLE BEST ANSWER (SBA) QUESTIONS

1. Which one of the following statements about angle X is LEAST accurate?

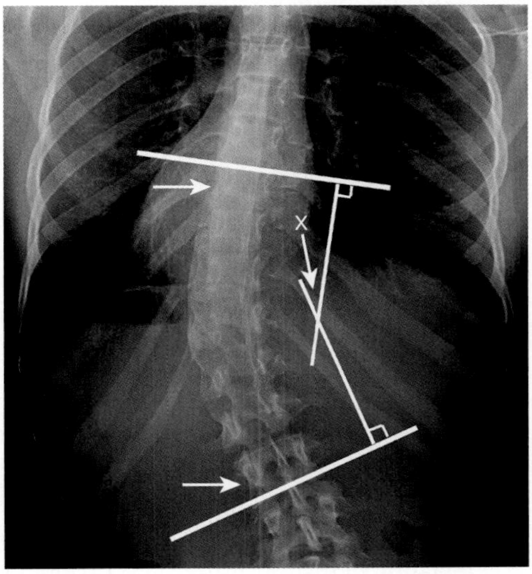

   a. Only applies to coronal plane deformity
   b. Requires identification of proximal and distal end vertebrae
   c. The largest angle defines the major (structural) scoliosis curve
   d. Can be reduced in a non-structural curve by side bending
   e. Is a reflection of the sagittal balance

2. Which one of the following statements regarding development of scoliosis in patients with neuromuscular disorders is most accurate?
   a. Neuromuscular curves tend to be longer and involve more vertebrae than idiopathic scoliosis curves
   b. Neuromuscular curves form due to the Heuter-Volkmann principle
   c. Neuromuscular scoliosis tends to develop later than most cases of idiopathic scoliosis
   d. Neuromuscular spinal deformities are less likely to progress in severity
   e. Neuromuscular curves are rarely associated with pelvic obliquity

3. Which one of the following statements regarding management of neuromuscular scoliosis is LEAST accurate?
   a. Neuromuscular curves do not respond well to orthotic treatment, and spinal surgery is frequently required
   b. Observation is reasonable for patients with small curves (30°)
   c. Surgery is not recommended before the age of 5
   d. Earlier surgical treatment is advised for patients with Duchenne's muscular dystrophy (when curves reach 20°)
   e. Curves up to 90° are most commonly treated with posterior spinal instrumentation and fusion

4. Which one of the following statements about infantile idiopathic scoliosis is LEAST accurate?
   a. Idiopathic adolescent curves are commonly right thoracic, whereas infantile scoliosis curves are left sided
   b. Genetic testing for scoliosis curve progression is currently not available
   c. Infantile scoliosis commonly affects girls, whereas adolescent idiopathic scoliosis predominantly affects boys
   d. Infantile scoliosis is associated with plagiocephaly
   e. A rib vertebral angle (RVA) of >20° is associated with curve progression

5. Which one of the following statements regarding juvenile idiopathic scoliosis is LEAST accurate?
   a. It shows increasing female predominance with older ages
   b. Refers to scoliosis presenting at age 4-10 years
   c. The majority of curves require treatment
   d. Surgical treatment is usually considered when curves reach 50-60°
   e. Single-staged posterior fusion procedures are the preferred surgical treatment

6. Which one of the following statements regarding adolescent idiopathic scoliosis is most accurate?
   a. Lumbar and thoracolumbar curves are more likely to progress than thoracic curves because they lack the inherent stability provided by the rib cage
   b. It is commoner in females and tends to have a right thoracic curve
   c. Female sex is not a risk factor for curve progression
   d. Genetic risk stratification is not an option
   e. Curves measuring 50-75° at maturity progress steadily at a rate of approximately 5° per year

7. Which one of the following statements regarding the management of adolescent idiopathic scoliosis is LEAST accurate?
   a. Untreated adult patients with a history of adolescent idiopathic scoliosis do not have increased mortality
   b. In the absence of hypokyphosis, cardiorespiratory complications occur with curves of 90° or more
   c. Bracing is contraindicated in the presence of skeletal maturity
   d. Observation is appropriate for curves less than 20°
   e. Skeletally mature adolescents with curves of >30° should undergo posterior instrumented fusion

8. Which one of the following statements regarding the Lenke classification of scoliosis curves is LEAST accurate?
   a. There are six types based on the number of structural and non-structural curves present
   b. It does not take into account thoracic kyphosis
   c. Curve types are subclassified by the relationship of the center sacral vertical line to the lumbar spine
   d. Curve classification takes the form of curve type, lumbar modifier and thoracic sagittal modifier
   e. Cervical curves are not included in the classification

9. A 12-year-old girl with scoliosis was found to have a fluid-filled cavity within the spinal cord on a routine preoperative MRI scan. Which one of the following statements is LEAST accurate?
   a. There is an increased risk of neurological deficit with spinal distraction and instrumentation in this patient
   b. A left-sided thoracic curve is more likely in this patient
   c. Scoliosis is reported in 25-85% of syringomyelia cases.
   d. She may have abnormal abdominal reflexes
   e. Decompression of the syrinx causes improvement of the scoliosis in most cases

10. Which one of the following statements regarding adult scoliosis is most accurate?
   a. Type 1 adult scoliosis is associated with degenerative disease of the spine
   b. Curves 30-50° at skeletal maturity progress on average 3° per year
   c. Curves between 50° and 75° progress at an average of 5° per year.
   d. Leg length discrepancy is a cause of Type 2 adult scoliosis
   e. Adult idiopathic scoliosis generally does not progress if curves are less than 50°

11. Which one of the following statements regarding congenital scoliosis is LEAST accurate?
   a. The defect arises between weeks 4 and 6 of embryogenesis.
   b. Fully segmented hemivertebrae results in rate of progression of 5° per year
   c. Block vertebrae are defects of segmentation
   d. Wedge vertebrae are defects of formation
   e. Incarcerated hemivertebrae produce little or no spinal deformity

12. Which one of the following is NOT included in the VACTERLS association?
   a. Eye abnormalities
   b. Tracheo-esophageal fistula
   c. Cardiac abnormalities
   d. Single umbilical artery
   e. Anorectal abnormalities, eye abnormalities

13. Which one of the following statements regarding sagittal plane deformities is LEAST accurate?
   a. Type I congenital kyphosis defects lead to a sharp angular kyphosis that may cause paraplegia
   b. Thoracolumbar kyphosis in achondroplasic dwarfs resolves in the majority of cases by 12-18 months of age
   c. Type II congenital kyphosis is due to a defect of vertebral body segmentation
   d. Posterior *in situ* fusion should be considered for a young child with a kyphosis measuring less than 50°
   e. Bracing prevents deformity progression and may provide long-term correction of a congenital kyphotic deformity in skeletally immature patients

14. A 15-year-old presents with back pain and kyphotic deformity in the thoracic spine with a Cobb angle of 60° between T5 and T12. He is unable to correct the deformity by active extension. Sagittal CT spine is shown. Which one of the following statements regarding this condition is LEAST accurate?

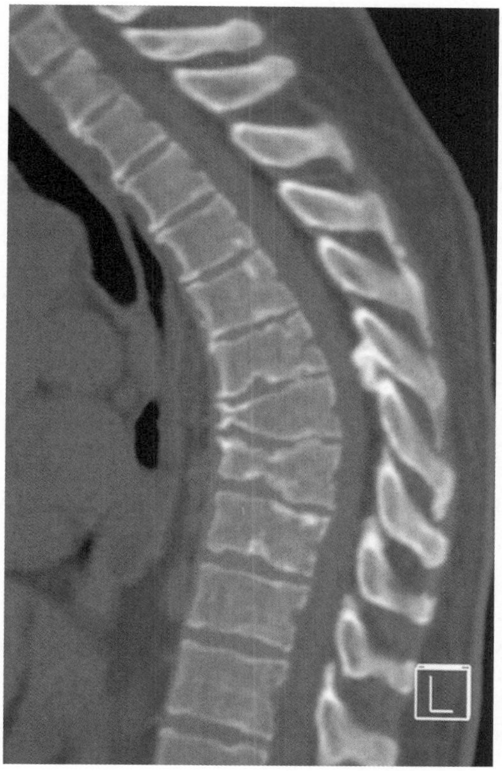

a. The condition is often accompanied by a lumbar hyperlordosis
b. This is the most common cause of thoracic back pain in adolescents
c. MRI spine should be performed preoperatively
d. Extension bracing is not appropriate even in skeletally immature patients
e. Ligamentum flavum excision should be performed at the apex of the curve during surgery

EXTENDED MATCHING ITEM (EMI) QUESTIONS

15. **Scoliosis terms:**
a. Center sacral vertebral line
b. Cobb angle
c. Coronal balance
d. Major curve
e. Minor curve
f. Non-structural curve
g. Rib-vertebral angle difference
h. Risser sign
i. Sagittal balance
j. Stable vertebra
k. Structural curve

For each of the following descriptions, select the most appropriate answer from the list shown above. Each answer may be used once, more than once or not at all.

1. Scoliosis curves that do not correct completely on bending
2. A useful guide to assessing skeletal maturity based on ossification of the iliac apophysis.
3. A vertical line extending cephalad from the center of the sacrum and through the S1 spinous process
4. The vertebra bisected by the center sacral line
5. Horizontal distance between a perpendicular line dropped from the center of the body of C7 to the floor and the posterior superior corner of the S1 segment

16. **Scoliosis management:**
a. Anterior or posterior fusion of the lumbar curve
b. Anterior release followed by posterior instrumentation of the thoracic curve
c. Boston brace (TLSO)
d. Fusion of the whole spine including pelvis
e. Growth rod application
f. Kyphectomy
g. Milwaukee brace (CTLSO)
h. Posterior instrumentation of curve
i. Posterior instrumented fusion of thoracic and lumbar curve

For each of the following descriptions, select the most appropriate answer from the list shown above. Each answer may be used once, more than once or not at all.

1. A 17-year-old girl presents with a right thoracic curve of 55° and a lumbar curve of 40°. On the bending views, the thoracic curve corrects to 33° and the lumbar to 18° with no significant apical vertebral rotation.
2. An 11-year-old premenarchal girl presents with a right low thoracic curve (apex at T10) of 38°. MRI spine and craniocervical junction are normal.
3. A 15-year-old boy wheelchair user with cerebral palsy presents with a 70° lumbar curve with associated pelvic obliquity.

SBA ANSWERS

1. **a**—Only applies to coronal plane deformity

The Cobb angle (X) is obtained on the frontal PA radiograph and is calculated by finding the vertebrae that are maximally tilted at the cranial and caudal portions of the curve being evaluated (proximal and distal end vertebrae). Lines are drawn parallel to the superior endplate of the proximal end vertebrae and parallel to the inferior endplate of the distal end vertebrae; 90° perpendicular lines are then drawn for each of these lines so that they intersect. The angle created by these two intersecting lines is the Cobb angle. The apex of a curve is the most lateral vertebral body on frontal radiographs and is considered cervical if its apex is between C2 and C6, cervicothoracic if between C7 and T1, thoracic if between T2 and T11, thoracolumbar if between T12 and L1, lumbar if between L2 and L4, or lumbosacral if at L5 or below. While there should not be any curve in the coronal place normally, the sagittal Cobb angle can be used to measure normal cervical lordosis, thoracic kyphosis and lumbar lordosis (40-60°) using a lateral radiograph.

Image with permission from Czervionke LF, Fenton DS. Imaging Painful Spine Disorders, Copyright © 2011, Mayo Foundation for Medical Education and Research. Published by Saunders, Elsevier Inc.

FURTHER READING

Czervionke LF, Fenton DS. Imaging Painful Spine Disorders. Copyright © 2011 by Mayo Foundation for Medical Education and Research Published by Saunders, Elsevier Inc.

2. **a**—Neuromuscular curves tend to be longer and involve more vertebrae than idiopathic scoliosis curves

The Heuter-Volkmann principle states that decreased loading across an epiphyseal growth plate inhibits growth and increased pressure tends to accelerate growth, hence imbalance of forces across vertebral end plates due to neuromuscular disease results in scoliosis. A wide spectrum of spinal deformities may develop including scoliosis (most common), hyperkyphosis, hyperlordosis, and complex multiplanar deformities. Neuromuscular curves are typically long, sweeping C-shaped curves that extend to the pelvic region. The curve apex is usually in the thoracolumbar or lumbar region. When secondary curves develop, they are usually unable to restore coronal balance. Significant sagittal plane deformity often accompanies coronal plane deformity. Pelvic obliquity is common and poses a major problem because it creates an uneven sitting base. Neuromuscular scoliosis develops at an earlier age than most cases of idiopathic scoliosis, often before age 10 and are more likely to progress in severity due to the early age of onset of neuromuscular disease. Neuromuscular causes of scoliosis may be myopathic or neuropathic. Myopathic causes include muscular dystrophies (Duchenne, limb-girdle, and fascioscapulohumeral), myotonic dystrophy and congenital hypotonia. Neuropathic causes may be upper motor neuron (cerebral palsy, Friderich's ataxia, syringomyelia, quadriplegia), lower motor neuron (spinal muscular atrophy, poliomyelitis, dysautonomia) or mixed. The prevalence of spinal deformities in different neuromuscular diseases is variable: cerebral palsy (25%), myelodysplasia (60%), spinal muscular atrophy (67%), Friedreich's ataxia (80%), Duchenne's muscular dystrophy (90%), and spinal cord injury before 10 years of age (100%).

FURTHER READING

Mardjetko S, Devlin VJ. Neuromuscular spinal deformities. In: Devlin VJ (Ed.), Spine Secrets Plus, 2nd ed., Elsevier, Mosby, 2012 [chapter 41].

3. **c**—Surgery is not recommended before the age of 5

Evaluation of neuromuscular scoliosis requires assessment of the spinal deformity as well as multidisciplinary evaluation of underlying neuromuscular disease (e.g. developmental, seizures, musculoskeletal, infections). Observation is reasonable for curves <30°, large curves without functional loss in severe developmental disability, and those not fit for major spinal reconstructive surgery. In most cases of neuromuscular scoliosis, a spinal orthosis will not prevent curve progression but serves to (i) help nonambulatory patients to sit and (ii) slows progression of spinal deformities until the onset of puberty (permits growth of the spine prior to definitive treatment with spinal instrumentation and fusion). Orthotic management is challenging in neuromuscular disorders because of poor muscle control, impaired sensation, pulmonary compromise, impaired gastrointestinal function, obesity, and difficulty with cooperating with brace wear. In general, operative treatment is considered when progressive curves exceed 40° or when patients develop trunk decompensation, and there is no absolute minimum age to consider surgery. Earlier surgical treatment is advised for patients with Duchenne's muscular dystrophy (when curves reach 20°) due to predictable pulmonary deterioration associated with further curve progression. It is not necessary to delay surgery until skeletal maturity. Curves up to 90° are most commonly treated with posterior spinal instrumentation and fusion. Curves exceeding 90° or curves with severe stiffness are considered for more complex procedures. Combined anterior (i.e. ATDF - anterior thoracic discectomy and fusion) and posterior approaches may help deformity correction, enhance fusion and avoid the crankshaft phenomenon (by destroying anterior growth plates in skeletally immature patients).

FURTHER READING

Mardjetko S, Devlin VJ. Neuromuscular spinal deformities. In: Devlin VJ (Ed.), Spine Secrets Plus, 2nd ed., Elsevier, Mosby, 2012 [chapter 41].

4. **c**—Infantile scoliosis commonly affects girls, whereas adolescent idiopathic scoliosis predominantly affects boys

The criterion for diagnosis of scoliosis is a coronal plane spinal curvature of 10° or more as measured by the Cobb method. Curves less than 10° are referred to as *spinal asymmetry*. MRI spine including craniocervical junction is required to exclude CNS causes (e.g. syrinx, Chiari malformation, tethered cord). Idiopathic scoliosis is defined as a spinal deformity characterized by lateral bending and fixed rotation of the spine in the absence of any known cause. Idiopathic scoliosis is classified according to age at onset into *infantile* (birth-3 years), *juvenile* (3-10 years), and *adolescent* (after 10 years) subtypes. An alternative classification distinguishes *early-onset scoliosis* (0-5 years) from *late-onset scoliosis* (after 5 years) due to increased cardiopulmonary risk associated with early-onset scoliosis due to rapid curve progression. In general, the younger the age at diagnosis, the more likely the deformity will progress and require treatment. Infantile idiopathic scoliosis is common in Europe but rare in the USA, and is characterized by male predominance, commonly a left thoracic curve, and is associated with plagiocephaly, developmental delay, congenital heart disease, and developmental hip dysplasia; it is divided into resolving (85%) and progressive (15%) types, with progression likely in those with a rib-vertebral angle difference >20° and increasing rib phase (overlap of rib head and apical vertebral body). Resolving curves are observed with advice to sleep in the prone position. Progressive curves are treated with serial derotational (plaster) casting followed by orthotic treatment with a Milwaukee brace. Curves that continue to progress despite orthotic treatment require surgery. Growth preserving options (permit delay of definitive fusion until the child has achieved additional growth) include posterior spinal instrumentation without fusion or the vertically expandable prosthetic titanium rib. Posterior spinal instrumented fusion is avoided due to: (1) restriction of thoracic cage and lung development, and (2) the risk of crankshaft phenomenon. In extreme cases, a combined anterior and posterior fusion procedure is an option but will consequently limit development of the thorax, lungs, and normal trunk height.

FURTHER READING

Devlin VJ. Idiopathic scoliosis. In: Devlin VJ (Ed.), Spine Secrets Plus, 2nd ed., Elsevier, Mosby, 2012 [chapter 39].

5. **e**—Single-staged posterior fusion procedures are the preferred surgical treatment

Juvenile idiopathic scoliosis represents a gradual transition from the characteristics of infantile idiopathic scoliosis to those of adolescent idiopathic scoliosis. It is less common than adolescent idiopathic scoliosis, increasing female predominance is noted with increasing age from 4- to 10-year-olds, and right thoracic and double major curve types are commonest. Approximately 70% of curves progress and require some forms of treatment (bracing or surgery). Orthotic treatment is initiated for curves in the 25-50° range. Surgical treatment is considered when curve magnitude exceeds 50-60°. Surgical decision making is complex in view of the wide age range of patients presenting in this group. Major concerns include the effect of treatment on remaining growth and potential for development of crankshaft phenomenon if a single-stage posterior fusion procedure is performed. Dual growing rod instrumentation is considered for early juvenile scoliosis patients. Combined anterior and posterior fusion with posterior instrumentation is an option for older patients.

FURTHER READING

Devlin VJ. Idiopathic scoliosis. In: Devlin VJ (Ed.), Spine Secrets Plus, 2nd ed., Elsevier, Mosby, 2012 [chapter 39].

6. **b**—It is commoner in females and tends to have a right thoracic curve

Adolescent idiopathic scoliosis is the most common type of scoliosis in children (prevalence is 3% in the general population), but few adolescent patients (0.3%) develop curves requiring treatment. Commonly patients are female (especially larger curves), have a right thoracic curve and do not have severe pain. Risk factors for curve progression in skeletally immature patients are future growth potential (e.g. age at onset, Risser stage, Tanner stage, menarche, peak height velocity, triradiate physeal closure, skeletal age as determined by hand radiographs), curve magnitude, curve pattern, female sex and genetic risk score. Curves measuring less than 30° at maturity are least likely to progress. Curves measuring 30-50° are likely to progress an average of 10-15°

over the course of a normal lifetime. Curves measuring 50-75° at maturity progress steadily at a rate of approximately 1° per year. Lumbar and thoracolumbar curves are more likely to progress than thoracic curves because they lack the inherent stability provided by the rib cage.

FURTHER READING

Devlin VJ. Idiopathic scoliosis. In: Devlin VJ (Ed.), Spine Secrets Plus, 2nd ed., Elsevier, Mosby, 2012 [chapter 39].

7. **e**—Skeletally mature adolescents with curves of >30° should undergo posterior instrumented fusion

The mortality rate of untreated adult patients with adolescent idiopathic scoliosis is comparable with that of the general population, unlike those with early-onset scoliosis (before age 5) who develop severe curves (90°) with cor pulmonale and right ventricular failure, resulting in premature death. Common reasons for presentation are back pain and cosmesis. The treatment options for adolescent idiopathic scoliosis include observation, orthoses, and operation. The purpose of observation for adolescent idiopathic scoliosis is to identify and document curve progression and thereby facilitate timely intervention. Bracing aims to prevent progression, and the general types of orthoses used for adolescent idiopathic scoliosis are CTLSO (Milwaukee brace, most efficacious for curve apex above T8), TLSO (e.g. Boston brace; curves with an apex at T8 or below; better tolerated), bending brace and flexible brace. Contraindications to brace treatment include skeletal maturity, curves >40°, thoracic lordosis (worsens cardiopulmonary restriction), not tolerating. Surgical decision making is based on the coronal Cobb angle, sagittal plane alignment, rotational deformity, the natural history of the patient's curve, and the patient's skeletal maturity.

Major Curve	Management
<20°	Observation
20-29°	If Risser 0-1, premenarchal: Immediate bracing If Risser 2: brace if progresses by 5° during observation
30-40°	Brace if skeletally immature
>40°	If skeletally immature and failed bracing, offer surgery If skeletally mature, wait till >50° before surgery

FURTHER READING

Devlin VJ. Idiopathic scoliosis, chapter 39. In: Devlin VJ (ed), Spine Secrets Plus, 2nd ed, 2012, Elsevier, Mosby.

8. **b**—It does not take into account thoracic kyphosis

The Lenke classification is based on assessment of PA, lateral, and side-bending radiographs (the latter aim to distinguish structural from non-structural curves) and measuring the Cobb angle of all curves present; the curve with the largest Cobb angle is the major curve, which is always structural, while other minor curves can be classified as structural or non-structural on the basis of Cobb angle >25° on side bending films and degree of kyphosis. Various combinations at proximal thoracic, main thoracic and thoracolumbar/lumbar levels result in 6 curve types: (1) main thoracic, (2) double thoracic, (3) double major, (4) triple major, (5) thoracolumbar/lumbar, and (6) thoracolumbar/lumbar-main thoracic. Next, a lumbar spine modifier is applied depending on the relationship of the center sacral vertebral line to the lumbar spine: (A) between pedicles, (B) touches apical body, and (C) completely medial. Finally, a thoracic sagittal modifier describes degree of T5-T12 kyphosis:— (hypo) if <10°, N (normal) if 10-40°, and + (hyper) if >40°. The classification takes the form of (1-6)+(A, B or C)+(−, N, +), e.g. 1BN.

FURTHER READING

Devlin VJ. Idiopathic scoliosis. In: Devlin VJ (Ed.), Spine Secrets Plus, 2nd ed., Elsevier, Mosby, 2012 [chapter 39].

9. **e**—Decompression of the syrinx resolves scoliosis in most cases

Syringomyelia, a fluid-filled cavity within the spinal cord, may lead to scoliosis that can be mistakenly attributed to idiopathic scoliosis. Associated spinal curvature has been reported in 25-85%. Syrinx related curves are rapidly progressive, atypical and usually left sided, and associated with abnormal abdominal reflexes. Other musculoskeletal features include pes cavus, wasting of intrinsic hand muscles and Charcot joints. A symptomatic syrinx requires surgical treatment, which may improve neurologic deficits and prevent curve progression. Surgical treatment (spinal distraction and instrumentation) of scoliosis without recognition of syringomyelia can result in increased neurological complications.

FURTHER READING

Kontio K, et al. Management of scoliosis and syringomyelia in Children. J Pediatr Orthopaed 2002;22(6):771-9.

10. **a**—Type 1 adult scoliosis is associated with degenerative disease of the spine

Adult scoliosis can be divided into type 1 adult scoliosis, which is degenerative; type 2 idiopathic adolescent scoliosis, which progresses into adulthood; and type 3 secondary adult scoliosis, which may be due to a leg length discrepancy, hip pathology, or may be secondary to a metabolic bone disease such as osteoporosis combined with asymmetric arthritic disease. Adult idiopathic scoliosis: curves <30° generally do not progress, curves 30-50° progress 10-15° during life, and curves 50-75° progress at 1° per year. Degenerative scoliosis usually develops after the age of 50 and is typically associated with disk degeneration, facet arthritis, thickening/hypertrophy of the ligamentum flava, loss of lumbar lordosis, and lateral listhesis. Degenerative scoliosis can lead to neurogenic claudication, radicular pain, and back pain.

FURTHER READING

Czervionke LF, Fenton DS. Imaging Painful Spine Disorders, Copyright © 2011 by Mayo Foundation for Medical Education and Research Published by Saunders, Elsevier Inc.

11. **b**—Fully segmented hemivertebrae results in rate of progression of 5° per year

Congenital scoliosis is due to vertebral anomalies that produce a frontal plane growth asymmetry. The anomalies are present at birth, but the curvature may take years to become clinically evident. During weeks 4-6 of the embryonic period. Defects of segmentation include block vertebra (bilateral failure of segmentation), unilateral bar alone, or unilateral bar with contralateral hemivertebra. Defects of formation include hemivertebra (unilateral complete failure of formation) or wedge vertebra (unilateral partial failure of formation). Most rapidly progressive deformities are unilateral unsegmented bar ± hemivertebra at 5-6° per year. Fully segmented hemivertebra progresses at 1-2° per year. Semi-segmented, incarcerated, and non-segmented hemivertebrae produce little or no deformity.

FURTHER READING

Karlin LI. Congenital spinal deformities. In: Devlin VJ (Ed.), Spine Secrets Plus, Elsevier, Mosby, 2012 [chapter 42].

12. **a**—VACTERL association is usually defined by the presence of 3 of: vertebral, anorectal, cardiac, tracheo-esophageal fistula, renal abnormalities and limb dysplasia. Extensions of the association include lung abnormalities and single umbilical artery, amongst others.

13. **e**—Bracing prevents deformity progression and may provide long-term correction of a congenital kyphotic deformity in skeletally immature patients.

Type I is a defect of vertebral body formation (hemivertebra), type II is a defect of vertebral body segmentation (block vertebra or bar), and type III is a mixed or combined lesion. Type I defects are more common and more serious because they lead to a sharp angular kyphosis that may cause paraplegia. Bracing does not prevent deformity progression or provide long-term correction of a congenital kyphotic deformity. Non-surgical management does not play a role in the treatment of congenital kyphosis. Congenital kyphosis does not respond to non-operative treatment. Posterior *in situ* fusion should be considered for a young child (1-5 years old) with a kyphosis measuring less than 50°. Kyphosis greater than 50° and older children require an anterior and posterior fusion. Symptomatic neural compression at the apex of the kyphosis requires decompression. In select deformities, circumferential decompression and fusion may be achieved through a single-stage posterior surgical approach. Extensive preoperative evaluation is required, including cardiopulmonary assessment, evaluation of the genitourinary system, detailed neurologic examination, MRI of the neural axis, and a computed tomography scan to define osseous abnormalities. Thoracolumbar kyphosis is the most common sagittal plane deformity among achondroplasic dwarfs. The kyphosis is generally evident at birth, progresses as the child begins to sit, and resolves in approximately 70% of cases with ambulation at 12-18 months. Radiographs show anterior wedging at the apex of the deformity. Progression can lead to a focal kyphosis and possible neural compression, which may be masked by the lumbar stenosis associated with achondroplasia. Anterior and posterior fusion is reserved for children with progressive deformity, thoracolumbar kyphosis greater than 50° at age older than 5 years, or neural compromise attributed to compression in the kyphotic region.

FURTHER READING

Gupta MC, Devlin VJ. Sagittal plane deformities in paediatric patients. In: Devlin VJ (Ed.), Spine Secrets Plus, Elsevier, Mosby, 2012 [chapter 40].

14. **d**—Extension bracing is not appropriate even in skeletally immature patients

Scheuermann's kyphosis is a kyphotic deformity of >45° in the thoracic spine with >5° of anterior wedging across three consecutive vertebrae, and is the commonest cause of thoracic back pain in children and adolescents. The exact cause is unknown but may involve avascular necrosis of the vertebral body ring apophysis. Type I Scheuermann's kyphosis is a rigid, angular thoracic kyphosis and has a hereditary component while type II is thoracolumbar, more painful, and affects predominantly athletes and laborers. A male or female approaching the end of skeletal growth presents with back deformity and/or pain. The increased thoracic kyphosis is accentuated with forward-bending, but not corrected by active extension (unlike in postural kyphosis). The condition is often associated with a lumbar hyperlordosis. Other radiological features include vertebral endplate irregularities, Schmorl's nodes, and decreased disk space height are additional radiographic findings that may be present. An MRI scan is indicated to look for disk herniation, cord abnormalities and spinal stenosis. Extension bracing is appropriate for curves between 45° and 74° with 2 years of growth remaining and greater than 5° wedging. An apex at T9 or above is traditionally treated with a Milwaukee type brace. A thoracolumbar orthosis (TLSO) is considered if the apex is below T9. Braces should be updated every 4-6 months to maximize deformity correction and weaned with skeletal maturity. Indications for surgery include (1) skeletally immature adolescent patients with painful kyphosis >75° with local wedging >10° not responsive to 6 months of bracing, (2) skeletally mature patients with painful deformity resistant to bracing, (3) curves >80° in skeletally mature patients. Surgery entails a posterior spinal fusion with dual-rod instrumentation/anterior release and interbody fusion. The fusion level should stop distally at the vertebra which is parallel to the floor (usually the L3 level). A ligamentum flavum excision should be performed at the apex to prevent buckling of the ligament and therefore decrease the risk of neurological deficit.

Image with permission from Waldman MD, Campbell RS. Imaging of Pain, Elsevier, Saunders, 2011.

FURTHER READING

Gupta MC, Devlin VJ. Sagittal plane deformities in paediatric patients. In: Devlin VJ (Ed.), Spine Secrets Plus, Elsevier, Mosby, 2012 [chapter 40].

EMI ANSWERS

15. 1—k, Structural curve; 2—h, Risser sign; 3—a, Center sacral vertebral line; 4—j, Stable vertebra; 5—i, Sagittal balance

Common Terms in Scoliosis Surgery

Major curve	The curve with the largest Cobb measurement and is always a structural curve
Minor curve	Other curves associated with the major curve, which can be either structural or nonstructural
Non-structural curve	Curves that correct completely when the patient bends toward the convexity of the curve. Nonstructural curves permit the shoulders and pelvis to remain level to the ground and permit the head to remain centered in the midline above the pelvis. For this reason, nonstructural curves are also referred to as compensatory curves
Structural curve	Curves that do not correct completely on bending (e.g. A 60° curve corrects to 45° on bending)
Sagittal balance (lateral radiograph)	Sagittal balance is the horizontal distance between a perpendicular line dropped from the center of the body of C7 to the floor and the posterior superior corner of the S1 segment (normally within ±2 cm). Relative to the posterior superior corner of S1, the C7 plumb line may fall posteriorly (negative sagittal balance), directly through it (neutral balance) or anteriorly (positive sagittal balance). Positive sagittal balance greater than 2 cm is more significantly associated with pain and disability than curve magnitude, curve location, or coronal imbalance.
Coronal balance (frontal radiograph)	The horizontal distance between a vertical plumb line drawn through the C7 vertebral body and the center sacral vertebral line. The C7 plumb line should normally pass within ±2 cm of the Centerl Sacral Vertical Line, either to the right (positive coronal balance), directly through it (neutral), or to the left (negative coronal balance)
Center sacral vertebral line	A vertical line extending cephalad from the center of the sacrum and through the S1 spinous process

Continued

Risser sign	Ossification of the iliac apophysis used as a guide to assessing skeletal maturity. The iliac crest is divided into quarters, and the stage of ossification is used as a guideline to assess skeletal maturity: grade 0 (absent), grade 1 (0-25%), grade 2 (26-50%), grade 3 (51-75%), grade 4 (76-100%), and grade 5 (fusion of apophysis to the ilium). Risser stage 4 correlates with the end of spinal growth in females, and Risser stage 5 correlates with the end of spinal growth in males. For the same curve angle, the risk of progression is lower with greater skeletal maturity (i.e. higher Risser stage)
Rib-vertebral angle difference	A line perpendicular to the endplate of the apical vertebra is bisected by a line drawn along the central axis of its rib, producing a smaller angle inferiorly and a lager angle superiorly (both adding to 180°). The difference between these two RVAs is calculated
Stable vertebra	The vertebra bisected by the center sacral line
Neutral vertebra	The first nonrotated vertebra at the caudal and cranial end of a curve. Rotation is assessed based on the radiographic appearance of the vertebral pedicle shadow

16. 1—i, Posterior instrumentation of thoracic curve. In this case of a skeletally mature patient with a non-structural minor curve (i.e. corrects to <25°) bracing is contraindicated and posterior instrumentation of the major curve is the optimal choice. 2—c, Boston brace. In this case of adolescent idiopathic scoliosis in a skeletally immature patient, bracing should be trialed given a curve of 30-40°. Skeletal maturity (Risser 5) is achieved at 16 years in females and 18 years in males, with Risser 1 stage appearing prepuberty/early puberty. 3—d, Spinal fusion down to pelvis. Due to pelvic obliquity any surgical treatment should include instrumentation of the pelvis.

CHAPTER 28

Spinal Trauma and Acute Pathology

SINGLE BEST ANSWER (SBA) QUESTIONS

1. Which one of the following statements regarding pre-hospital spinal immobilization is LEAST accurate?
   a. Pre-hospital spine immobilization should be routinely used in the setting of penetrating trauma
   b. Time spent on a spinal board is associated with pressure ulcer development in the next 8 days
   c. The probability of a noncontiguous spinal injury in the setting of a known injury is approximately 20%
   d. Firm application of a cervical collar may be associated with an ICP rise of 2-5 mmHg
   e. Pre-hospital selective spine immobilization protocols can be up to 99% sensitive in identifying trauma patients with cervical injuries requiring immobilization

2. Which one of the following statements regarding clinical assessment of SCI using the American Spinal Injury Association Scale is most accurate?
   a. ASIA E is where no sensory or motor function is preserved below the level of injury or in the sacral segments S4-S5
   b. ASIA D is where sensory but not motor function is preserved below the neurological level and includes the sacral segments S4-S5
   c. ASIA C describes preserved motor function below the neurological level, and more than half of key muscles below the neurological level have a muscle grade <3
   d. ASIA B describes preserved motor function below the neurological level, and at least half of key muscles below the neurological level have a muscle grade ≥ 3
   e. ASIA A describes normal sensory and motor function

3. Which one of the following statements regarding clearing the cervical spine in suspected spinal injury is most accurate?
   a. NEXUS low-risk criteria includes absence of a flexion-distraction mechanism of injury
   b. In awake, symptomatic patients three-view radiographs are the initial imaging study for cervical spine injury
   c. In obtunded or comatose patients a high-quality CT scan of the entire spinal axis is recommended
   d. Canadian C-spine rules require assessment of the range of movement of the cervical spine to justify not imaging the cervical spine
   e. STIR MRI is used to confirm spinal instability

4. An 18-year-old male is brought into the emergency room after diving into a shallow pool. He is awake and alert, has intact cranial nerves (CNs), and is able to move his shoulders, but has a flaccid quadriplegia and a sensory level at C5. Which one of the following statements regarding medical management of SCI is most accurate?
   a. Methylprednisolone should be administered if the injury was within 3 h of arrival to the emergency department (30 mg/kg bolus followed by a 5.4-mg/kg/h infusion for 24 h)
   b. Class II studies have shown therapeutic efficacy of methylprednisolone in improving motor function in acute spinal cord injury
   c. Class I studies have shown significant harmful side effects associated with methylprednisolone in spinal cord injury
   d. Maintenance of mean arterial pressure from 85 to 90 mmHg in the first 7 days may improve spinal cord perfusion and outcome after SCI
   e. Cardiovascular instability is unlikely to develop if the patient is initially stable on admission

5. A 21-year-old male is involved in an RTA. Examination shows that he is able to move over half of muscles but not against gravity (ASIA C) and CT trauma protocol shows a C4 burst fracture, 25% loss of vertebral body height, 70% encroachment of the spinal canal due to retropulsion. MRI shows evidence of injury to the posterior ligamentous complex and cervical cord compression. Which one of the following statements regarding the STASCIS trial is most accurate?
   a. The results are not applicable to traumatic cervical spinal cord injury
   b. Those with ASIA A injuries at presentation were excluded
   c. Early decompression (<24 h) was associated with significantly more patients with a ≥2 grade improvement in ASIA impairment scale at 6-month follow-up
   d. Early decompression (<24 h) was associated with significantly more patients with a only 1 grade improvement in ASIA impairment scale at 6-month follow-up
   e. Odds of a ≥2 grade improvement in ASIA impairment scale at 6-month follow-up were fourfold higher in the early decompression (<24 h) versus late decompression (>24 h) group

6. Which one of the following statements regarding spinal cord perfusion pressure (SCPP) and intradural spinal pressure (ISP) in spinal cord injury patients is most accurate?
   a. Inotropes cause an increase in ISP and MAP but with a net increase in SCPP
   b. Mannitol administration causes a reduction in ISP and increases MAP
   c. Reduction in $PaCO_2$ reduces ISP
   d. Sevoflurane increases ISP
   e. Laminectomy plus expansion duraplasty provided a higher ISP and SCPP

7. A 75-year-old man falls sustaining a hyperextension injury to his neck. On examination, he has 3/5 strength in his deltoids, elbow and wrist flexors and extensors bilaterally in the upper limbs. In the lower limbs, he has 4/5 strength in his hip flexors, knee flexors, extensors, ankle dorsiflexors and plantarflexors bilaterally. Sensation is intact throughout the limbs and saddle area. T2 weighted axial MRI is shown. Which one of the following is most likely?

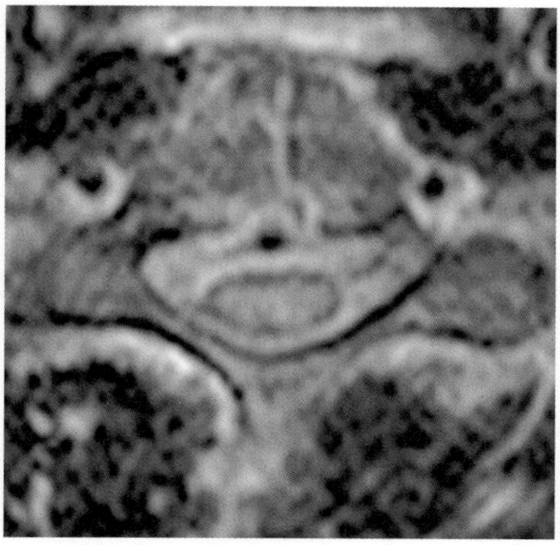

   a. Complete spinal cord injury
   b. Central cord syndrome
   c. Anterior cord syndrome
   d. Posterior cord syndrome
   e. Brown-Sequard syndrome

8. A patient develops Wallenberg syndrome 4 days after C5-C6 fracture dislocation: Which one of the following statements regarding further management is most accurate?
   a. CT head, CT angiogram and start anticoagulation
   b. Diffusion weighted MRI
   c. Clinical observation
   d. CT head and anticoagulation
   e. CT head and commence antiplatelet

9. Which one of the following statements regarding VTE prophylaxis in SCI is most accurate?
   a. Prophylactic IVC filter insertion is appropriate in those with complete SCI
   b. Low molecular weight heparin should be discontinued after 3 months post-injury in those without other risk factors for VTE
   c. Oral anticoagulation is the new standard of care for VTE prophylaxis in SCI in the first 28 days post-injury
   d. Patients tolerating mechanical DVT prophylaxis do not require anticoagulation
   e. SCI patients with retained lower limb function have similar DVT rate to those with complete injury

10. Regarding Punjabi and white stability criteria, which one of the following weightings is inaccurate?
    a. Anterior elements destroyed or unable to function (2 points)
    b. Posterior elements destroyed or unable to function (2 points)
    c. Relative sagittal plane translation >3.5 mm (or $>20\%$ AP vertebral width) on X-ray (2 points)
    d. Relative sagittal plane rotation $>11°$ on X-ray (2 points)
    e. Cord or root damage (2 points)

11. An 18-year-old male was admitted following a fall from a height of 20 m. His American Spinal Injury Association (ASIA) motor score was 43/100 and ASIA Impairment Scale (AIS) A. Cervical spine CT showed a C7/T1 flexion-distraction injury. MRI indicated complete disruption of discoligamentous complex with persistent spinal cord compression. Which one of the following is the most likely SLIC score?
    a. 7
    b. 8
    c. 9
    d. 10
    e. 11

12. Which one of the following statements regarding closed reduction of cervical fracture-dislocations is LEAST accurate?
    a. MRI is essential before attempted closed reduction of cervical fracture-dislocations
    b. MRI results should be available before open reduction of fractures as a significant disc herniation may favor an anterior cervical approach
    c. Closed reduction of cervical fracture-dislocations is safe in awake patients
    d. Risk of transient injury with closed reduction is 2-4%
    e. Risk of permanent neurological injury from closed reduction is 1%

13. Which one of the following is a reasonable guide for weight increments used in cervical traction with Gardener Wells tongs?
    a. 1 lb per level
    b. 5 lb per level
    c. 10 lb per level
    d. 15 lb per level
    e. 20 lb per level

14. Which one of the following statements regarding management of occipital condyle fractures is LEAST accurate?
    a. Occipito-cervical fusion is generally recommended in the context of bilateral fractures with overt instability
    b. Halo immobilization is not commonly used in the management of unilateral OC fractures
    c. Cervical collars are the mainstay of treatment
    d. Cervical collars are contraindicated in the presence of cranial nerve palsy after unilateral fracture
    e. MRI is recommended to assess the integrity of the craniocervical ligaments

15. A 16-year-old is brought into the emergency department intubated and ventilated after a high speed MVA. Which one of the following statements regarding the injury shown is LEAST accurate?

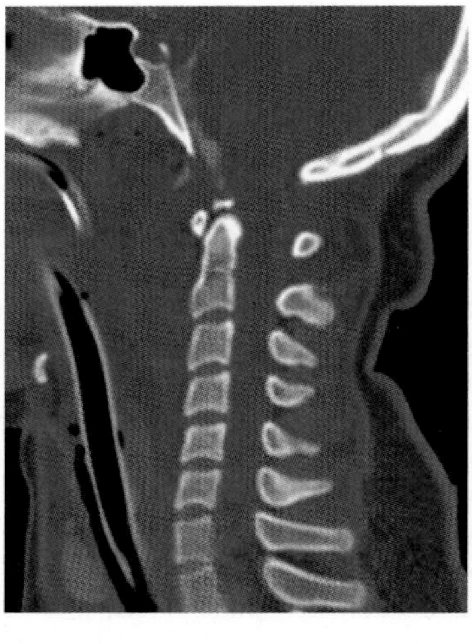

    a. Associated with a Power's ratio <0.8
    b. Associated with BAI or BDI >12 mm
    c. Associated with increased condyle-C1 interval in children
    d. Associated with a high mortality
    e. Associated with high speed motor vehicle accidents

16. A 21-year-old male complains of 1 year duration of neck pain. He denies any recent trauma. He has noticed intermittent episodes of gait imbalance and difficulty with buttoning his shirt over the past 3 months. Physical exam shows normal strength in all four extremities and hyper-reflexic patellar tendons. Neutral and flexion radiographs are awaited. Which one of the following is the most appropriate treatment?

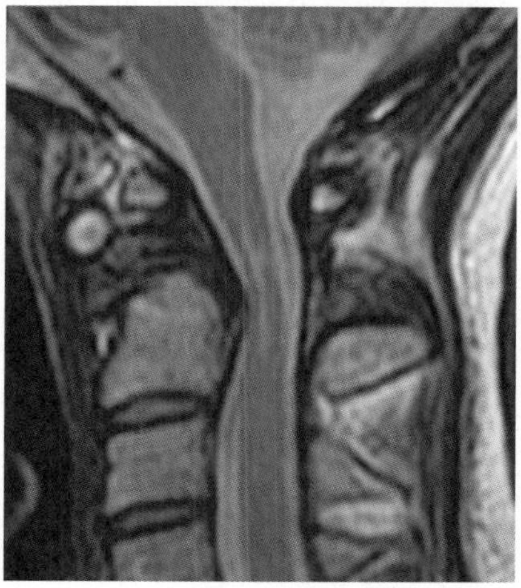

a. Physiotherapy
b. Conservative management with avoidance of contact sport
c. Soft collar during sports
d. Posterior C1-C2 fusion
e. Anterior C1-C2 fusion

17. A 76-year-old falls but does not lose consciousness, but does complain of neck pain. He is neurologically intact. CTs are shown and sum of displacement of C1 lateral masses on C2 is 9 mm.

Which one of the following would be appropriate management in this case?

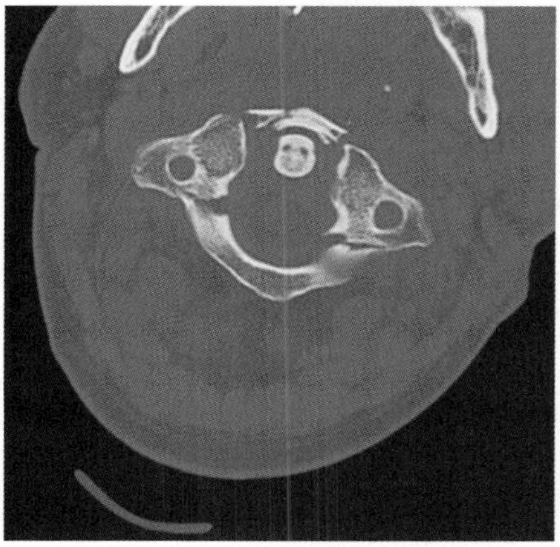

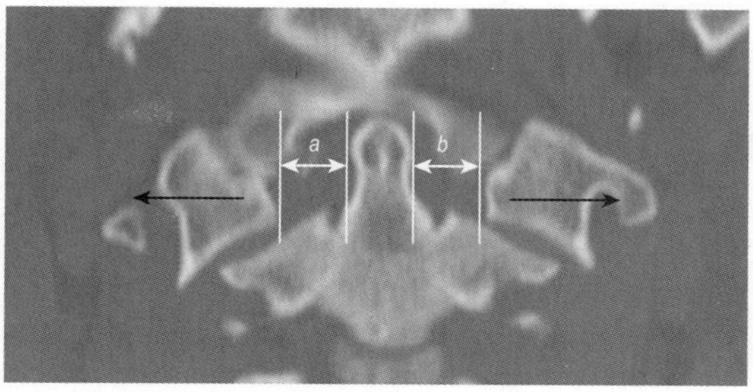

a. Conservative management
b. Cervical collar
c. Halo immobilization for 12 weeks
d. C1-C2 instrumented fusion
e. Minerva vest

QUESTIONS 18–37

Additional questions 18–37 available on ExpertConsult.com

EXTENDED MATCHING ITEM (EMI) QUESTIONS

38. **Spinal Fractures:**
a. Atlanto-occipital dissociation
b. Avulsion fracture
c. Burst fracture
d. Chance fracture
e. Clay-shoveler's fracture
f. Compression fracture
g. Extension teardrop fracture
h. Flexion teardrop fracture
i. Hangman's fracture
j. Jefferson's fracture
k. Occipital condyle fracture
l. Unilateral facet dislocation

For each of the following descriptions, select the most appropriate answers from the list above. Each answer may be used once, more than once, or not at all.

1. A 32-year-old male is transferred after accidentally diving into a shallow pool. He was found to be quadriplegic with loss of pain and temperature sensation. CT shows sustaining a highly unstable fracture at C4
2. An 11-year-old child is involved in a road accident and is found to be quadriplegic

at scene. CT of the cervical spine showed an increased Condyle-C1 interval and cranio-cervical subarachnoid hemorrhage

3. A 67-year-old female has significant neck pain after falling and striking her head. X-rays of the cervical spine demonstrated the bow tie sign at C5. Axial CT show an uncovered left C5 facet

39. **Mechanism of Injury:**
    a. Axial compression
    b. Extension
    c. Extension and axial compression
    d. Flexion
    e. Flexion and axial compression
    f. Flexion-distraction
    g. Rotational flexion-dislocation
    h. Rotational flexion-distraction
    i. Shear and rotation
    j. Tension

For each of the following descriptions, select the most appropriate answers from the list above. Each answer may be used once, more than once, or not at all.

1. Bilateral facet dislocation
2. Flexion teardrop
3. Jefferson's fracture
4. Hangman fracture

40. **Surgical approaches for spine trauma:**
    a. Anterior corpectomy and combined anterior-posterior instrumented fusion
    b. Anterior corpectomy, cage and plate
    c. Anterior discectomy and fusion
    d. Anterior odontoid screw
    e. C1-C2 posterior instrumented fusion
    f. Closed reduction with cervical traction
    g. Halo immobilization
    h. Posterior C2-C3 transarticular screws
    i. Posterior decompression without pedicle screw fixation
    j. Posterior wiring

For each of the following descriptions, select the most appropriate answers from the list above. Each answer may be used once, more than once, or not at all.

1. Jefferson's fracture in 57-year-old
2. Bilateral facet dislocation in patient with neurological compromise

41. **Craniocervical measurements:**
    a. Atlantodens interval (ADI)
    b. Basion axial interval (BAI)
    c. Basion dens interval (BDI)
    d. C1-Condyle interval (CCI)
    e. Chamberlain
    f. McGregor
    g. McRae
    h. Pavlov (torg) ratio
    i. Power's ratio
    j. Ranawat
    k. Space available for the cord (SAC)
    l. Wackenheim's line

For each of the following descriptions, select the most appropriate answers from the list above. Each answer may be used once, more than once, or not at all.

1. A value less than 0.80 is considered a risk factor for neurological injury after minor trauma.
2. A value less than 14 mm is considered a risk factor for neurological injury in patients with rheumatoid arthritis.
3. A line drawn from the center of the C2 pedicle to the C1 arch.

SBA ANSWERS

1. **e**—Pre-hospital spine immobilization should be routinely used in the setting of penetrating trauma

Penetrating trauma (stab and gunshot) rarely causes spinal instability even when specifically injuring the spine and those who are placed in spinal immobilization at scene are twice as likely to die as those who are not (due to proper application of spinal immobilization delaying patient resuscitation) hence routine use is not recommended. Pre-hospital spinal immobilization is advised when there is: (i) spinal pain or tenderness, including any neck pain with a history of trauma, (ii) significant multiple system trauma, (iii) severe head or facial trauma, (iv) numbness or weakness in any extremity after trauma, (v) loss of consciousness caused by trauma, (vi) mental status is altered (including drugs, alcohol, trauma) and no history is available, or the patient is found in a setting of possible trauma (e.g. lying at the bottom of stairs or in the street); or the patient experienced near drowning with a history or probability of diving, (vii) any significant injury distracting the patient from reporting spinal pain/symptoms. These criteria are 99% sensitive in identifying trauma patients with cervical injuries requiring immobilization, but extra vigilance is required in old (>67 years) and very young patients. As such, immobilization of trauma patients who are awake, alert, and are not intoxicated, who are without neck pain or tenderness, who do not have an abnormal motor or sensory examination and who do not have any significant associated injury that might detract from their general evaluation is not recommended. The probability of a noncontiguous spinal injury in the setting of a known injury is approximately 20%, necessitating the need for complete spinal immobilization. Limiting untoward spinal motion during transportation of patients with cervical spine injuries is considered essential to preserve neurological function and to limit further injury from spinal instability. Cervical SCIs have a high incidence of airway compromise and pulmonary dysfunction; therefore, respiratory support measures should be available during transport. Immobilization is associated with modest morbidity such as rises in ICP due to cervical collar placement, risk of pressure sores in the next 8 days (proportional to length of time on rigid spinal board; also if not turned in the first 2 h), risk of aspiration and impaired respiratory function, and must take into account pre-existing spinal deformity (e.g. ankylosing spondylitis, occipital recess in children)—favoring removal as soon as safe to do so.

FURTHER READING

Theodore N, et al. Prehospital cervical spinal immobilization after trauma. Neurosurgery. 2013;72 Suppl 3:22-34.

Theodore N, et al. Transportation of patients with acute traumatic cervical spine injuries. Neurosurgery. 2013;72 Suppl 2:35-39.

2. **c**—ASIA C describes preserved motor function below the neurological level, and more than half of key muscles below the neurological level have a muscle grade <3

American Spinal Injury Association Impairment Scale

ASIA A	No sensory or motor function is preserved below the level of injury or in the sacral segments S4-S5
ASIA B	Sensory but not motor function is preserved below the neurological level and includes the sacral segments S4-S5
ASIA C	Preserved motor function below the neurological level, and more than half of key muscles below the neurological level have a muscle grade <3
ASIA D	Preserved motor function below the neurological level, and at least half of key muscles below the neurological level have a muscle grade ≥3
ASIA E	Normal sensory and motor function

FURTHER READING

Hadley MN, Walters BC, Aarabi B, Dhall SS, Gelb DE, Hurlbert RJ, Rozzelle CJ, Ryken TC, Theodore N. Clinical assessment following acute cervical spinal cord injury. Neurosurgery. 2013;72 Suppl 2:40-53.

3. **c**—In obtunded or comatose patients a high-quality CT scan of the entire spinal axis is recommended

In awake trauma patients in the emergency department, cervical spine imaging is recommended unless they meet all of the NEXUS low-risk criteria: absent posterior midline cervical tenderness, no evidence of intoxication, a normal level of alertness and consciousness, absence of any focal neurological deficit, absence of any distracting injuries (painful enough to distract the patient from another, particularly cervical, injury e.g. long-bone fracture; a visceral injury; a significant laceration, degloving or crush, large burns). Alternatively, the Canadian C-spine rules can be applied to stable trauma patients with a GCS 15/15 to determine the need for imaging based on the presence/absence of high risk factors necessitating radiography (age >65, significant mechanism, paresthesias in extremities), presence or absence of low-risk factors allowing safe assessment of cervical ROM (simple rear-end collision, sitting up in ED, delayed onset of neck pain, absence of midline cervical tenderness) and (if safe to do so) the ability to rotate neck actively 45° to right and left. Imaging would need to be performed if (i) high risk factors are present, (ii) low-risk factors are absent, or (iii) if low-risk factors present but the physician is unable to complete the range of motion assessment. Although not 100% sensitive, clinicians can easily apply the NEXUS criteria or Canadian C-spine rules to deciding whether to request further cervical spine imaging for an awake and asymptomatic patient. In awake, symptomatic patients (neck pain and/or neurology) CT of the cervical spine should be the initial imaging study. Traditional three-view radiographs (anteroposterior, lateral and open-mouth odontoid view) should be obtained only if it is not possible to obtain a high-quality CT scan, but should be supplemented with CT as soon as it becomes available if there is high suspicion of injury or poor visualization on plain X-ray. If the CT scan is normal and the patient continues to have neck pain then several options exist: (i) continue cervical immobilization until asymptomatic, (ii) discontinue cervical immobilization after normal MRI (<48 h post-injury) and/or adequate dynamic flexion/extension radiographs, or (iii) discontinue immobilization at the discretion of the treating physician. MRI including short T1 inversion recovery (STIR) fat suppressed sequences to identify damaged ligaments that indirectly suggests potential laxity in the joints and vertebrae (i.e. potential instability), which could cause a subluxation and narrow the spinal canal. True cervical spinal instability can only be directly confirmed with cervical flexion-extension lateral radiographs. These films must be performed under controlled conditions to ensure that the patient does not move his/her neck past the point of worsening pain or symptoms, and the lateral views must include the C7-T1 disc space to ensure the entire cervical spine can be imaged. If CT, MRI and dynamic flexion/extension views are normal in a symptomatic patient (i.e. most likely muscle spasm or soft tissue trauma) one can either remove the collar or continue immobilization until the patient is reviewed in a few weeks, at which point the collar can be removed without further imaging if the patient has a stable and normal neurological examination or repeat dynamic X-rays if still symptomatic. In obtunded or comatose patients a high-quality CT scan of the entire spinal axis is recommended initially (as there is a risk of noncontiguous injury that would otherwise remain occult). If the CT scan is normal, MR imaging within 48 h may identify subtle signs of cervical spine injury. If the MR scan is normal or performed after 48 h, the clinician must determine whether to continue cervical collar immobilization on an individual patient basis.

FURTHER READING

Ryken TC, Hadley MN, Walters BC, et al. Radiographic assessment. Neurosurgery. 2013;72 Suppl 2:54-72. Doi:10.1227/NEU.0b013e318276edee. Review. PubMed PMID: 23417179.

Stiell IG, Wells GA, Vandeheem K, et al. The Canadian C-Spine rule study for alert and stable trauma patients. JAMA. 2001;286:1841-1848.

Stiell IG, Clement CM, McKnight RD, et al. The Canadian C-Spine rule versus the NEXUS low risk criteria in patients with trauma. New England Journal of Medicine. 2003;349:2510-2518.

4. **d**—Maintenance of mean arterial pressure from 85 to 90 mmHg in the first 7 days may improve spinal cord perfusion and outcome after SCI

Administration of methylprednisolone for the treatment of acute spinal cord injury is no longer recommended based on evidence, although variation in practice persists due to medicolegal and other contentions. There is no Class I or Class II medical evidence supporting clinical benefit in the treatment of acute SCI (e.g. NASCIS I and III), but Class I, II, and III evidence does exist suggesting that high-dose steroids are associated with harmful side effects including death, GI hemorrhage, pneumonia, steroid-induced myopathy and wound infection. A variety of Class III medical evidence (e.g. NASCIS II) has been published supporting the neuroprotective effect of methylprednisolone in SCI but generally, these studies suffer from 1 of 2 significant limitations: limited sample size derived retrospectively from much larger study populations and/or incomplete data reporting in which omitted data are likely to have negated the proposed beneficial effect. Additionally, the claimed beneficial effects have been inconsistent (e.g. sensory only, motor only, or other type of neurological recovery) and not necessarily clinically/functionally meaningful. For example, although NASCIS III was a randomised double-blind trial (without a placebo arm) assessing effect of starting steroids within 8 hours of SCI the only positive results came from an arbitrary post-hoc analysis (i.e. decision to split into <3 h and 3-8 h groups, which showed a 5-point motor improvement at 1 year in the latter group with a $p=0.053$) which cannot be classed as level I evidence. In light of both significant methodological errors and inconsistent neurological outcomes, the beneficial effects of MP can as easily be ascribed to random chance as to any true therapeutic effect. In head injured patients, the CRASH trial showed the administration of steroids led to a worse outcome and they should not be used in this context either. Where methylprednisolone is still given the accepted dose is a

30-mg/kg bolus followed by a 5.4-mg/kg/h infusion for either 24 h (if started <3 h post-injury) or 48 h (3-8 h post-injury). In general, ICU/HDU management of patients with an acute cervical spinal cord injury should include cardiac, hemodynamic, and respiratory monitoring to detect cardiovascular dysfunction and respiratory insufficiency. Hypotension, hypoxemia, pulmonary dysfunction, and cardiovascular instability, are frequent despite initial stable cardiac and pulmonary function. Life-threatening cardiovascular instability and respiratory insufficiency may be transient and episodic and may be recurrent in the first 7-10 days after injury. Prompt treatment of these events in patients with acute SCI reduces cardiac- and respiratory-related morbidity and mortality. Hypotension may be due to hypovolemia, direct severe spinal cord trauma itself, or a combination of the two and contributes to secondary injury after acute SCI by further reducing spinal cord blood flow and perfusion. Correction of hypotension in spinal cord injury (systolic blood pressure >90 mmHg) and volume expansion have improved ASIA scores in patients with acute SCI compared with historical controls. Maintenance of mean arterial blood pressure between 85 and 90 mmHg for the first 7 days is safe and may improve spinal cord perfusion and ultimately neurological outcome.

FURTHER READING

Hurlbert RJ, Hadley MN, Walters BC, et al. The acute cardiopulmonary management of patients with cervical spinal cord injuries. Neurosurgery. 2013;72 Suppl 2:84-92.

5. **c**—Early decompression (<24 h) was associated with significantly more patients with a ≥2 grade improvement in ASIA impairment scale at 6-month follow-up

There are currently no standards regarding the role, timing, and method of vertebral decompression in acute spinal cord injury. Options include closed reduction using traction and open surgical procedures. Goals for surgical intervention in TSCI include stabilization of the spine (preceded by closed or open reduction of dislocations if required) and decompression of neural elements. Neurologically intact patients are treated nonoperatively unless there is instability of the vertebral column. Indications for cervical spine surgery include significant cord compression with neurologic deficits, especially those that are progressive, that are not amenable or do not respond to closed reduction, or an unstable vertebral fracture or dislocation. Most penetrating injuries require surgical exploration to ensure that there are no foreign bodies imbedded in the tissue, and also to clean the wound to prevent infection. More contemporary studies suggest that medical complication rates are actually lower in patients who undergo early surgery, which allows for earlier mobilization and reduced length of intensive care unit and hospital stay. The nonrandomized, Surgical Timing in Acute Spinal Cord Injury Study (STASCIS), compared 6-month outcomes in those with acute cervical SCI (ASIA A-D) who received surgery within 24 h after injury ($n=131$) to those whose surgery was performed later ($n=91$). It found that 19.8% of patients undergoing early surgery showed a ≥2 grade improvement in ASIA impairment scale compared to 8.8% in the late decompression group. After adjusting for glucocorticoid treatment and injury severity, there was a 2.8-fold higher odds of ≥2 grade improvement in ASIA impairment scale with early surgery (but no difference between groups of patients with only 1 AIS grade improvement). Mortality and complications were similar in both patient groups. The role of early surgery with a complete TSCI (ASIA grade A) is debatable and although surgery to stabilize the spine is performed it is not immediate. Most clinicians consider deteriorating neurologic function after incomplete TSCI to be an indication to perform surgery as early as possible if there are no contraindications (e.g. hemorrhagic shock, blood dyscrasias) hence shorter time intervals (within 6-12 h) are preferred. Criticisms of the study include problems related to baseline differences in epidemiological characteristics of the groups under study (patient age, injury morphological subtype, steroid administration, and neurological status at admission), biases related to treatment peculiarities (patient allocation by different physicians' discretion and variations in surgical technique), and further concerns regarding data analysis (loss of follow-up, specific criteria for outcomes evaluation—such as AIS >2, and unclearly reported findings).

FURTHER READING

Fehlings MG, Vaccaro A, Wilson JR, et al. Early versus delayed decompression for traumatic cervical spinal cord injury: results of the Surgical Timing in Acute Spinal Cord Injury Study (STASCIS). PLoS One. 2012;7(2):e32037.

6. **a**—Inotropes cause an increase in ISP and MAP but with a net increase in SCPP

Intraspinal pressure (ISP) and spinal cord perfusion pressure (SCPP) at the site of injury in severe TSCI (ASIA grade A-C) has been monitored via laminectomy and insertion of a pressure transducer between the swollen spinal cord and the dura for up to 1 week. After severe TSCI, ISP is high (typically 20-40 mmHg) and SCPP low (typically 40-60 mmHg). Interestingly, although mannitol administration, reduction in $PaCO_2$, and increase in sevoflurane dose are known to have a major effect on intracranial pressure, they had little effect on ISP after TSCI. Increasing the dose of inotropes caused an increase in ISP and MAP but with a net increase in SCPP. By intervening to increase SCPP, we could improve outcome in some patients as assessed using motor evoked potentials and a limb motor score. In addition to bone, dura is a major cause of spinal cord compression after TSCI and may explain why studies of bony decompression without dural opening have not convincingly shown a beneficial effect on outcome. Spinal decompression combined with dural decompression (expansion duroplasty) safely and effectively improves ISP, SCPP and spinal cord pressure reactivity after TSCI. Compared with the laminectomy group, the laminectomy plus duroplasty group had greater increase in intradural space at the injury site and more effective decompression of the injured cord. In the laminectomy+duroplasty group, ISP was lower, SCPP higher, and sPRx lower, (i.e. improved vascular pressure reactivity), compared with the laminectomy group. Laminectomy + duroplasty caused cerebrospinal fluid leak that settled with lumbar drain in one patient and pseudomeningocele that resolved completely in five patients. Change in ASIA grade (ASIA grade at follow-up minus ASIA grade at presentation), walking ability, bladder function, and bowel function were better in the laminectomy+duroplasty versus the laminectomy group, though not significant ($p < 0.05$) and assessed at significantly different time points post-injury (10 months vs. 25 months post-injury, respectively).

FURTHER READING

Phang I, Werndle MC, Saadoun S, et al, Expansion duroplasty improves intraspinal pressure, spinal cord perfusion pressure, and vascular pressure reactivity index in patients with traumatic spinal cord injury: injured spinal cord pressure evaluation study. J Neurotrauma. 2015;32(12):865-874.

Werndle MC, Saadoun S, Phang I, et al, Monitoring of spinal cord perfusion pressure in acute spinal cord injury: initial findings of the injured spinal cord pressure evaluation study*. Crit Care Med. 2014;42(3):646-655.

Phang I, Papadopoulos MC. Intraspinal Pressure Monitoring in a Patient with Spinal Cord Injury Reveals Different Intradural Compartments: Injured Spinal Cord Pressure Evaluation (ISCoPE) Study. Neurocrit Care. 2015;23 (3):414-418.

7. **b**—Central cord syndrome

Acute traumatic central cord syndrome is an incomplete spinal cord injury in which the upper extremities are weaker, (at least 10 points in ASIA Motor Score) than the lower extremities with variable involvement of the sensory system and a variable effect on bladder function. Regardless of the mechanism, nearly 70% of patients suffering from incomplete spinal cord injuries will have central cord syndrome. Despite this, it is the mechanism and associated degree of instability, biomechanical failure, urgency of spinal cord decompression, and the need for internal fixation of a potentially unstable cervical spine which will influence management hence early CT and MRI are recommended. Approximately 10% of patients with ATCCS have MRI evidence of signal change within the spinal cord with no other radiographic abnormality. It is recommended that these patients be managed medically cardiac, hemodynamic, and respiratory monitoring, and maintenance of mean arterial blood pressure at 85-90 mmHg for the first week after injury to improve spinal cord perfusion. Roughly 20% of patients present with an acute disc herniation as the cause of ATCCS. Surgical intervention is recommended for this group. Nearly 30% of patients with ATCCS have cervical spine skeletal injuries in the form of fracture subluxation injuries. In this group of patients, early re-alignment of the spinal column (closed or open) with spinal cord decompression is recommended. The last group of patients (approximately 40%) have spinal stenosis without evidence of bony or ligamentous injury and management remains controversial due to the variable degree of spontaneous recovery of neurological function. Patients with central cord syndrome usually regain bowel and bladder function and their ability to ambulate. Return of upper extremity function is less reliable, and patients are often left with deficits in their upper extremity, worse distally, characterized by "clumsy" hands.

Image with permission from Fatterpekar GM, Naidich TP, Som PM. The Teaching Files: Brain and Spine, Elsevier, Saunders, 2012.

FURTHER READING

Aarabi B, Hadley MN, Dhall SS, Gelb DE, Hurlbert RJ, Rozzelle CJ, Ryken TC, Theodore N, Walters BC. Management of acute traumatic central cord syndrome (ATCCS). Neurosurgery. 2013;72 Suppl 2:195-204.

8. **a**—CT head, CT angiogram and start anticoagulation

The incidence of vertebral artery injury may be as high as 11% after nonpenetrating cervical spinal trauma in patients meeting specific clinical and physical exam criteria. The modified Denver Screening Criteria for BCVI are the most commonly used: lateralizing neurologic deficit (not explained by CT head), infarct on CT head scan, cervical hematoma (nonexpanding), massive epistaxis, anisocoria/Homer's syndrome, GCS <8 without significant CT findings, cervical spine fracture, basal skull fracture, severe facial fracture (LeForte II or III only), seatbelt sign above clavicle, and presence of cervical bruit or thrill. Gold standard of imaging is catheter angiography but there is Class I evidence supporting CTA as a highly accurate alternative to catheter angiography for screening for VAI in blunt injury trauma patients, with a very high negative predictive value. It appears that the majority of patients with VAI are asymptomatic, and those who with symptomatic VAI have neurological deficit attributable to the initial blunt traumatic injury; no definitive longitudinal study has defined the future stroke risk of either of these groups, with or without anticoagulation/antiplatelets. While no conclusive medical evidence supports treatment for VAI, most clinicians support treatment for patients with symptomatic VAI with either anticoagulation or antiplatelet therapy individualized based on the patient's vertebral artery injuries, associated traumatic injuries, and the relative risk of bleeding associated with that form of therapy. Because of an increased relative risk of hemorrhagic complications from anticoagulation therapy for VAI, without clear superior efficacy, anticoagulation therapy is not considered ideal treatment in multiple trauma patients with either symptomatic or asymptomatic VAI. Antiplatelet therapy (aspirin the most studied) appears to be a safe and comparable option for symptomatic patients with VAI after blunt trauma. For asymptomatic patients with documented VAI, no treatment is comparable to antiplatelet therapy but the potential to reduce future stroke risk favors the use of aspirin if there are no contraindications.

FURTHER READING

Rozzelle CJ, Aarabi B, Dhall SS, Gelb DE, Hurlbert RJ, Ryken TC, Theodore N, Walters BC, Hadley MN. Spinal cord injury without radiographic abnormality (SCIWORA). Neurosurgery. 2013;72 Suppl 2:227-233.

9. **b**—Low molecular weight heparin should be discontinued after 3 months post-injury in those without other risk factors for VTE

Thromboembolic disease is a common occurrence in patients who have sustained a cervical spinal cord injury and is associated with significant morbidity. Class I medical evidence exists demonstrating the efficacy of several means of prophylaxis for the prevention of thromboembolic events. Therefore, patients with SCI should be treated with a regimen aimed at VTE prophylaxis. Although low-dose heparin therapy has been reported to be effective as prophylaxis for thromboembolism in several Class III studies, other Class I, Class II, and Class III medical evidence indicates that better alternatives than low-dose heparin therapy exist. These alternatives include the use of low molecular weight heparin, adjusted dose heparin, or anticoagulation in conjunction with rotating beds, pneumatic compression devices or electrical stimulation. Oral anticoagulation alone does not appear to be as effective as these other measures used for prophylaxis. There appears to be a DVT prophylaxis benefit to early anticoagulation in acute spinal cord injury patients. Class II medical evidence supports beginning mechanical and chemical prophylaxis upon admission after SCI and holding chemical prophylaxis 1 day prior to and 1 day following surgical intervention. The incidence of thromboembolic events appears to decrease over time and the prolonged use of anticoagulant therapy is associated with a definite incidence of bleeding complications. There are multiple reports of the beneficial effects of the prophylaxis therapy for 6-12 weeks following spinal cord injury. Class II medical evidence indicates that the majority of thromboembolic events occur in the first 3 months following acute SCI and very few occur thereafter. For these reasons, it is recommended that prophylactic therapy be discontinued after 3 months unless the patient is at high risk for a future VTE event (previous thromboembolic events, obesity, advanced age). It is reasonable to discontinue therapy earlier in patients with retained lower extremity motor function after spinal cord injury, as the incidence of thromboembolic events in these patients is substantially lower than among those patients with motor complete injuries. Although the guidelines author group concluded that caval filters appeared to be efficacious for the prevention of PE in SCI patients in the 2002 guideline on this topic, more recent medical evidence suggests that prophylactic filters may be more morbid than initially believed. Caval filters still have a role for SCI patients who have suffered thromboembolic events despite anticoagulation, and for SCI patients with contraindications to anticoagulation and/or the use of pneumatic compression devices.

FURTHER READING

Dhall SS, et al. Deep venous thrombosis and thromboembolism in patients with cervical spinal cord injuries. Neurosurgery 72:244-54, 2013.

10. **e**—Cord or root damage (2 points)

In 1990, White and Punjabi described a formula for evaluating fracture stability in the subaxial cervical spine based on cadaveric studies utilizing radiographs. Under normal physiological conditions, cervical spine movements are smooth, effortless, pain-free, and do not produce neurological symptoms. One should consider the fact that White and Panjabi's stability checklist was based on radiographs (not CT/MRI) and that some suggested maneuvers, such as stretch testing or dynamic studies, may not be compatible with the present standards of cervical spine clearance in patients with traumatic brain or cervical spine injuries. The checklist has never been validated nor its reliability measured but it remains in use. A total of 5 points or more suggests spinal instability: anterior elements destroyed or unable to function [2 points], posterior elements destroyed or unable to function [2 points], relative sagittal plane translation >3.5 mm (or $>20\%$ AP vertebral width) on X-ray [2 points], relative sagittal plane rotation $>11°$ on X-ray [2 points], positive stretch test [2 points], cord damage [2 points], root damage [1 point], developmentally narrow spinal canal (sagittal <13 mm or Pavlov's ratio <0.8) [1 point], abnormal disc narrowing [1 point], dangerous loading anticipated [1 point].

FURTHER READING

Aarabi B, et al. Subaxial cervical spine injury classification systems. Neurosurgery. 2013;72:170-186.

11. **c**—9

The Subaxial cervical spine Injury Classification (SLIC) and severity scale (0-10) is recommended as a classification system for spinal cord injury. This system includes morphology of the anatomical injury, including the discoligamentous complex and neurological condition of the patient. The total score in this case was 9. The patient was treated with circumferential (anterior cervical discectomy and fusion and posterior spinal fusion) fusion of the cervical spine. Morphology in this case is eligible for a score of 4 (translation/rotation), DLC a score of 2 (complete disruption), and neurology a score of 2 for complete spinal cord injury (+1 for persistent). The Cervical Spine Injury Severity Score (CSISS) is limited to clinical trials rather than daily practice.

Subaxial Cervical Spine Injury Classification and Severity Scale (SLIC)

SLIC Scale	Points
Morphology	
No abnormality	0
Compression	1
Burst	+1 (=2)
Distraction (facet perch, hyperextension)	3
Rotation/translation (facet dislocation, unstable teardrop, advance stage flexion compression injury)	4
Discoligamentous complex	
Intact	0
Indeterminate (isolated interspinous widening, MRI signal change only)	1
Disrupted (widening of disc space, facet perch or dislocation)	2
Neurological status	
Intact	0
Root injury	1
Complete Cord Injury	2
Incomplete cord injury	3
Continuous cord compression in setting of neurological deficit (neuro modifier)	+1 (=1)

Continued

FURTHER READING

Vaccaro AR, Hurlbert RJ, Patel AA, et al.; Spine Trauma Study Group. The subaxial cervical spine injury classification system: a novel approach to recognize the importance of morphology, neurology, and integrity of the disco-ligamentous complex. Spine (Phila Pa 1976). 2007;32(21):2365-2374.

Arabi B, et al. Subaxial cervical spine injury classification systems. Neurosurgery. 2013;72:170-186.

12. **a**—MRI is essential before attempted closed reduction of cervical fracture-dislocations

Closed reduction of cervical fracture-dislocations may obviate surgery and promote neurologic improvement in some cases. Early reports raised a concern that closed reduction in the setting of associated disc disruption and/or herniation has the potential to exacerbate neurologic injury but studies have shown this not to be true in practice. In the clinical scenario of traumatic cervical spine fractures and cervical facet dislocation injuries, narrowing of the spinal canal caused by displacement of fracture fragments or subluxation of one vertebra over another frequently produces spinal cord compression and injury, necessitating urgent reduction of the dislocation which may improve neurologic outcome. Closed reduction of fracture/dislocation injuries of the cervical spine by traction-reduction appears to be safe and effective in awake patients. Approximately 80% of patients will have their cervical fracture dislocation injuries reduced with this technique. The overall permanent neurological complication rate of closed reduction is approximately 1%. The associated risk of a transient injury with closed reduction appears to be 2-4%. Closed traction-reduction appears to be safer than MUA. Pre-reduction MRI has not been shown to improve the safety or efficacy of closed traction-reduction of patients with acute cervical fracture dislocation injuries, hence may unnecessarily delay spinal column realignment for decompression of the spinal cord. The ideal timing of closed reduction of cervical spinal fracture dislocation injuries is unknown, but many investigators favor reduction as rapidly as possible after injury to maximize the potential for neurological recovery. Patients who fail attempted closed reduction of cervical fracture injuries have a higher incidence of anatomic obstacles to reduction, including facet fractures and disc herniations. Patients who fail closed reduction should undergo more detailed radiographic study/MRI before attempts at open reduction. The presence of a significant disc herniation in this setting is a relative indication for an anterior decompression procedure, either in lieu of or preceding a posterior procedure. Patients with cervical fracture dislocation injuries who cannot be examined because of head injury or intoxication cannot be assessed for neurological deterioration during attempted closed reduction. For this reason, an MRI before attempted reduction (open or closed) is recommended as a treatment option on the basis of Class III medical evidence.

FURTHER READING

Gelb DE et al. Initial closed reduction of cervical spinal fracture-dislocation injuries. Neurosurgery 72:73-83, 2013.

13. **b**—5 lb per level

This technique involves use of longitudinal traction using skull tongs or a halo headpiece. An initial weight of 5-15 pounds is applied; this is increased in 5 lb increments, taking lateral X-rays after each increment is applied. The more rostral the dislocation, the less weight is used, usually about three to five pounds per vertebral level. While weights up to 70 pounds are sometimes used, we suggest that after 35 pounds is applied, patients be observed for at least an hour with repeat cervical spine X-rays before the weight is cautiously increased further. Administration of a muscle relaxant or analgesic, such as diazepam or meperidine, may help facilitate reduction.

Position, correct bed type, angle of traction, X-ray check 15 min post adding weight. Repeat CT cervical spine 6-8 weeks.

14. **d**—Cervical collars are contraindicated in the presence of cranial nerve palsy after unilateral fracture

OCF is an uncommon injury (1-3% frequency of OCF in patients sustaining blunt craniocervical trauma) and requires CT imaging to establish the diagnosis. Patients sustaining high-energy blunt craniocervical trauma, particularly in the setting of loss of consciousness, impaired consciousness, occipito-cervical pain or motion impairment, and lower cranial nerve deficits, should undergo CT imaging of the craniocervical junction. Magnetic resonance imaging (MRI) is recommended to assess the integrity of the craniocervical ligaments. OCFs have been classified by Anderson and Montesano into three types: Type I (comminuted), Type II (extension of a linear basilar skull fracture), and Type III (avulsion of a fragment). Untreated patients with OCF can develop lower cranial nerve deficits that usually recover or improve with non-rigid external immobilization (cervical collar). Nonsurgical treatment with external cervical immobilization is sufficient to promote bony union/healing and recovery or cranial nerve deficit improvement in nearly all types of OCF. Bilateral OCF injuries should prompt consideration for more rigid external immobilization in a halo vest device. Surgical treatment (occipito-cervical instrumented fusion) may be indicated in patients with OCF who have overt instability, neural compression from displaced fracture fragments, or who have associated occipito-atlantal or atlanto-axial injuries (e.g. Atlanto-occipital dissociation).

FURTHER READING

Theodore N, et al. Occipital condyle fractures. Neurosurgery. 2013;72:106-113.

15. **a**—Associated with a Power's ratio <0.8

Atlanto-occipital dislocation (dissociation) accounts for <1% of all acute cervical spine injuries. It is usually seen in high-speed motor vehicle accidents and results from hyperextension and distraction of the cervical spine. Atlanto-occipital dislocation is more commonly seen in children because the pediatric occipital condyles are small, are almost horizontal, and lack inherent stability. Atlanto-occipital dislocation is often immediately fatal because of associated injury to the brainstem and there is a high incidence of neurologic deficits in survivors. Patients who survive AOD injuries often have neurological impairment including lower cranial nerve deficits, unilateral or bilateral weakness, or quadriplegia. Nearly 20% of patients with acute traumatic AOD will have a normal neurological examination on presentation. The lack of localizing findings and/or global neurological deficits from severe brain injury may impede/hinder the diagnosis of AOD in patients with normal-appearing initial cervical radiographs. A high index of suspicion must be maintained in order to diagnose AOD. Prevertebral soft tissue swelling on a lateral cervical radiograph should prompt CT imaging to rule out AOD. Commonly used radiological parameters suggesting AOD include: craniocervical subarachnoid hemorrhage, Powers ratio (basion-posterior atlas arch distance divided by the opisthion-anterior atlas arch distance) >1, basion axial interval or basion dental interval >12 mm (Harris rule of 12), Condyle-C1 interval (highest diagnostic sensitivity in pediatric AOD). AOD is classified into Type I (anterior), Type II (longitudinal), and Type III (posterior) dislocations. All patients with AOD should be treated with craniocervical fixation and fusion. Without treatment, nearly all patients developed neurological worsening, many of whom never fully recover. Treatment of AOD with traction is associated with 10% risk of neurological deterioration and external immobilization has a high failure rate.

Image with permission from Saraf-Lavi E. Spine Imaging: Case Review Series, 3rd ed., Elsevier, Saunders, 2014.

FURTHER READING

Theodore N, et al. The diagnosis and management of traumatic altanto-occipital dislocation injuries. Neurosurgery. 2013;72:114-126.

16. **d**—Posterior C1-C2 fusion

Os odontoideum is an ossicle with smooth circumferential cortical margins representing the odontoid process that has no osseous continuity with the body of C2. The origin of os odontoideum remains debated in the literature with evidence for both acquired and congenital causes. There are 3 groups of patients with os odontoideum: those with occipito-cervical pain alone, those with myelopathy, and those with intracranial symptoms or signs from vertebrobasilar ischemia. Patients with os odontoideum and myelopathy have been subcategorized further into those with transient myelopathy (commonly after trauma), those with static myelopathy, and those with progressive myelopathy. It is usually found on imaging for other causes, and plain cervical spine radiographs are sufficient to obtain a diagnosis but will necessitate dynamic flexion/extension views (plain film and dynamic CT). It may be orthotopic (moves with the anterior arch of C1 on flexion/extension) or dystopic (functionally fused to the basion, potentially subluxing anterior to the arch of C1). Plain dynamic radiographs in flexion and extension have been used to depict the degree of abnormal motion between C1 and C2 and narrowest canal diameter. Most often, there is anterior instability, with the os odontoideum translating forward in relation to the body of C2. However, at times, one will see either no discernible instability or "posterior instability" with the os odontoideum moving posteriorly into the spinal canal during neck extension. The degree of C1-C2 instability identified on cervical X-rays does not correlate with the presence of myelopathy. A sagittal diameter of the spinal canal at the C1-C2 level of 13 mm does correlate with myelopathy detected on clinical examination. MRI can depict spinal cord compression and signal changes within the cord that correlate with the presence of myelopathy. Management is surveillance or surgery based on degree of instability, neurological deficits or risk of future spinal cord injury. Patients who have no neurological deficit and no instability at C1-C2 on flexion and extension studies can be managed without operative intervention. However, many favor operative stabilization and fusion of C1-C2 instability associated with os odontoideum because of the increased likelihood of future spinal cord injury following minor trauma (if not already present). Posterior C1-C2 internal fixation with arthrodesis in the treatment of os odontoideum provides effective stabilization of the atlantoaxial joint in the majority of patients. Neural compression in association with os odontoideum has been treated with a reduction of deformity, dorsal decompression of irreducible deformity, and ventral decompression of irreducible deformity, each in conjunction with C1-C2 or occipito-cervical fusion with internal fixation. Each of these combined approaches has provided satisfactory results. Odontoid screw fixation has no role in the treatment of this disorder.

Image with permission from Brecknell JE, Malham GM. Os odontoideum: report of three cases, J Clin Neurosci. 2008;15(3):295-301.

FURTHER READING

Rozzelle CJ, et al. Os odontoideum. Neurosurgery. 2013;72:159-169. Doi:10.1227/NEU.0b013e318276ee69.

17. **d**—C1-C2 instrumented fusion

Fractures of C1 are usually classified by the Landell's and Von Petegham classification. A central issue in the management of atlas fractures has been the importance placed on the integrity of the transverse atlantal ligament. Criteria proposed to determine transverse atlantal ligament injury with associated C1-C2 instability include the sum of the displacement of the lateral masses of C1 on C2 of 6-9 mm on a plain open-mouth X-ray (or 8.1 mm, the rule of Spence corrected for magnification), a predental space of >5 mm in adults, and evidence of transverse atlantal ligament disruption or avulsion on MRI.

Management of Atlas (C1) Fractures

Atlas (C1) Fracture Type	Description	Treatment Options
Type I	Anterior or posterior arch fractures	Collar 8-12 weeks
Type II	Burst fracture of anterior and posterior arch at three or more points (Jefferson's fracture is 4 point break). Transverse atlantal ligament which is intact (stable) or disrupted (unstable)	If stable: Collar or Halo (10-12 weeks) If unstable: Halo (12 weeks) or C1-C2 stabilization and fusion
Type III	Unilateral C1 lateral mass fracture	Comminuted: Collar or Halo 8-12 weeks Transverse process: Collar

Consideration of the potential complications of halo immobilization, particularly in the elderly, is suggested and must be balanced against the potential morbidity/mortality associated with surgical treatment for these fracture injuries.

Image A with permission from Naidich TP. Imaging of the Spine, Elsevier, Saunders, 2011. Image B with permission from Dane B, Bernstein MP. Imaging of Spine Trauma, Seminars in Roentgenology, Elsevier, 2016, in press.

FURTHER READING

Ryken T, et al. Management of isolated fractures of the atlas in adults. Neurosurgery. 2013;72:127-131.

ANSWERS 18–37

Additional answers 18–37 available on ExpertConsult.com

EMI ANSWERS

38. 1—h, Flexion "teardrop" fracture, 2—a, Atlanto-occipital dissociation, 3—l, Unilateral facet dislocation.

39. 1—f, Flexion-distraction, 2—e, Flexion and axial compression, 3—a, Axial compression, 4—c, Extension and axial compression

Although there may be discrepancies in terminology depending on classification system, main causes are described below.

Initial Management of Spinal Fractures

Upper cervical spine			
Distraction	Atlanto-occipital	Unstable	Occipito-cervical fusion
Rotation	Atlanto-axial subluxation (rotatory fixation)	Potentially Unstable	Closed reduction and Halo immobilization for 8-10 weeks
Axial compression	Jefferson's fracture	Unstable	Halo immobilization
Hyperextension and axial compression	Hangman's fracture	Unstable	Halo immobilization
Flexion (or less commonly extension)	Odontoid peg fracture	Type II and III unstable	Halo immobilization (surgery in Type II if >50-years old)

Continued on following page

Initial Management of Spinal Fractures (Continued)

Subaxial cervical spine			
Axial compression	Burst fracture	Unstable	Anterior and posterior instrumented fusion
Hyperflexion	Clay shoveler's (spinous process avulsion)	Stable	Cervical collar
Flexion and axial compression	Compression (wedge)	Stable	Cervical collar
Flexion and axial compression (severe)	Flexion teardrop	Unstable	Open reduction and instrumented fusion
Flexion-distraction	Facet dislocation; posterior ligamentous injury	Unstable	Open reduction and instrumented fusion
Extension	Extension teardrop (avulsion)	Stable	Conservative or orthosis
	Spinous process/lamina fracture	Stable	Cervical collar
Extension and axial loading	Lateral mass/facet fracture	Stable or unstable	Stable—cervical collar 6 weeks Unstable—closed or open reduction and anterior/posterior/combined stabilization
Thoracolumbar spine			
Axial compression	Burst	Unstable	TLSO or Surgical stabilization
Flexion and axial compression	Compression (wedge)	Stable	Conservative or TLSO
Flexion and axial compression (severe)	Flexion teardrop	Unstable	Open reduction and surgical stabilization
Extension	Extension teardrop (avulsion)	Stable	Conservative or TLSO
Flexion	Chance fracture	Unstable	Surgical stabilization
Flexion-distraction	Facet dislocation; PLC injury	Unstable	Open reduction and surgical stabilization
Shear/rotation	Translocation (fracture dislocation)	Unstable	Open reduction and surgical stabilization

40. 1—j, Halo immobilization, 2—a, Anterior corpectomy and combined anterior-posterior instrumented fusion

41. 1—h, The Pavlov (or Torg) ratio, 2—k, Space available for the cord (SAC), 3—j, Ranawat's line

A number of radiological lines and spaces are used when assessing a rheumatoid cervical spine and relate to atlantoaxial subluxation and cranial settling (or basilar invagination). They include:

Radiological Lines Used to Assess Instability at the Craniocervical Junction

Line	Description	Utility
Power's ratio	Ratio of BC line (basion to anterior lamina of C1) to AO line (Posterior C1 anterior arch to posterior lip of foramen magnum)	Ratio ~1 is normal If >1.0 concern for anterior dislocation. If ratio <1.0 raises concern for posterior atlanto-occipital dislocation, odontoid fractures, ring of atlas fractures
Atlantodens interval (ADI)	Gap between anterior C1 arch and C2 dens. Assessed on both flexion and extension views	Instability is present when there is a 3.5-mm difference on each view; a 7-mm difference suggests disruption of the alar ligaments; a difference of more than 9-mm is associated with an increase in neurological injury and indication for surgery
Wackenheim's (clivus) line	A line extended inferiorly from the slope of the clivus	Normally should pass through C2 dens or be tangential to it. Abnormal in AOD or basilar invagination.
Space available for the cord (SAC)	Sagittal diameter of spinal canal. May change with flexion/extension if instability present.	Less than 14 mm is considered a risk factor for neurological injury and indication for surgery
Ranawat's line	Center of the C2 pedicle to the C1 posterior arch	Normally 17 mm; a distance less than 13 mm would suggest cranial settling
McRae's line	Foramen magnum line drawn from the anterior margin of the foramen to the posterior margin	The tip of the dens should not cross this line. If it does it suggests basilar invagination
McGregor's line	Hard palate to the posterior occipit curve	If tip of dens >4.5 mm above line suggests basilar invagination
Chamberlain's line	Posterior end of the hard palate to the posterior lip of the foramen magnum	Normally the tip of the dens is no more than 3 mm above this line. >3 mm suggest basilar invagination
Pavlov (torg) ratio	Ratio of sagittal canal diameter to total vertebral body width	Normally equals 1. A value less than 0.80 is considered a risk factor for neurological injury after minor trauma such as hyperextension.
Basion dens interval (BDI) or Basion axial interval (BAI)	Gap between basion and tip of dens or Gap between basion and posterior C2 (axial) line	Harris rule of 12: If BDI or BAI >12 mm suggest atlanto-occipital dissociation
C1-Condyle interval (CCI)	Distance between upper border of C1 and occipital condyle	Increased in atlanto-occipital dissociation
Sum of lateral mass displacement	Sum of overhang of C1 lateral masses on C2	If >8.1 mm in adults then a transverse ligament rupture is assured or C1 fracture and the injury pattern is considered unstable

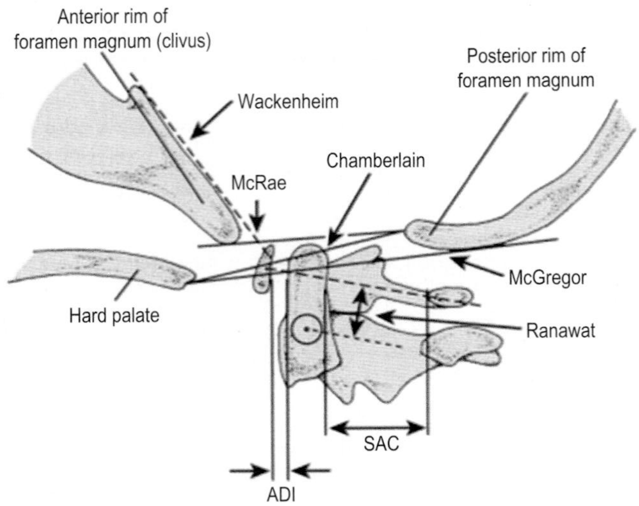

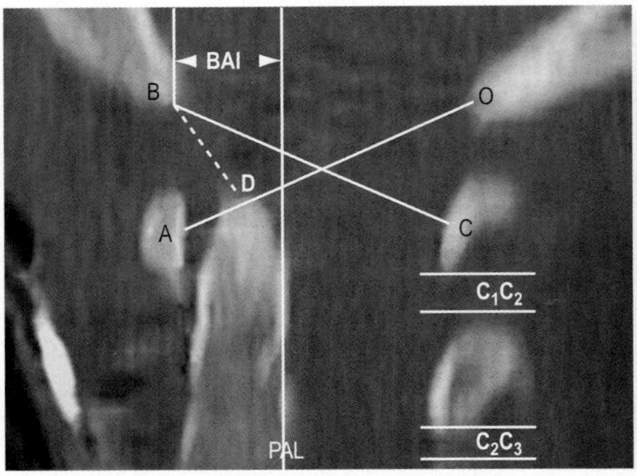

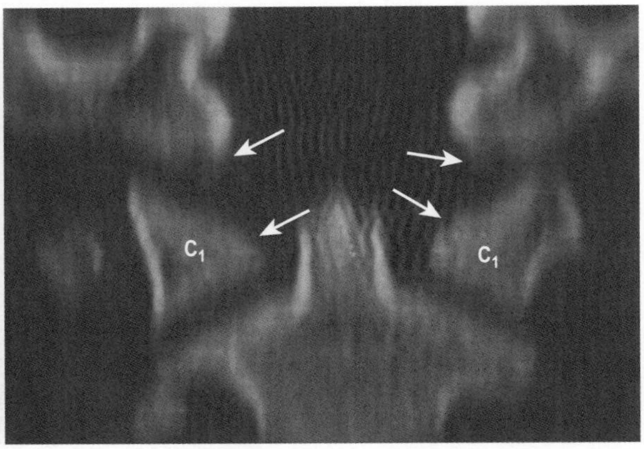

Image A with permission from Miller MD, Thompson SR. Miller's Review of Orthopaedics, 7th ed., Elsevier, 2016; Images B and C with permission from Winn, HR, Youman's Neurological Surgery, 4-Volume Set, 6th ed., 2011, Elsevier, Saunders.

CHAPTER 29

DEGENERATIVE SPINE

SINGLE BEST ANSWER (SBA) QUESTIONS

CERVICAL

1. A 56-year-old female presents with neck pain worsened by activity over the last 6 months. On examination, she has full power bilaterally in the upper and lower extremities. She has a normal gait and no difficulties with manual dexterity. Which one of the following is the most appropriate next step in management?

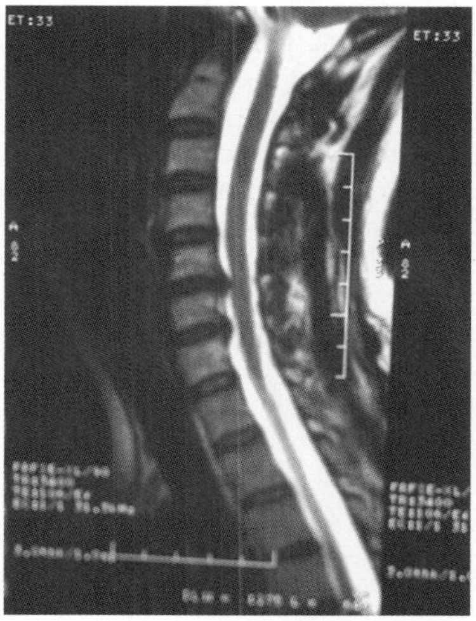

   a. Posterior laminectomy C5-C7
   b. Physiotherapy
   c. Cervical epidural injection
   d. C5/C6 ACDF
   e. C5/C6 foraminotomy

2. Which one of the following statements regarding nonoperative management of cervical disc and degenerative disorders is most accurate?
   a. Nonsteroidal anti-inflammatories should be avoided
   b. Neck pain related to cervical spondylosis improves in only one third of patients
   c. Cervical traction systems are generally recommended
   d. Use of soft cervical collars should not exceed 3 months
   e. Cervical epidural injections are more effective in those with neck pain and radiculopathy

3. A 41-year-old male presents with left arm pain of 4 weeks duration. On examination there is weakness of triceps and wrist flexion. Axial MRI is shown. Which level is the pathology shown likely to be at?

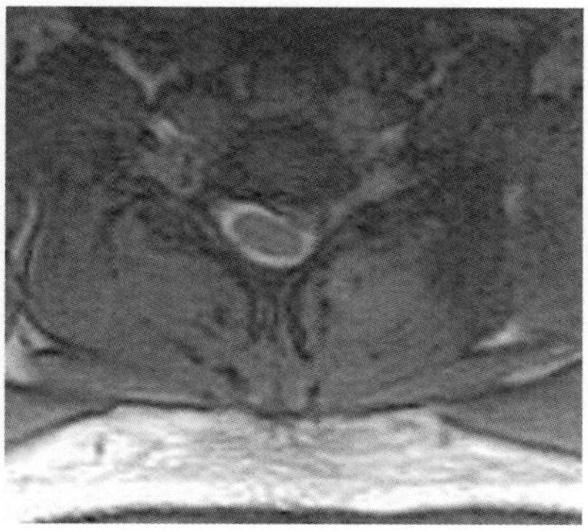

   a. C4/5
   b. C5/6
   c. C6/7
   d. C7/T1
   e. T1/T2

4. Which one of the following statements regarding radiculopathy is most accurate?
   a. Hoffman's sign is suggestive of C5 radiculopathy
   b. Spurling's test involves rotation, extension and axial compression applied to the cervical spine

c. Cervical foraminotomy is indicated in radiculopathy secondary to posterolateral disc protrusion
d. ACDF is not appropriate for patients presenting with radiculopathy and neck pain alone
e. Shoulder abduction test is positive if radiculopathic pain worsens

5. A 65-year-old male presents to your office with difficulty ambulating and buttoning his shirt. It started 2 years ago but has worsened significantly over the last year. On examination he is unable to perform a tandem gait and is Hoffman's sign positive bilaterally, but has flexor plantar reflexes bilaterally. He has 4/5 power in his hands, but 5/5 power in all other muscle groups. MRI sequences are shown. Which one of the following is the most appropriate next step in management?

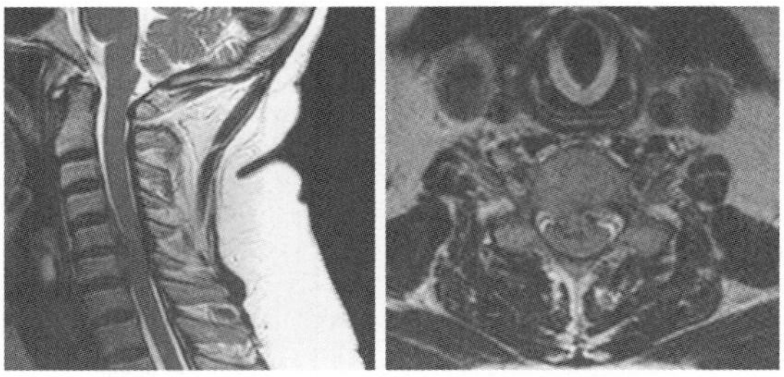

a. C5/6 ACDF
b. C5/6 and C6/7 ACDF
c. C6 corpectomy
d. C5-C6 laminectomy
e. C5-C6 laminectomy and instrumented fusion

6. A 55-year-old man presents to your office with difficulty ambulating and buttoning his shirt. It started 2 years ago but has worsened significantly over the last year. On physical exam he is unable to perform a tandem gait and has a positive Hoffman's sign bilaterally, however he has no ankle clonus and flexor plantars bilaterally. He has 4/5 strength in his hands, but 5/5 strength in all other muscle groups. Sagittal MRI is shown. Which one of the following is the most appropriate next step in management?

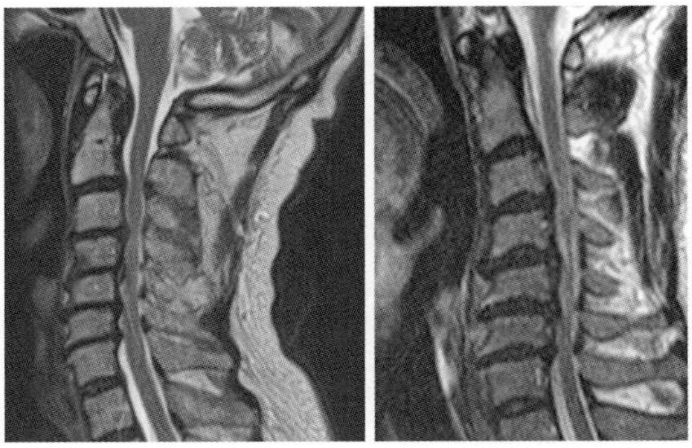

a. C3-C6 laminectomy with lateral mass screw fixation
b. C3-C6 ACDF without instrumentation
c. Cervical epidural steroid injection
d. C3-C6 laminectomy
e. C3-C6 bilateral foraminotomies

7. A 68-year-old female presents with progressive loss of ability to ambulate and dexterity problems with her hands. Six months ago she was able to walk with a cane, but now has difficulty with ambulating with a walker. She also reports difficulty with her hands and needs assistance with eating. Physical exam shows limited neck extension. Flexion extension X-rays do not show any dynamic instability. MRI is shown. Which one of the following is the most appropriate next step in management?

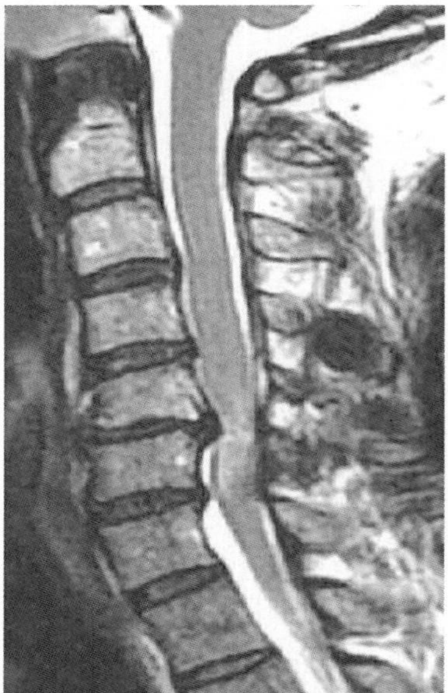

a. C5-C6 posterior decompression and instrumented fusion
b. Physiotherapy and NSAIDs

c. C5-C6 laminoplasty
d. C5-C6 decompressive laminectomy
e. C5/6 and C6/7 anterior cervical decompression and fusion with anterior plate fixation

8. A 44-year-old presents with worsening gait and loss of fine motor control in his hands. Examination reveals normal cranial nerve examination, negative jaw jerk, hyperreflexia in all four limbs, positive bilateral Hoffman's signs and Babinski positive. There is no evidence of dynamic instability on flexion/extension radiographs. MRI shown below. Which one of the following is the most appropriate next step in management?

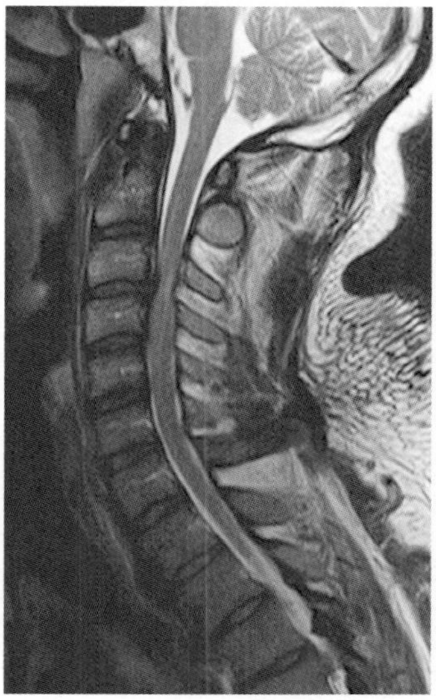

a. C3-C6 laminectomy
b. C3-C6 unilateral foraminotomy
c. C3-C6 bilateral foraminotomy
d. C3-C6 anterior cervical decompression
e. C3-C6 microdiscectomy

9. A 42-year-old with a 3-month history of shooting pains down his left arm which is still severe 7/10 and not improved with physiotherapy or epidural steroid injection. On examination, Spurling's sign is positive (left side), left wrist extensor weakness 4+/5, decreased sensation to pinprick in left C6 distribution. No hyperreflexia or Babinski sign. Cervical MRI shown below. Flexion/extension views do not show any evidence of instability. Which one of the following is the most appropriate next step in management?

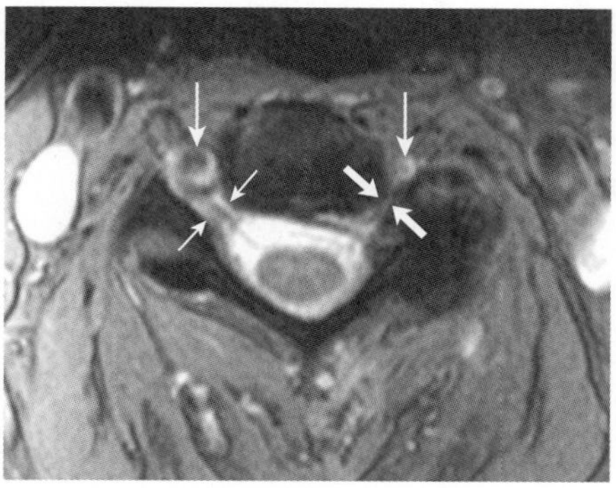

a. Posterior foraminotomy
b. Anterior cervical decompression
c. C6 laminectomy
d. C6 arthroplasty
e. C6 laminectomy and C5-C7 instrumented fusion

10. A 55-year-old presents with 4 months of gait impairment and sustains a fall. On examination, there is spastic tetraparesis 4-/5 globally without evidence of any cerebellar signs. MRI cervical spine is shown. Which one of the following is the most appropriate next step in management?

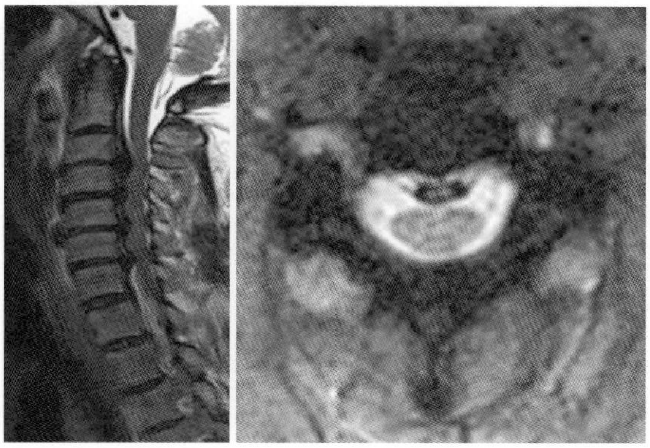

a. C3-C7 laminectomy
b. C3-C7 laminoplasty
c. C3/4, C4/5.C5/6, and C6/7 ACDF
d. C3-C5 corpectomy, srut graft, plates and screws
e. C3-C6 corpectomy, srut graft, plates and screws with resection of posterior longitudinal ligament

11. Postoperatively following C3/4 ACDF a patient notices decreased sweating on one side of her face and slight eyelid droop on the same side. Which one of the following is most likely?
    a. Retraction injury to vagus nerve in carotid sheath
    b. Intraoperative stroke due to disruption of carotid plaque
    c. Injury to sympathetic chain along longus colli muscle
    d. Traction injury to cutaneous cervical sensory nerves giving reduced sensation of sweating
    e. Thermal injury to branches of facial nerve within the parotid gland

12. Which one of the following have been associated with reduced risk of recurrent laryngeal nerve palsy?
    a. Left sided neck dissection
    b. Deflating ETT pressure after retractor insertion
    c. Same side approach for revision surgery
    d. Sharp dissection during exposure
    e. Anterior cervical plate fixation

13. A 54-year-old female undergoes an C6/7 ACDF via right sided approach and does not have any new postoperative deficits. Three days later, she develops burning pain to her left shoulder region followed by loss of shoulder abduction and weakness of elbow flexion. Post-operative MRI of the cervical spine was unremarkable. Which one of the following is most likely?
    a. Cage migration
    b. Epidural hematoma
    c. Traction injury to brachial plexus from taping of shoulders
    d. Parsonage-Turner syndrome
    e. C7 palsy

14. Six hours after a C5-C6 ACDF, the nurse calls you that the patient is having difficulty swallowing and breathing. By the time you arrive to the bedside, the patient is in distress, SOB, tachycardic, tachypneic, despite being on a nonrebreathe oxygen facemask. The hemovac drain reservoir showed minimal bloody drainage and the tubing appeared to be clotted and his neck is extremely tense and swollen. She appears cyanosed and SpO_2 is 79% and falling. Which one of the following is the most appropriate next step in management?
    a. Stat neck X-ray to look for cage migration
    b. Urgent neck CT
    c. Immediately reopen neck incision at the bedside
    d. Intramuscular adrenaline
    e. CT pulmonary angiogram

15. A 52-year-old female underwent a C5/6 ACDF for cervical radiculopathy through a left-sided approach 2 years ago. She has had an altered voice since this operation. Recently, the patient has developed myelopathic symptoms including gait instability and dexterity problems with her hands. Flexion extension X-rays do not reveal any dynamic instability. MRI is shown. Laryngoscopy demonstrates abnormal function of the vocal cords on the left hand side. Which one of the following is the most appropriate next step in management?

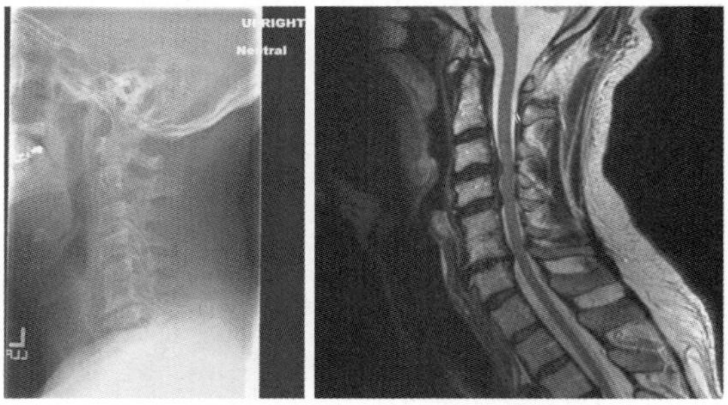

    a. C3/4 and C4/5 ACDF via right sided anterior approach
    b. C3/4 and C4/5 ACDF via left sided anterior approach
    c. C3-C7 laminectomy with instrumented fusion
    d. C3-C7 laminoforaminotomy
    e. C3-C5 laminoplasty

16. A 73-year-old female presents with neck pain and clumsiness in her hands. Past medical history includes rheumatoid arthritis. On exam she has 4+/5 power in the lower limbs, hyperreflexia and extensor plantars. Flexing her neck produces an electric shock-like sensation down her spine. Which one of the following is the most appropriate next step in management?

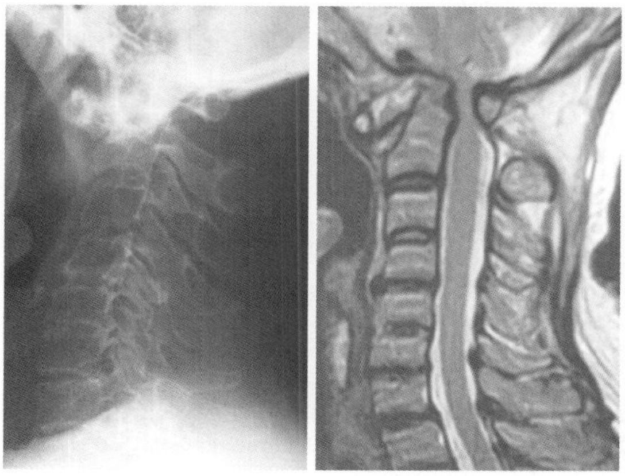

a. Rigid collar for 6-12 weeks
b. Halo immobilization for 12 weeks
c. Transoral odontoid resection
d. Anterior odontoid screw fixation
e. Posterior C1-C2 fusion

17. Which one of the following statements regarding the condition shown is LEAST accurate?

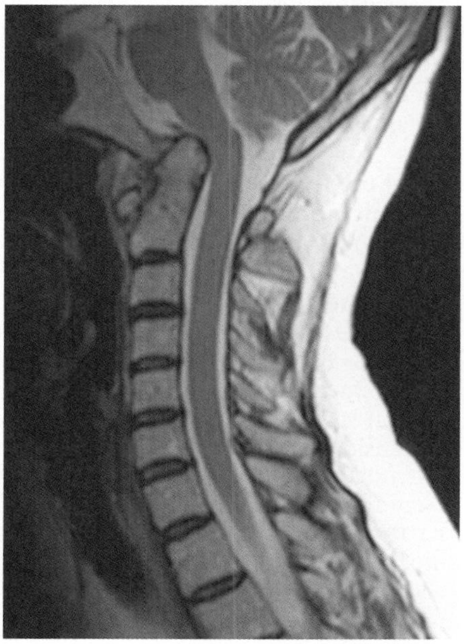

a. Transoral odontoid resection may be required in reducible migration
b. Cervicomedullary angle <135° suggests impeding neurological compromise
c. Occipitocervical (O-C2) fusion is usually appropriate if deformity reduction if possible
d. Ranawat C1-C2 index is the most reproducible radiological sign
e. The tip of the dens is >4.5 mm above McGregor's line

18. A 29-year-old male presents with numbness and tingling in his lower extremities and gait instability for 2 weeks. Physical exam shows 3+ brisk patellar reflexes. MRI is shown. Which one of the following is the LEAST appropriate next step in management?

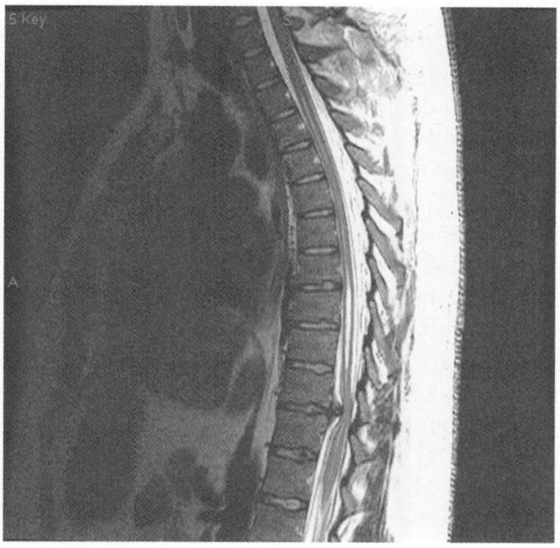

a. Laminectomy and discectomy
b. Anterior thoracic discectomy
c. Transpedicular approach and discectomy
d. Transcostovertebral approach and discectomy
e. Costotransversectomy and discectomy

19. A 35-year-old female presents for evaluation of new onset lumbar spine pain. Which one of the following physical exam findings is indicative of an organic cause of low back pain symptoms?
a. Superficial and nonanatomic tenderness
b. Pain with axial compression of the lumbar spine
c. Negative straight-leg raise with patient distraction
d. Regional disturbances which do not follow a logical dermatomal pattern
e. Nocturnal pain in the thoracic spine

20. A 35-year-old female presents for evaluation of new onset lumbar spine pain. Which one of the following is a yellow flag for back pain?
   a. Recent history of violent trauma
   b. Constant, progressive, nonmechanical pain
   c. Reduced activity levels due to avoidance
   d. Focal kyphosis
   e. Unexplained weight loss

QUESTIONS 21–34

Additional questions 21–34 available on ExpertConsult.com

EXTENDED MATCHING ITEM (EMI) QUESTIONS

35. **Back pain:**
   a. Ankylosing spondylitis
   b. Cauda equina syndrome
   c. Degenerative lumbar disc disease
   d. Destructive spondyloarthropathy
   e. Diffuse idiopathic skeletal hyperostosis (DISH)
   f. Mechanical back pain
   g. Ossification of the posterior longitudinal ligament (OPLL)
   h. Osteoporosis
   i. Rheumatoid arthritis
   j. Spinal stenosis
   k. Spondylolisthesis
   l. Vascular claudication

For each of the following descriptions, select the most appropriate answers from the list above. Each answer may be used once, more than once or not at all.

1. A 68-year-old male presents with buttock and bilateral leg pain made worse by walking and relieved on bending forward.
2. A 70-year-old diabetic male presents with back pain and stiffness. Plain radiographs of the thoracolumbar spine showed the presence of nonmarginal osteophytes at three successive levels.
3. A 48-year-old hemodialysis patient presents with back pain. Radiographs of the thoracolumbar spine showed a destruction of three adjacent vertebrae and two intervening discs.
4. A 38-year-old male presents with an insidious onset of back pain. Spine radiographs revealed the presence of vertical osteophytes giving a "bamboo" appearance.

36. **Neurological signs and tests:**
   a. Abdominal reflex
   b. Adam's test
   c. Babinski reflex
   d. Bowstring test
   e. Bulbocavernosus reflex
   f. Femoral stretch test
   g. Finger escape sign
   h. Hoffman's test
   i. Inverted radial reflex
   j. Lasegue's test
   k. Lhermitte's sign
   l. Oppenheim test
   m. Schober's test
   n. Spurling's test

For each of the following descriptions, select the most appropriate answers from the list above. Each answer may be used once, more than once or not at all.

1. Snapping or flicking the middle fingernail results in flexion of thumb.
2. Supinator reflex elicits finger flexion only
3. Scratch along the crest of the patient's tibia in a downward motion produces extensor plantar response
4. It is one of the first reflexes to return after spinal shock

37. **Intervertebral disc disease:**
   a. Central disc
   b. Disc bulge
   c. Disc extrusion
   d. Disc protrusion
   e. Far lateral disc
   f. Herniated disc
   g. Migrated disc
   h. Neural foraminal disc
   i. Paracentral disc
   j. Sequestered disc

For each of the following descriptions, select the most appropriate answers from the list above. Each answer may be used once, more than once or not at all.

1. A herniated disc where the base of the herniation is smaller than the anterior-posterior dimension
2. A herniated disc where the base of the herniation is wider than the anterior-posterior dimension
3. Extruded disc material that has broken away from the site of extrusion
4. Extruded disc material extending in the craniocaudal plane but still in continuity with disc

SBA ANSWER

1. **b**—Physiotherapy

Cervical spondylosis is characterized by degeneration of the disc, both facet joints and both uncovertebral joints of the cervical motion segment most commonly at C5/6 and C6/7 levels where the majority of flexion/extension occurs. Risk factors include age (5th decade onwards), males, excessive driving, smoking, lifting, and professional athletes (e.g. jockeys, rugby, gymnastics). It involves disc degeneration (loss of height, bulging, and herniation), joint degeneration (uncinate spurring, facet hypertrophy), ligamentous changes (thickening, infolding, bowstringing), and kyphosis. Presentation is usually with discogenic neck pain, radiculopathy or myelopathy. Nerve root compression may be due to foraminal stenosis due to spondylotic changes (e.g. chondrosseous spurs of facet and uncovertebral joints), posterolateral disc herniation or disc-osteophyte complex in the lateral recess, and foraminal soft disc herniation. Cervical cord compression due to central canal stenosis leads to a clinical picture of myelopathy and occurs with a canal diameter <13 mm (normal is 17 mm), worse during neck extension when the central cord becomes pinched between degenerative disc (anteriorly) hypertrophic facets and infolded ligamentum (posteriorly). X-rays may show degenerative changes of uncovertebral and facet joints, osteophyte formation, disc space narrowing, vertebral endplate sclerosis, sagittal canal diameter <13 mm and spondylolisthesis but often do not correlate with symptoms (70% of patients by 70 years of age will have degenerative changes). Flexion and extension views should be assessed for instability and compensatory subluxation above or below the spondylotic segment, and oblique views for foraminal stenosis. MRI can assess status of soft tissues and identifies neural compression (CT myelography in patients that cannot have an MRI). Nerve conduction studies may help in cases where clinical and imaging findings are unable to distinguish between central versus peripheral causes. Management in initially nonoperative (physiotherapy, NSAIDs, and a cervical collar) but can be escalated if this fails or the patient develops radiculopathy/myelopathy (e.g. foraminotomy, laminectomy, anterior cervical discectomy).

Image with permission from Miller, M, Hart, JA, MacKnight JM. Essential Orthopaedics, Saunders, Elsevier, 2010.

2. **e**—Cervical epidural injections are more effective in those with neck pain and radiculopathy

Many cases of acute neck pain may arise from soft tissue sprains and muscle strains, but ongoing neck pain is more suggestive of a spondylotic source. The natural histories of most nonmyelopathic spondylotic cervical disorders are statistically favorable, with 40-50% becoming pain free/no recurrence and 20-30% getting worse/persisting (i.e. 70-80% improve to varying degree). Modifiable factors have been identified, including smoking, obesity, occupational hazards, and psychological factors. Initial treatment of acute pain can include a brief trial of rest and immobilization with a soft cervical collar. Medications including narcotics, NSAIDs, oral steroids, and antidepressants can be beneficial. Although short-term (<2 weeks) use of cervical collars may be beneficial, prolonged immobilization should be avoided to prevent atrophy of the cervical musculature. Traction (at home) should be avoided in myelopathic patients to prevent stretching of a compromised spinal cord. Participation in an active rehabilitation protocol seems much more likely to be successful than use of passive modalities. Cervical manipulation should not be undertaken without an adequate radiographic examination to screen for potential instability, given complications that include radiculopathy, myelopathy, spinal cord injury, and vertebrobasilar artery injury. Cervical epidural injections, or selective root blocks, help most in those with neck pain and radiculopathy but it is unclear whether they alter the natural history of radiculopathy or surgical management. Complications of cervical steroid injections are rare but devastating when they occur (dural puncture, meningitis, epidural abscess, intraocular hemorrhage, adrenocortical suppression, and epidural hematoma). Patients with myelopathy, severe or progressive neurologic symptoms, or failure to improve with time are good candidates for surgery whereas those with axial neck pain alone from disc degeneration are not.

3. **c**—C6/7 (i.e. C7 radiculopathy)

Pedicle/nerve root mismatch between cervical and thoracolumbar spine is that in the cervical spine a given nerve root exits above the pedicle belonging to its named vertebra (e.g. C6 nerve root exits at the C5/6 intervertebral foramen). However, since C8 nerve root exits at C7/T1 level below this all names nerve roots exit below the pedicle of its named vertebrae (e.g. L5 nerve root exits at L5/S1 intervertebral foramen). As such, nerve roots in the cervical spine have a horizontal path whereas those in the lumbar spine are more vertically orientated. This is important, because of the resultant differential effect of posterolateral and foraminal disc herniations in the lumbar spine but not the cervical spine. For example, in the cervical spine at C5/6 either a posterolateral disc herniation or a foraminal disc herniation will cause a C6 radiculopathy. In contrast, in the lumbar spine at L4/5 a posterolateral disc herniation will affect the traversing nerve root (i.e. L5 nerve root) while foraminal disc will affect the exiting L4 nerve root. Central disc prolapses in the cervical or thoracic spine will result in myelopathy if significant, whereas in the thoracolumbar (T12-L2) and lower lumbar spine they may cause conus medullaris syndrome (mixture of UMN/LMN signs and bladder involvement) or cauda equina syndrome respectively. Common patterns of radiculopathy in the cervical spine include:

C5 radiculopathy leads to deltoid and biceps weakness,
C6 radiculopathy leads to brachioradialis and wrist extension weakness,
C7 radiculopathy leads to triceps and wrist flexion weakness, and
C8 radiculopathy leads to finger flexion weakness.

Image with permission from Saraf-Lavi E. Spine Imaging: Case Review Series, 3rd ed., Elsevier, Saunders, 2014.

4. **b**—Spurling's test involves rotation, extension and axial compression applied to the cervical spine

Incidence of cervical radiculopathy was found to be 83 per 100,000 population, with a peak incidence in the 6th decade of life. While central disc prolapses can cause myelopathy in cervical/thoracic spine, or conus medullaris/cauda equina syndromes in the lumbar spine. While in the lumbar spine posterolateral disc prolapse causes a radiculopathy affecting the traversing nerve root and far lateral/foraminal disc prolapses affect the exiting nerve root, both types of disc herniation affect the same nerve root in the cervical spine (as travel horizontally). The two major provocative tests for cervical radiculopathy include the Spurling test and the shoulder abduction test. They state that acute cervical radiculopathy has 75% rate of spontaneous improvement with nonsurgical treatment. If surgery is necessary, either anterior cervical discectomy and fusion (ACDF) or posterior laminoforaminotomy is warranted. Posterior cervical foraminotomy is highly effective in treating patients with cervical radiculopathy. The approach is effective in decompressing lateral spinal roots that are compromised by soft disc herniations or osteophytic spurs. It also reduces the risk of iatrogenic injury with anterior approaches. Long-term radiographic follow-up shows no significant trend toward kyphosis and improved long-term pain scores compared to nonoperative treatment. Advantages of ACDF include increased fusion rates (with graft insertion in the disc space) and decompression of the neural foramina by increasing its cephalocaudal dimension. On the other hand, the posterior approach maintains spinal alignment and does not require fusion, but increases risk of neck pain (from posterior muscle dissection).

5. **a**—C5/6 ACDF

The incidence of cervical myelopathy is difficult to ascertain due to subtly of early findings and overlap with features of "old age." The natural history of spondylotic cervical myelopathy is characterized by slow progression in a pattern of stepwise deterioration following periods of stable symptoms. Patients often complain of balance issues, numbness and weakness in their hands, and difficulty with fine motor tasks. Examination may reveal Hoffman's sign and finger escape sign in a myelopathic hand, and long tract signs in the legs (e.g. clonus, extensor plantar response), and difficulty with tandem gait. Factors that are associated with worse outcomes with nonoperative treatment include segmental kyphosis and circumferential spinal cord compression. Clinical classification systems for cervical myelopathy include Nurick, Ranawat, and the Japanese Orthopaedic Association. Imaging shows loss of the CSF signal around the cord, and intramedullary hyperintensity on T2 weighted imaging. Sometimes myelopathy may be due to dynamic cord compression, still producing high T2 signal in the cord, without cord compression in the neutral position hence flexion extension X-rays or dynamic imaging may be required. In this case, there is extrusion of the C5/6 disc with migration caudally and ACDF at this level is indicated.

Image with permission from Townsend CM, Beauchamp D, Evers BM, Mattox KL (Eds.), Sabiston Textbook of Surgery, 19th ed., Saunders, Elsevier, 2012.

6. **a**—C3-C6 laminectomy with lateral mass screw fixation

This patient has cervical myelopathy with multilevel anterior and posterior compression. Presence of a rigid kyphotic deformity favors use of an anterior approach (can correct kyphotic deformity as well as decompress cord; posterior surgery is unable to correct deformity and may make it worse if noninstrumented). Posterior laminectomy and instrumented fusion is preferable for patients with a lordotic cervical spine and either three or more levels of compression, primarily posterior compression or diffuse congenital stenosis.

Images with permission from (a) Quiñones-Hinojosa A. Schmidek and Sweet's Operative Neurosurgical Techniques, 6th ed., Saunders, Elsevier, 2012. (b) Du W, Zhang P, Shen Y, et al. Enlarged laminectomy and lateral mass screw fixation for multilevel cervical degenerative myelopathy associated with kyphosis, Spine J 14 (1);2014:57-64.

7. **e**—C5/6 and C6/7 anterior cervical decompression and anterior plate fixation

In patients with cervical myelopathy due to canal stenosis, surgical approach will be influenced by the sagittal alignment of the cervical spine. Lateral cervical radiographs in neutral position and flexion and extension can identify kyphotic deformity and determine whether it is rigid or not. The C2-C7 angle is determined by intersecting lines extended from the posterior borders of the C2 and C7 vertebral bodies respectively, whereas the local kyphotic angle is based on the posterior borders of the vertebral bodies that immediately flank the kyphotic segment. If patients have significant kyphosis, the spinal cord is draped over the anterior compressive elements, and a posterior approach alone is not recommended. The mainstay of treatment in most patients with multi-level disease would be laminectomy with posterior fusion or laminoplasty (if kyphosis is <10-13°) or a combined anterior and posterior approach (if kyphosis is >10-13°). Possible treatment options in this case could be (1) C5/6 and C6/7 anterior cervical decompression and fusion with anterior plate fixation, (2) C5 corpectomy with ACDF at C5/6 and anterior plate fixation, or (3) a C5 and C6 corpectomy, anterior plate fixation, followed by posterior decompression and instrumented fusion (any two level corpectomy needs to be stabilized posterior due to the high rate of graft migration).

Image with permission from Yeh KT, Lee RP, Chen IH. Laminoplasty with adjunct anterior short segment fusion for multilevel cervical myelopathy associated with local kyphosis. J Chin Med Assoc 2015;78(6):364-9.

8. **a**—C3-C6 laminectomy

This case shows cervica myelopathy due to canal stenosis at multiple levels without any kyphotic deformity. In this situation, the goal is decompression of the spinal cord which will only be adequate with laminectomy. Pre-operative flexion/extension films should be performed as if any evidence of instability this may favor instrumented fixation with lateral mass screws. Intraoperative concerns include maintaining MAP >70 mmHg in myelopathic patients, avoiding dural tears, ensuring sufficient width of the laminectomy (approx. 15 mm), avoiding violation of the facet joints (<50%) and minimizing risk factors for C5 palsy.

Image with permission from Saraf-Lavi E. Spine Imaging: Case Review Series, 3rd ed., Elsevier, Saunders, 2014.

9. **a**—Posterior foraminotomy

The case describes a left C6 radiculopathy which has failed conservative management, and MRI shows foraminal stenosis. As such posterior foraminotomy is the most appropriate first line operative treatment. The goal is to open the intervertebral foramen to decompress exiting nerve root, which can be done unilaterally or bilaterally at one or more levels for patients with radiculopathy. Care must be taken to avoid resecting over 50% of the facet otherwise this could lead to instability. The other choices are indicated when myelopathy is present due to canal stenosis/disc herniation.

Image with permission from Czervionke LF, Fenton DS. Imaging Painful Spine Disorders, 2011 by Mayo Foundation for Medical Education and Research, Published by Saunders, Elsevier.

10. **b**—C3-C7 laminoplasty

OPLL is a common cause of cervical myelopathy in the Asian population, men >women, C4-C6 levels Risk factors diabetes obesity high salt-low meat diet poor calcium absorption mechanical stress on posterior longitudinal ligament. Presentation may be with myelopathy, neck pain or asymptomatic. Lateral radiographs often shows ossification of PLL important to evaluate sagittal alignment of cervical spine. MRI is study of choice to evaluate spinal cord compression, whereas CT will delineate bony anatomy of ossified posterior longitudinal ligament. Given the propensity for progression, nonoperative management may only be indicated in those with mild symptoms and/or who are not candidates for surgery. Most symptomatic patients will undergo surgery, with anterior or posterior approaches. Anterior approaches may involves interbody fusion (limiting changes in sagittal canal diameter with flexion/extension hence best for dynamic myelopathy) or corpectomy with/without resection of the OPLL (can just be left to float in corpectomy site, and reduces risk of dural tear when trying to dissect PLL off thecal sac) and must be used in those with existing kyphotic deformity. Posterior laminoplasty or laminectomy with fusion is only appropriate in lordotic cervical spine and is safer and preferable approach due to the difficulty of resecting the OPLL off the dura from an anterior approach. Where laminectomy (rather than laminoplasty) is performed instrumented fusion to avoid post-operative kyphosis is recommended.

Image with permission from Jandial R, Garfin SR. Best Evidence for Spine Surgery: 20 Cardinal Cases, Saunders, Elsevier, 2012.

11. **c**—Injury to sympathetic chain along longus colli muscle (post-op Horner's syndrome)

Advantages of Anterior Approach	Disadvantages of Anterior Approach
Direct decompression of anterior pathology Muscle sparing approach Reduced blood loss, infection, LOS High fusion rate Access to multiple levels via small incision Good for correction of kyphotic deformity Transverse incision allows access up to three levels	Requires fusion Increased surgical time, and morbidity with multiple levels Risk of recurrent laryngeal nerve injury Risk of dysphagia Risk of injury to vascular/visceral structures Access limited to C2-T1 Visible scar Limited access after previous surgery/ radiotherapy

12. **a**—Left-sided neck dissection

Right recurrent laryngeal nerve ascends in the neck after passing around the subclavian vessels, courses medially and cranially at the C6-C7 level, often along with the inferior thyroid artery. In contrast, the left recurrent laryngeal nerve curves around the aortic arch and then ascends along the tracheoesophageal groove in a more midline and protected position. This has led some to suggest a left-sided approach is safer especially when lower cervical segments are approached, but studies favoring either a right- or a left-sided approach are found in the literature. Arguments supporting a left-sided approach have been based on anatomical factors described and the possible occurrence of a nonrecurrent inferior laryngeal nerve on the right, while proponents of a right-sided approach have argued that it is more comfortable for right-handed surgeons, that a left-sided approach puts the thoracic duct at risk (at C7-T1 level), and that the esophagus lies anatomically slightly to the left, which renders a right-sided approach safer.

13. **d**—Parsonage-Turner syndrome

The most common nerve injury with anterior and posterior cervical spine surgery is C5 nerve palsy, with an incidence of about 5%; decompressive procedures for myelopathy have the highest rate of this complication. Several theories potentially explain nerve root palsies, including direct trauma or a traction phenomenon from displacement of the spinal cord after decompression, or segmental cord gray matter dysfunction. Patients with C5 palsy generally present in a delayed fashion (within 1 week) postoperatively, sometimes even as long as 1 month postoperatively. The most common presentation is with deltoid and biceps weakness.

Generally, if a patient awakens from surgery with upper extremity weakness, the differential should include shoulder traction (diffuse distribution) caused by positioning or intraoperative nerve trauma (root and side specific). When presenting in a delayed fashion, the main differentials include compressive causes (cage/bone graft migration) which can be excluded on MRI, C5 nerve palsy and Parsonage-Turner syndrome (PTS). PTS is typically characterised by severe pain followed shortly by the onset of weakness, and the weakness, sensory deficit, and pain usually do not all correspond to the same nerve root or peripheral nerve distribution. By contrast, the C5 palsy is predominantly motor disturbance. EMG is useful at 1-4 weeks after onset to clarify distribution. If no compression is noted, patients are treated symptomatically with physical therapy and pain control. Given the lack of deltoid function and the possibility of a traction phenomenon, patients with C5 palsy are given a sling for comfort (steroids are not routinely given). Most patients recover within 6 months.

Common Complications of Cervical Spine Surgery

Anterior Approach	Posterior Approach
Hypoglossal nerve injury Superior laryngeal nerve injury Recurrent laryngeal nerve injury Sympathetic chain injury (Horner's syndrome ~1%) C5 palsy ~5%	C2 nerve root injury (C1 lateral mass screws) Third occipital nerve injury (occipital neuralgia) C5 nerve root palsy ~5% C8 nerve root palsy (C7/T1 osteotomy)

FURTHER READING

Brown JM, Yee A, Ivens RA, Dribben W, Mackinnon SE. Post-cervical decompression parsonage-turner syndrome represents a subset of C5 palsy: six cases and a review of the literature: case report. Neurosurgery. 2010 Dec;67(6): E1831-43; discussion E1843-4. doi: http://dx.doi.org/10.1227/NEU.0b013e3181f8254b. Review. PubMed PMID: 21107152.

14. **c**—immediately reopen neck incision at bedside

One of the most serious adverse events associated with anterior cervical spine surgery is postoperative airway obstruction due to wound hematoma. The reported incidence of this complication has varied from 0.2% to 1.9%. Hematoma following anterior cervical spine surgery may be the result of inadequate control of arterial or venous bleeding during the operation, and has been reported due to superior thyroid artery dissection. In other instances, a hematoma can form after surgery irrespective of adequate intraoperative hemostasis. Postoperative hemorrhage may occur secondary to coagulopathy, increased blood pressure during emergence from anesthesia, or elevated venous pressure due to the Valsalva effect of coughing at the time of extubation. There are two potential pathophysiologic mechanisms by which hematoma can produce airway compromise. The first is direct mechanical compression leading to reduction in the cross-sectional area of the airway lumen. The second mechanism involves the development of intrinsic airway edema in response to the mass effect of collected blood within the surgical wound impaired venous drainage (more likely as requires lower pressure to obstruct). Although delayed hematoma is possible beyond the first 12 h, alternative causes of airway obstruction (e.g. pharyngeal/prevertebral edema, spinal construct failure, cerebrospinal fluid collection or retropharyngeal abscess) become more probable. The primary treatment objective is to establish and maintain patency of the airway by placement of an endotracheal tube—in a noncritical airway this is attempted in the operating suite, whereas in the critical airway compromise (e.g. air hunger, excessive salivation, a rocking motion of the head and chest with the respiratory cycle, use of accessory muscles of respiration, inspiratory stridor and, eventually, central cyanosis) this is done at the bedside. Once definitive airway control is achieved, the patient can undergo wound exploration in theater. However, if the initial intubation attempt fails (or airway management equipment is not immediately available), the surgical wound should be opened and blood clot removed at the bedside followed by reassessment of airway and need for further intubation attempts/cricothyroidotomy.

FURTHER READING

Palumbo MA, et al. Airway compromise due to wound hematoma following anterior cervical spine surgery. Open Orthop J 6;2012:108-13.

15. **c**—C3-C7 laminectomy with instrumented fusion

Adjacent level disease is a relatively frequent clinical finding after cervical spine surgery (approx. 3%). Whenever possible, nonoperative treatment should be attempted, but it may be less successful than in de novo cervical spondylotic syndromes. If nonoperative treatment fails, radiculopathy or myelopathy caused by adjacent level disease can be treated operatively much in the same manner as de novo disease. Relevant considerations in the operative treatment of adjacent segment disease include anterior versus posterior approaches, fusion versus motion-preserving procedures, and single-level versus multilevel surgical procedures. Revision ACDF has good outcomes, but suspected pseudoarthrosis at the index level and recurrent laryngeal nerve status should be considered. The right and left recurrent laryngeal nerves innervate the posterior cricoarytenoid muscles which open the vocal cords. Injury to the ipsilateral recurrent laryngeal nerve can occur in 1.5-6% of patients after ACDF, with resultant unilateral paralysis of the posterior cricoarytenoid muscle. Although paralysis of this muscle unilaterally is usually benign, bilateral paralysis can lead to severe airway difficulties and the need for tracheostomy. If revision surgery is planned from the opposite side, the vocal cords need to be evaluated with laryngoscopy preoperatively. If there was asymptomatic/occult (left) RLN injury from the initial surgery, then the opposite side approach is inadvisable for fear of developing bilateral vocal cord paralysis and its catastrophic complications. Posterior decompression and fusion can provide a high fusion rate and avoid revision ACDF at the index level. Patients with multilevel spondylotic compression may also benefit from a posterior approach to address multiple levels of disease. Posteriorly based nonfusion options include laminoforaminotomy for single-level radiculopathic symptoms and laminoplasty for multilevel disease. Contraindications to laminoplasty include cervical kyphosis, which does not allow the spinal cord to drift posteriorly and be indirectly decompressed, and significant preoperative neck pain. The rate of postoperative neck pain after laminoplasty is high, and patients should be counseled accordingly. Given the relatively recent advent of cervical disc arthroplasty, clinical data are currently not sufficient to recommend for or against arthroplasty at a level adjacent to a fusion. This case describes myelopathy with evidence of multilevel disease, both above and below the fused segment, without any kyphotic deformity, but in the presence of an occult left recurrent laryngeal nerve palsy. These features favor a posterior approach from C3 to C7, which could be either laminoplasty or laminectomy with instrumented fusion.

Image with permission from Shen FH, et al. (Eds.), Textbook of the Cervical Spine, Saunders, Elsevier, 2015.

FURTHER READING

Regan C, Lim MR. Adjacent segment disease. In: Shen FH, et al. (Eds.), Textbook of the Cervical Spine, Saunders, Elsevier, 2015.

16. **e**—Posterior C1-C2 fusion

Although the occurrence of radiographic evidence of disease as atlantoaxial subluxation in asymptomatic patients is common, the most frequent presenting symptom is pain. It is usually a combination of occipital and neck pain that either is caused by mechanical instability or is radicular, as a result of compression of C1 and C2 nerves. A positive Sharp-Purser test is a clicking sensation in extension that results with spontaneous reduction of atlantoaxial subluxation. Neurologic manifestations are less common and are caused by mechanical neurovascular compression on the cervical spine and cervicomedullary junction. Patients may present with cervical myelopathy manifesting as gait dystaxia, hand clumsiness, and difficulty with dexterity. Objective findings of myelopathy include weakness, hyperreflexia, and positive Hoffmann, Babinski, and Lhermitte signs. Cruciate paralysis and even sudden death from respiratory arrest have also been reported. The deep tendon reflex may not be elicited in RA because of appendicular joint destruction. Anterior subluxation of the atlas on the axis results from weakening and disruption of the transverse ligament following joint inflammation around it. The subluxation can be anterior, posterior, lateral, or rotatory. An atlantoaxial subluxation occurs in 60-80% of cases of rheumatoid arthritis (RA) as the result of pannus formation at the synovial joints between the dens and the ring of C1. Patients with symptomatic instability or no symptoms but ADI > 10 mm and SAC < 14 mm are generally managed with operative stabilization. If the subluxation is reducible, a posterior approach and C1-C2 instrumented fixation are used. Occipitocervical fusion (O-C2) may be considered in this patient population if co-existent basilar invagination is present or likely in future, or if anterior compression from pannus requires C1 posterior arch resection. When the subluxation is not reducible or when it is associated with anterior pannus compressing the upper cervical spine, anterior release of odontoid is generally required before posterior fusion.

Image with permission from Ogihara N, Takahashi J, Hirabayashi H, et al. Long-term results of computer-assisted posterior occipitocervical reconstruction. World Neurosurg 2010;73(6):722-8.

17. **a**—Transoral odontoid resection may be required in reducible migration

With RA progression, the atlanto-occipital and atlantoaxial joints and lateral masses are destroyed, resulting in cranial migration of the odontoid process and hence "settling" and rheumatoid basilar invagination in 40%. This condition leads to variable degrees of neurovascular cervicomedullary compression. Multiplanar CT and MRI studies that delineate the bony and the neurovascular anatomy, respectively, should always be used during the workup because they also facilitate the diagnosis. Surgery is indicated when patients are symptomatic, when radiographic evidence of instability is present, or when

Radiological Features of Atlantoaxial Instability Versus Basilar Invagination

Atlantoaxial Instability/Subluxation Radiological Features	Basilar Invagination Radiological Features
ADI difference of >3.5 mm between flexion and extension suggests instability (not an indication for surgery)	Ranawat C1-C2 index <13 mm (most reproducible; normally 17 mm in men, 15 mm in women)
ADI >5 mm is diagnostic of subluxation	Tip of dens >4.5 mm above McGregor's line
ADI difference of >7 mm of motion may indicate disruption of alar ligament	Dens is above McRae's line
ADI difference of >10 mm motion of associated with increased risk of neurologic injury and an indication for surgery	Dens >3 mm above Chamberlain's line Cervicomedullary angle <135°
PADI (SAC) <14 mm associated with increased risk of neurologic injury and is an indication for surgery	
PADI (SAC) >13 mm may predict complete neural recovery after decompressive surgery	

the degree of compression of cervicomedullary junction is severe (cervicomedullary angle $<135^\circ$). The surgical approach depends on the ability to achieve reduction preoperatively. Flexion and extension imaging is helpful in determining the extent or absence of reduction. Often, preoperative traction can also be used in achieving reduction and is successful in 75% or 80% of the cases. When reduction occurs, dorsal occipitocervical fusion (O-C2), with or without suboccipital decompression, is sufficient. When the invagination is not reducible, transoral resection of the odontoid/pannus should precede dorsal occipitocervical fusion.

Image with permission from Saraf-Lavi E. Spine Imaging: Case Review Series, 3rd ed., Elsevier, Saunders, 2014.

18. **a**—Laminectomy and discectomy

The clinical presentation and imaging studies are consistent with a thoracic disc herniation with spinal cord compression causing symptoms of thoracic myelopathy. This is an indication for surgery. Thoracic level disc herniations are treated with anterior discectomy with or without fusion.

- Thoracic disc herniations, although uncommon, are encountered by spine surgeons. Relative immobility of the thoracic spine as compared with the cervical and lumbar regions and thus the low incidence of degenerative changes. The majority are T8-T11.
- Laminectomy is an unacceptable treatment for thoracic disc herniations due to high rates of paralysis and death in the earliest published studies (1950-1960s). Since the abandonment of laminectomy for thoracic disc herniations, morbidity and mortality rates have dropped significantly.
- Posterior techniques include the transpedicular, Stillerman's transfacet pedicle sparing, transcostovertebral, costotransversectomy, and lateral extracavitary.
- Posterior approaches are generally favored in cases of more lateral, noncalcified, extradural disc herniations and in those not fit enough for an anterior approach (e.g. pulmonary disease.
- Anterior approaches include the transthoracic (below T4), retropleural, and transsternal (above T4).
- Anterior techniques offer better ventral exposure for discs that are centrally located, calcified, and/or intradural.
- Complication rates for the common posterior and anterior procedures are similar.

Image with permission from Quiñones-Hinojosa A. Schmidek and Sweet's Operative Neurosurgical Techniques, 6th ed., Saunders, Elsevier, 2012.

FURTHER READING

Simmons NE. Surgical techniques in the management of thoracic disc herniations. In: Quiñones-Hinojosa A (Ed.), Schmidek and Sweet's Operative Neurosurgical Techniques, 6th ed., Saunders, Elsevier, 2012.

19. **e**—Nocturnal pain in the thoracic spine

Nonorganic signs of low back pain (i.e. Waddell Signs) include superficial and nonanatomic tenderness, pain with axial compression or simulated rotation of the lumbar spine, negative straight-leg raise with patient distraction, regional disturbances which do not follow a logical dermatomal pattern, and overreaction to physical examination. Nocturnal pain is a red flag symptom, especially considering the majority of spinal metastases are thoracic.

FURTHER READING

Waddell G, McCulloch JA, Kummel E, Venner RM. Nonorganic physical signs in low-back pain. Spine (Phila Pa 1976) 5 (2);1980:117-25.

20. **c**—Reduced activity levels due to avoidance

Red flags are indicators of serious spinal pathology: age of onset less than 20 years or more than 55 years, recent history of violent trauma; constant progressive, nonmechanical pain (no relief with bed rest); thoracic pain; past medical history of malignant tumor; prolonged use of corticosteroids; drug abuse, immunosuppression, HIV; systemically unwell; unexplained weight loss; widespread neurological symptoms (including cauda equine syndrome); spinal deformity; fever. Yellow flags are psychosocial factors indicative of long-term chronicity and disability: a negative attitude that back pain is harmful or potentially severely disabling; fear avoidance behavior and reduced activity levels; an expectation that passive, rather than active, treatment will be beneficial; a tendency to depression, low morale, and social withdrawal; social or financial problems.

ANSWERS 21–34

Additional answers 21–34 available on ExpertConsult.com

EMI ANSWER

35. 1—j, Spinal stenosis. Patients with neurogenic claudication improve with bending forward, and have pain radiating from proximally to distally. In contrast, claudication due to peripheral vascular disease usually comes on after walking a fixed distance, starts as a cramp or tightness in the calf and relieved by rest. 2—e, Diffuse idiopathic skeletal hyperostosis (DISH). Defined by the presence of nonmarginal osteophytes at three or more successive levels. 3—d, Destructive spondyloarthropathy. Seen in hemodialysis patients with chronic renal failure, it typically involves three adjacent vertebrae and their intervening disc spaces. 4—a, Ankylosing spondylitis. Vertical or marginal osteophytes produce a bamboo spine appearance.

36. 1—h, Hoffman's test; 2—i, Inverted radial reflex; 3—l, Oppenheim test; 4—e, Bulbocavernosus reflex

Neurological Examination Findings

Test or Sign	Technique and Interpretation
Babinski reflex	Extensor plantar response on stroking sole of foot suggesting UMN lesion
Spurling's test	Examiner turns the patient's head to the affected side while extending and applying downward pressure to the top of the patient's head (foraminal compression). A positive test (Spurling's sign) is when the pain arising in the neck radiates in the direction of the corresponding painful dermatome ipsilaterally
Hoffman's test	Quickly snapping or flicking the middle fingernail; if positive, the tip of the index finger, ring finger, and/or thumb suddenly flex in response, and this indicates cervical myelopathy
Inverted radial reflex	Said to be present when the supinator reflex associated with the brachioradialis muscle elicits finger flexion (abnormal) rather than elbow flexion (normal). This is due pathology causing to an absent biceps jerk (C5-C6) and an exaggerated triceps jerk (C7). It occurs because a lower motor neuron lesion of C5 root is combined with an upper motor neuron lesion affecting reflexes below C5
Finger escape sign	Ask the patient to hold fingers extended and adducted. Little finger spontaneously abducts and flexes due to weak intrinsic muscles indicating cervical myelopathy
Lhermitte's sign	Electric shock-like sensation shooting down the spine when flexing the cervical spine
Oppenheim test	Scratch along the crest of the patient's tibia in a downward motion. A normal (negative) response is no reaction. An abnormal (positive) response is an extensor plantar response suggesting upper motor neuron lesion
Adam's test	Not reliable in the presence of lower limb length discrepancy. The patient bends forward at the waist until the back comes in the horizontal plane, with feet together, arms hanging and knees extended. The palms are held together. The examiner looks from behind, along the horizontal plane of the column vertebrae. The examiner looks for indicators of scoliosis, such as spinal asymmetry, nonlevel shoulders, scapula asymmetry, nonlevel hips, the head that does not line up with the pelvis or a rib hump. An increased or decreased lordosis/kyphosis can also be a sign for scoliosis. The rotation deformity or rib hump can be measured with a scoliometer
Schober's test	A mark is made at the level of the posterior iliac spine on the vertebral column, i.e. approximately at the level of L5. The examiner then places one finger 5 cm below this mark and another finger at about 10 cm above this mark. The patient is then instructed to touch his toes. If the increase in distance between the two fingers on the patients spine is less than 5 cm then this is indicative of a limitation of lumbar flexion
Femoral stretch test	Knee is passively flexed and the hip is passively extended with the patient in the prone position. Test is positive if results in anterior thigh pain, most often in L2-L3 and L3-L4 disc herniation (less so or negative in L4/5 and L5/S1 herniation)
Lasegue's test	Straight leg raise. Positive for herniated disc if the patient experiences sciatica when the straight leg is at an angle of 30-70°

Continued

Test or Sign	Technique and Interpretation
Bowstring test	Performed after a positive straight leg raise is elicited; the angle of hip elevation is decreased to decrease the radicular pain and then pressure is applied to the popliteal fossa, over the nerve, to reproduce symptoms
Abdominal reflex	Stroke on the abdominal skin from lateral to the medial aspect in all four quadrants A normal positive response usually involves a contraction of the abdominal muscles, and the umbilicus moving towards the source of the stimulation. Polysynaptic T7-T12 reflex. Absence can be pathological or physiological (e.g. obesity, multiparity, tolerance, children)
Bulbocavernosus reflex	Polysynaptic S2-S4 reflex. Monitoring internal/external anal sphincter contraction in response to squeezing the glans penis or clitoris, or tugging on an indwelling Foley catheter. In the context of acute spinal cord injury, absence suggests spinal shock, whereas presence suggests a severed cord. It is one of the first reflexes to return after spinal shock at 48 h. Absence after lumbar trauma may be due to conus medullaris or cauda equina injury
Shoulder abduction test	Patients with radiculopathy have improvement of their symptoms with elevation of the arm above the head. This is an important test to distinguish cervical pathology from other sources of shoulder/arm pain

37. 1—d, Disc protrusion; 2—c, Disc extrusion; 3—j, Sequestered disc; 4—g, Migrated disc

Terminology Relating to Intervertebral Disc Pathology	
Herniated disc	A localized displacement of nucleus, cartilage, fragmented apophyseal vertebral bone, and/or annular tissue beyond the intervertebral disc space
Disc bulge	A disc which extends beyond the edges of the disc space, over greater than 50% (180°) of the circumference of the disc and usually less than 3 mm beyond the edges of the vertebral body apophyses
Disc extrusion	A herniated disc where the base of the herniation (transverse dimension) is smaller than the AP dimension
Disc protrusion	A herniated disc where the base of the herniation (transverse dimension) is wider than the AP dimension; >25% but <50% (180°) of disc herniation
Central disc	A disc that extrudes or protrudes in the midline
Paracentral disc	A disc that extrudes or protrudes just off the midline but still in the spinal canal (i.e. right central or left central)
Neural foraminal disc	A disc that extrudes or protrudes into the neural foramen
Far lateral disc	A disc that extrudes or protrudes anterolateral to the neural foramen outside of the spinal canal
Sequestered disc	A subtype of extruded disc that has broken away from the from the site of extrusion (i.e. free disc material in canal)
Migrated disc	A subtype of extruded disc that extends in the craniocaudal plane but still maintains continuity with the disc

CHAPTER 30

SPINAL INFECTION

SINGLE BEST ANSWER (SBA) QUESTIONS

1. A 39-year-old presents with 4 days of neck pain and unsteady gait. He had recently completed a course of antibiotics for cellulitis. On examination he was myelopathic, with sensory impairment below C4 level. Reflexes were brisk globally with upgoing plantars. He is pyrexial with a temperature of 38.2 °C. Blood cultures grow Staph aureus. T1 contrast MRI is shown. Which one of the following is most likely?

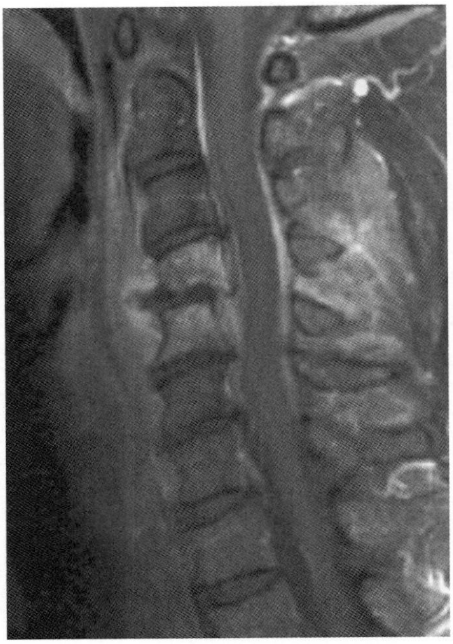

   a. Arachnoiditis
   b. Epidural abscess
   c. Epidural lipomatosis
   d. Epidural metastasis
   e. Subdural empyema

2. A 54-year-old renal transplant patient presents with back pain, fever, and a new thoracic kyphotic deformity. She is otherwise neurologically intact on examination. T2W MRI is shown. Which one of the following is most likely?

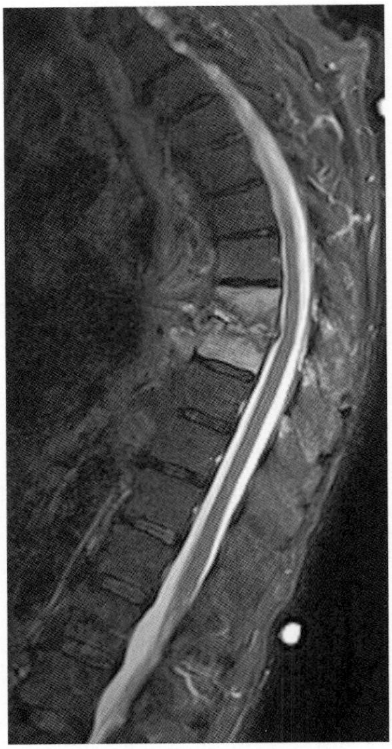

   a. Epidural abscess
   b. Intramedullary abscess
   c. Pyogenic vertebral osteomyelitis
   d. Spinal subdural empyema
   e. Tuberculosis spondylitis

3. Which one of the following factors is LEAST likely to predict good candidates for nonsurgical management of vertebral osteomyelitis?
   a. Over the age of 60
   b. Immunocompetent
   c. No neurological deficit
   d. No kyphotic deformity
   e. Cultures positive for *Staphylococcus aureus*
   f. Primarily discitis (minimal involvement of adjacent vertebrae)

4. Which one of the following statements about surgical management of vertebral osteomyelitis is LEAST accurate?
   a. Simple laminectomy is the primary procedure for emergency management of neural element compression in vertebral osteomyelitis
   b. Anterior or combined anterior-posterior approaches are required in the majority of cases
   c. Posterior approach alone can be considered if there is disc space infection below the conus without anterior column instability
   d. Refractory back pain after a period of nonoperative management is an indication for surgery
   e. Correction of progressive spinal deformity is an indication for surgery

5. A 32-year-old recent immigrant from Southeast Asia presents with back pain and a new kyphotic deformity after tripping up in his flat. T1 and T2 W MRI are shown. Which one of the following is most likely diagnosis?

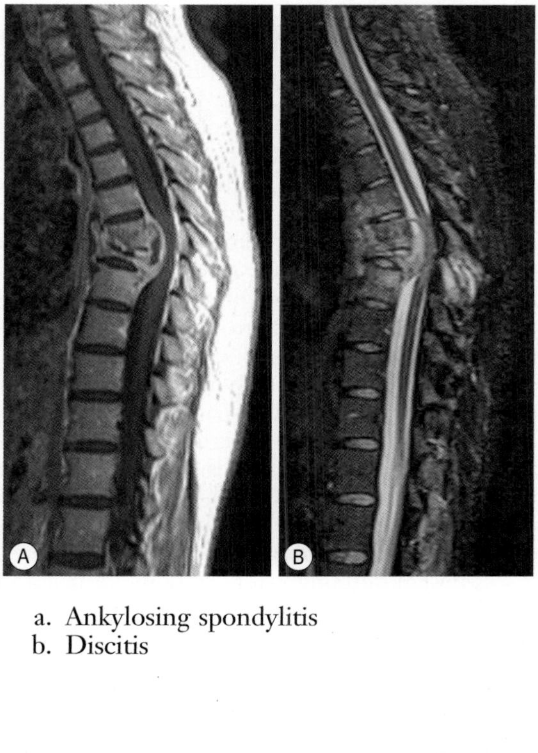

   a. Ankylosing spondylitis
   b. Discitis
   c. Multiple myeloma
   d. Pyogenic vertebral osteomyelitis
   e. Spinal tuberculosis

6. Which one of the following statements regarding spinal subdural empyema is most accurate?
   a. Two thirds are associated with discitis/osteomyelitis
   b. Are commoner than cranial subdural empyemas
   c. Lumbar puncture should be attempted before proceeding to open surgery
   d. MRI is definitive in distinguishing subdural empyema from epidural abscesses
   e. Commonly occur in adolescents

7. A 19-year-old male presents with neck pain, fever, and numbness in his legs and trunk up to his arm pits. His neurological examination is consistent with an upper motor neuron lesion, and you note a small midline sinus on the back of his neck. Blood cultures grow *Streptococcus epidermis*, T1 MRI with contrast is shown. Which one of the following is the next appropriate step?

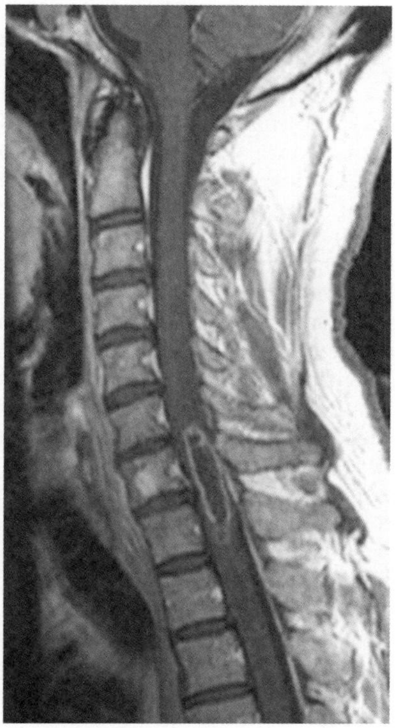

   a. MRI head with contrast
   b. CSF analysis
   c. Cardiac echo
   d. Dental examination
   e. Start IV antibiotics immediately

SBA ANSWERS

1. **b**—Epidural abscess

Epidural abscess can result from hematogenous spread, local extension, or direct inoculation. This condition is usually found in adults; risk factors include intravenous drug abuse, diabetes mellitus, prior spine trauma, renal failure, and pregnancy. The majority of cases are located in the thoracic spine. Causative organisms are *S. aureus* (70%), other staphylococcal species, aerobic streptococci, *Enterobacteriaceae* (mainly *E. coli*) *Pseudomonas* species mixed bacterial infections and fungi. The initial presentation includes localized pain and fever with elevation of the ESR, CRP, and leukocyte count. Blood cultures are positive in 60% of patients. MRI is able to visualize the degree of cord compression and extent of abscess in all directions, and discitis/vertebral osteomyelitis which commonly accompanies it. Areas of infection have characteristically high signal intensity on T2-weighted image. Without treatment, significant neurologic deficits occur and eventually paralysis may develop. Significant neurologic recovery is observed in patients with mild neurologic deficits or paralysis of less than 36 h duration who undergo surgical intervention. Complete paralysis of greater than 36-48 h duration has not shown recovery. The death rate associated with epidural abscess has been reported as 12%. The surgical approach is determined by the location of the epidural abscess. An abscess located posteriorly and extending over multiple levels is best treated by multiple-level laminotomies or laminectomy, taking care to preserve the facet joints. Alternatively, debridement of the spinal canal through fenestrations removing the ligamentum flavum and portions of adjacent lamina, and use of catheters can be considered. An abscess located anteriorly and associated with vertebral osteomyelitis is most directly treated with an anterior surgical approach. If an abscess involves both the anterior and posterior epidural space, an anterior and posterior approach combined with spinal stabilization using posterior instrumentation is considered. A symptomatic epidural abscess is considered a medical and surgical emergency. The combination of surgical and antibiotic treatment is required for a symptomatic epidural abscess. Nonoperative management is considered in patients who are extremely high-risk surgical candidates and in patients with an established complete neurologic deficit for greater than 72 h. In addition, neurologically intact patients without sepsis can be considered for a trial of culture-specific antibiotic therapy under close clinical supervision.

Image with permission from Herkowitz et al. Rothman-Simeone The Spine, 6th ed., Elsevier, Saunders, 2011.

FURTHER READING

Devlin VJ, Steinmann JC. Spinal infections. In: Devlin VJ (Ed.), Spine Secrets Plus, 2nd ed., Elsevier, Mosby, 2012 (Chapter 67).

2. **c**—Pyogenic vertebral osteomyelitis

Pyogenic vertebral osteomyelitis accounts for 2-7% of all osteomyelitis, and at-risk groups include the elderly, diabetics, AIDS, IV drug abusers, and the immunosuppressed. The most common method for bacteria to spread to the spine is by the hematogenous route. Common sources of infection include infected catheters, urinary tract infection, dental caries, IV drug use, and skin infections. The next most common route is local extension from an adjacent soft tissue infection or paravertebral abscess, followed by direct inoculation via trauma, puncture, or following spine surgery. The nucleus pulposus is relatively avascular, providing little or no immune response, and thus is rapidly destroyed by bacterial enzymes. The disc is nearly always involved in pyogenic vertebral infections, unlike in tuberculous spondylitis (granulomatous). The most consistent symptom is back or neck pain, fever, neurologic deficits, radicular pain, weight loss, and kyphosis. The spinal areas affected in descending order are lumbar, thoracic, and cervical. *Staphylococcus aureus* is the most common organism and has been identified in over 50% of cases. However, gram-negative organisms (*Escherichia coli*, *Pseudomonas* spp., *Proteus* spp.) are associated with spinal infections following genitourinary infections or procedures. Intravenous drug abusers have a high incidence of *Pseudomonas* infections. Anaerobic infections are common in diabetics and following penetrating trauma. Investigations should include FBC, CRP, ESR, and blood cultures. Vertebral body and adjacent discs appear hypointense on T1-weighted and hyperintense on T2 weighted MRI, and both enhance on T1 + contrast imaging. Positive radiographic findings are not evident for at least 4 weeks after the onset of symptoms: the earliest detectable finding is disc space narrowing, followed by localized osteopenia and finally destruction of the vertebral endplates. Technetium-99m bone scanning is valuable in the early diagnosis of pyogenic vertebral osteomyelitis because it demonstrates positive findings before X-ray changes. CT is best at defining extent of bony destruction and localization of lesions for biopsies. In the absence of positive blood cultures, biopsy of the site of presumed vertebral osteomyelitis or discitis is essential to provide a definitive diagnosis, identify the causative organism, and guide treatment. The biopsy ideally should be performed before initiation of antibiotics. If antibiotics have been given, they should be discontinued for 3 days before the biopsy. Computed tomography (CT)-guided, closed Craig needle biopsy is safe and effective and yields the etiologic organism in 70% of cases. If a closed biopsy is negative after two attempts, an open biopsy can be considered. Tissue samples should be sent for Gram stain, acid-fast stain, aerobic and anaerobic cultures, and fungal and tuberculosis (TB) cultures. Bacterial cultures should be observed for at least 10 days to detect low-virulence organisms. TB cultures may take weeks to grow. Histology studies should also be performed to detect neoplastic processes and to differentiate acute versus chronic infection. The goals in treating vertebral osteomyelitis include early definitive diagnosis, eradication of infection, relief of axial pain, prevention or reversal of neurologic deficits, preservation of spinal stability, and correction of spinal deformity.

Image with permission from Saraf-Lavi E. Spine Imaging: Case Review Series, 3rd ed., Elsevier, Saunders, 2014.

FURTHER READING

Devlin VJ, Steinmann JC. Spinal infections. In: Devlin VJ (Ed.), Spine Secrets Plus, 2nd ed., Elsevier, Mosby, 2012 (Chapter 67).

3. **a**—Over the age of 60

Nonoperative treatment includes antibiotic administration, treatment of underlying disease processes, nutritional support, and spinal immobilization with an orthosis. Antibiotic selection is based on identification and sensitivity testing. Consultation with an infectious disease specialist is recommended. Intravenous antibiotics generally should be continued for 6 weeks, provided that satisfactory clinical results and reduction in ESR and CRP occur. In the setting of a broadly sensitive organism and rapid clinical resolution, intravenous antibiotics may be replaced with oral antibiotics at 4 weeks. Relapse of infection has been reported in up to 25% of patients who receive intravenous antibiotic treatment for less than 4 weeks. Contemporary mortality rates resulting from pyogenic spinal infections range from 2% to 17%. Nonoperative treatment is reported as successful in up to 75% of appropriately treated patients when criteria for success focus on infection cure, infection recurrence, and neurologic status following treatment. The ideal patient for nonoperative treatment is a neurologically intact patient with primarily disc space involvement, minimal involvement of adjacent vertebrae, no kyphotic deformity, and who is not debilitated by systemic disease or immune suppression. The most consistent predictors of success for nonoperative treatment include:

- patients younger than 60 years
- patients who are immunocompetent
- infections with *Staphylococcus aureus*
- decreasing ESR and CRP with treatment.

FURTHER READING

Devlin VJ, Steinmann JC. Spinal infections. In: Devlin VJ (Ed.), Spine Secrets Plus, 2nd ed., Elsevier, Mosby, 2012 (Chapter 67).

4. **a**—Simple laminectomy is the primary procedure for emergency management of neural element compression in vertebral osteomyelitis

Indications for operative treatment of pyogenic vertebral osteomyelitis include: (1) need for open biopsy; (2) failure of nonsurgical management (high ESR/CRP, refractory back pain); (3) need for open drainage of abscess; (4) neural decompression; (5) spinal stabilization; and (6) correction of progressive spinal deformity. As such, the location of the infection, presence/absence of abscess, extent of bone destruction, and need for stabilization are key. Spinal discitis/osteomyelitis primarily affects the anterior spinal column, hence anterior only or combined anterior and posterior approaches are indicated in the majority of spinal infections. Posterior approaches may be considered in special circumstances such as posterior epidural abscesses, disc space infections below the conus with satisfactory anterior column support, and in the absence of significant paravertebral abscess. Laminectomy alone is associated with deformity progression, instability, and neurologic deterioration, hence it is not recommended. Surgery should achieve complete debridement of nonviable and infected tissue, decompression of neural elements, and long-term stability through fusion (use of autogenous graft material is gold standard). The surgical approach generally should include anterior debridement and grafting followed by a staged or simultaneous posterior spinal stabilization procedure. While placing implants in infected environments would normally be avoided, bone infections are better controlled with antibiotics and bone stabilization than with antibiotics alone in an unstable bony environment. Use of titanium alloys is preferable to stainless steel due to increased bacterial adherence to stainless steel implants. In this setting, advantages of posterior spinal instrumentation include:

1. preservation of spinal alignment and restoration of spinal stability following radical debridement

2. increased fusion rates
3. ability to correct kyphotic deformities
4. avoidance of graft collapse or dislodgement
5. rapid patient mobilization and early rehabilitation without the need for an external orthosis.

FURTHER READING

Devlin VJ, Steinmann JC. Spinal infections. In: Devlin VJ (Ed.), Spine Secrets Plus, 2nd ed., Elsevier, Mosby, 2012 (Chapter 67).

5. **e**—Spinal tuberculosis

Tuberculosis is the most common granulomatous infection of the spine. The three patterns of spinal involvement are peridiscal (commonest), central, and anterior. Peridiscal occurs adjacent to the vertebral endplate and spreads around a single intervertebral disc as the abscess material tracks beneath the anterior longitudinal ligament (the disc is usually spared unlike in pyogenic infections). Central involvement occurs in the middle of the vertebral body and eventually leads to vertebral collapse and kyphotic deformity. This pattern of involvement can be mistaken for a tumor. Anterior infections begin beneath the anterior longitudinal ligament, causing scalloping of the anterior vertebral bodies, and extend over multiple levels. The presentation is highly variable. Mild back pain is the most common symptom. Patients with tuberculous infections may present with malaise, fevers, night sweats, and weight loss. In addition, chronic infections may result in cutaneous sinuses, neurologic deficits (in up to 40% of patients), and kyphotic deformities. Certain factors define the high-risk population and should raise suspicion. Patients from countries with a high incidence of tuberculosis, such as Southeast Asia, South America, and Russia are considered high risk. Patients who live in confinement with others, such as homeless centers and prisons, are also at risk. Elderly adults, chronic alcoholics, patients with AIDS, and patients with a family member or a household contact with tuberculosis are additional high-risk groups. The leukocyte count may be normal or mildly elevated. The ESR is mildly elevated (typically <50), but may be normal in up to 25% of cases. Although the purified protein derivative (PPD) skin test may detect active infection or past exposure, this test is unreliable because false-negative results may occur in malnourished and immunocompromised patients. Anergy panel testing should be included for this reason. Urine cultures, sputum specimens, and gastric washings may be helpful for diagnosis if the primary source is unknown. The most reliable test for diagnosis is CT-guided biopsy. The characteristic finding on histology is a granuloma, which is described as a multinucleated giant-cell reaction surrounding a central region of caseating necrosis. Molecular detection of mycobacterium DNA or RNA is useful for rapid diagnosis and for determining drug resistance. Radiographs: A clue to diagnosis is the presence of extensive vertebral destruction out of proportion to the amount of pain. Typically, the intervertebral discs are preserved in the early stages of this disease. Chest radiographs can be useful in demonstrating pulmonary MRI: The imaging modality of choice for diagnosis of spinal TBCT: Plays a role in defining the extent of bony destruction and localization for biopsies. Chemotherapy (four-drug regimen, for a minimum of 6-month duration, includes isoniazid, rifampin, pyrazinamide, and ethambutol) and brace immobilization are the initial treatment except in patients presenting with neurologic deficit or progressive deformity. The indications for surgery and the principles of surgical reconstruction are similar to those advised for pyogenic spinal infections.

Image with permission from Saraf-Lavi E. Spine Imaging: Case Review Series, 3rd ed., Elsevier, Saunders, 2014.

6. **e**—Commonly occur in adolescents

Spinal subdural empyemas are uncommon and tend to occur in thoracolumbar spine, in those in 5th-7th decades. Suggestions for why they are less common than cranial subdural empyema and spinal epidural abscesses include the lack of air sinuses in the spine, the fact that the epidural space in the spine is an actual rather than potential space, and blood is directed centripetally in the spine, whereas it is directed centrifugally in the brain. The pathogenesis of these infections can be categorized into one of four major categories: hematogenous spread of primary infection, iatrogenic (lumbar puncture, spinal injections), direct extension into the subdural space (dysraphism, penetrating trauma, spinal infection), and cryptogenic. The most common organism is *Staphylococcus aureus*, other *Staphylococcus* species, *Streptococcus*, *Escherichia coli*, *Pseudomonas aeruginosa*, *Streptococcus pneumoniae*, and *Peptococcus magnus*. The classical presentation of an SSE includes fever, neck/back pain, followed by symptoms of spinal cord/cauda equina compression. Presence of spinal tenderness may favor epidural abscess rather than subdural empyema. Routine tests include FBC, ESR, CRP; lumbar puncture is not performed due to risks of contaminating deeper meningeal layers. Contrast MRI is imaging of choice as allows better visualization of the spinal cord, vertebrae, disc spaces, extent of lesion, and extent of compression. The major limitation of MRI, however, remains its inability to distinguish whether the lesion is intradural or extradural; the presence of discitis/osteomyelitis accompanies two thirds of SEAs. The mainstay of treatment for these infections is surgical decompression (laminectomy) with irrigation and drainage of the subdural space followed by appropriate antibiotic therapy. The exposure should encompass the extent of the abscess. After copious irrigation, most authors advocate the primary closure of the dura. The arachnoid should be preserved if possible. A significant indication for surgery is obtaining a definitive organism to treat; therefore cultures should be obtained before using antibiotic irrigation. The use of postoperative antibiotics should be based on the given organism found during surgery. Empiric antibiotic coverage for these infections must cover gram-positive cocci. Some advocate the additional use of corticosteroids (dexamethasone) during the perioperative period as a prophylaxis against the development of thrombophlebitis. Among the surgically treated group, 82.1% made a complete recovery or improved, whereas 17.9% died. In the conservatively treated group, 80% died (4 of 5 patients) and only 20% (1 of 5 patients) improved. On the basis of these numbers, the current recommendations are for aggressive surgical treatment followed by antibiotic therapy.

FURTHER READING

Javahery RJ, Levi AD. Spinal intradural infection. In: Herkowitz et al. (Eds.), Rothman-Simeone the Spine, 6th ed., Elsevier, Saunders, 2011 (Chapter 90).

7. **a**—MRI head with contrast

Intramedullary spinal cord abscesses (ISCAs) are rare, and patients are young. ISCAs occur throughout the spine, but they are most frequently found in the thoracic region. The pathogenesis of ISCA can be divided into two broad categories: hematogenous spread and direct implantation. The more complex of the two is hematogenous spread via arterial supply (septic emboli), venous drainage (increased intrathoracic/abdominal pressure causing backflow in low pressure spinal venous system), or lymphatics (draining mediastinum, abdomen connect with Virchow Robins paces in spinal cord via channels in spinal nerves). The most common primary infection is pulmonary, endocarditis, urinary tract infections, peritonitis, and peripheral skin infections. The other major route for the pathogenesis of ISCA is direct implantation via a congenital midline neuroectodermal defect (e.g. dermal sinus tract), postoperative, after penetrating trauma. Most commonly no cause is found (cryptogenic). Causative organisms are *Staphylococcus* and *Streptococci*, with other significant organisms *Actinomyces*, *Proteus mirabilis*, *Pneumococcus*, *Listeria monocytogenes*, Hemophilus, and *Escherichia coli.* Cases of contiguous spread via a dermal sinus tract are most commonly due to *Staphylococcus epidermidis*, *S. aureus*, *Enterobacteriaceae*, anaerobes, and *Proteus mirabilis*. Postsurgical (contiguous) cases are most often due to *S. epidermidis*, *S. aureus*, *Enterobacteriaceae*, and *Pseudomonas aeruginosa*. The cases that arise from hematogenous spread reflect the site of primary infection. The presenting signs and symptoms in patients with ISCAs almost always involve motor deficits, sensory impairment, loss of sphincteric control, pain, and fever. Acute infections (<2 weeks) partial transverse myelitis commonly associated with fever and leucocytosis, while subacute (2-6 weeks) and chronic (>6 weeks) present like intramedullary tumors. Investigations include WCC, CRP, ESR, CSF analysis (usually negative unless meningitis). Imaging of choice is contrast MRI which may differentiate between early and late myelitis. CT myelography may show widening of the cord at a focal segment with obstruction to CSF flow. X-rays are usually normal at presentation. Other features are osteomyelitis, spinal deformity, spinal stenosis, and spinal dysraphism, current recommendations are for immediate surgical treatment. The surgery should include laminectomies at the involved levels, intradural exploration, midline myelotomy, and irrigation and drainage of the abscess cavity. Aggressive treatment with antibiotics requires empirical therapy until an organism has been isolated. The choice of antibiotics for empirical therapy should be based on the suspected source of infection and then adjusted on the basis of the operative culture results. The current recommendation is a minimum of 4-6 weeks of parenteral therapy. Patients presenting with acute symptoms have a worse prognosis in terms of neurologic recovery. Overall, the death of a patient diagnosed with an ISCA is most frequently due to the presence of multiple CNS abscesses and, specifically, to brain or brainstem abscesses.

Image with permission from Saraf-Lavi E. Spine Imaging: Case Review Series, 3rd ed., Elsevier, Saunders, 2014.

FURTHER READING

Javahery RJ, Levi AD. Spinal intradural infection. In: Herkowitz et al. (Eds.), Rothman-Simeone the Spine, 6th ed., Elsevier, Saunders, 2011 (Chapter 90).

CHAPTER 31

SPINAL ONCOLOGY

SINGLE BEST ANSWER (SBA) QUESTIONS

1. Which one of the following statements regarding spinal tumors is most accurate?
   a. The commonest extradural tumor is an osteoid osteoma
   b. Intradural tumors in adults are predominantly intramedullary rather than extramedullary
   c. The commonest intramedullary tumor in adults is ependymoma
   d. Intramedullary metastases are more common than extradural metastases
   e. The commonest intramedullary tumor in children is ganglioglioma

2. Which one of the following groups of primary malignancies represents the most frequent causes of spinal column metastases?
   a. Breast, lung, kidney, melanoma, and colorectal
   b. Breast, lung, thyroid, melanoma, and colorectal
   c. Breast, lung, kidney, prostate, and thyroid
   d. Breast, lung, prostate, melanoma, and colorectal
   e. Breast, prostate, lung, kidney, thyroid

3. Which one of the following clinical presentations is most concerning for spinal metastatic disease?
   a. A 47-year-old with breast cancer treated with mastectomy and lymph node dissection, on tamoxifen, presents with moderate lower back pain worse at the end of the day, relieved by rest, not exacerbated by movement.
   b. A 54-year-old with previous Dukes B colorectal cancer who underwent bowel resection and end ileostomy, followed by chemotherapy presents with gait disturbance. On examination he has a stocking distribution of sensory loss in the lower limbs only.
   c. A 35-year-old with a past medical history of wide local excision of melanoma presents with mechanical back pain, stabbing in nature, which she is more aware of at night. On examination there is nonspecific tenderness in the mid-thoracic spine, but no focal neurological signs.
   d. A 79-year-old with a past medical history of benign prostatic hyperplasia presents with mechanical back pain after a fall. On examination there is tenderness in the paraspinal muscles, but no focal neurological signs.
   e. A 57-year-old with a past medical history of small cell lung cancer presents with mechanical back pain. On examination he appears kyphotic there is tenderness in the mid-thoracic spine. Neurological examination shows brisk reflexes and extensor plantars in both lower limbs.

4. Which one of the following statements regarding the imaging of spinal metastatic disease is LEAST accurate?
   a. Plain radiographs may only show changes in approximately half of affected vertebrae
   b. Nuclear scintigraphy detects areas of increased metabolic activity in bone but this is not specific to metastatic lesions.
   c. SPECT can be used to differentiate between malignant and benign lesions
   d. PET scans can be used to identify the biopsy site
   e. Angiography is not likely to be of benefit prior to resection of vertebral metastases from renal cell carcinoma

5. Which one of the following statements regarding prognostic scoring for patients presenting with metastatic disease of the spine is LEAST accurate?
   a. Tokuhashi score considers Karnofsky performance status, number of extraspinal metastases and neurological status whereas the Tomita score does not
   b. A lower Tomita score favors more aggressive surgical treatment

c. A higher Tokuhashi score predicts a poorer prognosis
d. Both Tokuhashi and Tomita scores consider the treatability of visceral metastases
e. Tokuhashi score assesses neurological status using the Frankel grading system

6. Which one of the following statements regarding management of pain related to spinal metastasis is most accurate?
a. Bisphosphonates have shown utility in management of pain resistant to conventional analgesia and/but not in reducing the risk of malignant spinal cord compression
b. Intrathecal morphine pump insertion is inappropriate in patients with intractable pain from spinal metastases
c. NSAIDs are inappropriate for management of pain related to spinal metastases due to their platelet inhibiting effect
d. Single fraction palliative radiotherapy for spinal metastases causing non-mechanical pain is not appropriate in those with complete paralysis
e. Vertebroplasty has been shown to be effective in the setting of pain from metastatic spinal cord compression in non-surgical candidates

7. A 57-year-old with who recently underwent right upper lobectomy for small cell lung cancer presents due to worsening back pain over the last 3 days. It initially started at night over the last 2 weeks or so, but is now exacerbated by physical movement. He denies any trauma. On examination he is tender to palpation in the mid thoracic spine. Neurological examination reveals mild weakness of both lower limbs bilaterally, brisk knee and ankle reflexes, and extensor plantars. Sensory examination reveals a sensory level at the umbilicus. Which one of the following would you do next?
a. Standing spine X-ray
b. MRI whole spine MRI and CT whole spine
c. ensure they are Nurse flat with neutral spine alignment
d. CT lumbar spine
e. Dexamethasone

8. Which one of the following statements regarding definitive oncological management of patients presenting with MSCC is LEAST accurate?
a. In patients who present with MSCC without a known diagnosis of malignancy radiotherapy can usually start sooner than chemotherapy
b. Preoperative radiotherapy should not be carried out on patients with MSCC if surgery is planned
c. Radiotherapy can be given as soon as there is suspected MSCC on imaging
d. Spinal instability is a relative contraindication to radiotherapy
e. Teratoma is one of the rare causes of spinal cord compression where chemotherapy is more effective than radiotherapy

9. Which one of the following statements regarding surgery in patients with metastatic disease of the spine is LEAST accurate?
a. Indicated in those with metastatic spinal cord compression who are ambulant and without significant neurological deficit if they are expected to survive greater than 3 months
b. Indicated in those with metastatic spinal cord compression with less than 24 h of complete paralysis who otherwise have a good prognosis
c. Indicated in those with spinal instability and evidence of structural spine failure to prevent malignant spinal cord compression, even if their pain is controlled
d. Indicated in those with spinal instability related mechanical back pain resistant to analgesia
e. Indicated only in those patients expected to survive at least 12 months

10. Which one of the following statements regarding the 2005 RCT (Patchell et al., Lancet 366:643-648) comparing decompressive resection plus adjuvant radiotherapy versus radiotherapy alone for metastatic spinal cord compression is LEAST accurate?
a. The surgical arm and radiotherapy only arm both received 30 Gy of external-beam radiation delivered in 10 fractions
b. The surgical arm did not have increased survival time compared to radiotherapy alone
c. The surgical arm had greater return of ambulation after treatment compared to radiotherapy alone
d. The surgical arm remained ambulatory for longer compared to radiotherapy alone
e. The surgical plus radiotherapy, and radiotherapy alone groups both excluded those with radio-sensitive tumors

11. Which one of the following statements regarding surgical management of spinal metastatic disease is LEAST accurate?
a. The goal of surgery is preservation of neurological function, pain relief, and mechanical stabilization

b. Expected patient survival should exceed 12 months before surgical treatment of spinal metastases is considered
c. Percutaneous biopsy (or excisional biopsy during surgery) often required for tissue diagnosis as 10-20% of spine metastases have no known source
d. Seeding and recurrence along the biopsy needle track can occur with some primary tumors, such as chordomas
e. Posterior and posterolateral approaches are preferred to deal with vertebral body tumor in the setting of spinal metastases where possible

12. Which one of the following statements regarding radiation myelopathy is LEAST accurate?
a. A history of radiation therapy in doses sufficient to result in injury must be present
b. The region of the irradiated cord must lie slightly below the dermatome level of expression of the radiation myelitis
c. Local tumor progression must be ruled out before a diagnosis can be made
d. A latent period from the completion of treatment to the onset of injury is usually within 20-30 months
e. The probability of dying from radiation myelopathy is approximately 70% with cervical lesions

13. A 31-year-old man presents with back pain and erectile dysfunction. MRI is performed. Which one of the following statements regarding further management is key?

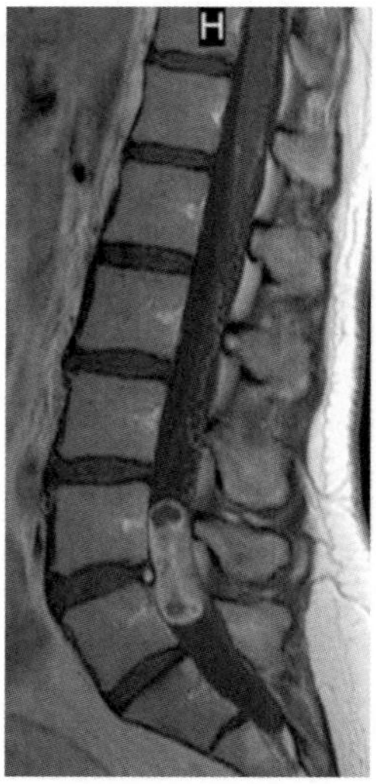

a. Gross total resection is the next appropriate step
b. Craniospinal axis MRI should be performed
c. External beam radiotherapy is critical after gross total resection
d. Etoposide chemotherapy is critical after subtotal resection
e. Conservative management with surveillance imaging is recommended

14. Which one of the following is most likely based on the T2-Weighted MRI shown below?

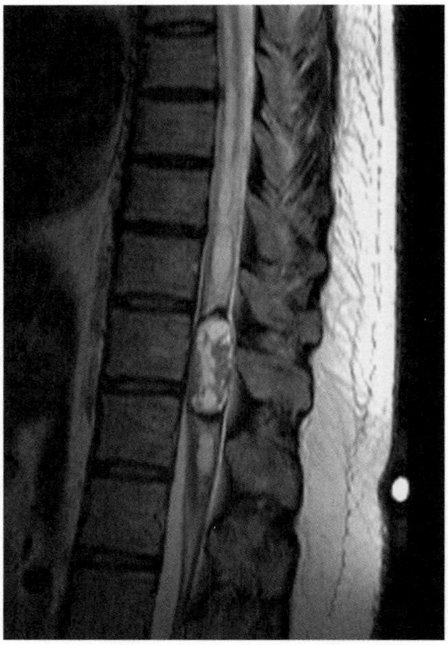

a. Ependymoma
b. Lipoma
c. Neurofibroma
d. Primary CNS lymphoma
e. Schwannoma

15. A 34-year-old male presents with a several month history of neck pain, with intermittent episodes of arm and leg numbness. MRI is shown. Which one of the following is most likely?

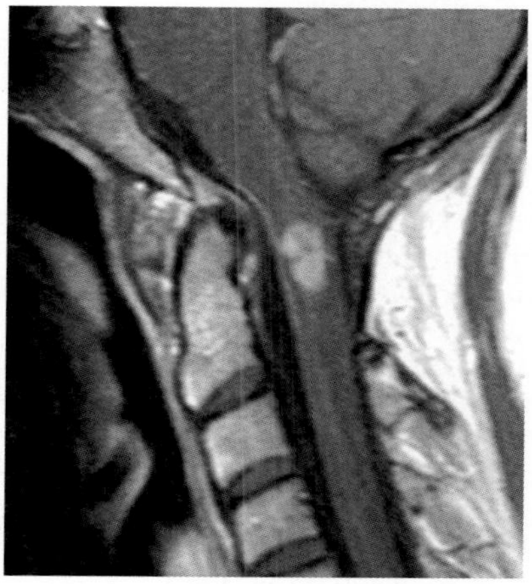

a. Ependymoma
b. Ganglioglioma
c. Meningioma
d. Neurofibroma
e. Schwannoma

16. A 21-year-old with asymmetrical, bilateral sensorineural hearing loss presents and progressive gait disturbance. T1-weighted MRI with gadolinium is shown. Which one of the following chromosomes is likely to be mutated?

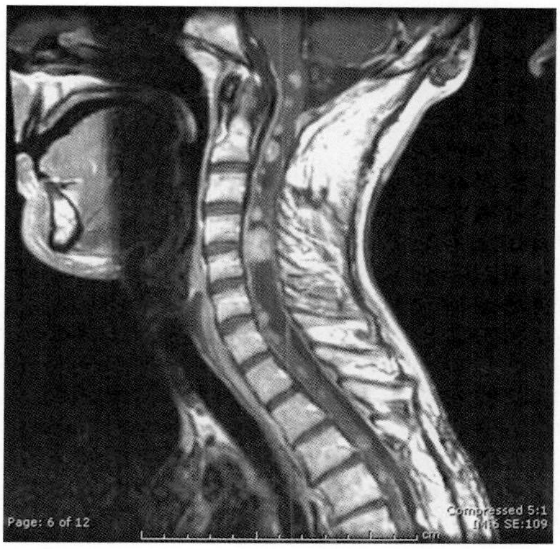

a. Chromosome 7
b. Chromosome 9
c. Chromosome 11
d. Chromosome 17
e. Chromosome 22

17. A 39-year-old presents with a 6-month history of tingling in her fingers and in the last few months, her legs. There is no bowel or bladder disturbance. On examination, there is cape-like pattern of pain and temperature loss in her upper limbs. Upper limbs are weak distally 4/5, and reflexes are globally brisk with extensor plantar responses bilaterally. MRI is shown. Which one of the following is most likely?

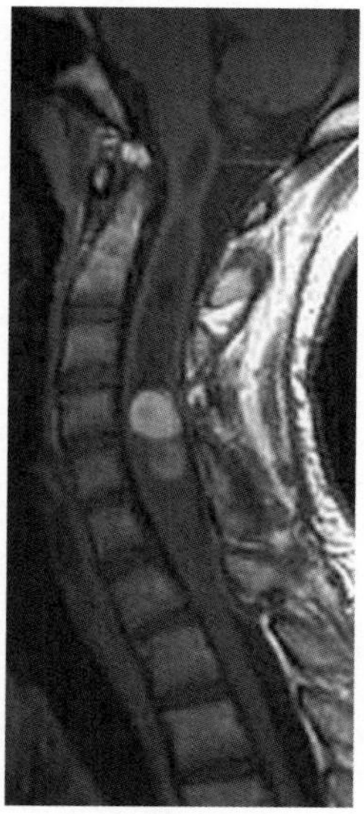

a. Astrocytoma
b. Ganglioglioma
c. Hemangioblastoma
d. Meningioma
e. Metastasis

QUESTIONS 18–24

Additional questions 18–24 available on ExpertConsult.com

EXTENDED MATCHING ITEM (EMI) QUESTIONS

25. **Intramedullary tumors:**
a. Astrocytoma
b. Ependymoma
c. Ganglioglioma
d. Hemangioblastoma
e. Hemangioma
f. Medulloblastoma
g. Oligodendroglioma
h. Teratoma
i. PCNSL
j. Metastasis

For each of the following descriptions, select the most appropriate answers from the list above. Each answer may be used once, more than once or not at all.

1. Commonest primary intramedullary tumor in adults
2. Second commonest intramedullary tumor in children

26. **Intradural extramedullary lesions:**
    a. Myxopapillary ependymoma
    b. Epidermoid
    c. Lipoma
    d. Meningioma
    e. Neurofibroma
    f. Paraganglioma
    g. Schwannoma
    h. Leptomeningeal drop metastasis
    i. Teratoma
    j. Arachnoid cyst

For each of the following descriptions, select the most appropriate answers from the list above. Each answer may be used once, more than once or not at all.

1. Important in risk stratification of patients presenting with PNETs
2. The commonest intradural, extramedullary lesion in China and Japan
3. The commonest intradural, extramedullary lesion in Western countries

27. **Extradural tumors:**
    a. Chordoma
    b. Chondrosarcoma
    c. Eosinophilic granuloma
    d. Hemangioma
    e. Multiple myeloma
    f. Metastasis
    g. Neuroblastoma
    h. Neurofibroma
    i. Osteoblastoma
    j. Osteochondroma
    k. Osteoid osteoma
    l. Osteosarcoma

For each of the following descriptions, select the most appropriate answers from the list above. Each answer may be used once, more than once or not at all.

1. A 37-year-old male sustained a wedge fracture of L1 following a fall down a flight of stairs. Jailhouse striations (honeycomb pattern) of the vertebra were also seen with a high signal on STIR MRI
2. A 7-year-old boy presents with mid-thoracic back pain. Spinal X-rays show a vertebra plana at T10
3. An 11-year-old boy has had back pain for the last 6 months that has failed to improve with observation and simple analgesia. X-rays showed a reactive bone around a 1 cm radiolucent nidus in the lamina of L1
4. A 49-year-old male presents with lower abdominal pain. X-rays and CT pelvis showed a lytic lesion of the anterior sacrum and histology after wide-margin surgical excision reveals cells with a foamy physaliferous appearance

SBA ANSWERS

1. **c**—The commonest intramedullary tumor in adults is ependymoma

Extradural tumors in adults: 90% metastatic tumors. The highest proportion of spinal metastatic deposits come from breast cancer (16.5%), lung cancer (15%), prostate cancer (10%), and renal cell carcinoma (7%) and 10-20% will have no known primary. Therefore primary extradural tumors only make up <10% of all spinal column tumors, and may be benign or malignant. The commonest benign lesions are osteoid osteomas, osteoblastomas, osteochondromas, aneurysmal bone cysts and hemangiomas (and Langerhans cell histiocytosis in children). The commonest malignant lesions are osteosarcoma, chondrosarcoma, malignant fibrous histiocytoma, giant cell tumor, plasmacytoma (solitary myeloma), Ewing's sarcoma and chordoma. In adults, approximately two thirds of intradural lesions are extramedullary and one third intramedullary (in children it is approximately equal)—with the incidence of intradural spinal cord tumors 3-10 per 100,000 per year. Intradural extramedullary lesions are most commonly thoracic, and most commonly meningiomas and nerve sheath tumors in equal proportions (spinal schwannomas are much more common than meningiomas in China and Japan). Intramedullary "lesions": ependymoma 41%, astrocytoma (WHO I-II) 15%, astrocytoma (WHO III-IV) 5%, ganglioglioma 3.2%, lipoma 2.8%, subependymoma 0.9%, metastasis 0.6%.

FURTHER READING

Petteys RJ et al. Epidural tumours and metastases. In: J-C Tonn et al. Oncology of CNS tumours. Springer-Verlag, Berlin, 2010, pp. 719-737.

Goldbrunner R. Intradural extramedullary tumours. In: J-C Tonn et al. Oncology of CNS tumours. Springer-Verlag, Berlin, 2010, pp. 709-718.

Westphal M. Intramedullary tumours. In: J-C Tonn et al. Oncology of CNS tumours. Springer-Verlag, Berlin, 2010, pp. 689-708.

2. **e**—Breast, prostate, lung, kidney, thyroid

The commonest cancers which metastasize to bone are breast, lung, prostate, kidney and thyroid (in contrast to brain metastasis where the commonest primary tumors are breast, lung, kidney, melanoma, and colorectal). Bony metastasis most commonly occur in the spine. At autopsy 30-90% of patients who die of cancer are found to have spinal metastases. Symptomatic secondary metastases are estimated to occur in approximately 10% of all cancer patients. Up to 50% of spinal metastases require some form of treatment, and 5-10% require surgical management. The highest incidence of spinal metastases is found in individuals 40-65 years of age, corresponding to the period of highest cancer risk. Males are slightly more prone to the development of spinal metastases, probably reflecting the slightly higher prevalence of lung cancer in men, and of prostate cancer over breast cancer. Metastatic spread is via hematogenous seeding, direct extension or invasion, and by seeding in the CSF. Hematogenous spread of tumors usually results in multicentric disease of the spine, which also occurs with CSF seeding (e.g. after surgical manipulation of cerebral or cerebellar metastatic or primary lesions). Spinal tumors may be extradural, intradural-extramedullary, and intramedullary; the overwhelming majority of all spinal metastases are found in the extradural compartment; that is, the bony spine and associated tissues. Metastases to the extradural compartment are found most commonly in the VB, with or without extension into the posterior elements, followed by the paravertebral regions and the epidural space, respectively. Intradural extramedullary and intramedullary metastases are very rare, and are often due to CSF seeding. The thoracic spine is by far the most frequent site for metastasis (70%), followed by the lumbar spine (20%), cervical spine, and sacrum, respectively.

FURTHER READING

Sciubba DM, Petteys RJ, Dekutoski MB, Fisher CG, Fehlings MG, Ondra SL, Rhines LD, Gokaslan ZL. Diagnosis and management of metastatic spine disease. A review. J Neurosurg Spine. 2010;13(1):94-108. doi: 10.3171/2010.3.SPINE09202. Review. PubMed PMID:20594024.

3. **e**—A 57-year-old with a past medical history of small cell lung cancer presents with mechanical back pain. On examination he appears kyphotic there is tenderness in the mid-thoracic spine. Neurological examination shows brisk reflexes and extensor plantars in both lower limbs

Symptoms associated with spinal metastatic disease may be systemic (weight loss, anorexia, organ dysfunction) or local (pain and/or neurology). The most common symptom is pain, which may predate neurological symptoms by weeks or months, and may even be the presenting symptom of an undiagnosed cancer. Three classically defined types of pain often affect patients with symptomatic spinal metastases, including local (periosteal stretching and inflammation due to tumor and often nocturnal, usually deep ache), mechanical (impending or established spinal instability due to deformity/collapse of vertebrae), and radicular pain (nerve root compression directly from tumor or narrowing of intervertebral foramen due to vertebral collapse). Neurological symptoms may be due to radiculopathy or metastatic spinal cord compression (MSCC). MSCC can present with motor, sensory or autonomic disturbance (bladder, bowel or sexual dysfunction or rarely even spinal shock) due to direct compression of neural structures by tumor, or to a pathological fracture that leads to retropulsion of bone fragments into the spinal canal or neural foramina. The patient's neurological function when a diagnosis of spinal cord compression is made usually correlates well with their prognosis. This observation underscores the importance of diagnosis before motor or autonomic deficits occur. Most patients will have pain before these deficits appear. However, because reports of back pain are very common in the general population, with a lifetime prevalence of up to 84% in some studies, a delay in diagnosis occurs in many cases of vertebral metastasis in which the initial complaint is one of new-onset back or neck pain.

FURTHER READING

Sciubba DM, Petteys RJ, Dekutoski MB, Fisher CG, Fehlings MG, Ondra SL, Rhines LD, Gokaslan ZL. Diagnosis and management of metastatic spine disease. A review. J Neurosurg Spine. 2010;13(1):94-108.

4. **e**—Angiography is not likely to be of benefit prior to resection of vertebral metastases from renal cell carcinoma

Plain radiographs are a useful screening test to identify lytic or sclerotic lesions, pathological fractures, spinal deformities, and large masses. Breast or prostate cancers may produce sclerotic or blastic lesions, but most spinal metastases are lytic, and plain radiographs may not reveal changes until up to half of the VB is affected. Due to this relative insensitivity, diagnosis is often obtained with other imaging techniques. Nuclear scintigraphy (bone scan) is a sensitive method for identifying areas of increased metabolic activity throughout the skeletal system. They are not specific for metastatic lesions, because this activity may be related to inflammation or infection. A more advanced form of nuclear bone scan, SPECT, provides 3D imaging of suspected vertebral metastases can be used to differentiate between metastatic and benign lesions. Positron emission tomography with FDG is also commonly used for whole-body surveillance in the detection of metastatic disease and cancer staging PET scans can also be used to identify cystic or necrotic areas of tumor, information that may increase the diagnostic yield of biopsy sampling and assist planning of surgical intervention. However, the resolution of PET is limited, and correlation with CT or MR imaging is required. Additionally, PET scanning is time-consuming and expensive. CT scanners provide highly detailed imaging of the osseous anatomy of the spine and the degree of tumor involvement, can aid surgical planning, and may be combined with CT angiography (vascular supply and tumor drainage) and myelography. MRI is most sensitive at detecting lesions within the vertebral column, The MR images also elucidate the bone- to soft-tissue interface, providing accurate anatomical detail of tumor invasion or related compression of osseous, neural, and paraspinal structures. Diffusion weighted studies, although not routinely used, may help distinguish benign and pathological compression fractures. Digital subtraction angiography is useful for lesions that originate from primary tumors with abundant vascularity (i.e. renal cell, thyroid, angiosarcoma, leiomyosarcoma, hepatocellular, and neuroendocrine tumors), knowledge of the vascular supply of metastases may prove invaluable if surgery is considered. Angiography may also permit preoperative embolization of metastases, which can be an effective alternative treatment for patients who are not candidates for surgical treatment. Embolization reduces intraoperative blood loss and facilitates complete resection of the lesion. In addition to limiting intraoperative hemorrhage, reducing the vascularity of metastases can also potentially shorten operating times and prevent the development of postoperative hematomas, which can cause wound breakdown and neurological decline.

FURTHER READING

Sciubba DM, Petteys RJ, Dekutoski MB, Fisher CG, Fehlings MG, Ondra SL, Rhines LD, Gokaslan ZL. Diagnosis and management of metastatic spine disease. A review. J Neurosurg Spine. 2010;13(1):94-108.

5. **c**—A higher Tokuhashi score predicts a poorer prognosis

Tokuhashi score for metastatic spine tumor prognosis (irrespective of treatment modality).

Modified Tokuhashi Score Criteria	Points
General condition (Karnofsky)	
Poor (10-40%)	0
Moderate (50-70%)	1
Good (80-100%)	2
Number of extra-spinal bone metastases foci	
≥3	0
1-2	1
2 points: 1	2
Number of metastases in the vertebral body	
≥3	0
1-2	1
1	2
Metastases to the major internal organs	
Unremovable	0
Removable	1
No metastases	2
Primary site of the cancer	
Lung, osteosarcoma, stomach, bladder, esophagus, pancreas	0
Liver, gallbladder, unidentified	1
Others	2
Kidney, uterus	3
Rectum	4
Thyroid, breast, prostate, carcinoid tumor	5
Palsy	
Complete (Frankel A, B)	0
Incomplete (Frankel C, D)	1
None (Frankel E)	2

Total score 0-8: 85% live <6 months thus conservative treatment or palliative surgery appropriate. Total score 9-11: 73% live >6 months (and 30% >1 year) thus palliative surgery or (exceptionally) excisional surgery an option. Total score 12-15: 95% live >1 year thus excisional surgery an option.

With permission from Tokuhashi Y, Matsuzaki H, Oda H, et al., A revised scoring system for preoperative evaluation of metastatic spine tumor prognosis, Spine (Phila Pa 1976). 2005;30(19):2186-2191.

Tomita Score Criteria	Points
Primary tumor	
Slow growth (e.g. breast, prostate, thyroid) Moderate growth (e.g. kidney, uterus)	1 2
Rapid growth (e.g. lung, liver, stomach, colon, primary unknown)	4
Visceral metastases	
No visceral metastases	0
Treatable	2
Untreatable	4
Bone metastases (including spine)	
Solitary/isolated	1
Multiple	2

Treatment goal & surgical strategy based on total score:

2-3 points: long-term local control (mean survival 50 months) → wide or marginal excision

4-5 points: middle-term local control (mean survival 23.5 months) → marginal or intralesional excision

6-7 points: short-term palliation (mean survival 15 months) → palliative surgery

8-10 points: terminal care (mean survival 6 months) → supportive care, no surgery

FURTHER READING

Tomita K, Kawahara N, Kobayashi T et al. Surgical strategy for spinal metastases, Spine (Phila Pa 1976). 2001;26(3):298-306.

6. **a**—Bisphosphonates have shown utility in management of pain resistant to conventional analgesia and but not in reducing the risk of malignant spinal cord compression

Offer conventional analgesia (including NSAIDs, non-opiate and opiate medication) as required to patients with painful spinal metastases in escalating doses as described by the WHO three-step pain relief ladder. Consider referral for specialist pain care including invasive procedures (such as epidural or intrathecal analgesia) and neurosurgical interventions for patients with intractable pain from spinal metastases (e.g. intrathecal morphine pump).

Bisphosphonates should only be used (if conventional analgesia fails) for pain relief in cases of vertebral metastases from breast, myeloma or prostate cancer only, and should not be used as prophylaxis for malignant spinal cord compression. Offer patients with spinal metastases causing non-mechanical spinal pain 8 Gy single fraction palliative radiotherapy even if they are completely paralysed, but not with the intention of preventing MSCC. In the absence of MSCC or spinal instability, consider vertebroplasty or kyphoplasty for patients who have vertebral metastases causing mechanical pain resistant to conventional analgesia, or vertebral body collapse.

FURTHER READING

Metastatic Spinal Cord Compression: Diagnosis and Management of Patients at Risk of or with Metastatic Spinal Cord Compression. NICE Clinical Guidelines, No. 75. National Collaborating Centre for Cancer (UK). Cardiff (UK): National Collaborating Centre for Cancer (UK); 2008 Nov.

7. **c**—Ensure he is nursed flat with neutral spine alignment

Acute management should include spinal precautions, steroids, and usually MR imaging. Patients with severe mechanical pain suggestive of spinal instability, or any neurological symptoms or signs suggestive of MSCC, should be nursed flat with neutral spine alignment (including "log rolling" or turning beds, with use of a slipper pan for toilet) until bony and neurological stability are ensured and cautious remobilization may begin. For patients with MSCC, once any spinal shock has settled and neurology is stable, carry out close monitoring and interval assessment during gradual sitting from supine to 60° over a period of 3-4 h. When patients with MSCC begin gradual sitting, if their blood pressure remains stable and no significant increase in pain or neurological symptoms occurs, continue to unsupported sitting, transfers and mobilization as symptoms allow. If a significant increase in pain or neurological symptoms occurs when patients with MSCC begin gradual sitting and mobilization, return them to a position where these changes reverse and reassess the stability of their spine. After a full discussion of the risks, patients who are not suitable for definitive treatment should be helped to position themselves and mobilize as symptoms permit with the aid of orthoses and/or specialist seating to stabilize the spine, if appropriate. Unless contraindicated (including a significant suspicion of lymphoma) offer all patients with MSCC a loading dose of at least 16 mg of dexamethasone as soon as possible after assessment, continue dexamethasone 16 mg daily in patients awaiting surgery or radiotherapy for MSCC. After surgery or the start of radiotherapy the dose should be reduced gradually over 5-7 days and stopped. If neurological function deteriorates at any time the dose should be increased temporarily. In those not proceeding to surgery or radiotherapy reduce gradually and stop dexamethasone as tolerated.

FURTHER READING

Metastatic Spinal Cord Compression: Diagnosis and Management of Patients at Risk of or with Metastatic Spinal Cord Compression. NICE Clinical Guidelines, No. 75. National Collaborating Centre for Cancer (UK). Cardiff (UK): National Collaborating Centre for Cancer (UK); 2008 Nov.

8. **c**—Radiotherapy can be given as soon as there is suspected MSCC on imaging

Start definitive treatment, if appropriate, before any further neurological deterioration and ideally within 24 h of the confirmed diagnosis of MSCC. In deciding on definitive treatment, establishing primary histology and staging (sites and extent of visceral and bony metastases) are key. Other important factors are the preferences of patients, neurological deficit, functional status, general health and fitness, previous treatments, magnitude of surgery, likelihood of complications, fitness for general anesthesia and overall prognosis. In particular, early decisions should be made about aggressiveness of MSCC treatment in those with (i) a poor performance status and widespread metastatic disease or (ii) completely paraplegic or tetraplegic for more than 24 h, and (iii) too frail or unfit for specialist treatment. Major surgical treatments should only be considered in those patients expected to survive 3 months or more, and use of the revised Tokuhashi scoring system and American Society of Anaesthetists (ASA) grading will help define its type and extent. Management options include mobilizing with bracing, palliation, radiotherapy (most common), chemotherapy (e.g. localized non-Hodgkin's lymphoma and germ cell tumors) and surgery. Consider patients with MSCC who have severe mechanical pain and/or imaging evidence of spinal instability, but who are unsuitable for surgery, for external spinal support (for example, a halo vest or cervico-thoraco-lumbar orthosis). In those with non-mechanical pain related to extradural spinal metastases only (i.e. without MSCC or spinal instability) offer fractionated radiotherapy as the definitive treatment. In those with MSCC confirmed on imaging there must be a cancer diagnosis established before radiotherapy can start. Relative contraindications to radiotherapy include no histological diagnosis of cancer, radio-resistant tumor if surgery is an option (renal cell carcinoma, sarcoma, melanoma etc.), vertebral displacement/spinal instability, poor general condition (irreversible) due to comorbidities, and previous radiotherapy (to cord tolerance) to same spinal site. Preoperative radiotherapy should not be carried out on patients with MSCC if surgery is planned, but postoperative fractionated radiotherapy should be offered routinely to all patients with a satisfactory surgical outcome once the wound has healed. In those with MSCC who are not suitable for surgery, urgent radiotherapy should be offered (<24 h) unless they have had complete tetraplegia or paraplegia for more than 24 h and their pain is already well controlled; or their overall prognosis is judged to be too poor. Chemotherapy is generally not indicated as the immediate treatment for malignant spinal cord compression and its main role is following the initial treatment with decompressive spinal surgery, or sometimes following local radiotherapy. Patients who present with malignant spinal cord compression, without a previous known malignancy, generally require a tissue diagnosis, and in most cases immediate surgery to decompress the spinal cord before the diagnosis is made, so that a biopsy would be obtained as part of the procedure. Rarely, radiological appearances may strongly suggest lymphoma, and needle biopsy, rather than immediate surgery is occasionally warranted, in which case immediate radiotherapy, rather than chemotherapy is given, as a provisional diagnosis can be obtained in an emergency within 24 h, and the correct chemotherapy usually requires a more detailed pathological diagnosis, which takes longer. Most chemo-sensitive tumors are also radio-sensitive, and it is often preferable to give local radiotherapy in such cases, to deal with the anatomical cause of the cord compression without having to consider the fitness of the patient for what may be life-threatening treatment with chemotherapy. Teratoma, yolk sac tumor, choriocarcinoma or a malignant molar pregnancy, are the (rare) causes of spinal cord compression where chemotherapy is more effective than radiotherapy, and should be the treatment of choice following initial tissue diagnosis.

FURTHER READING

Metastatic Spinal Cord Compression: Diagnosis and Management of Patients at Risk of or with Metastatic Spinal Cord Compression. NICE Clinical Guidelines, No. 75. National Collaborating Centre for Cancer (UK). Cardiff (UK): National Collaborating Centre for Cancer (UK); 2008 Nov.

9. **e**—Indicated in those patients expected to survive at least 12 months

To be considered for surgery the patient must be surgically fit, no pre-existing neurology, ambulant/weak/<24 h paralysis, single area of cord compression (this can include several contiguous spinal or vertebral segments), expected to survive 6 months or at least >3 months. Indications for surgery in the context of spinal metastastic disease will generally occur in the following scenarios: (i) to stabilize the spine and prevent MSCC in those with imaging evidence of structural spinal failure with spinal instability; (ii) to stabilize the spine in those with mechanical pain resistant to conventional analgesia, irrespective of neurological status, or (iii) to decompress the cord (usually with spinal stabilization if vertebral involvement) in those with MSCC who are can walk, have <24 h complete paralysis, or have little (but some) neurological function with very good prognosis giving them a chance of functional recovery. If surgery is appropriate in patients with MSCC attempt to achieve both spinal cord decompression and durable spinal column stability before they lose the ability to walk. If there is the slightest doubt as to the underlying pathology, particularly where there is a solitary bony lesion, further investigations including percutaneous bone biopsy should be carried out before definitive surgery. In those with a good prognosis but only residual distal sensory or motor function should still be offered surgery in an attempt to recover useful function, regardless of their ability to walk. Patients with MSCC who have been completely paraplegic or tetraplegic for more than 24 h should only be offered surgery if spinal stabilization is required for pain relief. Posterior decompression alone should not be performed in patients with MSCC except in the rare circumstances of isolated epidural tumor or neural arch metastases without bony instability. If spinal metastases involve the vertebral body or threaten spinal stability, posterior decompression should always be accompanied by internal fixation with or without bone grafting. Consider vertebral body reinforcement with cement for patients with MSCC and vertebral body involvement who are suitable for instrumented decompression but are expected to survive for less than 1 year. Consider vertebral body reconstruction with anterior bone graft for patients with MSCC and vertebral body involvement who are suitable for instrumented decompression, are expected to survive for 1 year or longer and who are fit to undergo a more prolonged procedure. En bloc excisional surgery with the objective of curing the cancer should not be attempted, except in very rare circumstances (e.g. confirmed solitary renal or thyroid metastasis following complete staging).

FURTHER READING

Metastatic Spinal Cord Compression: Diagnosis and Management of Patients at Risk of or with Metastatic Spinal Cord Compression. NICE Clinical Guidelines, No. 75. National Collaborating Centre for Cancer (UK). Cardiff (UK): National Collaborating Centre for Cancer (UK); 2008 Nov.

10. **b**—The surgical arm did not have increased survival time compared to radiotherapy alone

In 2005, Patchell et al. reported the results of the first prospective randomized controlled trial of direct decompressive resection plus adjuvant radiotherapy versus radiotherapy alone for metastatic spinal cord compression. Their study showed surgery plus radiotherapy to be far superior to radiotherapy alone, and the trial was stopped after 50% recruitment. Both groups of patients received 30 Gy of external-beam radiation delivered in 10 fractions, and the surgical group underwent operations intended to decompress the spinal cord, resect tumor bulk, and stabilize the spine. This approach was associated with statistically superior post-treatment ambulatory rate (84% vs. 57%, $p=0.001$), duration of ambulation (median 122 days vs. 13 days, $p=0.003$), maintenance of ambulation after treatment (94% vs. 74%, $p=0.024$), return of ambulation after treatment (62% vs. 19%, $p=0.012$), functional ability (Frankel scores), muscle strength (American Spinal Injury Association scores), continence, and survival time than those treated with radiotherapy alone. The median survival time in the surgery plus radiotherapy group was 126 days, versus 100 days in the radiotherapy alone group ($p=0.033$). However, those with highly radio-sensitive tumors (e.g. lymphoma, myeloma, and small cell lung carcinoma) were excluded from both groups hence it should be seen as proving the superiority of this approach for MSCC due to radio-resistant tumors. In patients with radio-sensitive primary tumors, radiotherapy alone is still indicated for MSCC presenting without spinal instability, rapidly progressive neurological decline without significant bone intrusion of the spinal canal, or with expected survival time <3 months. Surgical decompression and stabilization is indicated in patients with spinal instability, bony cord compression, rapid decline due to non-bony cord compression, recurrent tumor despite radiotherapy, MSCC caused by radio-resistant tumors, and cases in which tissue diagnosis is necessary. Total en bloc resection and spondylectomy may be indicated with curative resection possible for patients with solitary metastases of relatively indolent course, such as renal cell carcinoma without systemic metastases.

FURTHER READING

Patchell RA, Tibbs PA, Regine WF, et al. Direct decompressive surgical resection in the treatment of spinal cord compression caused by metastatic cancer. A randomised trial. Lancet 2005;366:643-648.

11. **b**—Expected patient survival should exceed 12 months before surgical treatment of spinal metastases is considered

Curative treatment is often not possible; therefore, therapeutic objectives are focused on preservation of neurological function, pain relief, and mechanical stabilization. Surgical intervention can successfully achieve these goals, but patient variables (such as age, tumor burden, life expectancy, and functional status) overwhelmingly influence the choice of therapy as much as stability and neurology. Developments in surgical technique and anterior and posterior stabilization of the spine that allow improved decompression and tumor resection with acceptable morbidity. Long-term disease-free survival is possible in some cases, specifically in solitary renal cell carcinoma metastases. Additionally, most clinicians would agree that the expected patient survival should exceed 3 months before surgical treatment of spinal metastases is considered. The principles used to develop these scoring systems were designed to assist surgeons in selecting patients who may benefit from surgical intervention and to determine the extent of surgical invasiveness that is appropriate. Practically speaking, the calculated scores from the Tomita and Tokuhashi systems are not binding in the choice of treatment, especially with the recent development of other treatment modalities like SRS. Moreover, once patients have been deemed appropriate candidates for surgical intervention, the determination of operative approach and stabilization requires a comprehensive understanding of the anatomy and histopathological features of the metastatic tumor and its surrounding structures, as well as the biomechanics of the spine and changes induced by vertebral metastases. Advances in imaging technology have improved the detection of cancerous lesions, but tissue from spinal masses is often still required for definitive diagnosis as 10-20% of spine metastases have no known source. If surgery and excisional biopsy are not immediately indicated, percutaneous biopsy may be required, because most treatment decisions will be dictated by the tumor histological findings. When a primary tumor is considered a possibility, the surgeon should be consulted in planning the biopsy procedure, because seeding and recurrence along the biopsy needle track can occur with some primary tumors, such as chordomas. The surgical approach to resection or decompression in spinal metastases is in large part determined by the spinal segment involved, the location of the tumor within the vertebra, the tumor's histological features, and the type of spine reconstruction necessary. The vertebral body is the most commonly affected portion of the spine in metastatic disease, and therefore, anterior approaches provide the greatest ability to resect the lesion and decompress the spinal canal. However, these approaches are associated with increased surgery-related morbidity and mortality, especially since the thoracic spine is the commonest site. Therefore, a transpedicular posterior or posterolateral approach is frequently used for T1-T4, Three-column decompression and stabilization can be achieved with this approach, especially with circumferential involvement and/or multiple levels. A right-sided thoracotomy, which minimizes risk to the great vessels and aortic arch, permits access to the mid-thoracic spine (T5-12). If, however, the majority of tumor bulk is on the left, a left-sided thoracotomy is indicated. Decompression of the thoracolumbar junction (T11-L1) may necessitate a combined thoracotomy and retroperitoneal approach. The lumbar spine (L2-5) and sacrum may be approached via anterior approaches, but posterior excision and stabilization is usually adequate in metastatic disease. Vertebral body resection requires subsequent reconstruction, often with titanium distractible or static mesh cages or with PMMA and anterolateral plating. Posterior stabilization with pedicle screw instrumentation is indicated for resections at high-stress areas, such as the cervicothoracic and thoracolumbar junction, and for patients with two or more adjacent vertebrectomies, kyphosis, or circumferential involvement.

FURTHER READING

Sciubba DM, Petteys RJ, Dekutoski MB, Fisher CG, Fehlings MG, Ondra SL, Rhines LD, Gokaslan ZL. Diagnosis and management of metastatic spine disease. A review. J Neurosurg Spine. 2010;13(1):94-108.

12. **b**—The region of the irradiated cord must lie slightly below the dermatome level of expression of the radiation myelitis

Radiation myelopathy may present as a transient early-delayed or late-delayed reaction. Transient (acute) radiation myelopathy is clinically manifested by Lhermitte's sign developing 3-4 months after treatment and spontaneously resolves over the following 3-6 months without therapy. It is attributed to transient demyelination caused by radiation-induced inhibition of myelin producing oligodendroglial cells in the irradiated spinal cord segment. Irreversible radiation myelopathy usually is not seen earlier than 6-12 months after completion of treatment. Typically, half of the patients who develop radiation-induced myelopathy in the cervical or thoracic cord region will do so within 20 months of treatment and 75% of cases will occur within 30 months. The signs and symptoms are typically progressive over several months, but acute onset of plegia over several hours or a few days is possible. It is thought to be multifactorial in origin, involving demyelination and white matter necrosis ultimately resulting from oligodendroglial cell depletion and microvascular injury. Radiation myelopathy is a diagnosis of exclusion with the following characteristics: (1) a history of radiation therapy in doses sufficient to result in injury must be present; (2) the region of the irradiated cord must lie slightly above the dermatome level of expression of the lesion; (3) the latent period from the completion of treatment to the onset of injury must be consistent with that observed in radiation myelopathy; and (4) local tumor progression must be ruled out. There are no pathognomonic laboratory tests or imaging studies that conclusively diagnose radiation myelopathy. MRI findings include swelling of the spinal cord with hyperintensity on the T2-weighted images with or without areas of contrast enhancement. There is no known consistently effective treatment for radiation myelitis. The probability of dying from radiation myelopathy is approximately 70% with cervical lesions and 30% with thoracic spinal cord injury. Radiation side effects in children include growth abnormalities such as decreased vertebral height, kyphosis, and scoliosis. Secondary malignant disease, including bone or soft-tissue sarcomas and glioblastoma, has been reported after irradiation of spinal cord tumors.

13. **b**—Craniospinal axis MRI should be performed

Myxopapillary ependymomas are most commonly benign and localize most often to the filum terminale and conus medullaris. They differ from other ependymomas morphologically and biologically and often resemble chordomas or chondrosarcomas; immunohistochemical analysis is frequently required for differentiation. Myxopapillary ependymomas manifest in younger individuals, in comparison with cellular ependymomas, and are also more common in male patients. They display large variations in size and are associated with scalloping of the vertebral body and enlargement of the neural foramina. On T1-weighted imaging, myxopapillary ependymomas are most often isointense or hypointense; however, in some instances, they have displayed hyperintensity on T1-weighted imaging because of hemorrhage or their mucin content. On T2-weighted imaging, these tumors are most often hyperintense. Polar cysts are also common findings in myxopapillary ependymomas. Myxopapillary ependymomas are low-grade tumors that typically occur in the lumbosacral region (filum terminale), are well-differentiated, and are often encapsulated but can seed the CSF, typically with "drop metastases" at the thecal sac. Myxopapillary ependymomas often progress slowly and cause milder-than-expected neurologic deficits for their size. These tumors represent a special variant of ependymoma found almost exclusively in the region of the filum terminale, although occasionally they have been found higher in the spinal cord or, rarely, in the brain. They may occur at any age, but most arise in the fourth decade. Myxopapillary ependymomas characteristically form a sausage-shaped mass in the lumbosacral region, displacing spinal nerve roots of the cauda equina. Their biologic behavior is usually benign, but because of their location they are often associated with significant compression-induced paralysis. Treatment consists of local excision, which must often be only partial because of the tumor's location; approximately 20% recur even after complete initial resection. Metastases infiltrating the CSF and extradural space may occur, but transformation to anaplastic variants is extremely rare. Myxopapillary subtypes appear to be associated with a favorable prognosis, potentially because of ease of resection because of their anatomic location. Patients who are able to achieve GTR have improved outcomes and the upfront addition of radiation therapy is of questionable benefit. However, one study suggests that pediatric patients with this tumor had higher recurrence rates, even in the setting of GTR, and appeared to benefit from postoperative irradiation. A retrospective review from the Rare Cancer Network suggests that higher postoperative radiation dose (>50.4 Gy) for the myxopapillary subtype may be associated with improved PFS.

Image with permission from Yachnis AT, Rivera-Zengotita ML, Neuropathology, High-Yield Pathology Series, Saunders, Elsevier, 2014.

14. **a**—Ependymoma

However, studies have shown that ependymomas have a predilection for the caudal spinal cord, with 50% of ependymomas arising in the lumbosacral cord or filum terminale and the remaining 50% occurring nonpreferentially along the cervical or thoracic spinal cord. On imaging, anaplastic ependymomas may be distinguished by their larger size, numerous cysts, and heterogeneous postcontrast enhancement. Anaplastic ependymomas are uncommon, comprising only 5% of all ependymomas, but they are characterized by anaplastic features (i.e. vascular proliferation, mitotic figures, cellular pleomorphism, and necrosis) on histologic analysis. Patients experience higher rates of tumor recurrence and decreased rates of survival. Classic radiographic features of spinal cord ependymomas include distinct tumor-spinal cord border, an associated syrinx, cysts within or adjacent to the mass, and hemosiderin deposits or "caps" near the poles of the tumor on T1 and T2. The treatment of choice is gross total surgical resection.

Image with permission from Herkowitz et al., Rothman-Simeone The Spine, 6th ed., Elsevier, Saunders, 2011.

15. **a**—Ependymoma

Ependymomas arise from ependymal cells and typically occur in the central canal of the spinal cord, the filum terminale, and the white matter adjacent to a ventricular surface. They are the commonest intramedullary spinal cord tumor in adults and commoner in males than females (the commonest intramedullary tumors in children are astrocytoma, ganglioglioma then ependymoma). The mean age at presentation is 30-40 years with long duration of symptoms (e.g. 2-4 years). Two thirds occur in the lumbosacral region (40% of these arise from the filum terminale (myxopapillary ependymoma). Because of the propensity of these tumors for seeding the craniospinal axis, CSF evaluation and MRI of the whole craniospinal axis is strongly recommended. The three main subsets of ependymomas are cellular (this case), myxopapillary, and anaplastic. Cellular ependymomas are most often located in the cervical spine. On T1-weighted MRI, they are isointense to hypointense, whereas on T2-weighted MRI, they are hyperintense and there may be a syrinx in 50% of cases. Factors prognostic for a favorable outcome include patient age younger than 40 years; tumors with a lumbosacral location, myxopapillary histologic findings, or a grade of WHO grade I; tumors amenable to GTR or STR; and good preoperative function of the patient. Whether volume of residual disease correlates with a worse outcome after EBRT is controversial. Most intradural extramedullary ependymomas are myxopapillary and are often amenable to complete surgical resection if they are not multifocal. The goal of surgery is GTR. Every attempt should be made to remove tumors as a whole as opposed to piecemeal removal, because of the risk of seeding, including upward seeding to the cranial nerves. Typically, complete resection is achievable in 80-100% of modern series, with 10-year survival for all spinal cord ependymomas is 70-100%. Postoperative EBRT appears to improve local control in patients with STR ependymomas and also for patients with high-grade lesions and those with neuraxis dissemination. In most but not all series, the outcome for STR followed by EBRT appears to be similar to that of complete resection. In patients with tumors at high risk of seeding, when pretreatment CSF cytologic studies reveal malignant cells, or if the spinal MRI scan shows evidence of leptomeningeal disease, the craniospinal axis should be treated. There is no strong body of evidence thus far demonstrating that the addition of chemotherapy to EBRT improves the outcome, but it is used in pediatric patients with anaplastic ependymoma or ependymoblastoma are routinely given chemotherapy.

Image with permission from Yachnis AT, Rivera-Zengotita ML, Neuropathology, High-Yield Pathology Series, Saunders, Elsevier, 2014.

16. **e**—Chromosome 22

MISME syndrome (multiple inherited schwannomas, meningiomas, and ependymomas) is seen in NF-2, which has a locus on chromosome 22. NF-1 gene locus is on chromosome 17, tuberous sclerosis on chromosomes 9 and 16, neuroblastoma on chromosome 11.

Image with permission from Holland K, Kaye AH, Spinal tumors in neurofibromatosis-2: management considerations—a review, J Clin Neurosci. 2009;16(2):169-177.

17. **a**—Astrocytoma

Astrocytomas are the second most common intramedullary spinal cord tumors in adults (30%), compared to children in which they are the commonest. Almost 60% of these tumors occur in the cervical and cervicothoracic region, and 20% have an associated syrinx. Back pain and motor deficits are the most common presenting symptom in astrocytomas. The most significant prognostic factors in patients with primary spinal cord astrocytoma are tumor histology, tumor grade, age, and performance status. Because of the rare nature of this disease, almost all data are based on retrospective reviews fraught with selection bias. Therefore, neither the extent of resection nor treatment with adjuvant irradiation appears to be prognostic, although this is controversial. The classic MRI appearance of intramedullary astrocytoma is cord enlargement with a central lesion with poorly defined margins, cysts, peritumoral edema and patchy enhancement (no enhancement in 30%). It is typically isointense to hypointense on T1-weighted images and hyperintense on T2-weighted images. The treatment of choice for intramedullary astrocytomas is complete excision of the tumor, when it can be safely accomplished without neurologic compromise. Otherwise, an incomplete excision is typically performed for grade I lesions, and biopsy alone is the surgical strategy for the non-exophytic component of an infiltrative glioma. GTR is typically extremely difficult to achieve because of the infiltrative nature of all but the pilocytic lesions, with most authors reporting a 0-50% likelihood of GTR for spinal cord astrocytoma. In patients with favorable prognostic factors (low-grade histologic findings, good performance status, and young age), observation with serial imaging studies, reserving irradiation for local recurrence, is an appropriate management option, particularly for young children. Radiation should be considered for high-grade tumors, inoperable tumors, tumors remaining after surgery, and recurring tumors. In the remainder of patients, adjuvant irradiation is usually recommended because progression of tumor in the spinal cord may lead to significant neurologic impairment. The overall outcomes are similar for patients with low-grade gliomas of the spinal cord treated either by GTR or STR or biopsy followed by external beam irradiation (EBRT), with most series reporting OS at 5 years of 55-100%. With high-grade tumors in adults and children, the median survival time is quite poor (4-10 months) despite surgery and EBRT. Extrapolating from the results of Stupp et al. for intracranial glioblastoma, temozolomide has emerged as a treatment strategy in high-grade intramedullary tumors.

Image with permission from Adam A et al. (Eds), Grainger & Allison's Diagnostic Radiology, 6th ed., 2014, Elsevier, Churchill Livingstone.

ANSWERS 18–24

Additional answers 18–24 available on ExpertConsult.com

EMI ANSWERS

25. 1—b, Ependymoma; 2—c, Ganglioglioma

26. 1—h, Leptomeningeal drop metastasis; 2—g, Schwannoma; 3—d, Meningioma

27. 1—c, Hemangioma; 2—c, Eosinophilic granuloma; 3 = k, Osteoid osteoma; 4—a, Chordoma

Summary of Epidemiology, Histology, and Imaging Findings of Primary Vertebral Tumors

Tumor	Behavior	Age Range	Sex Predilection	Associated Syndromes or Diseases	Location	Histological Findings	CT Findings	MRI Findings
Aneurysmal bone cyst	Benign	1st-3rd decades	Female (slight)		Posterior elements	"Blood-filled sponges" of cavernous cysts with walls of woven bone	"Soap bubble", lytic and multilobulated	Variable on T1 and T2; gadolinium enhances
Chondroma/ enchondroma	Benign	2nd-3rd decades	Male (2:1)	Olier syndrome, Maffucci syndrome	Cervical thoracic lumbar	Hypocellular, chondrocytes within lacunae	Calcified, lytic	T1 low to intermediate signal; T2 hyperintense
Eosinophillic granuloma	Benign	2nd decade	Male (2-5:1)	Langerhans cell histiocytosis	Thoracic lumbar; vertebral bodies and anterior elements	"Tennis racquet"-shaped Birbeck granules in cytoplasm, stains for CD1a	Lytic destruction of vertebral bodies may cause collapse (vertebra plana)	T1 isointense; T2 hyperintense with soft tissue swelling
Fibrous dysplasia	Benign	1st-2nd decades	Equal	McCune-Allbright syndrome	No preference	Sheets of broken or retracted fibroblasts with woven bone; foamy macrophages, cystic changes, hemorrhage	Lytic and expansive with "ground glass" and sclerotic margins	T1 and T2 with variable intensity
Hemangioma	Benign	4th-6th decades	Female (slight)		No preference; vertebral bodies	Multiple small vessels with sclerotic trabeculated bone	"Honeycomb" pattern on plain radiograph; polka dots of bone on CT	T1 isointense; T2 hyperintense gadolinium enhances
Osteoid osteoma	Benign	1st-2nd decades	Male (2-3:1)		Lumbar; posterior elements	"Cloudlike;" well-circumscribed hypodense tumor and surrounding normal trabecula (osteoblastomas similar appearing but >2 cm)	Low-attenuation nidus with sclerotic boarder	T1 nidus with intermediate signal intensity; T2 hypointense; gadolinium nidal enhancement

Chordoma	Locally aggressive (malignant)	4th-6th decades	Male (2:1)	Sacrum, cervical	"Physalipharous" bubble-containing cytoplasm and large, round cells; Brachyury, epithelial membrane antigen, 5-100 staining	Expansive, lytic, sclerotic	T1 isointense; T2 hyperintense gadolinium, variable
Giant cell tumor	Locally aggressive (malignant)	2nd-4th decades	Female (slight)	Sacrum	Multinucleated giant cells in spindle cell stroma	Lytic, cystic	T1 isointense; T2 hyperintense with areas of hemorrhage; gadolinium enhances
Chondrosarcoma	Malignant	4th decade	Male (2:1)	Thoracic	Large or binucleated pleomorphic cells with small nucleoli	Expansive and lytic; scalloping of cortex with cortical expansion	Markedly T2 hyperintense; gadolinium "rings and arcs" pattern
Ewing sarcoma	Malignant	1st-3rd decades	Male (slight)	Sacral	Small round cells with uniform nuclei; CD99 is sensitive nut not specific	Lytic	T1 isointense; T2 hyperintense to hyperintense gadolinium enhances
Multiple myeloma/ solitary plasmacytoma	Malignant	5th decade	Male (2:1)	Thoracic	Sheets of plasma cells, cytologic atypia	Lytic, osteoporotic	T1 isointense; T2 hyperintense gadolinium enhances
Osteosarcoma	Malignant	3rd-6th decades	Male (slight)	Sacrum	Spindle cells with nuclear pleomorphism; osteoid or bone production with the tumor	Lytic and destructive with matrix mineralization	T1 hypointense; T2 hyperintense

With permission from Ropper AE, Cahill KS, Hanna JW, et al., Primary vertebral tumors: a review of epidemiologic, histological, and imaging findings, Part I: benign tumors, Neurosurgery. 2011;69(6):1171-1180.

CHAPTER 32

SPINAL VASCULAR NEUROSURGERY

SINGLE BEST ANSWER (SBA) QUESTIONS

1. The artery of Adamkiewicz is best described as which one of the following?
   a. Centripetal artery
   b. Radiculomedullary artery
   c. Radiculopial artery
   d. Segmental artery
   e. Sulcocommissural artery (centrifugal)

2. Which one of the following best describes Foix-Alajouanine syndrome?
   a. Involves descending sensory loss
   b. Involves hemorrhage from multiple spinal AVMs
   c. Involves normal cerebrospinal fluid protein level
   d. Involves progressive paraparesis due to congestive myelopathy
   e. Involves spinal venous thrombosis on pathological examination

3. In the literature, Type II spinal Arteriovenous malformations (AVMs) generally refer to which one of the following?
   a. Conus medullaris AVM
   b. Dural arteriovenous fistula (AVF)
   c. Intradural perimedullary AVF
   d. Intramedullary glomus AVM
   e. Juvenile or mixed AVM

4. A 55-year-old male presents with progressive gait disturbance and impotence. Coronal Magnetic resonance angiogram and angiograms are shown in the lumbar spine. There is no evidence of hemorrhage. VHL screen is negative. Which one of the following diagnoses is most likely?

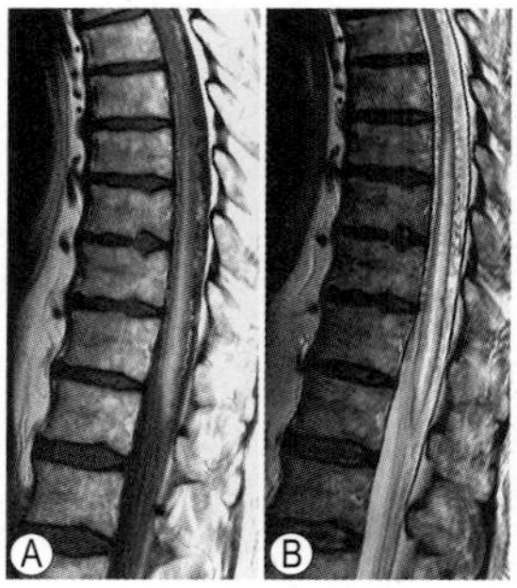

   a. Aneurysm of artery of Adamkiewicz
   b. Cavernoma
   c. Hemangioblastoma
   d. Type I Dural AVF
   e. Type II intramedullary glomus AVM

5. A 15-year-old boy presents with neck pain and bilateral upper limb weakness. MRI is shown below. Which one of the following is most likely?

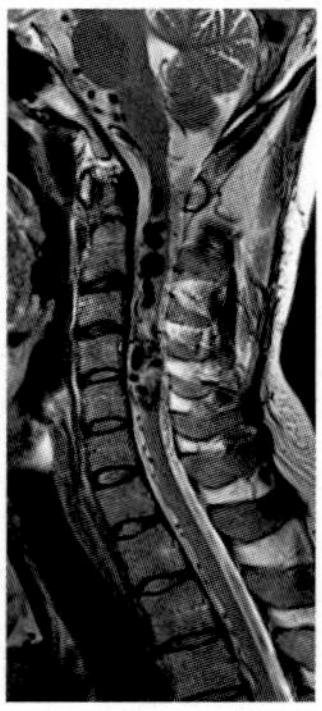

   a. Astrocytoma
   b. Ependymoma
   c. Transverse myelitis
   d. Type I Dural (dorsal intradural) AVF
   e. Type III juvenile (extradural-intradural) AVM

6. A 35-year-old with Osler-Weber-Rendu syndrome presents with gait disturbance. T2W MRI is shown below. Which one of the following is most likely?

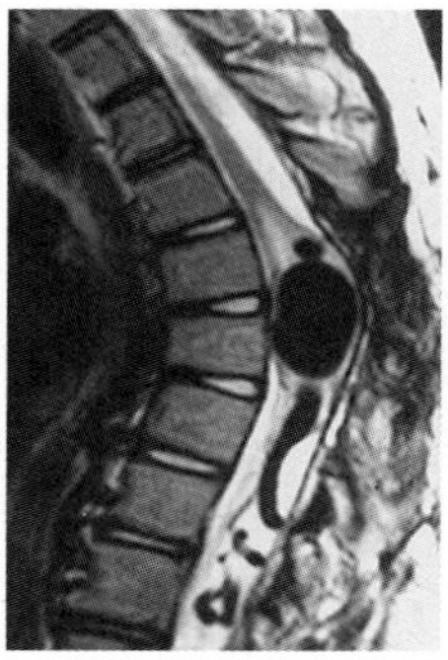

a. Hemangioblastoma
b. Neurenteric cyst
c. Spinal artery aneurysm
d. Type III juvenile (extradural-intradural) AVF
e. Type IV-C perimedullary (ventral intradural) AVF

7. Which one of the following is most likely from the images below?

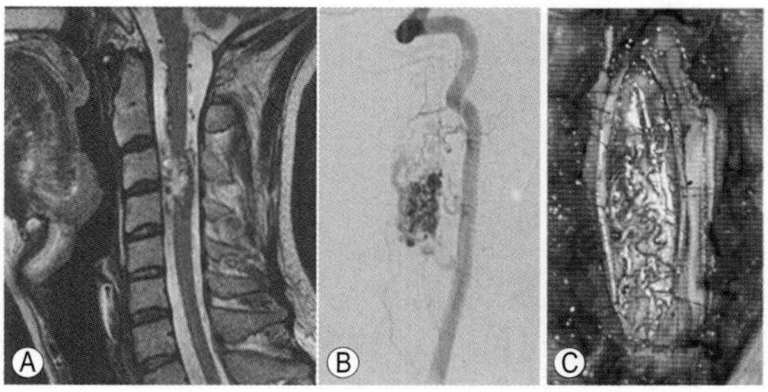

a. Cavernous angioma
b. Hemangioblastoma
c. Hemangioma
d. Type I dural (dorsal intradural) AVF
e. Type II intramedullary (Glomus) AVM

8. A 33-year-old presents with sudden onset neck pain. MRI is shown below. Which one of the following is most likely?

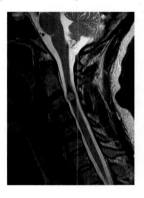

a. Cavernous angioma
b. Multiple sclerosis
c. Syringomyelia
d. Type I dural AVF
e. Type II intramedullary glomus AVM

9. A 54-year-old male presents with sudden onset stabbing neck pain two days ago, and is now has a left hemiparesis with impaired pain and temperature sensation on the contralateral side. Which one of the following would you consider the appropriate next management step?

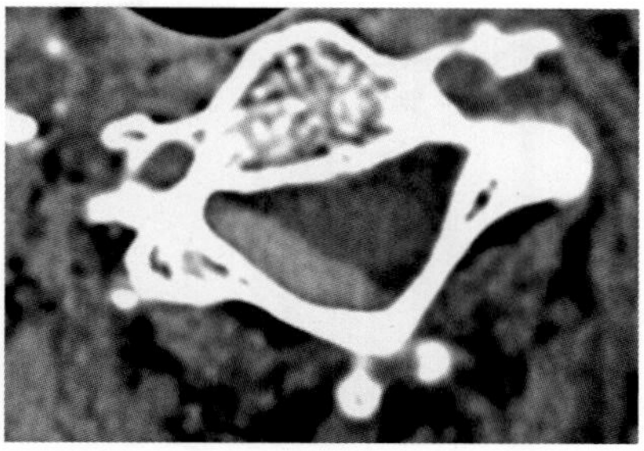

a. CT myelogram
b. Epidural hematoma
c. Prothrombin complex concentrate
d. Spinal angiogram
e. Spinal decompression
f. Spinal traction

QUESTIONS 10–11

Additional questions 10–11 available on ExpertConsult.com

12. A 54-year-old with a Type II glomus AVM who has been under surveillance presents with worsening myelopathy such that they are now unable to work. Repeat MRI shows increased T2 signal in the cord at the L1 level. Which one of the following would be appropriate next?
a. Embolization followed by surgical decompression at level of AVM only
b. Embolization followed by surgical excision with interruption of arterial side of AVM first
c. Embolization followed by surgical excision with interruption of venous side of AVM first
e. Endovascular obliteration of primary arterial feeders alone
f. Surveillance

EXTENDED MATCHING ITEM (EMI) QUESTIONS

13. **Arterial supply to spine:**

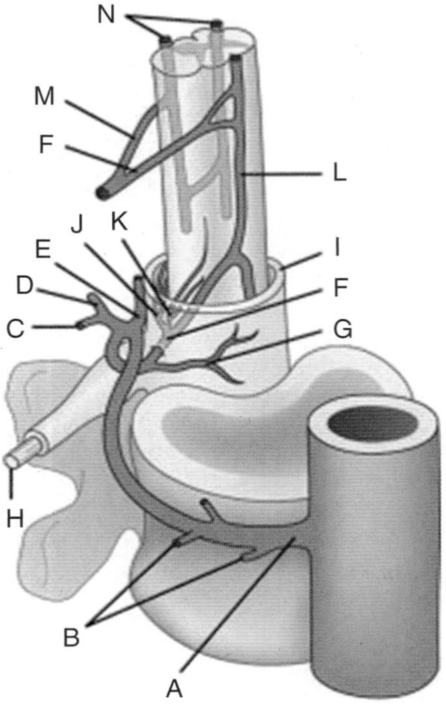

For each of the following descriptions, select the most appropriate answer from the image above. Each answer may be used once, more than once or not at all.

1. Anterior spinal artery
2. Paravertebral longitudinal anastamosis
3. Radiculomedullary artery
4. Radiculopial artery
5. Segmental artery

14. **Venous drainage of spine:**

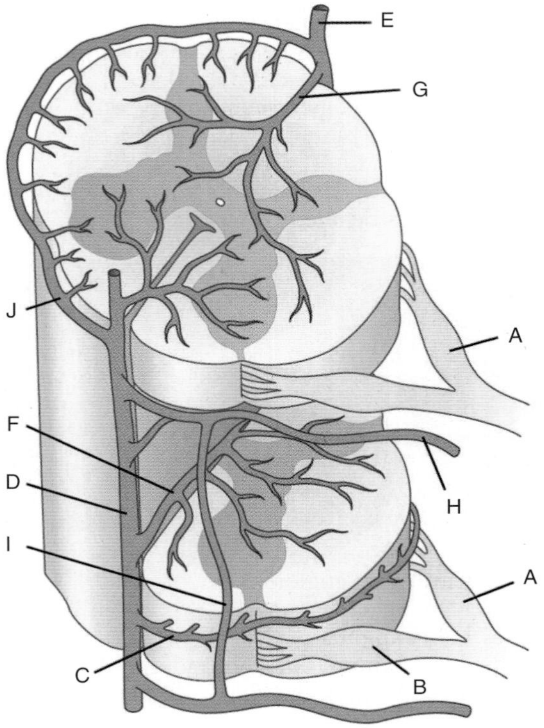

For each of the following descriptions, select the most appropriate answer from the image above. Each answer may be used once, more than once or not at all.

1. Anterior median vein
2. Coronal vein
3. Dorsal sulcal vein
4. Intramedullary anastamosis
5. Radiculomedullary vein

15. **Vascular disorders of the spine:**
    a. Cavernous angioma
    b. Conus medullaris AVM
    c. Dural AVF
    d. Extradural AVF
    e. Extradural-intradural (juvenile) AVM
    f. Hemangioblastoma
    g. Intradural dorsal (dural) AVF
    h. Intradural ventral (perimedullary) AVF

i. Intramedullary glomus AVM
j. Paraspinal AVM
k. Spinal artery aneurysm

For each of the following descriptions, select the most appropriate answer from the list above. Each answer may be used once, more than once or not at all.

1. Associated with hereditary hemorrhagic telangiectasia
2. Associated with Cobb syndrome

SBA ANSWERS

1. **b**—Radiculomedullary artery

The simplified algorithm for the vascular supply at each segmental level is *major arterial trunk* (vertebral artery, aorta) → *spinal/segmental artery* → *radicular branches which* give off branches to the paraspinous musculature, vertebral body, and dura before forming:

1. *Radiculopial arteries* supply the nerve roots by means of smaller branches and then run ventral to either the dorsal or ventral nerve root to supply the pial network. Although they anastomose with pial branches of the ASA, they do not supply the ASA directly. There are more dorsal than ventral radiculopial arteries, and the dorsal radiculopial arteries are the dominant supply to the PSA. Their number varies from three to four in the cervical region, from six to nine in the thoracic region, and from zero to three in the lumbosacral region.
2. *Radiculomedullary arteries* are the dominant supply to the ASA. After giving off their radicular branches to the nerve roots, they run along the ventral surface of the nerve root, occasionally give off pial collateral branches, and continue to the ASA. On average, there are two to four radiculomedullary arteries in the cervical region, two to three in the thoracic region, and zero to four in the lumbosacral region. The largest radiculomedullary artery of the thoracolumbar segment is also known as the artery of Adamkiewicz. In 75% of patients, the AKA arises between T9 and T12, more commonly on the left. When its origin is above T8 or below L2, another major contributor to the ASA can be found either cranially or caudally. In 30-50% of cases, it also contributes significantly to the PSA. Generally, a pair of arteries arises in the cervical region from the intradural segment of each vertebral artery that fuse to one "Y"-shaped ASA running in the subpial space in the ventral sulcus of the spinal cord (dorsal to the anterior spinal vein) to the terminal film. The typical hairpin anastomosis between the radiculomedullary arteries and the ASA is found angiographically at the lower thoracic and lumbar levels.

2. **d**—Involves progressive paraparesis due to congestive myelopathy

The exact etiology of the process which resulted in the progressive and fatal neurological deterioration the two patients described by Foix and Alajouanine in 1926 is still a cause for debate, leading to confusion about it's actual definition. Both patients presented with a progressive lower limb weakness, incontinence and sensory level; pathological examination in both cases revealed myelitis and spinal cord necrosis, with extensive hypertrophy of intradural vessels (veins on cord surface, extramedullary veins, intramedullary veins and to a lesser extent some arteries); histological analysis showed vessels endo-meso-vasculitis with necrotizing tendencies with widely patent vessel lumens. Despite the authors specifically excluding thrombosis on pathological examination, the Foix-Alajouanine syndrome was initially associated with spinal artery thrombosis leading to myelopathy. However, some patients diagnosed with Foix-Alajouanine syndrome improved, making thrombosis of the spinal artery an unlikely cause. Afterward, in 1989 Criscuolo et al. also pointed against its association with thrombosis and explained that the symptoms of this syndrome could be explained by congestive myelopathy, which is a reversible process. As such, nowadays it may also refer to spinal AVM (usually intradural AVF) patients with clinically subacute to chronic progressive neurological symptoms due to congestive myelopathy without hemorrhage.

FURTHER READING

Criscuolo GR, Oldfield EH, Doppman JL. Reversible acute and subacute myelopathy in patients with dural arteriovenous fistulas. Foix-Alajouanine syndrome reconsidered. J Neurosurg 1989;70(3):354-9.

Ferrell AS, Tubbs RS, Acakpo-Satchivi L, Deveikis JP, Harrigan MR. Legacy and current understanding of the often-misunderstood Foix-Alajouanine syndrome. Historical vignette. J Neurosurg 2009;111(5):902-6.

3. **d**—Intramedullary glomus AVM

Classification of spinal AVMs is another area of controversy. Two salient classifications for neurosurgeons are shown below:

FURTHER READING

Bao YH, Ling F. Classification and therapeutic modalities of spinal vascular malformations in 80 patients. Neurosurgery 1997;40(1):75-81.

Spinal Cord Vascular Lesions (Spetzler et al. 2002)

Modified Classification	Previous Name
AV fistulas	
Extradural AVF	Epidural AVF
Dorsal intradural AVF	Dural AVF (IA)
Ventral intradural AVF	Perimedullary AVF
Arteriovenous malformation	
Extradural-intradural AVM	Juvenile AVM
Intramedullary AVM	Glomus AVM
Conus medullaris AVM	-
Neoplastic vascular lesion	
Hemangioblastoma	-
Cavernous malformation	-
Spinal cord aneurysm	-

FURTHER READING

Spetzler RF, Detwiler PW, Riina HA, Porter RW. Modified classification of spinal cord vascular lesions. J Neurosurg 2002;96:145-56.

4. **d**—Type 1 Dural AVF

Dural arteriovenous fistulas comprise 80-85% of spinal AVMs. These lesions show a male predominance (80-90%) and generally present in late adulthood, ages 40-60. Presentation is generally with radiculomyelopathy, followed by slow but progressive neurological deterioration. Site of pathology in these lesions is within the dural root sleeve, where a direct arteriovenous fistula develops, generally with a single dural artery feeder vessel. Venous drainage of the AV fistula is by a high pressure, low-flow arterialized vein intradurally. Chronic venous hypertension yields chronic spinal cord ischemia, cell loss, and cord atrophy. Impaired autoregulation yields direct transmission of changes in systemic arterial pressure to the spinal cord without the normal dampening effect of the venous plexus. Goal of treatment is isolation and obliteration of the fistula and draining veins, which normalizes venous pressure and corrects venous hypertension.

Image with permission from Krings T, Lasjaunias PL, Hans FJ, et al. Imaging in spinal vascular disease. Neuroimaging Clin N Am 2007;17(1):57-72.

Classification of Spinal Vascular Malformations (Bao & Ling 1997)

Type	Name	Description	Age
I	Dural AVF	AVFs between a radicular or radiculomedullary artery and a medullary vein, with the fistulous connection located in the dural root sleeve. These malformations are likely often acquired and arise predominantly at thoracic and thoracolumbar levels, almost universally dorsal. Most authors have classified this lesion as type A if fed by a single arterial feeder and type B if fed by two or more feeders	40-60
II	Intramedullary glomus AVM	Well-defined, completely or partially intramedullary lesions consisting of a distinct conglomeration of dysmorphic arteries and veins in direct communication without an intervening capillary bed. Type II AVMs of the cervical spinal cord frequently have multiple feeding vessels of anterior spinal, posterior spinal, and radiculomedullary arteries, whereas Type II AVMs of the thoracic spinal cord or conus are often supplied via a single enlarged branch of the anterior spinal artery. Latent anastomotic channels invariably exist, however, which may emerge after proximal ligation or endovascular occlusion of the primary feeding vessel	20-30
III	Juvenile or mixed AVM	Rare. Consist of diffuse arteriovenous shunts with variable degrees of involvement of the spinal cord, vertebral, and paraspinal tissues. Other metameric anomalies of associated organs and the skin are commonly associated with these lesions	10-20
IV	Intradural perimedullary AVF	Most occur in the thoracolumbar region as a fistula between the anterior spinal artery (ASA) and vein (ASV) on the ventral spinal cord surface Type IV-A malformation is a small, simple direct fistula with a single ASA feeder Type IV-B lesions are medium-sized fistulas and have additional, smaller feeding vessels arising from either the ASA or posterior spinal artery (PSA) Type IV-C fistulas are giant sized and demonstrate several enlarged ASA and PSA feeding branches with dilated venous outflow	20-40

5. **e**—Type III juvenile (extradural-intradural) AVM

Juvenile spinal AVMs are extremely rare lesions. These lesions are again true AVMs, with an intramedullary nidus which may occupy the entire spinal canal at the involved level. Cord tissue is present within the AVM interspaces. Extramedullary and even extraspinal extension of the lesion is possible. Juvenile AVMs are large and complex lesions, with multiple arterial feeding vessels often arising from different cord levels. Hemodynamically, this lesion manifests both high flow and high pressure, often yielding an auscultatable spinal bruit over involved levels. They occur most commonly in adolescents and young adults. Presentation and treatment are similar to Type II AVMs; however, prognosis for these lesions, considering their size and vascular complexity, is understandably very poor. MR imaging typically demonstrates prominent flow voids suggestive of underlying vascular malformation. Edema or gliosis can also be seen on MR imaging.

Image with permission from Fatterpekar GM, Naidich TP, Som PM (Eds.), Teaching Files: Brain and Spine, Elsevier, Saunders, 2012.

6. **e**—Type IV-C perimedullary AVF

Perimedullary (ventral intradural) AVFs have a fistulous connection which is intradural but extramedullary, with feeding vessel(s) from the anterior spinal artery. Venous drainage is via an enlarged coronal venous plexus. These lesions may present in young adults, but presentation in the third to sixth decade is more likely. SAH is possible with subsequent acute neurologic deterioration, but a gradual progressive neurologic deterioration is common. Three subcategories of intradural spinal AV fistulas have been recognized, with different treatment options appropriate for each.

- Type IVa has a single feeding vessel, often the artery of Adamkiewicz, with low flow through the arteriovenous shunt and moderate venous enlargement. Endovascular techniques are difficult with these lesions due to the small size of feeding vessels hence surgical excision is often mandated.
- Type IVb AV fistulas are medium-sized, often with multiple feeding vessels, and more marked venous enlargement. Embolization in these lesions is easier, due to the increased size of feeding vessels. In cases of incomplete shunt obliteration with an endovascular approach, direct surgical excision may be necessary.
- Type IVc are giant, multipediculated, high-flow fistulas with large, tortuous draining veins. Spinal ischemia may develop in these lesions secondary to vascular steal. Due to the size of these lesions, surgery is technically difficult and may jeopardize the spinal cord. Treatment is hence through combination of endovascular ablation, followed by surgical excision of retained elements.

Image with permission from Krings T, Lasjaunias PL, Hans FJ, et al. Imaging in spinal vascular disease. Neuroimaging Clin N Am 2007;17(1):57-72.

7. **e**—Type II intramedullary (glomus) AVM

Type II intramedullary (glomus) AVMs are characterized by a compact intramedullary nidus, with feeding vessels arising from the anterior or posterior spinal arteries, or both, and drainage into an arterialized coronal venous plexus. Unlike spinal AV fistulas they are high pressure, low-flow lesions (rapid filling on angiogram and early venous drainage). Affect men and women equally, and mean age of presentation in 20s. The clinical course of these lesions is marked by progressive and fluctuating myelopathy, often overlaid by periods of acute neurologic deterioration secondary to hemorrhage within the AVM. Sudden apoplectic presentation, often with profound neurologic impairment and possible transverse myelopathy is common. SAH often occurs in these lesions, occurring in 50% of cases. True intramedullary AVMs occur throughout the cord hence presentation with upper extremity symptoms is possible. Imaging demonstrates intramedullary AVM at C3-C4 levels with associated hematoma and flow voids from arterialized coronal venous plexus of the spinal cord, while angiogram demonstrates feeders arising from the left vertebral artery. Treatment involves initial embolization of feeding vessels using particulate matter. Immediate clinical improvement is often noted after embolization, through reduction in arterial steal and improved cord perfusion; however, recanalization may occur over time, with continued risk of hemorrhage. Hence, surgical resection of residual nidus after embolization is generally reasonable.

Image with permission from Kim DH, et al. (Eds.), Surgical Anatomy and Techniques to the Spine, 2nd ed., Elsevier, Saunders, 2013.

8. **a**—Cavernous angioma

Central nervous system (CNS) cavernomas are rare vascular malformations consisting of closely packed large sinusoid-like vascular channels with little or no intervening nervous tissue. They can occur anywhere in the CNS but favor the cerebral hemisphere. Spinal cord cavernomas are uncommon, accounting for 3-5% of all cavernous malformations. Most commonly seen in the thoracic region (50%), they are uncommonly identified in the conus (10%); the cervical cord accounts for 40% of such lesions. Sudden onset paraplegia in a young adult. MR is the imaging modality of choice. The typical imaging features are of a well-defined lesion causing focal expansion of the cord with mixed signal intensity on T1WI and T2WI. These lesions are typically surrounded by a complete hypointense rim owing to hemosiderin deposition. Typically, no or only sparse edema is associated with this lesion. Enhancement following contrast administration is variable.

Image with permission from Fatterpekar GM, Naidich TP, Som PM (Eds.), Teaching Files: Brain and Spine, Elsevier, Saunders, 2012.

9. **e**—Spinal decompression

Epidural hematoma can occur secondary to trauma, iatrogenic procedures, or vascular malformation or sometimes can be seen as a spontaneous occurrence, such as in patients with coagulopathy. Spinal extradural haematoma (EDH) is seen to occur most commonly in the thoracic and lumbar region in adults, whereas in children, it is seen to occur in the cervicothoracic region. The dorsal aspect of the canal is the most common site for an epidural hematoma. Most spinal EDHs have a venous source of hemorrhage. Spinal hemorrhage (epidural, subdural or subarachnoid) presents with intense, stabbing pain at the location of the hemorrhage ("coup de poignard of Michon") that may be followed in some cases by a pain-free interval of minutes to days, after which there is progressive paralysis below the affected spinal level. CT scan will demonstrate lentiform or biconvex hyperdense collection with variable cord compression. MR will demonstrate a lentiform collection in the epidural compartment, the signal intensity of which will vary with the age of the hemorrhage (Fat-suppressed T1WI can be used to distinguish blood from fat). Early surgical decompression is standard, and if the exact location of the hematoma cannot be detected and confirmed by MRI, the dura should be opened to exclude a subdural hematoma. Conservative treatment has also been documented, usually when neurological deficits improved in the early phase or with the coexistence of coagulopathy and multilevel acute epidural hematomas.

FURTHER READING

Kreppel D, Antoniadis G, Seeling W. Spinal hematoma: a literature survey with metaanalysis of 613 patients. Neurosurg Rev 2003;26(1):1-49.

Image with permission from Fatterpekar GM, Naidich TP, Som PM (Eds.), Teaching Files: Brain and Spine, Elsevier, Saunders, 2012.

ANSWERS 10–11

Additional answers 10–11 available on ExpertConsult.com

12. **b**—Embolization followed by surgical excision with interruption of arterial side of AVM first

Summary of Management of Spinal Cord Vascular Lesions

Type	Management Notes
I (Dural AVF)	Surgical interruption of the intradural draining vein More complex/recurrent fistula excision definitively prevents re-establishment of retrograde intradural venous drainage through collateral longitudinal extradural venous channels at adjacent radicular levels. Several millimeters of the feeding radicular artery and intradural draining vein may be cauterized, divided, and contiguously excised along with a small window of dura on the root sleeve. Fistula obliteration rate is significantly lower with embolization, and progressive myelopathy is a risk due to delay in definitive treatment
II (Glomus AVM)	Classic AVM—require surgical excision with or without preoperative embolization. Interruption of the venous side of an AVM first can lead to hazardous elevations in pressure in the remaining venous drainage system, producing either excessive bleeding around the AVM or rupture of associated venous aneurysms
III (juvenile AVM)	Most difficult to treat—no well-defined margin for resection Partial treatment through embolization, surgical decompression and limited arterial clip ligation may produce some clinical benefit but it is unlikely to last and is not without significant risk
IV (perimedullary AVF)	Surgical ligation is definitive for small (Type IV-A) shunts For more complex, higher-flow lesions (Types IV-B and C), endovascular obliteration of the shunt may be the preferred primary treatment or at least a preoperative adjunct
Cavernoma	For pial-based lesions, a circumscribing pial incision allows detachment and delivery of the cavernoma from the superficial substance of the spinal cord. Deeper intramedullary lesions are exposed by a midline myelotomy. Although unencapsulated, these malformations are generally well circumscribed and present a clear dissection plane

Successful treatment of spinal vascular malformations requires the total obliteration or excision of the abnormal shunt. Procedures that only partially reduce the shunt or address only proximal feeders may provide temporary benefit but all too often lead to delayed recurrences and intervening neurological decline. Management options are outlined below, but surgery and/or endovascular approaches will be dictated by clinical, MRI and spinal angiography findings. Intraoperative angiography (or other vessel imaging) may be used to confirm shunt elimination, and electrophysiological monitoring may be useful in either setting. Whether endovascular techniques occupy a primary or adjunctive role depends not only on the type of vascular lesions but also on institutional experience.

EMI ANSWERS

13. 1 = L, 2 = E, 3 = F, 4 = M, 5 = A

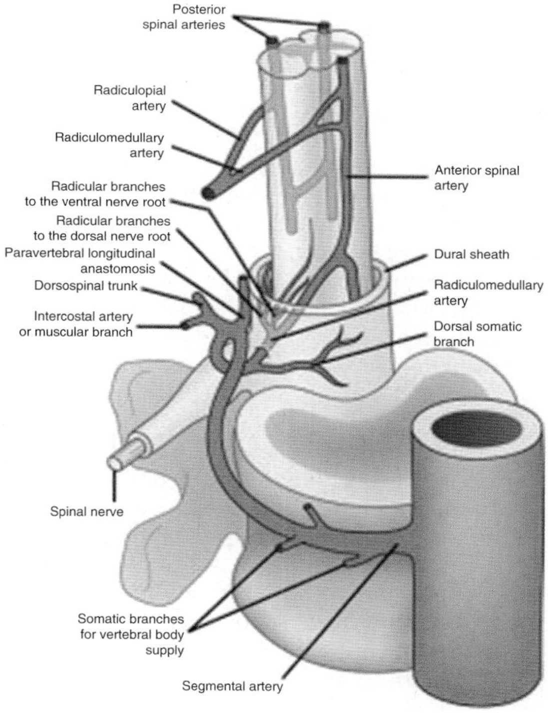

Image adapted with permission from Mathis JM, Shaibani A, Wakhloo AK. Spine anatomy. In Mathis JM (Ed.), Image-Guided Spine Interventions. New York, Springer-Verlag, 2004.

14. 1 = D, 2 = C or J, 3 = G, 4 = F, 5 = H

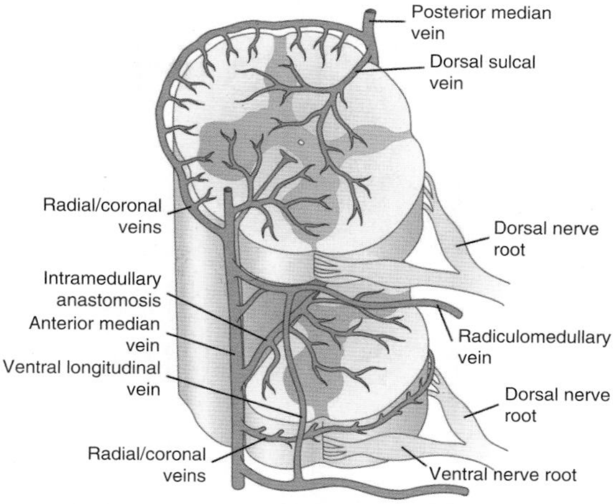

Image adapted with permission from Mathis JM, Shaibani A, Wakhloo AK. Spine anatomy. In: Mathis JM (Ed.), Image-Guided Spine Interventions. New York, Springer-Verlag, 2004.

15. 1 = h, Perimedullary AVF, 2 = d, Extradural-intradural (juvenile) AVF

Osler-Weber-Rendu syndrome (Hereditary Hemorrhagic Telangiectasia) is an autosomal dominant syndrome and consists of two genotypes (Types I and II). Type I is associated with mucocutaneous telangiectasia, pulmonary AVF, and arteriovenous shunts of the central nervous system. The associated spinal arteriovenous shunts are most often seen in the pediatric population and are always pial AVF (subtype C, ventral intradural AVF, or Type IV). The endothelial cells in this syndrome lack the molecule endoglin and form abnormal vessels, especially after injury.

Cobb syndrome is a synonym for the complete manifestation of the juvenile/metameric type of spinal vascular malformation where skin, muscle, bone, dura, and spinal cord are involved. Klippel-Trenaunay and Parkes-Weber syndromes consist of vascular malformations involving primarily the lower limbs, with the following dominant features: cutaneous capillary malformation, varicose veins, and limb hypertrophy. Klippel-Trenaunay syndrome is composed mainly of venous anomalies; Parkes-Weber syndrome has more arteriovenous shunts.

PART V
FUNCTIONAL NEUROSURGERY

CHAPTER 33

PAIN SURGERY

SINGLE BEST ANSWER (SBA) QUESTIONS

1. A 55-year-old male with known ischemic heart disease develops a crushing chest pain which radiates into his neck and left arm. The phenomenon of referred pain is best explained by which one of the following mechanisms?
   a. Pain transmission along a given afferent nerve is transferred to another afferent pathway due to ephaptic transmission
   b. Lateral inhibition of secondary afferent fibers by a single primary afferent
   c. Convergence of primary afferent fibers from a specific part of the body onto second-order neurons that normally receive primary afferents from a different body part
   d. Disruption of dorsal root ganglia
   e. The blockade of substance P and glutamate in the dorsal horn

2. The descending pathway for central control of nociception is best described as involving which one of the following structures?
   a. Anterior cingulate cortex fibers that synapse directly on dorsal horn neurons
   b. Periaqueductal gray fibers that synapse nucleus raphe magnus neurons, which in turn synapse on dorsal horn neurons
   c. Thalamic neurons that synapse upon red nucleus neurons, which in turn synapse upon dorsal horn cells
   d. Hypothalamic fibers that synapse upon neurons of the nucleus solitarius that then synapse upon neurons of the dorsal horn
   e. Thalamic fibers that synapse upon inhibitory interneurons in the dorsal horn

3. Which one of the following is not a potential site for ulnar nerve entrapment?
   a. Arcade of Struthers
   b. Heads of the flexor carpi ulnaris
   c. Intermuscular septum
   d. Osbourne's fascia
   e. Sublimis arch

4. A 43-year-old woman is referred with a 2-year history of sharp, shooting pains radiating into the right side of her jaw. Each attack lasts for a few seconds but they seem to merge together so it can seem like several minutes of pain. After this she may be pain free for several hours. It is often triggered by eating/drinking, brushing her teeth, touching her face, and talking. She denies any tearing, eye/eyelid changes or nasal congestion/rhinorrhea. There is no other past medical or family history. Neurological examination is normal and MRI head was unremarkable. Which one of the following is most appropriate first line therapy?
   a. Baclofen
   b. Carbamazepine
   c. Gabapentin
   d. Lamotrigine
   e. Pimozide

5. A 22-year-old female presents to her GP with a 3-month history of sharp, stabbing jaw pain and blurred vision on the right side. She is about to sit her examinations and is finding it difficult to study because of her symptoms. Which one of the following would you wish to exclude as a priority?

a. Tolosa-Hunt syndrome
b. Multiple sclerosis
c. Intracranial tumor
d. Classical trigeminal neuralgia
e. Psychogenic pain syndrome

6. Which one of the following statements regarding surgical treatments for trigeminal neuralgia is LEAST accurate?
  a. Microvascular decompression is a favored option for trigeminal neuralgia in MS
  b. Radiofrequency thermocoagulation of gasserian ganglion is most likely to cause anesthesia dolorosa
  c. Percutaneous destructive techniques directed at the gasserian ganglion may cause a trigemino-cardiac reflex
  d. Balloon compression is usually performed under general anesthetic
  e. Stereotactic radiosurgery of the trigeminal root only produces pain relief in a delayed fashion

7. Gate control theory of pain is best described by which one of the following statements?
  a. The thalamus gates pain perception in the cortex
  b. The substantia gelatinosa gates nociceptive signals before they reach the thalamus
  c. The dorsal root ganglion gates nociceptive signals before they reach the substantia gelatinosa
  d. The nociceptive nerve endings gate pain signals by altering the ratio of C and A-delta fibers activated
  e. The dorsal columns gate nociceptive signals by ephaptic transmission

8. Which one of the following is the commonest vessel thought to cause compression of the trigeminal root in cases of trigeminal neuralgia?
  a. Anterior inferior cerebellar artery
  b. Basilar artery
  c. Dandy's vein
  d. Posterior inferior cerebellar artery
  e. Superior cerebellar artery
  f. Vertebral artery

9. Which one of the following statements regarding intrathecal drug delivery systems is LEAST accurate?
  a. The intrathecal route results in higher subarachnoid drug concentrations, lower absolute drug doses, and avoidance of side effects associated with systemic dosing
  b. Ziconotide is exclusively intrathecal analgesic which blocks a N-type calcium channel
  c. Development of an catheter tip granuloma is particularly associated with morphine
  d. Intrathecal baclofen has a potent analgesic effect
  e. Indications for intrathecal drug delivery do not include patient preference.

10. Which one of the following statements regarding motor cortex stimulation for pain is LEAST accurate?
  a. Electrodes may be placed in the subdural or extradural space
  b. Subdural placement of electrodes may be required to achieve lower limb pain coverage
  c. Risk of seizures is highest intraoperatively and during programming
  d. Is appropriate for deafferentation pain syndromes
  e. Is not indicated in patients with multiple sclerosis related chronic pain syndromes due to high seizure risk

QUESTIONS 11–15

Additional questions 11–15 available on ExpertConsult.com

EXTENDED MATCHING ITEM (EMI) QUESTIONS

16. **Sensory disturbances:**
  a. Allodynia
  b. Analgesia
  c. Anesthesia dolorosa
  d. Causalgia
  e. Dysesthesia
  f. Hyperesthesia
  g. Hyperalgesia
  h. Hyperpathia
  i. Hypoesthesia
  j. Hypoalgesia
  k. Neuropathic pain
  l. Nociceptive pain
  m. Paresthesiae

For each of the following descriptions, select the most appropriate answers from the list above. Each answer may be used once, more than once or not at all.

1. An unpleasant abnormal sensation, whether spontaneous or evoked.
2. A painful syndrome characterized by an abnormally painful reaction to a stimulus, especially a repetitive stimulus, as well as an increased threshold.

3. A syndrome of sustained burning pain, allodynia, and hyperpathia after a traumatic nerve lesion, often combined with vasomotor and sudomotor dysfunction and later trophic changes.
4. Pain in an area or region which is anesthetic.
5. Pain due to a stimulus that does not normally provoke pain.

17. **Craniofacial pain syndromes:**
    a. Anesthesia dolorosa
    b. Cluster headache
    c. Geniculate neuralgia
    d. Glossopharyngeal neuralgia
    e. Migraine
    f. Occipital neuralgia
    g. Persistent idiopathic facial pain
    h. Temporomandibular joint disorder
    i. Tension-type headache
    j. Trigeminal neuralgia

For each of the following descriptions, select the most appropriate answers from the list above. Each answer may be used once, more than once or not at all.

1. A 58-year-old presents with paroxysmal attacks of stabbing pain in the throat which occasionally shoots to her right ear, usually lasting less than 1 min. She experiences some relief with cocainization of the right tonsil.
2. Brief paroxysms of pain felt deep in the auditory canal. A trigger area is present in the posterior wall of the auditory canal. May benefit from transection of nervus intermedius.
3. Pain attacks of severe or very severe unilateral orbital, supraorbital, and/or temporal pain lasting 15-180 min if untreated. May be accompanied by ipsilateral conjunctival injection and/or lacrimation, nasal congestion, and/or rhinorrhea, eyelid edema, forehead and facial sweating, miosis and/or ptosis and a sense of restlessness or agitation. Attacks have a frequency from 1 every other day to 8 per day.

18. **Spine and peripheral pain syndromes:**
    a. Brachial plexus avulsion
    b. Chronic low back pain
    c. CRPS
    d. Diabetic peripheral neuropathic pain
    e. Failed back surgery syndrome
    f. Phantom limb pain
    g. Post-herpetic neuralgia
    h. Post-spinal cord injury
    i. Post-thoracotomy pain syndrome
    j. Post-traumatic pain

For each of the following descriptions, select the most appropriate answers from the list above. Each answer may be used once, more than once or not at all.

1. Persistent or recurring low back pain, with or without sciatica, after one or more spine surgeries.
2. Pain after acute rash has healed accompanied by pain, allodynia, paresthesia, or dysesthesia. The pain usually affects a single dermatome.
3. Present with severe pain that is disproportionate to the inciting event, most commonly affecting the hand or foot but that can spread to other body regions. The affected body parts may display sensory disturbances, temperature changes, abnormal patterns of sweating, edema, reduced joint range of motion, movement abnormalities such as weakness, tremor, or dystonia, trophic changes such as skin atrophy or altered hair and nail growth, and localized osteoporotic changes.

19. **Surgical procedures for pain:**
    a. Anterolateral cordotomy
    b. Cingulotomy
    c. Deep brain stimulation
    d. DREZ lesions
    e. Intrathecal morphine
    f. Midline myelotomy
    g. Mesencephalic tractotomy
    h. Motor cortex stimulator
    i. Spinal cord stimulation
    j. Sympathectomy
    k. Thalamotomy

For each of the following descriptions, select the most appropriate answers from the list above. Each answer may be used once, more than once or not at all.

1. Involves disconnection of the anterior commissure
2. Involves lesioning Lissauer's tract
3. Involves a cord lesion just anterior to the dentate ligament
4. Involves a lesion of extralemniscal pathways lateral to the spinothalamic tract
5. Aims to treat the motivational-affective component of pain that contributes to fear, suffering, and anxiety.

SBA ANSWER

1. **c**—A convergence of primary afferent fibers from a given region onto second-order neurons that also normally receive primary afferents from a different body part

Referred pain is a phenomenon in which pain impulses, usually arising from primary visceral afferent fibers from one part of the body, terminate on dorsal horn projection neurons that normally receive cutaneous afferents from a different part of the body (such as the arm). It is the convergence of these distinctly different inputs onto the same projection neurons that provides the basis for this phenomenon. However, other theories including central sensitization, thalamic convergence, and hyperexcitability have also been proposed. Pain signaling in the spinal cord dorsal horn is via glutamate (C fibers and A-delta fibers) and substance P (C fibers). The opioid peptides (enkephalin and dynorphin) are released by inhibitory interneurons in the dorsal horns, medulla, and PAG and inhibit transmission of pain impulses.

2. **b**—Periaqueductal gray that synapse on neurons of the nucleus raphe magnus that then synapse on dorsal horn cells

Periaqueductal gray stimulation activates enkephalin-releasing neurons that project to the nucleus raphe magnus, 5-HT release activates projections to inhibitory interneurons in Laminae II (substantia gelatinosa). This results in release of either enkephalin or dynorphin (endogenous opioid neurotransmitters), which bind to mu opioid receptors on the axons of incoming nociceptive C and A-delta fibers, inhibiting the release of substance P/glutamate from then and activation of ascending pain pathways.

3. **e**—Sublimis arch (fibrous arch between flexor digitorum superficialis)

Ulnar nerve at the elbow lies in the postcondylar groove, then under the aponeurosis (Osbourne's fascia) then under the FCU itself. Initial benefit following ulnar nerve transposition at the cubital tunnel may be complicated by kinking at the arcade of Struthers more proximally, which may necessitate release at this level. Technique for ulnar nerve decompression ± transposition is: incision, identify, and protect/mobilize medial antebrachial cutaneous nerve, identify ulnar nerve proximal to Osbourne's fascia, decompress distally through leading edge of FCU (simple decompression); for transposition, extend decompression proximally by cutting intermuscular septum and arcade of Struthers if present; assess position in full range of motion to ensure no subluxation. Recurrence of symptoms after decompression alone may suggest kinking/tethering at the intermuscular septum (or arcade of Struthers if not divided initially) requiring release.

4. **b**—Carbamazepine

The history is suggestive of trigeminal neuralgia (tic douloureux). First line treatment is carbamazepine. Common side effects of CBZ: dizziness, vertigo, ataxia, diplopia, blood disorders, drowsiness, skin reactions. If CBZ not tolerated due to side effects could try oxcarbazepine (higher risk of hyponatremia), or if allergic start gabapentin. Other useful drugs include baclofen, phenytoin, and lamotrigine.

5. **b**—Multiple sclerosis

While the majority of cases of trigeminal neuralgia are due to vascular compression or idiopathic (Classical), in a small proportion of cases it may be the presenting feature of significant underlying condition such as multiple sclerosis (brainstem plaque causing ephaptic transmission), basilar artery aneurysms, acoustic schwannomas, and posterior fossa meningiomas, all of which may cause injury to the fifth cranial nerve by compression. Red flag symptoms which should be excluded include: sensory changes, deafness, difficulty achieving pain control, poor response to carbamazepine, history of skin or oral malignancy that could lead to perineural spread, symptoms in ophthalmic distribution (more likely herpes zoster), under age of 40, symptoms suggestive of optic neuritis, family history of MS. The Tolosa-Hunt syndrome is a presumably inflammatory disorder that produces ophthalmoplegia associated with headache and loss of sensation over the forehead. Pupillary function is usually spared, and the site of pathology is believed to be in the superior orbital fissure or the cavernous sinus. It is usually not associated with trigeminal neuralgia.

6. **a**—Microvascular decompression is a favored option for trigeminal neuralgia in MS

Microvascular decompression is the gold standard in good surgical candidates (i.e. classical trigeminal neuralgia, evidence of vascular compression on MRI, short duration of disease, no previous surgery); pain relief is usually immediate and 60-70% remaining pain free at 10-20 years. Indications include patients whose pain is no longer controlled by drugs and whose quality of life has markedly deteriorated, young patients, side effects from antiepileptic drugs. The procedure requires general anesthesia, and its adverse effects include aseptic meningitis, ipsilateral hearing loss (in less than 5%), CSF leak, low risk of sensory loss, and death (0.4%). Stereotactic radiosurgery targeting the trigeminal root does not require general anesthesia, but its pain-relieving effects are not immediate. Adverse effects include facial numbness, paresthesias, and sensory complications. Percutaneous destructive neurosurgical techniques (radiofrequency thermocoagulation, glycerol rhizolysis, or balloon compression) can achieve immediate pain relief and can therefore be considered for emergency management, but 50% of patients have recurrence at 5 years. Sedation or even GA is required, and it carries a risk of trigeminal-vagal reflex effects on the heart during lesioning and a very small risk of carotid injury or intracranial infection. Balloon compression carries a risk of temporary trigeminal motor dysfunction. Adverse effects include a facial numbness, corneal numbness (risk of keratitis), dysesthesias, and anesthesia dolorosa.

FURTHER READING

Zakrzewska Joanna M, Linskey Mark E. Trigeminal neuralgia. BMJ 2015;350:h1238.

7. **b**—The substantia gelatinosa gates nociceptive signals before they reach the thalamus

The 1965 gate control theory of pain by Melzack and Wall proposed that there were three spinal cord systems involved in pain transmission: the substantia gelatinosa, dorsal column fibers, and central transmission cells in the DH. The substantia gelatinosa functions as a gate that modulates signals before they reach the brain. Large diameter fibers have inhibitory effects to "shut the gate" whereas small diameter fibers carrying noxious stimuli open the gate to pain transmission. In a simplistic view of this model, rubbing of the injured area promotes proprioceptive (i.e. large diameter) fiber input and reduces pain perception. In the late 1990s, Melzack proposed the neuromatrix theory, adding higher cortical functions as key elements of pain transmission and interpretation. Today, the experience of pain is described as distributed in three dimensions: cognitive, affective, and sensory. Frontal and limbic areas are believed to subserve the cognitive-evaluative component of pain. Limbic cortex, cingulum, hypothalamus, thalamus, and various midbrain regions are thought to contribute to the motivational-affective component of pain. Primary somatosensory cortex, thalamus, spinothalamic tract, and local nerve endings are involved in the sensory component of pain.

FURTHER READING

Bourne S, et al. Basic anatomy and physiology of pain pathways. Neurosurg Clin N Am 2014;25:629-638.

8. **e**—Superior cerebellar artery

Neurovascular compression is found in ~88% of cases on imaging, but an average of 7% of explorations reveal no pathology intraoperatively. The superior cerebellar artery is the most common (70-80%), and is usually compressing the rostral and anterior portion of the nerve in patients with V2 or V3 symptoms. The anterior inferior cerebellar artery is the compressive vessel in 10% of cases and occurs in the caudal and posterior portion of the nerve closest to nerve VI, while veins impact the nerve in 5-13% of cases. Microvascular decompression involves separating offending vessels from the nerve and inserting a synthetic sponge or Teflon felt between them to maintain the separation. The trigeminal nerve must be carefully and circumferentially inspected along its entire intracranial course from the root entry zone to its entrance laterally into Meckel's cave. This procedure ordinarily provides pain relief without any facial sensory loss and has a greater potential for producing long-lasting pain relief. Interestingly, tic pain does not always stop immediately following a microvascular decompression, and nerve manipulation by itself (e.g. where no offending vessel found, or without moving the artery) transiently stops the tic pain although it will soon recur thereafter.

FURTHER READING

Grant GA, Loeser JD. Trigeminal neuralgia. In: Ellenbogen RG et al., editors. Principles of Neurological Surgery. 3rd ed. p. 729-736 (Chapter 48).

9. **a**—Intrathecal baclofen has a potent analgesic effect

The continuous administration of analgesics via the intrathecal route results in higher subarachnoid drug concentrations, lower absolute drug doses, and avoidance of side effects associated with systemic dosing (especially at high doses). Additionally, concerns about opiate diversion and analgesic compliance are reduced. Indications for intrathecal drug delivery for pain control:

1. An established pain diagnosis has been made classifying the symptoms as neuropathic, nociceptive, or mixed.
2. Pain is chronic or both chronic and progressive in nature owing to either a malignant or nonmalignant cause.
3. Pain should be present throughout nearly the entire day.
4. Patients have failed to achieve analgesia with conservative nonpharmacologic modalities.
5. Patient is refractory or intolerant to orally administered analgesics.
6. Corrective treatment addressing the pain generator is not warranted.
7. Surgical contraindications to implanting prosthetic hardware and accessing the intrathecal space are absent (e.g. bacteremia, anticoagulation).

Although several agents are commonly used for chronic intrathecal delivery, only three medications currently have FDA approval for long-term intrathecal use: baclofen, morphine, and ziconotide. Ziconotide is exclusively intrathecal form of ω-conotoxin MVIIa that blocks a N-type calcium channel on small myelinated and unmyelinated nociceptive afferents that are primarily localized in the superficial Rexed laminae (I and II). Intrathecal baclofen, a GABA-B agonist, is primarily used to treat spasticity but may help with pain associated with spasticity and dystonias. Intrathecal delivery of medications can result in several potential adverse events including sedation, cognitive impairment, nausea, vomiting, pruritus, urinary retention, constipation, hormonal dysfunction, and edema. The development of an inflammatory mass (granuloma) is particularly associated with morphine and increasingly hydromorphone, with high drug concentrations combined with low flow rate increase the risk of granuloma development. Presentation is with loss on pain control or new-onset pain complaints or progressive myelopathy. CT myelography or MRI with gadolinium contrast of the catheter tip region is necessary to confirm the diagnosis. In asymptomatic and nonprogressive patients, weaning of intrathecal medications and initiation of saline infusion can produce spontaneous disintegration of the mass. In patients with progressive or severe neurologic compromise, urgent surgical decompression and excision are recommended.

FURTHER READING

Bolash R, et al. Intrathecal pain pumps: indications, patient selection, techniques, and outcomes. Neurosurg Clin N Am 2014;25:735-742.

10. **e**—Is not indicated in patients with multiple sclerosis related chronic pain syndromes due to high seizure risk

Chronic stimulation of the precentral gyrus below the threshold to produce a motor response is able to alleviate certain types of deafferentation pain and MCS has shown efficacy for a number of deafferentation pain syndromes (e.g. trigeminal, central post-stroke pain, anesthesia dolorosa, post-herpetic neuralgia, multiple sclerosis, phantom limb pain, and spinal cord injury). The mechanism of action has been attributed to modulation of deafferentation-induced pathologic hyperactivity in thalamic relay nuclei and/or increased sensitivity of higher order pain pathway neurons. Intraoperatively, the central sulcus is localized using SSEPs and a contact paddle electrode is placed in the epidural space overlying the facial or upper extremity region of the motor cortex. The electrode is then used for motor evoked potentials with electromyography to confirm motor activity. Iced saline is prepared for irrigation if a seizure is induced. The minimum thresholds for motor activity and any seizure activity are noted. After confirmation, a paddle electrode is sutured to the dura over the precentral gyrus over the motor area that corresponds to the patient's pain distribution. Subdural placement is associated with greater energy efficiency, but also an increased rate of complications, including subdural hematomas and a higher reported rate of seizures. However, opening of the dura may be necessary anyway for coverage of lower extremity pain, which requires placement of an electrode along the medial part of the hemisphere. MCS has an overall complication rate of about 5%: wound breakdown or infection (5.1%), hardware breakage from trauma, and seizures (12%). Stimulation of the motor cortex is known to be associated with the potential to induce seizures, and most seizures observed during MCS occur during programming sessions.

FURTHER READING

Ostergard T, et al. Motor cortex stimulation for chronic pain. Neurosurg Clin N Am 2014;25:693-698.

ANSWERS 11–15

Additional answers 11–15 available on ExpertConsult.com

EMI ANSWER

16. 1—e, Dysesthesia; 2—h, Hyperpathia; 3—d, Causalgia; 4—c, Anesthesia dolorosa; 5—a, Allodynia

International Association for the Study of Pain Taxonomy:

Pain is an unpleasant sensory and emotional experience associated with actual or potential tissue damage, or described in terms of such damage.

Pain: Definitions

Term	Definition
Hypoesthesia	Decreased sensitivity to stimulation, excluding the special senses
Paresthesiae	An abnormal sensation, whether spontaneous or evoked (not unpleasant)
Dysesthesia	An unpleasant abnormal sensation, whether spontaneous or evoked
Hyperesthesia	Increased sensitivity to stimulation, excluding the special senses, includes both allodynia and hyperalgesia, but the more specific terms should be used wherever they are applicable
Allodynia	Pain due to a stimulus that does not normally provoke pain
Hyperalgesia	Increased pain from a stimulus that normally provokes pain
Hypoalgesia	Diminished pain in response to a normally painful stimulus
Hyperpathia	A painful syndrome characterized by an abnormally painful reaction to a stimulus, especially a repetitive stimulus, as well as an increased threshold
Neuropathic pain	Pain caused by a lesion or disease of the somatosensory nervous system. May be central or peripheral
Nociceptive pain	Pain that arises from actual or threatened damage to non-neural tissue and is due to the activation of nociceptors. Describes pain occurring with a normally functioning somatosensory nervous system to contrast with the abnormal function seen in neuropathic pain
Analgesia	Absence of pain in response to stimulation which would normally be painful
Anesthesia dolorosa	Pain in an area or region which is anesthetic
Causalgia	A syndrome of sustained burning pain, allodynia, and hyperpathia after a traumatic nerve lesion, often combined with vasomotor and sudomotor dysfunction and later trophic changes

FURTHER READING

http://www.iasp-pain.org/Education/

17. 1—d, Glossopharyngeal neuralgia; 2—c, Geniculate neuralgia; 3—b, Cluster headache

Craniofacial Pain Syndromes: Clinical Features and Management

Syndrome	Comments	Surgical Options
Cluster headache	Pain attacks of severe or very severe unilateral orbital, supraorbital, and/or temporal pain lasting 15-180 min if untreated. May be accompanied by ipsilateral conjunctival injection and/or lacrimation, nasal congestion, and/or rhinorrhea, eyelid edema, forehead and facial sweating, miosis and/or ptosis and a sense of restlessness or agitation. Attacks have a frequency from 1 every other day to 8 per day. Episodic form is six times more common than the chronic form (attacks occurring for >1 year without remission or with remissions lasting <1 month)	Occipital nerve stimulation Sphenopalatine ganglion stimulation Radiofrequency ablation of sphenopalatine ganglion Gamma knife SRS to trigeminal root Hypothalamic DBS Transection of nervus intermedius

Continued

Syndrome	Comments	Surgical Options
Migraine	Usually a throbbing headache with or without sensory aura	Botulinum toxin A prophylactic injections Trigger site deactivation surgery Occipital nerve stimulation
Occipital neuralgia	Paroxysmal stabbing pain, with or without persistent aching between paroxysms, in the distribution of the greater, lesser, and/or third occipital nerves	Peripheral neurectomy C2 dorsal root ganglionectomy Microvascular decompression (C2 root) Percutaneous neurolysis C2 root Occipital nerve stimulation RF lesioning of greater/lesser occipital nerves Pulsed RF treatment C2 dorsal root ganglion
Trigeminal neuralgia	Brief strong, sharp, unilateral shooting pain in one or more branches of trigeminal nerve. Combined V2 and V3 symptoms commonest, V1 symptoms alone rarest presentation	Microvascular decompression Gamma knife surgery to trigeminal DREZ Peripheral ablation of gasserian ganglion
Glossopharyngeal neuralgia	Paroxysmal attacks of facial pain lasting from a fraction of a second to 2 min. Characterized by unilateral, sharp, stabbing, and severe pain in the distribution within the posterior part of the tongue, tonsillar fossa, pharynx, or beneath the angle of the lower jaw and/or in the ear. Triggers include swallowing, chewing, talking, coughing, and yawning	MVD Rhizotomy of IX ($\pm$ upper rootlets of X) Gamma knife surgery Motor cortex stimulation Trigeminal tractotomy $\pm$ nucleotomy
Geniculate neuralgia	Brief paroxysms of pain felt deep in the auditory canal. A trigger area is present in the posterior wall of the auditory canal	Transection of nervus intermedius (with or without geniculate ganglion removal) Microvascular decompression
Persistent idiopathic facial pain	Persistent facial pain that does not have the characteristics of cranial neuralgias or cannot be attributed to another disorder. Usually a throbbing pain situated deep in the eye and malar region, often radiating to the ear, neck, and shoulders	CT-guided percutaneous trigeminal tractotomy-nucleotomy Nucleus caudalis DREZ lesioning pulsed radiofrequency to the sphenopalatine ganglion
Anesthesia dolorosa	Uncommon complication of surgical treatments for neuralgias: excruciating pain perceived in an insensate region of the face	Motor cortex stimulation Deep brain stimulation Nucleus caudalis DREZ lesioning
Temporomandibular joint disorder	Recurrent pain in one or more regions of the head and/or face precipitated by jaw movements and/or chewing of hard or tough food. Other findings are a reduced range of or irregular jaw opening, noise from one or both TMJs during jaw movements, tenderness of the joint capsule	Botulinum toxin Arthrocentesis/arthroscopy TMJ disc surgery or joint replacement Denervation of TMJ

FURTHER READING

Gutierrez, et al. Introduction to neuropathic pain syndromes. Neurosurg Clin N Am 2014;2:639-662.

18. 1—e, Failed back surgery syndrome; 2—g, Post-herpetic neuralgia; 3—c, Complex regional pain syndrome

Neuropathic Pain Syndromes: Features and Surgical Management

Syndrome	Comments	Surgical Options
Failed back surgery syndrome	Persistent or recurring low back pain, with or without sciatica, after one or more spine surgeries. Incidence of FBSS has increased with increasing rates of spine surgery: 10-40% patients may develop FBSS after lumbar spinal surgery. Success rate of lumbar spinal surgery falls with each successive surgery on the same patient	Lumbar epidural steroid injection Percutaneous epidural adhesiolysis Percutaneous ozone injection (intradiscal/paravertebral/intraforaminal) Facet joint rhizotomy Intrathecal drug delivery Peripheral nerve field stimulation Spinal cord stimulation Deep brain stimulation Revision surgery
Chronic low back pain	Chronic, recurrent, or long-lasting pain localized below the costal margin and above the inferior gluteal folds lasting for at least 6 months. Prevalence: 8.1-10.2% of the US population	Lumbar fusion Total disc replacement Spinal endoscopic adhesiolysis Caudal epidural steroid injection Spinal cord stimulation
Post-spinal cord injury	Neuropathic pain and dysesthesia in areas with sensory deficit and can be spontaneous or stimulus evoked. Quality can be burning, smarting, shooting, aching, pricking, and tingling ± paresthesia. Approximately 65-85% of people have pain (nociceptive and neuropathic) after spinal cord injury and it is severe in one third	DREZ lesion Spinal cord stimulation Cordotomy Intrathecal drug delivery Motor cortex stimulation
Post-herpetic neuralgia	Pain after acute rash has healed accompanied by pain, allodynia, paresthesia, or dysesthesia. The pain usually affects a single dermatome	Botulinum toxin A Sympathetic nerve block Spinal cord stimulation Gamma knife SRS (trigeminal/thalamic) Peripheral nerve stimulation DREZ lesioning
Post-thoracotomy pain syndrome	Pain that recurs or persists along a thoracotomy incision at least 2 months after the surgical procedure. The gentlest of stimulation can trigger intense burning and stabbing pain, with dysesthesia 5% of patients experience severe and disabling pain	Peripheral nerve field stimulation Peripheral nerve stimulation Intercostal nerve block Intercostal nerve cryoablation DREZ lesion Spinal cord stimulation Pulsed RF intercostal nerve or DRG
Brachial plexus avulsion	The typical root avulsion pain is a constant dull, crushing, or burning pain with superimposed lightening jolts of severe sharp pain shooting down the arm. Most occur as a consequence of motorcycle accidents. Prevalence of neuropathic pain ranges from 34% to 95% of cases, with a quarter of patients experience intractable long-term pain of the upper limb	DREZ lesion
Phantom limb pain	The pain presents as short-lasting and rarely occurring painful shocks or as constant, excruciatingly painful experience in the missing body part. Prevalence of phantom pain among amputated patients: 50-90%	Neurostimulation (e.g. dorsal root ganglion) Sympathectomy DREZ lesion Cordotomy Rhizotomy
Complex regional pain syndrome	CRPS type I (Reflex Sympathetic Dystrophy) has no definable nerve lesion, while a peripheral nerve lesion can be demonstrated in CRPS type II (causalgia). Present with severe pain that is disproportionate to the inciting event, most commonly affecting the hand or foot but that can	Epidural clonidine Regional anesthetic block Local anesthetic block ± Botox Intrathecal baclofen Sympathectomy Repair of injured nerve (CRPS II)

Continued

Syndrome	Comments	Surgical Options
	spread to other body regions. The affected body parts may display sensory disturbances, temperature changes, abnormal patterns of sweating, edema, reduced joint range of motion, movement abnormalities such as weakness, tremor, or dystonia, trophic changes such as skin atrophy or altered hair and nail growth, and localized osteoporotic changes. Alterations in body perception or schema may be present	Amputation Spinal cord stimulation TENS Repetitive TMS PNS Dorsal root ganglion stimulation DBS (for pain and dystonia) Motor cortex stimulation
Post-traumatic pain	Symptoms such as hypesthesia, paresthesia, allodynia, hyperpathia, and hyperalgesia may be seen within days of nerve damage or months later Post-traumatic neuropathic pain (from accidental or surgical injury) is one of the most common causes of chronic pain	Brachial plexus grafting Epidural steroid injection Nerve resection/end neuroma relocation/ neurolysis Spinal cord stimulation Motor cortex stimulation Deep brain stimulation Peripheral nerve stimulation DREZ lesion ± selective rhizotomy
Diabetic peripheral neuropathic pain	Presents with burning-type pain, paresthesia, and numbness of mild to moderate severity. These symptoms may be accompanied by loss of proprioception, temperature sensitivity, and eventually pain sensation. Prevalence among adults with diabetes in the US population: 27-50%. Of these, 11% have neuropathic pain	Surgical decompression Spinal cord stimulation

FURTHER READING

Gutierrez, et al. Introduction to neuropathic pain syndromes. Neurosurg Clin N Am 2014;25:639-662.

19. 1—f, Midline myelotomy; 2—d, DREZ lesion; 3—a, Anterolateral cordotomy; 4—g, Mesencephalic tractotomy; 5—b, Cingulotomy

Surgical Approaches for the Management of Neuropathic Pain	
DREZ lesions	DREZ lesioning can be thought of as a treatment for pain that is believed to be confined to a unilateral limb. The Lissauer tract is a key pathway that conducts nociceptive information at least two segments above and below the DREZ (hence pain could be arising up to two segments above or below an involved dermatomal segment). If dorsal root fibers are avulsed, as commonly seen in pain associated with brachial or lumbar-sacral plexus trauma anatomy is more difficult and complications more likely. Lesions that inadvertently are placed too far laterally and injure the corticospinal tract, resulting in permanent ipsilateral weakness below the lesion. Alternatively, if lesions deviate too medially from the DREZ, ipsilateral loss of proprioception and light touch may occur due to dorsal column injury
Anterolateral cordotomy	The spinothalamic tract lies just anterior to the dentate ligament and near the anterolateral surface of the cord, while the corticospinal tract is just posterior. The anterior spinal artery is a significant vascular structure whose midline position must be appreciated and avoided during open transection of the spinothalamic tract. Lesioning the spinothalamic tract removes pain below the level of the lesion, but levels of adequate pain control are several levels below the lesion. Good candidates are patients who experience severe pain that originates from cancer involving the pelvis, leg, hip, and lower trunk. Those with nonmalignant pain syndromes are not ideal due to recurrence rate of pain within a few years or the emergence of new central neuropathic pain (burning dysesthesias below the level of the lesion). Complications are urinary retention or incontinence, permanent dysesthesias, transient hemiparesis, and respiratory complications (cervical cordotomies). Mirror pain is a unique complication of open thoracic cordotomies in patients with cancer in which a similar pain develops contralaterally within weeks to months after the cordotomy. Other complications that are shared with open dural procedures and laminectomies include possible mechanical spinal instability, CSF leak, and meningitis

Continued on following page

Surgical Approaches for the Management of Neuropathic Pain (Continued)

Midline myelotomy (commissurotomy)	In patients with bilateral lower extremity pain and, in particular, with involvement of the pelvis and lower abdominal organs, a single lesion disconnecting the anterior commissure through a lower thoracic approach has been quite effective in relieving severe refractory pain. The typical patient is one with pelvic cancer or sarcoma that invades bilateral structures in the pelvis and lower extremities. Loss of bowel and bladder function, and proprioception with relative preservation of motor function (leg weakness in one third) may be acceptable in this group who may otherwise be bedridden with severe pain. The risks of respiratory and sympathetic damage (fibers located near the central gray matter) in creating a mid to upper cervical midline myelotomy are likely the reasons why this technique has not been used much for upper trunk and arm pain
Mesencephalic tractotomy	Mesencephalic tractotomy has been successfully used for the treatment of denervation pain, such as central dysesthesia, in the upper extremity, head, or neck. Potential candidates are those who fail medical management, neuromodulation, intrathecal infusions, and thoracic or cervical cordotomy, or those patients whose pain is from structures more superior than what cervical cordotomy can treat. In particular, neuropathic pain from head or neck malignancy could be a potential indication. Patients with chronic nonmalignant pain do not respond well to this technique. It involves a lesion of extralemniscal pathways lateral to the spinothalamic tract and medial lemniscus can result in relief of intractable pain without loss of sensation or dysesthesia
Cingulotomy	Because the motivational-affective component of pain contributes to the fear, suffering, and anxiety of pain, cingulectomy and cingulotomy were proposed to treat this component of chronic pain. The anterior midcingulate cortex is implicated as an area of overlap between negative affect, pain, and cognitive control based on functional MR imaging and DTI studies. The first open resection of 4 cm of the anterior cingulate gyrus for intractable pain, called cingulectomy. Unilateral and bilateral cingulotomies that affect a large volume of the cingulate fasciculus were subsequently developed, and more recently stereotactic cingulotomy. Its main success has been in malignant pain of the head and neck with associated sensations of respiratory distress, and for the discomfort of chronic dyspnea in a patient with malignant mesothelioma. Patients with significant preexisting brain disease, sociopathic personalities, or advanced age are generally not thought good candidates for cingulotomy

FURTHER READING

Konrad P. Dorsal root entry zone lesion, midline myelotomy and anterolateral cordotomy. Neurosurg Clin N Am 2014;25:699-722.

CHAPTER 34

ADULT AND PEDIATRIC EPILEPSY SURGERY

SINGLE BEST ANSWER (SBA) QUESTIONS

1. Which one of the following is the most epileptogenic primary brain tumor?
   a. DNET/ganglioglioma
   b. Glioblastoma
   c. Low grade glioma
   d. Meningioma
   e. Metastasis

2. Which one of the following types of epilepsy is LEAST likely to benefit from epilepsy surgery referral?
   a. Hemimegalencephaly
   b. Rasmussen's syndrome
   c. Rolandic epilepsy
   d. Sturge-Weber syndrome
   e. West syndrome with focal malformation of cortical development

3. A 37-year-old male with medically refractory epilepsy undergoes workup for surgery. MRI shows frontal cortical dysgenesis, and a concordant EEG shows that the seizure focus involves the posteriorly located motor cortex. Which one of the following operative approaches could you consider when seizure activity extends beyond the area of resection and into eloquent cortex?
   a. Corpus callosotomy
   b. Deep brain stimulation
   c. Hemispherectomy
   d. Multiple subpial transection
   e. Vagal nerve stimulation

4. Which one of the following is the best predictor for seizure-free outcome after epilepsy surgery (assuming total lesionectomy)?
   a. Preoperative EEG and MRI concordance
   b. Extratemporal seizure focus
   c. History of febrile seizures
   d. Mesial temporal sclerosis
   e. Low grade temporal glioma

5. The frequency of abnormal interictal EEG findings in the investigation of seizures is which one of the following?
   a. 10-20%
   b. 20-30%
   c. 30-40%
   d. 40-50%
   e. 50-60%

6. Which one of the following is most appropriate for predicting postoperative language and memory impairment in epilepsy surgery candidates?
   a. BOLD functional MRI
   b. EEG
   c. Hippocampal depth electrodes
   d. Ictal SPECT
   e. Video telemetry
   f. Wada test

7. Neuropsychological testing preoperatively is unable to:
   a. Aid lateralization of the epileptogenic zone
   b. Predict postoperative deficits
   c. Assess patients mental reserve capacity
   d. Define the epileptogenic zone preoperatively
   e. Assess for depression and anxiety

8. Prolonged delay between ictal behavior onset and first appearance of ictal EEG discharge during video telemetry (continuous video-EEG recording) is most likely due to:
   a. Malfunction of scalp electrodes
   b. Drowsy patient
   c. Remote/distant site of seizure onset
   d. Hyperventilation
   e. Withdrawal of antiepileptic medication

9. A 28-year-old male presents with intractable epilepsy. Sleep EEG is unable to localize the focus. Coregistered MRI and PET studies cannot identify an epileptic focus. Subtracted ictal and interictal SPECT was performed which showed a hypermetabolic focus in the left posterolateral temporal lobe. Which

one of the following statements are most appropriate in this patient?
a. The next appropriate step would be to place subdural grids/strips
b. The next appropriate step would be to perform a left insular corticectomy
c. The next appropriate step would be to perform multiple subpial resection
d. The next appropriate step would be to place depth electrodes (stereotactic EEG)
e. The next appropriate step would be to perform a left temporal lobectomy

10. Which one of the following is the commonest neurological complication after VNS?
a. Arrhythmia
b. Bradycardia
c. Dysphonia
d. Facial numbness
e. Hypotension

11. A 10-year-old child undergoes hemispherectomy. At 2 years post-op, he is only having nocturnal seizures now. Which one of the following Engel Epilepsy surgery outcome classes does he fall into?
a. I
b. II
c. III
d. IV
e. V

12. Which one of the following is an unlikely primary indication for using invasive EEG monitoring as part of evaluation for epilepsy surgery?
a. Seizure onsets are lateralized but not localized
b. Seizure onsets are localized but not clearly lateralized (i.e. bilateral)
c. Seizure onset near eloquent cortex however unknown focus
d. Dual pathology in opposite hemispheres
e. Multiple cortical lesions (e.g. tuberous sclerosis)
f. Predicting postoperative memory deficit

13. A 29-year-old man with a history of febrile seizures as a child has developed medication-refractory complex partial seizures within the past 2 years. EEG suggests a left temporal focus, with evidence of concordant PET imaging. An MRI as shown below, reveals the abnormality. Which one of the following is the next appropriate step in management?

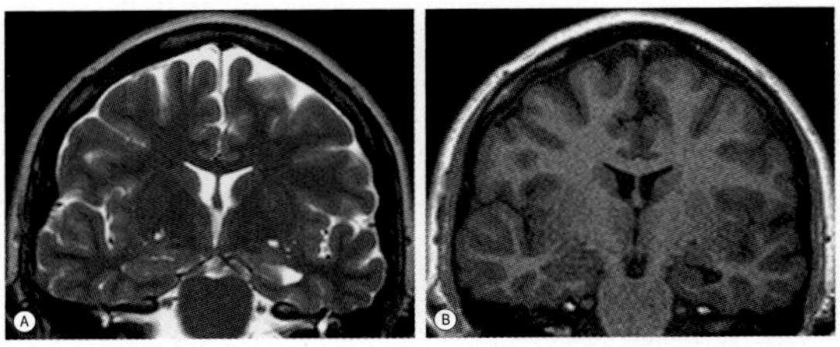

a. Depth electrodes
b. Subdural grid
c. Subdural strip
d. AVM resection
e. Temporal lobectomy

14. A 49-year-old woman is referred with a 1-year history of medically refractory epilepsy. Electrographically, both interictally and ictally, this patient's seizures were consistent with left mesial temporal onset. However, no definite abnormalities were observed on MRI. Assuming left hemisphere dominance for language, neuropsychological data were suggestive of left temporal lobe dysfunction. Some intact verbal memory scores raised a question that the left mesial temporal lobe structures were intact. Wada test: Language lateralized to the left hemisphere. She underwent invasive electrocorticographic (ECoG) monitoring with a left mesial temporal (LMT) strip, basal temporal strips (anterior, LAT and posterior, LPT), and an 8 × 8 electrode grid with the upper five rows located frontoparietally (contacts 1-40) and the lower three rows over the lateral temporal neocortex (contacts 41-64). All seizures were electrographically stereotyped. Electrographic onset preceded clinical onset and consisted of fast activity of 80-100 Hz isolated to the contact at LG41. Six to nine seconds later this abruptly transitioned to a 2.5-Hz spike and wave pattern involving the mesial and basal temporal contacts. Which one of the following statements is most accurate?

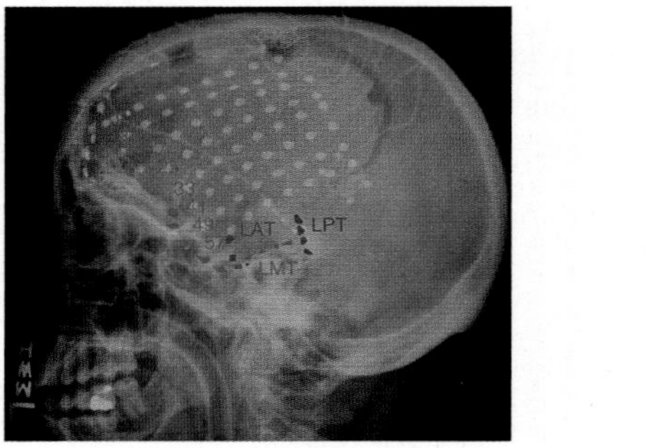

a. Seizure onset is from left mesial temporal structures
b. Seizures onset is from the left orbitofrontal region
c. Seizure onset is from the left anterior temporal pole
d. Seizure onset is from the left anterosuperior temporal gyrus
e. Hippocampal depth electrodes should have been placed

QUESTIONS 15–18

Additional questions 15–18 available on ExpertConsult.com

EXTENDED MATCHING ITEM (EMI) QUESTIONS

19. For each of the following descriptions, select the most appropriate answers from the image below. Each answer may be used once, more than once or not at all.

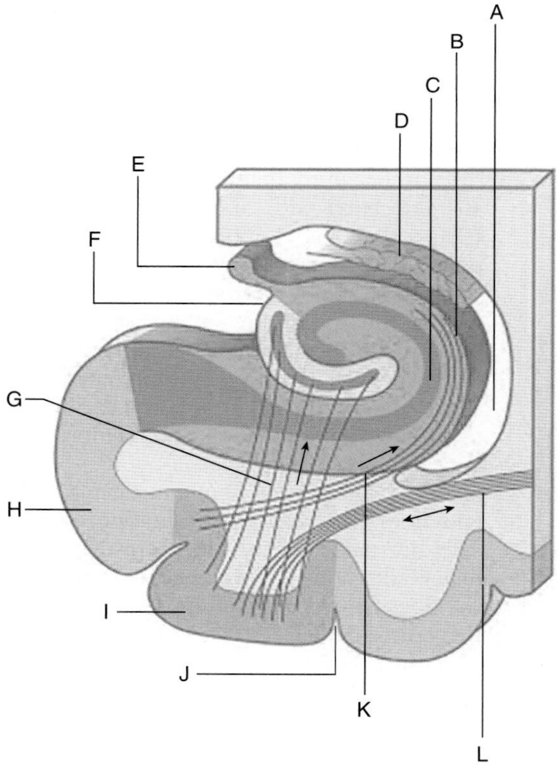

a. Choroid plexus
b. Dentate gyrus
c. Entorhinal cortex
d. Fimbria
e. Subiculum

20. **Imaging in epilepsy:**
   a. Arterial spin-labeling MRI
   b. Diffusion-tensor MRI
   c. Diffusion-weighted MRI
   d. FLAIR MRI
   e. Functional MRI
   f. Gradient echo MRI
   g. Ictal and interictal subtraction SPECT (SISCOM)
   h. MR spectroscopy
   i. PET imaging
   j. Susceptibility-weighted imaging MRI
   k. Volumetric T1 MRI

For each of the following descriptions, select the most appropriate answers from the list above. Each answer may be used once, more than once or not at all.
1. Increasingly being used to screen language lateralization
2. Sensitive for detection of hemosiderin deposition (e.g. cavernoma)
3. Best for identifying mesial temporal sclerosis

21. **Surgical options in epilepsy:**
   a. Anatomical hemispherectomy
   b. Corpus callosotomy
   c. Deep brain stimulation
   d. Functional hemispherectomy
   e. Multiple subpial transection
   f. Repetitive cortical stimulation
   g. Selective amygdalohippocampectomy
   h. Tailored temporal lobectomy
   i. Topectomy
   j. Vegal nerve stimulation
   k. Vertical parasagittal hemispherotomy

For each of the following descriptions, select the most appropriate answers from the list above.
1. Considered to be an established palliative surgical option for generalized seizures.
2. Intraoperative option when part of the epileptogenic zone overlaps an area of eloquent cortex
3. Classically associated with late postoperative complication of superficial cerebral siderosis
4. Temporal epilepsy with a lesion in lateral temporal lobe in the dominant hemisphere
5. Resection of cortex sparing underlying white matter often used in extratemporal lesions

22. **Epilepsy surgery workup:**
    a. Sleep-deprived EEG
    b. Video EEG
    c. MRI
    d. PET
    e. Neuropsychological testing
    f. Psychiatric evaluation
    g. Wada study
    h. Functional MRI
    i. Ictal and interictal subtraction SPECT (SISCOM)
    j. Magnetoencephalography
    k. Visual field testing

For each of the following descriptions, select the most appropriate answers from the list above. Each answer may be used once, more than once or not at all.

1. Aids in localizing language and motor function but not sufficient for predicting postoperative verbal memory impairment.
2. Important before resuming driving if seizure free after temporal lobectomy.
3. Suspicion of nonepileptic attack disorder.
4. Can help assess risk of postoperative amnesia and likelihood of seizure-free outcome
5. Epileptic focus often appears hypometabolic

23. **Seizure semiology:**
    a. Complex partial
    b. Epilepsia partialis continua
    c. Generalized tonic-clonic
    d. Generalized absence
    e. Jacksonian March
    f. Myoclonic
    g. Nonconvulsive status epilepticus
    h. Pseudoseizures
    i. Rolandic epilepsy
    j. Simple partial sensory
    k. Status epilepticus
    l. Uncinate seizures

For each of the following descriptions, select the most appropriate answers from the list above. Each answer may be used once, more than once or not at all.

1. A 37-year-old man develops involuntary twitching movements in his left thumb, which spread to his entire left hand and forearm and the left side of his face then blacked out. Witnesses report that he fell down and the entire left side of his body appeared to be twitching, followed by unresponsive episode for a few minutes and confusion for 15 min. During the episode, he bit the side of his tongue and was incontinent of urine.
2. A 17-year-old boy reports involuntary jerking movements in his arms when he awakens. This has occurred during the day after a nap as well as in the morning after a full night's sleep.
3. A 21-year-old man with septicemia induced DIC develops continuous rhythmic jerking of the right thumb and wrist lasting several hours. CT head shows a small hemorrhage in the left posterior frontal region. He is otherwise conscious and obeying commands.
4. A 21-year-old presents with unpleasant olfactory hallucinations.

24. **Medical treatment of epilepsy:**
    a. ACTH
    b. Clonazepam
    c. Ethosuximide
    d. Felbamate
    e. Levetiracetam
    f. Lorazepam
    g. Magnesium sulfate
    h. Phenobarbital
    i. Primidone
    j. Phenytoin
    k. Sodium valproate

For each of the following descriptions, select the most appropriate answers from the list above. Each answer may be used once, more than once or not at all.

1. A 7-month-old boy develops generalized limb extension and neck flexion spasms that occur more than 20 times daily and are associated with altered consciousness. EEG reveals diffuse, high-voltage, polyspike-and-slow-wave discharges between spasms and suppression of these bursts during the spasms. A sibling died with a brainstem glioma, and the father has several large areas of hypopigmented skin in the shape of ash leaves. The infant had obvious psychomotor retardation even before the appearance of the spasms.
2. A 5-year-old girl has frequent staring spells and does not respond when her mother calls her name during these episodes. She never falls down or bites her tongue, but she does have occasional lip smacking during episodes. EEG reveals a 3 Hz spike-and-wave pattern that occurs for less than 10 s at a time but several times an hour. The child has normal motor and cognitive development.
3. A 35-year-old pregnant woman at term is admitted to the hospital for delivery. She has headaches and visual blurring. Her blood pressure is 180/100. On examination,

she is edematous. Reflexes are increased. Protein is found in the urine. She then develops a generalized tonic-clonic convulsion.

4. A 19-year-old woman describes recurrent memory problems. Her fiancé reports that she seems to be inattentive for minutes at a time several times a week. She never injures herself during these episodes, but she cannot recall what happened, and, on one occasion, she became lost while walking home. An ambulatory EEG demonstrates evolving spike activity originating in the left temporal lobe during one of the episodes. The EEG pattern does not generalize. CT and MRI scanning of the brain reveal no structural abnormalities. Conversations with the woman's parents reveal that she had febrile seizures when she was 3 years old, which abated with antipyretic treatment alone.

SBA ANSWERS

1. **a**—DNET/ganglioglioma

The most epileptogenic tumors are DNET/gangliogliomas, but these are rare compared to meningiomas which are thus the commonest primary intracranial tumor (34%). However, brain metastases account for 50% of all intracranial mass lesions—with lung and breast metastasis making up the majority due to their prevalence, but melanoma having a higher propensity to metastasize to the brain (but is less common).

Tumor	% of Primary Brain Tumors (Adults and Children)	Approximate Seizure Frequency
DNET/ganglioglioma	1%	80-100%
Low grade glioma	9%	60-85%
Brain metastasis	N/A	24% (melanoma 67%)
Glioblastoma	17%	25-40%
Meningioma	34%	25-40%

FURTHER READING

Uptodate. Meningioma: clinical presentation and diagnosis. Topic 5220 Version 10.0.

Uptodate. Seizures in patients with primary and metastatic brain tumours. Topic 5181 Version 25.0.

American Brain Tumour Association. Brain tumour statistics.

2. **c**—Rolandic epilepsy

The catastrophic epilepsies of infancy and childhood (named due to the deleterious effect on development) are recognizable early and referral for surgical workup should not be deferred. They are characterized by multiple daily seizures, intractability to standard AEDs, developmental arrest or decline, and presumed/known epileptogenic pathology. Examples include Sturge-Weber syndrome, seizures due to malformations of cortical development, infantile spasms (West syndrome) due to malformations of cortical development and Rasmussen's syndrome. Rolandic epilepsy is benign and spontaneously remits in adolescence hence surgery is not indicated.

3. **d**—Multiple subpial transection

The technique of multiple subpial transections of cortex aimed to address the management of that portion of the epileptogenic zone that was electrocorticographically demonstrated to be functionally eloquent cortex. Instead of topectomy or cortical resection, the cortex is instead disrupted by parallel subpial cuts transecting the gray matter every 3-5 mm. The intention is to preserve centripetal axonal outflow while isolating silos of epileptogenic neurons by disrupting lateral dendritic communication across gyri, thereby preventing Jacksonian patterns of spreading cortical propagation of seizures. The benefit and indications of this technique remain controversial. A newer approach for treatment of focal epilepsy arising from eloquent cortex is chronic subthreshold subdural cortical stimulation.

FURTHER READING

Maciunas RJ. Surgical treatment of medically intractable epilepsy. In: Werz MA, editors. Epilepsy Syndromes. Elsevier, Saunders; 2010.

4. **e**—Low grade temporal glioma

In patients with intractable epilepsy it is important to determine if the seizures arise from the temporal lobes because temporal lobectomy is known to achieve seizure freedom in the majority of this group. A recent randomized trial by Wiebe and associates showed the superiority of temporal lobectomy to ongoing medication therapy, with about 60% becoming completely seizure free compared with 8% in those continuing on medical management with antiepileptic drugs. In this study, 70% of both groups had mesial temporal lobe epilepsy, compared to 10-15% who had a different temporal lesion (e.g. low grade glioma, cortical dysplasia, vascular malformation), and 10-15% who had a normal MRI. The only death in the study occurred in the medically managed group and was secondary to a seizure. However, in studies looking at surgery for low grade temporal lobe tumours specifically, gross total tumour resection results in seizure freedom in closer to 80% of patients. The most common complication of temporal lobectomy is a visual field defect caused by interruption of fibers from the optic tracts passing over the temporal horn of the lateral ventricles. Superior quadrantanopia is more common than hemianopsia. Some deficits may improve if the injury does not completely damage the nerves. Language deficits, particularly dysnomia, occur less frequently. Hemiparesis is uncommon (<2%), because the surgery is performed at a distance from the motor fibers of the corticospinal tract. Other neurological problems that can occur include diplopia caused by extraocular nerve deficits and facial paresis.

FURTHER READING

Wiebe S, Blume WT, Girvin JP, Eliasziw M. A randomized, controlled trial of surgery for temporal-lobe epilepsy. N Engl J Med 2001;345:311-318.

Englot DJ, Han SJ, Berger MS, Barbaro NM, Chang EF. Extent of surgical resection predicts seizure freedom in low-grade temporal lobe brain tumors. Neurosurgery. 2012 Apr;70(4):921-8; discussion 928. doi: 10.1227/NEU.0b013e31823c3a30. Review. PubMed PMID: 21997540.

5. **e**—50-60%, with further increase in yield by repeated or prolonged recordings that sample drowsiness and sleep. Routine EEGs aim to answer the following questions:
   1. Are there any interictal epileptiform discharges (IEDs; sharp waves, spikes, spike-and-wave complexes)?
   2. Are the IEDs diagnostic of an idiopathic generalized syndrome (i.e. not appropriate for surgery)?
   3. Are the IEDs confined to one hemisphere or bilateral?
   4. If unilateral, are IEDs confined to one area/lobe or are they multifocal?

6. **f**—Wada test

Mesial temporal structures, especially the hippocampal formation, are critical for the formation of new memories. Both sides are involved in memory consolidation, although the left may be more significant in verbal memories and the right in visuospatial (nonverbal) memories. Thus, removal of the mesial temporal structures in a temporal lobectomy may lead to memory decline. Many patients with temporal lobe epilepsy have bilateral disease, hence a unilateral temporal lobectomy in a patient with poor function on the contralateral side could have catastrophic results, such as an amnestic syndrome. The main means of assessing language dominance in epilepsy patients includes clinical presentation, neuropsychological assessment, functional MRI and Wada (sodium barbital infusion) test. While functional MRI and/or magnetoencephalography may aid in language lateralization, Wada is performed not only to demonstrate language dominance but also to assess the potential for verbal memory reduction postoperatively by evaluating the behavioral function of each brain hemisphere independent of the contralateral hemisphere. Injection of sodium amytal into a carotid artery transiently shuts down the hemisphere supplied, so that the memory and verbal function of the contralateral hemisphere can be assessed; usually the side of resection is injected first to determine the functioning of the nonresection side. Patients at high risk of postoperative memory impairment are those without MRI lesion, average-low average memory on preoperative neuropsychology, good memory when side contralateral to planned resection is injected (i.e. good memory on side of resection) and poor memory when side of planned resection is injected (i.e. poor memory on side to be preserved postoperatively). Equally, lower risk candidates are those with a unilateral mesial temporal sclerosis (MTS), poor material-specific memory on neuropsychological testing (i.e. poor verbal memory if left MTS, or visual memory if right MTS), good memory on injection of side to be resected and poor memory on injection of hemisphere to be preserved.

FURTHER READING

Shoenberg M. Intracarotid sodium amytal procedure (the Wada test). In: Werz MA, editors. Epilepsy Syndromes. Elsevier, Saunders; 2010.

7. **d**—Define the epileptogenic zone preoperatively

The neuropsychological evaluation can (1) assist in lateralizing and localizing brain dysfunction presumably related to the area of seizure origin, (2) predict cognitive risks from surgical treatment, (3) study the cognitive and behavioral effects of focal and generalized epilepsies over time, and (4) assess for cognitive and mood effects of antiepileptic medications. Mood can strongly impact on patient performance. Therefore, measures of mood and affect (e.g. anxiety and depression) are frequently administered as a measure of test validity/task engagement. Thus, the neuropsychological evaluation is to estimate the cognitive capabilities/reserve of the patient; to discern what cognitive risks may occur with the proposed surgical treatment for a patient with refractory epilepsy that combines results from neuropsychological evaluation, intracarotid sodium amobarbital procedure (Wada test), and structural neuroimaging. The epileptogenic zone is the zone whose resection or disruption is both necessary and sufficient to eliminate seizures and hence is not determinable preoperatively.

FURTHER READING

Schoenberg M. Neuropsychology in epilepsy. In: Werz MA, editors. Epilepsy Syndromes. Elsevier, Saunders; 2010.

8. **c**—Remote/distant site of seizure onset

The time taken for discharge to reach scalp surface electrode can vary depending on its distance from the site of ictal onset. Video EEG is done in conjunction with sleep deprivation and reduction/cessation of AEDs to maximize the chance of recording a seizure during the observation period. The goals of video EEG are to:

1. Further characterize the interictal discharges and correlate ictal EEG with behavior
2. Detect, characterize and quantify the patients habitual seizures—are they having more than one type?
3. Lateralize and localize seizure onset to allow comparison with neuroimaging findings

9. **a**—The next appropriate step would be to place subdural grid/strips

An epileptic focus appears as an area of hypometabolism on an interictal FDG-PET scan and surgical outcomes are better in patients with concordant PET and MRI foci. PET may be of more importance in extratemporal lobe epilepsy, where the proportion of patients with normal anatomic imaging is higher than in temporal lobe epilepsy. However, interictal PET for extratemporal epilepsy is less sensitive than in the temporal lobe. In general, the role of interictal PET in extratemporal epilepsy is to guide the surgeon in where to place electrodes for invasive EEG monitoring (electrocorticography). SPECT studies in epilepsy are for the evaluation of regional cerebral blood flow, which is decreased interictally and increased ictally (up to threefold) in the epileptic focus. The sensitivity of 99mTc-HMPAO SPECT in detecting abnormalities with interictal SPECT is about 70%, while ictal or early postictal imaging localizes epileptic foci in temporal lobe epilepsy between 80% and 90%. As with PET, extratemporal epileptic foci are not as easily localized and the response rate to surgery of extratemporal foci seen on SPECT is not as good as with temporal lobe foci. Additionally, SPECT is also technically difficult due to tracer half-life and need to inject the tracer within the first seconds of seizure onset to increase the likelihood of identifying just the area of seizure origin rather than the area of seizure propagation. PET has increased spatial resolution compared with SPECT and has a higher positive predictive value compared with SPECT in the interictal state. But interictal PET combined with ictal and interictal SPECT can result in a better identification of an epileptic focus than either alone. Coregistration of subtracted ictal and interictal SPECT data with MRI (SISCOM) will add to this armory

FURTHER READING

Faulhaber P. Nuclear imaging and epilepsy. In: Werz MA, editors. Epilepsy Syndromes. Elsevier, Saunders; 2010.

10. **c**—Dysphonia

The vagal nerve stimulator (VNS) may provide relief to patients who are not candidates for intracranial surgery, but at a cost of limited efficacy for complete seizure control and MRI incompatibility. VNS should not be viewed as a low-morbidity alternative to intracranial surgery, since it typically only offers a 50% reduction in seizure frequency in approximately two thirds of children and makes minimal difference in seizure control in about one fourth of patients (though a subset may experience a marked reduction in seizure frequency). The electrode is attached by three small flexible coils to the vagus nerve in the carotid sheath in the groove between the carotid artery and jugular vein, and connects to a generator placed in the anterior chest wall. The signal travels up the vagus nerve to the brain stem and spreads across the diencephalon and cerebral cortex. The VNS output is gradually ramped up at approximately 2-week intervals over a period of several months. Some children experience a mild cough or hoarse voice during the first day after the VNS is ramped up, but they quickly adapt to this. Typically, a few months are required before efficacy of the VNS for a particular patient will become evident. It is difficult to predict preoperatively who will obtain better seizure control, and while seizure frequency may not decrease overall it may become short enough to avoid emergency measures, or reduce the impact at school. The VNS generator typically has enough energy to last 3-5 years, depending on the settings and the amount of magnet usage. The VNS is not compatible with current model MRIs with risk of thermal injury to the vagus nerve. Thus, all patients should ideally have a relatively recent MRI before the VNS is implanted. The VNS is relatively contraindicated in patients with tumors that will require serial imaging, such as children with tuberous sclerosis. The overall morbidity of the surgical procedure is relatively low, with the most common risks being bleeding, infection, and nerve injury. A fracture in the lead is suggested when a previously effective VNS loses efficacy, adequate generator energy is present, and the DC current is high when the VNS is interrogated. The lead fracture is occasionally apparent on a plain radiograph but can be difficult to appreciate preoperatively. Removal of the lead and its replacement should only be considered for those children who have demonstrated a significant improvement in their quality of life, because the risks of bleeding and nerve injury are much higher than with the initial surgery. When a child undergoes other surgical procedures with anesthesia, it is generally recommended that VNS output current be set to zero with the programmer. In emergencies the magnet can be taped over the generator. Families need to be counseled to advise their other health care providers of the need to reprogram the VNS so arrangements can be made.

FURTHER READING

Robinson S. Pediatric epilepsy surgery. In: Werz MA, editors. Epilepsy Syndromes. Elsevier, Saunders; 2010.

11. **b**—II

The Engel Epilepsy surgery outcome scale is outlined below, however it is worth noting that the ILAE have introduced a newer postsurgical scale which may be more sensitive and reduce ambiguity.

Engel Class	Description	Comments
I	Free of disabling seizures	Completely seizure free; nondisabling, simple partial seizures only; some disabling seizures, but free of disabling seizures for at least 2 years; generalized convulsion with antiepileptic drug withdrawal only
II	Rare disabling seizures	Initially free of disabling seizures, but rare seizures now; rare disabling seizures since surgery; more than rare disabling seizures, but rare seizures for at least 2 years; nocturnal seizures only
III	Worthwhile improvement	Worthwhile seizure reduction; prolonged seizure-free intervals amounting to more than half the follow-up period, but not less than 2 years
IV	No worthwhile improvement	No significant seizure reduction; no appreciable change; seizures worse

12. **f**—Predicting postoperative language/memory deficit

Scalp electrodes give the best overview of interictal epileptiform activity because they sample extensive areas of the cranium, but they are limited by their low sensitivity due to intervening high-resistance tissue and poor ability to sample activity from deep structures. Invasive recordings resolve this limitation (improving both sensitivity and spatial localization) but have the risk of sampling error as a result of the limited spatial distribution selected for monitoring. Stereotactic implantation of depth electrode arrays to define the epileptogenic zone provides unparalleled sampling from deep cortical anatomy not directly accessible by other means, allowing for the definitive lateralization and localization of mesial temporal lobe, insular region, mesial frontoparietal and pericingulate, orbitofrontal, and submerged perisulcal cortical onset epilepsy. Bilateral temporal and frontal implantation of subdural electrode strips through enlarged bur holes, though less precise, are associated with a lower risk of intracerebral hemorrhage. If localization (rather than lateralization) is the priority, unilateral craniotomy for placement of subdural electrode grids allows one to achieve refined definition of the epileptogenic zone through localization of the irritative zone and the ictal onset zone, and also to carry out extraoperative cortical mapping for preoperative delineation of functionally eloquent cortex that must be spared at resection. However, this comes with the risks of craniotomy, mass effect from the grids and a higher infection risk, but the information gained can guide the choice between anterior temporal lobectomy and amygdalohippocampectomy and inform the tailoring of dominant temporal lobectomies to spare lateral cortical regions exhibiting speech arrest with stimulation (reducing postoperative language deficits while maximizing the extent of lateral temporal resection). Craniotomy and grid placement can be combined with subdural strip electrodes (passed around the temporal pole, underneath the temporal lobe, and under the orbitofrontal cortex) or frameless image-guided implantation of depth electrodes targeting the amygdala and hippocampus. Craniotomy for placement of subdural electrode grids and strips is frequently employed to guide tailored extra-temporal cortical resections.

13. **e**—Temporal lobectomy

Invasive monitoring is unnecessary when there is concordance between interictal and ictal video-EEG scalp recordings localizing to the nondominant temporal lobe, with ipsilateral mesial temporal sclerosis on MRI and contralateral language and memory dominance on Wada testing (with congruent neuropsychological testing), ipsilateral PET hypometabolism of the temporal lobe, and perhaps magnetoencephalographic data. In such cases where a safe resection is possible, proceeding directly to surgery is usually indicated. As many as 50-90% of such patients will be rendered free of seizures postoperatively. Anterior Medial Temporal Lobectomy represents the gold standard of surgical management of temporal lobe epilepsy. More lateral temporal resection is carried out with the intention of maximizing disruption of the circuit of the epileptogenic zone while sparing the superior temporal gyrus (and limiting middle temporal gyrus resection more on the dominant side) to minimizing interference with language function in the dominant hemisphere. Alternatively, awake intraoperative cortical stimulation producing speech arrest to map critical language regions can be used as a guide to tailor the extent of resection of the dominant temporal lobe. Resections that extend more posterior may be associated with an increased incidence of visual field deficits, ranging from contralateral superior quadrantanopia to hemianopsia due to disruption of Meyer's loop of visual fibers in the periventricular white matter surrounding the temporal horn of the lateral ventricle. More extensive resection of mesial temporal structures, including the amygdala and hippocampus has improved seizure control but injury to the anterior choroidal and posterior cerebral artery branches risks contralateral hemiparesis. Equally, some have advocated sparing of the lateral temporal neocortex in cases of epilepsy due to mesial temporal sclerosis (trans-sylvian amygdalohippocampectomy). Gamma Knife Radiosurgery targeting of mesial temporal lobe structures is available in some centers.

Image with permission from Loevner L. Brain Imaging: Case Review Series, 2nd ed. Elsevier, Mosby; 2009.

14. **d**—Seizure onset is from the left anterosuperior temporal gyrus

The epileptogenic zone is the zone whose resection or disruption is both necessary and sufficient to eliminate seizures hence is only determinable postoperatively once seizure freedom has been gained. As such, epilepsy surgery targets the ictal onset zone and areas involved in early seizure organization, which generally tend to coincide or intersect with the epileptogenic zone. The ictal onset zone is defined as the area where the ictal discharge is first detected, regardless of its morphology, before the clinical manifestations of the seizure. Identifying that area (using ECoG and/or nuclear imaging), a major prerequisite for successful resective epilepsy surgery, requires familiarity with electrographic ictal patterns. Early ictal patterns seen on the ECoG include rhythmic sinusoidal waves, irregular spike discharge, spike and wave activity, low-voltage fast activity, and high-frequency oscillations. An appropriate broad definition of an electrocorticographic ictal discharge is any electrodecremental or rhythmic pattern that represents a considerable deviation from the baseline, whether or not it contains apiculate waveforms. In general, it is believed that ictal onsets consisting of fast frequency activity indicate the proximity of the recording electrodes to the ictal onset zone whereas slower ictal onsets tend to represent propagated activity. In this case, seizure onset was from the anterosuperior temporal gyrus (LG41) with spread to the hippocampus (mesial and basal contacts). There are several caveats to this: the epileptogenic zone may be more extensive than the ictal onset zone hence resection may not eliminate seizures (or adjacent areas become capable of initiating seizures), the majority of epilepsy surgery patients only remain seizure free on antiepileptic drugs, the epileptogenic zone and the ictal onset zone may be separate, e.g. the epileptogenic zone in a "clinically silent" area and the seizure becomes clinically manifest only after it propagates to the temporal lobe (ECoG will localize ictal onset to temporal lobe but resection will not eliminate the seizure generator).

Image with permission from Werz MA. Epilepsy Syndromes. Elsevier, Saunders; 2010.

ANSWERS 15–18

Additional answers 15–18 available on ExpertConsult.com

EMI ANSWER

19. a—D, b—F, c—I, d—E, e—H

a—Lateral ventricle, b—Alveus, c—hippocampus, d—choroid plexus, e—fimbria, f—dentate gyrus, g—performant path, h—subiculum, i—entorhinal cortex, j—collateral sulcus, k—alvear path, l—two-way connections with sensory association areas

Image with permission from Mtui E, Gruener G, Dockery P. Fitzgerald's Clinical Neuroanatomy and Neuroscience, 7th ed. Elsevier; 2016.

20. 1—e, Functional MRI; 2—j, Susceptibility weighted MRI; 3—d, FLAIR MRI

21. 1—b, Corpus callosotomy; 2—e, Multiple subpial transection; 3—a, Anatomical hemispherectomy; 4—h, Tailored temporal lobe resections are directed by the results of the initial stage of depth or subdural grid electrode invasive monitoring. Because the cases typically involve discordant noninvasive findings, they are more likely to demonstrate complex pathologic findings, including purely lateral temporal lesions such as cortical dysplasia, tumors, vascular malformations, "dual pathology" of mesial temporal sclerosis plus another lesion, or the absence of any definitive pathologic etiologic diagnosis. 5—i, Topectomy. Extratemporal resections are tailored by the findings of invasive monitoring to include the epileptogenic lesion and the epileptogenic zone while sparing functionally eloquent cortical regions. Topectomy, or the resection of cortex sparing underlying white matter, is employed. Resection of epileptogenic cortex while incompletely removing the epileptogenic lesion is associated with a lower incidence of seizure control. On the other hand, resection of the lesion alone, whether tumor or vascular malformation, is associated with a lower incidence of seizure control than resection of the lesion plus surrounding epileptogenic zone. This surrounding epileptogenic zone may at times prove to contain cortical dysplasia on pathologic evaluation.

22. 1—h, functional MRI; 2—k, Visual field test; 3—f, Psychiatric evaluation; 4—g, Wada test; 5—d, PET imaging

Epilepsy Work-up: Rationale for Investigations

Investigation	Comments
Sleep-deprived EEG	Many routine EEGs are normal, especially if the patient has been taking antiepileptic medication before the study. A prolonged (1 h) sleep-deprived EEG may show epileptiform discharges during nonrapid-eye-movement sleep.
Video EEG	Admission for monitoring while medication is tapered with the aim of recording a minimum number of seizures. May also require sleep deprivation, hyperventilation, photic stimulation, caffeine, vigorous exercise. Sphenoidal electrodes should be placed when mesial temporal lobe origin is suspected. Can be complicated by concomitant nonepileptic seizures.
MRI	Standard sequences include T1, T2, and FLAIR with coronal sequences through mesial temporal lobe. Contrast is given if inflammatory, infectious or neoplastic etiology suspected.

Continued

Investigation	Comments
PET	Seizure focus is often hypometabolic on FDG-PET. In patients with frequent seizures, if a seizure happens immediately before or during the scan the epileptogenic focus may appear hypermetabolic and be missed—hence concurrent EEG should be used in these patients.
Neuropsychological testing	Identifies epileptogenic region (and associated dysfunctioning areas), lateralization/dominance of language and memory, prediction of postoperative deficits, and preoperative psychological issues needing treatment (depression, anxiety).
Psychiatric evaluation	Aim to identify and treat psychological problems which require surgery to be delayed/withheld or arise postoperatively, e.g. depression/anxiety, nonepileptic seizures, adjustment to seizure freedom.
Wada study	Indicated preoperatively in patients with TLE or involvement of areas critical for language. It aids localizing language and memory, assess risk of postoperative amnesia, risk of memory decline and likelihood of seizure-free outcome. Angiography must exclude cerebral vessel cross filling before injection of sodium amobarbital otherwise results will be affected. Ipsilateral carotid injection allows testing of contralateral hemisphere memory and language for 15 min.
fMRI	Aids in localizing language and motor function, and interictal spikes. Not sufficient for predicting postoperative verbal memory impairment.
Ictal SPECT with SISCOM	Technically difficult hence used when preceding workup has not identified an epileptogenic focus—usually in the case of extratemporal nonlesional epilepsy. Interictal SPECT is performed and then the patient undergoes video EEG. As soon as seizure onset is detected radioactive tracer injected which concentrates at the focus (delays in tracer injection result in poorer distinction between onset zone and propagation zone). Subtraction Ictal SPECT Coregistered to MRI (SISCOM) allows better localization of the seizure focus and operative targeting.
Magnetoencephalography	Records interictal magnetic brain waves and maps them in 3D onto MRI images of the patient's brain. Aids localization of seizure focus in extratemporal nonlesional epilepsy and preoperative functional mapping.
Visual field testing	Testing should be done where seizure foci are in temporal, parietal or occipital lobes; preoperative testing may reveal deficits unnoticed by patients, and new postoperative deficits.

23. 1—e, Jacksonian March. With a Jacksonian March, or sequential seizure, the patient develops focal seizure activity that is primarily motor and spreads. This type of seizure often secondarily generalizes, at which point the patient loses consciousness and may have a generalized tonic-clonic seizure. The hand is a common site for the start of a Jacksonian March. The face may be involved early because the thumb and the mouth are situated near each other on the motor strip of the cerebral cortex. 2—f, Myoclonic seizures may be generalized or partial benign juvenile myoclonic epilepsy (BJME). The episodes occur when the affected person wakes up rather than when he or she is falling asleep. Myoclonic jerks may be triggered by light flashes or loud sounds, and patients may also have generalized tonic-clonic seizures. 3—b, Epilepsia partialis continua is persistent focal motor seizure activity (i.e. a focal motor status epilepticus). The distal hand and foot muscles are most frequently affected. 4—l, Uncinate fits are characterized by seizure activity involving portions of the anterior aspect of the temporal lobe resulting in unpleasant olfactory hallucinations. The structures most often implicated include the uncus, parahippocampal gyrus, the region of the amygdala and adjoining tissue, and the piriform cortex.

24. 1—a, ACTH. This child has West syndrome, a generalized seizure disorder of infants characterized by recurrent spasms, the EEG pattern of hypsarrhythmia, and retardation. Several different diseases cause West syndrome. The family history in this case suggests tuberous sclerosis as the underlying problem. ACTH is the best of the given choices. 2—c, Ethosuximide. This girl has generalized absence attacks. This may be a manifestation of a more complex epilepsy syndrome or may occur as an isolated

finding. Generalized absence attacks have no aura and no postictal period. The affected child has no warning that an attack is about to occur and is usually unaware that one has occurred unless it is more than a few seconds long. In fact, generalized absence seizures are most often only a few seconds long. Ethosuximide is the drug of choice, but it may cause gastrointestinal distress. Divalproex sodium is effective in many of the children who cannot tolerate ethosuximide or who are not well controlled on that antiepileptic. If the absence seizures are associated with generalized tonic-clonic seizures, divalproex sodium is a better choice. Some antiepileptic drugs, such as the sodium channel blockers phenytoin and carbamazepine, can actually worsen generalized from onset seizures. 3—g, Magnesium sulfate. Recent studies have established that magnesium sulfate ($MgSO_4$) is the optimal treatment both to prevent seizures in women with hypertension at the time of admission for delivery (preeclampsia) and to treat seizures in established eclampsia. The dose is 4-5 g intravenously, followed by a 1 g/h intravenous infusion. Magnesium sulfate was shown to result in a reduction in recurrent seizures and in maternal morbidity and mortality compared with both diazepam and phenytoin. In addition, the fetus should be delivered as quickly as possible, using cesarean section if necessary. Eclampsia is an example of the posterior leukoencephalopathy syndrome. 4—e, Levetiracetam. This young woman is having complex partial seizures without secondary generalization. She has episodic altered consciousness associated with a temporal lobe seizure focus and antedated by febrile seizures. Levetiracetam is the best choice because of its relatively good efficacy and adverse effect profile. Felbamate, phenobarbital, primidone, and divalproex sodium may also be effective at controlling the seizures, but all have side effect profiles making them poor first choices in this case.

CHAPTER 35

ADULT MOVEMENT DISORDERS

SINGLE BEST ANSWER (SBA) QUESTIONS

1. A 40-year-old man has a family history of hereditary neurodegenerative disease and early death. His father died of a rapidly progressive dementia at the age of 50 and he has previously been told that he has the defective gene. He presents with personality change and non-purposeful, slow, rhythmic movements of his hands and face. A magnetic resonance imaging (MRI) indicates atrophy in the head of the caudate nucleus. Which one of the following neurotransmitter deficiencies is most likely to be responsible?
   a. Dopamine in the substantia nigra
   b. Substance P in the subthalamic nucleus
   c. Acetylcholine and gamma-aminobutyric acid in the striatum
   d. Serotonin in the globus pallidus
   e. Glutamate in the cortex

2. A 43-year-old man has a father who died from Huntington's disease. The son was tested and found to have the gene for Huntington's disease. Which one of the following is true regarding the offspring of those with Huntington's disease?
   a. All children are at risk only if the affected parent is male
   b. 1 in 10 are at risk only if the affected parent is female
   c. 1 in 8 are at risk for the disease
   d. 1 in 4 are at risk for the disease
   e. 1 in 2 are at risk for the disease

3. Damage to the subthalamic nucleus is associated with which one of the following
   a. Myoclonus
   b. Dystonic tremor
   c. Hemiballism
   d. Levodopa-induced dyskinesia
   e. Tardive dyskinesia

4. Tardive dyskinesia is most likely the result of receptor changes causing hypersensitivity to which one of the following neurotransmitters?
   a. Serotonin (5-HT)
   b. Acetylcholine
   c. Enkephalin
   d. Dopamine
   e. GABA

5. Which one of the following statements regarding dystonia is most accurate?
   a. Isolated foot dystonia is very rare and may suggest an underlying Parkinsonian disorder or brain structural abnormality
   b. Torticollis is the least common dystonia
   c. Segawa's disease is a primary dystonia responsive to antidopaminergic drugs
   d. Trihexyphenidyl is the primary treatment for drug-induced dystonia
   e. Blepharospasm is involuntary opening of eyelids resulting in paradoxical blinking

6. A 65-year-old man presents with difficulty getting out of chairs and problems walking over the last year with multiple falls. On examination, his face appeared mask-like with reduced blinking and slight drooling, and he had a pill-rolling tremor at rest bilaterally, and on passive movement demonstrated cogwheel rigidity. His handwriting became smaller towards the end of a sentence. There was no weakness, sensory problems, or abnormalities in his reflexes. There are no autonomic symptoms. He had a stooped posture and walked with a slow shuffling gait, with a noticeably reduced arm swing. Which one of the following statements regarding this condition is most accurate?
   a. It may present with a 3 Hz rest pill rolling tremor
   b. The major neuronal loss is in the substantia nigra pars reticularis
   c. It is associated with a fluent aphasia
   d. Loss of smell is a non-motor symptom of this disease
   e. Dyskinesias are common in non-medicated patients

7. Which one of the followings statements regarding Parkinson's plus syndromes is LEAST accurate?
   a. MSA-P (Striatonigral degeneration) is characterized by Parkinsonism with autonomic failure
   b. Dementia with Lewy bodies is often associated with detailed visual hallucinations
   c. Tremor is rare in progressive supranuclear palsy
   d. Corticobasal degeneration may include cortical sensory loss and apraxia
   e. MSA-C (olivopontocerebellar atrophy) is characterized by Parkinsonism with progressive ataxia

8. A 67-year-old man had idiopathic tremulous Parkinson's disease diagnosed 15 years ago, and has had a 10-year history of progressive worsening in wearing-off phenomenon. Despite increasing the dose and frequency of levodopa this had still deteriorated, and higher doses induced peak-dose dyskinesias. High-frequency stimulation of which one of the following brain structures is most likely to improve his symptoms?
   a. Unilateral STN
   b. Bilateral STN
   c. Unilateral Vim
   d. Bilateral Vim
   e. Bilateral GPi

9. A 25-year-old man has had motor tics since age 13. They seem to be getting worse, and now he also has involuntary obscene vocalizations. Which one of the following stimulation targets would you use in this patient?
   a. Centromedian nucleus-parafascicular complex of thalamus
   b. Vim thalamus
   c. Posterior hypothalamus
   d. Subthalamic nucleus
   e. Hippocampus

10. A 22-year-old male is involved in a road traffic collision and sustains a significant traumatic brain injury. CT head shows traumatic subarachnoid hemorrhage and hemorrhagic contusions extending into the basal ganglia. After a long period of rehabilitation he is left with a residual left arm tremor. Which one of the following could be considered to manage his tremor?
    a. Motor cortex stimulation
    b. VIM thalamic stimulation
    c. STN stimulation
    d. Red nucleus stimulation
    e. Ventral striatal/ventral internal capsule stimulation

11. Which one of the following targets is most commonly used for the treatment of dystonia?
    a. GPi
    b. Vim thalamus
    c. Vo thalamus
    d. STN
    e. Nucleus accumbens

12. Which one of the following statements regarding thalamotomy is LEAST accurate?
    a. It is most appropriate for those with predominantly unilateral symptoms
    b. Lesions placed to laterally may result in contralateral weakness
    c. Bilateral thalamotomy is the treatment of choice in bilateral tremor dominant Parkinson's disease when deep brain stimulation is not possible
    d. Speech disturbance is a common problem
    e. Lesions placed too posteriorly may cause numbness and paresthesias of the mouth

QUESTIONS 13–18

Additional questions 13–18 available on ExpertConsult.com

EXTENDED MATCHING ITEM (EMI) QUESTIONS

19. **Movement disorder signs:**
    a. Akithisia
    b. Asterixis
    c. Ataxia
    d. Athetosis
    e. Ballism
    f. Bradykinesia
    g. Chorea
    h. Clonus
    i. Dyskinesia
    j. Dystonia
    k. Myoclonus
    l. Rigidity
    m. Stereotypy
    n. Tic
    o. Tremor

For each of the following descriptions, select the most appropriate answers from the list above. Each answer may be used once, more than once or not at all.

1. A 5-year-old child with Rett syndrome exhibits hand wringing
2. A 45-year-old patient with hepatic encephalopathy exhibits sudden and involuntary relaxation of a dorsiflexed hand
3. A 35-year-old with personality change and jerky limb movements, which he often attempts to mask by incorporating them into seemingly purposeful actions
4. A 67-year-old presents with a reduction in movement velocity
5. A 70-year-old presents with involuntary, high-amplitude arm flinging episodes 3 months after an ischemic stroke
6. A 34-year-old schizophrenic started on an antipsychotic presents 3 months later with involuntary, non-suppressible lip smacking, pouting and tongue protrusion

20. **Tremor:**
    a. Cerebellar tremor
    b. Drug-induced tremor
    c. Dystonic tremor
    d. Essential tremor
    e. Holme's tremor
    f. Neuropathic tremor
    g. Palatal tremor
    h. Parkinsonian tremor
    i. Physiological tremor
    j. Primary orthostatic tremor
    k. Psychogenic tremor

For each of the following descriptions, select the most appropriate answers from the list above. Each answer may be used once, more than once or not at all.

1. A 40-year-old literary agent has had worsening tremor of the hands. This has been present for 2 years, but has increasingly impaired her work ability because she is frequently required to take her clients to lunch, and she is embarrassed by her inability to eat and drink normally. A glass of wine with the meal typically helps somewhat. On examination, there is a mild head tremor, but no rest tremor of the hands. When she holds a pen by the tip at arm's length, however, a coarse tremor is readily apparent. Examination is otherwise normal
2. A 64-year-old man has noticed dragging of the right leg and tremor and stiffness of the right hand. On examination, he has a tremor of the right hand, which disappears when he reaches to grab a pen. Movements are slower on the right than the left. He has cogwheel rigidity of the right arm
3. A 56-year-old presents 4 months after a thalamic stroke with a left arm 3 Hz action tremor with a "wing beating" appearance
4. A 47-year-old patient presents with a jerky, low-frequency 2 Hz high-amplitude action tremor. He also had impairment in finger-nose and heel shin testing

21. **Chorea, athetosis, and ballism:**
    a. Ataxia telangiectasia
    b. Benign hereditary chorea
    c. Cerebrovascular disease
    d. Chorea gravidarum
    e. Huntington's disease
    f. Mitochondrial disease (Leigh's disease)
    g. Neuroacanthocytosis
    h. Spinocerebellar ataxia
    i. Sydenham's chorea
    j. Wilson's disease

For each of the following descriptions, select the most appropriate answers from the list above. Each answer may be used once, more than once or not at all.

1. A 12-year-old girl presents with acute rheumatic fever develops rhythmic, writhing movements in all four limbs
2. A 35-year-old patient with Kaiser-Fleischer rings and a low serum ceruloplasmin
3. A 48-year-old patient with new onset atrial fibrillation who presents with hemichorea
4. A 19-year-old, left-handed woman has had several weeks of nausea, vomiting, and weight gain. She has been taking cyclizine with some reduction in vomiting. She has also noticed the recent onset of an involuntary relatively rapid and fluid, but not rhythmic, limb and trunk movements. Neurological examination is otherwise unremarkable. Which one of the following is the most likely diagnosis?
5. A 26-year-old presents with orofacial dystonia and psychiatric disturbance. Peripheral blood smear shows acanthocytes

22. **Dystonia:**
    a. DYT1 dystonia (Oppenheim's dystonia)
    b. DYT5 dystonia (Segawa's disease)
    c. DYT11 Myoclonic-dystonia
    d. Huntington's disease

e. Lesch-Nyhan syndrome
f. Meige syndrome
g. Multiple system atrophy
h. Neuroacanthocytosis
i. Spinocerebellar ataxia
j. Wilson's disease

For each of the following descriptions, select the most appropriate answers from the list above. Each answer may be used once, more than once or not at all.

1. A 53-year-old woman is unable to stop blinking forcefully and has frequent grimacing movements of the face. At times, she protrudes her tongue against her will. She has never taken any medications
2. A 14-year-old boy from an Ashkenazi Jewish family presents with dystonia affecting his right leg which is not responsive to levodopa
3. A 9-year-old boy presents with left foot dystonia which shows a diurnal fluctuation and improves with levodopa treatment

23. **Adverse Effects of DBS:**
a. Ataxia
b. Blepharospasm
c. Diplopia
d. Dysarthria
e. Infection
f. Intracranial hemorrhage
g. Microthalamotomy effect
h. Paresthesia
i. Photopsias
j. Tonic contraction

For each of the following descriptions, select the most appropriate answers from the list above. Each answer may be used once, more than once or not at all.

1. Overstimulation of the subthalamic nucleus
2. Stimulation posterior to subthalamic nucleus
3. Stimulation posteromedial to globus pallidus interna
4. Stimulation posterior to Vim thalamus
5. Stimulation anterior to Vim thalamus

24. **Medical therapy for Parkinson's disease:**
a. Amantidine
b. Apomorphine
c. Benztropine
d. Entacapone
e. Levodopa-carbidopa
f. Nortriptyline
g. Rivastigmine (or donepezil)
h. Ropinerole (or pramipexole)
i. Rotigotine
j. Selegiline

For each of the following descriptions, select the most appropriate answers from the list above. Each answer may be used once, more than once or not at all.

1. First line therapy for elderly patients presenting with Parkinson's disease
2. First line transdermal therapy for early onset Parkinson's disease
3. May have neuroprotective effect if given early in Parkinson's disease
4. Extending the duration of action of levodopa-carbidopa

25. **Motor complications in Parkinson's disease:**
a. Acute akinesia
b. Akathisia
c. Camptocormia
d. Diphasic dyskinesia
e. Dystonia
f. Freezing of gait
g. No-on phenomenon
h. Peak-dose dyskinesia
i. Unpredictable off periods
j. Wearing off phenomenon

For each of the following descriptions, select the most appropriate answers from the list above. Each answer may be used once, more than once or not at all.

1. A 72-year-old man presented with idiopathic Parkinson's disease has been on levodopa treatment for 5 years. His dose requirements have been steadily increasing, and after the most recent dose increase he complains of odd movements in his limbs about an hour after taking his tablets.
2. An 82-year-old with Parkinson's disease is admitted to hospital as her symptoms are so severe she is frozen and cannot take her levodopa dose. Her temperature is 38.6 °C (101.8 °F), RR 30, O2 Sat 91% (air) and CXR demonstrates right lower lobe consolidation
3. A 73-year-old patient diagnosed 4 years ago with Parkinson's disease and is currently taking levodopa-carbidopa every 4 h. He presents with recurrence of bradykinesia and tremor 3 h after each dose of levodopa
4. A 67-year-old patient on levodopa-carbidopa for Parkinson's disease diagnosed 7 years ago presents with early morning painful flexion and inversion postures of the feet and toes

SBA ANSWER

1. **c**—Acetylcholine and gamma-aminobutyric acid in the striatum

Huntington's disease is characterized by loss of striatal neurons resulting in reduced levels of choline acetyltransferase, glutamic acid decarboxylase, and GABA in the striatum resulting in a relative excess of dopamine causing a hyperkinetic movement disorder with writhing and jerking movements of the limbs (chorea). Dopamine antagonists, such as haloperidol, may be used to suppress chorea, but also carry the risk of provoking tardive dyskinesia. Dopaminergic drugs, such as L-dopa, bromocriptine, and lisuride, may unmask chorea but should not be used diagnostically as it may not abate.

2. **e**—1 in 2 are at risk for the disease

Huntington's disease is transmitted in an autosomal dominant fashion. The age at which the patient becomes symptomatic is variable and has no effect on the probability of transmitting the disease. The defect underlying this degenerative disease is an abnormal expansion of a triplicate repeat (CAG) sequence in the HTT gene on chromosome 4 (normally coding for the protein huntingtin). Normal individuals have between 6 and 34 copies of this CAG section; patients with Huntington's disease may have from 36 to more than 100 repeats. People with the adult-onset form of Huntington's disease typically have more than 36 CAG repeats in the *HTT* gene (although those with 36-39 still may not develop signs/symptoms) and those with the juvenile form of the disorder tend to have more than 60 CAG repeats. Individuals who have 27-35 CAG repeats in the *HTT* gene do not develop Huntington's disease, but they are at risk of having children who will develop the disorder. As the gene is passed from parent to child, the size of the CAG trinucleotide repeat may lengthen into the range associated with Huntington's disease (36 repeats or more). Once expanded beyond 40 copies, the repeats are unstable and may further increase as they are passed on from one generation to the next. An increased number of repeats in successive generations can lead to earlier disease onset, a phenomenon termed *anticipation*.

3. **c**—Hemiballism

A lesion of the subthalamic nucleus results in hemiballism, a form of dyskinesia in which the patient displays severe involuntary movements. It is believed to occur as a result of an imbalance in the output signals of the basal ganglia, with overactivity of the direct pathway relative to the indirect pathway. This is in contrast to Parkinson's disease, where overactivity of the indirect pathway relative to the direct pathway results in bradykinesia.

4. **d**—Dopamine

Tardive dyskinesia results from treatment with dopamine receptor blocking agents. Tardive syndromes are less frequently caused by atypical than by typical neuroleptics. The most common pattern of tardive dyskinesia is stereotyped and repetitive movement of the face (e.g., tongue-thrusting and involuntary chewing movements is often accompanied by a feeling of restlessness). This akathisia may be localized and reported as a "burning" sensation, often of the genitals or mouth.

5. **a**—Isolated foot dystonia is very rare and may suggest an underlying Parkinsonian disorder or brain structural abnormality

Focal dystonias produce abnormal sustained muscle contractions in a single region of the body:

- Neck (torticollis): most commonly affected site with a tendency for the head to turn to one side.
- Eyelids (blepharospasm): involuntary closure of the eyelids that leads to excessive eye blinking, sometimes with persistent eye closure and functional blindness.
- Mouth (oromandibular dystonia): involuntary contraction of muscles of the mouth, tongue, or face.
- Hand (writer's cramp).

Isolated foot dystonia is very rare and may suggest an underlying Parkinsonian disorder or brain structural abnormality. Generalized dystonia affects multiple areas of the body and can lead to marked joint deformities. Primary dystonia can be sporadic or heritable (e.g., DYT1 dystonia, Segawa's disease). Secondary dystonia results from basal ganglia insults (stroke, demyelination, hypoxia, trauma), Huntington's disease, Wilson's disease, Parkinson's syndromes, and lysosomal storage diseases. Acute or chronic (tardive) dyskinesias can occur with dopaminergic antagonists (e.g., antipsychotics, antiemetics). In addition to removing any offending drug, trihexyphenidyl is an anticholinergic drug which is used to manage chorea, dystonia and dyskinesias (by correcting the imbalance between dopamine and acetylcholine in the basal ganglia).

6. **d**—Loss of smell is a non-motor symptom of this disease

Idiopathic Parkinson's disease is a neurodegenerative condition caused by progressive loss of dopaminergic cells in the substantia nigra pars compacta projecting to the striatum. This produces a hypokinetic movement disorder characterized by bradykinesia, rigidity and resting tremor. More specific symptoms include: a slow shuffling gait with a tendency to move progressively faster (festinating gait); micrographia; mask-like facial expression with reduced eye blinking; and difficulty getting out of a chair; quiet monotonous voice (hypophonia); muscle rigidity (lead-pipe rigidity); pill-rolling rest tremor 4-8 Hz, which combines with rigidity to produce "cogwheeling" on passive flexion by the examiner. Non-motor symptoms may also have a major impact on quality of life: drooling (reduced swallowing), dementia, REM sleep disorders, loss of smell, constipation, mood disorder (especially depression), orthostatic hypotension, bladder and erectile dysfunction. Dopamine cannot cross the blood-brain barrier, hence medical therapy must increase striatal dopamine by other means (e.g., prevent catecholamine breakdown [MAOI-B], provide the immediate precursor to dopamine [levodopa], or other dopaminergic receptor agonists).

7. **e**—MSA-C (olivopontocerebellar atrophy) is characterized by Parkinsonism with progressive ataxia

Many other disorders present with Parkinsonian features early in their course, and the more characteristic features of some of these "Parkinson's plus" syndromes (e.g., gaze paralysis in progressive supranuclear palsy or autonomic dysfunction in multiple system atrophy) may not become apparent until several years after symptom onset. An incorrect diagnosis of early Parkinson's disease is probably made between 10% and 20% of the time, even among Parkinson's disease specialists. An accurate early diagnosis of Parkinson's disease is becoming increasingly important as the long-term effects of early treatment on natural history are better understood. Secondary Parkinsonism may be idiopathic, drug-induced, toxin-induced, due to cerebrovascular disease or structural lesions, or post-traumatic. Clinically similar to Parkinson's disease, symptomatic Parkinsonism may be identified by history (e.g., medication history or exposure to toxins) or by symptoms and signs consistent with an underlying disorder. Clues suggesting secondary Parkinsonism include acute/subacute onset, symmetric symptoms, rapid progression or static course, poor response to dopaminergic drugs, history of exposure to causative drugs/toxins/CNS infection/cerebrovascular disease, and signs of underlying metabolic or structural brain disease.

Parkinson's Plus Syndrome	Description
Multiple system atrophy (Shy-Drager syndrome)	Classified into MSA-P (striatonigral degeneration) and MSA-C (olivopontocerebellar atrophy) subtypes. Predominance of rapidly progressive Parkinsonian features (rigidity, postural instability, tremor and gait freezing) in MSA-P and cerebellar features (gait, limb, and speech ataxia) in MSA-C. Both are accompanied by autonomic failure (urinary and bowel dysfunction, impaired potency and libido, decreased sweating and orthostatic hypotension)
Progressive supranuclear palsy	Progressive supranuclear palsy, or Steele-Richardson-Olszewski syndrome, is a rare, progressive brain disorder that causes serious and permanent problems with control of gait and balance. In particular, ocular motor control problems (blurred vision and difficulties looking up or down/saccades) and problems with speech and swallowing are commonly seen in progressive supranuclear palsy. Tremor is rare in these patients. Often there is retrocollis (hence tend to fall backwards) and a characteristic wide-eyed/astonished facial expression
Corticobasal degeneration	Corticobasal degeneration is a progressive neurological disorder with symptoms similar to those of Parkinson's disease, such as poor coordination, akinesia, rigidity, impaired balance, and limb dystonia. Both cortex and basal ganglia affected—cortical sensory loss and apraxia are important clinical signs
Dementia with Lewy bodies	Neurodegenerative dementia associated with Parkinsonism. Well-formed and detailed visual hallucinations; may be accompanied by delusions

8. **b**—Bilateral STN

A number of prospective and randomized trials comparing STN and GPi DBS have contributed to a better definition of the differences between these two targets. STN stimulation is superior for rigidity, bradykinesia, cost (medication reduction and less frequent battery change) and is more popular for tremor due to proximity to zona incerta. GPi stimulation is superior for dyskinesia, dystonia (including levodopa-unresponsive; STN only works for levodopa-responsive), cognition, mood and apathy, axial motor symptoms, does not adversely affect speech/swallowing, can be implanted unilaterally, and requires less frequent programming (initially). The motor benefits can be similar with each target, but STN offers greater benefit for off-symptoms, facilitates medication dose lowering and is most cost efficient, whereas dyskinesia suppression and long-term effects on postural stability and cognitive function favor GPi. STN stimulation may risk behavior and impulse control disorders, but medication reduction reduces these.

FURTHER READING

Fasano A, Lozano AM. Deep brain stimulation for movement disorders: 2015 and beyond. Curr Opin Neurol 2015;28:423-36.

9. **a**—Centromedian-parafascicular nucleus of thalamus

Tourette's syndrome is defined by the onset of motor and vocal tics before 18 years of age that cannot be ascribed to another medical condition. Tics must occur multiple times over at least 1 year and must evolve over time. The first tics are usually observed around the age of 5 or 6, and tic severity peaks 4-5 years later, and is lowest in patients' early 20s, coincident with frontal lobe maturation. Tics are worsened by heightened emotional states, stress, and fatigue. The tics of Tourette's syndrome are commonly accompanied by attention-deficit/hyperactivity disorder (ADHD) and obsessive-compulsive disorder (OCD). In Tourette's syndrome, obsessions center on concerns with symmetry, fear of violent thoughts, and a need to perform activities in a particular manner (rather than fears of contamination and checking seen in primary OCD). These obsessions may lead to self-injurious behavior. There is evidence that it shows a sex-linked autosomal dominant mode of inheritance, and is due to dysfunction in the corticostriatal-thalamocortical loop. The most commonly used targets for DBS have been the thalamic nuclei (centromedian nucleus-parafascicular complex and ventral oral nuclei) followed by either the limbic (anteromedial) or motor (posteroventral) regions of GPi. A double-blind, randomized cross-over trial on GPi DBS has reported a significant improvement in tic severity, with an overall acceptable safety profile.

FURTHER READING

Fasano A, Lozano AM. Deep brain stimulation for movement disorders: 2015 and beyond. Curr Opin Neurol 2015;28:423-36.

10. **b**—VIM thalamic stimulation

DBS of the ventro-intermedius nucleus (Vim) of the thalamus is an effective treatment for essential tremor, tremor dominant PD and other types of tremor. In essential tremor, a loss of benefit is sometimes observed over time. In both short- and long-term studies, dysarthria and disequilibrium are the most frequent reported adverse effects, especially with bilateral stimulation. The very mild cerebellar ataxia displayed by ET patients may also be improved by the stimulation of the posterior subthalamic area (STA), beneath the inferior border of the Vim, where the dentato-thalamic tract runs—conversely strong stimulation worsens cerebellar side effects.

FURTHER READING

Fasano A, Lozano AM. Deep brain stimulation for movement disorders: 2015 and beyond. Curr Opin Neurol 2015;28:423-36.

11. **a**—GPi

GPi DBS in isolated dystonias (either generalized or segmental) is supported by strong evidence of success, with improvement. Improvement is sustained up to 10 years after surgery, although some patients need the implantation of additional GPi electrodes. In addition, there are encouraging results in cervical dystonia, myoclonus-dystonia and tardive dystonia, in which the outcome of DBS is usually excellent, rapid and sustained. Case reports have also shown that cranial/cervical dystonias may not recur when DBS has stopped working (for a variety of reasons) suggesting chronic changes to circuits.

FURTHER READING

Fasano A, Lozano AM. Deep brain stimulation for movement disorders: 2015 and beyond. Curr Opin Neurol 2015;28:423-36.

12. **c**—Bilateral thalamotomy is the treatment of choice in bilateral tremor dominant Parkinson's disease when deep brain stimulation is not possible

The best candidates for thalamotomy are patients with tremor-predominant PD or those with incapacitating benign essential tremor. Less predictable outcomes are seen with tremor and hemiballismus/chorea due to damage of the cerebellar tracts from cerebrovascular accidents, trauma or multiple sclerosis, and primary and secondary dystonias. It is important to confirm the clinical diagnosis of idiopathic PD or benign essential tremor since Parkinson's plus syndromes have a much poorer prognosis after thalamotomy. Evidence of cognitive decline, speech disorders, serious systemic disease, and advanced age are also considered contraindications to surgery. Specific complications of thalamotomy are due to inaccurate lesion placement or overly large lesions. Lesions placed too laterally may result in contralateral weakness due to injury of the posterior limb of the internal capsule (face and arm). Lesions placed too posterior may cause contralateral hemisensory deficits due to injury of the VC nucleus (e.g., numbness or paresthesias of the mouth or fingers). A significant proportion have transient dysarthria or dysphasia, and transient confusion and may persist permanently in some. Left thalamic lesions are associated with an increased risk for deficits in learning, verbal memory and dysarthria while right thalamic lesions are associated with impaired visuospatial memory and nonverbal performance abilities. Bilateral thalamotomies are associated with deficits in memory/cognition and speech problems (e.g., hypophonia, dysarthria, dysphasia, and abulia) in up to 60%, hence should not be undertaken routinely—where they must be done it should be staged and slight variation in the target coordinates between sides may reduce major side effects.

ANSWERS 13–18

Additional answers 13–18 available on ExpertConsult.com

EMI ANSWER

19. 1—m, Stereotypy; 2—b, Asterixis; 3—g, Chorea; 4—f, Bradykinesia; 5—e, Ballism; 6—i, Dyskinesia

Movement Disorder Symptoms

Bradykinesia	Bradykinesia refers to a decrease in movement velocity (a reduction in amplitude is termed hypokinesia). The term akinesia, when properly used, refers to a complete lack of movement or an inability to initiate movement
Rigidity	A function of enhanced static or postural reflexes and either a "lead pipe" or "cogwheel" quality (tremor superimposed on rigidity) and is typically asymmetric
Chorea	Chorea refers to an involuntary, continual, irregular hyperkinetic disorder in which movements or movement fragments with variable rate and direction occur unpredictably and randomly. All body parts may be involved, and usually worsen during attempted voluntary action. Individuals may generate semivolitional movements that attempt to mask the involuntary choreic movements or incorporate them into seemingly purposeful movements, such as touching the face (parakinesias)
Ballism	An involuntary, high-amplitude, flinging movements typically generated proximally. May be brief or continual and may occur with chorea. Where there is hemiballism (one side of the body affected, usually due to a STN lesion), it may become milder and evolve into chorea over time
Athetosis	Slow, writhing, continuous, involuntary movements (not sustained postures like dystonia). It often accompanies basal ganglia disorders producing chorea or dystonia
Akithisia	Akathisia refers either to an uncomfortable sensation of inner restlessness or to the voluntary activity performed to relieve that restlessness. It is often manifested by an inability to remain seated, crossing and uncrossing the legs, or pacing. Causes include neuroleptic medication, but may be difficult to distinguish from tics and restless legs syndrome (RLS)
Dystonia	Dystonia refers to a group of disorders characterized by involuntary muscle contractions (sustained or spasmodic) that lead to abnormal body movements or postures

Continued

Dyskinesia	Dyskinesia refers to any disordered (non-rhythmic) and involuntary, non-suppressible movement including chorea/athetosis/ballism (and to a lesser degree dystonia). The limbs, neck, and face are the most frequently affected, but axial symptoms may also occur. When dyskinesia occurs in the face, the features may appear wry or overanimated. Head bobbing, blinking, lip smacking, and tongue protrusion are common. When dyskinesia occurs in the limbs, the movements may be proximal or distal and of either high or low amplitude. The limbs may tap, whirl, or writhe. Dyskinesia syndromes include abdominal (belly dancer's) dyskinesia, levodopa-induced dyskinesia, tardive dyskinesia, and the paroxysmal dyskinesias
Tremor	Involuntary rhythmic oscillation of a body part about a set point. The tremor may be regular or irregular, unilateral or bilateral, symmetrical or asymmetric, and present in one or several body regions. The frequency and amplitude of a tremor depend heavily on its underlying cause
Myoclonus	A sudden, arrhythmic, involuntary movement that is "shock-like" in its rapidity. When multiple, these movements do not flow into one another, which distinguishes them from chorea. True myoclonus is due to brief synchronous firing of agonist and antagonist muscles. Positive myoclonus occurs with active muscle contraction (e.g., hypnic jerks, a sudden body-wide contraction that occurs as a person drifts between sleep and wakefulness). Myoclonus is most often encountered as one of a collection of symptoms rather than as a pathology's primary manifestation. Symptomatic myoclonus may be a feature of any process involving cortical, basal ganglionic, or cerebellar degeneration, such as Creutzfeldt-Jakob disease or PD; Hepatic, renal, endocrine, and other metabolic derangements; myoclonic epilepsies, periodic leg movements of sleep and others
Ataxia	Clumsy or poorly organized movements due to deficits in the cerebellar, vestibular, or proprioceptive pathways. It may affect speech, manual dexterity, or gait and patients often complain of feeling as though they are drunk. Pure ataxia is not associated with deficits in strength or motor planning. Movements are poorly aimed or timed; patients have difficulty properly estimating the distance required to reach a target or terminating an action at the proper moment
Clonus	Rhythmic movement from hyperactive stretch reflex
Asterixis	An example of negative myoclonus and consists of sudden and involuntary relaxation of a dorsiflexed hand or other body part. The EMG pattern of negative myoclonus is distinctive, with aperiodic electrophysiologic silences in the antagonist muscle groups
Tic	Brief movements (motor tic) that are commonly preceded by a feeling of discomfort that builds until the tic appears, followed by a temporary feeling of relief. These preceding "premonitory urges" may consist of a feeling of itching or tension in the affected body part (sensory tic). One of the hallmarks of tics is that they are temporarily suppressible, although they typically rebound with increased frequency and severity after conscious suppression. They are both purposefully executed but performed out of a feeling of need ("semivoluntary" or "involuntary"). Tics can be clonic (i.e., brief), dystonic (i.e., sustained), or phonic (vocal). Simple tics consist of isolated actions, such as throat clearing or winking. Complex tics consist of speech or coordinated actions. They sometimes include obscene gestures (copropraxia) or vocalizations (coprolalia)
Stereotypies	Stereotypies are repetitive movements or vocalizations that mimic a purposeful action, are performed outside that action's normal context, and are involuntary or semivoluntary (e.g., hand wringing of Rett's syndrome). Stereotypies should be differentiated from automatisms (epilepsy) and perseverative/repetitive behavior (e.g., ADHD, OCD)

FURTHER READING

Clinical overview of movement disorders, In: Winn HR (Ed.), Youman's Neurological Surgery, vol. 4, 6th ed., Elsevier, Saunders, 2011 [Chapter 75].

20. 1—d, Essential tremor; 2—h, Parkinsonian tremor; 3—e, Holmes' tremor; 4—a, Cerebellar tremor

Types of Tremor

Essential tremor	The most common tremor disorder and is a low-amplitude, bilateral action and postural tremor with a frequency of 6-8 Hz. The tremor usually has its onset in adulthood and worsens over time, but it may begin in childhood and can coexist with other movement disorders. ET involves the upper limbs in more than 90% of patients. It less commonly involves the head, legs, or voice. Patients commonly first complain of difficulty with tasks requiring fine coordination, such as threading a needle, tying knots, or writing. Alcohol may temporarily alleviate symptoms, and family history is often positive. May be due to nonstructural cerebellar dysfunction with ET patients commonly have an intention tremor and difficulty with tandem gait
Dystonic tremor	Dystonic tremor is a jerky postural and task/action 3-8 Hz tremor that is abolished by complete rest and occurs in a body part affected by dystonia (e.g., limbs, trunk, head, vocal cords, or face). This contrasts with essential tremor in which the kinetic component is more or less constant throughout all postures. Dystonic tremor may occur with other involuntary movements including blepharospasm, torticollis, or spasmodic dysphonia. Isolated head tremor can be particularly challenging to distinguish between essential tremor and dystonic tremor (the latter of which can be exquisitely responsive to pharmacological treatment or botulinum toxin injections). The tremor caused by cervical dystonia is usually present as "no-no" kind of head shaking
Physiological tremor	Non-pathologic postural tremor, which typically has a frequency of 8-12 Hz. Both ET and physiologic tremor can be elicited by posture, both are fairly symmetrical, and both occur predominantly in the arms. Observing the progression of a tremor over time will eventually reveal whether a given patient has ET or physiologic tremor
Holme's tremor	Although predominantly an action tremor, Holmes tremor frequently has a significant resting component. The amplitude of movement tends to be large and it can sometimes adopt a "wing-beating" appearance. It is also among the slowest tremors, with frequencies often less than 4 Hz. It can occur with lesions affecting not only the red nucleus and rubral spinal tract in the brainstem but also the cerebellum and thalamus. The tremor may appear weeks to months after a known lesion (e.g., stroke), and some patients may have associated dystonia
Neuropathic tremor	Tremor may accompany diseases of the anterior horn cell (e.g., amyotropic lateral sclerosis) and peripheral neuropathies. It is unclear whether tremor associated with peripheral neuropathy is due to enhanced physiologic tremor secondary to weakness, to an abnormality in the central nervous system, or both
Drug-induced tremor	The onset of tremor should be temporally related to drug ingestion and may be due to an enhancement of physiologic tremor (e.g., amiodarone, antidepressants, antiepileptic medications, beta-agonist bronchodilators, caffeine, lithium, neuroleptics, nicotine, steroids, and sympathomimetics) or production of cerebellar tremor (immunosuppressive agents and acute/chronic alcohol)
Psychogenic tremor	Clinical features suggesting psychogenic tremor include sudden onset with severe presentations, inconsistent combinations of resting and postural or kinetic tremor, entrainment (change in frequency of tremor to that of a task performed in another body part, e.g., a patient with left hand tremor who taps at various frequencies with the right hand will have a left hand that acquires those frequencies), and tremor that diminishes with distraction
Parkinsonian tremor	A 4-9 Hz low-amplitude rest tremor, often with a "pill-rolling" quality. A typical pattern of spread is for the dominant hand to be affected first, followed by the dominant foot and then the non-dominant hand. Re-emergent tremor occurs while sustaining a prolonged position and most likely represents a rest tremor that has been reset by the relative stasis of a persistent position. Postural tremor that begins immediately on adopting a position is seen in as many as 93% of patients with PD and correlates with the degree of functional disability. Treatment with levodopa improves bradykinesia and rigidity more reliably than it does tremor
Cerebellar tremor	Cerebellar tremor is characterized as a jerky, low-frequency (2-5 Hz), high-amplitude action tremor. This tremor may be accompanied by other cerebellar signs such as ataxia, dysdiadochokinesia, dysarthria, dysmetria, and telegraphic speech
Post-traumatic tremor	The character of the tremor depends on the region of the brain that is damaged. Damage to the brainstem may produce rest tremor if it affects the substantia nigra and related pathways. Damage to the cerebellum may result in a low-frequency

Continued

	action tremor. Because multiple regions are usually damaged, post-traumatic tremors are generally mixed in character. Post-traumatic tremor is often accompanied by myoclonus
Primary orthostatic tremor	Uncommon condition that starts in late adulthood with feeling of tremulousness in the legs when standing (but not sitting or lying). The diagnosis is helped by specific surface EMG showing a 14-18-Hz oscillating tremor in the musculature of the legs when standing, disappearing with rest or movement
Palatal tremor (Palatal myoclonus/nystagmus)	A rare disorder presenting as unilateral or bilateral rhythmic involuntary movements of the soft palate. The movement consists of repetitive rather than oscillatory movements of agonist muscles only, thus having some similarity with myoclonus. The tremors in essential palatal tremor produce audible click due to the contraction of the tensor valipalatini muscle which disappear during sleep, whereas in symptomatic palatal tremor there is no audible click but it continues during sleep

21. 1—i, Sydenham's chorea.

A delayed complication of infection with group A β-hemolytic streptococci that usually develops 4-8 weeks after the infection, and the most common cause of acute childhood chorea in the world. The typical age at onset of Sydenham's chorea is 8-9 years; it is rarely seen in children younger than 5 years. The chorea usually generalizes but some patients remain hemichoreic. Associated symptoms include tics, OCD, and ADHD. The disease is self-limited and spontaneously remits after 8-9 months in a large percentage of patients, but up to 50% may still have chorea 2 years after infection. Huntington's disease typically presents with neuropsychiatric symptoms that predate choreiform movements. 2—j, Wilson's disease. An autosomal recessive disorder of copper metabolism that causes both liver and basal ganglia damage (*hepatolenticular degeneration).* usually appear between the ages of 11 and 25. Patients typically have a Parkinsonian akinetic-rigid syndrome, generalized dystonia, or a proximal postural/action tremor with ataxia and dysarthria. Although pure chorea may be seen in Wilson's disease, it is an unusual manifestation of the syndrome. Psychiatric findings include pseudobulbar affect, impulsivity, and depression. Ceruloplasmin testing may be normal hence elevated 24-h urinary copper levels is diagnostic. The classic Kaiser-Fleischer rings—flecks of copper visible in the cornea under slit-lamp examination—are almost universally present in patients with neurological symptoms. 3—c, Cerebrovascular disease. 4—d, Chorea gravidarum. Chorea in pregnancy usually presents in the first or second trimester, and may be autoimmune in nature. The severity of the chorea tends to decrease as the pregnancy progresses. Approximately a third of patients see their symptoms resolve after delivery. 5—g, Neuroacanthosis. Includes *choreoacanthocytosis* and *McLeod's syndrome*, which both show acanthocytes on peripheral smear, peripheral neuropathy, psychiatric symptoms, and seizures. Choreoacanthocytosis is an autosomal recessive disease with an age at onset of 20-40 years and orofacial dystonia (e.g., lip and tongue biting, involuntarily push food out of their mouths with their tongue when eating), generalized chorea, dystonia, and tics can also occur. Abnormalities of saccadic eye movement may develop, similar to those in HD. Symptoms of McLeod's syndrome include limb weakness, chorea, cognitive decline, paranoia, and schizophrenia.

- Genetic causes include Huntington's disease, neuroacanthocytosis, and Wilson's disease.
- Infectious causes include rheumatic fever causing Sydenham's chorea, chorea gravidarum during pregnancy, and spongiform encephalopathy (e.g., prion disease).
- Drug-induced causes include oral contraceptives, tricyclic antidepressants, cimetidine, digoxin, verapamil, baclofen, steroids, and antiepileptics.
- Strokes in the thalamic area of the brain can also cause choreiform movements.

22. 1—f, Meige syndrome.

Meige syndrome is a form of focal dystonia characterized by blepharospasm, forceful jaw opening, lip retraction, neck contractions, and tongue thrusting. Sometimes these features are produced by phenothiazine or butyrophenone use, but they may also occur idiopathically, more often in women than men, with onset in the sixth decade. Botulinum toxin injection has been more effective in treatment than any oral medication. 2—a, DYT1 dystonia (Oppenheim's dystonia). Primary dystonias are either sporadic mutations or heritable. The most common cause of early-onset generalized dystonia is DYT1 dystonia (Oppenheim's dystonia). It occurs relatively frequently in the Ashkenazi Jewish population, with a prevalence of 1 in 2000. DYT1 is inherited in an autosomal dominant fashion with a penetrance of 30-40%. The onset of symptoms is usually in late childhood/early adolescence, and they generally begin in one leg and later generalize. Dystonia plus syndromes are conditions in which Parkinsonism, tremor, or myoclonus develop in addition to dystonia. Dystonia plus can be divided into dystonia-Parkinsonism (DYT3 and DYT12), dopa-responsive dystonia (DYT5), paroxysmal dystonia (DYT8, DYT9, and DYT10), and myoclonus-dystonia (DYT11). 3—b, DYT5 dystonia (Segawa's disease). DYT5, or Segawa's disease, is a childhood-onset levodopa-responsive dystonia. The initial symptom is generally foot dystonia, with a marked diurnal fluctuation that attenuates with age. A postural tremor typically develops in adulthood, followed later by bradykinesia. Rest tremor is absent. Response to levodopa is marked and sustained. Both autosomal dominant and autosomal recessive subtypes have been identified. DYT11 has its onset in childhood or adolescence and is manifested as dystonia with alcohol-responsive proximal myoclonic jerks. The dystonia is usually mild and present in 50% of patients. Cervical dystonia and writer's cramp are the most common. Many adults with myoclonus-dystonia syndrome report dramatic improvement in their symptoms with alcohol ingestion.

Secondary dystonia is caused by basal ganglia insults (stroke, demyelination, hypoxia, trauma), Huntington's disease, Wilson's disease, Parkinson's syndromes, drugs and lysosomal storage diseases.

23. 1—b, Blepharospasm; 2—h, Paresthesia; 3—j, Tonic contraction; 4—h, Paresthesias; 5—a, Ataxia

General risks of DBS surgery include infection, intracerebral hemorrhage, electrode malposition, and lead-related complications (fractures/infection). Stimulation related side effects related to direction of current spread and adjacent structures and are outlined below:

Target	Current Spread	Site Affected	Side Effect
STN	STN	STN	Blepharospasm
	Anterior	Corticospinal tract Hypothalamus	Tonic contractions Sweating/flushing
	Posterior	Medial lemniscus	Paresthesias
	Medial	Red nucleus	Ataxia
	Inferomedial	CNIII/Supranuclear oculomotor center	Diplopia
	Lateral	Corticobulbar tract	Dysarthria
GPi	Anterior	Optic tract	Photopsias
	Posterior	Medial lemniscus	Paresthesias
	Posteromedial	Internal capsule	Tonic contraction
VIM thalamus	Target	VIM thalamus	Microthalamotomy effect
	Anterior	Cerebellothalamic tract	Ataxia
	Posterior	VPL thalamus	Paresthesia
	Lateral	Internal capsule	Tonic contraction

24. 1—e, Levodopa-carbidopa; 2—i, Rotigotine; 3— j, Selegiline; 4—d, Entacapone

It is generally accepted that symptomatic therapy should start when a patient becomes functionally impaired, although functional impairment is highly individualized depending on symptoms and patient lifestyle. The activities of daily living subscale of the UPDRS is useful to assess disability. Current opinion is divided about when to start therapy with levodopa-carbidopa. Delay may minimize the risks of motor complications and theoretical progression of disease by oxidant radical formation from the metabolism of

Medical Management of Parkinson's Disease

Drug Class	Example	Role
MAOI-B	Selegiline Rasagiline	May have neuroprotective effect hence given early in disease. Selegiline blocks free radical formation during dopamine oxidation
Levodopa	Levodopa-carbidopa	Usually first line in elderly patients; can lead to motor complications with prolonged treatment. Conversion of L-dopa to dopamine occurs outside the CNS in a wide variety of tissues, but once converted to dopamine in the periphery, the drug becomes inaccessible to the brain. Peripheral conversion of L-dopa to dopamine is routinely inhibited by adding a dopa decarboxylase inhibitor (carbidopa). Because it is cannot cross the blood-brain barrier, carbidopa cannot inhibit the conversion of L-dopa to dopamine in the brain
Dopamine agonists	Pramipexole Ropinerole Rotigotine (transdermal)	Usually first line in young patients (early onset PD). For elderly patients, dopamine agonists are often a second-line option. The effects of these agents are independent of degenerating dopaminergic neurons. Therefore, the use of dopamine agonists may avoid problems associated with levodopa-carbidopa. The dopamine agonists do not, however, improve all types of symptoms and have specific dopaminergic adverse effects. Rotigotine is a dopamine agonist that is administered transdermally and offers continuous dopaminergic stimulation. It is approved by the FDA for early-stage idiopathic Parkinson's disease
	Apomorphine	For the treatment of acute, intermittent hypomobility and "off" episodes
NMDA antagonist	Amantidine	Potentiates dopaminergic response with a mild anticholinergic effect and can be used for early Parkinsonism, as well as for reduction of levodopa-induced dyskinesias associated with later-stage Parkinson's disease
Anticholinergic	Benztropine	Treatment of isolated tremor
COMT inhibitor	Entacapone	Reduce motor fluctuation by extending the duration of action of levodo pa-carbidopa, thus having a dose-sparing effect and reducing "off-time"
Antidepressant	SSRI and TCA	TCAs are contraindicated in patients taking MAOI
Cholinesterase inhibitor	Rivastigmine	Treatment of mild to moderate dementia includes improve cognition and activities of daily living in about 15% of patients

levodopa. Most specialists, in fact, delay its introduction, giving less potent medications a trial first, especially in younger patients. Levodopa-carbidopa is generally the first-choice medication for most elderly patients and is almost universally effective. Combination therapy begins with the addition of a COMT inhibitor to levodopa-carbidopa. Dopamine agonists and levodopa-carbidopa can be tried next. In some patients, it may be necessary to use all three agents. Parkinson's related depression is the most common nonmotor symptom in Parkinson's disease, affecting 40% of patients.

25. 1—h, Peak dose dyskinesia; 2—a, Acute akinesia; 3—j, Wearing-off phenomenon; 4—e, Dystonia

Motor fluctuations are alterations between periods of being "on," during which the patient experiences a positive response to medication, and being "off," during which the patient experiences a re-emergence of the Parkinson's symptoms. Levodopa-induced dyskinesia encompass a variety of involuntary movements, including chorea, dystonia, ballism, and myoclonus. Dyskinesia tend to appear when the patient is "on" and are usually choreiform. Dyskinesia in the "off" state is more commonly dystonic but can be any of those listed above. Early morning dystonic inversion of a foot (usually on the side of greater Parkinsonian involvement) occurs as a withdrawal reaction because of the long interval without medication overnight. Dyskinesia are sometimes mistaken for manifestations of progressive PD or confused with tremor by patients and their families, rather than recognized as

Motor Complications of Parkinson's Disease

Motor Phenomena in PD	Description
Wearing off phenomenon	Re-emergence of Parkinsonian motor problems as the effect of levodopa diminishes near the end of the dose interval (i.e., usually before 4 h)
Unpredictable off periods	Transitions from being "on" to being "off" bearing no obvious relationship with the time of levodopa administration. May be due to erratic absorption of levodopa from the gut and pharmacodynamic changes in the brain
Freezing of gait	Occurs as a transient "off" phenomenon or randomly at variable frequency in patients with advanced PD. Patients suddenly become immobilized for seconds to minutes at a time, usually when initiating walking, in a confined space such as a doorway or a closet, or when getting on or off an elevator and may cause falls. Random freezing is poorly responsive to anti-Parkinson's medications and DBS
No-on phenomenon	Lack of an "on" response following a dose of levodopa. May be due to delayed gastric motility, especially when no-on preceded by an excessively prolonged or severe "off" period
Acute akinesia	Sudden severe exacerbation of PD including an akinetic state that lasts for several days and does not respond to treatment with anti-Parkinson's medication. Commonly due to systemic infection or other intercurrent medical problem
Peak-dose dyskinesia	Peak dose or "on" dyskinesia is usually choreiform in type: appearance of restlessness and continuous jerky, involuntary movements of the extremities, head, face, trunk, or respiratory muscles, typically starting 30-90 min after a dose of levodopa. Remarkably well tolerated by most patients as prefer being "on" with dyskinesia to being "off," but severe dyskinesia may take the form of large amplitude, ballistic movements that interfere with function and become very disturbing to patients and their families
Diphasic dyskinesia	Uncommon form where dyskinesia peaks twice after each dose—first when patients turn "on" and again when they begin to turn "off." In the second phase, dyskinesia (often involving the legs) in one body part may coexist with the emergence elsewhere in the body of Parkinsonian signs such as tremor and bradykinesia
Dystonia	Dystonia can be a manifestation of early untreated PD or may appear as a complication of levodopa treatment. Dystonia in young-onset PD most commonly involves the foot, typically taking onset as exercise-induced cramp-like discomfort, first noticed in the toes and later evolving into inversion of the affected foot, sometimes bringing the person to a halt (kinesigenic foot dystonia). Dystonia is also common in non-medicated patients with Parkinson's plus syndromes (e.g., retrocollis, blepharospasm). Dystonia due to levodopa can occur either as a peak levodopa effect or during "off" periods due to levodopa withdrawal. Withdrawal dystonia most commonly occurs in the early morning when it produces painful flexion and inversion postures of the feet and toes
Akathisia	Another form of levodopa withdrawal is akathisia or motor restlessness, which may resemble restless legs syndrome, and usually occurs at night, several hours after the last dose of levodopa. This is managed by providing slow release levodopa or a dopamine agonist before retiring
Camptocormia	Camptocormia is an apparently fixed trunkal flexion deformity that disappears in recumbent position

reversible consequences of levodopa treatment. Dyskinesia occurs in 30-40% of patients treated with levodopa during the first 5 years of use and nearly 60% or more by 10 years. Management usually involves adjusting the levodopa doses and dosing schedule, adding an additional anti-Parkinsonian medication or manipulating dietary protein intake.

FURTHER READING

Motor fluctuations and dyskinesia in Parkinson disease. Uptodate. Topic 4893 Version 20.0.

CHAPTER 36

SURGERY FOR PSYCHIATRIC DISORDERS

SINGLE BEST ANSWER (SBA) QUESTIONS

1. In anorexia nervosa, which one of the following surgical targets has been most used?
   a. Anterior nucleus of thalamus
   b. Hypothalamus
   c. Inferior thalamic peduncle
   d. Subgenual anterior cingulate
   e. Subthalamic nucleus

2. In Alzheimer's disease, which one of the following targets for deep brain stimulation has shown promise?
   a. Caudate
   b. Fornix
   c. Globus pallidus externa
   d. Hippocampus
   e. Nucleus accumbens

3. Circuit pathophysiology in OCD has been localized to which one of the following?
   a. Corticoreticular circuit
   b. Corticostriatal-thalamocortical circuit
   c. Nigro-striatal circuit
   d. Nigro-pallidal circuit
   e. Thalamocortical circuit

4. Targets for deep brain stimulation for obsessive-compulsive disorder do not include which one of the following?
   a. Anterior limb of the internal capsule
   b. Centromedian-parafascicular nucleus of thalamus
   c. Inferior thalamic peduncle
   d. Subthalamic nucleus
   e. Ventral capsule/ventral striatum

5. Which one of the following targets is not currently used in deep brain stimulation for treatment-resistant depression?
   a. Anterior limb of the internal capsule
   b. Nucleus accumbens
   c. Subgenual anterior cingulate
   d. Subthalamic nucleus
   e. Ventral capsule/ventral striatum

6. Anterior cingulotomy involves which one of the following?
   a. Bilateral burr holes and thermocoagulation
   b. Parasagittal approach to cingulate gyrus
   c. Division of fibers connecting the orbital cortex to subcortical and limbic areas
   d. Exclusion of obsessive-compulsive symptoms preoperatively
   e. The target site for the lesion is 20-25 mm posterior to the anterior horn of the lateral ventricles, 7 mm from the midline and 20 mm above corpus callosum.

7. Which one of the following components is LEAST important in the mechanism of vagal nerve stimulation for treatment-refractory depression is most accurate?
   a. Amygdala
   b. Hippocampus
   c. Locus coereleus
   d. Prefrontal cortex
   e. Red nucleus

8. Which one of the following statements regarding indications for lesional neurosurgical procedures for mental disorder is most accurate?
   a. Cerebrovascular disease and pre-existing epilepsy are absolute contraindications
   b. Patients can be treated in their best interests with neurosurgery for mental disorder
   c. Used occasionally to control affective or obsessional symptoms due to active organic or degenerative brain disease
   d. Can be considered in personality disorder and schizophrenia if the aim of the surgery is restricted to chronic intractable affective or obsessional comorbid symptoms
   e. Not currently performed in a multidisciplinary team setting

EXTENDED MATCHING ITEM (EMI) QUESTIONS

9. **Surgery for psychiatric disorders:**
   a. Anterior capsulotomy
   b. Anterior cingulotomy
   c. Electroconvulsive therapy
   d. Limbic leucotomy
   e. Nucleus accumbens DBS
   f. Subcaudate tractotomy
   g. Subthalamic nucleus DBS
   h. Transcranial magnetic stimulation
   i. Vagal nerve stimulation
   j. Ventral capsule/Ventral striatum DBS

For each of the following descriptions, select the most appropriate answers from the list above. Each answer may be used once, more than once or not at all.

1. Generates a magnetic field that traverses the cranium and induces an electrical field in the cortex. Used for measuring and modulating cortical plasticity approved for use in medication-refractory depression.
2. Division of fibers connecting the orbital cortex to subcortical and limbic areas (e.g. thalamus, basal ganglia, amygdala). Lesions are placed in the white matter of the substantia innominata, below the head of the caudate nucleus.

SBA ANSWERS

1. **d**—Subgenual anterior cingulate

A number of small recent studies have described the possible use of DBS in the treatment of anorexia nervosa and associated mood include subgenual anterior cingulate and nucleus accumbens.

FURTHER READING

Fitzgerald PB, Segrave RA. Deep brain stimulation in mental health: review of evidence for clinical efficacy. Aust N Z J Psychiatry 2015. pii: 0004867415598011. [Epub ahead of print] Review. PubMed PMID: 26246408.

2. **b**—Fornix

The two targets being investigated clinically that hold promise for dementias are the fornix for Alzheimer's disease, and the nucleus basalis of Meynert for dementia with Lewy bodies.

FURTHER READING

Zhang Q, Kim YC, Narayanan NS. Disease-modifying therapeutic directions for Lewy-Body dementias. Front Neurosci 2015;9:293.

3. **b**—Corticostriatal-thalamocortical circuit

Functional neuroimaging studies have implicated corticostriatal-thalamocortical circuitry in the pathophysiology of OCD. More specifically, in patients with OCD, there is abnormal (predominately increased) metabolic activity in the orbitofrontal cortex (OFC), the anterior cingulate cortex (ACC), medial prefrontal cortex and the caudate nucleus, particularly its ventral division. OFC and caudate hyperactivity are directly correlated with symptom severity, and these changes partially normalize with successful treatment.

4. **b**—Centromedian-parafascicular nucleus of thalamus

OCD has a prevalence of 1-3% of the population and is characterized by recurrent, intrusive anxious thoughts (obsessions) accompanied by repetitive stereotyped behaviors or mental routines (compulsions) that are frequently performed in an effort to reduce distress caused by obsessions. These can significantly hinder interpersonal relationships, social and occupational functioning, and the ability to carry out basic activities of daily living; it is associated with a higher lifetime risk of suicide (up to 27% of patients), as well as major depression. Treatment for OCD typically involves pharmacotherapy (e.g. selective serotonin reuptake inhibitors) which is often combined with psychotherapy (e.g. cognitive behavioral therapy/exposure and response prevention). Up to half of OCD patients do not obtain adequate benefit with standard treatment approaches, and approximately 10% experience severe treatment-refractory symptoms. Identification of DBS targets for OCD has been based on a combination of experience from lesional psychosurgery procedures, following observations of response to surgery for other conditions (e.g. STN DBS for PD) as well as gradual target refinement following ongoing evaluation of clinical outcomes in relation to lead location. The neuroanatomical targets used for DBS in the treatment of OCD have included the anterior limb of the internal capsule, nucleus accumbens, ventral capsule/ventral striatum, STN, and the inferior thalamic peduncle.

FURTHER READING

Fitzgerald PB, Segrave RA. Deep brain stimulation in mental health: review of evidence for clinical efficacy. Aust N Z J Psychiatry 2015. pii: 0004867415598011 [Epub ahead of print] Review. PubMed PMID: 26246408.

5. **d**—Subthalamic nucleus

Depression is extremely common with a lifetime prevalence of 15-20%, with 30% of patients not responding to standard medications or psychotherapy. The management of treatment-resistant depression includes repeated trials of medication, psychotherapy, and forms of brain stimulation (transcranial magnetic stimulation and electroconvulsive therapy). However, there is a significant subgroup of patients (10-20%) who remain chronically treatment refractory, and relapse and development of resistance to ECT also poses problems. Targets for DBS applications in depression have been proposed based on (a) extrapolation from sites targeted in lesional psychosurgical procedures and (b) from the results of neuroimaging experiments. The majority of research to date has focused on DBS implantation in the white matter adjacent to the subgenual anterior cingulate and on stimulation of the anterior limb of the internal capsule and the associated ventral capsule/ventral striatum (including the nucleus accumbens). Less commonly described targets include superolateral branch of the median forebrain bundle, inferior thalamic peduncle, and lateral habenula.

FURTHER READING

Fitzgerald PB, Segrave RA. Deep brain stimulation in mental health: review of evidence for clinical efficacy. Aust N Z J Psychiatry 2015. pii: 0004867415598011. [Epub ahead of print] Review. PubMed PMID: 26246408.

6. **a**—Bilateral burr holes and thermocoagulation.

FURTHER READING

Christmas D, Morrison C, Eljamel MS, Matthews K. Neurosurgery for mental disorder. Adv Psychiatr Treat 2004;10:189-199

Lesional Surgery for Psychiatric Disorders

Procedure	Description	Indications
Anterior capsulotomy	Thermal damage or gamma knife surgery to target fibers connecting the ventromedial cortex, orbitofrontal cortex, and anterior cingulate gyrus with the thalamus, amygdala, and hippocampus. These fibers pass through the anterior one-third of the anterior limb of the internal capsule	Indications for anterior capsulotomy vary across Europe. In Sweden, it is used for generalized anxiety disorder, agoraphobia with panic disorder, and obsessive-compulsive disorder, whereas in the UK it is mainly used for depression and obsessive-compulsive disorder
Anterior cingulotomy	Targets are the supracallosal fibers of the cingulum bundle (part of the Papez circuit) as it travels through the anterior cingulate gyrus. The lesion procedure also results in damage to a localized area of anterior cingulate cortex. The target site for the lesion is 20-25 mm posterior to the anterior horn of the lateral ventricles, 7 mm from the midline and 2-3 mm above corpus callosum	Initially developed for the treatment of intractable pain, but its other indications include anxiety disorders, depressive disorders, and obsessive-compulsive disorder
Limbic leucotomy	The fibers targeted are those of the anterior cingulate cortex, the cingulum bundle, and frontostriatolimbic circuits. It is a combination of anterior cingulotomy and stereotactic subcaudate tractotomy, although the frontal lesions are slightly smaller than those conventionally created using stereotactic subcaudate tractotomy	Its main indications are for depression, obsessive-compulsive disorder, and anxiety disorder. Used as a treatment alternative where anterior cingulotomy has resulted in non-sustained or partial benefit
Stereotactic subcaudate tractotomy	Division of fibers connecting the orbital cortex to subcortical and limbic areas (e.g. thalamus, basal ganglia, amygdala). Lesions are placed in the white matter of the substantia innominata, below the head of the caudate nucleus. Typically, the lesions would be created using radioactive yttrium-90 rods inserted using stereotactic guidance	This procedure has been used to treat depression, obsessive-compulsive disorder, anxiety disorder, and chronic pain, although it is no longer offered within the UK

7. **e**—Red nucleus

Vagus nerve stimulation has become established for treatment-resistant, partial-onset seizure disorder. The vagus nerve is not only a parasympathetic efferent nerve—around 80% of its fibers are afferent sensory fibers transmitting information to the brain. There are sensory afferent connections of the vagus nerve in the nucleus tractus solitarius that, in turn, send ascending projections to the forebrain, mainly through the parabrachial nucleus and locus ceruleus. Further connections offer potential routes of communication with the amygdala, hippocampus, hypothalamus, insular cortex, dorsal thalamus, orbitofrontal cortex, and other important limbic regions linked to mood regulation. The initial rationale for using VNS for the treatment of refractory depression resulted from mood improvements in epilepsy patients treated with VNS, irrespective of the presence or absence of beneficial effects on seizure frequency. VNS demonstrated steadily increasing improvement of depressive symptoms with full benefit after 6-12 months, sustained for up to 2 years. These studies reported response rates of 30-40% and remission rates of 15-17% after 3-24 months of treatment. Preclinical animal studies may suggest that VNS exerts its antidepressant effects through a rapid increase in the concentration of the monoamines, which then enhance neuronal plasticity/neurogenesis in the hippocampus. Newborn cells could then functionally integrate and restore the disturbed corticolimbic networks in depressed patients, and may explain the therapeutic lag of VNS in the treatment of depression.

FURTHER READING

Grimonprez A, Raedt R, Baeken C, Boon P, Vonck K. The antidepressant mechanism of action of vagus nerve stimulation: evidence from preclinical studies. Neurosci Biobehav Rev 2015;56:26-34. doi:10.1016/j.neubiorev.2015.06.019 [Epub 2015 Jun 25]. Review. PubMed PMID: 26116875.

8. **d**—Can be considered in personality disorder and schizophrenia if the aim of the surgery is restricted to chronic intractable affective or obsessional comorbid symptoms

Neurosurgery for mental disorder has suffered historically from relatively "crude" lesional procedures (e.g. anterior cingulotomy, limbic leucotomy, subcaudate tractotomy), and a lack of rigorous investigation regarding both effectiveness and adverse effects on personality and cognition. Inclusion criteria are a secure diagnosis and the ability to provide informed consent. In all cases, such surgery can only be offered following careful and detailed consideration of the potential costs and benefits to the individual on a case-by-case basis by the multidisciplinary team. Obvious contraindications include patients with affective or obsessional symptoms due to active organic or degenerative brain disease, or where pervasive developmental disorder is likely (although cerebrovascular disease or pre-existing epilepsy is not an absolute contraindication). There is no evidence that personality disorders, anorexia nervosa, or schizophrenia respond to lesional neurosurgery and these patients should not be considered unless the aim of the surgery is restricted to chronic intractable affective or obsessional comorbid symptoms. Difficulties can arise in determining the suitability of patients where illness onset was at a sufficiently early age to have had an adverse impact on personality development. Neurosurgery for mental disorder is contraindicated if the patient is not fit for surgery because of a tendency to bleed, local infection, or a high anesthetic risk.

FURTHER READING

Christmas D, Morrison C, Eljamel MS, Matthews K. Neurosurgery for mental disorder. Adv Psychiatr Treat 2004;10:189-199

EMI ANSWERS

9. 1—h, Transcranial magnetic stimulation; 2—f, Subcaudate tractotomy

PART VI
PERIPHERAL NERVE SURGERY

CHAPTER 37

PERIPHERAL NERVE

SINGLE BEST ANSWER (SBA) QUESTIONS

1. Which one of the following type of nerve fiber carries fast pain and temperature sensation?
   a. Type A alpha
   b. Type A beta
   c. Type A delta
   d. Type A gamma
   e. Type B
   f. Type C

2. Which one of the following tests is best for confirming an isolated cervical radiculopathy?
   a. Compound muscle action potential (CMAP)
   b. F-wave
   c. H-reflex
   d. Insertional activity on EMG
   e. Sensory Nerve Action Potential (SNAP)

3. EMG abnormalities in which one of the following muscles is LEAST specific for C5 radiculopathy?
   a. Infraspinatus
   b. Levator scapulae
   c. Pronator teres
   d. Rhomboids
   e. Supraspinatus

4. Fibrillation potentials are an indicator of:
   a. Dorsal root ganglion injury
   b. Motor axon loss
   c. Muscle necrosis
   d. Reinnervation
   e. Sensory axon loss

5. Which one of the following is the earliest electrophysiological change seen in radiculopathy?
   a. Fibrillation potentials
   b. Increased number of motor unit potentials
   c. Positive sharp spikes
   d. Reduced CMAP
   e. Reduced interference pattern

6. Which one of the following best describes a motor unit potential?
   a. Sum of conduction velocities of motor neurons
   b. Seen during muscle necrosis
   c. Reinnervation potential
   d. Sensory axon loss
   e. Sum of electrical activity from muscle fibers supplied by the same motor neuron

7. The F-wave is useful when trying to confirm which one of the following:
   a. Bilateral carpal tunnel syndrome
   b. Isolated C7 nerve root lesion
   c. Isolated S1 nerve root lesion
   d. Multiple proximal motor root compromise
   e. Multiple sensory root compromise

8. The H-reflex is used in which one of the following scenarios:
   a. Suspected common peroneal nerve palsy
   b. Suspected L4 radiculopathy
   c. Suspected L5 radiculopathy
   d. Suspected lumbar plexopathy
   e. Suspected S1 radiculopathy

9. Which one of the following are features of a primarily demyelinating neuropathy?

a. Fibrillation potentials
b. Increased insertional activity
c. Polyphasic waves
d. Positive sharp spikes
e. Reduced conduction velocity

● 10. A 76-year-old woman presented with numbness and tingling of the hands that had persisted for the previous 5 weeks. Examination revealed mild limitation of neck movements. Strength and reflexes were normal. She had mild atrophy of the right thenar muscles. Pain sensation was decreased in the radial 3½ digits; Phalen's test was positive bilaterally. Neurologic examination was otherwise negative and the EMG was done.

Motor nerve studies

Nerve and Site	Latency (ms)	Amplitude (mV)	Conduction Velocity (m/s)
Median nerve R.	Normal ≤ 4.2	Normal ≥ 6	Normal ≥ 50
Wrist	7.8	1.7	-
Elbow	12.2	1.7	55
Ulnar nerve R.	Normal ≤ 3.6	Normal ≥ 8	Normal ≥ 50
Wrist	3.0	11	-
Elbow	6.4	10	56
Median nerve L.	Normal ≤ 4.2	Normal ≥ 6	Normal ≥ 50
Wrist	4.3	6	-
Elbow	8.4	6	55

F-wave studies

Nerve	Latency (ms)	Normal Latency ≤ (ms)
Median nerve R.	39.4	30
Ulnar nerve R.	27.2	30
Median nerve L.	28.1	30

Sensory nerve studies

Nerve	Onset Latency (ms)	Normal Onset Latency ≤ (ms)	Peak Latency (ms)	Normal Peak Latency ≤ (ms)	Amp (μV)	Normal Amp ≥ (μV)	Conduction Velocity (m/s)	Normal Conduction Velocity ≥ (m/s)
Median nerve R.	6.5	2.6	7.0	3.1	5	20	20	50
Ulnar nerve R.	2.4	2.6	2.9	3.1	25	13	50	50
Median nerve L.	3.4	2.6	3.9	3.1	26	20	38	50

EMG data

Muscle	Insert Activity	Fibs	Pos Waves	Fasc	Amp	Dur	Poly	Pattern
Brachioradialis R.	Norm	None	None	None	Norm	Norm	None	Full
Flexor carpi ulnaris R.	Norm	None	None	None	Norm	Norm	None	Full
Extensor digitorum communis R.	Norm	None	None	None	Norm	Norm	None	Full
Abductor pollicis brevis R.	Norm	None	None	None	Lg	Inc	None	Red
First dorsal interosseous R.	Norm	None	None	None	Norm	Norm	None	Full

Results from Bertorini TE. Neuromuscular Case Studies, 1st ed., Butterworth-Heinemann, Elsevier, Case 1, 2008.

Which one of the following explains her symptoms?
a. C6 and C7 radiculopathy
b. C6 radiculopathy
c. Carpal tunnel syndrome
d. Musculocutaneous nerve entrapment
e. Ulnar nerve entrapment

11. A 57-year-old man presented with an 8 week history of progressive weakness and wasting in the left hand and mild numbness in the little finger. His past medical history was positive for poliomyelitis as a child, which left residual weakness in both legs. He had an almost complete recovery except for a mild deformity of the left foot. He did have occasional fasciculations in the leg. On examination, the left hand interossei muscles were wasted but without fasciculations. He had a positive Froment's sign and a Tinel's sign below the left elbow. When extending his fingers, the last two digits had a tendency to remain flexed. He could not "cup" the left hand. Adson's maneuver was negative. There was decreased pain sensation in the left little finger and the ulnar half of the ring finger with equivocal decreased pain sensation in the ulnar aspect of the dorsum of the hand. All reflexes were mildly depressed.

Motor nerve studies

Nerve and Site	Latency (ms)	Amplitude (mV)	Conduction Velocity (m/s)
Median nerve L.	Normal ≤ 4.2	Normal ≥ 6	Normal ≥ 50
Wrist	4.7	11	-
Elbow	9.8	10	53
Ulnar nerve L.	Normal ≤ 3.6	Normal ≥ 8	Normal ≥ 50
Wrist	3.5	3	-
Below elbow	8.3	3	57
Above elbow	11.4	1	39
Axilla	13.2	1	67
Peroneal nerve L.	Normal ≤ 5.7	Normal ≥ 3	Normal ≥ 40
Ankle	5.2	4	-
Fibular head	12.3	4	44
Knee	14.3	4	50
Median nerve R.	Normal ≤ 4.2	Normal ≥ 6	Normal ≥ 50
Wrist	4.3	15	-
Elbow	9.3	14	54
Ulnar nerve R.	Normal ≤ 3.6	Normal ≥ 8	Normal ≥ 50
Wrist	2.7	10	-
Below elbow	7.2	10	58
Above elbow	9.6	10	50

F-wave studies

Nerve	Latency (ms)	Normal Latency ≤ (ms)
Median nerve L.	30.7	30
Ulnar nerve L.	33.0	30
Peroneal nerve L.	54.9	54
Median nerve R.	30.8	30
Ulnar nerve R.	32.1	30

Inching technique: ulnar nerve L.

Stimulation Site	Latency (ms)	Amplitude (mV)
4 cm below elbow	8.1	3.3
3 cm below elbow	8.3	3.1
2 cm below elbow	9.0*	1.4
1 cm below elbow	9.7*	1.3
Ulnar groove	9.8	1.3
1 cm above elbow	9.9	1.3
2 cm above elbow	10.0	1.1
3 cm above elbow	10.1	1.1

*0.2 ms difference allowed between stimulation sites.

Sensory nerve studies

Nerve	Onset Latency (ms)	Normal Onset Latency ≤(ms)	Peak Latency (ms)	Normal Peak Latency ≤(ms)	Amp (μV)	Normal Amp≥ (μV)	Conduction Velocity (m/s)	Normal Conduction Velocity≥(m/s)
Median nerve L.	3.2	2.6	3.7	3.1	11	20	41	50
Ulnar nerve L.	NR	2.6	NR	3.1	NR	13	NR	50
Dorsal ulnar cut. L.	NR	*	NR	2.3	NR	12	NR	*
Sural nerve L.	2.9	3.5	3.4	4.0	14	11	48	40
Median nerve R.	2.6	2.6	3.1	3.1	9	20	50	50
Ulnar nerve R.	2.1	2.6	2.6	3.1	5	13	57	50
Dorsal ulnar cut. R.	1.5	*	2.0	2.3	12	12	53	*

*Normal data not available.

EMG data

Muscle	Insert Activity	Fibs	Pos Waves	Fasc	Amp	Dur	Poly	Pattern
Biceps brachii L.	Norm	None	None	None	Norm	Norm	Few	Full
Triceps L.	Norm	None	None	None	Lg	Inc	None	Full
Flexor carpi radialis L.	Norm	None	None	None	Norm	Norm	None	Full
Flexor carpi ulnaris L.	Norm	None	None	None	Norm	Norm	None	Full
1st dorsal interosseous L.	Inc	2+	2+	None	Lg	Inc	None	Red
Abductor pollicis brevis L.	Norm	None	None	None	Norm	Norm	None	Full
Flexor digitorum profundus L.	Inc	2+	2+	None	Lg	Inc	None	Red
Vastus lateralis L.	Inc	None	2+	None	Lg	Inc	None	Red
Tibialis anterior L.	Norm	None	None	None	Lg	Inc	None	Red
Gastrocnemius L.	Inc	None	1+	None	Lg	Inc	None	Full

Results from Bertorini TE. Neuromuscular Case Studies, 1st ed., Butterworth-Heinemann, Elsevier, Case 7, 2008.

Which one of the following explains his acute symptoms?
a. Bilateral carpal tunnel syndrome
b. Diabetic neuropathy
c. Lower trunk brachial plexopathy
d. Poliomyelitis
e. Ulnar nerve entrapment below the elbow

12. A 46-year-old woman had a 4-month history of left shoulder and arm pain, and a 3-week history of numbness in the dorsum of the hand with some arm weakness and now wrist drop. She had severe weakness of the brachioradialis muscle, wrist, and finger extensors on the left. Strength of the triceps muscle was difficult to evaluate because of severe pain. The left brachioradialis reflex was absent, and ankle reflexes were diminished bilaterally; other reflexes were normal. There was decreased sensation in the left hand first web space. The remainder of her neurologic examination was normal.

Motor nerve studies

Nerve and Site	Latency (ms)	Amplitude (mV)	Conduction Velocity (m/s)
Median Nerve L.	Normal ≤ 4.2	Normal ≥ 6	Normal ≥ 50
Wrist	3.5	17	-
Elbow	6.8	16	61
Ulnar nerve L.	Normal ≤ 3.6	Normal ≥ 8	Normal ≥ 50
Wrist	3.0	14	-
Below elbow	6.4	14	57

F-wave studies

Nerve	Latency (ms)	Normal Latency ≤ (ms)
Median nerve L.	26.8	30
Ulnar nerve L.	25.6	30

Sensory nerve studies

Nerve	Onset Latency (ms)	Normal Onset Latency ≤(ms)	Peak Latency (ms)	Normal Peak Latency ≤(ms)	Amp (μV)	Normal Amp ≥ (μV)	Conduction Velocity (m/s)	Normal Conduction Velocity ≥ (m/s)
Median nerve L.	2.1	2.6	2.6	3.1	40	20	62	50
Ulnar nerve L.	2.1	2.6	2.6	3.1	26	13	57	50
Radial nerve L.	NR	2.6	NR	3.1	NR	30	NR	50
Radial nerve R.	2.3	2.6	2.8	3.1	36	30	60	50

EMG data

Muscle	Insert Activity	Fibs	Pos Waves	Fasc	Amp	Dur	Poly	Pattern
Cervical paraspinals L.	Norm	None	None	None	Norm	Norm	None	Full
Deltoid L.	Norm	None	None	None	Norm	Norm	None	Full
Biceps brachii L.	Norm	None	None	None	Norm	Norm	None	Full

Continued on following page

Muscle	Insert Activity	Fibs	Pos Waves	Fasc	Amp	Dur	Poly	Pattern
Flexor carpi radialis L.	Norm	None	None	None	Norm	Norm	None	Full
Brachioradialis L.	Inc	1+	1+	None	Norm	Norm	Few	Red
Extensor digitorum com. L.	Inc	3+	3+	None	*	*	*	*
Extensor carpi radialis L.	Inc	3+	3+	None	*	*	*	*
1st dorsal interosseous L.	Norm	None	None	None	Norm	Norm	None	Full

*No motor units recruited.
Results from Bertorini TE. Neuromuscular Case Studies, 1st ed., Butterworth-Heinemann, Elsevier, Case 9, 2008.

Abnormalities can be localized to which one of the following?
a. C7 nerve root
b. C8 nerve root
c. Median nerve
d. Radial nerve
e. Ulnar nerve

13. A 65-year-old woman developed pain in the right arm and shoulder with some neck discomfort. A few days later, she presented with a rash on the arm and could no longer raise the arm. Examination revealed an erythematous vesicular rash in the outer aspect of the right arm, and she had weakness of the right deltoid of 2/5. Supraspinatus were 5 −/5 and brachioradialis was 3/5. Biceps strength was 3/5; triceps, forearm, and hand muscles were normal. The left arm and leg strength were normal. The right biceps and brachioradialis reflexes were absent; the triceps was normal. Reflexes in the legs and left arm were normal. Sensory examination showed diffuse hypoalgesia in the right lower arm; the affected dermatome was hard to localize. The rest of the neurologic examination was normal.

Motor nerve studies

Nerve and Site	Latency (ms)	Amplitude (mV)	Conduction Velocity (m/s)
Median nerve R.	Normal ≤ 4.2	Normal ≥ 6	Normal ≥ 50
Wrist	4.1	10	-
Elbow	7.0	10	62
Ulnar nerve R.	Normal ≤ 3.7	Normal ≥ 8	Normal ≥ 50
Wrist	3.7	9	-
Below elbow	6.9	9	53
Above elbow	9.2	9	52

F-wave studies

Nerve	Latency (ms)	Normal Latency ≤ (ms)
Median nerve R.	26.4	30
Ulnar nerve R.	27.6	30

Sensory nerve studies

Nerve	Onset Latency (ms)	Normal Onset Latency ≤ (ms)	Peak Latency (ms)	Normal Peak Latency ≤ (ms)	Amp (μV)	Normal Amp ≥ (μV)	Conduction Velocity (m/s)	Normal Conduction Velocity ≥ (m/s)
Median nerve R.	2.4	2.6	2.9	3.1	25	20	54	50
Ulnar nerve R.	2.3	2.6	2.8	3.1	18	13	52	50

EMG data

Muscle	Insert Activity	Fibs	Pos Waves	Fasc	Amp	Dur	Poly	Pattern
Cervical paraspinals R.	Inc	2+	2+	None	Norm	Norm	Few	Full
Infraspinatus R.	Norm	None	None	None	Norm	Norm	None	Full
Rhomboids R.	Norm	None	None	None	Norm	Norm	None	Full
Deltoid R.	Inc	2+	2+	None	Lg	Inc	Few	Red
Biceps brachii R.	Inc	2+	2+	None	Lg	Inc	Few	Red
Brachioradialis R.	Inc	2+	2+	None	Lg	Inc	Few	Red
Extensor digitorum comm. R.	Norm	None	None	None	Norm	Norm	None	Full
Flexor carpi radialis R.	Norm	None	None	None	Norm	Norm	None	Full
Flexor carpi ulnaris R.	Norm	None	None	None	Norm	Norm	None	Full
First dorsal interosseous R.	Norm	None	None	None	Norm	Norm	None	Full

Results from Bertorini TE. Neuromuscular Case Studies, 1st ed., Butterworth-Heinemann, Elsevier, Case 15, 2008.

Which one of the following is most likely?
a. C5 radiculopathy
b. C6 radiculopathy
c. Musculocutaneous mononeuritis
d. Suprascapular neuropathy
e. Upper trunk brachial plexopathy

14. A 44-year-old woman came with nearly a year long history of neck pain radiating to the right arm. Neurologic examination showed normal mentation and cranial nerves. There was no weakness, but there was diminished brachioradialis reflex on the right compared with the left. Sensory examination was normal. The rest of the examination was also normal. EMG findings are shown.

Motor nerve studies

Nerve and Site	Latency (ms)	Amplitude (mV)	Conduction Velocity (m/s)
Median nerve R.	Normal ≤ 4.2	Normal ≥ 6	Normal ≥ 50
Wrist	3.6	13	-
Elbow	7.3	12	59
Ulnar nerve R.	Normal ≤ 3.6	Normal ≥ 8	Normal ≥ 50
Wrist	2.8	18	-
Below elbow	6.0	16	61

F-wave studies

Nerve	Latency (ms)	Normal Latency ≤ (ms)
Median nerve R.	23.4	30
Ulnar nerve R.	25.2	30

Sensory nerve studies

Nerve	Onset Latency (ms)	Normal Onset Latency ≤(ms)	Peak Latency (ms)	Normal Peak Latency ≤(ms)	Amp (μV)	Normal Amp≥ (μV)	Conduction Velocity (m/s)	Normal Conduction Velocity≥(m/s)
Median nerve R.	2.5	2.6	3.0	3.1	34	20	52	50
Ulnar nerve R.	2.1	2.6	2.6	3.1	33	13	57	50

EMG data

Muscle	Insert Activity	Fibs	Pos Waves	Fasc	Amp	Dur	Poly	Pattern
Cervical paraspinals R.	Norm	None	None	None	Norm	Norm	None	Full
Rhomboids R.	Inc	None	2+	None	Norm	Norm	None	Full
Supraspinatus R.	CRDs	None	None	None	Norm	Norm	None	Full
Infraspinatus R.	Inc	None	None	None	Norm	Norm	None	Full
Deltoid R.	Inc	None	1+	None	Norm	Norm	None	Full
Biceps brachii R.	Inc	None	2+	None	Norm	Norm	None	Red
Flexor carpi radialis R.	Norm	None	None	None	Norm	Norm	None	Full
Flexor carpi ulnaris R.	Norm	None	None	None	Norm	Norm	None	Full
Extensor dig. communis R.	Norm	None	None	None	Norm	Norm	None	Full
1st dorsal interosseous R.	Norm	None	None	None	Norm	Norm	None	Full

Results from Bertorini TE. Neuromuscular Case Studies, 1st ed., Butterworth-Heinemann, Elsevier, Case 16, 2008.

Which one of the following is most likely?
a. Axillary nerve pathology
b. C5 radiculopathy
c. C6 radiculopathy
d. Dorsal scapular nerve pathology
e. Musculocutaneous nerve pathology

QUESTIONS 15–20

Additional questions 15–20 available on ExpertConsult.com

21. Which one of the labels in the image below corresponds to the innervation from the lateral plantar nerve?

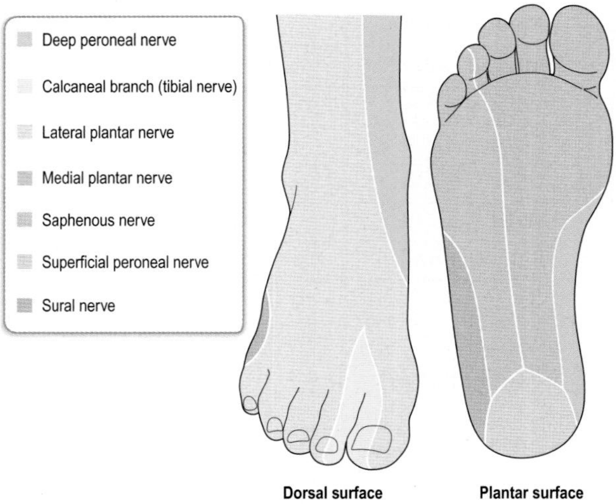

● 22. Which one of the following segments is responsible for finger extension?
a. C4,C5
b. C5,C6
c. C6,C7
d. C7,C8
e. C8,T1

EXTENDED MATCHING ITEM (EMI) QUESTIONS

● 23. **Brachial plexus:**

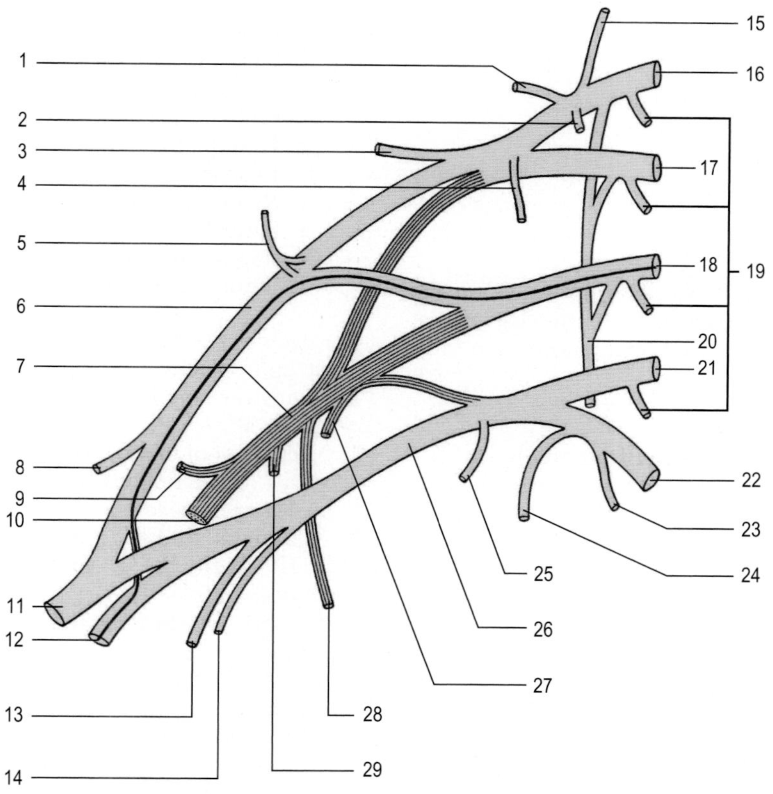

For each of the following descriptions, select the most appropriate answers from the list above. Each answer may be used once, more than once or not at all.
a. Long thoracic nerve
b. Musculocutaneous nerve
c. Radial nerve
d. Suprascapular nerve
e. Ulnar nerve

24. **Lumbar plexus:**

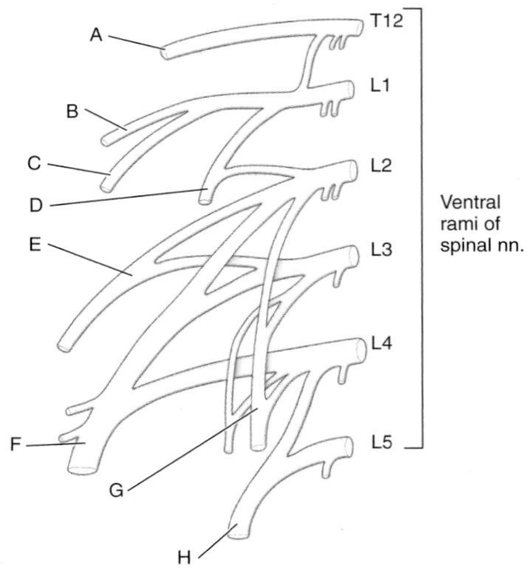

For each of the following descriptions, select the most appropriate answers from the list above. Each answer may be used once, more than once or not at all.

1. Femoral nerve
2. Genitofemoral nerve
3. Lateral cutaneous nerve of the thigh

25. **Sacral plexus:**

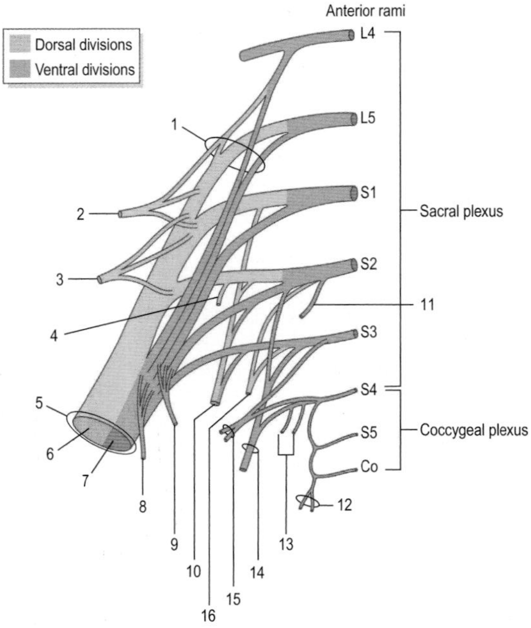

For each of the following descriptions, select the most appropriate answers from the list above. Each answer may be used once, more than once or not at all.

a. Common peroneal part of sciatic nerve
b. Nerve to piriformis
c. Inferior gluteal nerve
d. Pudendal nerve
e. Tibial part of sciatic nerve

26. **Upper limb nerve injuries:**

a. Anterior interosseous nerve syndrome
b. Carpal tunnel syndrome
c. Cheiralgia paresthetica
d. Cubital tunnel syndrome
e. Erb-Duchenne palsy
f. Guyon's canal syndrome
g. Klumpke's palsy
h. Pronator syndrome
i. Radial tunnel syndrome
j. Saturday night palsy
k. Supinator syndrome
l. Thoracic outlet syndrome

For each of the following descriptions, select the most appropriate answers from the list above. Each answer may be used once, more than once or not at all.

1. Weakness of elbow extension, wrist extension (wrist drop), finger extension and sensory loss in 1st web space.
2. Weakness in FPL, pronator quadratus and FDP (Digits 2 + 3); Abnormal pinch sign; no sensory loss.
3. Sensory loss in palmar ulnar 1½ fingers and hand (dorsal sensory branch arises before wrist); weakness and wasting of hypothenar, all interossei, lumbricals 3 + 4, deep head of FPB, adductor pollicis. Froment's sign due to weak thumb adduction (flexes IPJ instead). Clawing of 4 + 5th digits when attempting to extend fingers.

27. **Lower limb nerve entrapment:**

a. Anterior tarsal tunnel syndrome
b. Deep peroneal nerve entrapment
c. Distal tarsal tunnel syndrome
d. Exertional compartment syndrome
e. Femoral nerve compression syndrome
f. Fibular tunnel syndrome
g. Meralgia paresthetica
h. Obturator syndrome
i. Piriformis syndrome
j. Proximal tarsal tunnel syndrome

For each of the following descriptions, select the most appropriate answers from the list above. Each answer may be used once, more than once or not at all.

1. Entrapment of lateral cutaneous nerve of thigh (femoral n) under inguinal ligament. Sensory loss, burning dysesthesias in anterolateral thigh; no motor weakness.
2. Sensory loss anteromedial thigh; weakness and wasting of quadriceps femoris; point tenderness in groin; impaired knee jerk. Pain and numbness in saphenous nerve distribution (anterior knee, medial leg).
3. Pain and parasthesias in toes and sole of foot (heel spared as sensory branches arise proximal to tunnel), clawing of toes due to weakness of intrinsic foot muscles, typically worse at night. Tinel's test positive. Ankle eversion + dorsiflexion combined with toe dorsiflexion can reproduce pain (dorsiflexion-eversion test).

28. **Dermatomes:**
   a. C4
   b. C5
   c. C6
   d. C7
   e. C8
   f. T1
   g. L2
   h. L3
   i. L4
   j. L5
   k. S1
   l. S2
   m. S3

For each of the following descriptions, select the most appropriate answers from the list above. Each answer may be used once, more than once or not at all.

1. Obliquely from lateral thigh, lateral aspect of knee/calf, anterior shin and dorsum of foot including medial four toes and sole of foot including heel.
2. Medial arm, forearm and dorsal and palmar aspects of hand and ring + little fingers.
3. Lateral shoulder, arm, forearm, anatomical snuff box, thenar eminence and whole thumb.

29. **Innervation of the upper limb:**

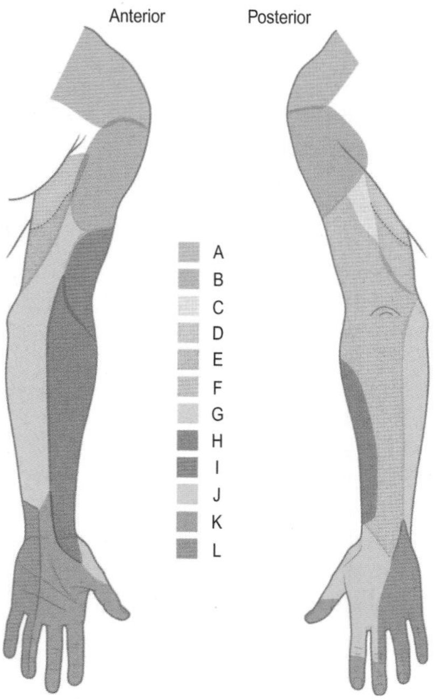

For each of the following descriptions, select the most appropriate answers from the list above. Each answer may be used once, more than once or not at all.

1. Ulnar nerve
2. Median nerve
3. Lateral cutaneous nerve of forearm
4. Superficial branch of radial

30. **Myotomes:**
   a. C3, C4
   b. C5, C6
   c. C6, C7
   d. C7, C8
   e. C8, T1
   f. L1, L2
   g. L2, L3
   h. L3, L4
   i. L4, L5
   j. L5, S1
   k. S1, S2

For each of the following descriptions, select the most appropriate answers from the list above. Each answer may be used once, more than once or not at all.

1. Wrist extension
2. Hip flexion
3. Ankle dorsiflexion

31. **Clinical signs:**
   a. Ape hand
   b. Claw hand
   c. Froment's sign
   d. Hand of benediction
   e. Hoffman's sign
   f. Hoover test
   g. Inverted radial reflex
   h. Lasegue's sign
   i. Lhermitte's sign
   j. Phalen's test
   k. Spurling's sign
   l. Tinel's test
   m. Volkman's contracture

For each of the following descriptions, select the most appropriate answers from the list above. Each answer may be used once, more than once or not at all.

1. Diminished brachioradialis reflex with reflex contraction of finger flexors.
2. On attempting to make a fist, only 4th and 5th digits flex at IPJs.
3. Loss of thumb opposition and abduction.

32. **Innervation of the lower limb:**

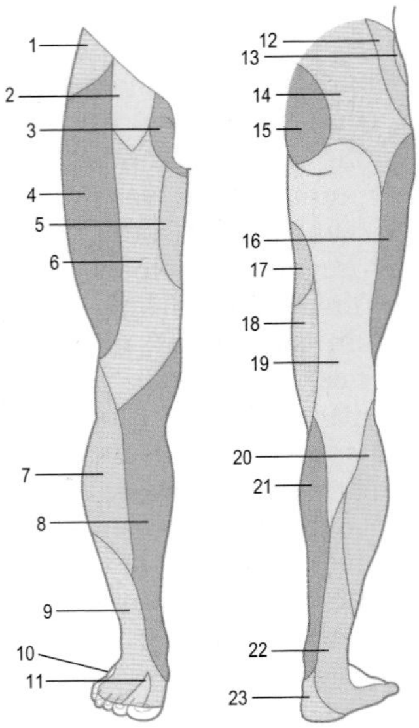

For each of the following descriptions, select the most appropriate answers from the list above. Each answer may be used once, more than once or not at all.

a. Saphenous nerve
b. Sural nerve
c. Obturator

SBA ANSWERS

1. **c**—Type A delta

	Diameter (μm)	Myelination	Conduction Velocity (m/s)	Modality
Type A alpha	13-20	Myelinated	70-120	Motor
Type A beta	6-12	Myelinated	30-70	Touch and pressure
Type A gamma	3-6	Myelinated	15-30	Proprioception
Type A delta	1-6	Myelinated	12-30	Fast pain and cold temperature
Type B		Myelinated	3-15	Autonomic, preganglionic sympathetic
Type C	0.5-1.5	Unmyelinated	0.5-2	Slow pain and warm temperature, autonomic, postganglionic sympathetic, polymodal receptors

2. **d**—Insertional activity on EMG (in a pattern excluding other root lesions)

Over 1-2 weeks denervated muscle fibers becomes progressively more mechanically irritable such that electrical discharges provoked by movement of the needle can be prolonged (increased insertional activity). Muscle fibers also become chemically sensitive to their microenvironment and their membranes can also become unstable enough to produce spontaneously activity (fibrillation potentials and positive sharp waves; disappear with complete degeneration of the denervated muscle fiber). The finding of fibrillations and positive sharp waves is the most reliable and objective test that there is for damage to motor axons to the muscle after 1 week at least up to 12 months after the damage. If there is ongoing damage such as in amyotrophic lateral sclerosis one can see ongoing denervation. Reinnervation of muscle is an ongoing process, occurring whenever a muscle is partially denervated. This process typically involves the development of sprouts from adjacent, unaffected motor nerve fibers that ultimately contact at least some of the denervated muscle fibers. These reinnervated muscle fibers cluster right in the area of other, normally innervated muscle fibers. This process results in the development of clumps of reinnervated muscle fibers attached to individual motor neurons, producing larger motor units more irregular potentials (polyphasic).This process takes months to develop and indicates the presence of chronic denervation.

3. **c**—Pronator teres (C6, C7)

The typical needle EMG examination requires sampling several muscles. Its ability to localize a lesion depends on sampling muscles innervated by the same nerve but different nerve roots, muscles innervated by the same nerve root but different nerves and muscles innervated at different locations along the course of the nerves. Paraspinal muscles can be very useful in this regard because nerve root damage will tend to produce abnormalities in these muscles as well as within the muscles of the limbs (helping to distinguish a radiculopathy from a plexopathy or peripheral neuropathy, for example). Sometimes precise localization can be difficult due to the overlap in innervation of the various nerve root levels.

4. **b**—Motor axon loss

5. **e**—Reduced interference pattern

During EMG assessment of a muscle during contraction, the electrical activity should fully obscure the baseline (termed a full interference pattern). Incomplete interference pattern is considered to be a reflection of loss of motor units in a muscle, though it can also be seen with diminished effort. The table below shows the sequence of EMG changes in radiculopathy:

Days After Onset of Radiculopathy	Electrophysiological Abnormalities
>0	Reduced number of MUPs (reduced interference pattern) Fasciculations H-reflex prolonged latency Reduced F waves
>1 week	Fibrillation potentials and positive sharp spikes in paraspinal muscles
>2 weeks	Fibrillation potentials and positive sharp spikes in proximal limb muscles
>3 weeks	Fibrillation potentials and positive sharp spikes in distal limb muscles

6. **e**—MUP is the sum of the electrical signals arising from the discharge of the several muscle fibers within recording distance of the tip of the needle that innervated by the same motor neuron. The amplitude of the MUP is dependent on the density of the muscle fibers attached to that one motor neuron (also to the proximity of the MUP). As the degree of contraction is slowly increased, more motor units are recruited.

7. **d**—Multiple motor root compromise

The F-wave (originally recorded in the foot, hence the name) is a late response that occurs in muscles during a motor nerve conduction study long after the initial contraction of the muscle (CMAP). CMAP usually appears within several milliseconds but another response can be normally recorded in the muscle slightly later (25-55 ms). The electrical impulse is transmitted proximally along the motor axon from the site of initiation of the action potential. When this antidromic depolarization reaches the motor neurons in the spinal cord, a percentage of these motor neurons are activated a second time. This results in an electrical signal being conducted in the normal (orthodromic) direction from the spinal cord to the muscles innervated by the nerve. This second, later activation produces a small muscle contraction that is termed the F-wave. Because the number of motor neurons that are re-activated is somewhat unpredictable, the amplitude of this signal is variable and, therefore, amplitude measurements are usually not used. However, delay in the F-wave indicates some slowing of conduction of the motor axon. Since the F-response traverses more proximal portions of the motor axons (twice) it may be useful in the investigation of proximal nerve pathology. Since the antidromic impulse in motor axons in a single peripheral nerve will test the multiple nerve roots forming it, F-wave is not useful for isolated radiculopathy but is valuable where multiple roots may be involved (e.g., Guillain-Barre syndrome, or chronic inflammatory demyelinating polyradiculopathy).

8. **e**—Suspected S1 radiculopathy

H-reflex is named in honor of Hoffmann, who first described this response in 1918. The H-reflex is most commonly tested by electrical stimulation of the tibial nerve, with recordings from the gastrocnemius/soleus muscle complex (triceps surae). Therefore, this response utilizes the same neural pathway as the ankle jerk reflex. Electrical stimulation will depolarize the largest, most heavily myelinated nerve fibers at a lower stimulus intensity than is required to activate other smaller nerve fibers. Since the largest nerve fibers in a peripheral nerve are those arising from muscle stretch receptors, there should be a stimulus intensity that activates muscle stretch afferent nerve fibers without directly activating many motor nerve axons eliciting a monosynaptic reflex contraction in the muscle. Because this response must traverse the sensory axon all the way back to the spinal cord before synapsing on the motor neuron, and since the motor response must then traverse the length of the motor axon to reach the triceps surae muscle, this reflex takes a long time (i.e., late). Theoretically, this reflex can be elicited from virtually any muscle but only the triceps surae muscle produces H-reflexes that are reliable enough to be clinically useful. Therefore H-reflex evaluates the integrity of the reflex arc from the tibial nerve, sciatic nerve, S1 sensory root, spinal cord, S1 motor root and back to the triceps surae. Damage to any portion of the reflex arc can result in loss or slowing of the reflex response. Since the H-reflex is mediated primarily over the S1 nerve root (just like the ankle jerk reflex), it is a sensitive test for S1 radiculopathy. However, once the reflex arc has been damaged, it often does not return to normal (making the test less useful in investigating the question of recurrent radiculopathy).

9. **e**—Reduced conduction velocity (or conduction block)

The table below shows general patterns of peripheral neuropathies due to demyelination versus those due to axonal degeneration, though in reality each can cause secondary damage to the other and electrophysiology may be mixed. Pathology which may affect both myelin and axons equally include diabetes, uremia and paraproteinemia. Radiculopathies (root lesions) and neuropathies (e.g., MND, herpes zoster) are not included in this table, although they may mimic peripheral neuropathy.

EMG/NCS	Focal (Mononeuropathy)	Multifocal (Mononeuritis Multiplex)	Generalized (Polyneuropathy)
Demyelination	Nerve entrapment	Paraproteinemia Diphtheria Leprosy	Guillain-Barre syndrome CIPD Lymphoma Multiple myeloma Amiodarone Hereditary
Axonal degeneration	Severe nerve entrapment	Diabetes Vasculitis Neoplastic HIV Sarcoidosis Amyloidosis Lyme disease	Diabetes Alcohol Drugs/toxin Critical illness Multiple myeloma Hereditary

10. **c**—Carpal tunnel syndrome

It showed prolonged median nerve distal motor latency on the right with low-amplitude compound muscle action potential (CMAP). The elbow to wrist conduction velocity was normal. The right ulnar conduction velocity, CMAP amplitude, and distal latency were normal. The right median sensory nerve action potential (SNAP) had a prolonged latency and slow conduction velocity. The left median CMAP distal latency was mildly prolonged and of normal amplitude; the conduction velocity was normal. The left median SNAP was prolonged and had slow conduction velocity. The ulnar SNAP was normal. The F-response on the right median nerve was prolonged, likely secondary to the prolonged distal motor latency. The needle test showed large motor units potentials only in the abductor pollicis brevis muscle. There was thus distal median nerve demyelination and chronic axonal degeneration in the right, causing a low-amplitude CMAP and large motor unit potentials with reduced recruitment. It was concluded that this patient had carpal tunnel syndrome from RA and likely also from a compression from the use of a walker.

11. **e**—Ulnar nerve entrapment below the elbow

Absent were the left digital ulnar and dorsal cutaneous SNAPs. The motor ulnar nerve conduction velocity from elbow to wrist was normal but was slow at 39 m/s across the elbow. Conduction velocity of less than 50 m/s, or 10 m/s slower than the elbow-wrist segment, or 10 m/s slower than the velocity across the elbow in the opposite side, are considered abnormal. The "inching," or short (1 cm) segment increment study, revealed a significant prolongation of 0.7 ms (normal, $\leq$0.5 ms) at 2 cm distal to the medial epicondyle where there was also a drop in amplitude over 50%. The needle EMG showed denervation potentials in the left ulnar-innervated intrinsic hand muscles, but not in the median-innervated muscles. There were also denervation potentials in the flexor digitorum profundus although not in the flexor carpi ulnaris. The test also showed electrophysiologic evidence of bilateral median neuropathy at the wrist. In addition, there were electrophysiologic findings consistent with the previous history of polio, characterized by large motor unit potentials in the lower extremities with mild active denervation in the gastrocnemius muscle.

12. **d**—Radial nerve

The left median and ulnar nerve SNAPs conduction velocities and amplitudes were normal, whereas the superficial radial SNAP was absent. Radial nerve motor conduction could not be studied because of discomfort. The needle test showed denervation potentials in radial-innervated muscles, including wrist extensor and the brachioradialis, indicating that the lesion occurred above the elbow. The normal median and ulnar-innervated muscles negate a C7 radiculopathy or a lesion of the middle trunk of the brachial plexus. The normal EMG of her deltoid is evidence against a posterior cord lesion. Denervation in the brachioradialis and extensor carpi radialis and the absent radial SNAP indicate that the main trunk of the radial nerve was affected with axonal degeneration.

13. **b**—C6 radiculopathy

The sensory and motor nerve conduction studies were normal. The needle test showed denervation potentials with reduced recruitment of motor units in the deltoid, biceps, brachioradialis, and cervical paraspinal muscles, indicating axonal degeneration of the C6 roots sparing the infraspinatus and rhomboids, as well as forearm and intrinsic hand muscles.

14. **a**—C5 radiculopathy

The median and ulnar motor conduction velocities, distal latencies, compound muscle action potential amplitudes, F-responses, and sensory nerve action potentials were normal. Needle EMG showed denervation potentials in the right biceps, deltoid, and rhomboids, and complex repetitive discharges in the supraspinatus muscle. The motor units appeared normal in these muscles. Paraspinal muscles were normal. This EMG was suggestive of a C5 radiculopathy (despite no paraspinal denervation). This was concluded because there was involvement of muscles innervated only by C5; in particular, the rhomboid that is innervated by the dorsal scapular nerve that originates directly from the C5 root and not the brachial plexus.

ANSWERS 15–20

Additional answers 15–20 available on ExpertConsult.com

21. **c**—appears to be superficial peroneal, query E?

Image with permission from Sen CK, Roy S. Wound healing. In: Neligan P (ed.), Plastic Surgery, 6 volumes, 3rd ed., Elsevier, 2013.

22. **d**—C7/C8 roots

Joint	Action	Segments	Major Muscle	Nerve	Reflex
Scapula	Elevation	C3,4	Upper trapezius Levator scapulae	Spinal acc. (XI) Dorsal scapular	
Shoulder	Flexion	C5,6	Deltoid Pectoral Coracobrachialis	Axillary Pectoral Musculocut.	
	Extension	C5,6	Deltoid Teres minor Infraspinatus Teres major Lat. dorsi	Axillary Suprascapular Lower subscap. Thoracodorsal	
	Adduction	C5,6	Pectoral Lat dorsi Coracobrachialis		
	Abduction	C5,6	Deltoid Supraspinatus		
	Internal rotation	C5,6	Subscapularis Teres major Lat dorsi Anterior deltoid		
	External rotation	C5,6	Infraspinatus Posterior deltoid Teres minor	Suprascapular Axillary	
Elbow	Extension Flexion	C6,7 C5,6	Triceps Biceps brachii Brachialis Brachioradialis	Radial Musculocutaneous	Triceps Biceps Brachioradialis
Wrist	Flexion	C6,7	FCR, PL FCU	Median Ulnar	
	Extension	C6,7	ECRL ECRB, ECU	Radial PIN	
Finger	Flexion Extension Abduction Adduction	C8,T1 C7,8 C8,T1 C8,T1	FDS,FDP,FPL ED, EI, EPL APB, dorsal interossei Palmar interossei	Ulnar/median Posterior interosseous Median/ulnar Ulnar	

EMI ANSWERS

23. a—20, b—8, c—10, d—3, e—12

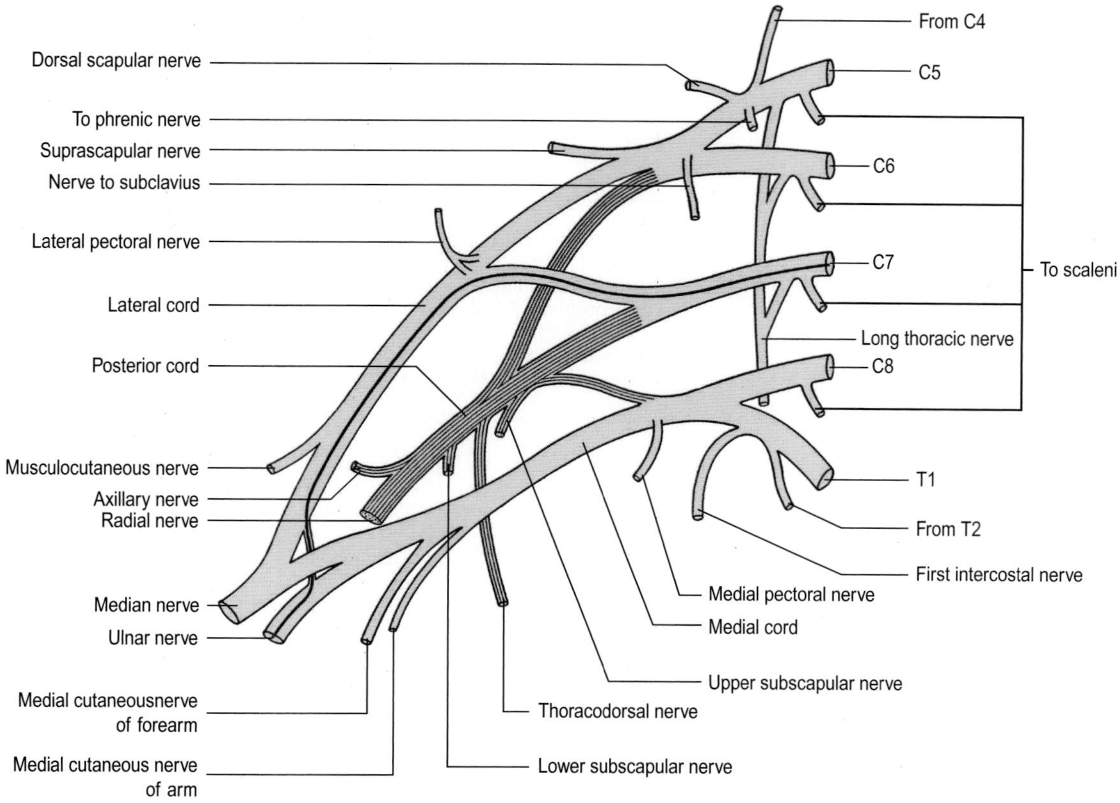

Image with permission from Mancall, Elliott L. Gray's Clinical Neuroanatomy: The Anatomic Basis for Clinical Neuroscience, Elsevier, Saunders, 2011.

Major Nerves	Roots	Cord	Important Motor Supply	Motor Test	Sensory Supply
Axillary	C5-6	Posterior	Deltoid Teres minor	Shoulder abduction	Superior lateral arm
Radial	C5-T1	Posterior	Triceps brachii Brachioradialis ECRL and ECRB *Posterior interosseous nerve* Forearm extensors: supinator, ECU, ED, EDM, APL, EPL, EPB, EI.	Elbow extension Brachioradialis jerk Wrist extension Finger extension	Dorsal hand and radial 3½ digits
Musculocutaneous	C5-7	Lateral	Coracobrachialis, biceps, brachioradialis	Elbow flexion	Lateral forearm

Continued on following page

Major Nerves	Roots	Cord	Important Motor Supply	Motor Test	Sensory Supply
Median	C6-T1	Lateral +Medial	Forearm flexors (PT, FDS, PL, FCR) Thenar (Lumbricals 1 +2, opponens pollicis, abductor pollicis, FPB) *Anterior interosseous nerve* Forearm flexors: median FDP, FPL, pronator quadratus	Forearm pronation Wrist flexion PIPJ flexion PIPJ extension (index, middle) DIPJ flexion (index, middle) Thumb abduction, opposition; Pinch sign;	Palmar aspect of radial 3½ digits and nailbeds
Ulnar	C7-T1	Medial	FCU FDP (ulnar: ring and little) Adductor pollicis Hypothenar: ADM, ODM, FDM Dorsal and palmar interossei, lumbricals 3+4	Wrist flexion and adduction, little finger abduction, MCPJ flexion (little finger), DIPJ flexion (little, ring fingers) finger adduction, Froment's sign	Palmar and dorsal aspects of ulnar 1½ fingers

24. 1—f, 2—d, 3—e

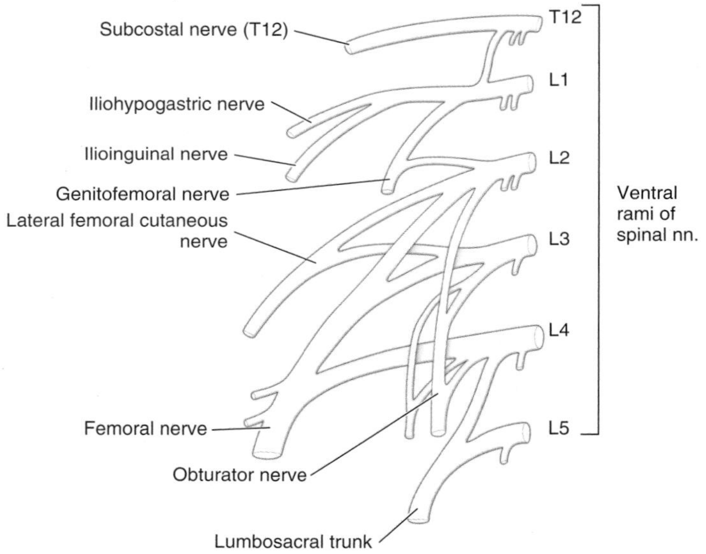

Image with permission from Waldman SD. Pain Review, Elsevier, Saunders, 2009.

Major Nerves	Important Motor Supply	Sensory
Iliohypogastric (L1)		Posterolateral buttock
Ilioinguinal (L1)		Inguinal and suprapubic
Genitofemoral (L1-2)	Genital branch to cremaster muscle	Femoral triangle
Lateral cutaneous nerve of thigh (L2-3)	-	Anterolateral thigh
Femoral nerve (L2-4)	Iliacus and quadriceps	Anterior thigh; saphenous nerve branch supplies medial leg/foot
Obturator nerve (L2-4)	Motor to thigh adductors	Medial thigh

25. a—5, b—4, c—3, d—14, e—7

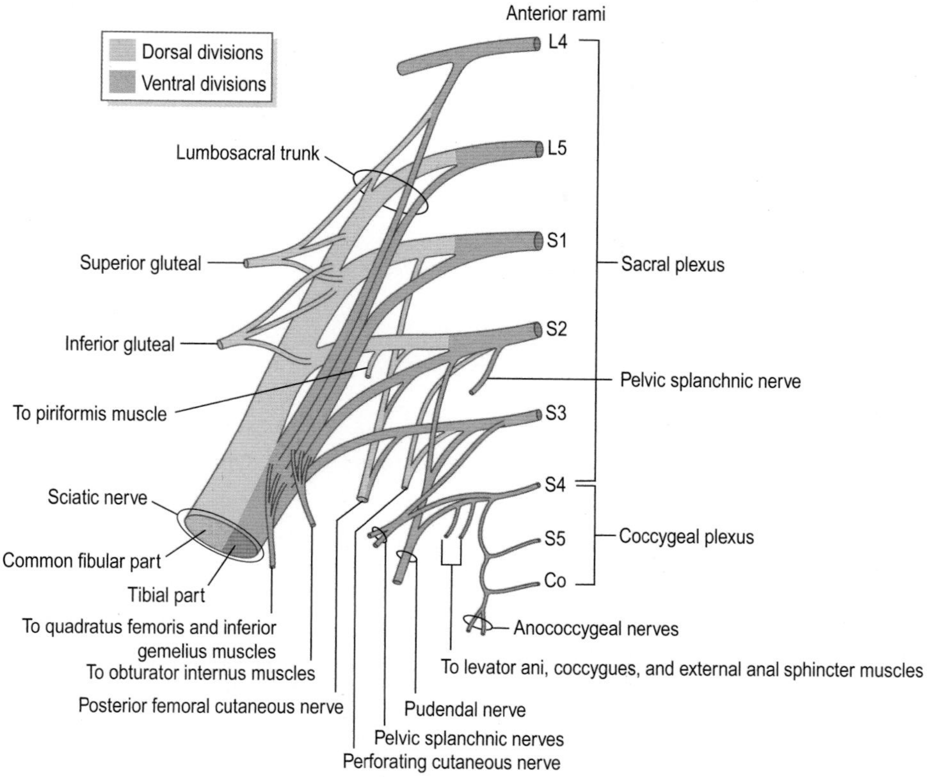

Major Nerves	**Important Motor Supply**	**Motor Test**	**Sensory Supply**
Superior gluteal	Gluteus medius Gluteus minimus Tensor fascia lata	Hip abduction; Trendelenburg sign	
Inferior gluteal	Gluteus maximus	Hip extension	
Sciatic Nerve (L4-S3)	Hamstrings Adductor magnus (medial)	Knee flexion	
Tibial nerve (L4-S3)	Gastrocneumius/soleus Tibialis posterior Flexor digitorum longus Flexor halluces longus *Medial and lateral plantar nerves* Intrinsic foot muscles	Ankle plantarflexion Ankle inversion	*Medial sural cutaneous* Lower posterolateral calf Lateral aspect of foot *Medial and lateral calcaneal* Heel of foot *Medial plantar* Digits 1-3 and medial sole of foot *Lateral plantar* 4th+5th digits and lateral sole of foot

Continued on following page

Major Nerves	Important Motor Supply	Motor Test	Sensory Supply
Common peroneal nerve (L4-S2)	*Superficial peroneal* Peroneus longus Peroneus brevis *Deep peroneal* Tibialis anterior EDL/EDB EHL/EDB Peroneus tertius		*Lateral sural cutaneous* Upper posterolateral calf *Superficial peroneal* Dorsum of foot and medial 3 toes *Deep peroneal* Space between 1st and 2nd toes
Pudendal nerve (S2-4)	*Inferior rectal nerve* External anal sphincter *Perineal nerve* External urethral sphincter, bulbospongiosus, ischiocavernosus		*Inferior rectal nerve* Below pectinate line *Perineal nerve* Posterior scrotum *Dorsal nerve of penis/clitoris* Skin of penis/clitoris

26. 1—j, Saturday night palsy, 2—a, Anterior interosseous nerve syndrome, 3—f, Guyon's canal syndrome

Entrapment Syndrome	Key Features
Klumpke's palsy	Lower brachial plexus injury—weakness and sensory loss in C8 and T1 distribution. Associated with Claw hand and Horner's syndrome
Erb-Duchenne palsy	Upper brachial plexus injury—C5 and C6 weakness and sensory loss predominantly affecting axillary nerve, musculocutaneous nerve and suprascapular nerve territories. At rest the arm hangs by the side, medially rotated, forearm extended and pronated resulting in "waiter's tip" posture
Radial nerve	
Saturday night/crutch palsy	Radial nerve compression against proximal humerus. Weakness of elbow extension, wrist extension (wrist drop), finger extension and sensory loss in first web space
Mid-arm	Radial nerve compression in spiral groove of humerus (after branch to triceps). Wrist drop, weakness finger extension, sensory loss first web space
Posterior interosseous nerve syndrome (radial tunnel syndrome)	Compression of posterior interosseous nerve (branch of radial nerve) at the lateral intermuscular septum of the arm. Pain in dorsal aspect of upper forearm and when extending middle finger against resistance
Supinator syndrome	Compression of posterior interosseous nerve (branch of radial nerve) at the arcade of Frohse. Sensory loss to area of superficial radial nerve supply with wrist drop
Cheiralgia paresthetica (Handcuff neuropathy)	Compression of superficial branch of radial nerve causing pain, paresthesias, numbness in first web space. No motor weakness
Median nerve	
Pronator syndrome	Median nerve entrapment in the proximal forearm. Proximal forearm pain and tenderness; FPL and abductor pollicis brevis weakness; paresthesias in radial 3½ digits; positive Tinel's sign
Anterior interosseous nerve syndrome	Entrapment of anterior interosseous nerve (branch of median nerve) causing weakness in FPL, pronator quadratus and FDP (Digits 2+3); Abnormal pinch sign; no sensory loss

Continued

Entrapment Syndrome	Key Features
Carpal tunnel syndrome	Median nerve entrapment at the wrist. Pain, paresthesias, numbness and reduced two-point discrimination in thumb and radial 2½ fingers; thenar weakness and wasting; positive Tinel's sign and Phalen's sign
Ulnar nerve	
Cubital tunnel syndrome	Ulnar nerve entrapment at the elbow. Sensory loss in ulnar 1½ fingers and ulnar aspect of hand; weakness and wasting of ulnar intrinsic hand muscles and FDP; positive Tinel's sign; ache in medial elbow and forearm
Guyon's canal syndrome	Ulnar nerve entrapment at the wrist. Sensory loss in palmar ulnar 1½ fingers and hand (dorsal sensory branch arises before wrist); weakness and wasting of hypothenar, all interossei, lumbricals 3+4, deep head of FPB, adductor pollicis. Froment's sign due to weak thumb adduction (flexes IPJ instead). Clawing of 4 +5th digits when attempting to extend fingers—MCPJ hyperextension due to intact long extensors, loss of interossei and lumbricals 3+4 (normally act to flex MCPJ, extend IPJs) means long flexors unopposed particularly in digits 4+5. Clawing less pronounced with higher ulnar nerve injuries due to weakness of ulnar half of FDP

27. 1—Meralgia paresthetica, 2—Femoral nerve entrapment, 3—Proximal tarsal tunnel syndrome

Meralgia paresthetica	Entrapment of lateral cutaneous nerve of thigh (femoral n) under inguinal ligament. Sensory loss, burning dysesthesias in anterolateral thigh; no motor weakness
Piriformis syndrome	Compression of sciatic nerve by piriformis muscle. Pain, tingling and sensory loss in the buttocks and sciatic nerve distribution
Obturator syndrome	Sensory loss superomedial thigh; weakness of thigh adduction
Femoral nerve entrapment	Sensory loss anteromedial thigh; weakness and wasting of quadriceps femoris; point tenderness in groin; impaired knee jerk. Pain and numbness in saphenous nerve distribution (anterior knee, medial leg)
Fibular tunnel syndrome	Common peroneal nerve entrapment/trauma, commonly at fibular head. Sensory loss of dorsal foot and lateral leg; foot drop; Tinel's sign over fibular head; anterior and lateral compartment atrophy
Exertional compartment syndrome	Exercise induced pain which is relieved by rest, and may be associated with weakness and paresthesia
Distal tibial tarsal tunnel syndrome	Tarsal tunnel syndrome due to entrapment of distal branches (medial and lateral plantar) of tibial nerve. Distal entrapment of lateral plantar nerve present with chronic heel pain (difficult to distinguish from plantar fasciitis)
Deep peroneal nerve entrapment	Can occur anywhere along its course, but compression at the ankle beneath the extensor retinaculum is termed anterior tarsal tunnel syndrome. Pain over dorsum of foot (possibly first web space); if proximal lesion foot drop or EHL weakness
Proximal tarsal tunnel syndrome	Entrapment of the tibial nerve anywhere along its course, but often seen in the tarsal tunnel (posterior and inferior to medial malleolus). Pain and paresthesias in toes and sole of foot (heel spared as sensory branches arise proximal to tunnel), clawing of toes due to weakness of intrinsic foot muscles, typically worse at night. Tinel's test positive. Ankle eversion+dorsiflexion combined with toe dorsiflexion can reproduce pain (dorsiflexion-eversion test)

28. 1—j, L5, 2—e, C8, 3—c, C6

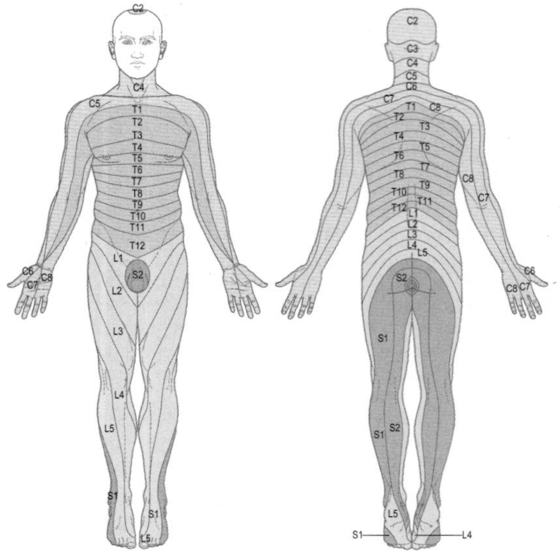

Image with permission from Standring S. Gray's Anatomy, 41st ed., Elsevier, 2015.

Spinal Nerve	Dermatome
C2	Occipital
C3	Upper neck
C4	Supraclavicular and acromioclavicular joint
C5	Clavicles, anterolateral aspect of arm and forearm until wrist.
C6	Lateral shoulder, arm, forearm, anatomical snuff box, thenar eminence and whole thumb
C7	Posterior arm, forearm, dorsum of hand, dorsal and palmar aspects of index and middle finger
C8	Medial arm, forearm and dorsal and palmar aspects of hand and ring + little fingers
T1	Anteromedial arm and forearm until wrist
T2	Chest and axilla
T4	Level of nipples/fourth intercostal space
T6	Level of the xiphoid process
T8	Level half way between xiphoid process and umbilicus
T10	Level of umbilicus
T12	Suprapubic level
L1	Inguinal and pubic levels
L2	Obliquely from upper lateral thigh to upper medial thigh (borders S2 dermatome posterior thigh)
L3	Obliquely from upper lateral thigh to lower medial thigh and medial aspect of knee
L4	Obliquely from lateral thigh, anterior aspect of knee, medial aspect of calf and medial side of foot
L5	Obliquely from lateral thigh, lateral aspect of knee/calf, anterior shin and dorsum of foot including medial 4 toes and sole of foot including heel
S1	Posterolateral aspect of buttock, thigh, popliteal fossa, calf and lateral aspect of ankle (lateral malleolus) and foot including little toe
S2	Posteromedial aspect of buttock, thigh, popliteal fossa, calf and heel; scrotum
S3	Perineum; glans penis/clitoris
S4/5	Perianal (S5 is within 1cm of mucocutaneous junction of anal canal)

Continued

29. 1—l, 2—k, 3—h, 4—j

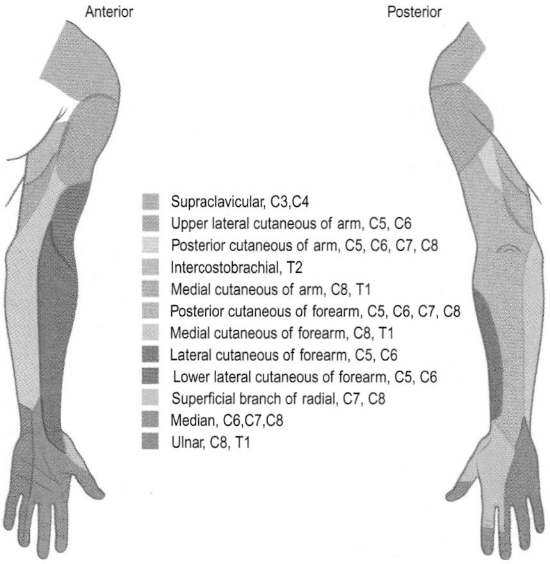

Image with permission from Mancall, Elliott L. Gray's Clinical Neuroanatomy: The Anatomic Basis for Clinical Neuroscience, Elsevier, Saunders, 2011.

30. 1—c, 2—f, 3—i

31. 1—g, Inverted radial reflex, 2—d, Hand of benediction, 3—a, Ape hand

Finding	Key Features
Ape hand	Loss of thumb opposition and abduction due to median nerve damage
Hand of benediction	On attempting to make a fist, only 4th and 5th digits flex at IPJs. Loss of flexion of digits 2+3 at MCPJ and IPJs due to median nerve palsy affecting lumbricals 1+2, median part of FDP
Volkman's contracture	Permanent flexion contracture of the hand at the wrist resulting in clawing of hand and fingers. Usually due to ischemia of long forearm flexors which then become fibrotic and short
Claw hand	On attempting to extend fingers, digits 4+5 remain in clawed position (MCPJ extension, flexed IPJs). Affects 4th and 5th digits with low ulnar nerve lesions (below mid-forearm), but complete claw hand can be seen if both low ulnar and median nerve injury occur together. Ulnar nerve lesions above mid-forearm do not produce clawing as there is also weakness of ulnar half of FDP
Hoover test	Aimed to distinguish organic from non-organic leg weakness using principle of synergistic contraction. Perform by holding the heel of the normal leg while asking patient to straight leg raise the weak leg against resistance. Normally examiner will feel heel push down as they try to raise the weak leg—absence suggests lack of effort to either leg
Tinel's test	Percussion over an (irritated) nerve elicits a sensation of pins and needles in the distribution of the nerve
Froment's sign	While grasping a piece of paper between thumb and index finger (palm flat) as it is pulled away, weakness of adductor pollicis (ulnar nerve) will result in compensatory flexion of thumb PIPJ to try and hold on to it
Hoffman's reflex	Tapping the nail or flicking the terminal phalanx of the middle/ring finger results in flexion of the terminal phalanx of the thumb. Suggests cervical cord pathology
Spurling's sign	Hyperextension of head and rotation towards symptomatic extremity (+/− pressing down on patients head) reproduces radicular symptoms due to narrowing of intervertebral foramina
Inverted radial reflex	Diminished brachioradialis reflex with reflex contraction of finger flexors. Suggests C5 pathology
Phalen's test	Holding wrist in complete forced flexion for up to 1 min, aiming to draw lumbricals into the carpal tunnel and compress the median nerve to reproduce symptoms. Reverse Phalen's test involves forced extension (prayer position)
Lasegue's sign	Straight leg raising test is considered positive if pain or paresthesia occur in a radicular distribution at less than 60° of elevation. Lowering the leg and dorsiflexing the ankle will exacerbate symptoms. Allowing the foot to rest on the table by flexing the knee will reduce pain (bowstring sign). Most specific for L5 or S1 root compression
Fajersztajn sign	Crossed straight leg raising test is usually positive with a large central disc protrusion. Raising the unaffected leg with patient supine produces radicular pain in the affected extremity
Femoral stretch test	Useful for distinguishing between sciatica involving L2 and L3 nerves and those involving L4 to S1. With the patient lying prone, the knee is passively flexed and the hip passively extended to elicit thigh pain
Pinch sign	Patient attempts to forcefully pinch the tips of index finger and thumb together to make an "OK" sign but AIN palsy causing weakness of FDP to digits 2+3 and FPL results in extension of terminal phalanges. As a result finger pulp rather than tips touch
Wartenberg's sign	Abducted little finger at rest due to weakness of 3rd palmar interosseous muscle in ulnar nerve palsy

32. a—8 & 21, b—10 & 22, c—5 & 17

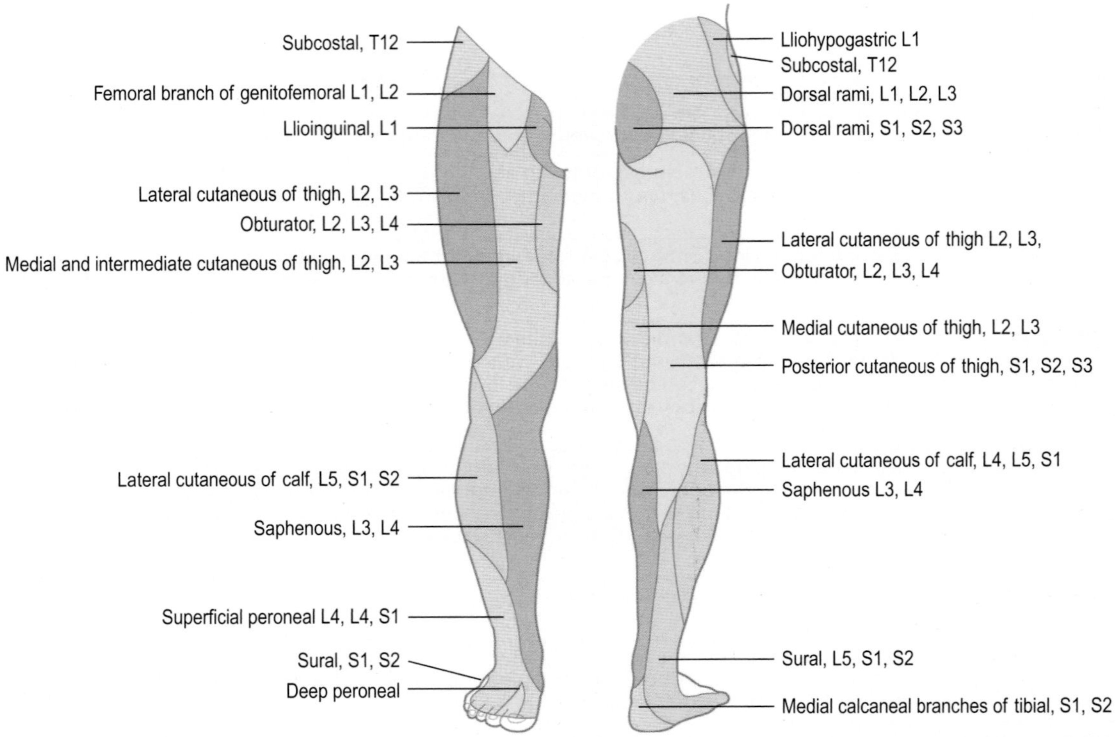

Image with permission from Mancall, Elliott L. Gray's Clinical Neuroanatomy: The Anatomic Basis for Clinical Neuroscience, Elsevier, Saunders, 2011.

PART VII
PEDIATRIC NEUROSURGERY

CHAPTER 38

Pediatric Neurosurgery: General Principles and Normal Development

SINGLE BEST ANSWER (SBA) QUESTIONS

1. Development of which one of the following domains has the best predictive value of future intelligence?
   a. Gross motor
   b. Adaptive
   c. Visuomotor
   d. Language
   e. Social

2. Which one of the following combinations of birthweight, height, and head circumference most likely represent normality?
   a. Weight 3500 g, height 50 cm, head circumference 35 cm
   b. Weight 3000 g, height 40 cm, head circumference 30 cm
   c. Weight 2500 g, height 50 cm, head circumference 40 cm
   d. Weight 2000 g, height 50 cm, head circumference 25 cm
   e. Weight 1500 g, height 30 cm, head circumference 20 cm

3. A neonate born at term has a weight of 3400 g, a length of 50 cm and a head circumference of 30 cm. There are no abnormal neurological findings or syndromic features. Which one of the following statements regarding the child's apparent microcephaly is true?
   a. He has a secondary microcephaly
   b. Microcephaly is due to the fact they are small for gestational age
   c. Cranial ultrasound should be performed as first choice for microcephaly
   d. Microcephaly is due to postnatal cause
   e. Isolated microcephaly

4. A 1-year-old infant has a head circumference in the 98th centile for age, he is at 75th centile for weight and height. At birth, his head circumference was just above the 95th centile. His father and mother have large heads. The child has achieved appropriate developmental milestones for age, and normal examination. Which one of the following is most accurate?
   a. He needs cranial ultrasound to rule out hydrocephalus
   b. He is likely to have subtle cerebral anomalies
   c. He is at risk for learning disabilities later in life
   d. He probably has familial macrocephaly and needs no further workup
   e. He is at risk for craniosynostosis

5. You are involved in a trauma call for a 2-year-old child fallen from a climbing frame and sustained a head injury. Hypotensive, and you are asked to prescribe a fluid bolus for him (he weighs 30 kg). What volume of fluid would you prescribe as per ATLS protocol?
   a. 600 ml
   b. 150 ml
   c. 300 ml
   d. 450 ml
   e. 900 ml

6. You are asked to prescribe maintenance fluids for an infant weighing 10 kg. Which

one of the following volumes of maintenance fluid should they receive over 24 h?
a. 1000 ml
b. 100 ml
c. 500 ml
d. 240 ml
e. 750 ml

7. What is the normal heart rate and respiratory rate for a child under 1 year?
a. HR < 100 and RR < 40
b. HR < 120 and RR < 30
c. HR < 160 and RR < 60
d. HR < 140 and RR < 50
e. HR < 150 and RR < 30

8. Which one of the following presentations most accurately suggests moderate blood volume loss (30-45%) in pediatric patients?
a. A 6-year-old child with increased HR, weak thready peripheral pulses, normal SBP, normal pulse pressure, confused, mottled skin, and capillary refill 3 s. Urine output is 0.5 ml/kg/h.
b. An 8-year-old child with markedly increased HR, weak thready central pulses, low normal SBP, normal pulse pressure, confused, prolonged CRT, and urine output 0.2 ml/kg/h.
c. A 5-year-old child with bradycardia, weak central pulses, hypotension, widened pulse, unresponsive to painful stimuli, cold, and anuric.
d. An 8-month-old child with increased HR, weak thready peripheral pulses, normal SBP, normal pulse pressure, irritable, mottled skin, and capillary refill 3 s. Urine output is 2 ml/kg/h.
e. An 8-year-old child with markedly increased HR, weak thready central pulses, low normal SBP, narrowed pulse pressure, dulled response to pain, markedly prolonged CRT, and urine output 0.2 ml/kg/h.

9. Which one of the following is NOT a feature of Down's syndrome?
a. Atrial septal defect
b. Occipital (and nasal) flattening
c. Brushfield spots
d. Epicanthic folds
e. Simian crease
f. Duodenal atresia
g. Clinodactyly
h. Butterfly erythema

10. Which one of the following statements about brain death in children is most accurate?
a. A single examination and confirmatory ancillary test are sufficient to make a diagnosis of brain death in most children
b. The diagnosis of brain death cannot be made in preterm infants less than 37 weeks of gestational age
c. MRI head is a commonly used ancillary test
d. Apnea testing must have been performed for a diagnosis of brain death
e. An observation period of 12 h is recommended between clinical examinations determining brain death

EXTENDED MATCHING ITEM (EMI) QUESTIONS

11. **Primitive reflexes:**
a. Asymmetric tonic neck
b. Babinski
c. Crossed extensor
d. Galant
e. Heel
f. Moro
g. Palmar grip
h. Plantar grip
i. Rossolimo
j. Suprapubic extensor

For each of the following descriptions, select the most appropriate answers from the list above. Each answer may be used once, more than once or not at all.
1. Scratching the skin of the infant's back from the shoulder downward, 2-3 cm lateral to the spinous processes results in incurvation of the trunk, with the concavity on the stimulated side.
2. Passive total flexion of one lower extremity results in extension of the other lower limb, with adduction and internal rotation into talipes equinus.
3. Sudden head extension produced by a light drop of the head results in abduction followed by adduction and flexion of upper extremities.

12. **Developmental milestones:**
a. 1 month
b. 2 months
c. 4 months
d. 6 months
e. 9 months
f. 12 months
g. 15 months
h. 18 months
i. 2 years

j. 3 years
k. 4 years
l. 5 years
m. 6 years

For each of the following descriptions, select the most appropriate answers from the list above. Each answer may be used once, more than once or not at all.

● 1. The child's parents report that she can ride a bicycle, write her own name, identifies written letters and numbers, knows right from left and knows all the color names.

● 2. The child's parents report that she can run, walks upstairs with her hand held, stoops and recovers, builds a three block tower, can use a spoon and scribbles spontaneously. Additionally, she uses up to 25 words, points to body parts when asked, uses words to communicate wants and needs, and plays near other children.

● 3. The child's parents report that she can sit but may need support, rolls in both directions, reaches with one hand, transfers object between hands, babbles and seems to recognize an object or person as unfamiliar.

● 4. The child's parents report that she raises her head slightly in the prone position, follows with her eyes to the midline only, her hands are tightly fisted, startles to sound and fixes on people's faces.

● 5. The child's parents report that she sits without support, crawls, pulls to stand, uses a pincer grasp, finger feeds, imitates speech sounds (nonspecific mama, dada), understands the meaning of "no," plays gesture games (pat-a-cake) and understands her own name. They have also noticed that she now knows hidden objects still remain there and is anxious around people she doesn't know.

SBA ANSWERS

1. **d**—Language

2. **a**—Weight 3500 g, height 50 cm, head circumference 35 cm

For the average term newborn:

- Weight is 3500 g (low birthweight is <2500 g, very low birthweight <1500 g and extremely low <1000 g). Neonates with birthweight below the 10th percentile are termed small for gestational age, and may be genetic or due to intrauterine growth restriction.
- Height is 50 cm
- Occipitofrontal head circumference (OFC) is 32.5-38 cm (mean 35 cm).

Head circumference increases approximately

- By 2 cm in first month
- By 6 cm in the first 4 months
- Approximately 1 cm/month during the first year of life
- Brain weight doubles by 4-6 months of age and triples by 1 year of age
- The majority of head growth is complete by 4 years of age

The measuring tape should encircle the head and include an area 1-2 cm above the glabella anteriorly and the most prominent portion of the occiput posteriorly. Measurement of OFC in the newborn may be unreliable until the 3rd or 4th day of life since it may be affected by caput succedaneum, cephalohematoma, or molding. It may be inappropriate to use a single head circumference standard for children in all countries or ethnic groups. The standard growth curves are not appropriate for monitoring the head size of children with certain medical conditions associated with macrocephaly (e.g. achondroplasia, neurofibromatosis) and other curves are available for these specific conditions.

FURTHER READING

Boom JA. Normal growth patterns in infants and prepubertal children. UpToDate Topic 2845 Version 15.0.

3. **e**—Isolated microcephaly

Microcephaly is generally defined as an occipitofrontal circumference more than 2 standard deviations (SD) below the mean for a given age, sex, and gestation (i.e. <3rd percentile); using this definition approximately 2% of the general population would be considered microcephalic even though many of these individuals are simply at the low end of the population distribution. Because head growth is driven by brain growth, microcephaly usually implies microencephaly (small brain size) except in cases of generalized craniosynostosis in which skull growth is restricted, but microencephaly may be present in children with normal OFC. In general, microencephaly can result either from abnormal brain development or insult to a previous normal brain. Multiple classifications: primary microcephaly is present at birth, while secondary develops postnatally; others include genetic vs. environments, isolated vs. syndromic, symmetric vs. asymmetric. The causes of microcephaly are summarized below:

Microcephaly: Causes

Genetic—isolated	Present at birth and uncomplicated by other anomalies; genetic failure to produce enough neurons, relatively normal brain anatomy, no neurological signs but some degree of learning difficulty
Genetic—syndromic	Down syndrome, Trisomy 18, Trisomy 13, Fetal alcohol syndrome, and many others
Genetic or other—CNS	Neural Tube Defect, holoprosencephaly, lissencephaly, schizencephaly, polymicrogyria, pachygyria, hydrancephaly, fetal brain disruption sequence
Metabolic	Aminoaciduria (e.g. phenylketonuria), storage disorders, and others
Environmental	Antenatal, perinatal, postnatal infection (e.g. TORCH), in utero drug/toxin exposure, hypoxic-ischemic insult, IVH/stroke, malnutrition

FURTHER READING

Boom JA. Microcephaly in infants and children: etiology and evaluation. UpToDate.

4. **d**—He probably has familial macrocephaly and needs no further workup

Head growth is affected by growth and alterations in the contents of the cranium and the timing of these changes in relation to closure of the fontanelles and sutures. Changes in the volume of any component before the closure of the fontanelles and sutures may alter the OFC. Evaluation for macrocephaly should be initiated when a single OFC measurement is abnormal, when serial measurements reveal progressive enlargement (i.e. crossing of one or more major percentile lines [e.g. 10th, 25th, 50th, 75th, 90th] between health supervision visits), or when there is an increase in OFC of >2 cm/month (for infants aged 0-6 months). Macrocephaly is defined as an OFC greater than two standard deviations (SD) above the mean for a given age, sex, and gestation (i.e. ≥97th percentile). The most common type of anatomic megalencephaly is benign familial megalencephaly where children are born with large heads and normal body size, and during infancy OFC increases to greater than the 90th percentile, typically 2-4 cm above, but parallel to, the 98th percentile; head growth velocity slows to a normal rate by approximately 6 months of age. In children with a normal neurologic examination, normal development, no clinical features suggestive of a specific syndrome, and no family history of abnormal neurologic or developmental problems, familial megalencephaly can be confirmed by measuring the patient's parents' head circumferences and by using Weaver curves. If the child's OFC falls within the normal ranges as estimated using the Weaver curves, radiologic evaluation is not necessary. Other causes of macrocephaly are summarized below:

Macrocephaly: Causes

Increased brain (megalencephaly)	Anatomic (increased cells): • Familial megalencephaly (commonest) • Neurophakomatoses • Autistic spectrum disorders • Achondroplasia • Cerebral gigantism (Sotos syndrome) • Fragile X syndrome • Cowden syndrome • Gorlin syndrome	Metabolic (deposition of substances in brain tissue): • Leukodystrophies • Lysosomal storage disorders
Increased CSF	Hydrocephalus Benign enlargement of subarachnoid space	
Increased blood	Hemorrhage (extradural, subdural, parenchymal, intraventricular). Arteriovenous malformation	
Increased bone	Thalassaemia (marrow expansion) Primary bone disorders	
Intracranial mass	Cyst, tumor, abscess	

FURTHER READING

Boom JA. Macrocephaly in infants and children: etiology and evaluation. UpToDate.

5. **a**—600 ml

Current ATLS protocol for fluid boluses in pediatric trauma is 20 ml/kg (0.9% saline or ringer's lactate). If hypotensive after two boluses of fluid, packed red cells should be administered (10 ml/kg).

6. **a**—1000 ml

In general, maintenance fluid requirement for children (excluding losses from drains, etc.) can be calculated as:

- 100 ml/kg/24 h for the first 10 kg of weight
- 50 ml/kg/24 h for the next 10 kg of weight
- 20 ml/kg/24 h for each kg over 20 kg

For example, in 24 h maintenance fluid requirement for a child weighing 25 kg would be: $(10\ \text{kg} \times 100\ \text{ml/kg}) + (10\ \text{kg} \times 50\ \text{ml/kg}) + (5\ \text{kg} \times 20\ \text{ml/kg}) = 1000\ \text{ml} + 500\ \text{ml} + 100\ \text{ml} = 1600\ \text{ml}$ (i.e. run at $1600/24 = 66.7$ ml/h)

7. **c**—HR < 160 and RR < 60

Normal Values in Children

Age	Weight Range	Heart Rate	BP	RR	Urinary Output
Infant (0-12 months)	0-10	<160	>60	<60	2.0 ml/kg/h
Toddler (1-2 years)	10-14	<150	>70	<40	1.5 ml/kg/h
Preschool (3-5 years)	14-18	<140	>75	<35	1.0 ml/kg/h
School age (6-12 years)	18-36	<120	>80	<30	1.0 ml/kg/h
Adolescent (>13 years)	36-70	<100	>90	<30	0.5 ml/kg/h

FURTHER READING

ATLS Student Course Manual: Advanced Trauma Life Support. J Am Coll Surg 2012; ISBN-10: 1880696029, ISBN-13: 978-1880696026.

8. **b**—An 8-year-old child with markedly increased HR, weak thready central pulses, low normal SBP, narrowed pulse pressure, dulled response to pain, markedly prolonged CRT, and urine output 0.2 ml/kg/h.

Hemorrhagic Shock in Children

System	Mild Blood Loss (<30%)	Moderate Blood Loss (30-45%)	Severe Blood Loss (>45%)
CVS	Increased HR Weak, thready peripheral pulses, normal SBP (80-90 + 2 × age in years), normal pulse pressure	Markedly increased HR Weak thready central pulses Low normal SBP (70-80 + 2 × age), narrowed pulse pressure	Tachycardia followed by bradycardia Weak/absent central pulses, hypotension (<70 + 2 × age), widened pulse pressure or undetectable diastolic pressure
CNS	Anxious, irritable, confused	Lethargic, dulles response to pain	Comatose
Skin	Cool, mottled, prolonged CRT	Cyanotic, markedly prolonged CRT	Pale and cold
Urine output	Low to very low	Minimal	Anuric

Continued

FURTHER READING

ATLS Student Course Manual: Advanced Trauma Life Support. J Am Coll Surg 2012; ISBN-10: 1880696029, ISBN-13: 978-1880696026.

9. **h**—Butterfly erythema

Down's syndrome affects 1 in 1000 births and is due to trisomy 21. Manifestations are various, systems are summarized (non-exhaustive) below:

Down Syndrome: Clinical Features

CNS	Mental retardation, early dementia, hearing impairment
Cardiac	Endocardial cushion defect: ASD, VSD, PDA, tetralogy of Fallot
Facial	Round face, occipital/nasal flattening, Brushfield spots (speckled iris), open mouth and protruding tongue, upslanting palpebral fissure, epicanthal folds
Hands and feet	Single transverse palmar (Simian) crease, short fingers, curved little finger (clinodactyly), sandal gap between big toe and adjacent toe
Spine/MSK	Hypotonia, atlanto-axial instability
GI	Duodenal atresia/stenosis, annular pancreas, omphalocele, Hirschsprung's disease, imperforate anus, tracheoesophageal fistula
Immune	Impaired cellular immunity (more infections), autoimmune disorders, increased childhood risk of AML-M7 and ALL
Endocrine	Hypo/hyperthyroidism, type 1 diabetes mellitus, infertility in males

10. **b**—The diagnosis of brain death cannot be made in preterm infants less than 37 weeks of gestational age

The most common causes of brain death in children are trauma, anoxic encephalopathy, infections, and cerebral neoplasms. In the UK, in children >2 months the criteria used to establish death should be the same as those in adults; it is also appreciated that between 37 weeks of gestation and 2 months of age, it is rarely possible confidently to diagnose death as a result of cessation of brainstem reflexes, and below 37 weeks of gestation the criteria to establish this cannot be applied. Although the definition of brain death and the declaration process in children is very similar to adult patients, there are several specific recommendations made by the American Academy of Pediatrics in 2011 (below). These guidelines are based in large part on consensus opinion as evidence is limited and committees in several countries decided to declare brain death only in children >2 months of age, while others requiring serial examinations in younger infants.

FURTHER READING

Spinello IM. Brain death determination. J Intens Care Med 2015;30(6):326-337;

Academy of Medical Royal Colleges. A code of practice for the diagnosis and confirmation of death; 2008;

Nakagawa TA, Ashwal S, Mathur M, Mysore M. Guidelines for the determination of brain death in infants and children: an update of the 1987 task force recommendations. Pediatrics 2011;128(3):e720-e740.

EMI ANSWERS

11. 1—d, Galant; 2—c, Crossed extensor; 3—f, Moro

Primitive reflexes are brainstem-mediated, complex, automatic movement patterns that commence as early as the 25th week of gestation, are fully present at birth in term infants, and disappear with central nervous system maturation (when voluntary motor activity and thus cortical inhibition emerges). Infants with cerebral palsy have been known to demonstrate persistence

American Academy of Pediatrics (2011) Guidlines for Determination of Brain Death in Children

Waiting period before initial brain death examination	24 h following cardiopulmonary resuscitation or severe acute brain injury is suggested if there are concerns about the neurologic examination or if dictated by clinical judgment
Clinical examination	Required
Core body temperature	>35 °C (95 °F)
Number of examinations	Two exams, irrespective of ancillary study results (if ancillary testing is being done in lieu of initial examination elements that cannot be safely performed, the components of the second examination that can be done must be completed)
Number of examiners	Two (different attending physicians must perform the first and second exam)
Observation interval between neurologic examinations	Age dependent Term newborn (37 weeks gestation) to 30 days of age: 24 h 31 days to 18 years: 12 h
Reduction of observation period between exams	Permitted for both age groups if EEG or CBF consistent with brain death
Apnea testing	Two apnea tests required unless clinically contraindicated
Final PCO_2 threshold for apnea testing	≥60 mmHg and ≥20 mmHg above the baseline $PaCO_2$
Ancillary study recommended	Not required except in cases where the clinical examination and apnea test cannot be completed • Term newborn (37 weeks gestation) to 30 days of age: EEG or CBF are less sensitive in this age group. CBF may be preferred. • >30 days to 18 years: EEG and CBF have equal sensitivity
Time of death	Time of the second examination and apnea test (or completion of ancillary study and the components of the second examination that can be safely completed)

of primitive reflexes or a delay in their disappearance. Persistence of obligatory primitive reflexes beyond 12 months of age is an indicator of a poor prognosis regarding ambulation. The major primitive motor reflexes or patterns that have been described include Moro, palmar and plantar grasp, rooting, sucking, placing, Moro, Galant (or truncal incurvation), asymmetric tonic neck reflex, crossed extensor, tonic labyrinthine reflex, and others. Special emphasis should be placed on the plantar response: different types of responses have been elicited in infants, varying from flexor to extensor according to the intensity of the stimulus used but it is generally accepted and that extensor plantar response matures to flexor by the end of the first year in most normal infants. The Babinski sign refers to the extensor toe response observed in corticospinal tract pathology but there is ongoing debate as to whether a true Babinski sign (dorsiflexion of the great toe and fanning of the remaining toes) is present as a primitive reflex in infants where it is part of flexion withdrawal of the leg.

Primitive Reflexes

Reflex	Position	Method	Response	Age at Disappearance
Palmar grip	Supine	Placing the index finger in the palm of the infant	Flexion of fingers, fist-making	6 months
Plantar grip	Supine	Pressing a thumb against the sole just behind the toes	Flexion of toes	15 months
Galant	Prone	Scratching the skin of the infant's back from the shoulder downward, 2-3 cm lateral to the spinous processes	Incurvation of the trunk, with the concavity on the stimulated side	4 months
Asymmetric tonic neck	Supine	Rotation of the infant's head to one side for 15 s	Extension of the extremities on the chin side and flexion of those on the occipital side	3 months
Suprapubic extensor	Supine	Pressing the skin over the pubic bone with the fingers	Reflex extension of both lower extremities, with adduction and internal rotation into talipes equinus	4 weeks
Crossed extensor	Supine	Passive total flexion of one lower extremity	Extension of the other lower limb, with adduction and internal rotation into talipes equinus	6 weeks
Rossolimo	Supine	Light tapping of toes 2-4 at their plantar surfaces	Tonic flexion of the toes at the first metacarpophalangeal joint	4 weeks
Heel	Supine	Tapping on the heel with a hammer, with the infant's hip and knee joints flexed and the ankle joint in neutral position	Rapid reflex extension of the lower extremity in question	3 weeks
Moro	Supine	Sudden head extension produced by a light drop of the head	Abduction followed by adduction and flexion of upper extremities	6 months
Babinski	Supine	Striking along the lateral aspect of the sole, extending from the heel to the head of the fifth metatarsal	Combined extensor response: simultaneous dorsiflexion of the great toe and fanning of the remaining toes	Presence always abnormal

FURTHER READING

Zafeiriou DI. Primitive reflexes and postural reactions in the neurodevelopmental examination. Pediatr Neurol 2004;31(1):1-8.

12. 1—m, 6 years; 2—h, 18 months; 3—d, 6 months; 4—a, 1 month; 5—e, 9 months

Normal Developmental Milestones in Children

Age	Gross Motor	Fine (Visual) Motor	Language	Social/Adaptive
1 month	Raises head slightly in prone position	Follows with eyes to midline only Hands tightly fisted	Alerts/startles to sound	Fixes on faces
2 months	Raises chest and head off bed in prone position	Regards object and follows 180 arc; briefly holds rattle	Coos and vocalizes reciprocally	Social smile, recognizes parent
4 months	Lifts onto extended elbows in prone position; steady head control with no head lag, rolls over front to back	Reaches for object with both hands together, bats at objects, grabs and retains objects	Orients to voice, laughs, and squeals	Initiates social interaction
6 months	Sits but may need support, rolls in both directions	Reaches with one hand, transfers object between hands	Babbles	Recognizes object or person as unfamiliar
9 months	Sits without support Crawls Pulls to stand	Uses pincer grasp, finger feeds	Imitates speech sounds (nonspecific mama, dada), understands meaning of "no"	Plays gesture games (pat-a-cake), understands own name, object permanence, stranger anxiety
12 months	Cruises furniture, stands alone, takes a few independent steps	Can voluntarily release items,	Discriminative use of mama, dada; one to four other words, follows command with gesture	Imitates, comes when called, cooperates with dressing
15 months	Walks well independently	Builds two block tower; throws ball underhand	Four to six more words; uses jargon; responds to one-step verbal command	Begins to use cup; indicates wants or needs
18 months	Runs; walks upstairs with hand held; stoops and recovers	Builds three block tower; uses spoon; spontaneous scribbling	Uses up to 25 words; points to body parts when asked; uses words to communicate wants and needs	Uses words to communicate wants and needs; plays near but not with other children
2 years	Walks unassisted up and down stairs; kicks ball; throws ball overhand; jumps with two feet off floor	Builds 4-6 brick tower, uses fork and spoon, copies a straight line	Uses 50+ words, two- and three-word phrases; uses I and me; 50% of speech intelligible to stranger	Removes simple clothing; parallel play
3 years	Pedals tricycle; broad jumps	Copies a circle	Uses 5-8 word sentences; 75% of speech intelligible to stranger	Knows age and gender, engages in group play, shares
4 years	Balances on one foot	Copies a cross; catches ball	Tells a story; 100% of speech intelligible to stranger	Dresses self, puts on shows, washes and dries hands, imaginative play
5 years	Skips with alternating feet	Draws person with six body parts	Asks what words mean	Names four colors; plays cooperative games; understands rules and abides by them
6 years	Rides a bicycle	Writes name	Identifies written letters and numbers	Knows right from left; knows all color names

FURTHER READING

Fine KS. Paediatric board recertification review. Lippincott, Williams and Wilkins; 2008. p. 2.

CHAPTER 39

CRANIOSYNOSTOSIS

SINGLE BEST ANSWER (SBA) QUESTIONS

1. Features demonstrated in the picture below are most likely the result of:

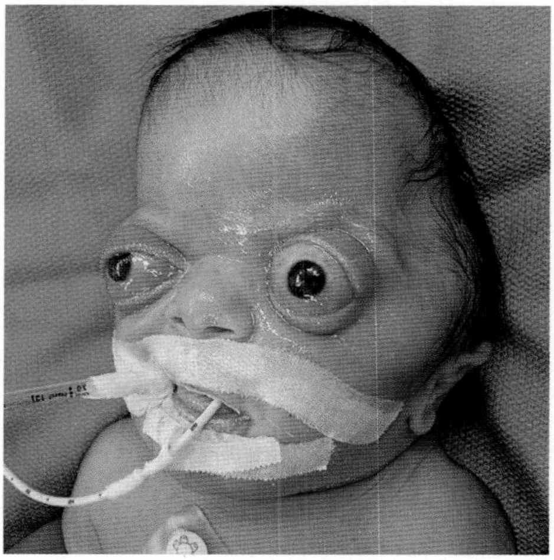

a. Anterior plagiocephaly
b. Deformational posterior plagiocephaly
c. Kleeblattschadel deformity
d. Oxycephaly
e. Turricephaly

2. What is the most likely craniosynostosis depicted in this image?

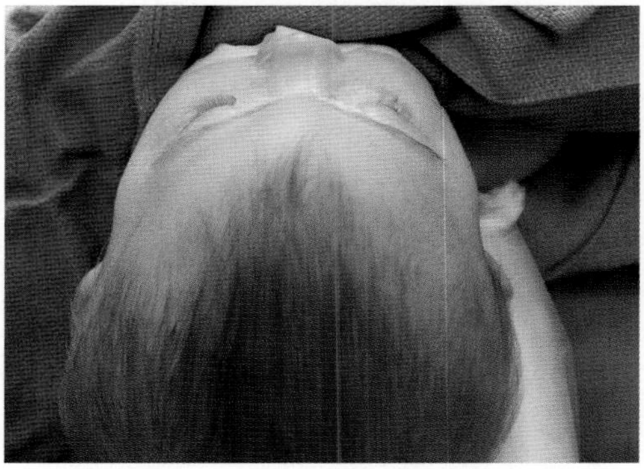

a. Bilateral Coronal synostosis
b. Cloverleaf (Kleeblattschadel)
c. Lambdoid synostosis
d. Metopic synostosis
e. Sagittal synostosis

3. Which one of the following most likely to cause the appearances shown below?

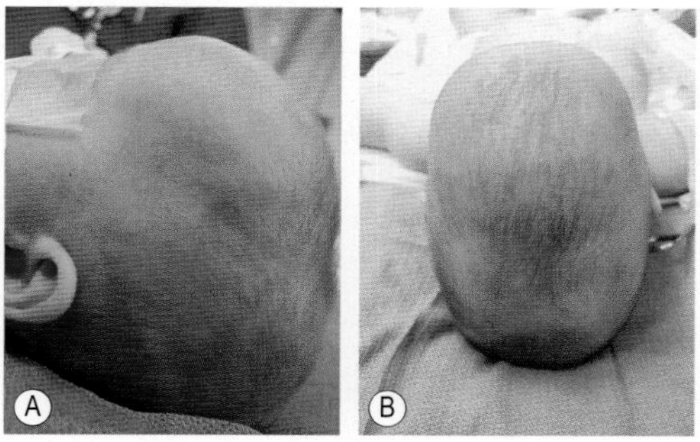

a. Bicoronal synostosis
b. Crouzon's syndrome
c. Metopic synostosis
d. Pierre-Robin sequence
e. Sagittal synostosis

4. Given the clinical features demonstrated in this 6-month-old child which one of the following is most likely:

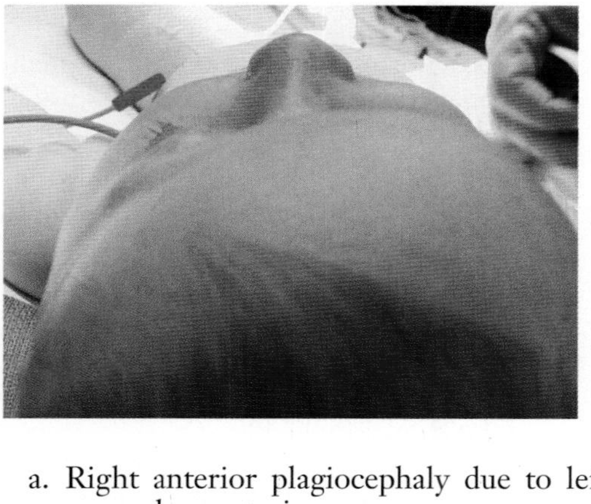

a. Right anterior plagiocephaly due to left coronal synostosis
b. Left anterior plagiocephaly due to left coronal synostosis
c. Right anterior plagiocephaly due to right coronal synostosis
d. Left anterior plagiocephaly due to right coronal synostosis

e. Left anterior plagiocephaly due to bilateral coronal synostosis
f. Right anterior plagiocephaly due to bilateral coronal synostosis

5. Features demonstrated in the bird's eye diagram below are most consistent with:

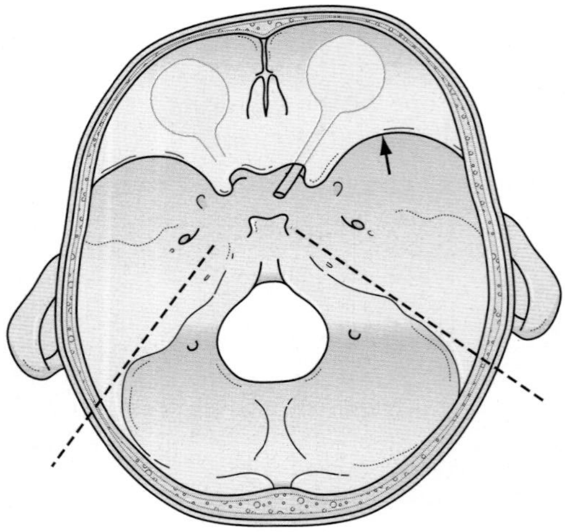

a. Right posterior plagiocephaly due to lambdoid synostosis
b. Left posterior plagiocephaly due to lambdoid synostosis
c. Right posterior plagiocephaly due to bilateral lambdoid synostosis
d. Right posterior deformational plagiocephaly
e. Left posterior deformational plagiocephaly
f. Left posterior plagiocephaly due to bilateral lambdoid synostosis

6. Craniosynostosis occurs in approximately how many live births?
a. 1/1000 to 1/1500
b. 1/1500 to 1/2000
c. 1/2000 to 1/2500
d. 1/2500 to 1/3000
e. 1/3000 to 1/3500

7. Frequency of different types of single suture synostoses is approximately:
a. Lambdoid 18%, Metopic 25%, Sagittal 60%, Unicoronal 3%
b. Lambdoid 18%, Metopic 60%, Sagittal 25%, Unicoronal 3%
c. Lambdoid 25%, Metopic 18%, Sagittal 3%, Unicoronal 60%
d. Lambdoid 3%, Metopic 25%, Sagittal 60%, Unicoronal 18%
e. Lambdoid 60%, Metopic 18%, Sagittal 3%, Unicoronal 25%

8. Virchow's law states
a. Skull growth is arrested in the direction perpendicular to the fused suture and reduced at the sites of unaffected sutures
b. Skull growth is arrested in the direction parallel to the fused suture and expanded at the sites of unaffected sutures
c. Skull growth is arrested in the direction perpendicular to the fused suture and expanded at the sites of affected sutures
d. Skull growth is arrested in the direction parallel to the fused suture and expanded at the sites of affected sutures
e. Skull growth is arrested in the direction perpendicular to the fused suture and expanded at the sites of unaffected sutures

9. Features of raised intracranial pressure on plain radiograph show:
a. Bilateral Harlequin sign
b. Copper beating
c. Frontal bossing
d. Temporoparietal bossing
e. Open fontanelle

10. Fronto-orbital advancement surgery is most likely considered in which one of the following scenarios
a. Apert's syndrome
b. Fibrous dysplasia
c. Paget's disease
d. Sagittal synostosis

11. Which one of the following most likely to cause the appearances shown below?

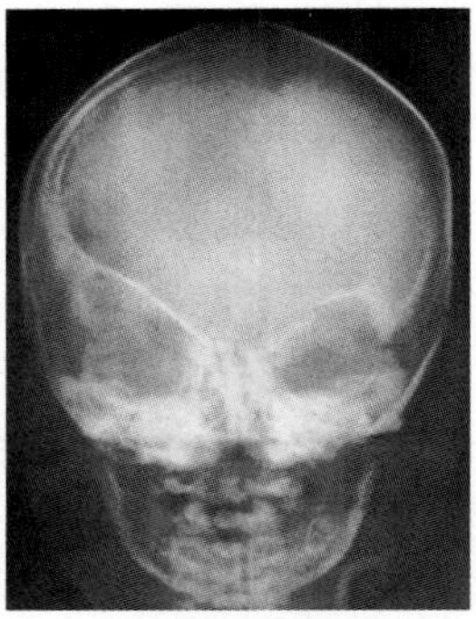

a. Lambdoid synostosis
b. Metopic synostosis
c. Positional plagiocephaly
d. Sagittal synostosis
e. Unicoronal suture synostosis

12. Which one of the following most likely to cause the appearances shown below?

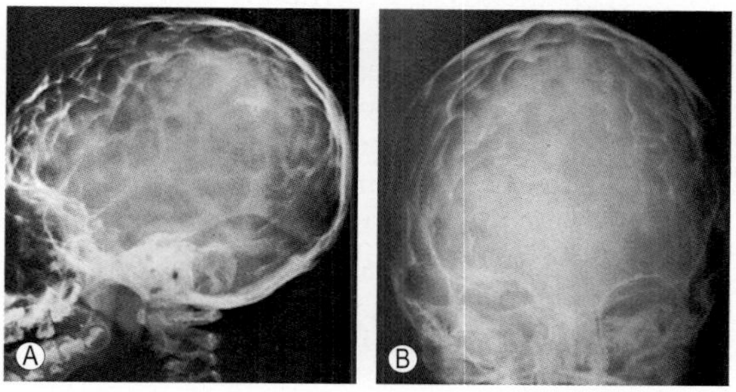

a. Aqueduct stenosis
b. Fibrous dysplasia
c. Hyperparathyroidism
d. Langerhan's histiocytosis
e. Multiple myeloma

13. Which one of the following most likely to cause the appearances shown below?

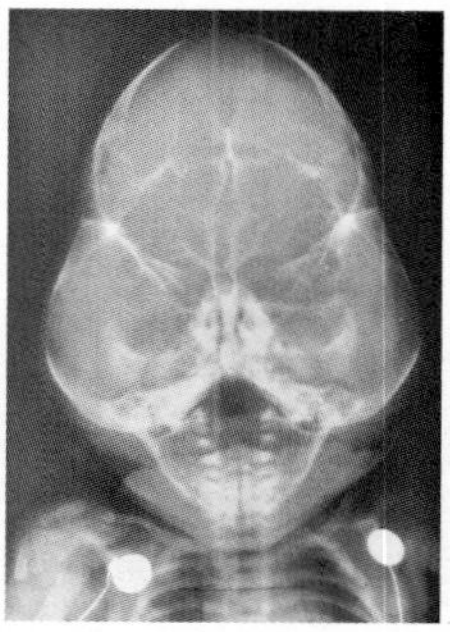

a. Hyperparathyroidism
b. Leukemia
c. Neurofibromatosis (NF)
d. Pfeiffer's syndrome
e. Saethre-Chotzen

14. Which one of the following most likely to cause the appearances shown below?

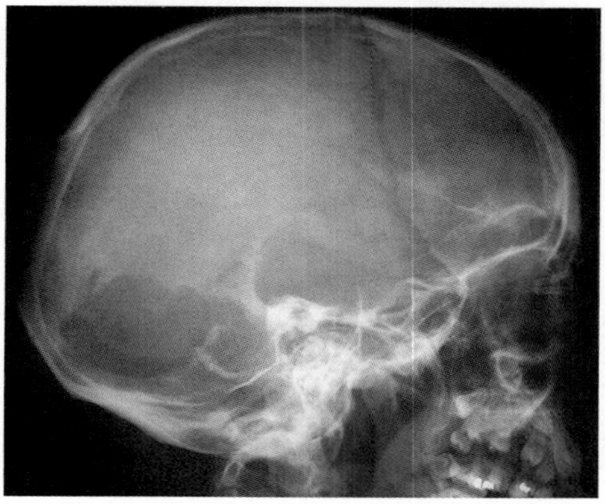

a. Cerebral abscess
b. Fibrous dysplasia
c. Multiple myeloma
d. Neurofibromatosis type 1
e. Raised intracranial pressure

15. Which one of the following most likely to cause the appearances shown below?

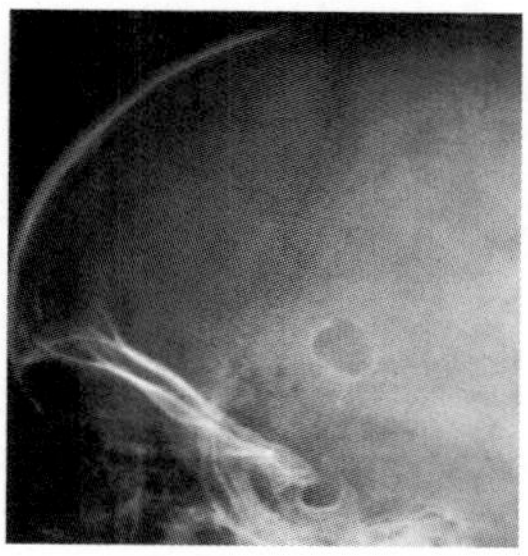

a. Arachnoid cyst
b. Epidermoid
c. Fibrous dysplasia
d. Leukemia
e. Raised intracranial pressure

16. Which one of the following most likely to cause the appearances shown below?

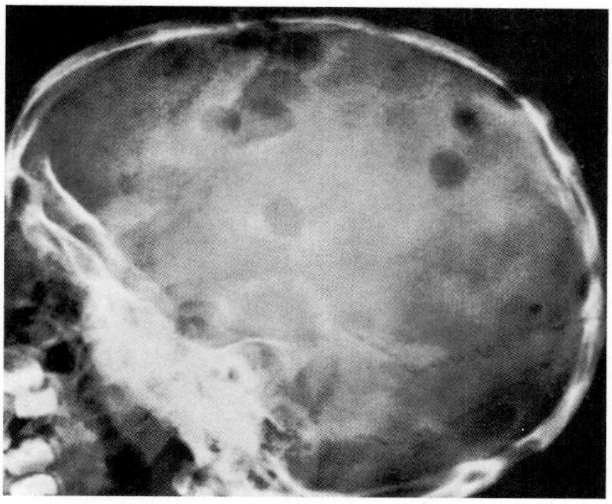

a. Dermoid
b. Epidermoid
c. Raised intracranial pressure
d. Saethre-Chotzen syndrome
e. Tuberculosis

EXTENDED MATCHING ITEM (EMI) QUESTIONS

17. **Craniofacial terminology:**
    a. Acrocephaly
    b. Anterior plagiocephaly
    c. Brachycephaly
    d. Cloverleaf skull
    e. Dolichocephaly
    f. Harlequin sign
    g. Oxycephaly
    h. Posterior plagiocephaly
    i. Scaphocephaly
    j. Trigonocephaly
    k. Turricephaly

For each of the following descriptions, select the most appropriate answers from the list above. Each answer may be used once, more than once or not at all.

1. Cephalic index <74
2. Cephalic index >83

18. **Causes of craniosynostosis:**
    a. Blood dyscrasias (e.g. thalassemia, sickle cell anemia, polycythemia vera)
    b. Fibroblast growth factor receptor mutations
    c. Holoprosencephaly
    d. Hyperthyroidism
    e. MSX-2 transcription factor
    f. Mucopolysaccharidoses (e.g. Hurler syndrome, Morquio syndrome)
    g. Overshunted hydrocephalus
    h. Rickets disease
    i. Teratogens (Valproic acid, Retinoic acid)
    j. Transforming growth factor-beta receptors
    k. TWIST transcription factor

For each of the following descriptions, select the most appropriate answers from the list above. Each answer may be used once, more than once or not at all.

1. Implicated in Crouzon, Apert, Pfeiffer and Jackson-Weiss syndromes
2. Implicated in intrauterine head constraint-related craniosynostosis—d
3. Implicated in Saethre-Chotzen syndrome—c

SBA ANSWERS

1. **c**—The picture demonstrates a newborn infant with cloverleaf skull deformity-frontal towering, bitemporal expansion, bilateral supraorbital recession (with proptosis), hypertelorism, and midface hypoplasia. One should also examine for broad great toe/thumb (Pfeiffer syndrome) and syndactyly (Apert's syndrome). It is caused by premature closure of sagittal, coronal, and lambdoid sutures and can occur in any severe craniosynostosis.

Image with permission from Ellenbogen RG, Abdulrauf SI, Sekhar LN. Principles of Neurological Surgery, 3rd ed., Elsevier, Saunders, 2012.

2. **d**—Metopic synostosis. Features demonstrated are trigonocephaly, significant ridging over the metopic suture, supraorbital recession and hypotelorism (see CT below). Due to reduced anterior cranial volume resulting in back pressure into the posterior fossa, there is an association with Type 1 Chiari malformations (30%). It is also associated with frontal dysmorphology-corpus callosum dysgenesis, holoproscencephaly.

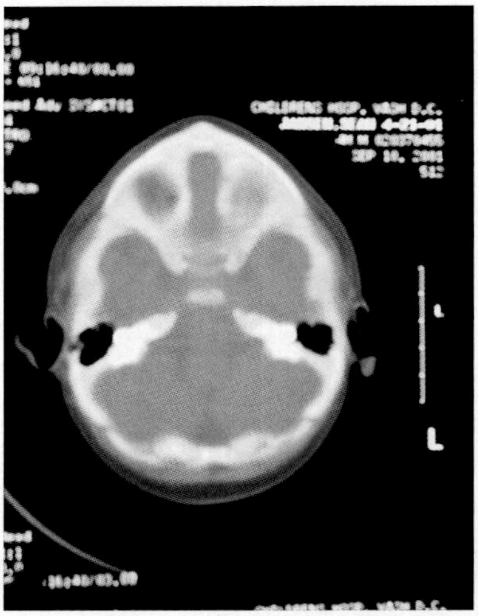

Image with permission from Ellenbogen RG, Abdulrauf SI, Sekhar LN. Principles of Neurological Surgery, 3rd ed., Elsevier, Saunders, 2012.

3. **e**—Sagittal synostosis

Image with permission from Ellenbogen RG, Abdulrauf SI, Sekhar LN. Principles of Neurological Surgery, 3rd ed., Elsevier, Saunders, 2012.

4. **b**—Left anterior plagiocephaly due to left coronal synostosis. Features seen are significant left supraorbital retrusion, left forehead flattening, and compensatory right frontal bossing. Other features to look for in unicoronal synostosis are ipsilateral perisutural ridging, ipsilateral nasal root displacement, anterior displacement of ipsilateral ear, contralateral chin deviation, and the pathognomonic feature of ipsilateral orbital elevation (harlequin sign). Strabismus is common (50-60%) due to mechanical effect on superior oblique, and anterior plagiocephaly is commoner on the right side (3:2).

Image with permission from Ellenbogen RG, Abdulrauf SI, Sekhar LN. Principles of Neurological Surgery, 3rd ed., Elsevier, Saunders, 2012.

5. **d**—Right posterior deformational plagiocephaly. Posterior deformational plagiocephaly is characterized by a parallelogram shaped head, anterior displacement of ipsilateral ear, and ipsilateral frontal bossing. In contrast, unilateral lambdoid synostosis is marked by a trapezoid shaped skull, posterior displacement of ipsilateral ear and contralateral occipital bossing.

Image with permission from Ellenbogen RG, Abdulrauf SI, Sekhar LN. Principles of Neurological Surgery, 3rd ed., Elsevier, Saunders, 2012.

6. **c**—1/2000 to 1/2500

7. **d**—Lambdoid 3%, Metopic 25%, Sagittal 60%, Unicoronal 18%. Sagittal (3.5-7:1) and metopic (75%) synostosis is commoner in boys, while unicoronal is commoner in girls (3:2). True lambdoid synostosis is rare, and must be distinguished from posterior deformational plagiocephaly (positional molding) where there is occipital flattening without suture fusion, possibly due to supine sleeping position instituted to reduce sudden infant death syndrome.

8. **e**—Skull growth is arrested in the direction perpendicular to the fused suture and expanded at the sites of unaffected sutures, leading to characteristic calvarial deformations

9. **b**—Copper beating. The thinned out skull is usually an indicator of chronic hydrocephalus.

10. **a**—Apert's syndrome

11. **e**—Unicoronal suture synostosis. The skull radiograph exhibits the classic 'harlequin' sign.

Image with permission from Coley BD. Caffey's Pediatric Diagnostic Imaging, 12th ed., Elsevier, Saunders, 2013.

12. **a**—Aqueduct stenosis. The appearances above are termed "copper beaten skull" associated with raised intracranial pressure in children. Common causes are craniosynostosis, obstructive hydrocephalus, intracranial masses and hypophosphatasia.

Image with permission from Coley BD. Caffey's Pediatric Diagnostic Imaging, 12th ed., Elsevier, Saunders, 2013.

13. **d**—Pfeiffer's syndrome (Cloverleaf skull).

Image with permission from Coley BD. Caffey's Pediatric Diagnostic Imaging, 12th ed., Elsevier, Saunders, 2013.

14. **d**—Angiomas and neurofibromas of the scalp may affect the underlying skull and cause deformities, bony defects, and regional hyperostoses. Plain film findings of NF include lytic defect in the lambdoid suture, absence of the orbital roof and floor, elevated lesser sphenoid wing, enlarged middle cranial fossa, enlarged cranial nerve foramina, unilateral orbital enlargement, and J-shaped sella turcica.

Image with permission from Coley BD. Caffey's Pediatric Diagnostic Imaging, 12th ed., Elsevier, Saunders, 2013.

15. **b**—Epidermoid

A small oval defect in the parietal bone with a sharply defined sclerotic border. Epidermoids are ectodermal rests or inclusions that may be located in the scalp, in the diploic spaces, or between the internal surface of the inner table and the dura. Epidermoids are usually benign and grow slowly. If they protrude into the cranial cavity, they may be the source of cerebral symptoms. When epidermoids grow within the bone or impinge on it, they produce local destruction of bone that appears radiographically as a sharply demarcated lucency surrounded by a smooth sclerotic margin, which sometimes may be scalloped. The margin is due to flaring of the edge of the bone into a marginal ridge. Most cases are found in children younger than 3 years. The lesions usually disappear within a few years of discovery.

Image with permission from Coley BD. Caffey's Pediatric Diagnostic Imaging, 12th ed., Elsevier, Saunders, 2013.

16. **e**—Multiple destructive tuberculosis foci in the calvaria of a 3-year-old girl. Tuberculosis of the calvaria usually manifests as a painless subgaleal scalp swelling with a discharging sinus. The lesions are usually either small, circumscribed, punched-out lytic areas or spreading, circumscribed sclerotic areas; or a combination of the two. The differential diagnosis of multiple lytic lesions in the skull—TB, multiple myeloma, Langerhans cell histiocytosis.

Image with permission from Coley BD. Caffey's Pediatric Diagnostic Imaging, 12th ed., Elsevier, Saunders, 2013.

EMI ANSWERS

17. 1—e, Dolichocephaly; 2—c, Brachycephaly

Cephalic index (CI) = biparietal diameter (BPD)/occipitofrontal diameter (OFD) × 100. Normal range 74-83, and it can be altered by breech presentation, ruptured membranes, twin pregnancy when measured intrauterine.

18. 1—b, Fibroblast growth factor receptor mutations; 2—j, Transforming growth factor-beta receptors; 3—k, TWIST transcription factor.

CHAPTER 40

Congenital Cranial and Spinal Disorders

SINGLE BEST ANSWER (SBA) QUESTIONS

1. Which one of the following is most likely based on the radiograph shown below?

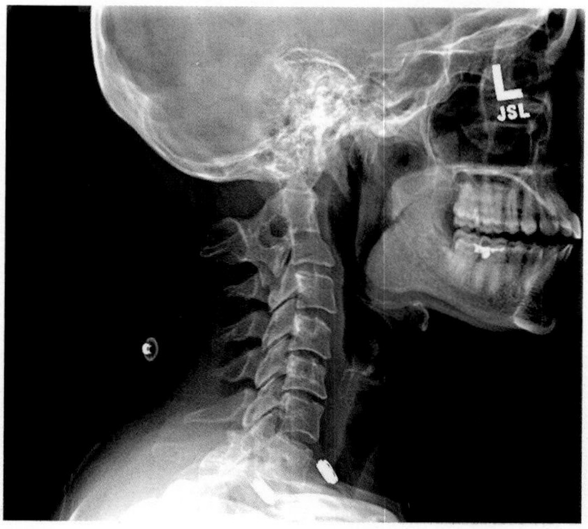

a. Achondroplasia
b. Klippel-Feil
c. Osteogenesis imperfecta
d. Posterior spina bifida
e. Segmental spinal dysgenesis

2. A young child with an FGFR-3 mutation is shown in the picture below. Which one of the following disorders is he NOT at increased risk of?
a. Cervicomedullary compression
b. Hydrocephalus
c. Posterior circulation aneurysms
d. Spinal canal stenosis
e. Thoracolumbar kyphosis

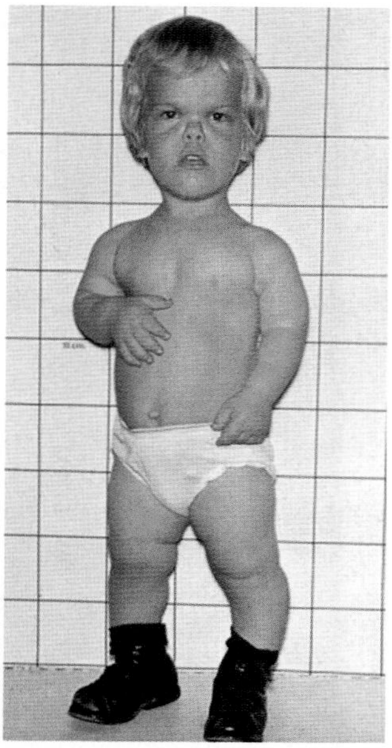

3. Which one of the following is most likely based on the MRI shown?

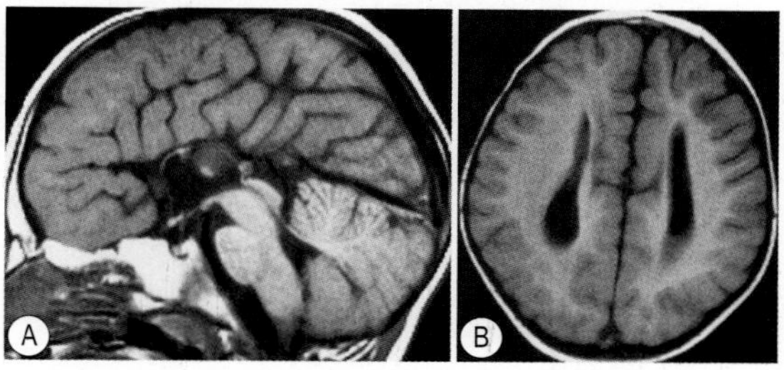

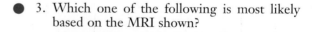

a. Basilar invagination
b. Corpus callosum agenesis
c. Hydrocephalus
d. Lissencephaly
e. Type II Chiari malformation

4. MRI shows the appearances below, and the lesion is bright on T2WI and dark on fat suppression sequences and does not show any contrast enhancement. Which one of the following is most likely?

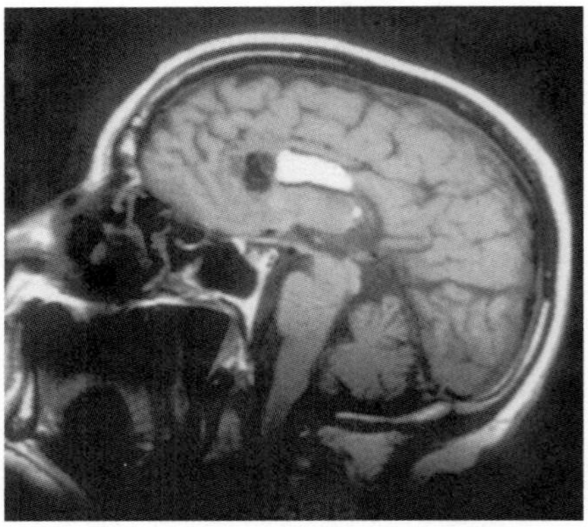

a. Colloid cyst
b. Craniopharyngioma
c. Intracranial lipoma
d. Intraventricular hemorrhage
e. Pericallosal aneurysm

5. Which one of the following is likely based on the MRI shown?

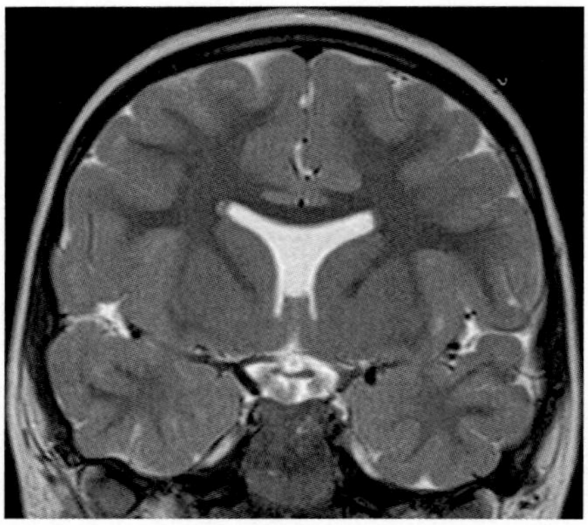

a. Closed-lip schizencephaly
b. Cobblestone cortex
c. Septo-optic dysplasia
d. Subcortical heterotopia
e. Tuberous sclerosis

6. Which one of the following is most likely based on the MRI shown?

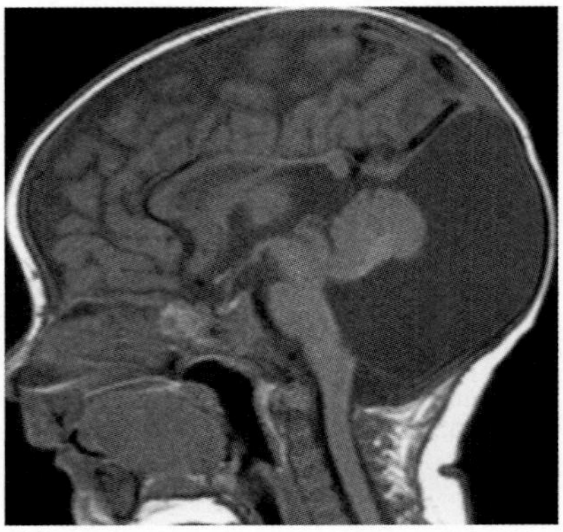

a. Blake's pouch cyst
b. Chiari III malformation
c. Dandy-Walker Malformation
d. Joubert's syndrome
e. Mega cysterna magna

7. Which one of the following is most likely based on the MRI shown?

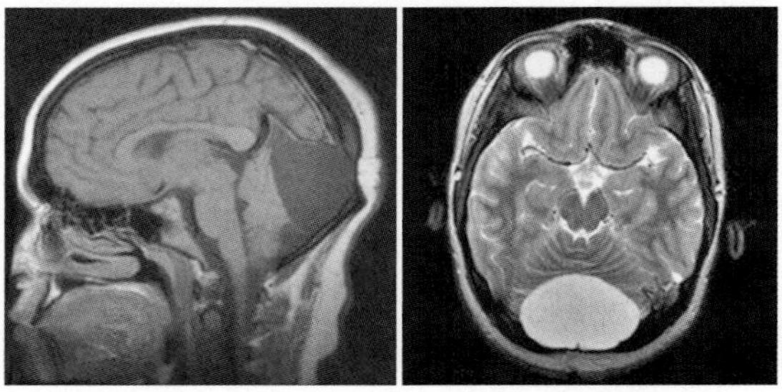

a. Arachnoid cyst
b. Dandy-Walker variant
c. Epidermoid cyst
d. Medulloblastoma
e. Type II Chiari malformation

8. A 31-year-old undergoes MRI for headache. On axial views the 4th ventricle is enlarged and on certain sequences choroid plexus can be seen under and posterior to the vermis entering the superior aspect of the lesion. There is no restricted diffusion. Which one of the following is most likely?

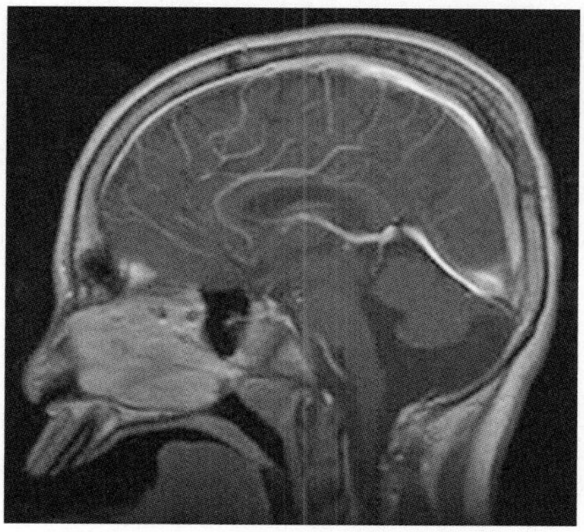

a. Arachnoid cyst
b. Blake's pouch cyst
c. Cystic metastasis
d. Epidermoid
e. Type II Chiari malformation

9. A child undergoes MRI scan as part of epilepsy evaluation after two seizures unrelated to febrile episodes. There are no symptoms of hydrocephalus. MRI appearances are shown, and there is no diffusion restriction. Which one of the following is most likely?

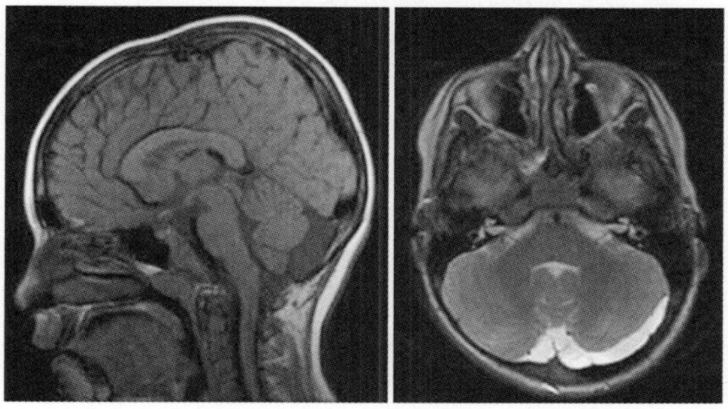

a. Arachnoid cyst
b. Dandy-Walker malformation
c. Epidermoid cyst
d. Mega cisterna magna
e. Type III Chiari malformation

10. Which one of the following is most likely based on the imaging shown?

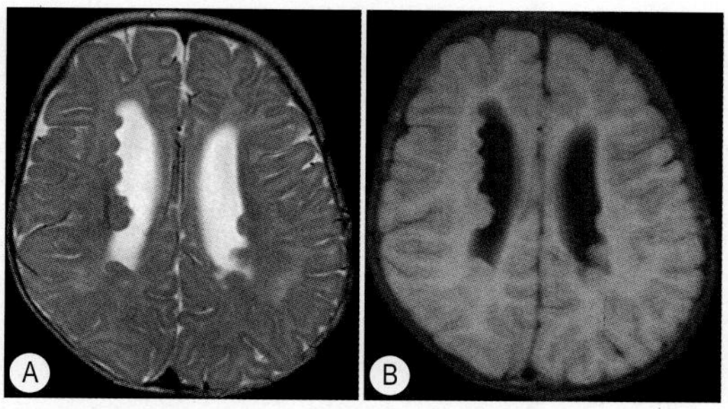

a. Band heterotopia
b. Marginal glioneuronal heterotopia
c. Subcortical heterotopia
d. Subependymal heterotopia
e. Type II lissencephaly

11. A 45-year-old woman with intractable structural epilepsy who had experienced partial complex and secondarily generalized seizures from the age of 8 years. Coronal FLAIR MRI is shown. Which one of the following is most likely?

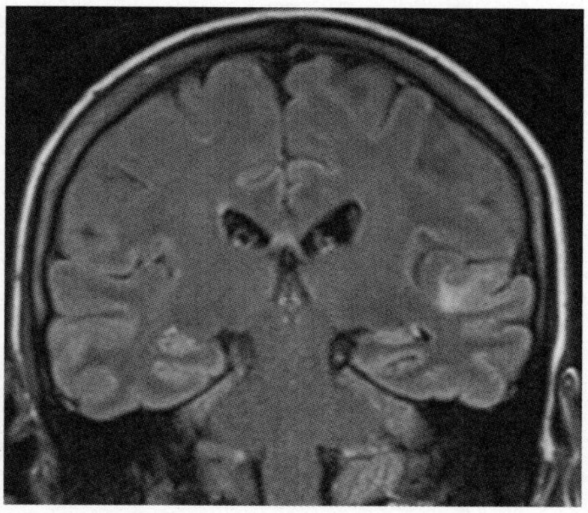

a. Abscess
b. Focal cortical dysplasia
c. Lissencephaly
d. Mesial temporal sclerosis
e. Tuberous sclerosis

12. Which one of the following is most likely based on the imaging shown below?

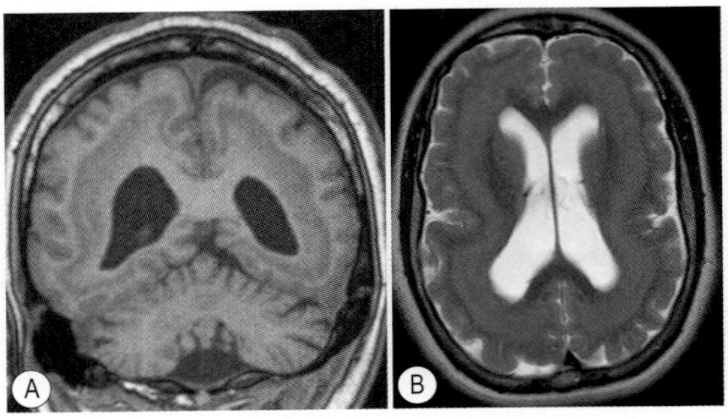

a. Cobblestone cortex
b. Focal cortical dysplasia
c. Hemimegalencephaly
d. Lissencephaly with band heterotopia
e. Periventricular nodular heterotopia

13. Which one of the following is most likely based on the imaging shown?

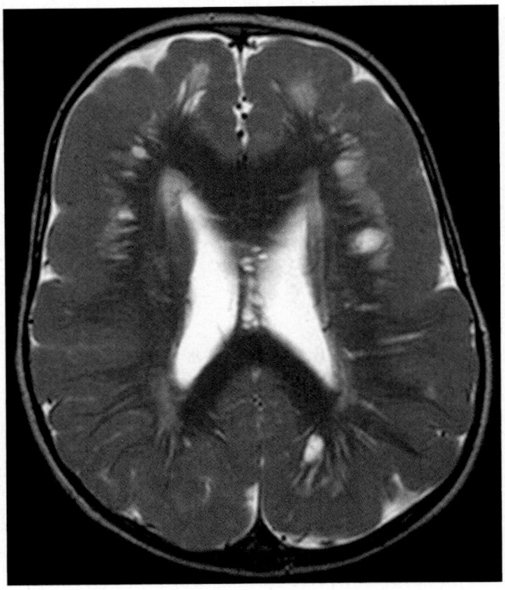

a. Cobblestone cortex
b. Focal cortical dysplasia
c. Lissencephaly with band heterotopia
d. Periventricular nodular heterotopia
e. Polymicrogyria

14. Which one of the following is most likely based on the imaging shown below?

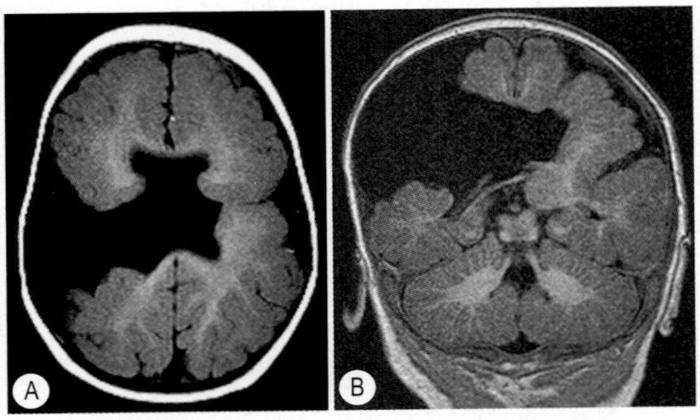

a. Lissencephaly with band heterotopia
b. Porencephalic cyst
c. Pachygyria
d. Schizencephaly
e. Semilobar holoprosencephaly

15. Which one of the following is most likely based on the imaging shown below?

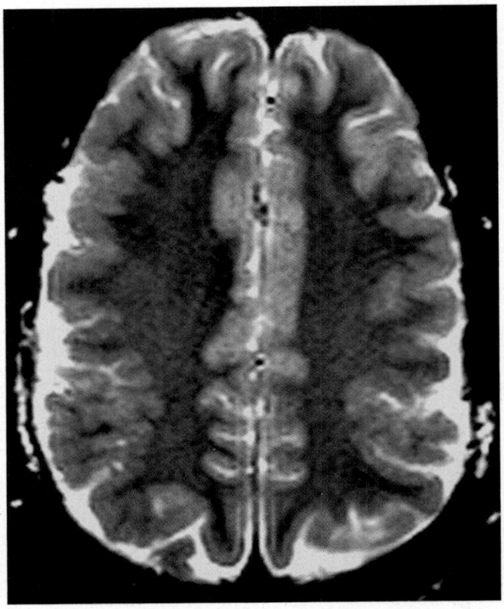

a. Agyria
b. Lissencephaly with band heterotopia
c. Pachygyria
d. Polymicrogyria
e. Walker-Warburg syndrome

16. Which one of the following is most likely based on the imaging shown?

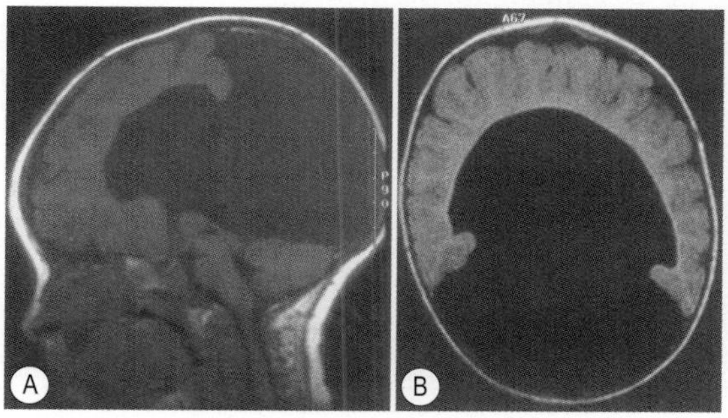

a. Alobar holoprosencephaly
b. Anencephaly
c. Dandy-Walker malformation
d. Porencephalic cyst
e. Schizencephaly

17. Which one of the following is most likely based on the imaging shown below?

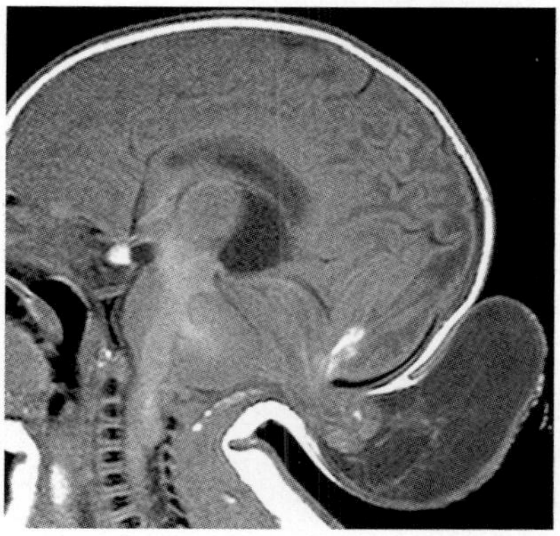

a. Atretic cephalocele
b. Encephalocele (meningoencephalocele)
c. Gliocele
d. Meningocele
e. Meningoencephalocystocele

18. A newborn infant has an apneic event with cyanosis and he was brought to the hospital. His evaluation was remarkable for developmental delay, bilateral lower-extremity frog-leg flaccid paralysis, with a large open defect in his lower back. At birth, the defect was covered by a transparent membrane, which subsequently ruptured and drained clear fluid for several weeks. Based on the imaging below, what is the cause of the infant's apneic events?

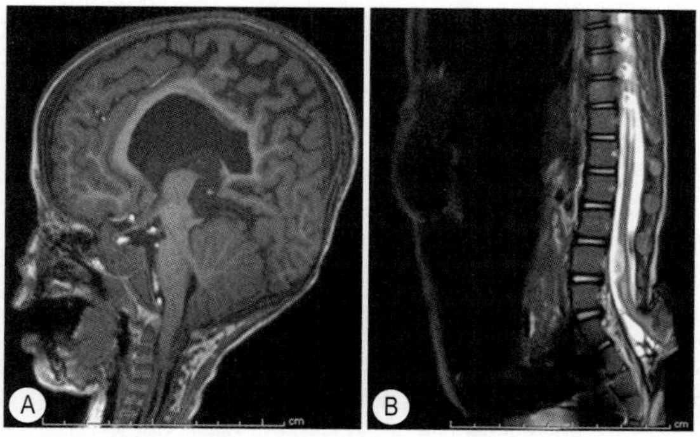

a. Dermal sinus tract
b. Dorsal enteric fistula
c. Lipomyelomeningocele
d. Myelocele
e. Type II Chiari malformation

19. The MRI shown below demonstrates features of which one of the following conditions?

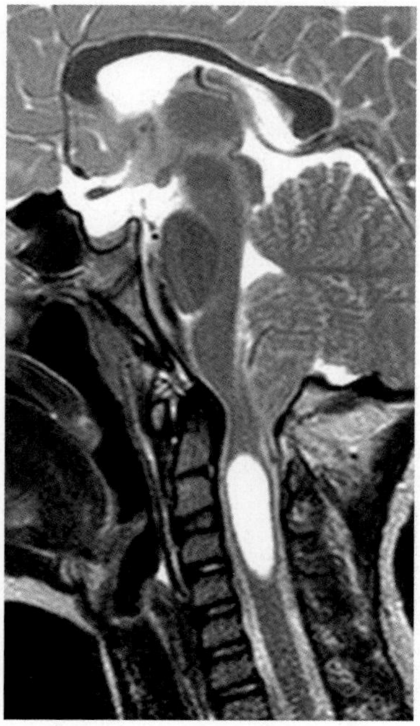

a. Chiari I malformation
b. Chiari II malformation
c. Chiari III malformation
d. Chiari IV malformation
e. Basilar invagination

20. You plan to perform a foramen magnum decompression on the patient shown below. Which one of the following investigations may be helpful?

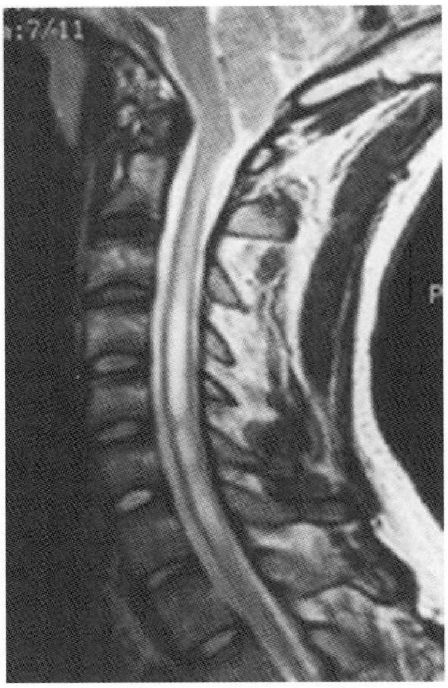

a. CSF flow study
b. CT cisternography
c. CT cervical angiogram
d. Flexion/extension X-rays
e. Nerve conduction studies

21. Which one of the following is most likely based on the clinical image shown below?

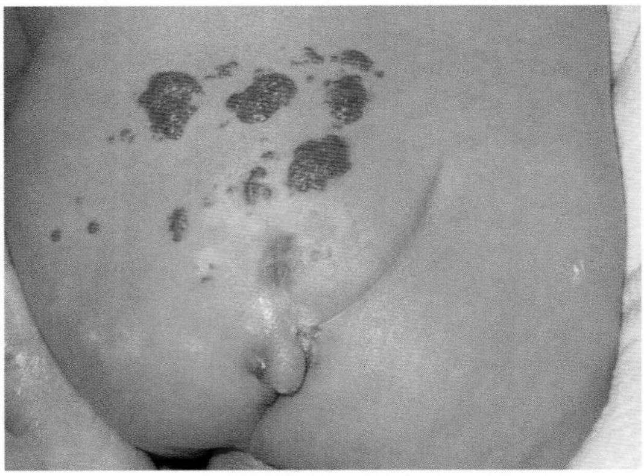

a. Achondroplasia
b. Closed spinal dysraphism
c. Klippel-Feil syndrome
d. Sturge-Weber syndrome
e. Wyburn-Mason syndrome

22. Which one of the following is likely to detect tethering of the spinal cord earliest?
a. Spinal CT
b. Spinal MRI
c. Spinal ultrasound
d. Spinal XR
e. Urodynamic testing

23. Which one of the following patients with tethered cord syndrome (TCS) is LEAST likely to benefit from detethering surgery?
a. A 1-day-old boy with bilateral 3/5 leg weakness and a midline open lumbar lesion leaking clear fluid.
b. A 6-week-old boy with static bilateral 3/5 leg weakness. Urodynamic testing shows evidence of neurogenic bladder which is being managed with intermittent catheterization.
c. A 2-year-old boy with a tuft of hair on his lumbar spine. He does not have any gross neurology in the lower limbs but MRI shows the conus at L2/3. Urodynamic testing shows evidence of neurogenic bladder disturbance.
d. A 9-year-old boy with progressive scoliosis. MRI shows a tight filum terminale.
e. A 12-year-old boy with back pain. MRI shows a tight filum terminale. Urodynamic testing is equivocal.

24. Which one of the following is most likely based on the findings in the image below?

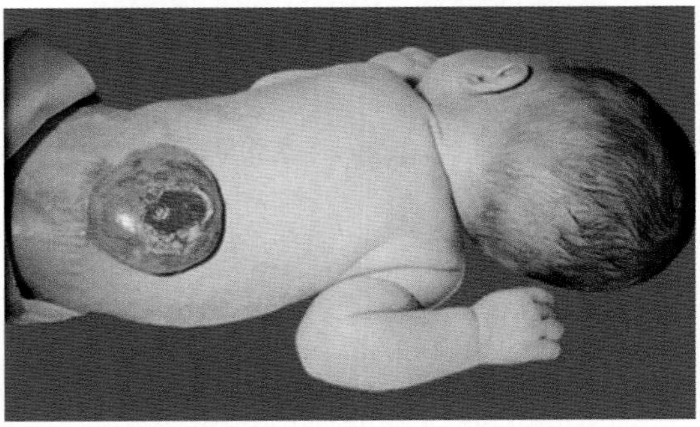

a. Lipomyelomeningocele
b. Meningocele
c. Myelocele
d. Myelocystocele
e. Myelomeningocele

QUESTIONS 25–33

Additional questions 25–33 available on ExpertConsult.com

EXTENDED MATCHING ITEM (EMI) QUESTIONS

34. **Spinal dysraphism:**
 a. Caudal agenesis
 b. Distematomyelia
 c. Dermal sinus
 d. Dorsal enteric fistula
 e. Filar lipoma
 f. Intradural lipo
 g. Hemimyelocele
 h. Hemimyelomeningocele
 i. Lipomyelocele
 j. Lipomyelomeningocele
 k. Meningocele
 l. Myelocele
 m. Myelocystocele
 n. Myelomeningocele
 o. Neurenteric cyst
 p. Persistent terminal ventricle
 q. Segmental dysgenesis
 r. Tight filum terminale

For each of the following descriptions, select the most appropriate answer from the list above. Each answer may be used once, more than once or not at all.

1. Epithelium-lined fistula which extends from skin to meninges within the spinal canal, possibly opening into the subarachnoid space or connecting to filum terminale, lipoma and may also be associated with a spinal dermoid.
2. Myelomeningocele affecting one of two hemicords in split cord malformation.
3. A subcutaneous lipoma tethers the spinal cord (lipoma-placode interface) inside the spinal canal via defect in vertebral elements.
4. Small ependymal lined cavity in the conus medullaris which may undergo cystic dilatation.
5. Cysts usually in intradural extramedullary plane of endodermal origin, usually lined with GI or respiratory epithelium.

35. **Congenital cranial abnormalities:**
 a. Adrenoleukodystrophy
 b. Arachnoid cyst
 c. Band heterotopia
 d. Blake's pouch cyst
 e. Chiari II malformation
 f. Dandy-Walker malformation
 g. Focal cortical dysplasia
 h. Holoprosencephaly
 i. Mega cisterna magna
 j. Porencephalic cyst
 k. Schizencephaly
 l. Subependymal heterotopia

For each of the following descriptions, select the most appropriate answer from the list above. Each answer may be used once, more than once or not at all.

1. An intraparenchymal vascular territory CSF cyst lined by white matter, communicating with the ventricles and/or subarachnoid space.
2. A full-thickness cerebral cleft extending from the pial surface of the cortex to the ependymal lining of the lateral ventricle, and is almost always lined by abnormal gray matter.

SBA ANSWERS

1. **b**—Klippel-Feil syndrome

KFS is a congenital anomaly that is caused by the failure of the spine to segment properly during embryonic development, resulting in fusion of two or more cervical vertebrae. Incidence is 1 in 40,000 with a slight female predominance (3:2). Clinically patients may have a shortened neck, a low posterior neckline, and limited neck mobility (less than half possess all three). Associated findings that may provide diagnostic clues include other skeletal abnormalities, orofacial anomalies, and visceral defects. Congenital fusions can occur at any level of the cervical spine, although 75% occur in the region of the first three cervical vertebrae. The most prevalent fusion is between C2 and C3. KFS is classified into three types: Type I—fusion of many cervical and upper thoracic vertebrae, Type II—fusion of 2-3 vertebrae with associated hemivertebrae/occipito-atlantal fusion/other abnormality, Type III—cervical fusion with lower thoracic/lumbar vertebral fusion. Fetal cervical vertebrae should be evaluated with ultrasound (US) for cervical fusions, blocking, and hemivertebrae. MRI can also be useful to determine whether the cervical malformation is causing compression of the brain, brainstem, or spinal cord. Treatment varies depending on the severity of the fusions, adjacent segment degenerative disease, degree of instability present and the underlying diagnosis. Isolated KFS is generally well tolerated. Initial treatment strategies include modification of activities, bracing, and traction, all of which may delay surgery and prevent neurologic compromise. Indications for surgical stabilization are symptomatic instability or neurologic compromise.

Image with permission from Dornbos D 3rd, Ikeda DS, Slivka A, Powers C. Vertebral artery dissection after neck extension in an adult patient with Klippel-Feil syndrome. J Clin Neurosci 2014;21(4):685-8.

2. **c**—Posterior circulation aneurysms

Achondroplasia is the most common form of human short-limbed dwarfism and is one of a spectrum of diseases caused by mutations in the FGFR3 gene. Occurs in 1 in 10,000-30,000 live births. The disease is autosomal dominant, but 80% of patients have new mutations. Classic features include a long, narrow trunk with short limbs, macrocephaly with frontal bossing/prominence and facial hypoplasia. Other features include hypotonia in infancy (motor delay), hyperextensible joints, short and broad trident hands, and thoracolumbar kyphosis. Abnormal compression at a number of levels along the neuraxis may result in hydrocephalus, cervicomedullary compression, spinal canal stenosis (both cervical and lumbar), syringomyelia, and spinal instability. Diminished growth of the skull base in achondroplasia results in cranial foraminal stenosis and intracranial venous hypertension resulting in impaired CSF absorption, macrocephaly; additionally, obstructive hydrocephalus may result from cervicomedullary compression. Monitoring of head growth should be performed at regular intervals and compared with control charts for children with achondroplasia to avoid unnecessary CSF shunting. If raised ICP is suspected, US can show ventricular size, but MRI will detect transependymal spread of CSF, assess craniocervical junction and venous stenosis. Despite mild-moderate ventriculomegaly, the majority of patients with macrocephaly stabilize spontaneously, and thus insertion of a VP shunt should be avoided if possible. Stress on the craniocervical junction by a large head with weak cervical musculature can produce cervicomedullary compression. Patients may present with neck pain, apneic episodes, bulbar dysfunction, bladder dysfunction, paresis, hyperreflexia, and hypertonia with clonus. Indeed, "normal" reflexes may reflect spasticity in normally hypotonic children with achondroplasia. Acute deterioration may occur after minor trauma and there is an increased incidence of sudden death at <4 years of age. Investigations include MR imaging and formal polysomnography. MRI may show tight foramen magnum, flexion/extension sequences may demonstrate transient cervicomedullary compression or CSF flow obstruction, and MRV may show a persistent occipital venous sinus preoperatively. The use of polysomnography to assess patients for the presence of central and/or obstructive sleep apnea has been reported to identify central/mixed apnea in up to 60% of unselected children with achondroplasia. Indications for surgery include myelopathy with upper motor neuron signs such as clonus and hyperreflexia, and/or central apnea as documented on polysomnography, or the presence of a syrinx, with evidence of a narrow foramen magnum and/or T2 signal change in the spinal cord on MR imaging.

Image with permission from Moore KL. Developing Human, 10th ed. Elsevier, 2016.

FURTHER READING

King JA, Vachhrajani S, Drake JM, Rutka JT. Neurosurgical implications of achondroplasia. J Neurosurg Pediatr 2009;4(4):297-306.

3. **b**—Corpus callosum agenesis

Complete corpus callosum agenesis is the most common type of commissural agenesis, and may be associated with absence of the hippocampal commissure; in partial agenesis, the genu and anterior body are formed, whereas portions that develop later like the posterior body, isthmus, and splenium are absent. Mid-sagittal MR images are diagnostic, and also show an everted cingulate gyrus and longitudinal Probst bundles containing non-crossing callosal axons, lateral ventricles are shifted laterally and closed medially by rolled up white matter lamina (which should be forming the leaf of the septum pellucidum). The inner walls of the lateral ventricles are concave medially as a result of encroachment of the Probst bundles on the ventricular lumen. In addition, the roof of the third ventricle bulges upward. The frontal horns of the lateral ventricles might be underdeveloped, whereas the dilated temporal horns invaginate into the core of the parahippocampal gyri because of decreased white matter. The lateral ventricles run parallel to each other, with marked dilation of the trigone and occipital horns (colpocephaly). Development of the cerebrum and cerebellar hemispheres occurs at the same time, hence associated Chiari malformation, Dandy-Walker malformation, neuronal migration anomalies, and midline facial anomalies (facial cleft, encephalocele). Periventricular or subcortical heterotopia may also be seen.

Image with permission from Loevner L. Brain Imaging: Case Review Series, 2nd ed. Elsevier, Mosby, 2009.

4. **c**—Intracranial lipoma

Intracranial lipomas are thought to be maldifferentiations of the meninx primitive (undifferentiated) mesenchyme that surrounds the developing brain. Evolution of the inner meninx primitiva leads to formation of the subarachnoid spaces, the pre-pontomedullary cistern is the first to develop, followed by cisterns around the brainstem and cerebral hemispheres, the quadrigeminal plate, and finally the suprasellar system. Meninx primitiva surrounding the dorsum of the lamina terminalis is the last to become evolved. The most common locations of an intracranial lipoma are in the deep interhemispheric fissure (40-50%), quadrigeminal plate cistern (30%), suprasellar/interpedicular cistern (10-20%), cerebellopontine angle cistern (10%), and sylvian fissures (5%). Because by embryologic definition lipomas occupy the subarachnoid space, blood vessels and cranial nerves course through them. Most intracranial lipomas are asymptomatic, so they are diagnosed incidentally. On CT scan, a lipoma is a well-defined, fat density mass within a cistern. MR appearances show T1 hyperintensity, T2 hyperintensity, fat suppression and no enhancement. Chemical shift artifact seen around the hyperintensity confirms the fatty origin of the mass as opposed to hemorrhage. Interhemispheric lipomas are invariably associated with hypogenesis of the corpus callosum. A pericallosal lipoma might also show multiple signal voids because of a combination of traversing vessels and calcification. Small lipomas might not demonstrate chemical shift artifact. In such cases, fat saturation can be very helpful in differentiating this lesion from other T1 bright lesions.

Image with permission from Perkin GD, et al. Atlas of Clinical Neurology, 3rd ed. Elsevier, Saunders, 2011.

5. **c**—Septo-optic dysplasia

Coronal T2-weighted MRI shows an absent septum pellucidum, right optic nerve hypoplasia, and "point-down" appearance of the frontal horns of the lateral ventricles. The main features of septo-optic-pituitary dysplasia include hypoplasia or absence of the septum pellucidum, optic nerve hypoplasia, and hypothalamic-pituitary dysplasia or dysfunction. SOPD is sporadic in most of the cases, with no etiologic factor identified although seen with maternal diabetes and intrauterine CMV infection. Clinical presentation is mainly related to seizures (50%), pituitary dysfunction or visual symptoms such as nystagmus or decreased visual acuity. Ophthalmoscopic examination shows optic nerve hypoplasia, a pale optic nerve head, and isolated tortuosity of the retinal vein. Fifty percent of patients might present with seizures. MRI may show corpus callosum agenesis lead to a box-like shape of the frontal horns in coronal planes, low-lying fornix (due to absent septum), pituitary hypoplasia/empty sella/ectopic posterior pituitary gland, hypothalamic hypoplasia, optic nerve and/or optic chiasm hypoplasia (visualization difficult as mild form—ophthalmological findings more reliable). In addition, the remainder of the brain parenchyma might have a variety of other congenital anomalies like malformations of cortical development (schizencephaly and gray matter heterotopia), olfactory hypoplasia (arrhinencephaly), hypoplasia of white matter, and/or ventriculomegaly.

Image with permission from Adam A, et al. (Eds.). Grainger & Allison's Diagnostic Radiology, 6th ed. Elsevier, Churchill Livingstone, 2014.

6. **c**—Dandy-Walker malformation

The classic triad of the full-blown Dandy-Walker malformation is complete or partial agenesis of the vermis, cystic dilation of the 4th ventricle, and an enlarged posterior fossa with upward displacement of the transverse sinuses, tentorium, and torcula. Hydrocephalus seen in 80% of cases but is not a part of the essential criteria. The presence of vermian agenesis and cystic dilatation of the fourth ventricle without an enlarged posterior fossa is termed Dandy-Walker variant, and remains in the Dandy-Walker spectrum of rhombencephalon roof development disorders (though hydrocephalus is less common). Failure of incorporation of the anterior membranous area (AMA) into the choroid plexus leads to its persistence between the caudal edge of the developing vermis and the cranial edge of developing choroid plexus. CSF pulsations cause the AMA to balloon out into a cyst that displaces the hypoplastic vermis superiorly so that it appears to be rotated in a counterclockwise fashion. The posterior membranous area can persist unopened or become patent, accounting for the reportedly variable patency of the foramen of Magendie and association of hydrocephalus. Global enlargement of the PF may result from arrested development of the tentorium, straight sinus and torcula, with failure of migration of the straight sinus from the vertex to the lambda, possibly because of the abnormal distention of the 4th ventricle. Imaging in the Dandy-Walker spectrum aims to distinguish a dilated 4th ventricle from extra ventricular cysts and assess hydrocephalus (the foramen of Magendie is usually not patent, whereas the foramina of Luschka generally are).

Image with permission from Loevner L. Brain Imaging: Case Review Series, 2nd ed. Elsevier, Mosby, 2009.

7. **a**—Arachnoid cyst

An arachnoid cyst usually is evident as a CSF isointense, non-enhancing, space-occupying cyst with walls that normally are too thin to visualize. It results from splitting of arachnoid membrane with inner and outer leaflet surrounding a cyst cavity which can undergo progressive expansion due to a ball-valve mechanism, fluid secretion by the cyst wall, or a small osmotic gradient. Arachnoid cysts are filled with CSF and do not communicate with the surrounding subarachnoid space and ventricular system; they usually are not associated with brain maldevelopment and may be present anywhere in the posterior fossa. When the arachnoid cyst is present inferior to the vermis, it may compress the inferior vermis, but identification of white matter to each vermian lobule suggests compression rather than vermian hypoplasia seen in Dandy-Walker spectrum. Confusion may arise when they are large and located posterior and inferior to the cerebellum. Imaging features suggestive of arachnoid cyst are similar intensity to CSF, mass effect, large cyst with obstructive hydrocephalus and scalloping of the occipital bone. The only definitive diagnosis of arachnoid cyst can be made with CT cisternography: arachnoid cysts should not demonstrate enhancement (or only after a delay), while cysts that fill with contrast immediately are regarded as diverticula of the subarachnoid space. Mega cisterna magna usually does not demonstrate mass effect on the cerebellum and vermis even if large, and hydrocephalus is generally absent. Arachnoid cysts are not associated with an enlarged 4th ventricle, whereas a persistent Blake's pouch is. It is essential to differentiate arachnoid cyst from epidermoid cyst which can be easily done with the use of FLAIR images and DWI (epidermoid cysts are diffusion restricting). Most arachnoid cysts are an incidental finding and patients are usually asymptomatic, but symptoms due to mass effect or hydrocephalus can be managed with fenestration or cystoperitoneal shunt.

Image with permission from Small JE, Schaefer PW (Eds.). Neuroradiology: Key Differential Diagnoses and Clinical Questions, Elsevier, Saunders, 2013.

8. **b**—Blake's pouch cyst

Blake's pouch is an embryologic midline evagination of the embryonic fourth ventricular roof lined by ependyma, glia, and choroid plexus. In normal early fetal development, this evagination along the inferior surface of the vermis ruptures and forms the foramen of Magendie that opens into the subarachnoid space. If the evagination fails to rupture, the diverticulum continues to expand and eventually forms an uncommon midline posterior fossa cyst (*Blake pouch* cyst) which looks virtually identical to an arachnoid cyst posterior and inferior to the vermis. However, the choroid plexus in a *Blake pouch* cyst at times may be identified as being displaced into the cyst along its superior wall (under and posterior to the vermis), though this can be mimicked by a prominent inferior vermian vein. No MRI sequence allows clear differentiation of a mega cisterna magna from a Blake pouch cyst, but generally it appears as a CSF collection with normal non-rotated cerebellar vermis, enlarged 4th ventricle (though may be normal at times) and brainstem compression, without other brain abnormalities.

Image with permission from Small JE, Schaefer PW (Eds.). Neuroradiology: Key Differential Diagnoses and Clinical Questions, Elsevier, Saunders, 2013.

9. **d**—Mega cisterna magna

The cisterna magna is a normal subarachnoid cistern located below the cerebellum and behind the medulla. Embryologically, it originates from the permeabilization of the Blake's pouch, which allows CSF flow out of the 4th ventricle via the foramen of Magendie. As such, it is in communication superiorly with the 4th ventricle and inferiorly with the peri-medullary subarachnoid spaces. The normal size limit is debated, but a mega cisterna magna refers to a cystic posterior fossa malformation that is characterized by large cisterna magna, an intact vermis, and absence of hydrocephalus. It is most likely the result of cerebellar volume loss and associated with cerebellar insults such as infection, infarction, and inflammation, as well as chromosomal abnormalities. The appearance is similar to a persistent Blake's pouch except for the consistent absence of hydrocephalus. The cerebellum and brainstem are typically normal. The vermis is intact, and there is usually no distortion of the cerebellum (unlike arachnoid cysts) though occipital scalloping may be seen when very large. Patients with mega cisterna magna do not usually have any neurological signs of involvement of PF. By itself mega cisterna magna is asymptomatic, and is usually discovered incidentally. The incidence is high and represents approximately 50% of all cystic PF malformations. The CSF in the enlarged cisterna magna freely communicates with the surrounding CSF spaces and does not obstruct CSF circulation and hence hydrocephalus is absent. If there is presence of hydrocephalus mega cisterna magna is not the correct diagnosis and it should then steer towards the diagnosis of a persistent Blake's pouch. There is no role for shunt surgery even if the cisterna magna is extremely large.

Image with permission from Small JE, Schaefer PW (Eds.). Neuroradiology: Key Differential Diagnoses and Clinical Questions, Elsevier, Saunders, 2013.

10. **d**—Subependymal heterotopia

Heterotopias are focal collections of morphologically normal neurons in abnormal locations secondary to interrupted neuronal migration from the ependyma of lateral ventricles to cortex. The most common clinical presentation is seizure disorder in the second or third decade. They are classified by location:

1. Subependymal heterotopia (commonest): unilateral or bilateral periventricular nodular heterotopia, the latter is X-linked dominant disorder only seen in females (lethal in males).
2. Subcortical heterotopia: no longer includes band heterotopia, which is included with lissencephaly due to common genetic background.
3. Marginal glioneuronal heterotopia—overmigration of neurons and glial cells into the leptomeninges but microscopic and not visible on imaging.

Imaging shows focal ovoid lesions which match the gray matter in signal intensity on all the sequences, lack edema and do not enhance with contrast. Differential diagnosis is subependymal hamartomas of tuberous sclerosis (irregular, iso- to hypointense to white matter, may enhance, associated tubers) and subependymal metastases.

Image with permission from Loevner L. Brain Imaging: Case Review Series, 2nd ed. Elsevier, Mosby, 2009.

11. **b**—Focal cortical dysplasia

FCD is the most commonly found malformation of cortical development in the surgical series and accounts for approximately 20-50% of all cases that have undergone epilepsy surgery. Attempts at classifying FCD have been incomplete and unsatisfactory because of the absence of a scientifically proven etiology. The latest classification system uses a multimodality approach which includes a combination of histopathological examination, imaging, and genetic findings. The most common clinical presentation is partial seizures with an otherwise normal neurological examination. The classical imaging features of FCD seen on T2 or FLAIR images is focal cortical thinning with hyperintensity and volume loss of the underlying white matter. High resolution thin section images may show focal blurring of the gray-white matter junction. Rarely, FCD may be associated with neuroglial tumors, such as dysembryoplastic neuroepithelial tumor and ganglioglioma and may also be seen in association with mesial temporal sclerosis.

Image with permission from Nowacki A, Seidel K, Schucht P, et al. Induction of fear by intraoperative stimulation during awake craniotomy: case presentation and systematic review of the literature. World Neurosurg. 2015;84(2):470-4.

12. **d**—Lissencephaly with band heterotopia

As progenitor cells begin to proliferate, they normally migrate outward from the germinal matrix to form the cortex. Lissencephaly is a severe form of abnormal neuronal migration characterized by an absence of gyri with a thickened cortex (agyria) or the presence of few broad fat gyri with a thickened cortex (pachygyria), both leading to a relatively smooth featureless brain. Classical lissencephaly presents with diffuse hypotonia, early developmental delay, spastic quadriplegia, opisthotonus, and severe mental retardation. Development of medically refractory epilepsy at a very early age with increasingly complex seizure patterns is very common. There are two main types:

1. Type 1 "classical" lissencephaly (lissencephaly with band heterotopia): only four cortical layers.
2. Type 2 lissencephaly (cobblestone cortex): no cortical layers.

Two separate mutations, a hemizygous mutation in the *DCX/XLIS* gene on chromosome Xq22.3q23 and a heterozygous (dominantly inherited) mutation in the *LIS1* gene on chromosome 17p13.3 can lead to classical lissencephaly. The DCX mutation also results in subcortical band heterotopia consists of a discrete extensive plate or band of gray matter situated between the cortex and the lateral ventricle. On imaging, classical lissencephaly shows a smooth brain with vertical orientation of the sylvian fissures giving the cerebrum a "figure 8" appearance on axial images, while band heterotopia shows a very characteristic layered pattern from cortex to midline: normal thickness cortex with shallow sulci, a variable thickness white matter band, an interposing gray matter band (the heterotopic band), and a deeper white matter layer extending to the ventricular margin or midline.

Image with permission from Loevner L. Brain Imaging: Case Review Series, 2nd ed. Elsevier, Mosby, 2009.

13. **a**—Cobblestone cortex

In cobblestone cortex (Type 2 lissencephaly) the brain surface is irregular because of the presence of heterotopic tissue which results from overmigration of glioneural elements. In general, this malformation shows a cobblestone cortex, dilated ventricles, abnormal white matter, a small brainstem, a hypoplastic vermis, and cerebellar polymicrogyria. It is associated with eye malformations as well as congenital muscular dystrophy, e.g., Walker-Warburg syndrome, Muscle-eye-brain disease, Fukuyama congenital muscular dystrophy.

Image with permission from Coley BD. Caffey's Pediatric Diagnostic Imaging, 12th ed. Elsevier, Saunders, 2013.

14. **d**—Schizencephaly

Schizencephaly (clefted brain) is a brain malformation characterized by a full-thickness cerebral cleft. This cleft extends from the pial surface of the cortex to the ependymal lining of the lateral ventricle, and is almost always lined by abnormal gray matter (polymicrogyria). Schizencephaly may result from disruption of any of the three phases of cortical development (proliferation, migration, and organization), but polymicrogyric cortex surrounding the cleft suggests that it is a disorder of cortical organization, probably secondary to hypoperfusion or ischemic cortical injury. As such, it may represent a spectrum where mild damage results in polymicrogyria while severe damage may involve the deep radial-glial fibers and result in schizencephaly. It may be unilateral (60%) or bilateral, and either:

1. Closed-lip schizencephaly (left hemisphere in MRI shown), the margins of the cerebrospinal fluid (CSF)-filled, gray matter lined cleft are closely opposed to one another along the entire length of the cleft. A small dimple is often seen in the ventricular wall where the cleft enters.
2. Open lip schizencephaly (right hemisphere in MRI shown) the cleft margins are widely separated, lined with polymicrogyria, absent septum pellucidum, dilated ventricles, scalloping and thinning of the inner vault of the calvarium (direct transmission of CSF pulsations), and the contralateral cerebral cortex may be dysplastic. On T2WI, a large vessel may be seen traversing the CSF cleft.

Unilateral closed-lip schizencephaly commonly presents with epilepsy, while open lip schizencephaly generally presents with microcephaly, contralateral hemiparesis, and mental retardation. Bilateral schizencephaly manifests as severe mental retardation with early onset epilepsy. Blindness because of optic nerve hypoplasia may be seen in 30% of cases. Porencephalic cysts are intraparenchymal and lined by white matter.

Image with permission from Kanekar S, Gent M. Malformations of cortical development. Semin Ultrasound CT MR 2011;32(3):211-27.

15. **d**—Polymicrogyria

Polymicrogyria (multiple malformed convulsions) is caused by disturbances in the late stages of neuronal migration or in the early stages of cortical organization (typically between 17 and 25-26 weeks of gestation). These disturbances result in the abnormal development of the deep layer of cerebral cortex which manifests as multiple small gyri separated by small sulci generating an irregular bumpy cortical surface. Causes include intrauterine ischemia, intrauterine infection (CMV or toxoplasmosis), metabolic disorders (e.g., peroxisomal storage disorders, pyruvate dehydrogenase deficiency), or genetic syndromes (e.g., Aicardi syndrome, DiGeorge syndrome, and Warburg Micro syndrome). The most common sites for PMG are the sylvian cortex (80%) and frontal lobes (70%) followed by the parietal, temporal and occipital lobes. Involvement may be either bilateral (60%) or unilateral (40%), focal or diffuse, symmetric or asymmetric. MRI shows a bumpy irregular appearance of the outer surface of the cortex because of multiple small gyri, diffuse cortical thickening, and an irregular corrugated appearance of the inner cortical surface (gray-white matter junction). Most common presentation is seizures (80%), but diffuse polymicrogyria can present with microcephaly, hypotonia, and infantile seizures with marked developmental delay (also possibly contralateral hemiplegia).

Image with permission from Kanekar S, Gent M. Malformations of cortical development. Semin Ultrasound CT MR 2011;32(3):211-27.

16. **a**—Alobar holoprosencephaly

Holoprosencephaly (HPE) is the most common developmental defect of the forebrain, with a live birth prevalence of approximately 1 in 10,000. The formation of two hemispheres from a single telencephalic vesicle begins around the 37th embryonic day. This division takes place as a result of induction by bone morphogenetic protein from the midline roof plate. The etiology of HPE is heterogeneous and might be due to either genetic causes (Sonic hedgehog pathway most common) or environmental factors, including maternal diabetes and exposure to teratogens such as alcohol. SHH is a protein that encodes a morphogen which mediates notochordal-ventral neural tube and development of craniofacial structures (facial deformities are also seen in association with the HPE spectrum). In HPE, the forebrain fails to divide into two separate hemispheres; rather, it develops into a single, unpaired forebrain called the holoprosencephalon. The degree of failure of hemisphere cleavage is classified as alobar, semilobar, and lobar HPE. Alobar HPE is the most common and most severe form, resulting in either stillbirth or a very short lifespan. In alobar HPE, the holosphere remains undivided as a single flattened mass of brain surrounding a midline holoventricle that is large and shaped like an inverted "U" or crescent. It is usually associated with severe facial deformities like premaxillary agenesis, cleft lip/palate, ocular hypotelorism, ethmocephaly (proboscis between the eyes), and in severe cases, cyclopia. On imaging, the holosphere is noted to be displaced in the most cephalad part of the intracranial cavity. There is complete absence of the interhemispheric fissure, falx cerebri, and corpus callosum. The gyri recti are also absent. This is associated with aplasia of the olfactory bulbs and optic nerves. The basal ganglia and thalami are fused and located in the floor of the holoventricle. The sylvian fissures and third ventricle are not present. A dorsal cyst is frequently seen communicating with the monoventricle.

Image with permission from Winn HR. Youman's Neurological Surgery, vol. 4, 6th ed. Elsevier, Saunders, 2011.

17. **b**—Encephalocele

Cephaloceles are complex neural axis malformations which manifest as herniation of the meninges and often cerebral tissue through a defect in the calvarium. Incidence is 1 in 10,000—1 in 1000 depending on series. They are usually midline, but vary in location with occipital (75%) site commonest in Europe and North America. They are thought to be attributable to nonseparation of neural and surface ectoderm leading to defective formation of the occipital bone. They can be classified by contents:

1. Meningocele: contains CSF and lined by meninges.
2. Gliocele: contains CSF and lined by glial tissue.
3. Encephalocele (meningoencephalocele): contains CSF and brain.
4. Meningoencephalocystocele: contains CSF, brain and ventricles.
5. Atretic cephalocele: small nodule of fibrous fatty tissue.

Occipital cephaloceles are often large but usually covered with normal skin and hair, with herniation of the infra and/or supratentorial structures through a narrow pedicle. Herniated brain tissue may be normal, dysplastic, or may show new/old ischemic or hemorrhagic changes because of strangulation of the blood vessels at the neck of the sac. The tentorium is frequently reduced into crescentic folds and is inserted inferior to the petrous ridge, leading to a narrow, funnel-shaped lower posterior fossa. The falx is usually thin, hypoplastic, and may either attach to the superior margin of the defect or herniate into the encephalocele. Because of traction, the cerebral parenchyma is pulled posteriorly, and nonherniated brain may assume abnormal positions in the skull. The anterior commissure, septum pellucidum, and fornices are absent in 80% of cases. Hydrocephalus may affect the entire ventricular system or it may be limited to the extracranial portion of the ventricles. Other associated anomalies like cerebellar cortical dysplasia, heterotopias, Chiari or Dandy-Walker malformation, and partial/complete absence of corpus callosum may be seen. By definition, Type III Chiari malformation includes an occipital or cervicooccipital encephalocele with herniation of the medulla, 4th ventricle and cerebellum, and sometimes the occipital lobes (rare).

Image with permission from Coley BD. Caffey's Pediatric Diagnostic Imaging, 12th ed. Elsevier, Saunders, 2013.

18. **e**—Type II Chiari malformation

MRI depicting cerebellar vermian displacement, downward displacement of cerebellar tonsils and brainstem, cervical hydrosyrinx, ventriculomegaly, and pachygyria. (Right) T2-weighted MRI of the lumbosacral spine depicting hydrosyrinx, tethered cord, and unrepaired lumbosacral myelomeningocele. In a Chiari II malformation, there is displacement of the cerebellum, part of the brainstem, and the fourth ventricle into the cervical canal (below the basion-opisthion line). A lumbar myelomeningocele is seen in almost all the cases. Several prominent theories exist regarding etiology:

1. Traction theory: primary defect is tethering of the spinal cord which leads to abnormal traction and pulling of the posterior fossa contents into the cervical canal.
2. Crowding theory: primary defect is in the mesodermal development involving the cranial base rather than neuroectodermal tissue, resulting in a smaller posterior fossa, underdevelopment of the occipital bone, and basal chondrocranium, which is unable to accommodate rapidly developing neural tissue which herniates through the foramen magnum.
3. Unified Theory/Hydrodynamic Oligo-CSF states that neurulation is the primary defect. There is lack of expression of the specific surface molecules required for neural tube closure, leading to incomplete occlusion of the neural tube and leakage of CSF through the neural tube. Subsequent hypotension

develops within the ventricular system. This disruption in the CSF dynamics has an effect all along the neural tube (from rostral to the caudal). At the level of lateral ventricle, the germinal matrix is disrupted, leading to malformation of the cortical development. At the level of the third ventricle, there is enlargement of massa intermedia because of extended contact between the thalami. In the posterior fossa, the rhombencephalic vesicle fails to expand, therefore stopping the induction of the perineural mesenchyma of the posterior fossa. All of this leads to a smaller posterior fossa, which is unable to accommodate the developing rhombencephalon. The result is displacement of cerebellum and brainstem into the cervical canal.

4. Primary defect in the genetic programming of hindbrain segment and growth associated structures of chondrocranium.

Image with permission from Kaye E. Apnea in a refugee child. Pediatr Neurol 2014;50(1):119-20.

Chiari II Malformation: Imaging

Location	Main Imaging Findings
Posterior fossa	1. Small posterior fossa with low-lying tentorium and torcula 2. Herniation of the cerebellar tonsils and vermis through widened foramen 3. Brainstem appears pulled down with elongated 4th ventricle 4. Tectal beaking: inferior colliculus elongated posteriorly causing angulation and stenosis of aqueduct resulting in hydrocephalus 5. Cervicomedullary kinking (as dentate ligament stops cord descending further) 6. Scalloping of petrous temporal bone
Supratentorial	1. Obstructive hydrocephalus 2. Corpus callosal agenesis and absent septum pellucidum 3. Stenogyria/polymicrogyria 4. Fenestration of falx cerebri with interdigitation of gyri
Spinal	1. Myelomeningocele 2. Syringohydromyelia 3. Klippel-Feil syndrome, scoliosis

19. **a**—Chiari I malformation

Chiari Malformation: Terminology

Accepted terms	
Chiari I	Downward herniation of cerebellar tonsils through the foramen magnum
Chiari II	Herniation of medulla, 4th ventricle and cerebellar vermis through the foramen magnum associated with myelomeningocele
Chiari III	Herniation of medulla, 4th ventricle and cerebellum into an occipitocervical encephalocele
Uncommon terms	
Chiari IV	Primary cerebellar aplasia/hypoplasia without hindbrain herniation
Chiari V	Herniation of occipital lobe through foramen magnum (absent cerebellum)
Chiari 0	Symptoms without 5 mm cerebellar tonsillar descent
Chiari 1.5	Downward herniation of cerebellar tonsils, medulla and 4th ventricle through the foramen magnum

Chiari I malformation is defined as inferior displacement of the cerebellar tonsils below the basion-opisthion line. Tonsillar herniation can be due to multiple causes:

1. Intracranial pressure: both intracranial hypertension and intracranial hypotension.
2. Congenital or acquired osseous anomaly or pathology of the posterior fossa and craniovertebral junction caused by softening of the skull base, leading to a decrease in the size of the posterior fossa (e.g., osteogenesis imperfecta, Paget's disease, platybasia, or basilar invagination).
3. Congenital causes: mesodermal abnormalities leading to a short clivus, reduced height of the supraocciput, and increased slope of tentorium severely reduce posterior fossa volume with subsequent overcrowding of the contents and inferior displacement of the tonsils and/or vermis.

Stridor and hindbrain dysfunction are the most common clinical presentations during the first 3 months in a child with a type I Chiari malformation. The stridor usually disappears by 3 months of age. Another common clinical presentation in children is a headache, which may be generalized, or can be localized to occipital region. In children, this headache becomes exacerbated by physical exercise, straining, or coughing. Other symptoms related to cerebellar or brainstem dysfunction, such as cranial nerve palsy or otoneurologic disturbances, such as tinnitus, vertigo, and dizziness, dysmetria (tremors and down-beating nystagmus). Disorders of motor, sensation, and reflexes are seen when there is an associated syrinx in the cervical/thoracic cord. MRI is done to assess whether clinically significant hindbrain herniation is present and likely cause; normal tonsillar descent below the basion-opisthion line is up to 6 mm in 5- to 15-year-olds and up to 5 mm in anyone over 15 years. Secondary features include a pointed appearance of the cerebellar tonsils, compression of cerebellar cistern (demonstrated by effacement of vallecula and cisterna magna), retroflexion of the odontoid process, compression of the fourth ventricle, and syringohydromyelia.

Image with permission from Coley BD. Caffey's Pediatric Diagnostic Imaging, 12th ed. Elsevier, Saunders, 2013.

20. **a**—CSF flow study

Syringohydromyelia may be seen in the cervical cord in 30-50% of Chiari I malformations. In healthy patients, an increase in the cerebral blood volume during the cardiac systole causes displacement of the corresponding amount of CSF from the basal cistern into the cervical subarachnoid space. In diastole with cerebral venous outflow, there is a caudo-cranial diastolic CSF wave. In hindbrain herniation, syrinx formation may occur due to partial obstruction of the CSF flow channel around the craniocervical junction and Venturi effect with enhanced intramedullary pulse pressure causing extracellular fluid accumulation in the distended cord. The syrinx may form anywhere along the cord, hence whole spine MRI is advised in patients with tonsillar herniation symptoms, such as sensori-motor weakness of the extremities, and/or loss of bladder/bowel control. MRI CSF flow studies can also be performed to study the CSF motion in and around the foramen magnum to predict likely benefits of decompressive surgery. In addition, before surgical intervention, a low tentorium should be evaluated with MR venography to document a low-lying torcula and transverse sinus to avoid damage during decompressive surgery.

Image with permission from Grainger RG, et al. (Eds.). Grainger and Allison's Diagnostic Radiology: A Textbook of Medical Imaging, 4th ed. Harcourt, London, 2001.

21. **b**—Closed spinal dysraphism (spina bifida occulta)

This infant displays segmental infantile hemangiomas, a dimple, a pseudotail, and a deviated gluteal cleft suggesting the presence of a closed (occult) spinal dysraphism. Other midline lesions to look for include a. The clinical presentation varies to some degree by age. Younger children tend to present with cutaneous markers that lead to an evaluation for CSD, but on formal testing, most have mild signs of lower motor neuron dysfunction and abnormalities on urodynamic testing. Older children and adolescents tend to present with either cutaneous stigmata or with progressive neurologic deficits. Some affected individuals remain asymptomatic into adulthood, at which time they may develop back pain with or without radiculopathy and perineal dysesthesias. Features associated with closed spinal dysraphism are summarized below:

Closed Spinal Dysraphism: Features

Cutaneous	Lipoma (most common sign of spinal dysraphism), faun's tail (V shaped patch of long silky hair), dermal sinuses (hair at ostium), true tails, telangiectasias, capillary malformations, aplasia cutis congenita, naevi, pigmentation abnormalities and other subcutaneous masses
Neurological	Autonomic dyfunction, sphincteric dysfunction, sensori-motor deficits in legs, meningitis (ruptured dermal sinus/cyst); if symptoms progressive rather than static more likely to be due to TCS or compression by mass lesion
Urological	Neurogenic bladder dysfunction (TCS) or urogenital malformations. Diagnosis of bladder dysfunction is often not recognized in pre-toilet trained children
Orthopedic	Scoliosis, kyphosis, lordosis, leg length discrepancy, and foot deformities
Gastrointestinal	Imperforate anus

If present, clinical evaluation for TCS should be performed as far as possible given the age of the patient. If there is a high clinical suspicion (or age >3-5 months or bulky lesion precluding USS) spinal MRI should be performed and depending on significance of findings, referral to neurosurgeon or neurologist made. Spinal US can be performed in those under 3-5 months and low clinical suspicion of TCS, but inappropriate visualization will necessitate MRI.

Image with permission from Bolognia J, et al. Dermatology Essentials, Elsevier, 2014.

22. **e**—Urodynamic testing

TCS is stretch-induced dysfunction of the caudal spinal cord and conus, caused by attachment of the filum terminale to inelastic structures caudally. TCS may occur independently (primary) or secondary to spinal dysraphism (open or closed), spinal cord trauma or other pathology. The filum terminale is normally viscoelastic in nature, and serves to dampen movements of the spine during flexion and extension, without applying undue traction to the moving spinal cord. In TCS, the spinal cord is attached to abnormally inelastic structures caudally, such as a fibrous or fat-infiltrated filum, tumor, meningoceles or myelomeningoceles, scars, or septa (as seen in SSCM). This causes the caudal portion of the spinal cord to stretch between the point of tethering and the dentate ligaments that fix the cord proximally. Progressive dysfunction occurs because of repeated extension or flexion of the spine and/or differential growth of the vertebral column as compared to the spinal cord. The clinical presentation of TCS is broad and varies with age at presentation as well as features associated with the underlying cause (e.g., cutaneous lesions of closed spinal dysraphism). Features commonly described as a direct cause of cord tethering are:

- Neurological—back pain, leg weakness, progressive gait disturbance, calf muscle atrophy, absent deep tendon reflexes, dermatomal sensory loss. The TCS causes spinal dysfunction caudal to the T12/L1spinal level, and does not explain upper motor neuron signs
- Urological—neurogenic bladder dysfunction
- Orthopedic—progressive scoliosis and foot deformities

In the classic progression of symptoms with TCS, children begin to stumble after they have learned to walk normally. Then they start dribbling urine after having achieved successful toilet training. Later, they develop musculoskeletal signs and symptoms; common findings include foot drop, painless sores, and scoliosis. Older children will often complain of back pain exacerbated by exercise, while younger children tend to have increased irritability and refuse to perform certain activities and movements, though without a frank complaint of pain. Back pain, leg pain, and scoliosis are the primary symptoms of TCS in adults, and these may be difficult to distinguish from other more common causes of chronic back pain. The earliest sign of motor dysfunction in the older child and adult with TCS is usually weakness of ankle dorsiflexion. Sensory symptoms usually are patchy and vague, especially when related to TCS. Imaging modality of choice is MRI, with US playing a role prior to ossification of posterior elements (<4 m) and plain films/CT for evaluation of bony abnormalities. MRI may show a low-lying conus medullaris but can also be normal. Urodynamic testing can detect preclinical urologic dysfunction in children with CSD. Urodynamic testing is often used for preoperative evaluation of children who might benefit from neurosurgery for tethered cord release.

23. **b**—A 6-week-old boy with static bilateral 3/5 leg weakness. Urodynamic testing shows evidence of neurogenic bladder which is being managed with intermittent catheterization.

Although no clear consensus exists, the main indication for neurosurgery is new onset or progression of neurologic symptoms related to the CSD or TCS. Early neurosurgical intervention also is warranted for severe neonatal symptoms such as bowel obstruction. Additional indications for neurosurgical intervention include cases where the spinal cord is internally exposed to decrease the risk of infection and meningitis, spinal instability or for pain relief. In contrast, severely disabled patients with static deficits related to CSD are unlikely to benefit from surgery. More controversial indications for surgical intervention include radiographic demonstration of a tethered cord in asymptomatic patients, or abnormal findings on urodynamic studies in a patient with CSD. The rationale for surgery in such cases is that even infants and children who are asymptomatic or mildly symptomatic may go on to develop progressive and irreversible neurologic deficits. Conservative management with watchful monitoring is also an acceptable approach in patients who are asymptomatic or mildly symptomatic, given the highly variable natural history of CSD. In CSD cases associated with cord tethering, surgery involves removal of any anatomic structure that is acting to tether the spinal cord, and may include transection of the filum, resection of transitional lipoma, lysis of adhesions, and excision of dermal sinus tracts. In addition, some data suggest that fashioning a large intradural compartment, with duraplasty if needed, is associated with a reduced risk of developing arachnoid adhesions and cord Asymptomatic patients with CSD who do not have surgery still require close monitoring to watch for the onset of neurologic, genitourinary or gastrointestinal symptoms, especially with respect to incontinence or constipation. Patients who have surgery for CSD should remain under close monitoring because of the risk of future worsening, which can occur with spinal cord retethering or progression of a preexisting syrinx. The earliest indication of retethering is usually urologic symptoms. In addition, non-neurological symptoms may continue to progress postoperatively, as can be seen with preexisting scoliosis and pain. Urodynamics are generally considered to be a good monitoring tool for both nonoperative patients and postoperative patients, and particularly for early detection of cord retethering.

FURTHER READING

Khoury C. Closed spinal dysraphism: pathogenesis and types. Uptodate, 2015.

24. **e**—Myelomeningocele

Open spinal dysraphism (OSD) is a clinical diagnosis and a neurosurgical emergency. Myelomeningocele accounts for 99% of OSD, myelocele is rare, and hemimyelocele and hemimyelomeningocele extremely rare. In all cases there is defective closure of the primary neural tube (primary neurulation) resulting in the neural placode being exposed through a midline skin defect on the back. In myelomeningocele, neural placode protrudes above skin surface, whereas in myelocele, the placode is flush with skin surface. The abnormality is most commonly found at lumbosacral region and a Chiari II malformation is invitable due to CSF leak. Surgical repair and closure of the defect is required as soon as possible. While imaging is not necessarily required before closure, MR imaging should be performed to assess for associated pathology at other levels (e.g., split cord malformation, lipoma, dermoid/epidermoid, Chiari II malformation) and is crucial in patients presenting with progressive neurological deficits postoperatively (e.g., exclude cord ischemia, arachnoid cyst, scar tethering).

Image with permission from Carlson BM. Human Embryology and Developmental Biology, 5th ed. Elsevier, Saunders, 2014.

ANSWERS 25–33

Additional answers 25–33 available on ExpertConsult.com

EMI ANSWERS

34. 1—c, Dermal sinus; 2—h, Hemimyelomeningocele; 3—i, Lipomyelocele; 4—p, Persistent terminal ventricle; 5—o, Neurenteric cyst

Spinal Dysraphism: Classification

Type	Description	Stage Affected
Open spinal dysraphism		
Myelomeningocele	Abnormal spinal cord exposed in the midline via defect in the dura, posterior vertebral elements, facia and skin. Defect produces Chiari II malformation in all cases and hydrocephalus. Neurosurgical emergency due to CSF leak and hydrocephalus	Primary neurulation
Myelocele	As myelomeningocele, but subarachnoid space ventral to placode is not expanded resulting in a lesion flush with skin	
Hemimyelocele	Myelocele affecting one of two hemicords in split cord malformation	Gastrulation and primary neurulation
Hemimyelomeningocele	Myelomeningocele affecting one of two hemicords in split cord malformation	
Closed spinal dysraphism with subcutaneous mass		
Lipomyelomeningocele	A subcutaneous lipoma tethers the spinal cord (lipoma-placode interface) outside the spinal canal via defect in vertebral elements	Primary neurulation
Lipomyelocele	A subcutaneous lipoma tethers the spinal cord (lipoma-placode interface) inside the spinal canal via defect in vertebral elements	

Continued on following page

Spinal Dysraphism: Classification (Continued)

Type	Description	Stage Affected
Meningocele	Posterior—Herniation of CSF-filled meningeal sac through posterior bony defect (may contain nerve roots but not spinal cord). Dura may have defect but overlying skin is intact. Anterior meningoceles are part of the caudal regression syndrome	Unknown
Terminal myelocystocele	Expansion of terminal central canal (syringocele) surrounded by a meningocele with no communication between two components. Syringocele is caudal to the meningocele and herniates through a wide spina bifida to cause a intergluteal cystic swelling	Secondary neurulation and retrogressive differentiation
Closed spinal dysraphism without subcutaneous mass		
Simple dysraphic state		
Posterior spina bifida	Simple defect of fusion of posterior neural arch of a vertebra, usually at L5 or S1	
Intradural lipoma	Lipomas originate from early disjunction between neuroectoderm and ectoderm—the surrounding mesenchyme creeps between and adheres to primitive ependyma which induces it to transform into fat	Primary neurulation
Filum terminale lipoma	Fibrolipomatous thickening of the filum terminale	Secondary neurulation and retrogressive differentiation
Tight filum terminale	Short, hypertrophic filum terminale producing tethering and impaired ascent of conus	
Persistent terminal ventricle	Small ependymal lined cavity in the conus medullaris which may undergo cystic dilatation	
Complex dysraphic state		
Split cord malformation	Type 1—bony midline septum dividing cord into two separate cords in own dural sleeves Type 2—single thecal sac containing split cords with an intervening fibrous band	Gastrulation (notochordal integration)
Neurenteric cyst	Cysts usually in intradural extramedullary plane of endodermal origin, usually lined with GI or respiratory epithelium	
Dorsal enteric fistula	Most severe. Cleft connecting the bowel with dorsal skin surface through the prevertebral soft tissues, split vertebral bodies and spinal cord, neural arch, subcutaneous tissue	
Dermal sinus	Epithelium-lined fistula which extends from skin to meninges within the spinal canal, possibly opening into the subarachnoid space or connecting to filum terminale, lipoma and may also be associated with a spinal dermoid	
Caudal regression syndrome	Agenesis of spinal column, imperforate anus, genital anomalies, bilateral renal dysplasia, pulmonary hypoplasia and lower limb abnormalities. Syndromic associations include OEIS, VACTERL and Currarino triad	Gastrulation (notochordal formation)
Segmental dysgenesis	Segmental agenesis of thoracolumbar spine: vertebral, segmental spinal cord hypoplasia/aplasia with caudal bulkiness, congenital paraparesis, lower limb deformities	

FURTHER READING

Tortori-Donati P, Rossi A, Cama A. Spinal dysraphism: a review of neuroradiological features with embryological correlations and proposal for a new classification. Neuroradiology. 2000;42(7):471-91.

35. 1—j, Porencephalic cyst

Porencephalic cysts are due to an encephaloclastic insult (e.g., intrauterine infections and ischemia), lined by white matter, and communicate with the ventricles and/or the subarachnoid space. They commonly become symptomatic in the 1st year of life with evidence of spasticity, seizures, and developmental delay. Imaging Well-defined CSF cyst (T1 hypointense, T2 hyperintense, FLAIR dark, no restricted diffusion, no enhancement) and often corresponds to a vascular territory. The cyst is lined by white matter, which may or may not demonstrate evidence of gliosis (this depends on the age at which the insult occurred). Importantly the cyst is not lined by gray matter, helpful in distinguishing them from arachnoid cysts and schizencephaly. Typically the cyst seen to communicate with the ventricles and/or the subarachnoid space and there is no mass effect. Management is supportive.

2—k, Schizencephaly

CHAPTER 41

PEDIATRIC NEUROSURGERY: GENERAL AND HYDROCEPHALUS

SINGLE BEST ANSWER (SBA) QUESTIONS

1. Which one of the following statements LEAST accurately describes CSF production?
   a. Neonates produce CSF at a rate of 25 ml/day
   b. Infants have a total CSF volume of 25 ml
   c. Adults produce CSF at a rate of approximately 0.5 ml/min
   d. Ventricles contain 25 ml of CSF
   e. Raised intracranial pressure does not affect formation of CSF at the choroid plexus

2. The estimated frequency of hydrocephalus in children is which one of the following?
   a. 1 in 100
   b. 1 in 250
   c. 1 in 500
   d. 1 in 1500
   e. 1 in 5000

3. An infant has a head CT performed because of a large head and failure to thrive. The diagnosis of hydrocephalus is made. Congenital hydrocephalus is most commonly caused by which one of the following maternal infections?
   a. Toxoplasmosis
   b. Rubella
   c. Influenza
   d. HIV
   e. Group B Streptococci

4. An 18-month-old child presents with poor feeding, and motor delay. Papilledema is present on fundoscopy. CT head shows a heterogeneously enhancing midline posterior fossa mass suspicious of medulloblastoma causing severe obstructive hydrocephalus. This child's risk of developing chronic hydrocephalus at 6 months postoperatively is which one of the following?
   a. 7%
   b. 19%
   c. 42%
   d. 56%
   e. 80%
   f. 97%

5. A 9-year-old child with VP shunt comes with headache and lethargy. CT head, blood, unchanged and shunt series are normal. Risk of CSF infection secondary to percutaneous shunt tap is which one of the following?
   a. 0.0002%
   b. 0.002%
   c. 0.02%
   d. 0.2%
   e. 2%

6. Which one of the following statements regarding the management of pediatric hydrocephalus is LEAST accurate?
   a. Preoperative antibiotics reduces the risk of subsequent shunt infection in patients with hydrocephalus
   b. There is insufficient evidence to recommend the routine use of endoscopic guidance in ventricular shunt placement
   c. There is insufficient evidence to recommend occipital over frontal point of entry for ventricular catheters
   d. There is no clear advantage for one shunt valve type over another
   e. Antibiotic-impregnated shunt tubing may be associated with a lower risk of shunt infection compared to conventional silver-impregnated hardware

7. Which one of the following statements regarding the choice of endoscopic third ventriculostomy or ventriculoperitoneal shunt CSF diversion in children is LEAST accurate?
   a. ETV is the standard of care for post-hemorrhagic hydrocephalus in infants (<24 months old)
   b. VP shunt is usually most appropriate for communicating hydrocephalus
   c. ETV should be considered first for hydrocephalus due to congenital aqueduct stenosis
   d. Late ETV failure (2 years) is less common than late VP shunt failure
   e. Majority of ETV failure occurs in the first 3 months

8. An 8-month-old previously healthy child presents with macrocephaly and delayed milestones. MRI is shown below. Which one of the following is his most likely ETV success score?

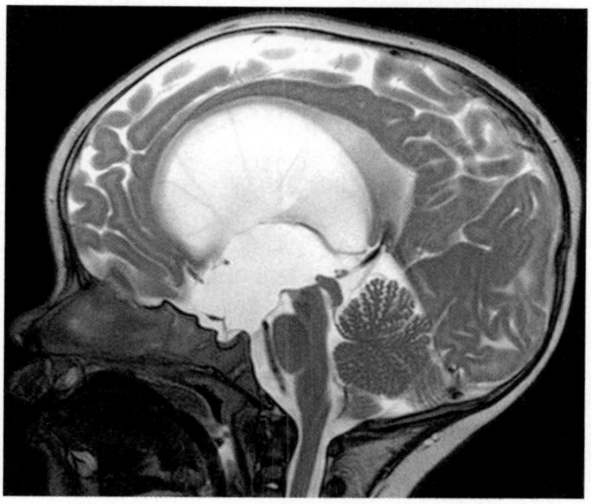

   a. 40
   b. 50
   c. 60
   d. 70
   e. 80

9. A preterm neonate is born at 28 weeks gestation with a birth weight of 1000 g. Cranial US performed in the first 24 h of birth due to a bulging fontanelle and episodes of apnoea revealed Papile grade III germinal matrix hemorrhage with hydrocephalus. Which one of the following statements is most accurate?
   a. The majority of intraventricular hemorrhage in low birthweight preterm infants is Grade III and IV
   b. The proportion of infants with post-hemorrhagic hydrocephalus who require permanent shunt placement is lower in preterm than term births
   c. Sunset phenomenon consists of impaired downgaze
   d. Term infants usually present with spontaneous apnea or bradycardia in the first 24 h after IVH
   e. The rate of intraventricular hemorrhage in both term and preterm babies is 30%, but the mean Papile grade is higher in preterms

10. Which one of the following statements regarding the management of post-hemorrhagic hydrocephalus LEAST correct:
   a. Ventriculosubgaleal shunts increase the need for daily CSF aspiration compared with ventricular access devices
   b. The use of prophylactic serial lumbar puncture is not recommended as it does not reduce the need for shunt placement or avoid the progression of hydrocephalus in premature infants compared to observation alone
   c. Intraventricular thrombolytic agents are not recommended as methods to reduce the need for shunt placement in premature infants with PHH
   d. Acetazolamide and furosemide are not recommended as methods to reduce the need for shunt placement in premature infants with PHH
   e. There is insufficient evidence to recommend a specific infant weight or CSF parameter to direct the timing of shunt placement in premature infants with PHH
   f. There is insufficient evidence to recommend the use of endoscopic third ventriculostomy (ETV) in premature infants with PHH

11. Which one of the following statements regarding the treatment of CSF shunt infection is most accurate?
   a. Evidence recommends shunt externalization over complete shunt removal as the preferred surgical strategy in management of CSF shunt infection
   b. Evidence recommends the combination of intrathecal and systemic antibiotics for patients with CSF shunt infection when the infected shunt hardware cannot be fully removed
   c. Evidence recommends the combination of intrathecal and systemic antibiotics for patients with CSF shunt infection when caused by gram-negative organisms
   d. Evidence recommends supplementation of antibiotic treatment with partial (externalization) or with complete shunt hardware removal
   e. Evidence recommends the combination of intrathecal and systemic antibiotics for patients with CSF shunt infection when the shunt must be removed and immediately replaced

12. A 4-month-old child with a history of *Escherichia coli* neonatal meningitis returns with poor feeding and a bulging fontanelle. CT head is done which shows hydrocephalus and MRI is done for surgical planning. Which one of the following is likely to be the surgical goal in this patient?

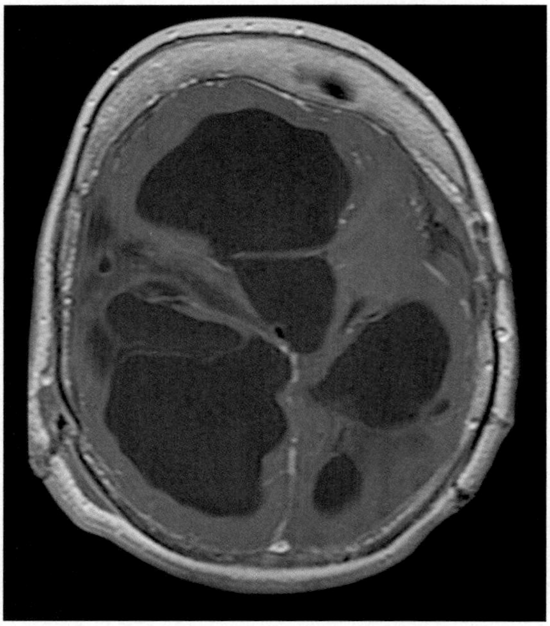

a. Complex VP shunt with at least two proximal catheters
b. Single VP shunt following endoscopic fenestration of loculations
c. ETV and endoscopic fenestration of loculations
d. Endoscopic aqueductoplasty
e. Ventriculocisternal shunt

13. Which one of the following statements regarding Lundberg waves seen during ICP monitoring is most accurate?
a. They represent aortic valve closure seen in normal patients
b. They are dicrotic representing arterial pulsation seen in normal patients
c. B wave is mean ICP with pressure 20-50 mmHg lasting 30 s to a few minutes during sleep
d. A waves represent the cyclic variation in systolic pressure due to oscillations in autoregulation
e. C waves suggest ICP exceeding limits of cerebral compliance

14. A 16-year-old child presents with cough related headache and sensory changes in her hands. Neurological examination is otherwise normal and there is no papilledema. MRI head and spine show a Chiari I malformation with 8 mm tonsillar decent and a small cervical syrinx at C3//4. Which one of the following statements regarding surgical management is most accurate?
a. Durotomy and tonsillectomy would be mandatory in this case
b. C1-C3 laminectomy should also be performed in this case to treat the syrinx adequately
c. Due to minimal tonsillar descent, primary treatment should be directed towards the syrinx (e.g. syringostomy) if her symptoms progress
d. Lumbar puncture should be performed to exclude neurological cause of her symptoms
e. Intraoperature ultrasound is less accurate at predicting those who do not need durotomy in the presence of tonsillar descent below C1 lamina

15. An 18-month old is treated for meningitis. After initially improvement, becomes less responsive on day 10 and imaging is performed. Which one of the following is LEAST appropriate?

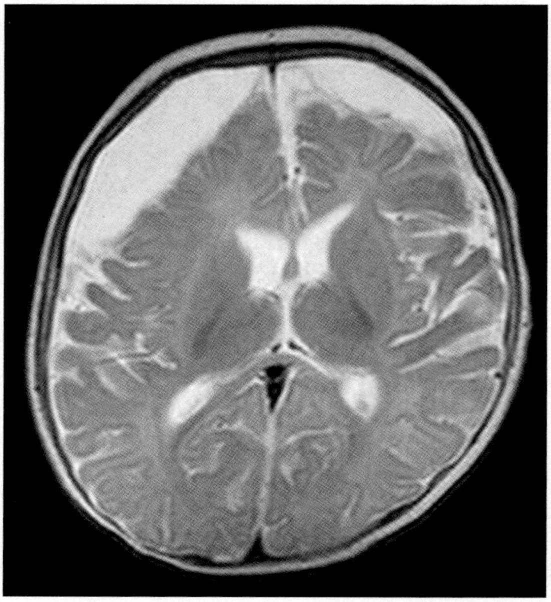

a. Subduroperitoneal shunt
b. Percutaneous needle drainage
c. Transventricular tap
d. External subdural drain
e. Burr hole drainage

QUESTIONS 16–25

Additional questions 16–25 available on ExpertConsult.com

EXTENDED MATCHING ITEM (EMI) QUESTIONS

26. **Congenital and Genetic hydrocephalus:**
 a. Arachnoid cyst
 b. Aqueduct stenosis
 c. Chiari malformation
 d. Dandy-Walker
 e. Foramen of Monro atresia
 f. Joubert syndrome
 g. Neural tube defect
 h. Posterior fossa defect
 i. VACTERL-H
 j. Walker-Warburg syndrome
 k. X-linked hydrocephalus

For each of the following descriptions, select the most appropriate answers from the list above. Each answer may be used once, more than once or not at all.

1. An infant presents with the most common heritable non-syndromic from of hydrocephalus, usually with mutation in LCAM1 gene.
2. An infant presents with hypotonia, sleep apnea, developmental delay. MRI head demonstrates midline cerebellar vermis hypoplasia with deepened interpeduncular fossa (Molar tooth sign) and thick elongated superior cerebellar peduncles.

27. **Shunt complications:**
 a. Abdominal pseudocyst
 b. Acute overdrainage
 c. Chronic overdrainage
 d. CSF ascites
 e. CSF infection
 f. Disconnection
 g. Erosion into abdominal viscus
 h. Migration of distal catheter
 i. Proximal catheter obstruction
 j. Shunt site infection
 k. Silicone allergy

For each of the following descriptions, select the most appropriate answers from the list above. Each answer may be used once, more than once or not at all.

1. A 7-year-old boy with a VP shunt in situ presents to the emergency department after being found by his parents unconscious in his room after 2 days of a headache and vomiting. His pupils are 5 mm and sluggish bilaterally, and he is hypertensive with bradycardia of 38 bpm. Shunt reservoir tap is unable to aspirate CSF.
2. An 8-month-old infant presents 1 month after VP shunt for post-hemorrhagic hydrocephalus with swelling over abdominal wound, without erythema or heat. XR shunt series shows that the shunt is in continuity and a bird's nest arrangement of the peritoneal catheter.
3. A 9-year-old boy presents with a fixed pressure VP shunt inserted for symptomatic aqueduct stenosis which was inserted several months ago. He has been experiencing intermittent headaches on standing for the last few weeks, and feeling nauseous. Now the headaches have become permanent even when lying flat and he is finding it difficult to keep food down. Shunt reservoir is filling adequately.

28. **Neonatal meningitis:**
 a. *Citrobacter koseri*
 b. Coagulase negative staphylococcus
 c. *Escherichia coli*
 d. *Hemophilus influenza*
 e. *Listeria monocytogenes*
 f. *Neisseria meningitidis*
 g. *Proprionobacter*
 h. *Staphylococcus epidermis*
 i. *Streptococcus pneumonia*
 j. *Tuberculosis*

For each of the following descriptions, select the most appropriate answers from the list above. Each answer may be used once, more than once or not at all.

1. Highest risk of associated brain abscess
2. Multiple tiny parenchymal nodules and basal meningeal enhancement

SBA ANSWERS

1. **b**—Infants have a total CSF volume of 25 ml

Infants have a total CSF volume of 50 ml (150 ml in adults), and in both infants and adults there is 25 ml of CSF in the ventricles. Neonates produce CSF at a rate of 25 ml/day, which increases to two thirds of the adult capacity as an infant. Adults produce CSF at a rate of 0.35 ml/min = 20 ml/h (approximately 500 ml/day).

FURTHER READING

Hdeib A, Cohen, AR. Hydrocephalus in Children and Adults. In: Ellenbogen RG, editor. Principles of Neurological Surgery, 3rd ed. Saunders, Elsevier; 2012.

2. **c**—1 in 500

It is estimated that hydrocephalus may occur with the frequency of 1 in every 500 children. Causes include genetic (e.g. X-linked aqueduct stenosis), other congenital causes (e.g. myelomeningocele and Chiari malformation) and more common acquired causes such as intraventricular hemorrhage, trauma, tumors, and infection.

FURTHER READING

Flannery AM, et al. Pediatric hydrocephalus: systematic literature review and evidence-based guidelines. Part 1: Introduction and methodology. J Neurosurg Pediatr 2014;14 Suppl. 1:3-7.

3. **a**—Toxoplasmosis

Congenitally acquired TORCHES infections (Toxoplasma, Other, Rubella, CMV, HErpes, Syphilis) are known to cause intrauterine growth restriction, microcephaly, intracranial calcifications, conjunctivitis, hearing loss, rash, hepatosplenomegaly and thrombocytopenia. Post-infectiouscauses of intrauterine and neonatal hydrocephalus due to aqueduct stenosis are also in this group, with Toxoplasma being the most frequent intrauterine infection associated with it, and viral causes including mumps and CMV.

Canadian Preoperative Prediction Rule for Hydrocephalus in Children with Posterior Fossa Neoplasms

Predictor	Score	Risk of Hydrocephalus at 6 Months by Score
Age <2	3	0 points = 7%,
Papilledema	1	1 = 11%, 2 = 19%,
Moderate to severe hydrocephalus present	2	3 = 29%, 4 = 42%, 5 = 56%, 6 = 69%, 7 = 80%, 8 = 88%,
Cerebral metastasis	3	9 = 93%, 10 = 96%
Likely Diagnosis of medulloblastoma, ependymoma, or dorsally exophytic brainstem glioma	1	

4. **e**—80%

Propensity of midline, and mostly posterior fossa, tumors in children causes a high incidence of hydrocephalus. Preoperative shunting is no longer routine, and most surgeons opt to remove the tumor and monitor for the development of hydrocephalus. External ventricular drain insertion at the time of tumor removal is common for tumors within the fourth ventricle but may be avoided in cerebellar hemispheric tumors. While preoperative ETV can reduce hydrocephalus and does not burden the child with hardware, some of these third ventriculostomies may be unnecessary because a proportion of children will not develop progressive hydrocephalus after tumor removal. The validated Canadian preoperative prediction rule for hydrocephalus in children with posterior fossa neoplasms predicts the risk of developing postoperative hydrocephalus based on age, papilledema, severity of hydrocephalus, metastatic disease, and estimated preoperative tumor type. Evaluating these factors allows a more informed discussion with patients and families and possibly the selective use of endoscopic third ventriculostomy before tumor surgery. Following surgery for tumors in the lateral ventricle that are associated with hydrocephalus, the surgical tract may lead to postoperative decompression of the hydrocephalus into the subdural space. When this collection persists as a subdural hygroma, it may require treatment with a subdural shunt.

FURTHER READING

Kestle JD. Hydrocephalus in children: approach to the patient. In: Winn RH, editor. Youmans Neurological Surgery, 6th ed. Saunders, Elsevier; 2011.

Riva-Cambrin J, Lamberti-Pasculli M, Armstrong D, et al. The validation of a preoperative prediction score for chronic hydrocephalus in pediatric patients with posterior fossa tumours. J Neurosurg 2005;102:A798.

5. **d**—0.2%

In a recent study, of 542 shunt taps performed in 266 children using a standard protocol (by neurosurgical department personnel only), there were 14 infected shunts but only one child (with redness over shunt track) whose first CSF tap was negative but then returned 11 days later with fever and irritability and whose repeat CSF tap grew *Staphylococcus aureus*. They state: "Assuming that this patient's shunt infection was secondary to the shunt tap, the infection rate would be 1 (0.18%) in 542. If one removes the 14 infected shunts, because theoretically a shunt tap leading to another infection might be masked by the antibiotics used to treat the first diagnosed infection, the rate would be 1 (0.19%) in 528. Because there were often multiple taps in the same patient, the incorporation of a time separation between the first and second tap can be used to ensure that the second tap was indeed negative. If one assumes a reasonable time interval to be 3 months, that would eliminate 162 taps, changing the incidence to 1 (0.27%) in 366."

FURTHER READING

Spiegelman L, Asija R, Da Silva SL, Krieger MD, McComb JG. What is the risk of infecting a cerebrospinal fluid-diverting shunt with percutaneous tapping? J Neurosurg Pediatr 2014;14(4):336-9. http://dx.doi.org/10.3171/2014.7.PEDS13612. Epub 2014 Aug 8. PubMed PMID: 25105511.

6. **e**—Antibiotic-impregnated shunt tubing may be associated with a lower risk of shunt infection compared to conventional silver-impregnated hardware

FURTHER READING

Baird LC, Mazzola CA, Auguste KI, Klimo P Jr, Flannery AM; Pediatric Hydrocephalus Systematic Review and Evidence-Based Guidelines Task Force. Pediatric hydrocephalus: systematic literature review and evidence-based guidelines. Part 5: Effect of valve type on cerebrospinal fluid shunt efficacy. J Neurosurg Pediatr 2014;14 Suppl. 1:35-43. http://dx.doi.org/10.3171/2014.7.PEDS14325. Review. PubMed PMID: 25988781.

Kemp J, et al. Pediatric hydrocephalus: systematic literature review and evidence-based guidelines. Part 9: Effect of ventricular catheter entry point and position. J Neurosurg Pediatr 2014;14 Suppl. 1:72-6. PubMed PMID: 25988785.

Flannery AM, et al. Pediatric hydrocephalus: systematic literature review and evidence-based guidelines. Part 3: Endoscopic computer-assisted electromagnetic navigation and ultrasonography as technical adjuvants for shunt placement. J Neurosurg Pediatr 2014;14 Suppl. 1:24-9. PubMed PMID: 25988779.

Klimo P Jr, et al. Pediatric hydrocephalus: systematic literature review and evidence-based guidelines. Part 6: Preoperative antibiotics for shunt surgery in children with hydrocephalus: a systematic review and meta-analysis. J Neurosurg Pediatr 2014;14 Suppl. 1:44-52. PubMed PMID: 25988782.

Klimo P Jr, et al. Pediatric hydrocephalus: systematic literature review and evidence-based guidelines. Part 7: Antibiotic-impregnated shunt systems versus conventional shunts in children: a systematic review and meta-analysis. J Neurosurg Pediatr 2014;14 Suppl. 1:53-9. Review. PubMed PMID: 25988783.

7. **a**—ETV is the standard of care for post-hemorrhagic hydrocephalus in infants (<24 months old)

The optimum treatment for hydrocephalus is controversial. Aside from obstructive hydrocephalus in children older than 2 years and adults, in whom ETV is often used, VPS placement remains the standard of care. But the indications for performing ETV have recently broadened to communicating types of hydrocephalus and the success of ETV in young infants for all causes of hydrocephalus has been increased by the addition of choroid plexus cauterization. No completed randomized trials have compared endoscopic and shunt treatment for pediatric hydrocephalus, and the International Infant Hydrocephalus Study is ongoing (direct comparisons of VPS versus ETV for infants [≤24 months of age] with aqueduct stenosis). Another randomized prospective trial is currently underway at CURE Children's Hospital of Uganda to compare ETV plus CPC versus VPS alone in infants younger than 6 months of age with post-infectious hydrocephalus. The best criteria to determine optimum hydrocephalus treatment are not known, since while acute symptoms may be alleviated ventriculomegaly may not completely resolve and continue to cause subtle white matter injury or impair cognitive outcome, hence brain volume may correlate better with cognitive outcome better than CSF volume.

FURTHER READING

Kahle KT, et al. Hydrocephalus in children. Lancet 2015, http://dx.doi.org/10.1016/S0140-6736(15)60694-8.

Limbrick DD Jr, Baird LC, Klimo P Jr, Riva-Cambrin J, Flannery AM. Pediatric Hydrocephalus Systematic Review and Evidence-Based Guidelines Task Force. Pediatric hydrocephalus: systematic literature review and evidence-based guidelines. Part 4: Cerebrospinal fluid shunt or endoscopic third ventriculostomy for the treatment of hydrocephalus in children. J Neurosurg Pediatr 2014;14 Suppl. 1:30-4. http://dx.doi.org/10.3171/2014.7.PEDS14324. Review. PubMed PMID: 25988780.

8. **d**—70

Most ETV failures occur within the first 6 months of surgery. ETV success score is a simple means to predict 6-month success rate of ETV, with scores ranging from 0 (meaning virtually no chance of ETV success) to 90 (meaning a roughly 90% chance of ETV success). ETVSS is calculated as Age Score + Etiology Score + Previous Shunt Score from the table above, and has demonstrated internal and external validity.

ETV Success Score

Score	Age	Etiology	Previous Shunt
0	<1 month	Post-infectious	Yes
10	1 month to <6 months	–	No
20	–	Myelomeningocele, IVH, non-tectal tumor	–
30	6 months to 1 year	Aqueduct stenosis, tectal tumor, other	–
40	1 year to <10 years	–	–
50	>10 years	–	–

Image with permission from Kahle KT, Kulkarni AV, Limbrick DD Jr, Warf BC. Hydrocephalus in children, Lancet 2015. pii:S0140-6736(15)60694-8.

FURTHER READING

Kulkarni AV, Riva-Cambrin J, Browd SR. Use of the ETV Success Score to explain the variation in reported endoscopic third ventriculostomy success rates among published case series of childhood hydrocephalus. J Neurosurg Pediatr 2011;7(2):143-6.

9. **b**—The proportion of infants with post-hemorrhagic hydrocephalus who require permanent shunt placement is lower in preterm than term births

The incidence of IVH increases inversely with decreasing birthweight or EGA. In extremely low birthweight preterm infants who survived and could be followed up, 33% had a history of intraventricular hemorrhage (IVH) of which 40% was Grade III or IV but eventually only 3% required VP shunt placement for post-hemorrhagic hydrocephalus (PHH). In term babies, 15% had peri/intraventricular hemorrhage and nearly all have grade I/II IVH. In preterm babies, most IVH occurs within the first 72 h of life and is diagnosed by bedside cranial US due to deterioration over several days. Infants with IVH should be observed closely with daily measurement of the occipitofrontal circumference (OFC): increase in growth rate from 0.5 to 1 cm/day for 2-3 consecutive days often suggests symptomatic hydrocephalus. Other features include bulging fontanelle and splayed sutures, episodes of spontaneous apnea or bradycardia, refractory seizures, lethargy, and impaired upward gaze ("sunset" phenomenon). Term infants with IVH typically present with lethargy or seizures, but a subset of infants presents with distress at birth, and the remainder often present within the first week. In contrast to ELBW preterm infants, many term infants have no or transient ventricular dilation in the period immediately after IVH but significant proportion may eventually require a shunt, usually during the first year of life.

FURTHER READING

Mazzola CA, et al. Pediatric hydrocephalus: systematic literature review and evidence-based guidelines. Part 2: Management of posthemorrhagic hydrocephalus in premature infants. J Neurosurg Pediatr 2014;14 Suppl. 1:8-23.

Hu YC, et al. Infantile posthemorrhagic hydrocephalus. In: Winn RH, editor. Youmans Neurological Surgery, 6th ed. Saunders, Elsevier; 2011.

10. **a**—VSG shunts increase the need for daily CSF aspiration compared with VADs

Preterm infants with higher grade (II/IV) IVH are also usually the smallest and have the most comorbidities; they are poor surgical candidates due to poor nutrition, immature immune system, and other comorbidities (e.g. anemia of prematurity treated with erythropoietin, red blood cell, and platelet transfusion). Interventions for symptomatic hydrocephalus are offered in a stepwise progression to identify patients in whom permanent CSF diversion is not required. This process allows surgery to be avoided in all but the few who definitely need it. Lumbar punctures are useful for drawing off CSF as an immediate treatment for elevated intracranial pressure or CSF sampling in infants with communicating PHH, but routine use of LP (to reduce CSF blood load) does not eliminate the need for a VP shunt hence should not be performed. Diuretic therapy, including acetazolamide and furosemide, is not effective in this population and may increase the risk of nephrocalcinosis and other complications, and intraventricular streptokinase is also not effective. Temporary surgical approaches (e.g. ventricular access device, ventriculosubgaleal shunt) should be used in those that do not show stabilization of the head circumference on a reasonable growth curve and stabilization/reduction of ventriculomegaly on cranial US. In these cases, temporary shunts are used to treat symptomatic hydrocephalus and allow the infant to grow and recover from other complications of prematurity before undergoing definitive surgical therapy. Ventricular taps are reserved for life-threatening emergencies because they are associated with a markedly increased risk of infection and loculated hydrocephalus in childhood. EVDs have a much higher risk of complications in preterm infants than in older neurosurgical patients. Definitive surgery (permanent ventriculoperitoneal shunts) are required in only a small minority of preterm infants who suffer IVH. These children are prone to cerebral palsy, epilepsy, cognitive delay, and behavioral abnormalities regardless of whether the CSF diversion is effective. Permanent shunt insertion at an older age in the neonatal period also likely decreases the need for shunt revisions throughout childhood.

FURTHER READING

Hu YC, et al. Infantile posthemorrhagic hydrocephalus, In: Winn RH, editor. Youmans Neurological Surgery, 6th ed. Saunders, Elsevier; 2011.

Mazzola CA, et al. Pediatric hydrocephalus: systematic literature review and evidence-based guidelines. Part 2: Management of posthemorrhagic hydrocephalus in premature infants. J Neurosurg Pediatr 2014;14 Suppl. 1:8-23.

11. **d**—Supplementation of antibiotic treatment with partial (externalization) or with complete shunt hardware removal is the standard of care

Current management of CSF shunt infection is dictated not by evidence, but rather by physician preference and other possibly relevant patient-level factors (for example, patient surgical risk, ventricle size, and complexity of the shunt system). It is not surprising that there is significant variation in CSF shunt infection treatment protocols between centers. An infected ventricular shunt, as an infected foreign body, is difficult if not impossible to sterilize using antibiotics alone. We therefore accept not only that shunt removal (and eventual replacement once CSF sterility is achieved) requires multiple surgeries, but also the risk of introducing secondary infection during a variable period of external drainage. Variations in whether the infected shunt was externalized or completely removed, and whether supplemental intrathecal antibiotics were administered contribute to significant between-study heterogeneity. Shunt infection should be ideally managed with antibiotics, complete shunt removal, and placement of a temporary external ventricular drain, followed by reimplantation after CSF sterilization (48 h after last negative CSF). Although intrathecal administration of antibiotics appears to make theoretical sense because of enhanced CSF antibiotic concentrations, its practical application is controversial, owing in large part to the potential adverse effects of intrathecal therapy, including neurotoxicity. The indications for intrathecal therapy are not well established and presently range from use in any shunt infection, use in only those infections in which the CSF cannot be sterilized by systemic antibiotics alone (for example, persistent positive cultures), or use in those ventricular shunt infections caused by specific organisms (for example, gram-negative infections).

FURTHER READING

Tamber MS, et al. Pediatric hydrocephalus: systematic literature review and evidence-based guidelines. Part 8: Management of cerebrospinal fluid shunt infection. J Neurosurg Pediatr 2014;14 Suppl. 1:60-71.

12. **b**—Single VP shunt following endoscopic fenestration of loculations

Given the high risk of failure of an ETV due to age and post-infectious etiology (ETVSS = 10), a VP shunt is more acceptable in this case but endoscopic fenestration could reduce the number of proximal catheters required for adequate drainage of CSF to one (as well as reducing the odds of shunt failure as there are less catheters/connection points). Patients with both multiloculated and uniloculated hydrocephalus, isolated lateral and fourth ventricles, arachnoid cysts, and slit ventricle syndrome have not always responded to simple shunting systems. The ventricular system may become trabeculated and encysted following bacterial meningitis or germinal matrix hemorrhage. Hydrocephalus arising from intraventricular septations is known as complex or loculated. The lateral ventricle may become trapped due to obstruction of the Monro foramina by noncolloid neuroepithelial cysts (ependymal, choroid plexus, or arachnoid), termed unilocular hydrocephalus, and in other cases there may be multiple encysted compartments (multilocular). Traditional treatment is by placement of multiple shunts or multiperforated catheters which were multiple shunt revisions and high morbidity and mortality rates. Multiple shunts have increased the risks of infection and mechanical obstruction, and their removal has been problematic, with its associated risk of intraventricular hemorrhage. Transcallosal fenestration via craniotomy may reduce shunt revision rates or achieve shunt independence in both multiloculated hydrocephalus and uniloculated hydrocephalus, but craniotomy itself carries concomitant risks. The specific risks associated with the transcallosal approach include venous infarction from sacrificed bridging veins, damage to the pericallosal arteries, disconnection syndromes after splitting the corpus callosum, and damage to the fornices and subcortical nuclei. Authors of many reports stress the operative simplicity of the stereotactic procedure in uniloculated hydrocephalus; however, it was associated with a high recurrence rate (up to 80%) because the cyst wall could not be widely fenestrated, making it unsuitable in cases of multiloculated hydrocephalus. In the present day where endoscopic fenestration (of loculations, cyst walls, septum pellucidum, etc.) is available, the aim of surgery is to control hydrocephalus, simplify complex shunts, reduce the shunt revision rate, avoid implanting a shunt if possible, and decrease operative morbidity. Fenestration of the septum pellucidum is indicated when there is an obstruction of one foramen of Monro causing the ipsilateral ventricle to dilate from trapped CSF. Membranous/parenchymal obstructions of the foramen of Monro causing unilateral hydrocephalus have been reported and endoscopic foraminoplasty =/- stent can be considered.

Image with permission from Winn RH, editor. Youmans Neurological Surgery, 6th ed. Saunders, Elsevier; 2011.

FURTHER READING

Teo C, et al. Endoscopic management of complex hydrocephalus. World Neurosurg 2013;79 (2S):S21.e1-7.

El-Ghandour NMF. Endoscopic cyst fenestration in the treatment of multiloculated hydrocephalus in children. J Neurosurg Paediatr 2008;1(3):217-22.

13. **c**—B wave is mean ICP with pressure 20-50 mmHg lasting 30 s to a few minutes during sleep

Lundberg ICP Waves

Lundberg Type	Criteria	Pathophysiology
A wave	Mean wave ICP >50 mmHg lasting 5-20 min before returning to elevated baseline	Low CPP results in vasodilatation (raised CBV and ICP) and ischemia (Cushing response to restore CPP). Suggests ICP exceeding limits of cerebral compliance, and ongoing ischemia.
B wave	Mean wave ICP 20-50 mmHg lasting 30 s to 3 min	Seen in sleep; respiratory changes and variations in CBF. Suggests qualitative rise in ICP and that A waves may form.
C wave	Mean wave ICP <20 mmHg occurring every 10 s	ICP transmission of cyclic Traube-Hering-Meyer variation in SBP due to oscillations in baroreceptor and chemoreceptor control. Sometimes seen in normal ICP waveform

Each individual ICP waveform has three peaks: percussion wave (P1) representing arterial pulsation, tidal wave (P2) representing intracranial compliance and dicrotic wave (P3) representing aortic valve closure. Lundberg waves describe patterns of mean ICP in patients.

14. **e**—Intraoperature ultrasound is less accurate at predicting those who do not need durotomy in the presence of tonsillar descent below C1 lamina

Chiari malformation Type I (CM-I) is a craniocervical junction disorder that is associated with deformity and elongation of the cerebellar tonsils and is specifically characterized by tonsils' descent of more than 5 mm below the foramen magnum into the spinal canal—a change in the flow of CSF at the level of the foramen magnum is frequently associated with development of syringomyelia. Patients with Chiari I malformation commonly undergo foramen magnum/suboccipital decompression (FMD) in order to restore free flow of CSF across the craniocervical junction, treating symptoms either related to raised ICP, brainstem compression or syringomyelia. There is no consensus on surgical indication, but a lower threshold may be expected in symptomatic hindbrain herniation with syringomyelia compared to asymptomatic hindbrain hernia with syrinx or symptomatic hindbrain herniation without syrinx. Variation in FMD technique is also possible at multiple stages: extent of bony decompression, indication for opening the dura and arachnoid, need for tonsils coagulation and dural closure. A recent review of all published studies of surgical treatment of Chiari I showed that there was slight variation in pediatric (97% FMD, 81% dural opening, 47% arachnoid opening/dissection and 21% tonsillar resection) versus adult (100% FMD, 97% dural opening, 70% arachnoid opening/dissection and 16% tonsillar resection) practice. In series reporting on syrinx association, the incidence was 69% in adult series, 40% in pediatric series, and 78% in mixed series. The traditional operation for CM-1 is FMD with bony decompression and dural opening with or without duraplasty. Some have contended that not all patients with CM-1 need durotomy, with bony decompression alone having been demonstrated as adequate/efficacious in a proportion of patients with CM-1, possibly as the dura of children may still have some elasticity and expand following bony decompression, leading to better CSF dynamics at the craniocervical junction. The main advantage of not needing to open the dura is that complications such as pseudomeningocoele, CSF leak, meningitis and hydrocephalus are reduced.

Preoperative and intraoperative prediction of those who could be adequately treated without durotomy/duraplasty (or conversely those who definitely should have it) would ensure the efficacy of the surgical intervention while minimizing the rate of complications and need for reoperation. Adequacy of cerebellar tonsillar or CSF pulsation at the craniocervical junction as judged on intraoperative ultrasound may be of value in this respect, although may be less reliable in predicting patients who will do well with bony decompression alone when there is moderate (below C1 lamina)/severe (below C2 lamina) tonsillar descent.

FURTHER READING

Arnautovic A, Splavski B, Boop FA, Arnautovic KI. Pediatric and adult Chiari malformation Type I surgical series 1965-2013: a review of demographics, operative treatment, and outcomes. J Neurosurg Pediatr 2015;15(2):161-77. http://dx.doi.org/10.3171/2014.10.PEDS14295. Epub 2014 Dec 5. PubMed PMID: 25479580.

McGirt MJ, Attenello FJ, Datoo G, Gathinji M, Atiba A, Weingart JD, Carson B, Jallo GI. Intraoperative ultrasonography as a guide to patient selection for duraplasty after suboccipital decompression in children with Chiari malformation Type I. J Neurosurg Pediatr 2008;2(1):52-7.

15. **c**—Transventricular tap

Subdural effusion occurs in 40-60% of infants and young children with proven meningitis. Small collections generally subside with observation alone and surgical drainage is only required when if symptomatic or causing mass effect. Options include serial percutaneous needle drainage, burr hole drainage, external subdural drain and subduroperitoneal shunt (SDP). External drains were placed whenever the fluid was purulent, when the collection was estimated to be too large to be cured with SDP alone, or when raised ICP recurred after SDP, and be kept in place for 1-2 weeks until fluid becomes clearer. At the end of that period, whenever the patient was dependent on the external drain, a subduroperitoneal drain was inserted. Removal of internal subdural shunts should ideally be after a few months. In rare cases of obstruction of the drainage associated with thick subdural membranes exerting a mass effect on the brain, craniotomy with membrane resection can be performed.

Image with permission from Khanna PC, Shaw DWW. Neuroimaging. In: Fuhrman BP, editor. Pediatric Critical Care, 4th ed. Mosby, Elsevier; 2011.

FURTHER READING

Vinchon M, Joriot S, Jissendi-Tchofo P, Dhellemmes P. Postmeningitis subdural fluid collection in infants: changing pattern and indications for surgery. J Neurosurg 2006;104:383-7.

ANSWERS 16–25

Additional answers 16–25 available on ExpertConsult.com

EMI ANSWERS

26. 1—k, X-linked hydrocephalus; 2—f, Joubert syndrome

Infants may have hydrocephalus at birth, caused by a congenital malformation that prevents adequate circulation of cerebrospinal fluid. Acquired hydrocephalus may arise after infection, intracranial hemorrhage, or structural or mass lesions. Most patients with non-syndromic congenital hydrocephalus have aqueduct stenosis. Of these, X-linked hydrocephalus is the most common heritable form, accounting for about 10% of cases in boys. Mutations in L1CAM, encoding the L1 cell adhesion molecule, are the most common cause. Primary ciliopathies such as Joubert's syndrome and Meckel-Gruber syndrome are associated with congenital hydrocephalus in human beings.

27. 1—i, Proximal catheter obstruction. Children with treated hydrocephalus face many potential long-term complications, often relating to treatment. Shunt failure, usually from mechanical obstruction, needing some form of intervention occurs in 40% of children within the first 2 years after original placement with continued risk of failure thereafter. Failure is diagnosed by imaging evidence of increased ventricle size compared with baseline (although this is not always the case) with symptoms of headache, vomiting, irritability, decreased level of consciousness, and, in infants, bulging fontanel and accelerated head growth. Evidence suggests that the type of shunt valve used has no effect on failure incidence. Shunt obstruction is treated with urgent surgery, either EVD (if in extremis) or shunt revision in patients with near normal preoperative GCS. In situations in which symptoms are more subtle (e.g. chronic headache or deteriorating school performance) intracranial pressure monitoring can sometimes be helpful to establish if shunt obstruction is the cause. 2—h, Migration of distal peritoneal catheter. Swelling over the abdominal wound is most likely a CSF seroma due to migration of the distal catheter out of the peritoneal cavity and into

subcutaneous tissues (producing a bird's nest pattern of coiled distal catheter). CSF ascites arises due to malabsorption of CSF by peritoneum, and may require needle paracentesis to exclude infection, whereas abdominal pseudocysts also present with abdominal pain and distension but, by definition, form around the distal catheter in the peritoneal cavity (perhaps due to low virulence organisms like *Proprionobacter* and *Corynebacterium*) and often require removal or the shunt and antibiotic treatment. 3—b, Acute overdrainage. If drainage of CSF occurs too rapidly, collapse of the ventricular system and brain may occur along with the creation of a potential space between the dura and the cortical surface of the brain. Extra-axial CSF collections may develop, but if bridging cortical veins are disrupted, subdural hemorrhage can occur. These collections may respond to conservative measures, but some necessitate draining the extra-axial collections, revising the shunt valve to one with higher resistance, or both. Approximately 40-60% of children with CSF shunts develop small, slit-like ventricles, which can be appreciated on radiographic imaging after CSF diversion. Over time with chronic overdrainage 10% of these patients may develop what is known as slit ventricle syndrome—typically presenting with cyclical signs and symptoms consistent with increased ICP, with slit-like ventricles unchanged from prior imaging studies. Intermittent obstruction of the proximal catheter and loss of the ability to compensate for transient changes in intracranial volume may underlie this picture.

FURTHER READING

Lee P, et al. Evaluation of suspected cerebrospinal fluid shunt complications in children. Clin Pediatr Emerg Med 2008;9:76-82.

28. 1—a, *Citrobacter koseri*; 2—j, *Tuberculosis*

CHAPTER 42

Pediatric Neuro-Oncology

SINGLE BEST ANSWER (SBA) QUESTIONS

1. Which one of the following lists of primary brain tumors in children is from most common to LEAST common (all age groups combined)?
   a. Astrocytoma, craniopharyngioma, medulloblastoma, ependymoma, germ cell tumors
   b. Astrocytoma, medulloblastoma, craniopharyngioma, ependymoma, germ cell tumors
   c. Ependymoma, astrocytoma, medulloblastoma, craniopharyngioma, germ cell tumors
   d. Medulloblastoma, astrocytoma, craniopharyngioma, ependymoma, germ cell tumors
   e. Medulloblastoma, craniopharyngioma, ependymoma, astrocytoma, germ cell tumors

2. Which one of the following is associated with the highest incidence of brain metastases in children?
   a. Neuroblastoma
   b. Sarcoma
   c. Wilms tumor
   d. Leukemia
   e. Lymphoma

3. Which one of the following statements regarding posterior fossa tumors in children is LEAST accurate?
   a. Pilocytic astrocytomas account for 35% of posterior fossa tumors in children
   b. Medulloblastoma account for 30% of posterior fossa tumors in children
   c. Ependymomas account for 20-30% of posterior fossa tumors in children
   d. Brainstem gliomas account for 10-20% of posterior fossa tumors in children
   e. Hemangioblastomas account for 10% of posterior fossa tumors in children

4. A 17-year-old boy patient presents with left arm clumsiness. MRI is shown. Which one of the following is most likely?

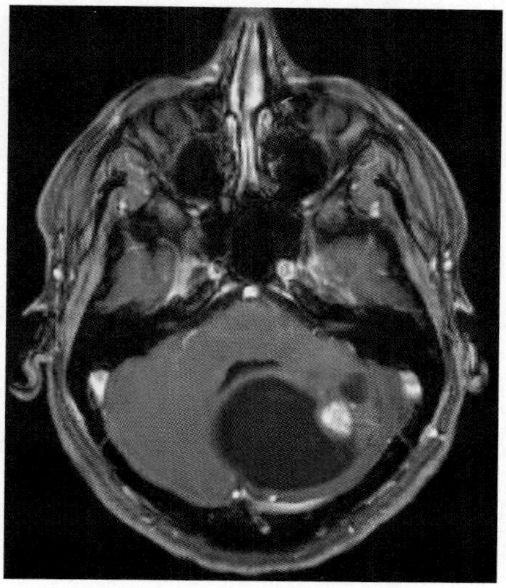

   a. Hemangioblastoma
   b. Medulloblastoma
   c. Neuroblastoma metastasis
   d. Pilocytic astrocytoma
   e. Vestibular schwannoma

5. A 5-year-old with features of NF-1 presents with visual disturbance. T1 postcontrast MRI is shown. Which one of the following statements regarding management of these lesions is most accurate?

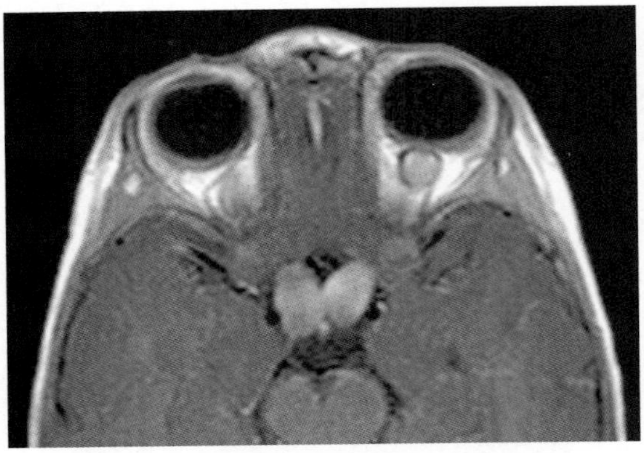

a. Surgical decompression is prophylactic to save bilateral vision
b. Chemotherapy is second line management in children under 9 years old
c. Biopsy should only be performed if there are features of NF-1
d. Somatostatin has been shown to improve outcome
e. Cranial irradiation is contraindicated in this case

6. A 16-year-old male patient who previously underwent excision of a right temporo-occipital lesion 7 years previously, with good control of seizures since, presents with increased frequency of tonic-clonic seizures and headaches. Neurological examination was unremarkable. MRI is shown. Which one of the following is most likely?

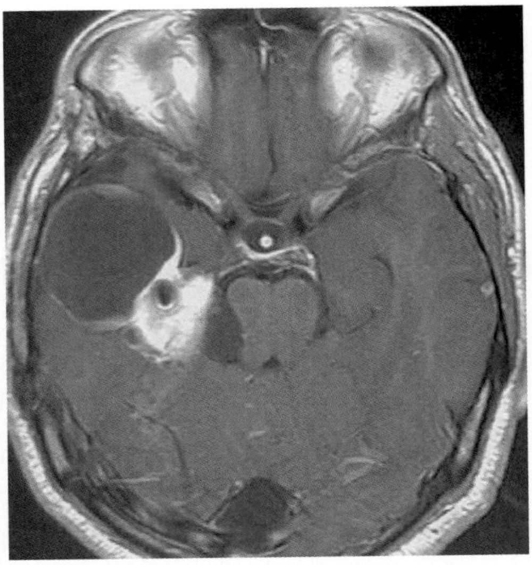

a. Diffuse astrocytoma
b. DNET
c. GBM
d. Pilocytic astrocytoma
e. Pleomorphic xanthoastrocytoma

7. A 2-year-old presents after his mother noted an abnormal white reflection in his right eye. MRI is shown. Which one of the following would you look for?

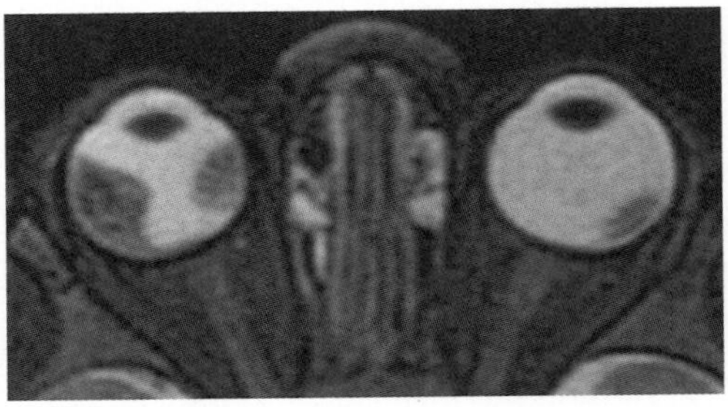

a. AT/RT
b. Hypothalamic hamartoma
c. Optic glioma
d. Pineoblastoma
e. Pontine glioma

8. A 4-year-old presents with torticollis, facial asymmetry and ophthalmoparesis. Which one of the following is appropriate next management?

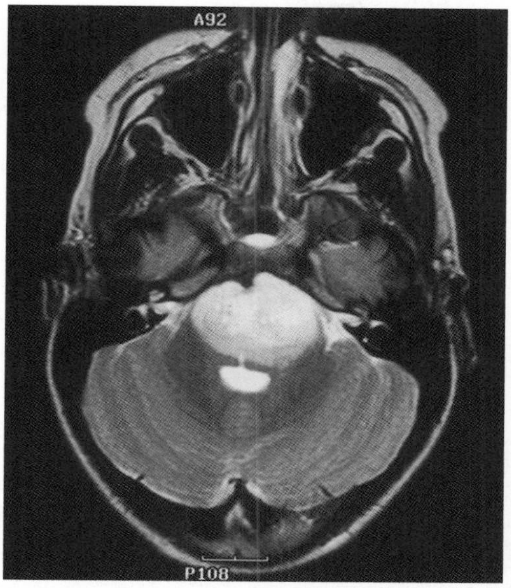

a. Biopsy
b. Radiotherapy
c. Chemotherapy
d. Midline suboccipital resection
e. Transoral resection

9. Which one of the following conditions is most likely?

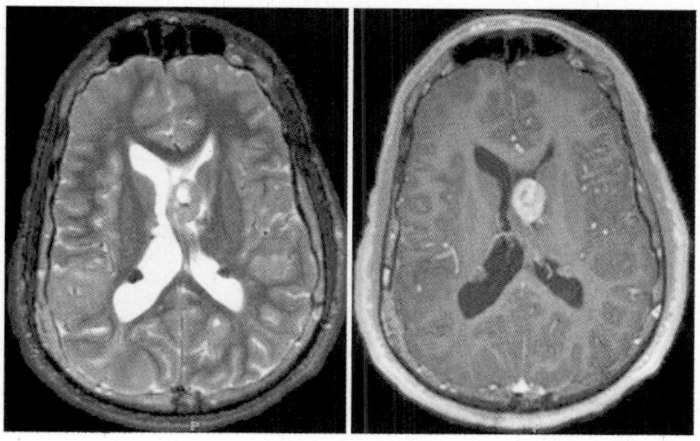

a. NF-1
b. NF-2
c. Tuberous sclerosis
d. Li-Fraumeni syndrome
e. Cowden syndrome

10. A 5-year-old child presents with gait ataxia. MRI is shown. Which one of the following management strategies is appropriate in this case?

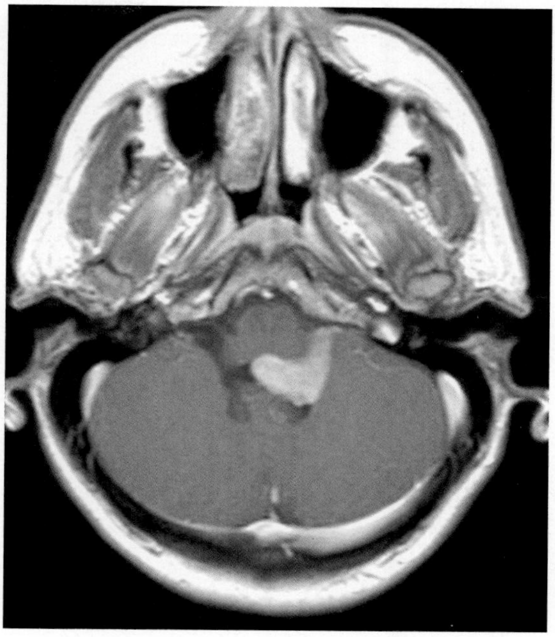

a. Complete resection followed by surveillance
b. Complete resection followed by focal radiotherapy boost
c. Neoadjuvant chemotherapy followed by resection and postoperative adjuvant chemotherapy
d. Debulking surgery followed by craniospinal irradiation
e. Stereotactic radiosurgery

11. A 9-year-old girl presents with headache and vomiting. On examination there is bilateral papilledema but she is otherwise neurologically stable. MRI is performed. Which one of the following is the next appropriate step?

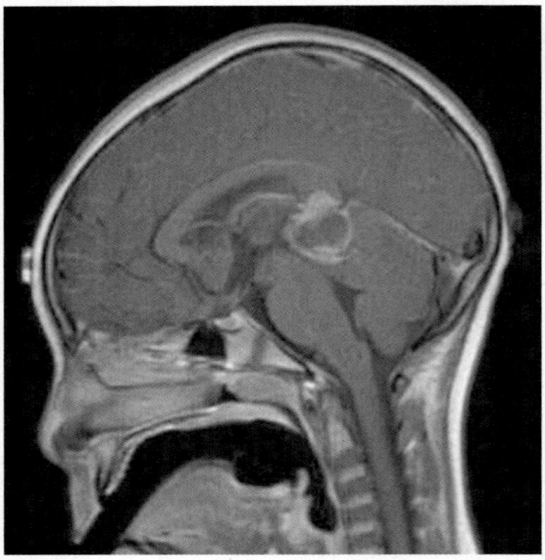

a. ICP monitoring
b. Lumbar puncture
c. Serum AFP and HCG
d. External ventricular drain
e. Endoscopic third ventriculostomy and biopsy of lesion

12. A 13-year-old presents with polydipsia and polyuria. Clinical examination is unremarkable. Serum blood tests show a Na 149 mEq/l and serum osmolality is 315 mOsm/kg H_2O, with urine osmolality of 115 mOsm/l. MRI is shown. Subsequent serum AFP and BHCG are within normal limits. Which one of the following is most likely?

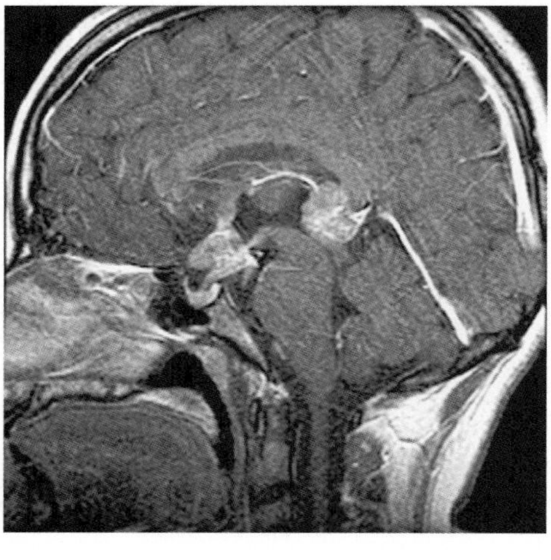

a. Craniopharyngioma
b. Germinoma
c. Langerhans cell histiocytosis
d. NGGCT
e. Pineoblastoma

13. A 12-year-old boy presents with precocious puberty and headache. CT head demonstrates obstructive hydrocephalus and pineal region mass on CT. Serum HCG is 8178 IU/l, AFP is 5 ng/ml. What would be the most appropriate next step in management?
a. Stereotactic biopsy
b. Endoscopic biopsy
c. Endoscopic third ventriculostomy without biopsy
d. Tumor debulking
e. Ventriculoperitoneal shunt

14. An 8-year-old girl presents with symptoms of raised intracranial pressure over the last 2 weeks. T1 + GAD MRI is shown. Which one of the following is most likely?

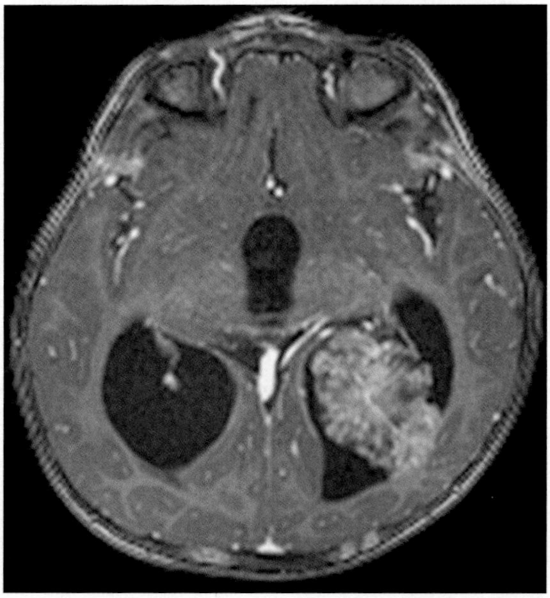

a. Arachnoid cyst
b. AT/RT
c. Choroid plexus papilloma
d. DNET
e. Medulloblastoma

15. A 6-year-old child presents with clumsiness and slurred speech. On examination and papilledema. CT head is abnormal therefore MRI of the craniospinal axis is performed showing the lesion above. Spinal MRI is normal. Which one of the following best describes conventional treatment?

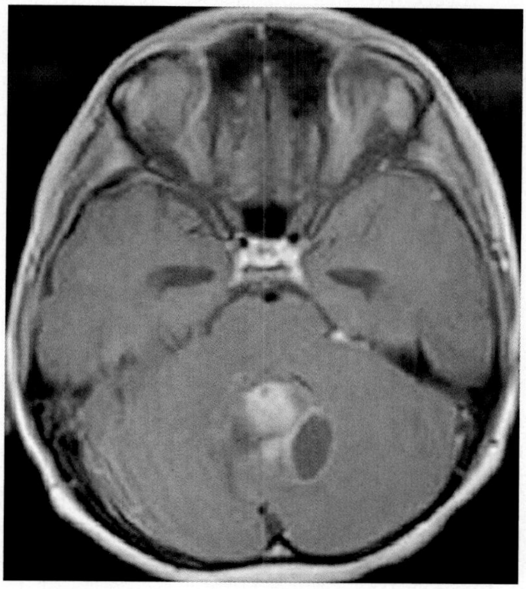

T1 Post

a. Neoadjuvant chemotherapy, surgical resection, postoperative focal radiotherapy
b. Surgical resection followed by focal radiotherapy plus craniospinal irradiation
c. Surgical resection followed by focal radiotherapy plus adjuvant chemotherapy
d. Surgical resection followed by chemotherapy
e. Surgical resection followed by craniospinal irradiation and focal radiotherapy with concurrent chemotherapy

QUESTIONS 16–21

Additional questions 16–21 available on ExpertConsult.com

EXTENDED MATCHING ITEM (EMI) QUESTIONS

22. For each of the following descriptions, select the most appropriate answer from the image below. Each answer may be used one, more than once, or not at all.

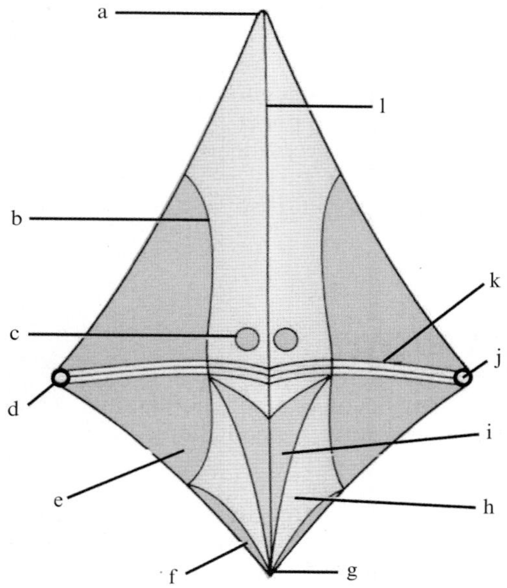

1. Striae medullaris
2. Sulcus limitans
3. Area postrema
4. Facial colliculus
5. Median sulcus

23. **Pediatric posterior fossa tumors:**
   a. Atypical teratoid/rhabdoid tumor
   b. Dermoid
   c. Diffuse intrinsic pontine glioma
   d. Ependymoma
   e. Epidermoid
   f. Hemangioblastoma
   g. Medulloblastoma
   h. Meningioma
   i. Pilocytic astrocytoma
   j. Sarcoma metastases
   k. Vestibular schwannoma

For each of the following descriptions, select the most appropriate answer from the list above. Each answer may be used one, more than once, or not at all.

1. A 15-year-old boy with multiple angiomatoses of the retina and cysts of the kidney and pancreas.

2. An 11-year-old presents with features of hydrocephalus. Imaging shows a cystic mass with an enhancing mural nodule, which lacks flow voids.

24. **Pediatric sellar and pineal lesions:**
 a. Arachnoid cyst
 b. Craniopharyngioma
 c. Germinoma
 d. Histiocytosis X
 e. Hypothalamic hamartoma
 f. Optic pathway glioma
 g. Pituitary adenoma
 h. Pituitary macroadenoma
 i. PNET
 j. Rathke's cleft cyst

For each of the following descriptions, select the most appropriate answer from the list above. Each answer may be used one, more than once, or not at all.

1. A 9-year-old developmentally delayed girl has precocious puberty and poorly controlled seizures. Her seizures are typically preceded by episodes of uncontrollable laughter.
2. An 11-year-old presents with hydrocephalus and diabetes insipidus. MRI shows an enhancing lesion in the pineal region and another in the suprasellar region.
3. A 5-year-old boy with neurofibromatosis 1 presents with visual field defect and pendular nystagmus.

SBA ANSWER

1. **b**—Astrocytoma, medulloblastoma, craniopharyngioma, ependymoma, germ cell tumors

Overall incidence approximately 5 per 100,000 persons per year (compared to 20-30 per 100,000 in adults). Incidence rates of tumor types vary by age, hence although posterior fossa tumors are much more common in children than adults, in children infratentorial tumors may only be commoner than supratentorial tumors within certain age groups (e.g. 4-10 years of age). Roughly 60-70% are gliomas; specific frequency of tumor types is astrocytomas 30%, medulloblastoma (15-20%), craniopharyngioma (10-15%), ependymomas (5-10%), germ cell tumors (5-10%). Commonest tumors vary by age (see below). Incidence in 19 years or younger in the Central Brain Tumor Registry of the United States:

FURTHER READING

Uptodate. Epidemiology of central nervous system tumours in children. Topic 6251 Version 17.0.

Epidemiology of Childhood Brain Tumours

Primary childhood CNS tumors incidence by WHO group	**Primary childhood CNS tumor incidence by diagnosis**
Neuroepithelial tissue 3.7 per 100,000 - Astrocytic 1.3 per 100,000 per year - Ependymoma 0.28 per 100,000 per year Sellar region 0.73 per 100,000 per year Embryonal CNS tumors 0.65 per 100,000 per year Neuronal and mixed neuronal-glial 0.37 per 100,000 per year Unclassified 0.3 per 100,000 per year Cranial and paraspinal nerves 0.27 per 100,000 per year Meninges 0.22 per 100,000 per year Germ cell tumors and cysts 0.21 per 100,000 per year Lymphoma and hemopoetic 0.03 per 100,000 per year	Pilocytic astrocytoma 0.84 per 100,000 per year Medulloblastoma/PNET 0.65 per 100,000 per year Pituitary and craniopharyngioma 0.73 per 100,000 per year Ependymoma 0.28 per 100,000 per year

0-4 years	**5-9 year**	**10-14 years**	**15-19 years**
Gliomas (excluding PA) Pilocytic astrocytoma Medulloblastoma PNET **Pituitary tumors**	Gliomas (excluding PA) Pilocytic astrocytoma Medulloblastoma **Pituitary tumors** PNET	Gliomas (excluding PA) Pilocytic astrocytoma **Pituitary tumors** Medulloblastoma PNET	Gliomas (excluding PA) **Pituitary tumors** Pilocytic astrocytoma Medulloblastoma PNET

2. **b**—Sarcoma

The commonest primary neoplasms in children uncommonly demonstrate hematogenous seeding resulting in brain metastasis—the overall rate approximates 4% in patient followed up >10 years. In a pooled analysis of multiple studies in over 2000 children, cerebral hematogenous metastases were reported in 4.4% of 429 patients with neuroblastoma, 1.9% of 574 rhabdomyosarcoma patients, 6.5% of 386 patients with osteosarcoma, 3.3% of 487 Ewing sarcoma patients, 3.6% of 44 melanoma patients, 13.5% of 37 patients with germ cell tumors, and 1.3% of the 78 patients with Wilms tumor.

Epidemiology of Childhood Cancer

Commonest cancers in <1 year	Commonest cancers 1-10 years	Commonest cancers >10 years
(1) Neuroblastoma (2) Leukemia (3) Germ cell tumors (4) CNS tumors (5) Wilms tumor	Leukemias CNS tumors Neuroblastoma Wilms tumor Germ cell tumors/Soft tissue sarcoma	Leukemias CNS tumors Lymphoma Bone tumors/Soft tissue sarcomas Germ cell tumors

FURTHER READING

Curless RG, Toledano SR, Ragheb J, Cleveland WW, Falcone S. Hematogenous brain metastasis in children. Pediatr Neurol 2002 Mar;26(3):219-21. Review. PubMed PMID: 11955930.

Uptodate. Epidemiology of central nervous system tumours in children. Topic 6251 Version 17.0.

Graphic 99680 Version 1.0.

3. **e**—Hemangioblastomas account for 10% of posterior fossa tumors in children

4. **d**—Pilocytic astrocytoma

Pilocytic astrocytomas are the most frequent posterior fossa tumors in children (approximately 35%). Peak age is 5-13 years; approximately half arise in the midline vermis and half from the cerebellar hemispheres. They are circumscribed, discrete, slow-growing lesions, often associated with cysts within and around the tumor. On CT they are large cystic lesions with a hypodense solid component which enhances avidly on contrast administration. On T1WI, the solid component tends to be iso- to hypointense and on T2WI it is hyperintense, with heterogeneity is due to microcystic and necrotic areas. The solid and mural components enhance prominently. Enhancement of the cyst wall suggests tumor infiltration of the capsule. They maintain their WHO grade I status for years; they only rarely show malignant transformation (anaplastic pilocytic astrocytomas). A large percentage of pilocytic astrocytomas, particularly those arising within the cerebellar hemisphere, have demonstrated alterations in the BRAF gene but this is not prognostically significant. Resection is the treatment of choice for well-circumscribed lesions and extent of resection most strongly associated with outcome. Gross total resection leads to over 90% long-term survival. Cerebellar lesions are generally completely resectable hence adjuvant therapy is not indicated, whereas. Those arising from the brainstem are often not and require adjuvant chemotherapy, usually including carboplatin and vincristine, and consideration of radiotherapy at progression. Trials of BRAF and MAPK pathway inhibitors, and antiangiogenic agents bevacizumab and linalidomide are ongoing. The main differential diagnosis is hemangioblastoma, which usually presents in young adults but may present in children with VHL but these may be multiple, show greater vascularity/abnormal vessels associated with enhancing portion/nodule, are usually abutting a pial surface, and have a considerably higher rCBV than pilocytic astrocytomas on perfusion imaging.

Image with permission from Perry A, Brat DJ. Practical Surgical Neuropathology: A Diagnostic Approach, Churchill Livingstone, Elsevier, 2010.

FURTHER READING

Aquilina K. Posterior fossa tumours in children. ACNR 2013:13:4:24-8.

5. **e**—Cranial irradiation is contraindicated in this case

Optic pathway gliomas are congenital WHO grade I astrocytoma of optic nerves or chiasm, and may be associated with NF-1 (50-60%) or be sporadic. Sporadic tumors typically arise within the chiasmatic-hypothalamic region or in other brain structures adjacent to, or involving the optic tract, and do not typically involve the optic nerves. In contrast, OPG associated with neurofibromatosis type 1 characteristically involve optic nerve, chiasm and optic radiation, including the geniculate ganglion. Tumors involving optic chiasm and hypothalamus are of a higher histologic grade (grade 2) than tumors confined to optic nerve and may cause considerable morbidity and even death. Usually discovered during first decade due to visual impairment, endocrine deficit, focal neurological deficit, hypothalamic behavioral disturbance (appetite, rage, obesity), stationary or progressive visual loss in one eye or both. Examination may show iris hamartomas (Lisch nodules) and/or eyelid plexiform neurofibromas, visual acuity and/or visual field loss, afferent pupil defect, pendular (monocular or seesaw) nystagmus, optic disc abnormality, proptosis if large intraorbital component. MRI shows intrinsic mass of optic nerves, optic chiasm, optic tracts, or hypothalamus and may also show hamartomas elsewhere that are typical of neurofibromatosis type 1. By definition, due to their location, surgery will inevitably damage the optic nerve or pathway (plus risk vascular supply to hypothalamus and pituitary) and biopsy cannot usually be justified if imaging is diagnostic (it is done only if imaging is non-diagnostic/atypical), and where useful vision is maintained ipsilateral to tumor debulking or resective surgery seems unnecessary. However, when there is unilateral failing or useless vision debulking, resective surgery may be appropriate to protect vision on the good side, potentially controlling hydrocephalus and delaying radiotherapy in what is often a young patient group. Surgical treatment may also be offered for optic nerve gliomas causing disfiguring proptosis in a blind eye (excision of optic nerve only). Chemotherapy is used for patients under age 9 with glioma involving the chiasm and/or hypothalamus and who have severe or worsening visual or hypothalamic dysfunction or signs of tumor growth (to delay radiotherapy and neurocognitive side effects, or in NF-1 for additional risk of secondary moyamoya disease and intracranial tumors). Cranial radiation is contraindicated in NF-1 but may have a vision sparing effect in sporadic tumors in older children and adults. Visual function often stable in untreated patients, but visual decline may result from tumor progression.

Image with permission from Trobe JD, Rapid Diagnosis in Ophthalmology: Neuro-Ophthalmology, Elsevier, 2008.

6. **e**—Pleomorphic xanthoastrocytoma

Pleomorphic xanthoastrocytoma is a very rare brain tumor accounting for only 1% of all brain neoplasms. It is however important to be familiar with the radiological findings of this tumor because it has a characteristic imaging appearance and is highly amenable to surgical resection with a good prognosis. PXAs predominantly occur in children and young adults and there is no gender predilection. PXA predominately affects the cerebral hemispheres, showing mainly involvement of the temporal and parietal lobes. The most common clinical presentation of this tumor is seizures, whilst increased intracranial pressure appears to be a less frequent finding. On CT, PXAs are usually seen as well-defined, partially cystic masses of various sizes, which show enhancement after contrast administration. The solid component of the neoplasm tends to be heterogeneous and isodense to gray matter, and calcification may be present. MRI reveals that most of these tumors are predominately superficial, cortical, partially cystic masses which are hypo- to isointense to gray matter on unenhanced T1-weighted images while mildly hyperintense on T2-weighted images. Gadolinium-enhanced T1-weighted images typically show marked enhancement of the solid component. The most consistent findings are peripheral location of the tumor, leptomeningeal contact of the tumor and marked enhancement of the solid tumor component. The radiologic differential diagnosis of PXAs includes mainly other astrocytomas, ganglioglioma, meningioma, meningiosarcoma and fibrous xanthoma. The treatment of choice for pleomorphic xanthoastrocytomas is complete surgical excision which is favored by the superficial location, relative circumscription, and cyst/mural nodule architecture of the tumor.

Image with permission from Douis H, Andronikou, S, von Bezing, H. Pleomorphic xanthoastrocytoma: case series with radiologic-pathological correlation and review of the literature, Eur J Radiol Extra 2008;68(1): pp.5-8.

7. **d**—Pineoblastoma.

The T2-weighted MRI shows left sided retinoblastoma. Retinoblastomas are bilateral in 30-40% of cases, and may be associated with pineoblastoma ("trilateral retinoblastoma" as the pineal gland has been historically labeled as the "inner/third eye") in 15% of cases.

Image with permission from LaPlante JK, Pierson NS, Hedlund GL. Common pediatric head and neck congenital/developmental anomalies, Radiol Clin North Am 2015 Jan;53(1):181-96.

8. **b**—Radiotherapy (diffuse intrinsic pontine glioma)

Brainstem gliomas account for 10-20% of all CNS tumors in children. They are broadly classified into diffuse or focal. Diffuse intrinsic pontine gliomas are high-grade fibrillary astrocytomas with median overall and progression-free survival of up to eleven and nine months respectively. They present with a short history, often characterized by cranial nerve palsies and ataxia. They are diagnosed radiologically and when typical, do not require biopsy. They are hyperintense on T2- and hypointense on T1-weighted images, with ill-defined boundaries and diffuse enlargement of the brain stem. They generally do not enhance with contrast. Surgical resection has no role in these tumors. Radiation is indicated to the tumor with a margin to a dose of approximately 54 Gy. Symptoms generally resolve with treatment. Unfortunately, duration of symptom relief is usually short lived, on the order of 6 months. This disease is uniformly fatal, and the median survival for these children is 1 year. Despite several clinical trials over the last fifteen years, based on various chemotherapeutic agents and radiotherapy delivery techniques, there has been no improvement in clinical outcome. Focal brainstem tumors are well-circumscribed masses that may be intrinsic, exophytic or cervicomedullary, solid or cystic, under 2 cm in diameter, and are commonly low grade astrocytomas. In one retrospective study of focal brainstem gliomas, following 52 children over a mean of ten years, the survival rate was 98% at five years and 90% at ten years; 36. 5% underwent gross or near total resection. If there is clinical or MRI progression, options include resection (for accessible tumors where the patient and family understand the high risk of new neurological deficit) or stereotactic biopsy followed by radiation.

Image with permission from Kaye AH. Brain Tumors an Encyclopedic Approach, 3rd ed. Elsevier, 2012.

FURTHER READING

Aquilina K. Posterior fossa tumours in children. ACNR 2013;13:4:24-28.

Klimo P Jr et al. Management and outcome of focal low-grade brainstem tumors in pediatric patients: the St. Jude experience. J Neurosurg Pediatr 2013.

9. **c**—Tuberous sclerosis

Tuberous sclerosis complex (TSC) is a genetic, multi-organ condition characterized by the development of benign tumors in the brain, heart, kidneys, liver, and lungs. Subependymal giant cell astrocytomas (SEGAs), develop in 10-15% of individuals with TSC. SEGAs can be unilateral or bilateral, developing from those benign subependymal nodules (hamartomas) located near the foramen of Monro. SEGA development is a gradual process that generally occurs within the first 2 decades of life. These are slow-growing, glial neuronal tumors, usually developing over 1-3 years. SEGAs are usually asymptomatic until they block circulation of cerebrospinal fluid (CSF), leading to increased intracranial pressure and hydrocephalus. Typically, serial neuroimaging is performed every 1-3 years in pediatric TSC patients and until the mid-20s, even in the absence of SEGA symptoms. Options include surgery or pharmacotherapy. Surgical tumor resection has traditionally been the standard therapy for SEGA and earlier intervention has been proposed to avoid sequelae of hydrocephalus. Indications for surgery include: asymptomatic SEGAs with documented tumor growth or enlargement of the ventricles is observed; symptomatic SEGA (e.g. behavioral changes, worsening of seizures, symptoms of raised ICP). Prognosis is good, particularly in cases where surgery is performed early for small lesions; in most cases resection is curative if tumor removal is complete. The goal of pharmacotherapy with mTOR pathway inhibitor (everolimus) is to shrink or stabilize the tumor in adults and children 3 years or older with SEGA associated with TSC who require therapeutic intervention but are not amenable to surgery (e.g. contraindications exist for anesthesia or surgery in general, total resection unlikely to be possible, or in rare cases of bilateral fornix lesions with high risk of morbidity). Treatment reduces tumor size, and the effect is sustained in EXIST-1 trial. The role of stereotactic radiosurgery has not yet been fully elucidated.

Image with permission from Perry A, Brat DJ. Practical Surgical Neuropathology: A Diagnostic Approach, Churchill Livingstone, Elsevier, 2010.

FURTHER READING

Jóźwiak, Sergiusz; Nabbout, Rima; Curatolo, Paolo. Management of subependymal giant cell astrocytoma (SEGA) associated with tuberous sclerosis complex (TSC): clinical recommendations. Eur J Paediatr Neurol 2013;17(4):348-52.

10. **b**—Complete resection followed by focal radiotherapy boost

Ependymoma is the third most common pediatric brain tumor; over 50% of cases arise in children under 5 years of age. Chromosomal abnormalities include 22q; chromosome 1q gain has been found in up to 22% of childhood ependymomas, and is associated with posterior fossa location, anaplastic features and a poor prognosis. Infratentorial ependymomas in children are classified as WHO grade 2 or 3 (grade 1 being reserved only for subependymoma and myxopapillary ependymoma). Infratentorial ependymomas arise from the floor or roof of the fourth ventricle and grow into the ventricular lumen. They have a propensity to extend through the foramen of Luschka into the cerebellopontine cistern and around the brainstem, as well as down through the foramen magnum. They are well-delineated, soft, heterogeneous tumors, often with cystic, necrotic and hemorrhagic elements. On CT, ependymomas are iso- or hyperdense lesions, up to 50%

have punctate calcification, and they enhance heterogeneously on contrast administration. On MRI, they are iso- to hypointense on T1-weighted sequences and hypointense on T2 but calcification, cysts, areas of necrosis and hemorrhage cause heterogeneity within the tumor mass on enhanced and non-enhanced sequences. Leptomeningeal dissemination at presentation is less common than in medulloblastoma; full spinal MRI at diagnosis is imperative as part of the staging process. The extent of surgical resection is a major determinant of outcome. In historical series, five-year overall survival for ependymoma has ranged from 50 to 64%. Despite several multi-institutional studies, mostly including platinum-based agents, no single chemotherapeutic regimen has demonstrated significant survival benefit for ependymoma. The role of chemotherapy alongside postoperative radiotherapy remains unclear. In a recent single-institution study, conformal radiotherapy, administered immediately after surgery, led to better overall survival rates, up to 85% at five years, compared to earlier studies with up to 73% at five years. This may be partly attributable to the high rate of gross total resection (82%) and use of radiotherapy for the first time in children under three years.

Image with permission from Yachnis AT, Rivera-Zengotita ML. Neuropathology, High-Yield Pathology Series, Saunders, Elsevier, 2014.

FURTHER READING

Aquilina K. Posterior fossa tumours in children. ACNR 2013;13(4):24-28.

Merchant TE, Li C, Xiong X, Kun LE, Boop FA, Sanford RA. Conformal radiotherapy after surgery for pediatric ependymoma: a prospective study. Lancet Oncol 2009;10:258-66.

11. **c**—Serum AFP and HCG

Pineal region masses have a wide differential diagnosis, and considering she is neurologically stable, the priority is to narrow the differential diagnosis ideally before any surgical intervention is required. In general germ cell tumors account for 60%, pineal parenchymal tumors for 30%, supporting cells/meninges for 10%, and cysts, vascular lesions and metastases. Approximately 60-70% of germ cell tumors are highly radiosensitive germinomas, while the rest are classed as non-germinomatous germ cell tumors (NGGCT: teratoma, choriocarcinoma, embryonal carcinoma, yolk sac tumors). The main question is whether the lesion is likely to be a germinoma (requiring non-surgical treatment with craniospinal irradiation), a NGGCT (requiring neoadjuvant chemotherapy, followed by surgery and radiotherapy), or another pineal region tumor (e.g. pineoblastoma requiring surgery followed by radiotherapy). The tumor markers alpha-fetoprotein (AFP), human chorionic gonadotropin (HCG), placental alkaline phosphatase, and lactic dehydrogenase isoenzymes are useful in the diagnosis and treatment monitoring of germ cell tumors. Elevations in levels of AFP alone in cerebrospinal fluid (CSF) and serum are found in pure endodermal sinus tumor, and may or may not be seen in mature teratomas. Elevated levels of both HCG and AFP are found in embryonal carcinoma, and high levels of HCG alone are found in choriocarcinoma. The serum and CSF levels in cells of AFP may be 10-100 times baseline. Serum HCG levels may be 100 times baseline, and there may be a CSF/serum gradient, especially when lumbar CSF is assayed. Normal levels are generally thought to be less than 1.5 IU/l or 1 IU/l for β-hCG, however, and less than 1.5 ng/ml for AFP. Modest elevations of HCG may be found in germinoma (CSF more likely), usually in the presence of elevated placental alkaline phosphatase and/or lactic dehydrogenase isoenzymes, whereas a serum or CSF HCG >50 IU/l and/or an AFP >25 ng/ml in the presence of a midline CNS tumor is supportive of a diagnosis of NGGCT. Germinomas may secrete low levels of B-HCG if it contains some syncytiotrophoblasts (unlike the very high levels secreted by choriocarcinomas >2000 IU/l) but pure germinomas do not, although they may secrete placental alkaline phosphatase. In this situation, biopsy of the tumor is required to distinguish between germinoma/non-secreting germ cell tumor and a pineal parenchymal tumor. This is ideally done at the same time as endoscopic third ventriculostomy. Additionally, endodermal sinus tumors secrete alpha fetoprotein, and embryonal carcinomas secrete a mixture of beta human chorionic gonadotropin and alpha fetoprotein. Pineal germinomas most often occur in male patients, pineal parenchymal neoplasms occur with equal frequency in male and female patients. Both tumors can arise at any age, but pineoblastomas peak during the first decade of life, whereas pineocytomas peak during the second and third decades. On CT imaging, pineal parenchymal tumors classically demonstrate a rim of "exploded" calcification that can be helpful in distinguishing them from germ cell tumors which have a central calcified pineal gland. Teratomas possess unique imaging characteristics because of fat and calcium, and choriocarcinomas may hemorrhage; these characteristics help identify these entities. The remainder of the NGGCTs have no unique characteristics that can be used to confidently distinguish them.

Image with permission from Quiñones-Hinojosa A. Schmidek and Sweet's Operative Neurosurgical Techniques, 6th ed. Saunders, Elsevier, 2012.

12. **b**—Germinoma

This child is presenting with features of diabetes insipidus, with MRI evidence of enhancing lesions in the hypothalamus-sellar area and the pineal region consistent with bifocal (synchronous) germinoma. Typical neuroimaging findings of CDI include absence of the posterior pituitary hyperintensity and normal or thickened infundibulum but they are nonspecific as they may progress to develop germinoma, Langerhans cell histiocytosis, or lymphocytic hypophysitis. Less common causes include lymphoma and granulomatous diseases (such as tuberculosis and sarcoidosis). Germ cell tumors are the most common neoplasm arising from the pineal region, accounting for roughly two thirds of pineal region neoplasms. They are much more common in people of Asian descent within the second and third decades of life, with men affected 10 times more frequently than women. The majority arise in the pineal region, and the rest are suprasellar or in the basal ganglia. On imaging, they classically engulf calcification, enhance avidly, and demonstrate intrinsic hyperdensity on CT and isointensity to gray matter on most MRI sequences. Because they are histologically unencapsulated, they sometimes invade the adjacent thalamus or tectum and disseminate via the CSF. For this reason, imaging of the entire neural axis for detection of metastases is vital during the initial workup. Pure germinomas are very radiosensitive, and patients typically have an excellent prognosis.

Image with permission from Perry A, Brat DJ. Practical Surgical Neuropathology: A Diagnostic Approach, Churchill Livingstone, Elsevier, 2010.

13. **c**—Endoscopic third ventriculostomy without biopsy

The history is suggestive of a non-germinomatous germ cell tumor, given the precocious puberty and raised serum HCG (e.g. choriocarcinoma). As such, tumor biopsy is not necessary in the initial management of this patient (but may be required later if there is no response to therapy). Instead, initially endoscopic third ventriculostomy can be performed and CSF samples taken for cytology and tumor markers to further stratify treatment. Beyond this, NGGCT treatment requires neoadjuvant chemotherapy followed by resective surgery and postoperative radiation to the tumor bed with or without craniospinal irradiation.

14. **c**—Choroid plexus papilloma.

Choroid plexus papillomas and carcinomas represent 0.4-0.6% of all intracranial tumors. They are more common in the pediatric population and account for approximately 3% of childhood brain tumors. More commonly, the lesions are seen in the lateral and third ventricle, but 30% are seen in the fourth ventricle, and less than 5% occur in the cerebellopontine angle. The lesions usually present with obstruction of the CSF pathways as well as overproduction of CSF with resultant hydrocephalus. These lobulated intraventricular masses may have internal small flow voids and possibly calcifications. Choroid plexus carcinomas are more heterogeneous in appearance than are choroid plexus papillomas and usually extend beyond the margins of the ventricle. CT shows an iso- to hyperdense mass with punctate calcification and homogeneous enhancement. On MRI the papillomas appear as lobulated, intraventricular masses of heterogeneous, predominantly intermediate signal intensity on both T1 and T2 images, with intense contrast enhancement. Choroid plexus carcinomas are rare, highly malignant tumors that invade the adjacent brain parenchyma to a greater degree than papillomas. On MR spectroscopy, choroid plexus papillomas tend to have an elevated myoinositol peak, whereas choroid plexus carcinomas are more often associated with an elevated choline peak.

Image with permission from Koob M, Girard N. Cerebral tumors: specific features in children, Diagn Interv Imaging 2014 Oct;95(10):965-83.

15. **e**—Surgical resection followed by craniospinal irradiation and focal radiotherapy with concurrent chemotherapy

Medulloblastoma is a primitive neuroectodermal tumor (PNET) arising from aberrant proliferation of granule neuron precursor cells that go on to constitute the external granular layer of the cerebellum. It represents 30% of posterior fossa tumors and is the commonest malignant brain tumor in children with an incidence of 6.5 per 1,000,000 children per year. It is a WHO grade 4 tumor and has a propensity to leptomeningeal dissemination. Associations include familial cancer syndromes such as Gorlin syndrome, Li-Fraumeni syndrome, Turcot syndrome, Gardner syndrome, and Cowden syndrome. It is a midline lesion in 75%—a cerebellar location is associated with older age and desmoplastic histology. The mass is hypointense on T1- and T2-weighted images; it enhances heterogeneously on gadolinium administration, may have cysts, and is diffusion restricting on DWI (due to hypercellularity). Leptomeningeal disease is identified as enhancing nodules on the surface of the brain and spinal cord ("sugar coating"). Histologically, medulloblastoma is composed of small blue round cells with a high nuclear to cytoplasmic ratio in four distinct pathological subgroups: classical (65-80%), desmoplastic/nodular (15-25%), medulloblastoma with extensive nodularity (15-25%), and an anaplastic/large cell variant (4-5%). The desmoplastic variant is commoner in older children and is associated with a better prognosis. The large cell and anaplastic variants are associated with a poor prognosis. Molecular classification is based on Wnt and SHH signaling abnormalities, which confer a very good and intermediate prognosis respectively. Treatment is maximal safe resection (including via transvermian, transcortical, or telovelar-cerebellar) followed by further adjuvant treatment depending on whether they are classified/staged as standard or high-risk cases based on preoperative craniospinal axis MRI (macroscopic metastases) and lumbar CSF cytology two weeks postoperatively to avoid false positives early after resection (microscopic metastases). High-risk patients include all children <3 years, those with positive CSF, macrometastases on MRI, and >1.5 cm of residual tumor visible on postoperative MRI (done within 24-72 h). Children older than three with anaplastic histology or c-myc amplification are also considered high risk. Children >3 years old classified as standard risk undergo craniospinal irradiation (23.4 Gy), commenced within 40 days of surgery with a posterior fossa boost to a total dose of 54-55.8 Gy and concurrent chemotherapy once weekly ("PACKER" regime, consisting of cisplatin, vincristine, CCNU) which yields a 5-year event-free survival of up to 80%. In children with high-risk disease, 5-year progression-free survival has historically been approximately 40% but in recent studies using a higher dose to the craniospinal axis, hyperfractionated radiotherapy with higher posterior fossa boosts, and myoablative myeloablative courses of chemotherapy followed by peripheral blood stem cell rescue, 5-year progression-free survival of up to 73% has been seen. Furthermore, as the neurocognitive sequelae of radiotherapy are more severe in young children repeated cycles of chemotherapy have been used after surgery in those <3 years in an attempt to prevent progression until they become eligible for radiotherapy.

Image with permission from Kumar Selvarajan S, Hsu L. Intraventricular posterior fossa yumors. In: Small JE, Schaefer PW, editors, Neuroradiology: Key Differential Diagnoses and Clinical Questions, Saunders, Elsevier, 2013.

FURTHER READING

Aquilina K. Posterior fossa tumours in children. ACNR 2013;13(4):24-8.

Gandola L, et al. Hyperfractionated accelerated radiotherapy in the Milan strategy for metastatic medulloblastoma. J Clin Oncol 2009;27:566-71.

Gajjar A, et al. Risk-adapted craniospinal radiotherapy followed by high-dose chemotherapy and stem-cell rescue in children with newly diagnosed medulloblastoma (St Jude Medulloblastoma-96): long-term results from a prospective, multicentre trial. Lancet Oncol 2006;7:813-20.

ANSWERS 16–21

Additional answers 16–21 available on ExpertConsult.com

EMI ANSWER

22. a—11, b—2, c—6, d—3, e—12

1—Rostral apex, 2—Sulcus limitans, 3—Facial colliculus, 4—Lateral aperture, 4—Vestibular area, 5—Area postrema, 6—Caudal apex (obex), 7—Vagal trigone, 8—Hypoglossal trigone, 9—Acoustic tubercle, 10—Striae medullaris, 11—Median sulcus

Image modified from Cohen AR. Surgical Disorders of the Fourth Ventricle, Cambridge, MA: Blackwell Science; 1996

23. 1—f, Hemangioblastoma, 2—i, Pilocytic astrocytoma

24. 1—e, Hypothalamic hamartoma, 2—c, Germinoma (bifocal), 3—f, Optic pathway glioma

Grossly, they can be classified as follows:

1. Sellar tumors: Pituitary adenoma (0.5-2.5%), arachnoid cyst;
2. Sellar-suprasellar tumors and cysts: Craniopharyngiomas (6-9%), Rathke's cleft cyst, arachnoid cysts;
3. Suprasellar tumors: Chiasmatic/hypothalamic glioma (4-8%), arachnoid cyst;
4. Lesions of the stalk: Germ cell tumors (1-2%), histiocytosis X;
5. Miscellaneous lesions: Hypothalamic hamartoma, metastatic lesions, PNET.

CHAPTER 43

PEDIATRIC HEAD AND SPINAL TRAUMA

SINGLE BEST ANSWER (SBA) QUESTIONS

1. You see a 9-month-old girl in the emergency department after she slipped out of her father's arms, falling 4 ft and hit her head on a hard floor. There is a tense bruise over the occiput. She is moving all four limbs spontaneously but intermittently, inconsistently inconsolable, moaning, and opens eyes to voice. Which one of the following best describes her Glasgow Coma Scale (GCS)?
   a. 9
   b. 10
   c. 11
   d. 12
   e. 13

2. A 12-year-old child sustains a head injury and is found to have evidence of venous sinus thrombosis on cranial imaging. Prior to discharge home, he is started on aspirin 25 mg od by the neurologist and the parents are advised that he is at increased risk of Reye syndrome if he develops a febrile illness or viral infection. Which one of the following best describes Reye syndrome?
   a. Vomiting, encephalopathy, and hepatic dysfunction
   b. Rash, encephalopathy, and renal dysfunction
   c. Encephalopathy, renal dysfunction, and hepatic dysfunction
   d. Wheeze, encephalopathy, and hepatic dysfunction
   e. Vasculitis, encephalopathy, and renal dysfunction

3. Which one of the following statements regarding the US PECARN pediatric head trauma algorithm is LEAST accurate?
   a. It aims to calculate the likelihood of clinically important traumatic brain injury needing computed tomography (CT) imaging based on the age group
   b. The likelihood of clinically important traumatic brain injury in children with GCS14/15, altered mental status or palpable skull fracture is approximately 4%
   c. In a child under 2 years, likelihood of clinically important traumatic brain injury without a scalp hematoma, LOC >5 s, altered behavior, or severe mechanism of injury is <0.02%
   d. Severe mechanism of injury include falls of more than 2 ft if <2 years old or 6 ft if >2 years old
   e. In a child over 2 years, CT head or observation are appropriate if the child has severe headache

4. Which one of the following risk factors in the UK NICE head injury guidelines for children is not sufficient alone to justify CT head scan within 1 h when identified?
   a. Suspicion of non-accidental injury
   b. Post-traumatic seizure but no history of epilepsy
   c. GCS less than 14/15, or for children under 1 year GCS less than 15/15 on initial assessment
   d. At 2 h after the injury, GCS less than 15
   e. Witnessed loss of consciousness lasting more than 5 min

5. In a ventilated infant following closed head injury which one of the following ICP monitoring values is considered the upper limit of normal?
   a. 5 mmHg
   b. 7.5 mmHg
   c. 10 mmHg
   d. 12.5 mmHg
   e. 15 mmHg

6. An 11-month-old girl was admitted to the hospital because of blunt head trauma. Her initial neurological examination was completely normal except that a depressed fracture was palpated in her right parietal region. CT of the head is shown.

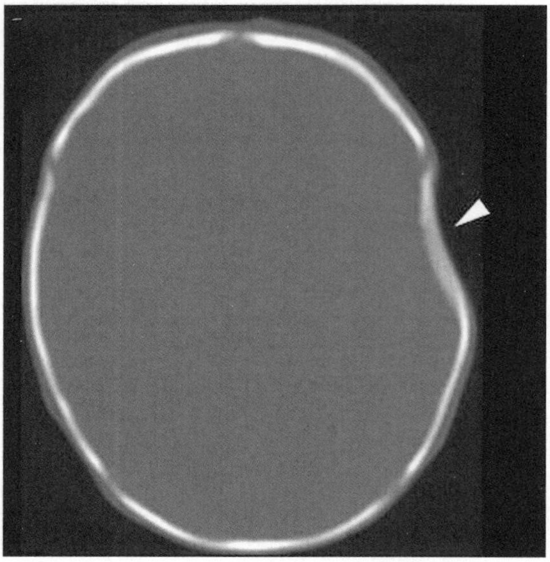

a. Comminuted fracture
b. Growing skull fracture
c. Linear skull fracture
d. Ping-pong fracture
e. Positional plagiocephaly

7. An 8-month-old female child who previously fell from a changing table. She presented on referral from her pediatrician for evaluation of a left frontoparietal mass. Which one of the following management strategies is most appropriate?

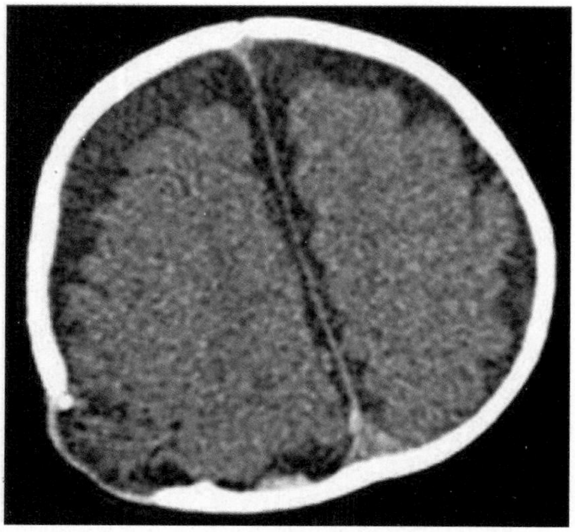

a. Cranioplasty
b. Conservative management
c. Dural repair
d. Duraplasty and autologous cranioplasty
e. Head bandage

8. Brain trauma foundation guidelines for medical management of TBI in children, which one of the following statements is incorrect:
a. Rewarming after hypothermia should not occur faster than 1 °C/h
b. A minimum CPP of 40 mmHg may be considered
c. 3% hypertonic saline should be considered for the treatment of intracranial hypertension
d. Continuous infusion of propofol for either sedation or the management of refractory intracranial hypertension should be avoided
e. The use of corticosteroids is not recommended to improve outcome or reduce ICP

9. Regarding Brain Trauma Foundation guidelines for surgical management of TBI in children which one of the following is LEAST accurate?
a. ICP should be treated when exceeding 15 mmHg in children
b. Simultaneous EVD and lumbar drainage of CSF can be used in refractory intracranial hypertension
c. Decompressive craniectomy should only be considered after the onset of late signs of neurologic deterioration
d. Decompressive craniectomy improves long-term neurological outcome compared to aggressive medical management of raised ICP
e. ICP monitor placement is recommended for early detection of expanding intracerebral hematomas in coagulopathic children

10. A 4-month-old girl presenting with apnea and loss of consciousness. CT head scan is shown. Which one of the following is most likely?

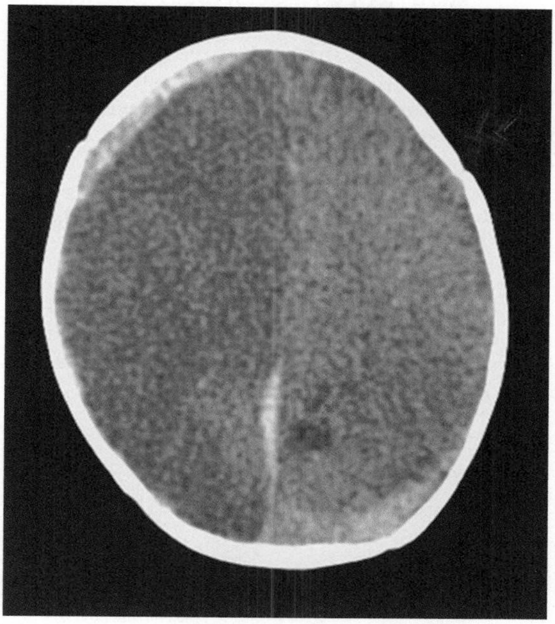

a. Fall from 3 ft height
b. Moya disease
c. Traumatic vertebral artery dissection
d. Shaken baby syndrome
e. Benign enlargement of the subdural space

11. Which one of the following is not a sensitive finding of non-accidental injury in children?
a. A fractured femur in a pre-mobile child.
b. Bruising away from bony prominences
c. Torn labial frenulum in a mobile child
d. Genital and perineal burns
e. Multiple fractures and/or fractures of different ages

12. A 12-year-old child is brought to the emergency department following an occipital head injury without loss of consciousness, but complains of significant headache and has vomited twice. The parents are concerned that he requires a scan. Which one of the following statements regarding the risk of cancer from CT scans in general is most accurate?
a. For a cumulative dose of between 50 and 60 mGy to the head there is a fivefold increase in the risk of brain tumors
b. For a cumulative dose of between 50 and 60 mGy dose to bone marrow there is a fivefold increase in the risk of leukemia
c. The lifetime additional risk of cancer due to CT scans in children is 1 extra case for 10,000 children scanned
d. The baseline incidence of any form of cancer in a child (before the age of 14) is 1 in 1000
e. The baseline incidence of any form of cancer is 1 in 20 in men before the age of 50.

13. Which one of the following factors does not predispose children to cervical cord injuries above C4 level?
a. Large head-to-body ratio
b. Horizontal, shallow facet joints
c. Ligamentous laxity
d. Increased spinal column elasticity
e. Age over 9 years

14. Which one of the following statements regarding history of spine trauma is LEAST accurate?
a. In young children aged 0-9 years, the predominant cause of injury is falls and automobile-versus-pedestrian accidents (>75%)
b. In children aged 10-14 years, motor vehicle accidents (40%) are the major cause of lumbar fractures, and falls and automobile-versus-pedestrian accidents are less prevalent
c. In children 15-17 years of age, motor vehicle and motorcycle accidents become the leading cause of spine injuries (>70%), and there is also an increase in sports-related spine trauma
d. SCI should be suspected if the child reports transient neurological symptoms at the time of injury, even if they are now resolved
e. Children with Down's syndrome are at higher risk of cervical injuries as it is associated with congenital fusion of cervical vertebrae

15. A 9-year-old girl is involved in a MVA and experiences a hyperflexion injury to the neck. She develops numbness and tingling in her arms and legs which progressed to an incomplete quadraparesis. GCS is 15/15. CT cervical spine does not show any fracture. MRI is shown below, and STIR sequences do not show any ligamentous disruption. Which one of the following statements is most accurate?

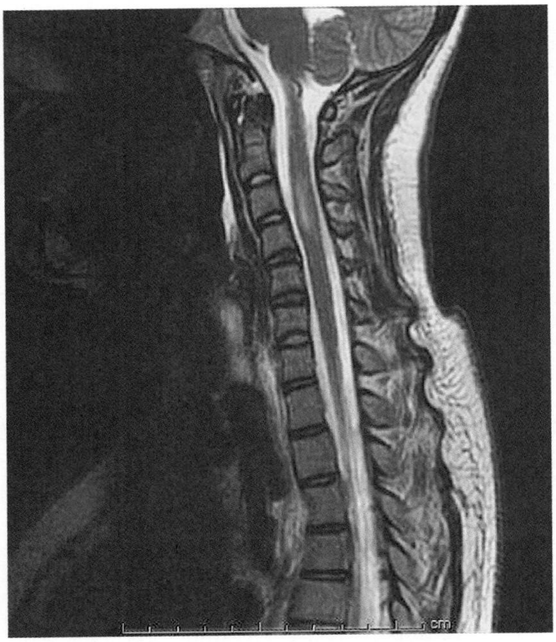

a. She should be managed in halo immobilization
b. Flexion-extensions should be done at the earliest opportunity
c. Somatosensory evokes potentials are likely to be of value in localizing the injury
d. Spinal angiography should be performed to exclude dissection
e. In the presence of normal dynamic cervical X-rays, cervicothoracic bracing for 12 weeks is appropriate initially

16. Which one of the following is not a normal variant seen in the pediatric cervical spine?
a. Pseudosubluxation of C2 on C3
b. Localized kyphosis in mid-cervical area
c. Overriding C1 over tip of odontoid peg in extension
d. Persistence of basilar odontoid synchondrosis
e. Anterior wedging of vertebral bodies

17. Which one of the following statements regarding imaging of the cervical spine after trauma in children is most accurate?
a. Overriding of the anterior atlas in relation to the odontoid on extension is a normal finding on cervical radiographs in young children
b. In children older than 9 years, open mouth X-ray views are not recommended
c. Children over 3 years of age should not have cervical spine imaging if they are alert, have no neurological deficit, no midline cervical tenderness, no painful distracting injury, no unexplained hypotension, and are not intoxicated.
d. In a child under 3 years of age with a GCS of 14/15 cervical spine imaging is mandatory after trauma
e. If gross ligamentous instability is suspected on static radiographs MRI should be performed urgently

18. A 10-year-old child presents with an abnormal head posture as shown below after a recent respiratory tract infection. Which one of the following is most likely?

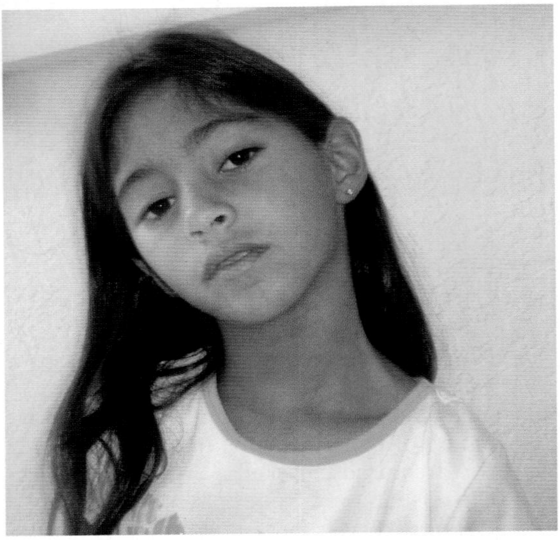

a. Atlanto-occipital dislocation
b. DYT-1 dystonia
c. Atlanto-axial rotatory subluxation (or fixation)
d. Odontoid epiphysiolysis
e. Subaxial cervical subluxation

QUESTIONS 19–27

Additional questions 19–27 available on ExpertConsult.com

EXTENDED MATCHING ITEM (EMI) QUESTIONS

28. **Pediatric injuries:**
    a. Cephalhematoma
    b. Copper deficiency
    c. Disseminated intravascular coagulation
    d. Fibrous dysplasia
    e. Idiopathic thrombocytopenic purpura (ITP)
    f. Mongolian blue spot
    g. Non-accidental injury
    h. Osteogenesis imperfecta
    i. Osteomalacia
    j. Preterm birth and osteopenia
    k. Rickets

For each of the following descriptions, select the most appropriate answers from the list above. Each answer may be used once, more than once or not at all.

1. A 1-week-old infant of African origin presents to you for the first time with a large, fairly well-defined, purple lesion over the buttocks bilaterally. The lesion is not palpable, and it is not warm or tender. This otherwise well-appearing infant is growing and developing normally and appears normal upon physical examination.
2. A 6-month-old infant is brought in 3 days after a fall due to reduced conscious level. On examination there is a bulging anterior fontanelle, and retinal hemorrhages. CT head demonstrates subdural hematoma adjacent to the falx and over the tentorium.
3. A 1-day-old healthy infant with a superficial swelling over the right parietotemporal region that does not cross the suture lines and without bruising.
4. Two weeks after a viral syndrome, a 2-year-old child develops bruising and generalized petechiae, more prominent over the legs. No hepatosplenomegaly or lymph node enlargement is noted. The examination is otherwise unremarkable. Laboratory testing shows the patient to have a normal hemoglobin, hematocrit, and white blood count and differential. The platelet count is 15,000/μL.
5. A 2-year-old child is rushed into hospital in circulatory shock has multiple nonblanching purple lesions of various sizes scattered about on the trunk and extremities; petechiae are noted, and oozing from the venepuncture site has been observed.

29. **Pediatric spinal injury:**
    a. Atlanto-occipital dislocation (dissociation)
    b. Atlanto-axial instability
    c. Atlas (C1) Fracture
    d. C2-C3 subluxation and dislocation
    e. Hangman fracture
    f. Odontoid epiphysiolysis
    g. Pseudosubluxation
    h. Thoracolumbar burst fracture
    i. Thoracolumbar compression fracture
    j. Thoracolumbar flexion-distraction

For each of the following descriptions, select the most appropriate answers from the list above. Each answer may be used once, more than once or not at all.

1. A 4-year-old falls from a climbing frame and complains of persistent neck pain. Lateral c-spine films show anterior displacement of C2 on C3 of up to 4 mm or 40% displacement.
2. A 10-year-old who underwent tonsillectomy 3 days ago presents to the emergency department with his head fixed in a "cock-robin" position.
3. A 6-year-old is involved in a high-speed RTA and has an incomplete quadraparesis on examination. CT cervical spine demonstrates a basion dens interval (BDI) is 14 mm, Power's ratio is 1.2 and C1-condyle interval of 9 mm.

SBA ANSWERS

1. **d**—12 (E3V3M6)

Pediatric GCS score applies to children under the age of 5 years

Eyes Opening	Verbal Response	Best Motor Response
4—Spontaneous 3—To voice 2—To pain 1—No response	5—Smiles, oriented to sounds, follows objects 4—Cries (but consolable), inappropriate interactions 3—Inconsistently inconsolable, moaning 2—Inconsolable (persistently), agitated 1—No response	6—Spontaneous and purposeful 5—Withdraws from touch 4—Withdraws from pain 3—Flexion to pain 2—Extension to pain 1—No response

2. **a**—Vomiting, encephalopathy, and hepatic dysfunction

Reye syndrome occurs most frequently after a viral illness and is characterized by the onset of severe vomiting followed by the development of encephalopathy and hepatic dysfunction. The onset of these symptoms typically occurs within several days after the onset of the viral illness and commonly during a period when the child seems to be recovering from this illness. In association with severe—often projectile—vomiting, which occurs for a transient period, are progressive encephalopathic changes that may follow stages from delirium through confusion, agitation, and lethargy to coma if untreated. It is associated with the ingestion of aspirin during the antecedent viral illness, hence aspirin is no longer recommended or used for the treatment of febrile illnesses in children. Alternative antipyretics, including nonsteroidal anti-inflammatory drugs and acetaminophen (Tylenol), have replaced aspirin as the primary therapy for such illnesses. Children with some disorders, including juvenile rheumatoid arthritis and Kawasaki disease, continue to be given aspirin to treat these disorders (and in this case CVST). Efforts to reduce the risk for development of Reye syndrome in these children have included influenza vaccination annually and vaccination against chickenpox. Careful monitoring of these children also is necessary to ensure early recognition and treatment of Reye syndrome should it occur.

3. **d**—Severe mechanism of injury include falls of more than 2 ft if <2 years old or 6 ft if >2 years old.

For children presenting after head injury with GCS 14 or 15 the PECARN algorithm may be used to calculate likelihood of clinically important TBI (ciTBI) and need for CT imaging. CT is recommended in all children with GCS 14 or altered mental status (agitation, somnolence, repetitive questioning, slow response to verbal communication) or palpable skull fracture—4.3-4.4% risk of ciTBI. If these are not present, criteria for scanning are based on age of patient. In those under 2 years old, inpatient observation or CT head should be considered if there is occipital/parietal/temporal scalp hematoma, LOC for >5 sec, not acting normally according to parent, or a severe mechanism of injury (e.g. motor vehicle crash with patient ejection, death of another passenger, or rollover; pedestrian/cyclist without helmet struck by motor vehicle; fall of more than 3 ft if <2 years or 5 ft if >2 years old; head struck by a high impact object). In those over 2 years old, inpatient observation or CT head should be considered if there is history of LOC, or vomiting, or a severe mechanism of injury, or severe headache. In the absence of any of these age-group specific criteria, the risk of clinically important TBI is <0.02% (under 2) and <0.05% (over 2) and CT head is not recommended. Decisions regarding whether to observe or scan a patient should be based on clinical experience, multiple findings rather than isolated, worsening condition, age <3 months and parental preference.

FURTHER READING

Kuppermann N, Holmes JF, Dayan PS, et al. Pediatric Emergency Care Applied Research Network (PECARN). Identification of children at very low risk of clinically-important brain injuries after head trauma: a prospective cohort study. Lancet 2009;374(9696):1160-70.

4. **e**—Witnessed loss of consciousness lasting more than 5 min

In the UK, NICE guidelines (CG176) cover criteria for CT scanning in children with head injuries

Risk Factors	Actions Required
Suspicion of non-accidental injury Post-traumatic seizure but no history of epilepsy On initial assessment, GCS less than 14, or for children under 1 year GCS (pediatric) less than 15. GCS less than 15 at 2 h after the injury. Suspected open or depressed skull fracture or tense fontanelle. Any sign of basal skull fracture (hemotympanum, "panda" eyes, cerebrospinal fluid (CSF) leakage from the ear or nose, Battle's sign). Focal neurological deficit. For children under 1 year, presence of bruise, swelling or laceration of more than 5 cm on the head	CT head scan within 1 h if any one risk factor present
Loss of consciousness lasting more than 5 min (witnessed). Abnormal drowsiness. Three or more discrete episodes of vomiting. Dangerous mechanism of injury (high-speed road traffic accident either as pedestrian, cyclist or vehicle occupant, fall from a height of greater than 3 m, high-speed injury from a projectile or other object). Amnesia (antegrade or retrograde) lasting more than 5 min.	CT head scan within 1 h if more than one risk factor present Observe for 4 h if only one risk factor present, but CT head within 1 h if develops GCS <15, further vomiting or further episode of abnormal drowsiness
Head injury (without other risk factors) on warfarin	CT head scan within 1 h

5. **a**—5 mmHg

The upper limit of normal when measuring ICP in a child (aged 4-16 years) using lumbar puncture is generally considered to be 18 cm CSF (12.9 mmHg). However, this applies to children who are comfortable in the lateral decubitus position with the knees flexed. A crying, distressed child will cause the ICP to rise and will be difficult to interpret. In an infant undergoing ICP measurement in the horizontal position while ventilated following acute head injury, an upper limit of 5 mmHg is considered normal. An older child with a closed skull with the same circumstances and in the same position will have ICP values similar to an adult with an upper limit of normal of 10 mmHg.

FURTHER READING

Wiegand C, Richards P. Measurement of intracranial pressure in children: a critical review of current methods. Dev Med Child Neurol 2007;49(12):935-41. Review. PubMed PMID: 18039242.

6. **d**—Ping-pong fracture

Depressed skull fractures occur in 7-10% of the children admitted to hospital with a head injury. Depressed skull fractures that occur in children younger than 1 year forms an inward buckling of the bones forming a "cup shape," termed a "ping-pong fracture." In the neonate, ping-pong ball or pond fractures occur with indentation of the bone surface without disruption of the continuity of the bone (similar to green stick fractures of the long bones). Typically the outer table is fractured around the periphery, while the inner table fractures at the center. In newborns, the main cause of the depressed fractures is birth trauma, which includes various perinatal factors such as sacral promontory, uterine fibroids, exostosis of the lumbar vertebra, symphysis pubis, and ischial spine. However, in the postnatal period, the main cause is head trauma. For children without evidence of neurological or radiographic intracranial lesions, there is no differences between conservative and surgical management strategy in terms of future neurological sequels or seizures. The natural history of these depressed skull fractures is variable, with some elevating spontaneously over time and others remaining depressed. Several nonsurgical elevation techniques that use the fact that the bone is in partial continuity have been demonstrated; these techniques include elevation using digital pressure, and vacuum devices such as a breast pump and a vacuum extractor which carry the disadvantages of patient discomfort, inability to obtain complete correction of the depression, and creation of local cephalhematoma with the procedure. It has been demonstrated that the deeper the depressed bone (>1 cm), the higher the risk of dural laceration and cortical laceration in adults and older children, but less clear in neonate and infant populations. Surgical treatment is required in cases where the fragments are depressed to the depth of at least one thickness of the skull, and in those with intracranial hematoma, dural laceration/CSF leak, cosmetically deforming defects, gross wound contamination, and established wound infection.

Image with permission from Law M, Som P, Naidich T. Problem Solving in Neuroradiology, Saunders, Elsevier; 2011.

FURTHER READING

Zalatimao O, et al. Treatment of depressed skull fractures in neonates using percutaneous microscrew elevation. J Neurosurg Pediatrics 2012;9(6):676-9.

7. **d**—Duraplasty and autologous cranioplasty

A rare complication after linear skull fracture in young children (usually younger than 2 or 3 years) is a "growing" skull defect at the fracture site. In these cases, the dura is torn under a linear skull fracture and a pouch of arachnoid passing through the defect and expands, acting as a one-way valve that traps CSF and causes progressive pressure erosion of the fractured edges to enlarge the fracture. Brain growth which produces pulsating, spreading tensile pressure forces on the edges of an unrepaired dural laceration may also contribute to enlargement of the skull defect, such that cerebral herniation through it causes a new neurological deficit. Presentation is with scalp swelling at the site of the fracture, skull defects, persistent or progressive neurological deficits, and seizures. Ideally, young children with a linear skull fracture managed conservatively should be followed up (e.g. at 1 year) to exclude the development of a growing skull fracture. Once the diagnosis of growing skull fracture is made management is surgical resection of the leptomeningeal cyst and degenerated brain tissue, water-tight repair of the dural defect (either primary or with duraplasty) and closure of the bony skull defect. The dural defect may be larger than the bone defect, such that sinus bleeding/injury at one or both ends of the dural tear. In late stages of growing skull fractures, the size of the bone defect increases and the deformity of the bone near the fracture is usually severe. In younger children (especially infants) it is technically difficult to split the skull bone to make enough materials for closure of the defect. Issues around cranioplasty which are controversial: age of the patient, timing, cranioplasty type, and resorption of the autologous bone. If GSF is diagnosed in the early stages, especially the prephase of GSF, these problems can be easily resolved.

Image with permission from Carter R, Anslow P. Imaging of the calvarium. Semin Ultrasound CT MR 2009;30 (6):465-91.

FURTHER READING

Liu X. Growing skull fracture stages ad treatment strategy. J Neurosurg Pediatrics 2012;9:670-5.

8. **a**—Rewarming after hypothermia should not occur faster than 1 °C/h

Therapy	Guidance
CPP	A minimum CPP of 40 mmHg may be considered in children with TBI A CPP threshold of 40-50 mmHg may be considered; there may be age-specific thresholds with infants at the lower end and adolescents at the upper end of this range
Brain oxygenation	If brain oxygen monitoring is used, maintenance of oxygen tension ≥10 mmHg may be considered
Hyperosmolar therapy	3% hypertonic saline (0.1-1 ml/kg of body weight per hour) should be considered for the treatment of intracranial hypertension
Hyperventilation	Avoidance of prophylactic severe hyperventilation to a PaCO2 < 30 mmHg may be considered in the initial 48 h after injury If hyperventilation is used in the management of refractory intracranial hypertension, advanced neuromonitoring for evaluation of cerebral ischemia may be considered
Temperature control	Moderate hypothermia (32-33 °C) beginning early after severe TBI for only 24-h duration should be avoided Moderate hypothermia (32-33 °C) beginning within 8 h after severe TBI for up to 48-h duration should be considered to reduce intracranial hypertension If hypothermia is induced for any reason, rewarming at a rate of >0.5 °C/h should be avoided

Continued

Therapy	Guidance
Barbiturates	High-dose barbiturate therapy may be considered in hemodynamically stable patients with refractory intracranial hypertension despite maximal medical and surgical management When high-dose barbiturate therapy is used to treat refractory intracranial hypertension, continuous arterial blood pressure monitoring and cardiovascular support to maintain adequate cerebral perfusion pressure are required
Corticosteroids	The use of corticosteroids is not recommended to improve outcome or reduce ICP for children with severe TBI
Anesthetic drugs	Etomidate may be considered to control severe intracranial hypertension; however, the risks resulting from adrenal suppression must be considered Thiopental may be considered to control intracranial hypertension As stated by the FDA, a continuous infusion of propofol for either sedation or the management of refractory intracranial hypertension in infants and children with severe TBI is not recommended
Antiseizure drugs	Prophylactic use of antiseizure therapy is not recommended for children with severe TBI for preventing late post-traumatic seizures Prophylactic antiseizure therapy may be considered as a treatment option to prevent early post-traumatic seizures in young pediatric patients and infants at high risk of seizures after head injury
Nutrition	Evidence does not support the use of immune-modulating diet to improve outcome

Adapted from Kochanek PM, Carney N, Adelson PD, et al. Guidelines for the acute medical management of severe traumatic brain injury in infants, children, and adolescents—second edition. Pediatr Crit Care Med. 2012;13(Suppl. 1):S1-82.

9. **c**—Decompressive craniectomy should only be considered after the onset of late signs of neurologic deterioration.

Consider ICP monitoring in infants and children with severe TBI and treating when ICP exceeds 20-25 mmHg. The presence of coagulopathy would contraindicate the placement of an ICP monitor, in which situation the Cushing reflex and autonomic dysfunction might be the only indicators of increased ICP. CSF drainage through an external ventricular drain may be considered in the management of increased ICP, with optional addition of a lumbar drain in refractory intracranial hypertension despite a functioning external ventricular drain, open basal cisterns, and no evidence of a mass effect. CSF drainage via EVD resulted in ICP control in 87% of pediatric patients. These three studies also confirmed that refractory raised ICP is associated with poor outcome, with 100% mortality in all patients with refractory intracranial hypertension after CSF drainage. Decompressive craniectomy with duraplasty may be considered for patients who are showing early signs of neurologic deterioration or herniation or are developing intracranial hypertension refractory to medical management during the early stages of their treatment. Multiple small case series also show that craniectomy is an effective rescue intervention in patients with sustained ICP greater than 20 mmHg, clearly demonstrating craniectomy has a role in ICH management. Certain questions are still unanswered, including the ideal timing and method of craniectomy, as well as its impact on long-term outcome.

FURTHER READING

Kochanek PM, Carney N, Adelson PD, et al. Guidelines for the acute medical management of severe traumatic brain injury in infants, children, and adolescents—second edition. Pediatr Crit Care Med 2012;13(Suppl. 1):S1-82.

10. **d**—Shaken baby syndrome

Abusive head trauma (shaken baby syndrome) remains the most common cause of death in children who are victims of non-accidental injury (NAI), and this usually occurs during the first year of life. The diagnosis is often missed since no history of head trauma is provided, and the signs and symptoms the child displays may be non-specific, such as vomiting, poor feeding, irritability or lethargy. Primary injuries (consequence of the initial trauma or impact of force) include epidural hemorrhages, subdural hemorrhages, subarachnoid hemorrhages, skull fractures, intraventricular hemorrhages, cortical contusions, diffuse axonal injury (DAI) and intraparenchymal hematomas. Epidural hemorrhages in children require a direct impact of forces and are generally venous bleeds which result from tears in the dural sinus or diploic veins. Subdural hemorrhages do not require direct impact and may result from inertial shearing or rotational forces but most commonly result from abrupt deceleration. Subdural hemorrhages occur in a space created by the traumatic separation of the arachnoid from the dura mater and are caused by bleeding from bridging veins. Subdural hematoma suggestive of abuse may be acute, subacute or chronic, frequently bilateral, closely related to the falx, layering over the tentorium and accompanied by hemispheric hypodensity (HH; hypodense edematous cortex and underlying white matter in multiple cerebrovascular territories) due to secondary insults (e.g. cardiac arrest, hypoxia and hypotension). DAI results from sudden acceleration and deceleration forces which may be combined with rotational forces, which disrupts fiber tracts. Infants are more susceptible to DAI due to their large head-to-body ratio, weak neck musculature and thinner skull. DAI typically affects subcortical white matter, the corpus callosum, the brainstem and internal capsule. Intraparenchymal hematomas can result from shearing-straining injuries due to rupture of small intraparenchymal blood vessels and typically occurs in the frontotemporal white matter. The differential diagnosis of a child with intracranial hemorrhage includes accidental trauma or NAT, birth trauma, coagulopathy, congenital vascular malformations, spontaneous SDH (related to benign enlargement of the subdural space), and metabolic deficiencies such as glutaric aciduria type I. Associated ocular findings which increase the likelihood of NAI (in the absence of verifiable history) include retinal hemorrhage, periorbital hematoma, eyelid laceration, subconjunctival/intraocular hemorrhage, subluxed or dislocated lens, cataracts, glaucoma, anterior chamber angle regression, iridiodialysis, retinal dialysis or detachment, intraocular hemorrhage, optic atrophy or papilledema. Multiple mechanisms of retinal hemorrhage have been postulated, including direct tracking of blood from intracranial hemorrhage, hemorrhage secondary to raised intracranial pressure or retinoschisis.

Image with permission from Adam D, editor. Grainger & Allison's Diagnostic Radiology, 6th ed. Churchill Livingstone, Elsevier; 2014.

FURTHER READING

Paul AR, Adamo MA (n.d.). Non-accidental trauma in pediatric patients: a review of epidemiology, pathophysiology, diagnosis and treatment. Transl Pediatr. Retrieved from http://www.thetp.org/article/view/4150/5031.

11. **c**—Torn labial frenulum in a mobile child

Abuse can be classified broadly as physical, emotional, sexual and neglect, with overlaps occurring in most cases. It has been estimated that 10-15% of childhood injuries resulting in emergency department visits are caused by abuse. Fractures are the second most common presentation after soft-tissue injury and bruising. In general, any delay in presentation, any injury that does not fit with the explanation offered or the developmental stage of the child, or a changing or conflicting account should raise suspicion. Important differential diagnosis of NAI includes accidental injury, osteogenesis imperfecta, ITP, Mongolian blue spot, and scalded skin syndrome.

Non-accidental Injury: Clinical Features

Extra-CNS Signs of Physical Abuse	Situations Highly Suspicious of NAI
Fractures	• children under 18 months with a fracture • where the fracture is inconsistent with the developmental stage of the child • multiple fractures and/or fractures of different ages • rib fractures in children with normal bones and no history of major trauma • a fractured femur in a pre-mobile child.
Bruises	Bruises cannot be aged accurately. Bruising that suggests the possibility of physical abuse includes: • bruising in children who are not independently mobile • bruising in babies • bruising away from bony prominences • bruising to the face, back, abdomen, arms, buttocks, ears, and hands • multiple bruises in clusters • multiple bruises of uniform shape • bruising that carries an imprint (of an implement or cord).
Oral injuries and bites	There is not enough evidence in the literature to support the view that a pre-mobile child with a torn labial frenum in isolation is diagnostic of child abuse. A full assessment should be performed. • 1% of emergency department attendances are due to bites. • Human bites can be distinguished from animal bites.

Continued

Extra-CNS Signs of Physical Abuse	Situations Highly Suspicious of NAI
Burns	A high percentage of childhood burns are due to abuse (2-35% overall; up to 45% for genital and perineal burns). The two kinds of burns most often seen in abused children are scald burns (from contact with hot liquids) and thermal burns (contact with hot objects). In accidental burns, the head, neck, anterior trunk, and arms are the most often affected. In cases of abuse, hands, legs, feet, and buttocks were more likely to be involved. The anterior aspect of the hand was more likely to be involved in accidental burns and the dorsum of the hand was more likely involved in abuse cases. Suspicious burns include patterned contact burns in clear shape of hot object (fork, clothing iron, curling iron, cigarette lighter) and classic forced immersion burn patterns with sharp stocking-and-glove demarcation and sparing of flexed protected areas. In addition, splash/spill burn patterns in children which is not consistent with the history of the child's developmental level should be considered suspicious. Cigarette burns should always raise concern for abuse, as should any evidence of delay in seeking medical treatment

FURTHER READING

Roderick C, Davies E, Rabb L, Bowley DM. What does the surgeon need to know about safeguarding children? How to spot signs of abuse. RCS Bull 2015;349-532. http://dx.doi.org/10.1308/rcsbull.2015.345.

12. **c**—The lifetime additional risk of cancer due to CT scans in children is 1 extra case for 10,000 children scanned.

Children are considerably more sensitive to radiation than adults, have a longer life expectancy than adults (a larger window of opportunity for expressing radiation damage), and may receive a higher radiation dose than necessary if CT settings are not adjusted for their smaller body size. For a cumulative dose of between 50 and 60 mGy to the head (i.e. 2-3 CT head scans), the investigators reported a threefold increase in the risk of brain tumors; the same dose to bone marrow (i.e. 5-10 CT head scans) resulted in a threefold increase in the risk of leukemia. However, it is important to stress that the absolute additional cancer risks associated with CT scans (1 additional case for every 2000 people scanned) are small compared to the baseline cancer risk (i.e. 1 in 35 (men) or 1 in 20 (female) risk of cancer before the age of 50, or 1 in 5 lifetime risk). In children, the lifetime extra risk of cancer from a single CT scan was small—about one case of cancer for every 10,000 scans performed on children (baseline 1 in 500 risk of developing some form of cancer before the age of 14).

FURTHER READING

http://www.cancer.gov/about-cancer/causes-prevention/risk/radiation/pediatric-ct-scans.

Berrington de Gonzále A, Mahesh M, Kim KP, Bhargavan M, Lewis R, Mettler F, Land C. Projected cancer risks from computed tomographic scans performed in the United States in 2007. Arch Intern Med 2009;169:2071-7.

Cancer Research UK, http://www.cancerresearchuk.org/health-professional/cancer-risk-statistics; 2016 [accessed 01.02.16].

Pearce MS, Salotti JA, Little MP, et al. Radiation exposure from CT scans in childhood and subsequent risk of leukemia and brain tumors: a retrospective cohort study. Lancet 2012;380(9840):499-505.

Mathews JD, Forsythe AV, Brady Z, et al. Cancer risk in 680,000 people exposed to computed tomography scans in childhood or adolescence: data linkage study of 11 million Australians. Br Med J 2013;346:f2360.

13. **e**—Age over 9 years

The pediatric cervical spine does not become adult like until about the age of 8 years. These factors increase the risk of injury/instability to the levels of C1-C3 include large head-to-body ratio, ligamentous laxity, relative paraspinal muscle weakness, horizontal/shallow facets. Cervical spine injuries occur mainly in the upper cervical spine above C4 in patients 8 years of age or younger which most often involve the occiput, C1, and C2 complex and thus carries increased risk of fatality. Patients older than 8 years of age typically sustain more injuries below C4 and carry a much lower fatality rate. Because of these biomechanical differences, younger children (0-8 years) tend to have fewer fractures and greater incidence of SCIWORA (spinal cord injury without radiographic abnormality).

14. **e**—Children with Down's syndrome are at higher risk of cervical injuries as it is associated with congenital fusion of cervical vertebrae.

Spine fractures are usually the result of high-speed and impact injuries such as a motor vehicle accident or a fall from great height. Spine fractures in children represent 1-3% of all pediatric fractures. The incidence of pediatric spine injuries peaks in 2 age groups; children <5 years old and children >10 years old. There is a seasonal peak of pediatric spinal injuries from June to September, during summer break. There is another seasonal peak in the 2 weeks surrounding the Christmas holiday. The mechanism of injury in the pediatric population varies with age. In young children aged 0-9 years, the predominant causes of injury are falls and automobile-versus-pedestrian accidents (>75%). In children aged 10-14 years, motor vehicle accidents (40%) are the major cause of lumbar fractures, and falls and automobile-versus-pedestrian accidents are less prevalent. In children 15-17 years of age, motor vehicle and motorcycle accidents become the leading cause of spine injuries (>70%), and there is also an increase in sports-related spine trauma. A spinal cord injury should be suspected if the child has a history of numbness, tingling, or brief paralysis even if it has recovered subsequently. Some children are predisposed to cervical injuries more than others includes children with Down's Syndrome (atlanto-axial instability), Klippel-Feil syndrome (congenital fusion of cervical spine), previous cervical spine surgery, and other syndromes affecting the cervical spine. Hyperflexion injuries are most common and are associated with wedge fractures of the anterior cervical bodies with disruption of posterior aspects. The classic triad of symptoms of cervical spine injury is localized neck tenderness, muscle spasm and decreased range of motion.

FURTHER READING

Rozzelle CJ, et al. Management of pediatric cervical spine and spinal cord injuries. Neurosurgery 2013;72:205-26.

15. **e**—In the presence of normal dynamic cervical X-rays, cervicothoracic bracing for 12 weeks is appropriate initially

SCIWORA is a widely recognized form of spinal cord injury, occurring almost exclusively in children (due to relative elasticity of the spinal column relative to the spinal cord), and is characterized by objective signs of myelopathy as a result of trauma in the absence of any radiographically evident fracture, dislocation, or ligamentous instability (on static or dynamic X-rays or CT). Children presenting with a history of transient neurological signs or symptoms referable to the spinal cord after a traumatic event but normal neurological examination can develop delayed onset SCIWORA, hence there is debate as to whether they should just be managed as such initially despite the absence of objective signs. By definition, normal acute flexion/extension X-rays are required for a diagnosis of SCIWORA. If paraspinous muscle spasm, pain, or uncooperation prevents dynamic studies, they recommended external immobilization until the child can cooperatively flex and extend the spine for dynamic X-ray assessment. Although concern exists for the late development of pathological intersegmental motion in children with SCIWORA following normal flexion and extension studies, there has been no documentation of such instability ever developing. MRI is recommended in children with potential SCIWORA as it may include identifying signal change or intramedullary injury (prognostic value), excluding compressive lesions of the cord/roots needing surgery, exclude spinal ligamentous disruption that might warrant surgical intervention (in situations where dynamic flexion/extension radiographs cannot be done or would be superfluous preoperatively), guiding treatment regarding length of external immobilization (e.g. evidence of residual ligamentous injury), and/or determining when to allow patients to return to full activity.

Pang has also recommended somatosensory evoked potential (SSEP) screening of children with presumed SCIWORA to detect subtle posterior column dysfunction when clinical findings are inconclusive, evaluating head-injured, comatose, or pharmacologically paralyzed children, distinguishing between intracranial, spinal, or peripheral nerve injuries, and/or providing a baseline for comparison with subsequent evaluations. Neither spinal angiography nor myelography is recommended in the evaluation of patients with SCIWORA. Because subluxation and/or malalignment/ligamentous instability are, by definition, absent in SCIWORA, the mainstay of treatment has been immobilization and avoidance of activity that may either lead to exacerbation of the present (ligamentous and spina cord) strain/injury or increase the potential for recurrent injury. Medical management issues such as blood pressure support and pharmacological therapy apply. Treatment consisting of cervicothoracic bracing for patients with cervical-level SCIWORA for 12 weeks and avoidance of activities that encourage flexion and extension of the neck for an additional 12 weeks (i.e. 6 months total) has not been associated with recurrent injury. Patients with normal MRI and SSEP findings following transient deficits or "symptoms only" may be managed with a cervical collar for 1-2 weeks. Despite this, it is unclear what role immobilization plays given that dynamic radiographs have confirmed the absence of instability required for diagnosing SCIWORA, and furthermore, that follow-up with dynamic radiographs in these children has not shown development of delayed pathological intersegmental motion. However, if (normal) physiological motion of the spinal column can potentiate spinal cord injury in these patients when there is no malalignment, subluxation, or lesion causing cord compression, then immobilization may be warranted.

Image with permission from Klimo Jr P, Ware ML, Gupta N, Brockmeyer D. Cervical spine trauma in the pediatric patient. Neurosurg Clin N Am 2007;18 (4):599-620.

FURTHER READING

Rozzelle CJ, et al. Spinal cord injury without radiographic abnormality (SCIWORA). Neurosurgery 2013;72:227-33.

16. **b**—Localized kyphosis in mid-cervical area

Ten unique features of the pediatric cervical spine that can cause confusion during the trauma evaluation: (1) the apical ossification center can be mistaken for a fracture; (2) the synchondrosis at the base of the odontoid can be mistaken for a fracture; (3) vertebral bodies appear rounded-off or wedged, simulating a wedge compression fracture; (4) secondary centers of ossification at the tips of the spinous processes can be mistaken for a fracture; (5) the odontoid may angulate posteriorly in 4% of children; (6) C2-C3 pseudosubluxation (can be assessed with Swischuk's line); (7) the ossification center of the anterior arch of C1 may be absent in the first year of life; (8) the atlanto-dens interval may be as wide as 4.5 mm and still be normal; (9) the width of the prevertebral soft tissues varies widely, especially with crying, and may be mistaken for swelling; and (10) horizontal facets in young children can be mistaken for a fracture.

17. **c**—Children over 3 years of age should not have cervical spine imaging if they are alert, have no neurological deficit, no midline cervical tenderness, no painful distracting injury, no unexplained hypotension, and are not intoxicated.

Anteroposterior (AP) and lateral cervical spine radiography (plus open mouth views if >9 years old) or high-resolution CT is recommended to assess the cervical spine in children. High-resolution CT scan with attention to the suspected level of neurological injury, radiographic abnormality or area not adequately visualized on plain films. Flexion and extension cervical radiographs or fluoroscopy are recommended to exclude gross ligamentous instability if suspected following static radiographs/CT. MRI is recommended to exclude spinal cord or nerve root compression, evaluate ligamentous integrity, or provide information regarding neurological prognosis. Common normal findings on cervical spine radiographs obtained on young children which may be mistaken for acute traumatic injuries are pseudosubluxation of C2 on C3, overriding of the anterior atlas in relation to the odontoid on extension, exaggerated atlanto-dens intervals, and the radiolucent synchondrosis between the odontoid and C2 body.

Cervical Spine Imaging in Children: Indications

Do not image cervical spine under 3 years of age who have experienced trauma and who:	Do not image cervical spine over 3 years of age who have experienced trauma and who:
• have a GCS greater than 13, • have no neurological deficit, • have no midline cervical tenderness, • have no painful distracting injury, • are not intoxicated, • do not have unexplained hypotension (i.e. due to SCI), • and do not have motor vehicle collision (MVC), a fall from a height >10 ft, or non-accidental trauma (NAT) as a known or suspected mechanism of injury.	• are alert, • have no neurological deficit, • have no midline cervical tenderness, • have no painful distracting injury, • do not have unexplained hypotension, • and are not intoxicated.

FURTHER READING

Rozzelle CJ, et al. Management of pediatric cervical spine and spinal cord injuries. Neurosurgery 2013;72:205-26.

18. **c**—Atlanto-axial rotatory subluxation (or fixation)

Fixed rotatory subluxation of the atlanto-axial complex (AARF) is not unique to children but is more common during childhood. AARF may present following minor trauma (30%), in association with an upper respiratory infection, or without an identifiable inciting event. It is associated with Down's syndrome, Morquio syndrome, spondyloepiphyseal dysplasia, Larsen's syndrome, achondroplasia and Grisel's syndrome (post-inflammatory). The head is rotated to one side with the head tilted to the other side (due to SCM spasm) causing the so-called "cock-robin" appearance mimicking torticollis, unable to turn his/her head past the midline, attempts to move the neck are often painful and usually there is no neurological deficit. Plain cervical spine radiographs may reveal the lateral mass of C1 rotated anterior to the odontoid on a lateral view. Fielding and Hawkins type I rotatory subluxation is characterized by rotatory fixation without anterior shift of the atlas (transverse ligament intact), type II consists of rotatory subluxation with an anterior shift (ADI) of greater than 3 mm but less than 5 mm due to transverse ligament compromise and may also be associated with spinal instability. Type III involves rotatory subluxation with an ADI of greater than 5 mm. Type IV is a rare and usually fatal injury that involves rotatory fixation with a posterior shift. If the diagnosis of AARF is suspected after clinical examination and plain radiographic study, a dynamic CT study should be obtained (three-position CT with C1-C2 motion analysis). The longer AARF is present before attempted treatment, the less likely reduction can be accomplished or maintained. Acute AARF (<4 weeks since onset) that has not reduced spontaneously should undergo attempted reduction with manipulation or halter traction. Chronic AARF (4 weeks duration or more since onset) should undergo attempted reduction with halter or skull tong/halo traction. Reductions achieved with manipulation or halter traction should be immobilized with a cervicothoracic (Minerva) brace, while those requiring tong/halo traction should be immobilized in a halo. Length of immobilization should be proportional to the length of time that the subluxation was present before treatment. Surgical arthrodesis can be considered for those with irreducible subluxations, recurrent subluxations, or subluxations present for 3 months' duration.

Green's skeletal trauma in children. Fielding and Hawkins classification of atlanto-axial rotatory displacement.

Image with permission from Klimo Jr P, Ware ML, Gupta N, Brockmeyer D. Cervical spine trauma in the pediatric patient. Neurosurg Clin N Am 2007;18 (4):599-620.

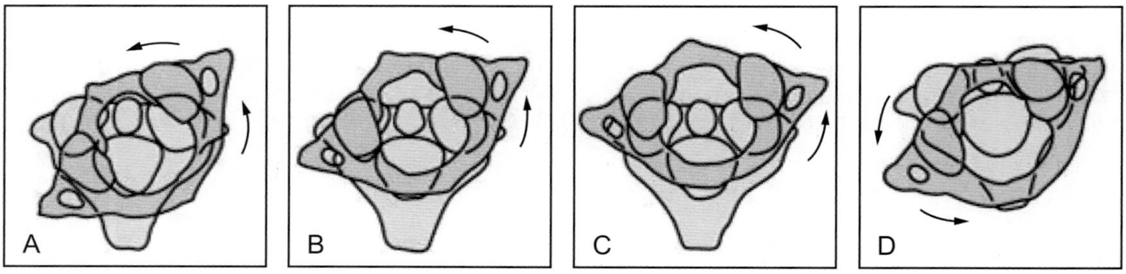

A, Type I, no anterior displacement, and the odontoid acts as pivot. B, Type II, anterior displacement of 3-5 mm and one lateral articular process acting as the pivot. C, Type III, anterior displacement of more than 5 mm. D, Type IV, posterior displacement. (With permission from Dormans JP. Evaluation of children with suspected cervical spine injury. Instr Course Lect 51:407, 2002.)

FURTHER READING

Rozzelle CJ, et al. Management of pediatric cervical spine and spinal cord injuries. Neurosurgery 2013;72:205-26.

ANSWERS 19–27

Additional answers 19–27 available on ExpertConsult.com

EMI ANSWERS

28. 1—f, Mongolian blue spots. These are bluish-gray lesions located over the buttocks, lower back, and occasionally, the extensor surfaces of the extremities. They are common in infants of African, Asian, and Latin American origin. They tend to disappear by 1-2 years of age, although those on the extremities may not fully resolve. 2—g, Non-accidental injury. This case is suspicious due to the delayed presentation, retinal hemorrhage and distribution of the subdural hemorrhage on CT scan. 3—a, Cephalhematomas. These are subperiosteal hematomas which thus do not cross the suture line, do not discolor the scalp, and swelling usually progresses over the first few hours of life. Most cephalhematomas resolve within the first few weeks or months of life without residual findings. By contrast, caput succedaneum is soft-tissue swelling of the scalp involving the presenting delivery portion of the head. This lesion is sometimes ecchymotic and can extend across the suture lines. The edema resolves in the first few days of life. 4—e, Idiopathic thrombocytopenic purpura (ITP). This is the most common form of thrombocytopenic purpura, usually triggered by a viral infection causing immune-mediated sequestration and destruction of platelets in the spleen. Treatment for ITP consists of observation and/or gamma globulin and steroids. Splenectomy is reserved for the most severe and chronic forms. 5—c, Disseminated intravascular coagulation. The disorder, which can be triggered by a variety of disorders (e.g. endotoxin shock, trauma, malignancy) results in microvascular thrombosis causing a consumptive coagulopathy and hemorrhage. Clotting studies show prolonged PT and PTT, decreased fibrinogen concentration, and an increase in fibrin degradation products. Blood film will show fragmented cells and few platelets. Microvascular thrombosis (fibrin clot formation) can lead to tissue ischemia and necrosis, further capillary damage, release of thromboplastic substances, and worsen DIC. Simultaneous activation of the fibrinolytic system produces increased amounts of fibrin degradation products, which inhibit thrombin activity. Treatment of the precipitating cause is critical.

29. 1—g, Pseudosubluxation. Normal anterior translation that can occur between C2 and C3 and less frequently between C3 and C4 in patients younger than 8 years. May be seen in 40% of children at C2-C3 level and in 14% of children at the C3-C4 level occurs because of increased ligamentous laxity, more horizontal nature of facet joint (30° versus 60-70° in adult); in children, fulcrum of motion that is relatively greatest at C2-C3 level (compared w/C5-C6 in the adult). The posterior cervical line (spinolaminar line of Swischuk) is used to distinguish pathologic displacement from normal anterior displacement. A line is constructed connecting the anterior aspect of the spinous processes of C1-C3. If the anterior aspect of the spinous process of C2 is more than 1.5 mm from this line, an injury should be suspected. 2—b, Atlanto-axial instability. The history is that of atlanto-axial rotatory subluxation, which is termed Grisel's syndrome if secondary to inflammatory conditions in the neck. 3—a, Atlanto-occipital dislocation (dissociation).

CHAPTER 44

PEDIATRIC VASCULAR NEUROSURGERY

SINGLE BEST ANSWER (SBA) QUESTIONS

1. Which one of the following pathologies is most likely to produce the ultrasound appearance seen below?

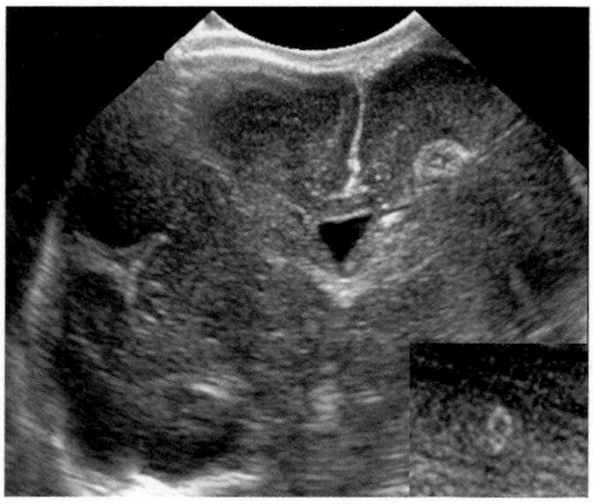

a. Band heterotopia
b. Germinal matrix hemorrhage
c. Hydrocephalus
d. Schizencephaly
e. Subependymal nodules

2. Which one of the following is most likely in a child with the below MRI appearance presenting with increasing head circumference and shortness of breath?

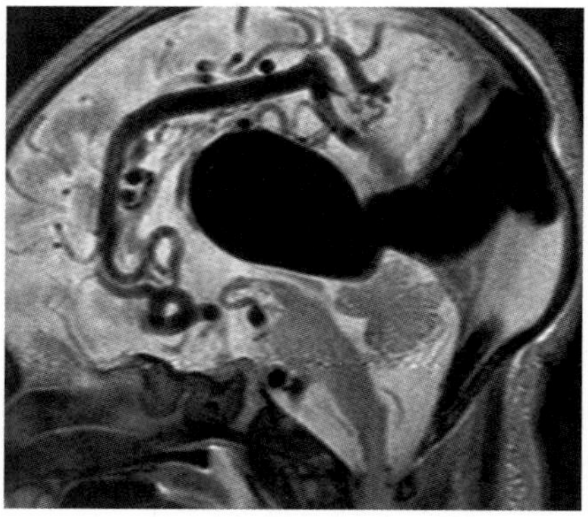

a. Cavernous malformation
b. Developmental venous anomaly
c. Dural AV fistula
d. Tentorial AVM
e. Vein of galen malformation

3. This 14-year-old presented with intraventricular hemorrhage. Which one of the following management options is likely to be discussed based on this right ICA angiogram?

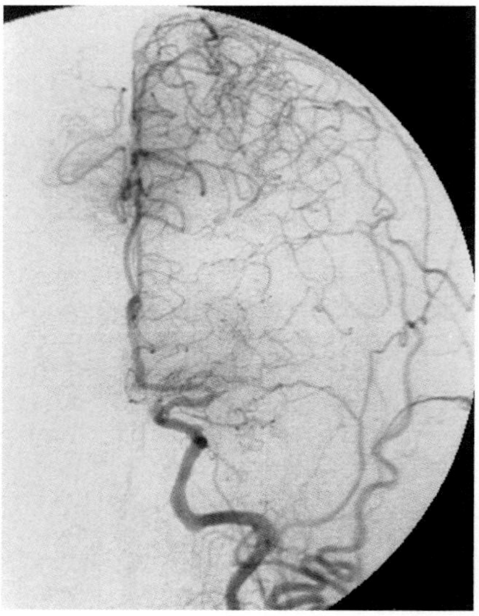

a. Coil embolization
b. Extracranial-Intracranial Bypass
c. Intravenous antibiotics
d. Onyx embolization
e. Stereotactic radiosurgery

4. Choroidal vein of Galen malformations present most commonly as:
a. Congestive heart failure
b. Delayed developmental milestones
c. Focal neurological deficit
d. Increasing head circumference
e. Subarachnoid hemorrhage

5. Which treatment would be preferred in a vein of Galen malformation patient with a extremely high flow shunt and in which perforating arteries are of small caliber?
   a. Surgical excision
   b. Transfemoral transarterial embolization
   c. Transfemoral transvenous embolization
   d. Transtorcula
   e. VP shunting

6. Wyburn-Mason syndrome is most accurately described by which one of the following statements?
   a. Facial angioma and ipsilateral parietooccipital AVM
   b. Multiple visceral, muscosal, and cerebral AVM
   c. Optic tract glioma and midbrain AVM
   d. Retinal angiomatosis, facial hemangioma, and midbrain AVM
   e. Retinal angioma and posterior fossa hemangioblastoma

7. Which one of the following statements about pediatric intracranial aneurysms is NOT likely?
   a. Infectious aneurysms are more common in children than adults
   b. Internal carotid bifurcation aneurysms are the commonest type
   c. Posterior circulation aneurysms are more common that anterior circulation aneurysms
   d. There is an association with coarctation of the aorta
   e. They occur more commonly in males than females

8. The approach LEAST likely to be utilized during surgery for a dorsolateral brainstem cavernous malformation is:
   a. Anterior petrosectomy
   b. Retrosigmoid
   c. Suboccipital
   d. Supracerebellar infratentorial
   e. Transcallosal

9. A 9-year-old boy sustains a left sided penetrating brain injury secondary to air rifle accident. Initial CT head shows traumatic SAH and hemorrhagic contusion in the left temporal lobe. GCS recovers to 15 and he is discharged after 7 days. He is readmitted 5 days later with intermittent dysphasia and right facial weakness. Which one of the following surgically treatable conditions are you concerned about?
   a. Enlarging aneurysm
   b. Hydrocephalus
   c. Maturation of hemorrhagic contusion
   d. Meningitis
   e. Vasospasm

10. A 22 month old male child with a history of iron deficiency anemia developed progressive lethargy and vomiting over several days, culminating in flaccid quadriparesis. Brain MRI and MRV confirmed cerebral venous sinus thrombosis with subcortical white matter infarction. Lumbar puncture revealed elevated opening pressure, normal cerebrospinal fluid cell count, protein and glucose. Laboratory studies showed Hb 7.5 mg/dl with iron deficiency, and a positive lupus anticoagulant. The most appropriate management strategy is:
   a. IV rehydration
   b. IV rehydration and systemic heparin
   c. IV rehydration and thrombolysis
   d. IV rehydration and warfarinization
   e. IV rehydration and venous stenting

11. Which one of the following extracranial to intracranial bypass grafts is LEAST likely to be possible in children?
   a. Encephaloduroarteriosynangiosis
   b. Encephalomyoarteriosynangiosis
   c. Encephalomyosynangiosis
   d. Superficial temporal artery to MCA
   e. Transposed temporalis muscle forms an anastomosis

12. Small, deep-seated pediatric arteriovenous malformations may be most appropriately treated with which one of the following?
   a. Endovascular coil embolization
   b. Fractionated stereotactic radiotherapy
   c. Proton beam therapy
   d. Stereotactic radiosurgery
   e. Surgical excision

EXTENDED MATCHING ITEM (EMI) QUESTIONS

13. **Pediatric Vascular Pathology:**
   a. Autosomal Dominant Polycystic Kidney Disease
   b. Coarctation of the aorta
   c. Ehlers-Danlos syndrome
   d. Fibromuscular dysplasia
   e. Klippel-Trenaunay syndrome
   f. Marfan's syndrome
   g. Osler-Weber-Rendu syndrome
   h. Parkes-Weber syndrome
   i. Pseudoxanthoma Elasticum

j. Sturge-Weber syndrome
k. Tuberous Sclerosis
l. Wyburn-Mason syndrome

For each of the following descriptions, select the most appropriate answers from the list above. Each answer may be used once, more than once or not at all.

1. Characterized by spontaneous recurrent epistaxis, telangiectasias and AVM affecting lung, liver, brain, and spine.
2. Characterized by arachnodactyly, lens dislocation, spontaneous pneumothorax, mitral valve prolapse and associated with intracranial aneurysms.
3. Characterized by facial angioma and ipsilateral parietooccipital AVM.

SBA ANSWERS

1. **b**—Grade IV germinal matrix hemorrhage

Papile's classification:
Grade I—hemorrhage is confined to the germinal matrix
Grade II—intraventricular hemorrhage without ventricular dilatation
Grade III—intraventricular hemorrhage with ventricular dilatation
Grade IV—intraventricular rupture and hemorrhage into the surrounding white matter

Image with permission from Coley BD. Caffey's Pediatric Diagnostic Imaging, 12th ed. Elsevier, Saunders, 2013.

FURTHER READING

Papile LA, Burstein J, Burstein R, Koffler H. Incidence and evolution of subependymal and intraventricular hemorrhage: a study of infants with birth weights less than 1,500 gm. J Pediatr 1978 Apr;92(4):529-34.

2. **e**—Vein of Galen Malformation

Persistence of the single median prosencephalic vein of Markowski into fetal life results in a dilated venous sac in the midline, the Vein of Galen malformation. Normal deep veins are absent and venous drainage is routed through the median prosencephalic vein (or primitive internal cerebral vein). This temporary vein drains the choroid plexus from both sides almost between 5th and 10th week of fetal life. With simultaneous development of basal ganglia, thalamus, and cerebral vascularization, paired internal cerebral veins appear to progressively annex the venous drainage of the midline structures. The falcine sinus becomes the normal outlet for the persistent median prosencephalic vein, with the straight sinus hypoplastic or stenosed. Such persistence of fetal pattern maintains the fetal hemodynamics and as a result some dural sinuses may fail to develop altogether.

Image with permission from Loevner L. Brain imaging: case review series, 2nd ed. Elsevier, Mosby, 2009.

3. **b**—Extracranial-Intracranial Bypass

Adult moyamoya patients often present with hemorrhage, leading to rapid diagnosis. In contrast, children usually present with TIAs or strokes. Other symptoms include seizures, headache, choreoatheform movements, ICH/ICH. Risk factors include Asian origin, cranial radiotherapy, NF-1, Down's syndrome among others. Moyamoya syndrome should be considered and diagnostic evaluation begun in any child who presents with symptoms of cerebral ischemia, especially if the symptoms are precipitated by physical exertion, hyperventilation, or crying. Hemorrhage from moyamoya vessels can be readily diagnosed on head CT, with the most common sites of hemorrhage being the basal ganglia, ventricular system, medial temporal lobes, and thalamus. Most suggestive of moyamoya on MRI is the finding of diminished flow voids in the internal carotid and middle and anterior cerebral arteries coupled with prominent collateral flow voids in the basal ganglia and thalamus. The diagnosis of moyamoya is said to require bilateral symmetrical stenosis or occlusion of the terminal portion of the intracranial carotid arteries as well as the presence of dilated collateral vessels that develop at the base of the brain producing the classic "puff of smoke" appearance on angiography. External carotid imaging is essential to identify pre-existing collateral vessels, so that surgery, if performed, will not disrupt them. Aneurysms or arterio venous malformations (AVMs), known to be associated with some cases of moyamoya, can also be best detected by conventional angiography.

Image with permission from Loevner L. Brain imaging: case review series, 2nd ed. Elsevier, Mosby, 2009.

4. **a**—Congestive heart failure

In the Lasjaunicas classification, VGMs are divided into choroidal or mural types. In choroidal type VGMs, the arteriovenous shunt is subarachnoid located in the tela choroidea along the cisterna velum interpositum with arterial feeders (choroidal arteries, thalamo-perforator arteries, and pericallosal artery) entering the anterior segment of the median prosencephalic vein. Multiple high-flow fistulas (large volume of shunt) results in cardiac failure in neonates. The aggressive volume overload results in cerebral ischemia and encephalomalacia.

In mural type VGMs, a single arteriovenous fistula is situated in the inferolateral wall of the median prosencephalic vein fed by collicular or posterior choroidal arteries (i.e. fewer fistulas, low-flow). They present later in infancy or early childhood with failure to thrive and macrocephaly due to hydrocephalus. Hydrocephalus develops mainly due to impaired absorption because of absence or stenosis of dural sinuses.

FURTHER READING

Rao VR, Mathuriya SN. Pediatric aneurysms and vein of Galen malformations. J Pediatr Neurosci 2011 Oct; 6(Suppl. 1):S109-17.

5. **c**—Transfemoral transvenous embolization

Surgical treatment and natural history are associated with high morbidity and mortality. Adjuvant ventricular shunting is not necessary unless definitive endovascular treatment is unavailable immediately. Emergency embolization is indicated in infants with refractory cardiac failure, acute or symptomatic hydrocephalus, rapid neurological deterioration or when parenchymal calcifications appear on follow-up scanning of brain. Neonates or infants having encephalomalacia or severe brain damage or severe parenchymal loss do not need any aggressive treatment because of poor clinical outcome in spite of successful closure of the shunt by embolization. Transarterial embolization is employed when the diagnostic angiogram demonstrates accessible feeding arterial branches from the choroidal and perforator arteries having sufficient caliber to permit navigation of the microcatheters. Transvenous technique is particularly employed when the perforating arteries are not of sufficient caliber to permit negotiation of the microcatheters. If the shunt is very large with extremely high flow the venous approach is preferred to avoid migration of the embolic material when delivered by the transarterial route. Occasionally it is necessary to use a combination of both techniques. In high flow choroidal malformations with no accessible femoral approach, occipital bone over the torcular is penetrated with a large bore needle for catheterization of the varix in neonates. However it is necessary to make a burr-hole in older children. The goal of treatment is to reduce the volume load initially and attempt to finally obliterate the shunt completely. In the majority of infants and children, it becomes necessary to stage the embolization ranging from a few weeks to a few months based on the angioarchitecture and clinical status. The follow-up endovascular approach is based on the residual shunt and the architecture of the malformation. Occlusive venopathy is a well-known delayed event causing progressive neurological deterioration. The acquired venopathy may be fatal. It is postulated that too long intervals between the embolization procedures would result in high venous pressures in the dural sinuses and cortical veins. The high flow venopathy is transmitted to the medullary veins and cortical veins which would result in progressive parenchymal calcifications and refractory seizures.

6. **d**—Retinal angiomatosis, facial hemangioma, and midbrain AVM

7. **c**—Posterior circulation aneurysms are more common that anterior circulation aneurysms.

8. **e**—Transcallosal

Common approaches to the dorsolateral brainstem:

Lesion location	Approach
Dorsal midbrain	Supracerebellar infratentorial
Lateral midbrain	Subtemporal; orbitozygomatic
Floor of 4th ventricle	Suboccipital
Lateral pons	Anterior/posterior petrosectomy and retrosigmoid
Dorsolateral medulla	Suboccipital and far lateral

9. **a**—Enlarging aneurysm

Traumatic aneurysms account for 14-39% of all pediatric aneurysms. Children with neurological deterioration after head injury should be suspected to have these lesions and investigated accordingly. These aneurysms can result from direct trauma (gunshot wounds, stab wounds, or surgical procedures). Indirect causes are trauma by falcine edge, sphenoid ridge, and sharp edge of fractured bone. The patient can present with devastating hemorrhage in 50%. It could be SAH, subdural hematoma (SDH), ICH or extradural hematoma (EDH). Aneurysm can bleed 5 h to 10 years after trauma with a mean of 3 weeks. The patient can present with irritability/unconsciousness or focal signs due to enlargement of aneurysm. Infraclinoid aneurysm can present with diabetes insipidus, cranial nerve deficits, unilateral blindness, recurrent massive epistaxis, and features of carotid-cavernous fistula. Rupture carries mortality of 32-50%.

10. **b**—IV rehydration and systemic heparin therapy

Symptoms of cerebral venous sinus thrombosis are diverse and nonspecific, including most commonly the triad of headache, vomiting, and depressed mental status. Seizures are common, especially in neonates. Clinical signs include reduced GCS, papilledema, cranial nerve abnormalities (6th nerve palsy), hemiparesis, quadriparesis, ataxia, and hyper-reflexia. In neonatal CSVT, the most common signs and symptoms are lethargy, vomiting, a full fontanelle, and seizures. In newborns, acute systemic illness with dehydration and infection are the most common predisposing conditions. Among previously healthy children, acute head and neck infections, dehydration, and iron deficiency anemia are common. Chronic diseases associated with childhood CSVT include inflammatory bowel disease, cancer, autoimmune disorders, and chronic liver or renal disease. Specific prothrombotic abnormalities that have been explored in pediatric CSVT include factor V Leiden and prothrombin gene mutations, protein C, S and antithrombin deficiencies, antiphospholipid antibodies, lipoprotein (a), methyl tetrahydrofolate reductase mutations, homocysteine, fibrinogen, plasminogen, factor VIII, and heparin cofactor II. While CT imaging is fast and convenient, this modality may miss the diagnosis of CSVT in up to 40% of cases, and is best identified using MRI with MR venogram (MRV). Ultrasound is convenient in infants with an open fontanel but is less sensitive than either CT or MRI. Primary treatment for CVST is anticoagulation with heparin. Additional therapies for CSVT include thrombolysis or surgical thrombectomy, but are associated with intracranial hemorrhage hence usually used when there is a failure to respond to anticoagulation.

FURTHER READING

Witmer C, Ichord R. Crossing the blood-brain barrier: clinical interactions between neurologists and hematologists in pediatrics—advances in childhood arterial ischemic stroke and cerebral venous thrombosis. Curr Opin Pediatr 2010 Feb;22(1):20-7.

11. **d**—Superficial temporal artery to MCA

In moyamoya disease, surgery is generally recommended for the treatment of patients with recurrent or progressive cerebral ischemic events and associated reduced cerebral perfusion reserve. Many different operative techniques have been described, all with the main goal of preventing further ischemic injury by increasing collateral blood flow to hypoperfused areas of cortex, using the external carotid circulation as a donor supply. Direct anastomosis procedures, most commonly superficial temporal artery (STA) to middle cerebral artery (MCA) bypasses, may achieve instant improvement in focal cerebral perfusion, but these procedures are often technically difficult to perform because small pediatric patients often do not have a large enough donor scalp artery or recipient middle cerebral artery to allow for a anastomosis large enough to supply a significant amount of additional collateral blood supply. A variety of indirect anastomotic procedures have been described: encephaloduroarteriosynangiosis (EDAS) whereby the STA is dissected free over a course of several inches and then sutured to the cut edges of the opened dura; encephalomyosynangiosis (EMS) in which the temporalis muscle is dissected and placed onto the surface of the brain to encourage collateral vessel development; and the combination of both, encephalomyoarteriosynangiosis (EMAS). Moyamoya patients are at particular risk of ischemic events in the perioperative period. Crying and hyperventilation, common occurrences in children at times during hospitalization, can lower $PaCO_2$ and induce ischemia secondary to cerebral vasoconstriction. Any techniques to reduce pain—including the use of perioperative sedation, painless wound dressing techniques, and absorbable wound suture closures—helped to reduce the incidence of strokes, TIAs, and length of stay in a recent study. A further perioperative consideration is the use of monitoring, such as intraoperative EEG or near-infrared spectroscopy, used to identify and ameliorate ischemic events detected while the patient is under general anesthesia.

FURTHER READING

Smith ER, Scott RM. Surgical management of moyamoya syndrome. Skull Base. 2005 Feb;15(1):15-26.

12. **d**—Stereotactic radiosurgery

EMI ANSWERS

13. 1—g, Osler-Weber-Rendu syndrome (HHT), 2—f, Marfan's syndrome, 3—j, Sturge-Weber syndrome

FURTHER READING

Xu HW, Yu SQ, Mei CL, Li MH. Screening for intracranial aneurysm in 355 patients with autosomal-dominant polycystic kidney disease. Stroke 2011 Jan; 42(1):204-6.

CHAPTER 45

Pediatric Movement Disorders and Spasticity

SINGLE BEST ANSWER (SBA) QUESTIONS

1. Spasticity is best described as:
   a. Velocity-dependent resistance to passive muscle stretch usually due to upper motor neuron lesion
   b. Velocity-dependent resistance to active muscle stretch usually due to upper motor neuron lesion
   c. Velocity-dependent resistance to passive muscle stretch usually due to lower motor neuron lesion
   d. Force-dependent resistance to passive muscle stretch usually due to upper motor neuron lesion
   e. Force-dependent resistance to active muscle stretch usually due to lower motor neuron lesion
   f. Force-dependent resistance to passive muscle stretch usually due to lower motor neuron lesion

2. The most common cause of spasticity in children is likely to be:
   a. Cerebral palsy
   b. Multiple sclerosis
   c. Stroke
   d. Traumatic spinal injury
   e. Wilson's disease

3. You see a 4-year-old child in clinic with a right spastic hemiparesis from a previously ruptured left basal ganglia cavernoma. She is currently taking oral baclofen and gabapentin. On examination, the right upper limb has increased tone throughout the range of movement but is easy to move, while the right leg has a considerable increased in muscle tone with passive movement being difficult. What are the Modified Ashworth scale grades for the right arm and leg?
   a. Right arm = 1, Right leg = 2
   b. Right arm = 1 +, Right leg = 2
   c. Right arm = 1 +, Right leg = 3
   d. Right arm = 2, Right leg = 3
   e. Right arm = 3, Right leg = 4

4. Which one of the following is LEAST likely to be a therapeutic end goal for intrathecal baclofen?
   a. Absence of limb spasticity
   b. Facilitating care
   c. Increasing range of motion
   d. Reducing painful muscle spasms
   e. Slowing the development of muscle contractures

5. Intrathecal baclofen treatment in children with cerebral palsy is most commonly associated with?
   a. Increased generalized itching
   b. Increased headache
   c. Increased progression of scoliosis
   d. Increased seizure frequency
   e. Reduced physostigmine requirements

6. A 27-year-old patient with spastic diplegia presents 2 years after baclofen pump insertion with increasing baclofen requirements. Until 6 months ago he had been stable for 1 year with a requirement of 300 μg/day. On the X-ray image of his baclofen pump below, which port would allow you to determine catheter patency?

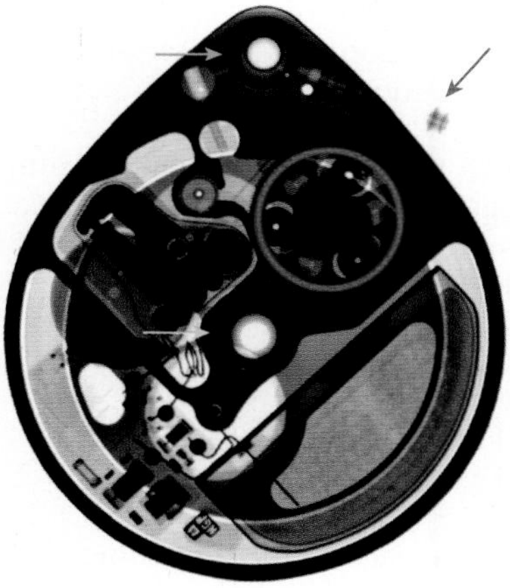

a. Blue arrow
b. Purple arrow
c. Red circle
d. Yellow arrow
e. Access port is usually in-line with catheter in lumbar region

7. The fluoroscopic image below most likely shows:

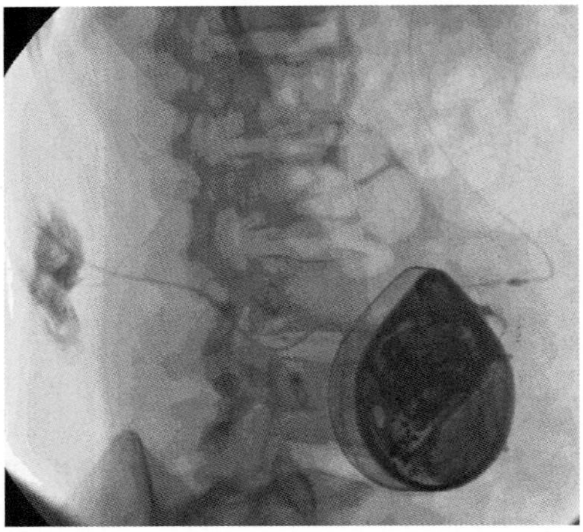

a. Catheter leak
b. Curling of catheter in subcutaneous tissues
c. Disconnection at pump catheter
d. Extradural position of catheter
e. Kinking of catheter

8. Selective dorsal rhizotomy for spastic cerebral palsy works by:
a. Electrical stimulation of dorsal root entry zone
b. Interruption of a subset of alpha-motor neurons
c. Interruption of gamma-motor neurons
d. Interruption of the spinal reflex arc
e. Restoration of GABAergic inhibition of alpha-motor neurons

9. Which one of the following treatments for pediatric dystonia works via vesicular monoamine transporter inhibition?
a. Baclofen
b. Carbamazepine
c. Carbidopa-levodopa
d. Clonazepam
e. Tetrabenazine
f. Trihexiphenidyl

10. The surgical treatment of choice for primary dystonia is likely to be:
a. Bilateral GPi DBS
b. Epidural motor cortex stimulation
c. Intrathecal baclofen pump
d. Pallidotomy
e. Selective dorsal rhizotomy

11. A child with cerebral palsy and a long-term intrathecal infusion pump presents with fever, seizures, and rebound spasticity. This is most likely to be:
a. Acute dystonic reaction
b. Baclofen withdrawal
c. Malignant hyperthermia
d. Neuroleptic malignant syndrome
e. Status dystonicus

EXTENDED MATCHING ITEM (EMI) QUESTIONS

12. **Drug treatment of spasticity:**
a. Carbidopa-levodopa
b. Cyproheptadine
c. Dantrolene
d. Diazepam
e. Gabapentin
f. Intrathecal baclofen
g. Oral baclofen
h. Physostigmine
i. Pregabalin
j. Tetrabenazine
k. Tizanidine
l. Trihexyphenidyl

For each of the following descriptions, select the most appropriate answers from the list above. Each answer may be used once, more than once or not at all.
1. Half-life is 4-5 h, therefore 24 h is required to achieve steady-state concentration after a change in dosage
2. Reduces intracellular calcium by binding ryanodine receptor in skeletal muscle
3. Alpha2 adrenergic antagonist

13. **Dystonia:**
a. Dopa-responsive dystonia (Segawa's disease)
b. Dystonic cerebral palsy
c. DYT-1 dystonia
d. Gangliosidoses
e. Glutaric aciduria
f. Leigh's disease
g. Mitochondrial disorders
h. Pantothenate kinase-associated neurodegeneration
i. Post-head injury dystonia
j. Post-stroke dystonia
k. Rett's syndrome
l. Wilson's disease

For each of the following descriptions, select the most appropriate answers from the list above. Each answer may be used once, more than once or not at all.

1. Dystonia worse in late afternoon, parkinsonism, and spastic gait but no history consistent with cerebral palsy, low biopterin and homovanillic acid levels
2. Childhood onset dystonia associated with TorsinA gene mutation

14. **Neuromodulation:**
    a. Anterior limb of internal capsule
    b. Anterior thalamic nucleus
    c. Cingulate cortex
    d. Globus pallidus internus
    e. Globus pallidus externus
    f. Nucleus accumbens
    g. Pedunculopontine nucleus
    h. Posterior hypothalamic
    i. Subgenual cortex
    j. Subthalamic nucleus
    k. Ventral PL thalamus

For each of the following descriptions, select the most appropriate answers from the list above. Each answer may be used once, more than once or not at all.

1. Primary generalized dystonia
2. Epilepsy

SBA ANSWERS

1. **a**—Velocity-dependent resistance to passive muscle stretch usually due to upper motor neuron lesion. Symptoms include muscle tightness, cramping/pain, and fatigue. It is due to a loss of descending GABA inhibition of muscle groups resulting in hypertonia (co-activation of agonist and antagonist muscles during volitional movement).

2. **a**—Cerebral palsy. Occurs in 1.5-3 per 1000 and accounts for 75% of spasticity in children. This is defined as a range of non-progressive syndromes of posture and motor impairment due to an insult to the developing nervous system. It is often accompanied by disturbances in sensation (visual and tactile), cognition/behavior, communication, and epilepsy (30%). CP is classified into spastic, dyskinetic, or mixed. Spastic CP is the most common and divided into spastic quadraplegia, diplegia, hemiplegia, or monoplegia. Severity of spasticity is graded according to Ashworth or Modified Ashworth scales. Dyskinetic cerebral palsy can be divided into dystonic and choreoathetoid forms.

Ashworth	Modified Ashworth
0 = Normal muscle tone	0 = Normal muscle tone
1 = Slight increase/catch when limb moved passively	1 = Slight increase/catch and release/minimal resistance at end of ROM
2 = More marked increase but limb easily flexed	1+ = Slight increase/catch and minimal resistance <50% of ROM
3 = Considerable increase in muscle tone	2 = More marked increase through most of ROM but affected parts easily moved
4 = Limb in rigid flexion or extension	3 = Considerable increase, passive movement difficult 4 = Affected parts in rigid flexion or extension

3. **d**—Right arm = 2, Right leg = 3. Generally patients with an Ashworth score of 3 are candidates for intrathecal baclofen, although those with less severe spasticity may also benefit depending on the clinical context. Additionally, during ITB test dose (25-50 μg in children) for spasticity an improvement of one point or greater is considered positive.

4. **a**—Absence of limb spasticity. This is because spasticity can help people with standing, walking or transferring and complete removal of spasticity can result in loss of function in some patients and thus intrathecal baclofen pump insertion is inappropriate.

5. **e**—Headache. CSF leaks occur in 5-15% of children with cerebral palsy, compared to 3% in adults. This is thought to be due to smaller size, thinner tissues, malnutrition of chronically disabled children and occult hydrocephalus in cerebral palsy.

6. **a**—Blue arrow. The general parts in the most commonly used pump (Medtronic Synchromed) consist of pump roller (red ring), pump reservoir port for filling (yellow arrow), catheter access port (blue arrow) and pump-catheter connector (purple arrow). In general, catheter malfunction can be assessed with plain radiographs (disconnection, kinking, migration) and either fluoroscopic or CT imaging after injection of contrast material via the catheter access port (catheter leak or extrathecal catheter-see image below).

Image with permission from Miracle AC, Fox MA, Ayyangar RN, et al. Imaging evaluation of intrathecal baclofen pump-catheter systems, AJNR Am J Neuroradiol Aug;32(7):1158-64, 2011.

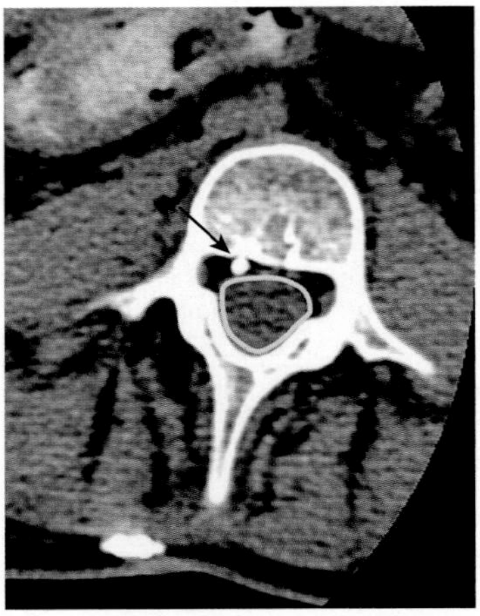

Image with permission from Miracle AC, Fox MA, Ayyangar RN, et al. Imaging evaluation of intrathecal baclofen pump-catheter systems, AJNR Am J Neuroradiol Aug;32(7):1158-64, 2011.

7. **a**—Catheter leak

Image with permission from Winn HR. Youman's Neurological Surgery, 4-Volume Set, 6th ed., Elsevier, Saunders, 2011.

8. **d**—Interruption of the spinal reflex arc. Deficient descending inhibition of spinal reflexes leads to hyperreflexia, hypertonia hence selective interruption of afferent fibers from spastic muscles will stop this. Briefly, in SDR (see diagram below) the conus is exposed and L2-S2 dorsal roots separated from motor roots using a silastic sheet, Each dorsal root is divided into 3-5 fascicles using a Scheer needle, and each of these is examined with EMG. Only rootlets which display a significant EMG response after stimulation are sectioned, while others are spared. L1 rhizotomy is required to reduce spasticity in hip flexors.

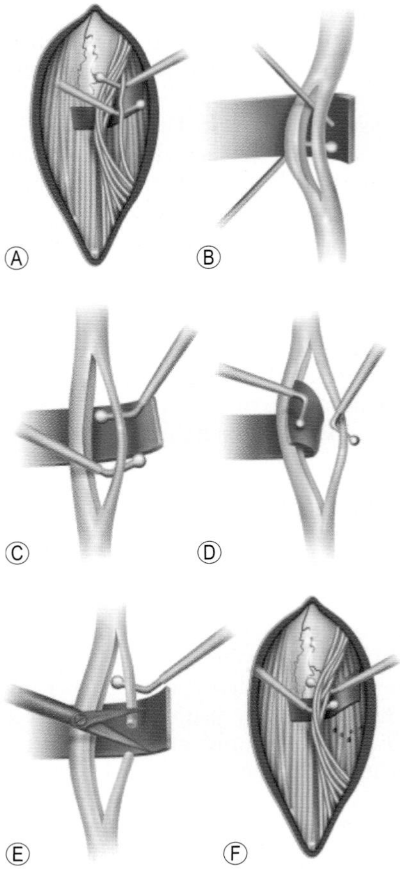

Image with permission from Winn HR. Youman's Neurological Surgery, 4-Volume Set, 6th ed., Elsevier, Saunders, 2011.

9. **e**—Tetrabenazine

10. **a**—Bilateral GPi DBS

11. **b**—Baclofen withdrawal

EMI ANSWERS

12. 1—f, Intrathecal baclofen, 2—c, Dantrolene, 3—k, Tizanidine.

13. 1—a, Dopa-responsive dystonia, 2—c, DYT-1 dystonia.

14. 1—d, Globus pallidus internus, 2—b, Anterior thalamic nucleus.

CHAPTER 46

NEUROSURGERY AND PREGNANCY

SINGLE BEST ANSWER (SBA) QUESTIONS

1. Which one of the following best describes the risk of subarachnoid hemorrhage during pregnancy?
   a. Lowest during the first trimester
   b. Highest during the puerperium
   c. Highest during the second trimester
   d. Lowest during the third trimester
   e. Highest during labor
   f. Not increased during pregnancy, labor, or puerperium

2. A 28-year-old left-handed female who is 14 weeks pregnant presented to the emergency department with worsening headache, vomiting and drowsiness. CT head scan showed a large right frontal tumor with significant edema. After 48 h of dexamethasone her headache has improved but she still has a mild left-sided arm weakness. Which one of the following would be most appropriate?
   a. Permit gestational advancement to second trimester
   b. Craniotomy and tumor resection followed by chemoradiotherapy
   c. Cesarean section followed by neurosurgery
   d. Iatrogenic termination followed by neurosurgery
   e. Radiotherapy alone until fetal maturity established

3. At what gestational age is it generally accepted that a ruptured cerebral aneurysm should be managed by cesarean section under general anesthesia followed by immediate aneurysm exclusion?
   a. 26 weeks
   b. 28 weeks
   c. 30 weeks
   d. 32 weeks
   e. 34 weeks

4. According to available evidence, which one of the following statements is most correct regarding the timing of cerebral arteriovenous malformation rupture during pregnancy?
   a. Most AVMs rupture during the first and second trimesters
   b. Most AVMs rupture during the puerperium
   c. Most AVMs rupture during the second trimester
   d. Most AVMs rupture during the second and third trimesters
   e. Most AVMs rupture during labor
   f. Same rate of AVM rupture throughout pregnancy and puerperium

5. Back pain in pregnancy is most likely due to the action which one of the following hormones?
   a. FSH
   b. Oestrodiol
   c. Oxytocin
   d. Progesterone
   e. Relaxin

6. A 36-year-old female who is 20 weeks pregnant presents with sciatica, saddle anesthesia and urinary incontinence. MRI of the lumbosacral spine reveals a significant L5/S1 disc prolapse with compression of cauda equina nerve roots. What would be your preferred option?
   a. Anterior discectomy in supine position with 30° lateral decubitus tilt
   b. Discectomy in lateral decubitus position
   c. Discectomy with patient prone on four-poster frame
   d. Iatrogenic termination and proceed to discectomy in prone position
   e. Laminectomy only in lateral decubitus position

7. The additional risk of childhood cancer above the natural risk (1 in 500) per CT head performed on a pregnant female is approximately:
   a. Less than 1 in 1,000,000
   b. 1 in 1,000,000 to 1 in 100,000
   c. 1 in 100,000 to 1 in 10,000
   d. 1 in 10,000 to 1 in 1000
   e. 1 in 1000 to 1 in 200

8. A 31-year-old female who is 34 weeks pregnant is involved in a high-speed RTA. She is immobilized by paramedics at the scene and transferred to your emergency department. She is GCS 15/15 but becomes hypotensive and tachycardic. What action would you take immediately?
   a. Place in left lateral position
   b. Manually push the uterus to the left
   c. Start a vasopressor
   d. Intermittent fetal monitoring
   e. Continuous cardiotocography
   f. Fetal blood sampling

9. Which one of the following is a major potential risk to the fetus exposed to MRI sequences employing time-varying gradient electromagnetic fields?
   a. Developmental delay
   b. Acoustic noise damage
   c. Magnetophosphenes
   d. Peripheral nerve and muscle stimulation
   e. Implant

10. A 31-year-old female who is 28 weeks pregnant presents to your emergency department with a self-terminating tonic-clonic seizure and currently has postictal confusion. She is under close monitoring for her hypertension and proteinuria. Which one of the following would you administer first?
    a. Lorazepam
    b. Diazepam
    c. Valproate
    d. Magnesium
    e. Phenytoin
    f. Levetiracetam

11. Women with aneurysmal subarachnoid hemorrhage 10 weeks pregnant and oculomotor palsy. She agrees to DSA and coil embolization and the aneurysm is secured. Postoperatively she asks about the possibility of terminating her fetus due to the probable harmful effects of the radiation exposure required in her treatment. Which one of the following actions would you take in the first instance?
    a. Organize a medical termination while she is still an inpatient
    b. Explain that the likely dose was much lower than the generally accepted threshold for causing fetal harm
    c. Recommend amniocentesis
    d. Advise her to discuss the risks with a medical physicist
    e. Arrange an obstetric review

EXTENDED MATCHING ITEM (EMI) QUESTIONS

12. **Shunt malfunction in pregnancy:**
    a. Cesarean section under epidural anesthesia
    b. Cesarean section under GA
    c. CT or MRI during pregnancy
    d. Induced hypocarbia
    e. Magnesium sulfate
    f. Preconception CT or MRI
    g. Prophylactic antibiotics
    h. Revision of ventriculoperitoneal shunt
    i. Shunt tap for pressure and CSF MCS
    j. Vaginal delivery with assisted second stage
    k. Ventriculoatrial shunt or third ventriculostomy

For each of the following descriptions, select the most appropriate answers from the list above. Each answer may be used once, more than once or not at all:

1. A 32-year-old with VP shunt placement 8 years ago for hydrocephalus following foramen magnum decompression is considering pregnancy.
2. A 36-year-old with VP shunt is undergoing a planned vaginal delivery with assisted second stage.
3. A 23-year-old with VP shunt develops headache, nausea, vomiting and a single generalized tonic-clonic seizure which self-terminates after 1 min. She does not have a pre-existing diagnosis of epilepsy and is not on antiepileptics. Blood pressure is 140/90 and urine dip shows 2+ leukocytes, negative nitrites, no ketones and no protein.

13. **Neurological disease in pregnancy:**
    a. Cerebral venous sinus thrombosis
    b. Choriocarcinoma
    c. Chorea gravidarum
    d. Idiopathic intracranial hypertension
    e. Lymphocytic hypophysitis
    f. Lymphoma
    g. Pituitary macroadenoma
    h. Pre-eclampsia/Eclampsia
    i. Reversible posterior leukoencephalopathy syndrome
    j. Sheehan's syndrome

For each of the following descriptions, select the most appropriate answers from the list above.

Each answer may be used once, more than once or not at all:

1. A 32-year-old female with a previous history of molar pregnancy 6 months ago presents with a generalized tonic-clonic seizure. CT head shows a right frontal hemorrhagic space occupying lesion and CT chest shows multiple pulmonary lesions.
2. A 27-year-old female who is 3 months postpartum presents with headache, fatigue and polyuria. Her past medical history includes with systemic lupus erythematosus. Initial investigations reveal sodium 155 and a diagnosis of diabetes is made after further workup. MRI shows a homogeneously enhancing sellar mass with thickening of the pituitary stalk producing a "pear-shaped" appearance.

SBA ANSWERS

1. **f**—Not increased during pregnancy, labor, or puerperium.

FURTHER READING

Algra AM, et al. Female risk factors for subarachnoid haemorrhage: a systematic review. Neurology 2012;79(12):1230-6.

2. **b**—Craniotomy and tumor resection

Treatment should adhere to the treatment options as in nonpregnant women. The optimal time to perform the procedure during pregnancy is still a matter of debate. It is recommended to delay surgery if possible until after the first trimester to reduce the miscarriage risk—surgery during the second and third trimesters surgery is considered safe. Delay can cause progressive neurologic deterioration and increasing risk of urgent intervention (resection and cesarean section). Due to the significant complications of prematurity (e.g. respiratory diseases, bradycardia, necrotizing enterocolitis, intraventricular hemorrhage, hypoglycemia and feeding problems, sepsis and seizures) iatrogenic preterm birth should be avoided whenever possible by postponing or continuing treatment until a term delivery can be achieved. The decision of performing an elective cesarean section preterm is often based upon the risk of increased intracranial pressure associated with bearing-down efforts during the second stage of labor. Nonetheless, if patients are clinically stable and carefully discussed, and the individual risk of rapid tumor growth has been evaluated, gestational advancement until fetal maturity should be considered, as well as the attempt to have a vaginal delivery. Balance between waiting for fetal maturation and risk of intrauterine death (secondary to maternal death) remains difficult in patients with highly malignant tumors.

A recent study summarized long-term data of children after antenatal exposure to chemotherapy (and/or radiotherapy) found a cardiac outcome equal to the general population, and no adverse effects of treatment on the general health and age-appropriate neurocognitive (IQ, attention, behavior, memory) development. Estimations of the absorbed fetal dose were between 0.01 and 0.1 Gy (10-100 mGy) for patients who received whole brain RT by a 3D conformal technique and many of the toxic effects will only be induced above the deterministic threshold of 0.1 Gy. Most studies reporting on the administration of radiotherapy to brain tumors showed that the fetal exposure never exceeded this threshold dose. These radiotherapy schedules are therefore considered safe. Still, proper shielding should always be used to further reduce the fetal dose and it is recommended to discuss treatment with a radiation physicist and to use a phantom to estimate the fetal dose as accurate as possible in order to counsel parents on the potential risks of radiation-induced toxicity.

FURTHER READING

Tewari KS, Cappuccini F, Asrat T, et al. Obstetric emergencies precipitated by malignant brain tumors. Am J Obstet Gynecol 2000;182:1215-21; Verheecke M, Halaska MJ, Lok CA, et al. Primary brain tumours, meningiomas and brain metastases in pregnancy: report on 27 cases and review of literature. Eur J Cancer 2014;50(8):1462-71; Amant F, Van Calsteren K, Halaska MJ, et al. Long-term cognitive and cardiac outcomes after prenatal exposure to chemotherapy in children aged 18 months or older: An observational study. Lancet Oncol 2012;13(3):256-64.

3. **e**—34 weeks

For ruptured cerebral aneurysms in pregnant women generally the aneurysm should be treated first and the pregnancy allowed to continue to term, except in cases of rupture during labor when delivery should be completed prior to aneurysm treatment. For gestational ages less than 26 weeks, proceed as best for the mother and if aneurysm treatment is successful vaginal delivery should be attempted. For gestational ages beyond 34 weeks, cesarean section under general anesthesia, followed immediately by aneurysm exclusion, is advised. Between 26 and 34 weeks, aneurysm exclusion should proceed and, if the fetus is stable, pregnancy allowed to continue to term. Deciding whether to undertake endovascular coiling or surgical clipping is difficult. In view of the progressive hormonal and hemodynamic changes in pregnancy, ISAT data may not be applicable; additionally complications such as coil prolapse require antiplatelet agents that need to be considered in unexpected labor or emergency cesarean section soon after coiling. Such issues certainly require detailed discussion between the neurosurgeon, neuroanesthetist, obstetrician and patient.

FURTHER READING

Ng J, Kitchen N. Neurosurgery and pregnancy. JNNP 2008;79:745-52.

4. **a**—Most occur during the second and third trimesters

It is accepted that the overall rate of hemorrhage from cerebral AVMs is not increased during pregnancy compared to nonpregnant periods of life. However, in pregnant patients with intracranial AVMs it is important to know that most ruptures occur in the second and third trimester, and not during the first trimester, labor or puerperium. The definitive management of AVMs in pregnancy thus follows standard neurosurgical guidelines. In general, those with fully treated AVMs before 35 weeks gestation unassisted vaginal delivery should be possible. In those with unruptured intracranial AVM, the risk of hemorrhage during vaginal delivery is recognized to be low with the use of epidural analgesia and an assisted second stage. In contrast, elective cesarean section has been advocated for women with an untreated or partially treated AVM, especially if it has bled during pregnancy.

FURTHER READING

Ng J, Kitchen N. Neurosurgery and pregnancy. JNNP 2008;79:745-52; Liu XJ, Wang S, Zhao YL, et al. Risk of cerebral arteriovenous malformation rupture during pregnancy and puerperium. Neurology 2014;82(20):1798-803.

5. **e**—Relaxin

This is a hormone released during pregnancy to cause ligamentous laxity in preparation for parturition. Women with severe pelvic girdle pain in pregnancy have significantly higher serum levels of relaxin than those who are pain free.

FURTHER READING

MacLennan AL, Nicholson R, Green RC, et al. Serum relaxin and pelvic pain of pregnancy. Lancet 1986;2:243-5.

6. **c**—Discectomy with patient prone on four-poster frame

Pregnant women who have progressive neurological deficit at 34-36 weeks' gestation or later should undergo induction of delivery or cesarean section before, or at the same time as, they undergo spinal surgery; pre-partum surgical treatment should be considered in patients who develop progressive neurological deficits before 34 weeks. The decision regarding timing of spinal surgery should be made in close consultation with the obstetrician, as uncertain dating of gestational age could greatly affect the infant's outcome. In addition, inducing labor before the neurological injury is treated could cause increased neurological injury in the patient because of the rise in epidural venous pressure that occurs during labor. In cases of true cauda equina syndrome or severe motor weakness occurring at later gestational ages ($\geq$34 weeks), cesarean delivery should be strongly considered over induction of labor to avoid more severe neurological deficits after delivery. Brookfield et al. used the prone position in pregnant patients with lumbar disc herniation after 20- and 32-weeks' gestation by use of a four-poster laminectomy frame to provide pressure relief over the abdomen; it is unnecessary to use the technically difficult lateral decubitus position. Diagnostic imaging in women of child-bearing age is limited to MRI scanning as the initial, and when possible the only, confirmatory and surgical planning diagnostic procedure. Intraoperative fluoroscopy is unlikely to deliver teratogenic fetal radiation doses but if any question about termination of pregnancy arises input from both an obstetrician and a medical physicist who can accurately calculate the exact dose of radiation to which the fetus was exposed. In the pregnant patient, only the surgical procedure that is necessary to alleviate neurological deficit should be performed.

FURTHER READING

Brookfield KF, Brown MD. How should pregnant women with spinal disease be managed? Nat Clin Pract Neurol 2008 Dec;4(12):652-3.

7. **a**—Less than 1 in 1,000,000

Fetal radiation doses of less than 50 mGy are not associated with increased fetal anomalies or fetal loss throughout pregnancy; fortunately, radiation doses of all diagnostic imaging examinations using ionizing radiation routinely used in a trauma evaluation should be well below this threshold (by comparison fetal dose from natural background radiation during pregnancy is 0.5-1.0 mGy):

Maternal Examination	Typical Fetal Dose (mGy)	Additional Risk of Childhood Cancer per Examination
XR Skull, CT head	0.001-0.01	<1 in 1,000,000
CT Pulmonary angiogram Cerebral angiography	0.01-0.1	1 in 1,000,000 to 1 in 100,000
XR Abdomen, XR Hip, XR pelvis, CT chest	0.1-1.0	1 in 100,000 to 1 in 10,000
XR lumbar spine, CT lumbar spine, CT abdomen	1.0-10	1 in 10,000 to 1 in 1000
CT pelvis, CT pelvis-abdomen	10-50	1 in 1000 to 1 in 200

Body CT examinations of pregnant trauma patients should be performed with intravenous iodinated contrast as it improves detection of both maternal and fetal injuries by providing vascular contrast in organs and opacification of vascular structures, including the placenta. The use of iodinated contrast material to obtain one diagnostic CT study is preferable to obtaining a nonenhanced CT study that may be nondiagnostic and necessitate repeat imaging. In a seriously injured pregnant patient, multiple or repeat imaging examinations could result in a fetal radiation dose that exceeds 50 mGy. In these situations, it is important to recognize the risks of ionizing radiation to the fetus, which depend on the stage of the pregnancy:

Gestation	Fetal Radiation Dose (mGy)	Risks
<2 weeks	50-100	Failure of blastocyst implantation (if survives, no other deleterious effect expected)
2-20 weeks	50-150	Teratogenesis
Any time	50	Carcinogenesis: doubles risk of fatal childhood cancer (from 1 in 500 to 1 in 250) Increases overall lifetime risk of cancer by 2%

FURTHER READING

Health Protection Agency. RCE-9: protection of pregnant patients during diagnostic medical exposures to ionizing radiation: advice from the Health Protection Agency, The Royal College of Radiologists and the College of Radiographers. March 2009; Raptis CA, Mellnick VM, Raptis DA, et al. Imaging of trauma in the pregnant patient. Radiographics 2014;34 (3):748-63.

8. **a**—Left lateral position

Trauma, which affects 5-7% of all pregnancies, is the leading cause of nonobstetric maternal mortality. Fetal loss rates approach 1-5% in minor injuries and 40-50% in life-threatening trauma, but as minor trauma is much more common it is the major cause of fetal loss. Stabilization of the mother involves resuscitation used with any trauma patient, bearing in mind that if she is more than 20 weeks pregnant, she should be placed in the 30° left lateral decubitus position to prevent systemic hypotension caused by compression of the inferior vena cava by the gravid uterus. For imaging studies that require the patient to lie flat for an extended time, use of the 30% left lateral decubitus position during imaging should be strongly considered. In addition, blood products should be administered to maintain a hematocrit level higher than 30% for optimal fetal oxygenation. After the patient has been stabilized, ultrasound should be performed to determine the gestational age of the fetus and whether a fetal heart rate is present. For a fetus older than 24-26 weeks of gestational age, continuous external fetal monitoring (cardiotocography; CTG) should be used as it would be viable outside the uterus and should be delivered if there is evidence of fetal distress.

FURTHER READING

Raptis CA, Mellnick VM, Raptis DA, Kitchin D, et al. Imaging of trauma in the pregnant patient. Radiographics 2014;34 (3):748-63.

9. **b**—Acoustic noise damage

MRI Field Type	Risks
Static field	Vertigo, nausea, magnetophosphenes, metallic taste, projectiles, implant malfunction and movement, monitoring device malfunction and movement
Radiofrequency pulse	Heating effect (specific energy absorption rate, SAR), Induced current burns
Time-varying gradient EMF	Acoustic noise damage, peripheral nerve stimulation, muscle stimulation (arrhythmia in extreme cases)

To minimize these potential risks, it is recommended that MR imaging of pregnant patients is performed at field strengths of 1.5 T or less. In addition, MR imaging protocols for pregnant patients should be tailored to include the minimum number of sequences required to answer the particular clinical question. Gadolinium is considered a pregnancy category C drug by the FDA, which means that animal studies have shown adverse effects but adequate data are not available in humans, and the potential benefits may warrant its use in pregnant women if it is considered critical for evaluation. Typically, the use of gadolinium-based contrast material is not necessary in pregnant trauma patients because essential clinical information can be obtained with nonenhanced MR imaging. Gadolinium-based contrast material can be used for imaging pregnant trauma patients in rare circumstances when it is believed to be absolutely necessary for diagnosis.

FURTHER READING

Raptis CA, Mellnick VM, Raptis DA, et al. Imaging of trauma in the pregnant patient. Radiographics 2014;34(3):748-63.

10. **d**—Magnesium

Empirical evidence supports the effectiveness of magnesium sulfate in preventing and treating eclamptic seizures. Therapeutic levels of magnesium can be obtained by administering a 6-g intramuscular loading dose followed by 2 g/h intravenous infusion, or alternatively with a 2- to 4-g intravenous bolus followed by a 1 g/min infusion, or a combination of both. The goal serum concentration is considered to be 4-8 mg/dL (2.0-3.5 mol/L). Magnesium is excreted in the urine; thus, impaired renal function may affect serum levels. Magnesium therapy has a narrow therapeutic index and symptoms of toxicity include loss of deep tendon reflexes at blood levels of 8-12 mg/dL, respiratory depression at concentrations of >14 mg/dL, muscular paralysis and respiratory arrest at levels >15-17 mg/dL. Cardiac arrest can occur above 30 mg/dL. Recommended treatment for toxicity includes calcium gluconate.

FURTHER READING

The Eclampsia Trial Collaborative Group. Which anticonvulsant for women with eclampsia? Evidence from the Collaborative Eclampsia Trial. Lancet 1995;345(8963):1455-63.

11. **b**—Explain that the likely dose was much lower than the generally accepted threshold for causing fetal harm.

Aneurysms are diagnosed by digital subtraction angiography (DSA) or, increasingly, by CT angiography. Furthermore, coil embolization requires prolonged use of DSA. Concerns exist regarding fetal radiation exposure. A phantom study has demonstrated that the effective radiation dose to the fetus during DSA for coil embolization is so small that it confers no additional risk to the fetus. If there is still concern then a medical physicist should be consulted.

FURTHER READING

Marshman LA, Rai MS, Aspoas AR. Comment to "Endovascular treatment of ruptured intracranial aneurysms during pregnancy: report of three cases". Arch Gynecol Obstet 2005;272:93.

EMI ANSWERS

12. 1—f, Preconception CT or MRI, 2—g, Prophylactic antibiotics, 3—i, Shunt tap for pressure and CSF MCS

Pregnancy is associated with a higher incidence of shunt complications, and more women with shunts are surviving into child-bearing age. Other causes of raised intracranial pressure (e.g. CVST) should also be excluded in the workup. General management is outlined below.

Preconception management

1. Baseline CT/MRI should be done in those considering pregnancy with a shunt *in situ*.
2. Review potentially teratogenic medications (e.g. anticonvulsants).
3. If shunt was inserted for a neural tube defect, there is a 2-3% chance that the baby will also have a neural tube defect. Therefore, relevant patients require genetic counseling and judicious measures taken to limit the risk factors for neural tube defects (e.g. folate supplementation)

Management during pregnancy

1. Raised ICP can mimic pre-eclampsia/eclampsia and a low index of suspicion is required.
2. If increasing intracranial pressure is suspected, a CT or MRI brain should be performed and compared with the baseline. If there is no change from preoperative imaging, the shunt should be tapped, the ICP measured and cerebrospinal fluid samples taken for culture.
3. If intracranial pressure is normal, and cultures are negative, physiological changes may be responsible. Treatment is bed rest

and the shunt may be pumped to aid cerebrospinal fluid flow.

4. If there is an increase in ventricle size or if intracranial pressure is raised on shunt tap, shunt revision is required. In the first and second trimesters, this may be performed as in the nonpregnant. In the third trimester, a ventriculoatrial shunt or third ventriculostomy may be considered as an alternative, thereby avoiding the risks of uterine trauma or induction of labor.

Intrapartum management

1. Prophylactic antibiotics are recommended during labor and delivery. Antibiotics should cover coliforms and be in accordance with local guidelines. Colonization with group B streptococcus has been associated with postpartum shunt infection following cesarean section and extended antibiotic regimens should be considered in such cases.
2. If the patient has no symptoms of raised intracranial pressure, vaginal delivery is safe and the preferred option, as there is a lower risk of adhesions, which may subsequently result in shunt malfunction and shunt infection. A shortened second stage is suggested, as increases in cerebrospinal fluid pressure at this time is greater than during any other Valsalva maneuver and may lead to functional shunt obstruction.
3. If a patient becomes symptomatic during labor, cesarean section under general anesthesia is indicated: epidural anesthesia is contraindicated with elevated intracranial pressure.

FURTHER READING

Ng J, Kitchen N. Neurosurgery and pregnancy. JNNP 2008;79:745-52; Wisoff JH, Kratzert KJ, Handwerker SM, et al. Pregnancy in patient with cerebrospinal fluid shunts: report of a series and review of the literature. Neurosurgery 1991;29:827-31.

13. 1—b, Choriocarcinoma, 2—e, Lymphocytic hypophysitis

Choriocarcinoma is a rare tumor of trophoblastic origin; 90% have lung metastasis at presentation and cerebral metastases are a common manifestation. Approximately 15% of tumors follow normal pregnancies, but most are discovered months after pregnancies characterized by spontaneous abortion or by vaginal bleeding, premature labor, and an enlarged uterus due to a molar pregnancy. Women with cerebral metastases present with seizures, hemorrhage, infarction, or gradually progressive deficits. The tumor may invade the sacral plexus, cauda equina, or spinal canal. A ratio of serum: CSF hCG of >1:60 suggests the presence of choriocarcinoma brain metastasis.

A pituitary mass presenting in late pregnancy or up to 1 year postpartum may be lymphocytic hypophysitis and is also associated with other autoimmune disease. Presentation is with headache, panhypopituitarism (as inflammation damages anterior pituitary, posterior pituitary and pituitary stalk equally unlike in adenomas) and pressure effects on the chiasm/cavernous sinus. MRI shows a homogeneously enlarged pituitary gland and stalk, often with a pear-shaped appearance. First-line treatment is with steroids and correction of endocrine abnormalities.

INDEX

Note: Page numbers followed by *f* indicate figures, and *t* indicate tables.

A

B

C

G

H

T